FSTA™ THESAURUS

NINTH EDITION

FSTA – FOOD SCIENCE AND TECHNOLOGY ABSTRACTS®

ifis
INTERNATIONAL FOOD
INFORMATION SERVICE

FSTA Thesaurus

Ninth Edition

Compiled by Members of the IFIS Editorial and Production team
IFIS Publishing
Lane End House
Shinfield Road
Shinfield, Reading RG2 9BB, UK

INTERNATIONAL FOOD INFORMATION SERVICE

IFIS Publishing

Reading · 2011

Published by
IFIS Publishing, Lane End House, Shinfield Road, Shinfield, Reading RG2 9BB, UK

Tel: + 44 118 988 3895
Fax: +44 118 988 5065
E-mail: ifis@ifis.org
Web: www.FoodScienceCentral.com

Charity Registration No. 1068176; Limited Company No. 3507902

ISBN 978-0-86014-195-2

British Library Cataloguing-in-Publication Data
A catalogue record for this book is available from the British Library

Typeset by IFIS Publishing

Printed in Great Britain by Lightning Source UK Ltd., Milton Keynes

Contents

Foreword

This is the ninth edition of the *FSTA Thesaurus*, and, in keeping with the previous editions, this revision has been the result of a concerted team effort.

The ninth edition contains 366 new terms which reflect the developments in food science, food technology, and human and pet nutrition that have taken place during the period since the eighth edition was published in 2007. Substantial revisions of the existing hierarchies have also been implemented to improve searchability and record retrieval. The thesaurus has, therefore, been brought fully up to date, and remains an indispensable aid for searching the database *FSTA – Food Science and Technology Abstracts®*.

Users should also be aware that a related dictionary is available in print and on IFIS' own version of the database, *FSTA Direct.* The dictionary comprises definitions of all the salient thesaurus terms.

I very much hope that users in the food community will continue to find the *FSTA Thesaurus* a valuable tool in their day-to-day work.

Richard Hollingsworth
Managing Director, IFIS Publishing
Shinfield, January 2011

Introduction

Background

This is the ninth edition of the thesaurus which has been compiled specifically as a companion and user aid to facilitate searching of the bibliographic database *FSTA – Food Science and Technology Abstracts*®. The database and thesaurus are both produced by IFIS (International Food Information Service), which was founded in 1968. IFIS is both a not for profit organisation (Charity No. 1068176) and a company limited by guarantee (Company No. 3507902).

FSTA is IFIS's best-known product. It is the world's leading database of information on food science, food technology, and food-related human and pet nutrition. *FSTA* was first published in 1969. It now contains approximately 910,000 records and electronic formats continue to grow at a rate of approximately 45,000 records per year. *FSTA* is available in printed and electronic formats. The database is updated monthly in print, and weekly or monthly online depending upon the platform of choice.

FSTA is comprised of records which are prepared from all the world's literature (journals, books, reports, conference proceedings, patent literature, standards, legislation, and theses, originating from a total of 90 countries and in 40 languages) of relevance to food science, food technology, and food-related human and pet nutrition. In general, records contain a bibliographic citation plus an abstract (summary) of the source document. The abstracts are either written by IFIS's editorial staff (who are also fully trained scientists) or, when appropriate, authors' summaries are reproduced from consenting primary journals. All records are indexed with terms (keywords) sourced from the *FSTA Thesaurus*. In common with its eight predecessors (published in 1977, 1981, 1992, 1996, 1998, 2000, 2004 and 2007), the ninth edition has its origins in the original IFIS word list which was based on the frequency of occurrence of terms in the *FSTA* subject index; the word list first appeared in 1970. All the revisions of the thesaurus have continued to be based on the frequency of occurrence of terms in *FSTA*. A list of new terms in this most recent edition of the thesaurus is given at Appendix I.

Structure and terminology

Terms appearing in the thesaurus are divided into specific types to describe their functionality as follows:

Heading — a subset of descriptors at the top or at least part-way up a given hierarchy which are included to assist with accumulation of narrower terms both during searching and within the printed index; headings are indicated in the printed version of the thesaurus by shading.

Descriptor — a term currently used in indexing which is indicated in the printed version of the thesaurus by bold print.

Non-descriptor — a term not currently used in indexing but which may have been used in the past; does not appear in bold print in the printed thesaurus.

The following terms and abbreviations are used throughout the thesaurus as follows:

HN history note (giving the background and usage of a specific term).

SN scope note (describing particular use of a term in *FSTA* - also used for Enzyme Commission (EC) numbers and to list terms synonymous (see *syn.,* below) with the term in question.

BT broader term (numbered BT1....BT9 as appropriate, numbers relating to level of proximity in meaning to the original term).

NT narrower term (numbered NT1...NT9 as appropriate, numbers relating to level of proximity in meaning to the original term).

RT related term (describing a term that does not fall within the direct hierarchy of another term but which might be considered when developing a search strategy).

UF use for indicates non-descriptors (non-preferred terms) for which the descriptor (preferred term) should be used.

USE indicates the descriptor to use in preference to the non-descriptor in question.

syn. synonym (used in SN (see above)) for terms synonymous with the descriptor, which may be used as descriptors in their own right.

abbrev. abbreviation.

Please see below for examples relating to usage of the above terms and abbreviations.

English spelling and internationally recognised chemical conventions for spelling, chemical symbols, SI units and widely recognised abbreviations for biochemicals, etc. are used throughout *FSTA* and the thesaurus.

Layout

The ninth edition contains 10,571 terms, including over 350 new terms (see Appendix I).

Typical examples of thesaurus entries illustrating layout and terminology are as follows:

Example 1

Descriptor	**Batters**
Scope note defining use in the FSTA database	SN for meat batters see Meat or specific type of meat
	BT1 Bakery products
	BT2 Cereal products
	BT3 Plant foods
	BT4 Foods
	BT1 Coatings
	RT Cake batters

Example 2

Descriptor/Heading **Venison**

History note giving period of time as a heading HN heading from vol. 30 (1998); under Meat specific up to vol. 29 (1997)
BT1 Meat specific
BT2 Meat
BT3 Animal foods
BT4 Foods
NT1 Deer carcasses
RT Deer
Non-descriptor UF Deer meat

Example 3

Non-descriptor Vitamin B_1

HN used in the index up to vol. 35, issue 6 (2003)
SN obsolete name for thiamin
Descriptor USE **Thiamin**

How to use the thesaurus

The thesaurus indicates the use of a term (keyword) in the *FSTA* subject index (displayed in the keyword or descriptor fields in electronic formats). If the term is a non-descriptor (i.e. it does not appear in bold print in the printed thesaurus), the corresponding (preferred) descriptor to use in searching will be indicated. For example:

Drinks
USE **Beverages**

The reciprocal relationship for descriptors and commonly used synonyms is also indicated by the 'use for' acronym, UF. For example:

Corn
UF Maize

If the term is a descriptor, then it will be found in the subject index (keyword or descriptor field). When searching the printed format of *FSTA*, a descriptor that is not a heading (appearing in bold but not in shading in the thesaurus) may be found in the index under a heading appearing as a broader term in its hierarchy. For example, if records on Cheddar cheese are required, the thesaurus will show the relationship:

Cheddar cheese
BT1 Cheese varieties

In this example, Cheddar cheese is not in itself a heading but the broader term at level 1 (Cheese varieties) is, and consequently this is the heading under which any records on Cheddar cheese will be found.

The inclusion of related terms in a search strategy may also enhance the efficiency of retrieving records of interest; relevant related terms are always given in the thesaurus.

The Dictionary of Food Science and Technology

The *Dictionary of Food Science and Technology* was first published by Blackwell in 2005, with a second edition in 2009 (ISBN: 978-1-4051-8740-4). Both editions were compiled by IFIS using the thesaurus as the source of terms to be defined. Many definitions are specific to food science and technology, covering sensory analysis, consumer research, food composition, nutrition (food related not clinical aspects), catering and food safety; however, the *Dictionary* is also augmented by definitions from cognate disciplines including chemistry, biochemistry, physics, microbiology, public health, economics, engineering and packaging. The *Dictionary* also contains a large number of definitions covering food commodities of every description including processed and prepared foods of all types together with: alcoholic and non-alcoholic beverages; fruits; vegetables; nuts; cocoa, chocolate and sugar confectionery products; sugars; syrups; starches; cereals and bakery products; fats; oils; margarine; milk and dairy products (including cream, butter, cheese, cultured milk products etc.); eggs and egg products; fish and marine products; meat; poultry; game; additives; spices; and condiments. The *Dictionary* was designed to appeal to a wide range of users and compliments both the thesaurus and database acting as a companion to both products.

Other references

A Dictionary of Food and Nutrition. 3rd Edition. 2009. Bender, D. A.; Oxford University Press, Oxford, UK.

All about cheese. http://www.cheese.com.

Benders' dictionary of nutrition and food technology. Eighth edition. 2006. Bender, D. A; Woodhead Publishing, Cambridge, UK.

Comparative Toxigenomics Database. http://ctd.mdibl.org/.

Compendium of Pesticide Common Names. http://www.alanwood.net/pesticides/index.html.

Dictionary of Dairy Terminology. 2nd Edition 1996. International Dairy Federation (Compiler). Elsevier Science B. V., Amsterdam, Netherlands.

Dictionary of Food Ingredients. 4th Edition. 2001. Igor, R. S.; Hui, Y. H.; Aspen Publishers, Inc., Gaithersburg, MD, USA.

Dictionary of Food Science & Technology. 2nd Edition. 2009. International Food Information Service. Wiley-Blackwell, Chichester, UK.

Documentation – Guidelines for Establishment and Development of Monolingual Thesauri. 2nd Edition. 1986. International Standard ISO 2788. International Organization for Standardization.

Elsevier's Dictonary of Edible Mushrooms. 1989. Chandra, A. (compiler). Elsevier Science Publishers B. V. Physical Sciences and Engineering Division, Amsterdam, Netherlands.

Enzyme Nomenclature. Recommendations of the Nomenclature Committee of the International Union of Biochemistry and Molecular Biology on the Nomenclature and Classification of Enzymes by the Reactions they Catalyse. http://www.chem.qmul.ac.uk/iubmb/enzyme. World Wide Web version prepared by G. P. Moss, School of Biological and Chemical Sciences, Queen Mary University of London, Mile End Road, London E1 4NS, UK; e-mail: g.p.moss@qmul.ac.uk.

FishBase. Froese, R.; Pauly, D. (Editors). http://www.fishbase.org.

Food Microbiology: Fundamentals and Frontiers. 3rd Edition. 2007. Doyle, M. P.; Beuchat, L. R. (Editors). ASM Press, Washington, D.C., USA.

Handbook of Nuts. 2000. Duke, J. A. CRC Press Inc., Boca Raton, Florida, USA.

International Union of Pure and Applied Chemistry. Recommendations on Organic & Biochemical Nomenclature, Symbols and Terminology etc. http://www.chem.qmul.ac.uk/iupac.

List of Prokaryotic names with Standing in Nomenclature. http://www.bacterio.net.

The Merck Index. An Encyclopedia of Chemicals, Drugs and Biologicals. 14th Edition. 2006. O'Neil, M. J. (Editor). Merck & Co Inc., Whitehouse Station, New Jersey, USA.

Multilingual Multiscript Plant Name Database. http://www.plantnames.unimelb.edu.au/Sorting/List_bot.html.

NCBI Taxonomy Database. www.ncbi.nlm.nih.gov/taxonomy.

The Official Website of the Mycoses Study Group. http://www.doctorfungus.org/.

The Oxford Companion to Food. 2006. Davidson, A. Oxford University Press, Oxford, UK.

PAN Pesticide Database. http://www.pesticideinfo.org/.

Pesticides: An International Guide to 1800 Pest Control Chemicals. 2nd Edition. 2004. Milne, G. W. A. (Editor). Ashgate Publishing Ltd., Aldershot, UK.

Species 2000 & ITIS Catalogue of Life. 2nd October 2010. Bisby, F.A.; Roskov, Y. R.; Orrell, T. M.; Nicolson, D.; Paglinawan, L. E.; Bailly, N.; Kirk, P. M.; Bourgoin, T.; Baillargeon, G.; Ouvrard, D. (Editors) http://www.catalogueoflife.org/col.

Structured Vocabularies for Information Retrieval – Guide – Part 2: Thesauri. BS 8723-2:2005. BSI, London, UK.

The Universal Virus Database of the International Committee on Taxonomy of Viruses. http://www.ictvdb.org/.

USDA, ARS, National Genetic Resources Program. *Germplasm Resources Information Network – (GRIN)* [Online Database]. National Germplasm Resources Laboratory, Beltsville, Maryland, USA. http://www.ars-grin.gov/cgi-bin/npgs/html/taxgenform.pl.

Additional information

For additional information on thesaurus usage, or to make comments/suggestions for subsequent revisions, or for more information about other IFIS products and services please contact IFIS by email at ifis@ifis.org. Alternatively, please visit our website at www.Food.ScienceCentral.com.

Alphabetical Thesaurus

A

AAS
SN index heading is Atomic absorption spectroscopy
BT1 Atomic absorption spectroscopy
BT2 Spectroscopy
BT3 Analytical techniques
UF Atomic absorption spectrophotometry

Abalones
BT1 Gastropods
BT2 Molluscs
BT3 Shellfish
BT4 Animals
BT4 Sea foods
BT5 Aquatic foods
BT6 Animal foods
BT7 Foods
UF Pauas

Abate
USE **Temephos**

Abattoirs
BT1 Slaughterhouses

Abondance cheese
BT1 Cheese varieties
BT2 Cheese
BT3 Dairy products
BT4 Animal foods
BT5 Foods

Abrasion
BT1 Damage

Abscisic acid
BT1 Plant growth regulators
BT2 Cultivation
BT3 Agriculture

Absidia
BT1 Fungi
BT2 Microorganisms
NT1 *Absidia corymbifera*

Absidia corymbifera
BT1 *Absidia*
BT2 Fungi
BT3 Microorganisms

Absinthe
BT1 Spirits
BT2 Alcoholic beverages
BT3 Beverages alcoholic
BT4 Beverages

Absorbents
BT1 Absorption
BT2 Sorption

Absorption
BT1 Sorption
NT1 Absorbents
RT Oil absorption capacity

Acacia
BT1 Plants
RT Gum acacia
RT Gum arabic

Acai
HN introduced from vol. 39, issue 1 (2007)
BT1 Fruits specific
BT2 Fruits
BT3 Crops
BT4 Plants
BT3 Plant foods
BT4 Foods
BT1 Palms
BT2 Plants

Acanthamoeba
HN introduced from vol. 39, issue 1 (2007)
BT1 Amoebae
BT2 Parasites
BT3 Pests

Acaricides
BT1 Pesticides
BT2 Biocides
BT2 Residues
NT1 Aldicarb
NT1 Amitraz
NT1 Azinphos-methyl
NT1 Bromocyclen
NT1 Camphechlor
NT1 Carbaryl
NT1 Carbofuran
NT1 Carbophenothion
NT1 Chlordimeform
NT1 Chlorfenvinphos
NT1 Chlorobenzilate
NT1 Chlorpyrifos
NT1 Chlorpyrifos-methyl
NT1 Coumaphos
NT1 Crotoxyphos
NT1 Cyhexatin
NT1 Cypermethrin
NT1 DDT
NT2 DDE
NT2 TDE
NT1 Deltamethrin
NT1 Demeton
NT1 Demeton-*S*-methyl
NT1 Dialifos
NT1 Diazinon
NT1 Dichlorobenzene
NT1 Dichlorvos
NT1 Dicofol
NT1 Dimethoate
NT1 Dioxathion
NT1 Disulfoton
NT1 Endosulfan
NT1 Ethion
NT1 Fenazaflor
NT1 Fenthion
NT1 Fenvalerate
NT1 Fluvalinate
NT1 Formothion
NT1 HCH
NT1 Malathion
NT2 Malaoxon
NT1 Methamidophos
NT1 Methomyl
NT1 Mevinphos
NT1 Monocrotophos
NT1 Naled
NT1 Omethoate
NT1 Oxamyl
NT1 Parathion
NT2 Paraoxon
NT1 Parathion-methyl
NT1 Permethrin
NT1 Phorate
NT1 Phosalone
NT1 Phosmet
NT1 Phoxim
NT1 Pirimiphos-methyl
NT1 Propargite
NT1 Propoxur
NT1 Quinalphos
NT1 Quinomethionate
NT1 Tetrachlorvinphos
NT1 Tetradifon
NT1 Triazophos
NT1 Trichlorfon

ACC
HN used as abbrev. for 1-aminocyclopropane-1-carboxylic acid from vol. 25 (1993)
BT1 Ethylene
BT2 Gases
BT3 Physical phases
BT4 Chemistry
BT5 Science
BT2 Hydrocarbons
BT3 Organic compounds
BT2 Plant growth regulators
BT3 Cultivation
BT4 Agriculture
UF 1-Aminocyclopropane-1-carboxylic acid

Acceptability
BT1 Consumer response
NT1 Consumer acceptability

Acceptable daily intake
USE **ADI**

Acceptance
BT1 Consumer response
NT1 Consumer acceptance

ACC oxidases
USE **1-Aminocyclopropane-1-carboxylate oxidases**

Accreditation
RT Certification

ACC synthases
USE **1-Aminocyclopropane-1-carboxylate synthases**

ACE inhibitors
HN introduced from vol. 39, issue 1 (2007)
BT1 Enzyme inhibitors
BT2 Enzymes
RT Antihypertensive activity
RT Peptidyl-dipeptidase A

Acephate
BT1 Organophosphorus insecticides
BT2 Insecticides
BT3 Pesticides
BT4 Biocides
BT4 Residues
BT2 Organophosphorus pesticides
BT3 Pesticides
BT4 Biocides
BT4 Residues

Acerola
USE **Barbados cherries**

Acesulfame K
HN heading from vol. 30 (1998); under Sweeteners up to vol. 29 (1997)
BT1 Sweeteners
BT2 Additives
NT1 Sunett

Acetaldehyde
SN syn. ethanal
BT1 Aldehydes
BT2 Carbonyl compounds
BT3 Organic compounds
BT1 Aroma compounds
BT2 Flavour compounds
BT2 Volatile compounds
NT1 Ethanal

Acetals
BT1 Aldehydes
BT2 Carbonyl compounds
BT3 Organic compounds
BT1 Aroma compounds
BT2 Flavour compounds
BT2 Volatile compounds

Acetates
HN under Salts up to vol. 42 (2010)
SN includes both salts and esters
NT1 Butyl acetate
NT1 Cellulose acetate
NT1 Ethyl acetate
NT1 Geranyl acetate
NT1 Hexyl acetate
NT1 Isoamyl acetate
NT1 Linalyl acetate
NT1 Polyvinyl acetate
NT1 Sodium acetate
NT1 Sodium diacetate
NT1 Terpinyl acetate
NT1 Vitamin E acetate
RT Acetic acid
RT Esters
RT Salts

Acetic acid
BT1 Organic acids
BT2 Acids
RT Acetates
RT Acetic fermentation
RT Sodium acetate
RT Vinegar

Acetic acid bacteria
HN under Pseudomonadaceae up to vol. 24 (1992)
BT1 Bacteria
BT2 Microorganisms
RT *Gluconobacter*

Acetic fermentation
BT1 Fermentation
RT Acetic acid

Acetobacter
HN heading from vol. 25 (1993); under Pseudomonadaceae up to vol. 24 (1992)
BT1 Bacteria
BT2 Microorganisms
NT1 *Acetobacter aceti*
NT1 *Acetobacter diazotrophicus*
NT1 *Acetobacter pasteurianus*
NT1 *Acetobacter suboxydans*
NT1 *Acetobacter xylinum*

Acetobacter aceti
BT1 *Acetobacter*
BT2 Bacteria
BT3 Microorganisms

Acetobacter diazotrophicus
SN synonymous with Gluconacetobacter diazotrophicus
BT1 *Acetobacter*
BT2 Bacteria
BT3 Microorganisms

Acetobacter pasteurianus
BT1 *Acetobacter*
BT2 Bacteria
BT3 Microorganisms

Acetobacter suboxydans
SN synonymous with Gluconobacter oxydans
BT1 *Acetobacter*
BT2 Bacteria
BT3 Microorganisms

Acetobacter xylinum
SN synonymous with Gluconobacter xylinus
BT1 *Acetobacter*
BT2 Bacteria
BT3 Microorganisms

Acetoin
SN syn. 3-hydroxy-2-butanone; syn. acetylmethylcarbinol
BT1 Aroma compounds
BT2 Flavour compounds
BT2 Volatile compounds
BT1 Ketones
BT2 Carbonyl compounds
BT3 Organic compounds
NT1 Acetylmethylcarbinol
NT1 3-Hydroxy-2-butanone

α-Acetolactate
HN also under Flavour compounds up to vol. 42 (2010)
BT1 Aroma compounds
BT2 Flavour compounds
BT2 Volatile compounds
BT1 Ketones
BT2 Carbonyl compounds
BT3 Organic compounds

Acetolactate decarboxylases
SN EC 4.1.1.5
BT1 Decarboxylases
BT2 Lyases
BT3 Enzymes

Acetolactate synthases
HN introduced from vol. 39, issue 1 (2007)
SN EC 2.2.1.6
BT1 Transferases
BT2 Enzymes

Acetomonas
HN under Pseudomonadaceae up to vol. 24 (1992)
SN obsolete name for Gluconobacter
BT1 *Gluconobacter*
BT2 Bacteria
BT3 Microorganisms

Acetone
SN syn. propanone
BT1 Ketones
BT2 Carbonyl compounds
BT3 Organic compounds
BT1 Solvents

Acetonitrile
BT1 Cyanides
BT2 Salts
BT1 Organic nitrogen compounds
BT1 Solvents

Acetophenone
BT1 Aroma compounds
BT2 Flavour compounds
BT2 Volatile compounds
BT1 Aromatic compounds
BT2 Organic compounds
BT1 Ketones
BT2 Carbonyl compounds
BT3 Organic compounds

Acetylacetone
HN also under Flavour compounds up to vol. 42 (2010)
SN syn. pentanedione
BT1 Pentanedione
BT2 Aroma compounds
BT3 Flavour compounds
BT3 Volatile compounds
BT2 Ketones
BT3 Carbonyl compounds
BT4 Organic compounds

Acetylation
BT1 Modification

Acetylcholinesterases
SN EC 3.1.1.7
BT1 Esterases
BT2 Hydrolases
BT3 Enzymes

Acetyl-CoA carboxylases
SN EC 6.4.1.2
BT1 Ligases
BT2 Enzymes

_N_-Acetyl-L-cysteine
HN introduced from vol. 41, issue 1 (2009)
BT1 Antioxidants
BT2 Additives
BT1 Cysteine
BT2 Amino acids
BT3 Nutrients
BT3 Organic acids
BT4 Acids
BT3 Organic nitrogen compounds

Acetylene
BT1 Gases
BT2 Physical phases
BT3 Chemistry
BT4 Science
BT1 Hydrocarbons
BT2 Organic compounds
BT1 Plant growth regulators
BT2 Cultivation
BT3 Agriculture

_N_-Acetylglucosamine
BT1 Amino sugars
BT2 Sugars
BT3 Carbohydrates
BT4 Nutrients
BT4 Organic compounds
BT3 Plant foods
BT4 Foods

Acetylglucosaminidases
SN EC 3.2.1.50; EC 3.2.1.96
BT1 Glycosidases
BT2 Hydrolases
BT3 Enzymes

β-_N_-acetylhexosaminidases
HN introduced from vol. 41, issue 1 (2009)
SN EC 3.2.1.52
BT1 Glycosidases
BT2 Hydrolases
BT3 Enzymes

N-Acetyllactosamine synthases
USE **Lactose synthases**

Acetylmethylcarbinol
SN syn. acetoin
BT1 Acetoin
BT2 Aroma compounds
BT3 Flavour compounds
BT3 Volatile compounds
BT2 Ketones
BT3 Carbonyl compounds
BT4 Organic compounds

_N_-Acetylneuraminic acid
SN syn. sialic acid
BT1 Organic acids
BT2 Acids

Acetyltransferases
HN introduced from vol. 41, issue 1 (2009)
SN EC 2.3.1
BT1 Acyltransferases
BT2 Transferases
BT3 Enzymes

Acha
BT1 Cereals
BT2 Crops
BT3 Plants
BT2 Seeds
BT3 Plant foods
BT4 Foods

Achillea millefolium
BT1 Yarrow
BT2 Plants

Achromobacter
BT1 Bacteria
BT2 Microorganisms

Acid casein
BT1 Casein
BT2 Milk proteins
BT3 Proteins milk
BT4 Animal proteins
BT5 Proteins animal
BT6 Proteins
BT7 Nutrients

Acid curd cheese
BT1 Cheese varieties
BT2 Cheese
BT3 Dairy products
BT4 Animal foods
BT5 Foods

Acidification
HN heading from vol. 25 (1993)
BT1 Processing
BT2 Technology
RT Acids
RT pH

Acidity
BT1 Physical properties
NT1 Acid values
NT1 Titratable acidity
RT Alkalinity
RT Neutralization

Acidocins
BT1 Bacteriocins
BT2 Antibiotics
BT3 Drugs
BT4 Residues
RT *Lactobacillus acidophilus*

Acidolysis
HN introduced from vol. 39, issue 1 (2007)
BT1 Esterification

Acidophilin
BT1 Fermented milk
BT2 Fermented dairy products
BT3 Dairy products
BT4 Animal foods
BT5 Foods
BT3 Fermented foods
BT4 Processed foods
BT5 Foods
BT2 Milk
BT3 Dairy products
BT4 Animal foods
BT5 Foods

Acidophilus milk
HN under Milk up to vol. 42 (2010)
BT1 Fermented milk
BT2 Fermented dairy products
BT3 Dairy products
BT4 Animal foods
BT5 Foods
BT3 Fermented foods
BT4 Processed foods
BT5 Foods
BT2 Milk
BT3 Dairy products
BT4 Animal foods
BT5 Foods

Acidophilus pastes
HN under Dairy products up to vol. 42 (2010)
BT1 Fermented dairy products
BT2 Dairy products
BT3 Animal foods
BT4 Foods
BT2 Fermented foods
BT3 Processed foods
BT4 Foods

Acid phosphatases
SN EC 3.1.3.2
BT1 Phosphatases
BT2 Esterases
BT3 Hydrolases
BT4 Enzymes

Acid rain
BT1 Weather

Acids
NT1 Acids resistance
NT1 Bile acids
NT1 Boric acid
NT1 Carbonic acid
NT1 HCl
NT1 H_2SO_4
NT1 Inorganic acids
NT1 Nitric acid
NT1 Nitrous acid
NT1 Organic acids
NT2 Acetic acid
NT2 *N*-Acetylneuraminic acid
NT2 Aconitic acid
NT2 Adipic acid
NT2 Amino acids
NT3 Alanine
NT3 D-Amino acids
NT3 Arginine
NT3 Asparagine
NT3 Aspartic acid
NT3 Canavanine
NT3 Citrulline
NT3 Cysteine
NT4 *N*-Acetyl-L-cysteine
NT3 Cystine
NT3 DOPA
NT3 Glutamic acid
NT4 Poly(γ-glutamic acid)
NT3 Glutamine

NT3 Glycine
NT3 Histidine
NT3 Homocysteine
NT3 Homoserine
NT3 Hydroxyproline
NT3 Isoleucine
NT3 Lanthionine
NT3 Leucine
NT3 Lysine
NT4 Polylysine
NT3 Methionine
NT4 *S*-Adenosyl-L-methionine
NT4 *S*-Methylmethionine
NT4 Selenomethionine
NT3 Methylhistidine
NT3 Octopine
NT3 Ornithine
NT3 Phenylalanine
NT3 Pipecolic acid
NT3 Proline
NT3 Pyroglutamic acid
NT3 Serine
NT3 Taurine
NT3 Theanine
NT3 Threonine
NT3 Tryptophan
NT3 Tyrosine
NT3 Valine
NT2 Aminobenzoic acid
NT2 Aminobutyric acid
NT2 Anthranilic acid
NT2 Barbituric acid
NT2 Benzoic acid
NT2 Bitter acids
NT3 α-Acids
NT4 Humulones
NT5 Adhumulone
NT5 Cohumulone
NT5 Humulinic acid
NT3 β-Acids
NT4 Hulupones
NT4 Lupulones
NT5 Colupulone
NT3 Iso-α-acids
NT4 Isohumulones
NT3 Lupulin
NT2 Caffeic acid
NT2 Carboxylic acids
NT2 Chlorogenic acid
NT3 Caffeoylquinic acid
NT2 Cinnamic acid
NT2 Citramalic acid
NT2 Citric acid
NT2 Cyclamic acid
NT2 Dehydroacetic acid
NT2 Diethylpyrocarbonate
NT2 Dipicolinic acid
NT2 EDTA
NT2 Ellagic acid
NT2 Erythorbic acid
NT2 Fatty acids
NT3 Branched chain fatty acids
NT4 Isobutyric acid
NT4 Isocaproic acid
NT4 Isovaleric acid
NT3 Cyclic fatty acids
NT3 Eicosanoids
NT4 Prostaglandins
NT3 Malvalic acid
NT3 Saturated fatty acids
NT4 Arachidic acid
NT4 Behenic acid
NT4 Butanoic acid
NT5 Butyric acid
NT4 Decanoic acid
NT5 Capric acid
NT4 Dodecanoic acid
NT5 Lauric acid
NT4 Heptadecanoic acid
NT5 Margaric acid
NT4 Heptanoic acid
NT4 Hexadecanoic acid
NT5 Palmitic acid
NT4 Hexanoic acid
NT5 Caproic acid
NT4 Lignoceric acid
NT4 Myristic acid
NT4 Octadecanoic acid
NT5 Stearic acid
NT6 Hydroxystearic acid
NT4 Octanoic acid
NT5 Caprylic acid
NT4 Pentanoic acid
NT5 Valeric acid
NT3 Sterculic acid
NT3 Unsaturated fatty acids
NT4 Essential fatty acids
NT4 Monounsaturated fatty acids
NT5 Decenoic acid
NT5 Docosenoic acid
NT6 Erucic acid
NT5 Eicosenoic acid
NT5 Hexadecenoic acid
NT6 Palmitoleic acid
NT5 Octadecenoic acid
NT6 Elaidic acid
NT6 Oleic acid
NT6 Petroselinic acid
NT6 Vaccenic acid
NT5 Ricinoleic acid
NT4 PUFA
NT5 Conjugated fatty acids
NT6 CLA
NT6 Eleostearic acid
NT5 Eicosatetraenoic acid
NT6 Arachidonic acid
NT5 ω-3 Fatty acids
NT6 Docosahexaenoic acid
NT6 Docosapentaenoic acid
NT6 Eicosapentaenoic acid
NT6 α-Linolenic acid
NT6 Stearidonic acid
NT5 ω-6 Fatty acids
NT6 Arachidonic acid
NT6 Linoleic acid
NT7 CLA
NT6 γ-Linolenic acid
NT5 Linolenic acid
NT6 Eleostearic acid
NT6 α-Linolenic acid
NT6 γ-Linolenic acid
NT4 *trans* Fatty acids
NT5 Elaidic acid
NT5 Vaccenic acid
NT3 Volatile fatty acids
NT4 Short chain fatty acids
NT5 Butanoic acid
NT6 Butyric acid
NT5 Hexanoic acid
NT6 Caproic acid
NT5 Hydroxybutyric acid
NT5 Isobutyric acid
NT5 Isocaproic acid
NT5 Isovaleric acid
NT5 Pentanoic acid
NT6 Valeric acid
NT2 Ferulic acid
NT2 Feruloylquinic acid
NT2 Formic acid
NT2 Fumaric acid
NT2 Gallic acid
NT2 Gluconic acid
NT2 Glutaric acid
NT2 Glycolic acid
NT2 Hippuric acid
NT2 Humic acids
NT2 Hydroxybenzoic acid
NT2 Hydroxycinnamic acid
NT3 Coumaric acid
NT2 Hydroxycitric acid
NT2 Isochlorogenic acid
NT2 Isocitric acid
NT2 Itaconic acid
NT2 Keto acids
NT2 α-Ketoglutaric acid
NT2 Lactic acid
NT2 Lactobionic acid
NT2 α-Lipoic acid
NT2 Maleic acid
NT2 Malic acid
NT2 Malonic acid
NT2 Mevalonic acid
NT2 Mucic acid
NT2 5-Nitrofurylacrylic acid
NT2 Nucleic acids
NT3 DNA
NT4 cDNA
NT4 Mitochondrial DNA
NT4 RAPD
NT3 RNA
NT4 mRNA
NT4 rRNA
NT2 Oleanolic acid
NT2 Orotic acid
NT2 Oxalic acid
NT2 Oxaloacetic acid
NT2 Peracetic acid
NT2 Phenylacetic acid
NT2 Phosphatidic acid
NT2 Phthalic acid
NT2 Propionic acid
NT2 Protocatechuic acid
NT2 Pyruvic acid
NT2 Quinic acid
NT2 Salicylic acid
NT2 Shikimic acid
NT2 Sialic acid
NT2 Sinapic acid
NT2 Sorbic acid
NT2 Succinic acid
NT2 Syringic acid
NT2 Tannins
NT3 Ellagitannins
NT3 Proanthocyanidins
NT4 Procyanidins

NT3 Tannic acid
NT2 Tartaric acid
NT2 Thioglycolic acid
NT2 Uronic acids
NT3 Galacturonic acid
NT3 Glucuronic acid
NT3 Polyuronides
NT2 Ursolic acid
NT2 Vanillic acid
NT1 Phosphoric acid
NT1 Silicic acid
NT1 Sulfurous acid
RT Acidification

α-Acids
BT1 Bitter acids
BT2 Bitter compounds
BT3 Flavour compounds
BT2 Organic acids
BT3 Acids
NT1 Humulones
NT2 Adhumulone
NT2 Cohumulone
NT2 Humulinic acid

β-Acids
BT1 Bitter acids
BT2 Bitter compounds
BT3 Flavour compounds
BT2 Organic acids
BT3 Acids
NT1 Hulupones
NT1 Lupulones
NT2 Colupulone

Acids resistance
BT1 Acids

Acidulants
BT1 Additives
NT1 Adipic acid

Acid values
BT1 Acidity
BT2 Physical properties
RT Fatty acids
RT Rancidity

Acid whey
BT1 Whey
BT2 Dairy products
BT3 Animal foods
BT4 Foods

Acinetobacter
HN heading from vol. 25 (1993); under Bacteria up to vol. 24 (1992)
BT1 Bacteria
BT2 Microorganisms
NT1 *Acinetobacter calcoaceticus*
NT1 *Acinetobacter haemolyticus*
NT1 *Acinetobacter radioresistens*

Acinetobacter calcoaceticus
BT1 *Acinetobacter*
BT2 Bacteria
BT3 Microorganisms

Acinetobacter haemolyticus
BT1 *Acinetobacter*
BT2 Bacteria
BT3 Microorganisms

Acinetobacter radioresistens
BT1 *Acinetobacter*
BT2 Bacteria
BT3 Microorganisms

Ackee
BT1 Fruits specific
BT2 Fruits
BT3 Crops
BT4 Plants
BT3 Plant foods
BT4 Foods

Aconitic acid
BT1 Flavourings
BT2 Additives
BT1 Organic acids
BT2 Acids

Acorns
BT1 Nuts
BT2 Fruits
BT3 Crops
BT4 Plants
BT3 Plant foods
BT4 Foods
BT2 Oilseeds
BT3 Seeds
BT4 Plant foods
BT5 Foods

Acorus calamus
USE **Calamus**

Acoustics
BT1 Analytical techniques
RT Sound

Acquired immunodeficiency syndrome
USE **AIDS**

Acremonium
SN synonym for the obsolete genus Cephalosporium
BT1 Fungi
BT2 Microorganisms
NT1 *Acremonium cellulolyticus*
NT1 *Cephalosporium*

Acremonium cellulolyticus
BT1 *Acremonium*
BT2 Fungi
BT3 Microorganisms

Acrocomia
BT1 Palms
BT2 Plants

Acrolein
SN syn. propenal
BT1 Aldehydes
BT2 Carbonyl compounds
BT3 Organic compounds
NT1 Propenal
RT Acrylamide
RT Taints

Acrylamide
BT1 Amides
BT2 Organic nitrogen compounds
RT Acrolein

Acrylonitrile
BT1 Fumigants
BT2 Biocides
BT1 Plastics
BT2 Packaging materials

Actidione
USE **Cycloheximide**

F-actin
BT1 Actins
BT2 Animal proteins
BT3 Proteins animal
BT4 Proteins
BT5 Nutrients
BT2 Globulins
BT3 Proteins
BT4 Nutrients

Actinidains
SN EC 3.4.22.14
BT1 Proteinases
BT2 Hydrolases
BT3 Enzymes
UF Actinidins

Actinidia arguta
BT1 Fruits specific
BT2 Fruits
BT3 Crops
BT4 Plants
BT3 Plant foods
BT4 Foods
RT Kiwifruit

Actinidia chinensis
BT1 Kiwifruit
BT2 Fruits specific
BT3 Fruits
BT4 Crops
BT5 Plants
BT4 Plant foods
BT5 Foods

Actinidia deliciosa
BT1 Kiwifruit
BT2 Fruits specific
BT3 Fruits
BT4 Crops
BT5 Plants
BT4 Plant foods
BT5 Foods

Actinidia polygama
BT1 Kiwifruit
BT2 Fruits specific
BT3 Fruits
BT4 Crops
BT5 Plants
BT4 Plant foods
BT5 Foods

Actinidins
USE **Actinidains**

Actinobacillus
HN introduced from vol. 42, issue 1 (2010)
BT1 Bacteria
BT2 Microorganisms

Actinobacteria
HN introduced from vol. 43, issue 1 (2011)
SN new name for Actinomycetes
BT1 Bacteria
BT2 Microorganisms
NT1 Actinomycetes

Actinomucor
BT1 Fungi
BT2 Microorganisms
NT1 *Actinomucor elegans*

Actinomucor elegans
HN introduced from vol. 39, issue 1 (2007)
BT1 *Actinomucor*
BT2 Fungi
BT3 Microorganisms

Actinomyces
BT1 Bacteria
BT2 Microorganisms

Actinomycetales
HN heading up to vol. 24 (1992)
BT1 Bacteria
BT2 Microorganisms

Actinomycetes
SN obsolete name for Actinobacteria
BT1 *Actinobacteria*
BT2 Bacteria
BT3 Microorganisms

Actinomycin
BT1 Antibiotics
BT2 Drugs
BT3 Residues

Actinoplanes
BT1 Bacteria
BT2 Microorganisms

Actinospectacin
USE **Spectinomycin**

Actins
BT1 Animal proteins
BT2 Proteins animal
BT3 Proteins
BT4 Nutrients
BT1 Globulins
BT2 Proteins
BT3 Nutrients
NT1 F-actin

Activated C
HN C activated also used in the index up to vol. 29 (1997)
BT1 Carbon
BT2 Elements
BT3 Minerals
BT4 Nutrients
NT1 Activated carbon
RT Adsorbents
RT Charcoal

Activated carbon
BT1 Activated C
BT2 Carbon
BT3 Elements
BT4 Minerals
BT5 Nutrients
RT Charcoal

Activation energy
BT1 Physical properties

Active packaging
BT1 Packaging
BT2 Technology
RT Antimicrobial packaging films

Active sites
RT Enzymes
RT Proteins

Actomyosin
BT1 Animal proteins
BT2 Proteins animal
BT3 Proteins
BT4 Nutrients
BT1 Globulins
BT2 Proteins
BT3 Nutrients

Acylamidases
USE **Amidases**

Acylases
USE **Amidases**
USE **Aminoacylases**

Acylation
BT1 Modification

Acylglycerols
SN syn. glycerides
BT1 Glycerides
BT2 Emulsifiers
BT3 Additives
BT2 Fatty acid esters
BT3 Esters
BT4 Organic compounds
BT2 Lipids
BT3 Nutrients

Acyltransferases
HN introduced from vol. 39, issue 1 (2007)
BT1 Transferases
BT2 Enzymes
NT1 Acetyltransferases
NT1 Alcohol *O*-acetyltransferases
NT1 Fatty acid synthases
NT1 γ-Glutamyltransferases
NT1 Protein-glutamine γ-glutamyltransferases

Additives
NT1 Acidulants
NT1 Adjuvants
NT1 Anardana
NT1 Anticaking agents
NT1 Antifoaming agents
NT1 Antioxidants
NT1 Aroma concentrates
NT1 Bakery additives
NT1 Binders
NT1 Binding agents
NT1 Bodying agents
NT1 $CaCl_2$
NT1 Chelating agents
NT1 Clouding agents
NT1 Colorants
NT1 Cryoprotectants
NT1 Defoaming agents
NT1 Degumming agents
NT1 EDTA
NT1 Emulsifiers
NT1 Flavourings
NT1 Food additives
NT1 Fumaric acid
NT1 Glucono-δ-lactone
NT1 Humectants
NT1 Improvers
NT1 $MgCl_2$
NT1 Oxidizing agents
NT1 Pet food additives
NT1 Polydimethylsiloxane
NT1 Preservatives
NT1 Reducing agents
NT1 Sequestrants
NT1 Softeners
NT1 Stabilizers
NT1 Sucrose polyesters
NT1 Sweeteners
NT1 Tartaric acid
NT1 Thickeners
NT1 Trilon B
NT1 Whiteners

Adenine
BT1 Purines
BT2 Heterocyclic compounds
BT2 Organic nitrogen compounds

Adenosine
BT1 Nucleosides
NT1 *S*-Adenosyl-L-methionine

Adenosine diphosphate
USE **ADP**

Adenosine monophosphate
USE **AMP**

Adenosinetriphosphatases
USE **ATPases**

Adenosine triphosphate
USE **ATP**

***S*-Adenosyl-L-methionine**
HN introduced from vol. 41, issue 1 (2009)
BT1 Adenosine
BT2 Nucleosides
BT1 Coenzymes
BT2 Enzymes
BT1 Methionine
BT2 Amino acids
BT3 Nutrients
BT3 Organic acids
BT4 Acids

BT3 Organic nitrogen compounds
BT2 Organic sulfur compounds

Adenoviruses
BT1 Viruses
BT2 Microorganisms
NT1 Mastadenovirus
NT2 Human adenovirus

Adherence
BT1 Virulence factors
RT Adhesins
RT Colonization
RT Colonization factors
RT Fimbriae
RT Intimins
RT Pili

Adhesins
BT1 Microbial proteins
BT2 Microorganisms
BT2 Proteins
BT3 Nutrients
BT1 Virulence factors
RT Adherence
RT Fimbriae
RT Intimins

Adhesion
BT1 Physical properties
NT1 Sticking
RT Adhesives

Adhesives
RT Adhesion
RT Packaging

Adhumulone
BT1 Humulones
BT2 α-Acids
BT3 Bitter acids
BT4 Bitter compounds
BT5 Flavour compounds
BT4 Organic acids
BT5 Acids

ADI
RT Nutrition
UF Acceptable daily intake

Adipic acid
BT1 Acidulants
BT2 Additives
BT1 Flavourings
BT2 Additives
BT1 Organic acids
BT2 Acids

Adipocytes
HN introduced from vol. 39, issue 1 (2007)
BT1 Cells
RT Adipogenesis
RT Adipose tissues

Adipogenesis
HN introduced from vol. 39, issue 1 (2007)
BT1 Physiology
BT2 Science
RT Adipocytes
RT Adipose tissues

Adiponectin
HN introduced from vol. 41, issue 1 (2009)
BT1 Hormones
BT2 Residues

Adipose tissues
BT1 Animal fats
BT2 Fats animal
BT3 Animal foods
BT4 Foods
BT3 Fats
BT4 Lipids
BT5 Nutrients
RT Adipocytes
RT Adipogenesis
RT Body fats

Adjunct cultures
HN introduced from vol. 37, issue 5 (2005)
BT1 Starters
BT2 Bacteria
BT3 Microorganisms
RT Cheesemaking

Adjuvants
BT1 Additives

Adlay
USE **Jobs tears**

Adolescents
BT1 Population groups
UF Teenagers

ADP
BT1 Nucleotides
UF Adenosine diphosphate

ADP-glucose pyrophosphorylases
USE **Glucose-1-phosphate adenylyltransferases**

Adrenaline
BT1 Catecholamines
BT2 Biogenic amines
BT3 Amines
BT4 Organic nitrogen compounds
BT2 Hormones
BT3 Residues
UF Epinephrine

β-Adrenergic agonists
BT1 Drugs
BT2 Residues
NT1 Cimaterol
NT1 Clenbuterol
NT1 Propranolol
NT1 Ractopamine
NT1 Salbutamol

Adsorbents
BT1 Adsorption
BT2 Sorption
RT Activated C

Adsorption
BT1 Sorption
NT1 Adsorbents

Adulteration
RT Contamination
RT Purity

Adults
HN introduced from vol. 43, issue 1 (2011)
BT1 Population groups

Advertising
BT1 Marketing
BT2 Economics
RT Information

Adzuki beans
BT1 Legumes
BT2 Vegetables specific
BT3 Vegetables
BT4 Crops
BT5 Plants
BT4 Plant foods
BT5 Foods

Aerated confectionery
BT1 Sugar confectionery
BT2 Plant foods
BT3 Foods

Aeration
BT1 Processing
BT2 Technology
RT Air
RT Bubbles
RT Carbonation
RT Whipping

Aerobacter
HN under Enterobacteriaceae up to vol. 24 (1992)
SN obsolete genus, now Klebsiella or Enterobacter spp.
USE ***Enterobacter***
USE ***Klebsiella***

Aerobes
BT1 Microorganisms

Aerococcus
BT1 Bacteria
BT2 Microorganisms

Aerolysins
BT1 Microbial proteins
BT2 Microorganisms
BT2 Proteins
BT3 Nutrients
BT1 Toxins
BT2 Residues
BT1 Virulence factors

Aeromonas
HN heading from vol. 25 (1993); under Pseudomonadaceae up to vol. 24 (1992)
BT1 Bacteria
BT2 Microorganisms
NT1 *Aeromonas caviae*
NT1 *Aeromonas hydrophila*

Aeromonas caviae
SN synonymous with Aeromonas punctata
BT1 *Aeromonas*
BT2 Bacteria
BT3 Microorganisms

Aeromonas hydrophila
BT1 *Aeromonas*
BT2 Bacteria
BT3 Microorganisms

Aerosol packs
BT1 Packs
BT2 Containers
RT Aerosols

Aerosols
BT1 Dispensers
BT2 Equipment
BT3 Technology
RT Aerosol packs

Afalon
USE **Linuron**

Affination
BT1 Refining
BT2 Purification
BT3 Processing
BT4 Technology

Affinity chromatography
BT1 Chromatography
BT2 Analytical techniques

Afghanistan
BT1 Asia

Aflatoxicosis
BT1 Mycotoxicosis
BT2 Diseases
BT2 Poisoning
RT Aflatoxins
RT *Aspergillus*

Aflatoxin B_1
BT1 Aflatoxins
BT2 Mycotoxins
BT3 Toxins
BT4 Residues

Aflatoxin B_2
BT1 Aflatoxins
BT2 Mycotoxins
BT3 Toxins
BT4 Residues

Aflatoxin B_3
BT1 Aflatoxins
BT2 Mycotoxins
BT3 Toxins
BT4 Residues
UF Parasiticol

Aflatoxin D_1
BT1 Aflatoxins
BT2 Mycotoxins
BT3 Toxins
BT4 Residues

Aflatoxin G_1
BT1 Aflatoxins
BT2 Mycotoxins
BT3 Toxins
BT4 Residues

Aflatoxin G_2
BT1 Aflatoxins
BT2 Mycotoxins
BT3 Toxins
BT4 Residues

Aflatoxin M_1
BT1 Aflatoxins
BT2 Mycotoxins
BT3 Toxins
BT4 Residues

Aflatoxin M_2
BT1 Aflatoxins
BT2 Mycotoxins
BT3 Toxins
BT4 Residues

Aflatoxin P_1
BT1 Aflatoxins
BT2 Mycotoxins
BT3 Toxins
BT4 Residues

Aflatoxin Q_1
BT1 Aflatoxins
BT2 Mycotoxins
BT3 Toxins
BT4 Residues

Aflatoxins
BT1 Mycotoxins
BT2 Toxins
BT3 Residues
NT1 Aflatoxin B_1
NT1 Aflatoxin B_2
NT1 Aflatoxin B_3
NT1 Aflatoxin D_1
NT1 Aflatoxin G_1
NT1 Aflatoxin G_2
NT1 Aflatoxin M_1
NT1 Aflatoxin M_2
NT1 Aflatoxin P_1
NT1 Aflatoxin Q_1
RT Aflatoxicosis
RT *Aspergillus*
RT Carcinogens
RT Hepatotoxins

AFLP
BT1 Genetic techniques
BT2 Genetics

Africa
HN heading up to vol. 24 (1992)
NT1 Central Africa
NT2 Burundi
NT2 Central African Republic
NT2 Chad
NT2 Democratic Republic of the Congo
NT2 Gabon
NT2 Rwanda
NT2 Zaire
NT1 East Africa
NT2 Djibouti
NT2 Eritrea
NT2 Ethiopia
NT2 Kenya
NT2 Somalia
NT2 Sudan
NT2 Tanzania
NT2 Uganda
NT1 North Africa
NT2 Algeria
NT2 Egypt
NT2 Libya
NT2 Morocco
NT2 Tunisia
NT1 Seychelles
NT1 Southern Africa
NT2 Angola
NT2 Botswana
NT2 Comoros
NT2 Lesotho
NT2 Madagascar
NT2 Malawi
NT2 Mauritius
NT2 Mozambique
NT2 Namibia
NT2 Reunion
NT2 South Africa
NT2 Swaziland
NT2 Zambia
NT2 Zimbabwe
NT1 West Africa
NT2 Benin
NT2 Burkina Faso
NT2 Cameroon
NT2 Cape Verde
NT2 Cote d'Ivoire
NT2 Equatorial Guinea
NT3 Bioko
NT2 Gambia
NT2 Ghana
NT2 Guinea
NT2 Guinea-Bissau
NT2 Liberia
NT2 Mali
NT2 Mauritania
NT2 Niger
NT2 Nigeria
NT2 Republic of the Congo
NT2 Senegal
NT2 Sierra Leone
NT2 Togo
RT Middle East

African breadfruit seeds
BT1 Seeds
BT2 Plant foods
BT3 Foods
RT *Treculia africana*

African locust beans
BT1 Oilseeds
BT2 Seeds
BT3 Plant foods
BT4 Foods
NT1 Dawadawa
NT1 Iru

African mangoes
BT1 Mangoes

BT2 Fruits specific
BT3 Fruits
BT4 Crops
BT5 Plants
BT4 Plant foods
BT5 Foods

African mango seeds
SN syn. dika nuts
BT1 Oilseeds
BT2 Seeds
BT3 Plant foods
BT4 Foods
NT1 Dika nuts

African nutmeg
BT1 Spices
BT2 Flavourings
BT3 Additives

African oil beans
BT1 Legumes
BT2 Vegetables specific
BT3 Vegetables
BT4 Crops
BT5 Plants
BT4 Plant foods
BT5 Foods
BT1 Oilseeds
BT2 Seeds
BT3 Plant foods
BT4 Foods
NT1 Ugba

African yam beans
BT1 Legumes
BT2 Vegetables specific
BT3 Vegetables
BT4 Crops
BT5 Plants
BT4 Plant foods
BT5 Foods

Afromomum danielli
BT1 Spices
BT2 Flavourings
BT3 Additives

Aftertaste
BT1 Flavour
BT2 Sensory properties

Afuega'l Pitu cheese
BT1 Cheese varieties
BT2 Cheese
BT3 Dairy products
BT4 Animal foods
BT5 Foods

Ag
HN under Minerals up to vol. 42 (2010)
BT1 Metals
BT2 Elements
BT3 Minerals
BT4 Nutrients
UF Silver

Agar
HN heading from vol. 25 (1993); under Agar-agar up to vol. 24 (1992)
BT1 Polysaccharides
BT2 Carbohydrates
BT3 Nutrients
BT3 Organic compounds
BT1 Stabilizers
BT2 Additives
BT1 Thickeners
BT2 Additives
NT1 Agar gels
NT1 Agarose
RT Media
RT Plate counts
RT Seaweeds
UF Agar-agar

Agar-agar
HN heading up to vol. 24 (1992)
USE **Agar**

Agarases
BT1 Glycosidases
BT2 Hydrolases
BT3 Enzymes

Agar gels
BT1 Agar
BT2 Polysaccharides
BT3 Carbohydrates
BT4 Nutrients
BT4 Organic compounds
BT2 Stabilizers
BT3 Additives
BT2 Thickeners
BT3 Additives
BT1 Gels
BT2 Physical phases
BT3 Chemistry
BT4 Science

Agaricus
HN heading from vol. 30 (1998); under Fungi edible up to vol. 29 (1997)
BT1 Edible fungi
BT2 Fungi edible
BT3 Vegetables specific
BT4 Vegetables
BT5 Crops
BT6 Plants
BT5 Plant foods
BT6 Foods
NT1 *Agaricus bisporus*
NT1 *Agaricus blazei*

Agaricus bisporus
BT1 *Agaricus*
BT2 Edible fungi
BT3 Fungi edible
BT4 Vegetables specific
BT5 Vegetables
BT6 Crops
BT7 Plants
BT6 Plant foods
BT7 Foods

Agaricus blazei
BT1 *Agaricus*
BT2 Edible fungi
BT3 Fungi edible
BT4 Vegetables specific
BT5 Vegetables
BT6 Crops
BT7 Plants
BT6 Plant foods
BT7 Foods

Agaritine
BT1 Carcinogens
BT2 Mutagens
BT1 Mycotoxins
BT2 Toxins
BT3 Residues
BT1 Organic nitrogen compounds

Agarose
BT1 Agar
BT2 Polysaccharides
BT3 Carbohydrates
BT4 Nutrients
BT4 Organic compounds
BT2 Stabilizers
BT3 Additives
BT2 Thickeners
BT3 Additives

Agastache
HN introduced from vol. 39, issue 1 (2007); under Spices up to vol. 42 (2010)
BT1 Herbs
BT2 Spices
BT3 Flavourings
BT4 Additives

Agave
BT1 Plants
NT1 *Agave tequilana*

Agave tequilana
BT1 Agave
BT2 Plants

Age
RT Ageing
UF Maturity

Ageing
RT Age
RT Ripening
UF Maturation

Agglomerates
BT1 Agglomeration

Agglomeration
NT1 Agglomerates
NT1 Aggregation
NT2 Agglutination
NT3 Haemagglutination
RT Granules

Agglutination
BT1 Aggregation
BT2 Agglomeration
NT1 Haemagglutination

Agglutination tests
BT1 Immunological techniques
BT2 Analytical techniques

Agglutinins
HN heading up to vol. 24 (1992)
USE **Lectins**

Aggregation
BT1 Agglomeration
NT1 Agglutination
NT2 Haemagglutination

Agitation
BT1 Mixing
BT2 Processing
BT3 Technology

Aglycones
BT1 Glycosides
BT2 Carbohydrates
BT3 Nutrients
BT3 Organic compounds

Agmatine
BT1 Amines
BT2 Organic nitrogen compounds

Agricultural produce
BT1 Crops
BT2 Plants

Agricultural products
BT1 Crops
BT2 Plants

Agriculture
NT1 Apiculture
NT1 Cultivation
NT2 Canopy
NT2 Crops rotation
NT2 Defoliation
NT2 Fertilizers
NT3 Foliar sprays
NT2 Girdling
NT2 Hydroponics
NT2 Irrigation
NT3 Water stress
NT2 Mulching
NT2 Plant density
NT2 Plant growth regulators
NT3 Abscisic acid
NT3 Acetylene
NT3 Aminoethoxyvinylglycine
NT3 Antisprouting agents
NT4 Maleic hydrazide
NT3 Antitranspirants
NT3 Auxins
NT4 Indole acetic acid
NT5 Indol-3-ylacetic acid
NT4 Naphthaleneacetic acid
NT5 2-(1-Naphthyl)acetic acid
NT5 (2-Naphthyloxy)acetic acid
NT3 Chlormequat
NT3 CPTA
NT3 Cytokinins
NT4 Benzyladenine
NT5 6-Benzylaminopurine
NT4 Kinetin
NT4 Thidiazuron
NT4 Zeatin
NT3 Daminozide
NT3 Ethylene
NT4 ACC
NT4 Ethephon
NT3 Gibberellins
NT4 Gibberellic acid
NT3 Growth promoters (plant)
NT3 1-Methylcyclopropene
NT3 Methyl jasmonate
NT4 Jasmonic acid
NT3 Paclobutrazol
NT3 Phytohormones
NT3 Propylene
NT3 Triiodobenzoic acid
NT2 Planting
NT2 Pruning
NT2 Rootstocks
NT2 Shading
NT2 Soils
NT2 Sowing
NT2 Thinning
NT2 Viniculture
NT2 Viticulture
NT1 Harvesting
NT2 Mechanical harvesting
NT2 Picking
NT2 Threshers
NT1 Horticulture
NT1 Housing
NT2 Lairage
NT1 Husbandry
NT2 Milking
NT2 Stocking density (husbandry)
NT1 Rearing
RT Environment
RT Feeds
RT Pesticides

Agrobacterium
BT1 Bacteria
BT2 Microorganisms
NT1 *Agrobacterium tumefaciens*
NT2 *Agrobacterium radiobacter*

Agrobacterium radiobacter
HN introduced from vol. 39, issue 1 (2007)
SN synonymous with Agrobacterium tumefaciens
BT1 *Agrobacterium tumefaciens*
BT2 *Agrobacterium*
BT3 Bacteria
BT4 Microorganisms

Agrobacterium tumefaciens
SN synonymous with Agrobacterium radiobacter
BT1 *Agrobacterium*
BT2 Bacteria
BT3 Microorganisms
NT1 *Agrobacterium radiobacter*

Agrocybe
BT1 Edible fungi
BT2 Fungi edible
BT3 Vegetables specific
BT4 Vegetables
BT5 Crops
BT6 Plants
BT5 Plant foods
BT6 Foods

Ahasverus advena
BT1 Beetles
BT2 Insects
BT3 Pests

Aichi virus
HN introduced from vol. 43, issue 1 (2011)
BT1 Kobuvirus
BT2 Viruses
BT3 Microorganisms

AIDS
BT1 Diseases
UF Acquired immunodeficiency syndrome

Aiele fruits
BT1 Fruits specific
BT2 Fruits
BT3 Crops
BT4 Plants
BT3 Plant foods
BT4 Foods
BT1 Oilseeds
BT2 Seeds
BT3 Plant foods
BT4 Foods

Air
BT1 Gases
BT2 Physical phases
BT3 Chemistry
BT4 Science
NT1 Airborne
NT1 Air conditioning
NT1 Air speed
NT1 Atmosphere
RT Aeration
RT Air pollutants
RT Ventilation

Airborne
BT1 Air
BT2 Gases
BT3 Physical phases
BT4 Chemistry
BT5 Science

Air conditioning
BT1 Air
BT2 Gases
BT3 Physical phases
BT4 Chemistry
BT5 Science

Air cooling
HN introduced from vol. 39, issue 1 (2007)
BT1 Cooling
BT2 Thermal processing
BT3 Processing thermal
BT4 Processing
BT5 Technology

Aircraft
BT1 Transport

Air drying
HN drying air also used in the index up to vol. 29 (1997)
BT1 Drying
BT2 Thermal processing

BT3 Processing thermal
BT4 Processing
BT5 Technology

Airflow properties
BT1 Mechanical properties
BT2 Physical properties

Airline meals
BT1 Meals
BT2 Processed foods
BT3 Foods

Air pollutants
BT1 Air pollution
BT2 Environmental pollution
BT3 Pollution
BT4 Contamination
BT1 Pollutants
BT2 Pollution
BT3 Contamination
NT1 Exhaust gases
NT1 Factory fumes
RT Air
RT Air quality

Air pollution
BT1 Environmental pollution
BT2 Pollution
BT3 Contamination
NT1 Air pollutants
NT2 Exhaust gases
NT2 Factory fumes
RT Air quality
RT Fallout

Air quality
RT Air pollutants
RT Air pollution

Air speed
HN introduced from vol. 39, issue 1 (2007)
BT1 Air
BT2 Gases
BT3 Physical phases
BT4 Chemistry
BT5 Science

Ajowan
BT1 Spices
BT2 Flavourings
BT3 Additives

Akara
BT1 Cowpeas
BT2 Legumes
BT3 Vegetables specific
BT4 Vegetables
BT5 Crops
BT6 Plants
BT5 Plant foods
BT6 Foods

Al
BT1 Aluminium
BT2 Metals
BT3 Elements
BT4 Minerals
BT5 Nutrients
BT2 Packaging materials
RT Al compounds
RT Al foils

Alachlor
BT1 Herbicides
BT2 Pesticides
BT3 Biocides
BT3 Residues

Alanine
HN heading from vol. 25 (1993); under Amino acids up to vol. 24 (1992)
BT1 Amino acids
BT2 Nutrients
BT2 Organic acids
BT3 Acids
BT2 Organic nitrogen compounds

Alar
USE **Daminozide**

Alaska pollack
HN heading from vol. 30 (1998) to vol. 42 (2010); under Fishes up to vol. 29 (1997); under Alaska pollock from vol. 43 (2011)
SN syn. walleye pollack
BT1 Alaska pollock
BT2 Marine fish
BT3 Fish
BT4 Animals
BT4 Sea foods
BT5 Aquatic foods
BT6 Animal foods
BT7 Foods

Alaska pollock
HN introduced from vol. 43, issue 1 (2011); heading
BT1 Marine fish
BT2 Fish
BT3 Animals
BT3 Sea foods
BT4 Aquatic foods
BT5 Animal foods
BT6 Foods
NT1 Alaska pollack
NT1 *Theragra chalcogramma*
NT1 Walleye pollack
RT Pollock

Albacore
SN syn. white tuna
BT1 White tuna
BT2 Tuna
BT3 Marine fish
BT4 Fish
BT5 Animals
BT5 Sea foods
BT6 Aquatic foods
BT7 Animal foods
BT8 Foods
BT3 Oily fish
BT4 Fish
BT5 Animals
BT5 Sea foods
BT6 Aquatic foods
BT7 Animal foods
BT8 Foods

Albania
BT1 Europe

Albendazole
BT1 Anthelmintics
BT2 Drugs
BT3 Residues

Albumen
USE **Egg whites**

Albumins
BT1 Proteins
BT2 Nutrients
NT1 Bovine serum albumin
NT1 Conalbumin
NT1 Lactalbumins
NT2 α-Lactalbumin
NT1 Ovalbumins

Alcaligenes
BT1 Bacteria
BT2 Microorganisms
NT1 *Alcaligenes eutrophus*
NT1 *Alcaligenes faecalis*
NT1 *Alcaligenes xylosoxydans*

Alcaligenes eutrophus
SN synonymous with Cupriavidus necator
BT1 *Alcaligenes*
BT2 Bacteria
BT3 Microorganisms

Alcaligenes faecalis
BT1 *Alcaligenes*
BT2 Bacteria
BT3 Microorganisms

Alcaligenes xylosoxydans
SN synonymous with Achromobacter xylosoxidans
BT1 *Alcaligenes*
BT2 Bacteria
BT3 Microorganisms

Alcohol
SN syn. ethanol
BT1 Ethanol
BT2 Alcohols
BT2 Solvents
RT Alcoholic beverages

Alcoholacetyltransferases
USE **Alcohol *O*-acetyltransferases**

Alcohol dehydrogenases
SN EC 1.1.1.1
BT1 Dehydrogenases
BT2 Oxidoreductases
BT3 Enzymes

Alcohol free beverages
BT1 Alcohol low beverages
BT2 Beverages alcohol low
BT3 Beverages

Alcoholic beverages
SN index heading is Beverages alcoholic
BT1 Beverages alcoholic

BT2 Beverages
NT1 Alcoholic soft drinks
NT1 Aperitifs
NT1 Beer
NT2 Alcohol low beer
NT2 Ale
NT2 Bouza
NT2 Draught beer
NT2 Happoshu
NT2 Lager
NT2 Lambic
NT2 Malt beverages
NT2 Merissa
NT2 Pito
NT2 Pombe
NT2 Shandy
NT2 Sorghum beer
NT2 Stout
NT2 Wheat beer
NT1 Boza
NT1 Cereal wines
NT2 Rice wines
NT3 Sake
NT4 Ginjoshu
NT4 Narazuke
NT3 Takju
NT3 Yakju
NT1 Cider
NT1 Cocktails
NT1 Egg nog
NT1 Fruit wines
NT2 Apple wines
NT2 Apricot wines
NT2 Orange wines
NT1 Kvass
NT1 Liqueurs
NT2 Anisette
NT2 Cordials
NT2 Cream liqueurs
NT2 Fruit liqueurs
NT3 Cassis
NT3 Cherry brandy
NT3 Limoncello
NT2 Pernod
NT1 Mead
NT1 Melomel
NT1 Perry
NT1 Pulque
NT1 Spirits
NT2 Absinthe
NT2 Aquavit
NT2 Arak
NT2 Awamori
NT2 Brandies
NT3 Armagnac
NT3 Brandy
NT3 Cognac
NT3 Eau de vie
NT3 Fruit brandies
NT4 Apple brandy
NT5 Calvados
NT4 Kirsch
NT4 Rakia
NT4 Slivovitz
NT3 Grappa
NT3 Pisco
NT2 Distillates
NT3 Wine distillates
NT2 Gin
NT2 Grape spirits
NT2 Lambanog
NT2 Mezcal
NT2 Ouzo
NT2 Raki
NT2 Rum
NT2 Schnapps
NT2 Shochu
NT2 Sugar cane spirits
NT3 Cachaca
NT2 Tequila
NT2 Vodka
NT2 Whiskies
NT3 Whiskey
NT4 Bourbon whiskey
NT3 Whisky
NT4 Scotch whisky
NT1 Wines
NT2 Alcohol low wines
NT2 Aromatized wines
NT3 Retsina
NT3 Sangria
NT3 Vermouths
NT3 Wine coolers
NT2 Dessert wines
NT2 Fortified wines
NT3 Madeira
NT3 Marsala
NT3 Port
NT3 Sherry
NT2 Ice wines
NT3 Eiswein
NT2 Red wines
NT2 Rose wines
NT2 White wines
NT2 Wines sparkling
NT3 Sparkling wines
NT4 Cavas
NT4 Champagne
NT4 Sekts
NT1 Wines palm
NT2 Palm wines
NT3 Coconut toddy
NT3 Toddy
NT3 Tuba
RT Alcohol
RT Alcohol-related disorders

Alcoholic fermentation
SN syn. ethanolic fermentation
BT1 Fermentation

Alcoholic soft drinks
BT1 Alcoholic beverages
BT2 Beverages alcoholic
BT3 Beverages
UF Alcopops

Alcohol low beer
BT1 Alcohol low beverages
BT2 Beverages alcohol low
BT3 Beverages
BT1 Beer
BT2 Alcoholic beverages
BT3 Beverages alcoholic
BT4 Beverages
UF Alcohol reduced beer
UF Low alcohol beer

Alcohol low beverages
SN heading is Beverages alcohol low
BT1 Beverages alcohol low
BT2 Beverages
NT1 Alcohol free beverages
NT1 Alcohol low beer
NT1 Alcohol low wines
RT Lite beverages
UF Alcohol reduced beverages
UF Low alcohol beverages

Alcohol low wines
BT1 Alcohol low beverages
BT2 Beverages alcohol low
BT3 Beverages
BT1 Wines
BT2 Alcoholic beverages
BT3 Beverages alcoholic
BT4 Beverages
UF Alcohol reduced wines
UF Low alcohol wines

Alcohol *O*-acetyltransferases
SN EC 2.3.1.84
BT1 Acyltransferases
BT2 Transferases
BT3 Enzymes
UF Alcoholacetyltransferases

Alcoholometers
BT1 Ethanol
BT2 Alcohols
BT2 Solvents

Alcohol oxidases
HN introduced from vol. 41, issue 1 (2009)
SN includes EC 1.1.3.13 (alcohol oxidase) and other alcohol oxidases
BT1 Oxidases
BT2 Oxidoreductases
BT3 Enzymes
NT1 Aryl-alcohol oxidases

Alcohol reduced beer
USE **Alcohol low beer**

Alcohol reduced beverages
USE **Alcohol low beverages**

Alcohol reduced wines
USE **Alcohol low wines**

Alcohol-related disorders
HN introduced from vol. 40, issue 4 (2008)
SN includes alcohol dependence, alcoholic liver diseases, etc.
BT1 Diseases
RT Alcoholic beverages

Alcohols
NT1 Aminoethanol
NT1 Amyl alcohol
NT2 Pentanol
NT1 Benzyl alcohol
NT1 Butanol
NT2 Butyl alcohol
NT1 Cafestol
NT1 Carnosol
NT1 Citronellol
NT1 Decanol

NT1 Diols
NT1 Ethanol
NT2 Alcohol
NT2 Alcoholometers
NT1 Ethanolamine
NT1 Farnesol
NT1 Flavonols
NT2 Dihydroquercetin
NT2 Fisetin
NT2 Isorhamnetin
NT2 Kaempferol
NT2 Morin
NT2 Myricetin
NT2 Quercetin
NT2 Quercitrin
NT2 Rutin
NT1 Fusel oils
NT1 Geosmin
NT1 Geraniol
NT1 Glycols
NT2 1,3-Butylene glycol
NT2 2,3-Butylene glycol
NT2 Diethylene glycol
NT2 Ethylene glycol
NT2 Polyethylene glycol
NT2 1,2-Propanediol
NT2 Propylene glycol
NT1 Hexanol
NT1 Isoamyl alcohol
NT2 Isopentyl alcohol
NT2 Methyl butanol
NT1 Isobutanol
NT2 Isobutyl alcohol
NT2 Methyl propanol
NT1 Isopropanol
NT1 Isopropyl alcohol
NT1 Kahweol
NT1 Linalool
NT1 Menthol
NT1 Methanol
NT1 Methionol
NT1 Nerol
NT1 Octanol
NT1 1-Octen-3-ol
NT1 Phenols
NT2 Alkylphenols
NT2 Alkylresorcinols
NT2 Anisole
NT2 Arbutin
NT2 Avenanthramides
NT2 Bisphenol A
NT2 Bisphenol A diglycidyl ether
NT2 Bisphenol F diglycidyl ether
NT2 Bromophenols
NT2 Caffeic acid
NT2 Carvacrol
NT2 Catechols
NT3 Catechin
NT3 Epicatechin
NT3 Epicatechin gallate
NT3 Epicatechol
NT3 Epigallocatechin
NT3 Epigallocatechin gallate
NT3 Gallocatechin gallate
NT3 Pyrocatechol
NT2 Chlorogenic acid
NT3 Caffeoylquinic acid
NT2 Chlorophenol
NT2 Cinnamic acid
NT2 Coumarins
NT3 Coumarin
NT3 Coumestrol
NT3 Esculetin
NT3 Furocoumarins
NT4 Bergapten
NT4 Psoralens
NT4 Xanthotoxin
NT3 Scopoletin
NT2 Cresols
NT2 Curcuminoids
NT3 Curcumin
NT2 Ellagic acid
NT2 Ellagitannins
NT2 Estragole
NT2 Eugenol
NT2 Ferulic acid
NT2 Feruloylquinic acid
NT2 Gingerols
NT2 Guaiacol
NT2 4-Hexylresorcinol
NT2 Hydroquinone
NT2 Hydroxycinnamic acid
NT3 Coumaric acid
NT2 Hydroxytyrosol
NT2 Isochlorogenic acid
NT2 Isoeugenol
NT2 Lignans
NT3 Sesamin
NT3 Sesamolin
NT2 Naphthol
NT2 Nordihydroguaiaretic acid
NT3 NDGA
NT2 Oleuropein
NT2 Phenylpropanoids
NT2 Phloroglucinol
NT2 Polyphenols
NT2 Protocatechuic acid
NT2 Pyrogallol
NT2 Resorcinol
NT2 Rosmarinic acid
NT2 Sesamol
NT2 Stilbenes
NT3 Piceatannol
NT3 Piceid
NT3 Resveratrol
NT2 Syringic acid
NT2 Thymol
NT2 Tyrosol
NT2 Vanillic acid
NT2 Vanillin
NT2 Zingerone
NT1 Phenylethanol
NT2 Phenethyl alcohol
NT1 Policosanols
NT1 Polyols
NT2 Alditols
NT2 Arabitol
NT2 Dulcitol
NT2 Erythritol
NT2 Galactitol
NT2 Glycerol
NT3 Glycerin
NT3 Glycerine
NT2 Inositol
NT3 Inositol phosphates
NT3 Phytates
NT3 Phytic acid
NT2 Lactitol
NT2 Maltitol
NT2 Mannitol
NT2 Sorbitol
NT2 Sugar alcohols
NT2 Xylitol
NT1 Propanol
NT2 Chloropropanols
NT1 2-Propanol
NT1 Propyl alcohol
NT1 Stearyl alcohol
NT1 Sterols
NT2 Avenasterol
NT2 Brassicasterol
NT2 Campesterol
NT2 Cholesterol
NT3 Cholesterol low foods
NT3 Cholesterol oxidation products
NT4 Cholesterol oxides
NT2 Cucurbitacins
NT2 Desmosterol
NT2 Ergosterol
NT2 Phytosterols
NT2 Sitosterol
NT2 Stanols
NT3 Phytostanols
NT4 Sitostanol
NT3 Stanol esters
NT2 Sterol esters
NT2 Stigmastadienes
NT2 Stigmasterol
NT1 Terpineol
NT1 Tryptophol
NT1 Veratryl alcohol
RT Aroma compounds
RT Thiols

Alcoholysis
HN introduced from vol. 39, issue 1 (2007)
BT1 Esterification
NT1 Glycerolysis
NT1 Methanolysis

Al compounds
BT1 Aluminium
BT2 Metals
BT3 Elements
BT4 Minerals
BT5 Nutrients
BT2 Packaging materials
RT Al
UF Aluminium compounds

Alcopops
USE **Alcoholic soft drinks**

Aldehyde dehydrogenases
SN include members of subclass EC 1.2
BT1 Dehydrogenases
BT2 Oxidoreductases
BT3 Enzymes

Aldehyde reductases
SN EC 1.1.1.21
BT1 Dehydrogenases
BT2 Oxidoreductases
BT3 Enzymes
UF Xylose reductases

Aldehydes
BT1 Carbonyl compounds
 BT2 Organic compounds
NT1 Acetaldehyde
 NT2 Ethanal
NT1 Acetals
NT1 Acrolein
 NT2 Propenal
NT1 Alkanals
NT1 Anisaldehyde
NT1 Benzaldehyde
NT1 Butanal
NT1 Butyraldehyde
NT1 Cinnamaldehyde
NT1 Citral
 NT2 Geranial
 NT2 Neral
NT1 Citronellal
NT1 Cuminaldehyde
NT1 Decanal
NT1 Formaldehyde
 NT2 Formalin
 NT2 Formol
 NT2 Methanal
NT1 Fural
NT1 Furaldehyde
NT1 Furfural
NT1 Glutaraldehyde
NT1 Glyceraldehyde
NT1 Glycolaldehyde
NT1 Glyoxal
NT1 Heptenal
NT1 Hexanal
NT1 Hexenal
NT1 5-(Hydroxymethyl)-2-furaldehyde
NT1 Hydroxymethylfurfural
NT1 3-Hydroxypropionaldehyde
NT1 Isobutyraldehyde
 NT2 2-Methylpropanal
NT1 Malonaldehyde
NT1 Malondialdehyde
NT1 Methional
NT1 3-Methylbutanal
 NT2 Isovaleraldehyde
NT1 Methylglyoxal
NT1 Nonanal
NT1 Nonenal
NT1 Octanal
NT1 Paraformaldehyde
NT1 Pentanal
 NT2 Valeraldehyde
NT1 Phenylacetaldehyde
NT1 Propanal
 NT2 Propionaldehyde
NT1 Pyruvaldehyde
NT1 Reuterin
NT1 Safranal
RT Aroma compounds
RT Off odour

Aldicarb
BT1 Acaricides
 BT2 Pesticides
  BT3 Biocides
  BT3 Residues
BT1 *N*-Methylcarbamate insecticides
 BT2 Insecticides
  BT3 Pesticides
   BT4 Biocides
   BT4 Residues
 BT2 *N*-Methylcarbamate pesticides
  BT3 Carbamate pesticides
   BT4 Pesticides
    BT5 Biocides
    BT5 Residues
BT1 Nematocides
 BT2 Pesticides
  BT3 Biocides
  BT3 Residues
UF Temik

Alditols
BT1 Polyols
 BT2 Alcohols
 BT2 Carbohydrates
  BT3 Nutrients
  BT3 Organic compounds

Aldolases
USE **Fructose-bisphosphate aldolases**

Aldose 1-epimerases
SN EC 5.1.3.3
BT1 Epimerases
 BT2 Isomerases
  BT3 Enzymes
UF Mutarotases

Aldoses
HN introduced from vol. 43, issue 1 (2011)
BT1 Monosaccharides
 BT2 Sugars
  BT3 Carbohydrates
   BT4 Nutrients
   BT4 Organic compounds
  BT3 Plant foods
   BT4 Foods

Aldrin
BT1 Organochlorine insecticides
 BT2 Insecticides
  BT3 Pesticides
   BT4 Biocides
   BT4 Residues
 BT2 Organochlorine pesticides
  BT3 Pesticides
   BT4 Biocides
   BT4 Residues

Ale
BT1 Beer
 BT2 Alcoholic beverages
  BT3 Beverages alcoholic
   BT4 Beverages

Aleurone
RT Cereals

Alewife
BT1 Marine fish
 BT2 Fish
  BT3 Animals
  BT3 Sea foods
   BT4 Aquatic foods
    BT5 Animal foods
     BT6 Foods
UF Alewives

Alewives
HN used up to vol. 29 (1997)
USE **Alewife**

Alexandrium
BT1 Dinoflagellates
 BT2 Microalgae
  BT3 Algae
   BT4 Microorganisms
NT1 *Alexandrium catenella*
NT1 *Alexandrium minutum*
NT1 *Alexandrium tamarense*

Alexandrium catenella
BT1 *Alexandrium*
 BT2 Dinoflagellates
  BT3 Microalgae
   BT4 Algae
    BT5 Microorganisms

Alexandrium minutum
BT1 *Alexandrium*
 BT2 Dinoflagellates
  BT3 Microalgae
   BT4 Algae
    BT5 Microorganisms

Alexandrium tamarense
BT1 *Alexandrium*
 BT2 Dinoflagellates
  BT3 Microalgae
   BT4 Algae
    BT5 Microorganisms

Alfalfa
SN syn. lucerne
BT1 Legumes
 BT2 Vegetables specific
  BT3 Vegetables
   BT4 Crops
    BT5 Plants
   BT4 Plant foods
    BT5 Foods
NT1 Alfalfa seeds
NT1 Lucerne
NT1 *Medicago sativa*
RT Alfalfa sprouts

Alfalfa seeds
BT1 Alfalfa
 BT2 Legumes
  BT3 Vegetables specific
   BT4 Vegetables
    BT5 Crops
     BT6 Plants
    BT5 Plant foods
     BT6 Foods

Alfalfa sprouts
BT1 Legume sprouts
 BT2 Legumes
  BT3 Vegetables specific
   BT4 Vegetables
    BT5 Crops
     BT6 Plants
    BT5 Plant foods
     BT6 Foods
 BT2 Sprouts

BT3 Vegetables specific
BT4 Vegetables
BT5 Crops
BT6 Plants
BT5 Plant foods
BT6 Foods
RT Alfalfa

Al foils
BT1 Foils
BT2 Packaging materials
RT Al
UF Aluminium foils

Algae
BT1 Microorganisms
NT1 Microalgae
NT2 *Chlamydomonas*
NT2 *Chlorella*
NT3 *Chlorella vulgaris*
NT2 *Chlorococcum*
NT2 *Crypthecodinium*
NT3 *Crypthecodinium cohnii*
NT2 Dinoflagellates
NT3 *Alexandrium*
NT4 *Alexandrium catenella*
NT4 *Alexandrium minutum*
NT4 *Alexandrium tamarense*
NT2 *Dunaliella*
NT3 *Dunaliella salina*
NT2 *Euglena*
NT3 *Euglena gracilis*
NT2 *Haematococcus*
NT3 *Haematococcus pluvialis*
NT2 *Nitzschia*
NT3 *Nitzschia laevis*
NT2 *Phaeodactylum*
NT3 *Phaeodactylum tricornutum*
NT2 *Porphyridium*
NT2 *Scenedesmus*
NT1 Seaweeds
NT2 *Caulerpa*
NT2 *Chondrus*
NT3 *Chondrus crispus*
NT2 *Cystoseira*
NT2 Dulse
NT3 *Palmaria palmata*
NT2 *Ecklonia*
NT2 *Eucheuma*
NT2 *Fucus*
NT2 *Furcellaria*
NT2 *Gigartina*
NT2 *Gracilaria*
NT2 *Hizikia*
NT2 *Iridaea*
NT2 *Laminaria*
NT3 Kombu
NT2 Laver
NT2 *Macrocystis*
NT2 Onigusa
NT2 *Phyllophora*
NT2 *Porphyra*
NT3 Nori
NT3 *Porphyra yezoensis*
NT2 *Sargassum*
NT2 *Ulva*
NT3 Sea lettuces
NT3 *Ulva lactuca*
NT2 *Undaria*
NT3 *Undaria pinnatifida*
NT3 Wakame
RT Algal oils
RT Aquaculture
RT Blue green algae
RT Cyanobacteria
RT Eukaryotes

Algal oils
HN introduced from vol. 41, issue 1 (2009)
BT1 Oils
BT2 Lipids
BT3 Nutrients
RT Algae

Algeria
BT1 North Africa
BT2 Africa

Algicides
BT1 Pesticides
BT2 Biocides
BT2 Residues

Alginate gels
BT1 Alginates
BT2 Polysaccharides
BT3 Carbohydrates
BT4 Nutrients
BT4 Organic compounds
BT2 Salts
BT2 Stabilizers
BT3 Additives
BT2 Thickeners
BT3 Additives
BT1 Gels
BT2 Physical phases
BT3 Chemistry
BT4 Science

Alginate lyases
USE **Poly(β-D-mannuronate) lyases**

Alginates
BT1 Polysaccharides
BT2 Carbohydrates
BT3 Nutrients
BT3 Organic compounds
BT1 Salts
BT1 Stabilizers
BT2 Additives
BT1 Thickeners
BT2 Additives
NT1 Alginate gels
NT1 Alginic acid
RT Seaweeds

Alginic acid
HN under Polysaccharides and Thickeners up to vol. 42 (2010)
BT1 Alginates
BT2 Polysaccharides
BT3 Carbohydrates
BT4 Nutrients
BT4 Organic compounds
BT2 Salts
BT2 Stabilizers
BT3 Additives
BT2 Thickeners
BT3 Additives

Alicyclobacillus
BT1 Bacteria
BT2 Microorganisms
NT1 *Alicyclobacillus acidocaldarius*
NT1 *Alicyclobacillus acidoterrestris*

Alicyclobacillus acidocaldarius
BT1 *Alicyclobacillus*
BT2 Bacteria
BT3 Microorganisms

Alicyclobacillus acidoterrestris
BT1 *Alicyclobacillus*
BT2 Bacteria
BT3 Microorganisms

Alimentary pastes
BT1 Pasta
BT2 Cereal products
BT3 Plant foods
BT4 Foods

Aliphatic compounds
BT1 Organic compounds
RT Hydrocarbons

Alitame
BT1 Sweeteners
BT2 Additives

Alkalies
NT1 $Ca(OH)_2$
NT1 KOH
NT1 Lyes
NT1 NaOH
RT Alkalization
RT Hydroxides

Alkaline phosphatases
SN EC 3.1.3.1
BT1 Phosphatases
BT2 Esterases
BT3 Hydrolases
BT4 Enzymes

Alkalinity
HN heading up to vol. 24 (1992)
BT1 Physical properties
RT Acidity
RT Neutralization

Alkalization
BT1 Processing
BT2 Technology
RT Alkalies
RT pH

Alkaloids
BT1 Organic nitrogen compounds
NT1 Caffeine
NT1 Carbolines
NT1 Ergotamine
NT1 Glycoalkaloids
NT2 Chaconine

NT2 Solanine
NT1 Harman
NT1 Lupanine
NT1 Methylxanthines
NT1 Nicotine
NT1 Norharman
NT1 Piperine
NT1 Pyrrolizidine alkaloids
NT1 Quinine
NT1 Sanguinarine
NT1 Solanidine
NT1 Theanine
NT1 Theobromine
NT1 Theophylline
NT1 Tomatine
NT1 Trigonelline
RT Coffee
RT Glycosides
RT Indoles
RT Mycotoxins
RT Tea
RT Toxins

Alkanals
BT1 Aldehydes
BT2 Carbonyl compounds
BT3 Organic compounds

Alkanes
BT1 Hydrocarbons
BT2 Organic compounds

Alkenes
HN introduced from vol. 39, issue 1 (2007)
BT1 Hydrocarbons
BT2 Organic compounds

Alkylcyclobutanones
HN introduced from vol. 39, issue 1 (2007)
BT1 Ketones
BT2 Carbonyl compounds
BT3 Organic compounds

Alkylphenols
HN introduced from vol. 39, issue 1 (2007)
BT1 Phenols
BT2 Alcohols
BT2 Aromatic compounds
BT3 Organic compounds
RT Endocrine disrupters

Alkylresorcinols
BT1 Antioxidants
BT2 Additives
BT1 Phenols
BT2 Alcohols
BT2 Aromatic compounds
BT3 Organic compounds

Allantoin
HN introduced from vol. 39, issue 1 (2007)
BT1 Imidazoles
BT2 Heterocyclic compounds
BT2 Organic nitrogen compounds

Alleles
BT1 Genes
BT2 Chromosomes
BT3 Genetics
BT2 Genomes
BT3 Genetics

Allergenicity
BT1 Allergies
BT2 Diseases
BT1 Immunology

Allergens
BT1 Allergies
BT2 Diseases
BT1 Immunology

Allergies
HN heading from vol. 25 (1993); under Allergy up to vol. 24 (1992)
BT1 Diseases
NT1 Allergenicity
NT1 Allergens
NT1 Anaphylaxis
RT Antiallergic activity
RT Cross-reactivity
RT Food intolerance
RT Hypoallergenic foods
RT Immunotherapy
RT Intolerance
RT Metabolic disorders
UF Allergy

Allergy
HN heading up to vol. 24 (1992)
USE **Allergies**

Allethrin
BT1 Pyrethroid insecticides
BT2 Insecticides
BT3 Pesticides
BT4 Biocides
BT4 Residues

Allicin
BT1 Aroma compounds
BT2 Flavour compounds
BT2 Volatile compounds
BT1 Organic sulfur compounds
BT1 Pungent principles
BT2 Flavour compounds
RT Garlic

Alligator meat
BT1 Meat specific
BT2 Meat
BT3 Animal foods
BT4 Foods

Alligator pears
USE **Avocados**

Alliin
HN also under Flavour compounds up to vol. 42 (2010)
BT1 Aroma compounds
BT2 Flavour compounds
BT2 Volatile compounds
BT1 Organic sulfur compounds
RT Garlic

Alliinases
USE **Alliin lyases**

Alliin lyases
SN EC 4.4.1.4
BT1 Lyases
BT2 Enzymes
UF Alliinases

Allium
BT1 Vegetables specific
BT2 Vegetables
BT3 Crops
BT4 Plants
BT3 Plant foods
BT4 Foods

Allspice
BT1 Spices
BT2 Flavourings
BT3 Additives
UF Pimento

Allura Red
BT1 Colorants
BT2 Additives

***S*-Allylcysteine**
BT1 Organic sulfur compounds

Allyl isothiocyanate
HN also under Flavourings up to vol. 42 (2010)
BT1 Aroma compounds
BT2 Flavour compounds
BT2 Volatile compounds
BT1 Isothiocyanates
BT2 Organic nitrogen compounds
BT2 Organic sulfur compounds
BT2 Volatile sulfur compounds
BT3 Volatile compounds
BT1 Pungent principles
BT2 Flavour compounds

Allyl sulfides
HN introduced from vol. 41, issue 1 (2009)
BT1 Aroma compounds
BT2 Flavour compounds
BT2 Volatile compounds
BT1 Organic sulfur compounds
BT1 Sulfides
BT2 Salts
NT1 Diallyl disulfide

Almond oils
BT1 Nut oils
BT2 Vegetable oils
BT3 Oils vegetable
BT4 Oils
BT5 Lipids
BT6 Nutrients
BT4 Vegetable products
BT5 Plant foods
BT6 Foods

Almonds
HN heading from vol. 30 (1998); under Nuts up to vol. 29 (1997)
BT1 Nuts

BT2 Fruits
BT3 Crops
BT4 Plants
BT3 Plant foods
BT4 Foods
BT2 Oilseeds
BT3 Seeds
BT4 Plant foods
BT5 Foods
NT1 Sweet almonds

Aloe
BT1 Plants
NT1 *Aloe vera*
RT Aloin

Aloe vera
HN introduced from vol. 42, issue 1 (2010)
BT1 Aloe
BT2 Plants

Aloin
BT1 Ketones
BT2 Carbonyl compounds
BT3 Organic compounds
RT Aloe

Alternan
BT1 Glucans
BT2 Polysaccharides
BT3 Carbohydrates
BT4 Nutrients
BT4 Organic compounds
RT *Alternaria*

Alternansucrases
HN introduced from vol. 37, issue 5 (2005)
SN EC 2.4.1.140
BT1 Glycosyltransferases
BT2 Transferases
BT3 Enzymes

Alternaria
BT1 Fungi
BT2 Microorganisms
NT1 *Alternaria alternata*
NT1 *Alternaria citri*
RT Alternan
RT Alternariol

Alternaria alternata
BT1 *Alternaria*
BT2 Fungi
BT3 Microorganisms

Alternaria citri
BT1 *Alternaria*
BT2 Fungi
BT3 Microorganisms

Alternariol
HN introduced from vol. 39, issue 1 (2007)
BT1 Mycotoxins
BT2 Toxins
BT3 Residues
RT *Alternaria*

Alteromonas
BT1 Bacteria
BT2 Microorganisms

Altitude
HN introduced from vol. 42, issue 1 (2010)
RT Environment

Alum
BT1 Salts

Aluminium
HN heading up to vol. 24 (1992) for packaging materials and from vol. 30 (1998)
SN symbol Al also used in the index
BT1 Metals
BT2 Elements
BT3 Minerals
BT4 Nutrients
BT1 Packaging materials
NT1 Al
NT1 Al compounds

Aluminium compounds
USE **Al compounds**

Aluminium foils
USE **Al foils**

Aluminium phosphide
SN syn. phostoxin
BT1 Fumigants
BT2 Biocides

Alveograms
BT1 Analytical techniques
RT Alveographs

Alveographs
BT1 Apparatus
BT2 Technology
RT Alveograms
RT Dough

Alzheimer's disease
USE **Neurodegenerative diseases**

Amadori compounds
BT1 Maillard reaction

Amala
BT1 Yams
BT2 Vegetables specific
BT3 Vegetables
BT4 Crops
BT5 Plants
BT4 Plant foods
BT5 Foods

Amanita
BT1 Edible fungi
BT2 Fungi edible
BT3 Vegetables specific
BT4 Vegetables
BT5 Crops
BT6 Plants
BT5 Plant foods
BT6 Foods
NT1 *Amanita phalloides*

Amanita phalloides
BT1 *Amanita*
BT2 Edible fungi
BT3 Fungi edible
BT4 Vegetables specific
BT5 Vegetables
BT6 Crops
BT7 Plants
BT6 Plant foods
BT7 Foods

Amanitins
BT1 Amatoxins
BT2 Mycotoxins
BT3 Toxins
BT4 Residues

Amaranth
BT1 Colorants
BT2 Additives

Amaranth flour
BT1 Amaranth grain
BT2 Pseudocereals
BT3 Seeds
BT4 Plant foods
BT5 Foods
BT1 Cereal flours
BT2 Flours cereal
BT3 Cereal products
BT4 Plant foods
BT5 Foods

Amaranth grain
HN heading from vol. 30 (1998); under Pseudocereals from vol. 25 (1993) up to vol. 29 (1997)
BT1 Pseudocereals
BT2 Seeds
BT3 Plant foods
BT4 Foods
NT1 Amaranth flour
NT1 Amaranth starch
NT1 *Amaranthus*
NT1 Grain amaranth

Amaranth starch
BT1 Amaranth grain
BT2 Pseudocereals
BT3 Seeds
BT4 Plant foods
BT5 Foods
BT1 Starch
BT2 Glucans
BT3 Polysaccharides
BT4 Carbohydrates
BT5 Nutrients
BT5 Organic compounds
BT2 Thickeners
BT3 Additives

Amaranthus
HN Amaranthus seeds or grain under Cereals, Seeds or Grain up to vol. 24 (1992)
BT1 Amaranth grain
BT2 Pseudocereals
BT3 Seeds
BT4 Plant foods
BT5 Foods
BT1 Vegetables specific

BT2 Vegetables
BT3 Crops
BT4 Plants
BT3 Plant foods
BT4 Foods

Amasi
BT1 Fermented milk
BT2 Fermented dairy products
BT3 Dairy products
BT4 Animal foods
BT5 Foods
BT3 Fermented foods
BT4 Processed foods
BT5 Foods
BT2 Milk
BT3 Dairy products
BT4 Animal foods
BT5 Foods

Amatoxins
BT1 Mycotoxins
BT2 Toxins
BT3 Residues
NT1 Amanitins

Ambaritsa
BT1 Sausages
BT2 Meat products
BT3 Animal foods
BT4 Foods

Amberjack
USE **Yellowtail**

Ambient storage
HN introduced from vol. 39, issue 1 (2007)
BT1 Storage

America
HN heading up to vol. 24 (1992)
NT1 Central America
NT2 Belize
NT2 Costa Rica
NT2 El Salvador
NT2 Guatemala
NT2 Honduras
NT2 Mexico
NT2 Nicaragua
NT2 Panama
NT1 Latin America
NT1 North America
NT2 Bermuda
NT2 Canada
NT2 Greenland
NT2 United States of America
NT1 South America
NT2 Argentina
NT2 Bolivia
NT2 Brazil
NT2 Chile
NT2 Colombia
NT2 Ecuador
NT2 Falkland Islands
NT2 French Guiana
NT2 Guyana
NT2 Paraguay
NT2 Peru
NT2 South Georgia
NT2 Surinam
NT2 Uruguay
NT2 Venezuela
NT1 West Indies
NT2 Antigua and Barbuda
NT2 Bahamas
NT2 Barbados
NT2 Cayman Islands
NT2 Cuba
NT2 Curacao
NT2 Dominica
NT2 Dominican Republic
NT2 Grenada
NT2 Guadeloupe
NT2 Haiti
NT2 Jamaica
NT2 Martinique
NT2 Puerto Rico
NT2 Trinidad and Tobago
NT2 Windward Islands

American groundnuts
BT1 Legumes
BT2 Vegetables specific
BT3 Vegetables
BT4 Crops
BT5 Plants
BT4 Plant foods
BT5 Foods

American lobsters
BT1 Lobsters
BT2 Crustacea
BT3 Shellfish
BT4 Animals
BT4 Sea foods
BT5 Aquatic foods
BT6 Animal foods
BT7 Foods

American Samoa
BT1 Oceania

Ames test
BT1 Microbiological techniques
RT Carcinogenicity testing
RT Mutagenicity

Amiben
USE **Chloramben**

Amidases
SN EC 3.5.1.4
BT1 Hydrolases
BT2 Enzymes
UF Acylamidases
UF Acylases

Amidation
HN introduced from vol. 41, issue 1 (2009)
BT1 Modification

Amides
BT1 Organic nitrogen compounds
NT1 Acrylamide
NT1 Avenanthramides
NT1 Azodicarbonamide
NT1 Capsaicinoids
NT2 Capsaicin
NT1 Carbamide
NT1 Dimethylformamide
NT1 Formamide
NT1 Urea
RT Amino acids

Amine oxidases
SN (flavin-containing) EC 1.4.3.4; (copper-containing) EC 1.4.3.6
BT1 Oxidases
BT2 Oxidoreductases
BT3 Enzymes
UF Diamine oxidases
UF Monoamine oxidases

Amines
BT1 Organic nitrogen compounds
NT1 Agmatine
NT1 Aminoethanol
NT1 Aniline
NT1 Anisidine
NT1 Benzidine
NT1 Biogenic amines
NT2 Cadaverine
NT2 Catecholamines
NT3 Adrenaline
NT3 Noradrenaline
NT2 Choline
NT2 Dopamine
NT2 Histamine
NT2 Hordenine
NT2 5-Hydroxytryptamine
NT2 Putrescine
NT2 Serotonin
NT2 Skatole
NT2 Spermine
NT2 Tryptamine
NT2 Tyramine
NT1 Chloramines
NT2 Monochloramine
NT1 Cyclohexylamine
NT1 Diethylamine
NT1 Dimethylamine
NT1 Ethanolamine
NT1 Ethylamine
NT1 Ethylenediamine
NT1 Heterocyclic amines
NT1 Heterocyclic aromatic amines
NT1 Hexylamine
NT1 Hydroxylamine
NT1 Isoamylamine
NT1 Methylamine
NT1 Morpholine
NT1 Nitrosamines
NT2 Diethylnitrosamine
NT2 Dimethylnitrosamine
NT2 *N*-Nitrosodiethylamine
NT2 *N*-Nitrosodimethylamine
NT1 Polyamines
NT2 Putrescine
NT2 Spermidine
NT2 Spermine
NT1 Propylamine
NT1 Trimethylamine
RT Amino acids
RT Carcinogens

Amino acid oxidases
HN introduced from vol. 41, issue 1 (2009)

SN includes both D-amino-acid oxidase (EC 1.4.3.3) and L-amino-acid oxidase (EC 1.4.3.2)
BT1 Oxidases
BT2 Oxidoreductases
BT3 Enzymes

Amino acids
BT1 Nutrients
BT1 Organic acids
BT2 Acids
BT1 Organic nitrogen compounds
NT1 Alanine
NT1 D-Amino acids
NT1 Arginine
NT1 Asparagine
NT1 Aspartic acid
NT1 Canavanine
NT1 Citrulline
NT1 Cysteine
NT2 *N*-Acetyl-L-cysteine
NT1 Cystine
NT1 DOPA
NT1 Glutamic acid
NT2 Poly(γ-glutamic acid)
NT1 Glutamine
NT1 Glycine
NT1 Histidine
NT1 Homocysteine
NT1 Homoserine
NT1 Hydroxyproline
NT1 Isoleucine
NT1 Lanthionine
NT1 Leucine
NT1 Lysine
NT2 Polylysine
NT1 Methionine
NT2 *S*-Adenosyl-L-methionine
NT2 *S*-Methylmethionine
NT2 Selenomethionine
NT1 Methylhistidine
NT1 Octopine
NT1 Ornithine
NT1 Phenylalanine
NT1 Pipecolic acid
NT1 Proline
NT1 Pyroglutamic acid
NT1 Serine
NT1 Taurine
NT1 Theanine
NT1 Threonine
NT1 Tryptophan
NT1 Tyrosine
NT1 Valine
RT Amides
RT Amines
RT Aminobutyric acid
RT Sequencing

D-Amino acids
BT1 Amino acids
BT2 Nutrients
BT2 Organic acids
BT3 Acids
BT2 Organic nitrogen compounds

Aminoacylases
SN EC 3.5.1.14
BT1 Hydrolases
BT2 Enzymes
UF Acylases

Aminobenzoic acid
BT1 Organic acids
BT2 Acids
BT1 Organic nitrogen compounds

2-Aminobutane
SN syn. butylamine
BT1 Fungicides
BT2 Pesticides
BT3 Biocides
BT3 Residues

Aminobutyric acid
BT1 Organic acids
BT2 Acids
BT1 Organic nitrogen compounds
RT Amino acids

1-Aminocyclopropane-1-carboxylate oxidases
SN EC 1.14.17.4. Accepted name now aminocyclopropanecarboxylate oxidases
BT1 Oxidases
BT2 Oxidoreductases
BT3 Enzymes
UF ACC oxidases

1-Aminocyclopropane-1-carboxylate synthases
SN EC 4.4.1.14
BT1 Lyases
BT2 Enzymes
UF ACC synthases

1-Aminocyclopropane-1-carboxylic acid
HN abbrev. ACC used from vol. 25 (1993)
USE **ACC**

Aminoethanol
SN syn. ethanolamine
BT1 Alcohols
BT1 Amines
BT2 Organic nitrogen compounds

Aminoethoxyvinylglycine
BT1 Plant growth regulators
BT2 Cultivation
BT3 Agriculture

Aminoglycoside antibiotics
HN introduced from vol. 43, issue 1 (2011)
BT1 Antibiotics
BT2 Drugs
BT3 Residues
NT1 Dihydrostreptomycin
NT1 Gentamicin
NT1 Hygromycins
NT1 Kanamycin
NT1 Neomycin
NT1 Spectinomycin
NT1 Streptomycin

Amino N
BT1 Nitrogen
BT2 Elements
BT3 Minerals
BT4 Nutrients
NT1 α-Amino N

α-Amino N
BT1 Amino N
BT2 Nitrogen
BT3 Elements
BT4 Minerals
BT5 Nutrients

Aminopeptidases
SN EC 3.4.11
BT1 Proteinases
BT2 Hydrolases
BT3 Enzymes

Amino sugars
HN heading from vol. 25 (1993); under Sugars specific up to vol. 24 (1992)
BT1 Sugars
BT2 Carbohydrates
BT3 Nutrients
BT3 Organic compounds
BT2 Plant foods
BT3 Foods
NT1 *N*-Acetylglucosamine
NT1 Furosine
NT1 Hexosamines
NT2 Galactosamine
NT2 Glucosamine

Aminotransferases
BT1 Transferases
BT2 Enzymes
RT Transaminases

Aminotriazole
USE **Amitrole**

Amitraz
BT1 Acaricides
BT2 Pesticides
BT3 Biocides
BT3 Residues
BT1 Insecticides
BT2 Pesticides
BT3 Biocides
BT3 Residues

Amitrole
BT1 Herbicides
BT2 Pesticides
BT3 Biocides
BT3 Residues
UF Aminotriazole

Amla
BT1 Fruits specific
BT2 Fruits
BT3 Crops
BT4 Plants
BT3 Plant foods
BT4 Foods
UF Aonla

Ammonia
SN symbol NH3 is also used in the index
BT1 Gases
BT2 Physical phases
BT3 Chemistry
BT4 Science
BT1 Inorganic compounds
NT1 NH_3
RT Ammonium compounds

Ammonium compounds
NT1 Betaine
NT1 Glycine betaine
NT1 Quaternary ammonium compounds
RT Ammonia
RT Disinfection

Amnesic shellfish poisoning
BT1 Diseases
BT1 Poisoning
RT Sea foods

Amoebae
BT1 Parasites
BT2 Pests
NT1 *Acanthamoeba*
RT Amoebiasis

Amoebiasis
BT1 Diseases
BT1 Poisoning
RT Amoebae

Amoxicillin
BT1 Penicillins
BT2 β-Lactam antibiotics
BT3 Antibiotics
BT4 Drugs
BT5 Residues
UF Amoxycillin

Amoxycillin
USE **Amoxicillin**

AMP
BT1 Nucleotides
UF Adenosine monophosphate

Amperometry
BT1 Analytical techniques

Ampicillin
BT1 Penicillins
BT2 β-Lactam antibiotics
BT3 Antibiotics
BT4 Drugs
BT5 Residues

Amprolium
BT1 Coccidiostats
BT2 Drugs
BT3 Residues

Amycolatopsis
HN introduced from vol. 37, issue 5 (2005)
BT1 Bacteria
BT2 Microorganisms

Amygdalin
BT1 Glycosides
BT2 Carbohydrates
BT3 Nutrients
BT3 Organic compounds

Amyl alcohol
SN syn. pentanol
BT1 Alcohols
BT1 Aroma compounds
BT2 Flavour compounds
BT2 Volatile compounds
NT1 Pentanol

Amylases
BT1 Glycosidases
BT2 Hydrolases
BT3 Enzymes
NT1 α-Amylases
NT1 β-Amylases
NT1 Amylolytic enzymes
NT1 Diastatic activity
NT1 Glucan 1,4-α-glucosidases
NT1 Isoamylases

α-Amylases
SN EC 3.2.1.1
BT1 Amylases
BT2 Glycosidases
BT3 Hydrolases
BT4 Enzymes
UF Diastases

β-Amylases
SN EC 3.2.1.2
BT1 Amylases
BT2 Glycosidases
BT3 Hydrolases
BT4 Enzymes

Amylases inhibitors
BT1 Antinutritional factors
BT2 Nutritional values
BT1 Enzyme inhibitors
BT2 Enzymes
NT1 α-Amylases inhibitors

α-Amylases inhibitors
BT1 Amylases inhibitors
BT2 Antinutritional factors
BT3 Nutritional values
BT2 Enzyme inhibitors
BT3 Enzymes

Amylodextrins
HN introduced from vol. 39, issue 1 (2007)
BT1 Dextrins
BT2 Starch
BT3 Glucans
BT4 Polysaccharides
BT5 Carbohydrates
BT6 Nutrients
BT6 Organic compounds
BT3 Thickeners
BT4 Additives

Amyloglucosidases
USE **Glucan 1,4-α-glucosidases**

Amylograms
BT1 Analytical techniques
RT Amylographs

Amylographs
BT1 Apparatus
BT2 Technology
RT Amylograms
RT Flour

Amylolytic enzymes
BT1 Amylases
BT2 Glycosidases
BT3 Hydrolases
BT4 Enzymes

Amylomyces
HN introduced from vol. 43, issue 1 (2011)
BT1 Fungi
BT2 Microorganisms
NT1 *Amylomyces rouxii*

Amylomyces rouxii
HN introduced from vol. 39, issue 1 (2007)
SN synonymous with Mucor rouxii
BT1 *Amylomyces*
BT2 Fungi
BT3 Microorganisms

Amylopectins
BT1 Starch
BT2 Glucans
BT3 Polysaccharides
BT4 Carbohydrates
BT5 Nutrients
BT5 Organic compounds
BT2 Thickeners
BT3 Additives
RT Amyloses

Amyloses
BT1 Starch
BT2 Glucans
BT3 Polysaccharides
BT4 Carbohydrates
BT5 Nutrients
BT5 Organic compounds
BT2 Thickeners
BT3 Additives
RT Amylopectins

Amylovorins
BT1 Bacteriocins
BT2 Antibiotics
BT3 Drugs
BT4 Residues
RT *Lactobacillus amylovorus*

Amyrin
BT1 Triterpenoids
BT2 Terpenoids
BT3 Lipids
BT4 Nutrients

An
USE **Ann**

Anabaena
BT1 Cyanobacteria

BT2 Bacteria
BT3 Microorganisms
RT Anatoxins

Anabolic agents
BT1 Drugs
BT2 Residues
RT Anabolic steroids

Anabolic steroids
BT1 Drugs
BT2 Residues
NT1 Trenbolone acetate
RT Anabolic agents

Anacystis
USE ***Synechococcus***

Anaemia
HN introduced from vol. 39, issue 1 (2007)
BT1 Diseases

Anaerobes
BT1 Microorganisms

Anaerobic digestion
HN introduced from vol. 39, issue 1 (2007)
BT1 Bioremediation
BT2 Biotechnology
BT3 Technology

Analogues
BT1 Simulated foods
BT2 Processed foods
BT3 Foods

Analysers
BT1 Apparatus
BT2 Technology

Analysis
BT1 Analytical techniques

Analytical methods
USE **Analytical techniques**

Analytical techniques
NT1 Acoustics
NT1 Alveograms
NT1 Amperometry
NT1 Amylograms
NT1 Analysis
NT1 Assay
NT1 Bioassay
NT1 Calorimetry
NT1 Candling
NT1 Chromatography
NT2 Affinity chromatography
NT2 Capillary electrochromatography
NT2 Column chromatography
NT2 Countercurrent chromatography
NT2 Gas chromatography
NT3 Gas solid chromatography
NT3 GC
NT3 GC-MS
NT3 GLC
NT2 Gel filtration
NT2 Gel permeation chromatography
NT2 High performance liquid chromatography
NT3 HPLC
NT3 LC
NT3 LC-MS
NT3 Supercritical HPLC
NT3 UPLC
NT2 Immunoaffinity chromatography
NT2 Ion chromatography
NT2 Ion exchange chromatography
NT2 Micellar electrokinetic chromatography
NT2 Paper chromatography
NT2 Size exclusion chromatography
NT2 Supercritical fluid chromatography
NT2 Thin layer chromatography
NT3 HPTLC
NT3 TLC
NT1 Colorimetry
NT2 Colorimeters
NT2 Photocolorimetry
NT1 Complexometry
NT1 Conductimetry
NT1 Coulometry
NT1 Cryoscopy
NT1 Crystallography
NT2 X-ray crystallography
NT1 Densitometry
NT1 Differential thermal analysis
NT1 Dilatometry
NT1 DSC
NT1 Dye binding tests
NT1 Electrophoresis
NT2 Capillary electrophoresis
NT2 Gel electrophoresis
NT3 PFGE
NT2 IEF
NT2 Immunoelectrophoresis
NT2 Isotachophoresis
NT2 PAGE
NT2 SDS-PAGE
NT1 Enzymic techniques
NT1 Evaluation
NT1 FIA
NT1 Fibre optics
NT1 Filth tests
NT1 Fluorescence
NT2 Autofluorescence
NT2 Bioluminescence
NT2 Chemiluminescence
NT2 Green fluorescent protein
NT2 Luminescence
NT3 Phosphorescence
NT2 Thermoluminescence
NT1 Fluorodensitometry
NT1 Fluorometry
NT2 Spectrofluorometry
NT2 Spectrophotofluorometry
NT2 X-ray fluorescence spectroscopy
NT1 Granulometry
NT1 Gravimetry
NT1 Headspace analysis
NT1 Hydrometry
NT1 Image analysis
NT1 Imaging
NT1 Immunological techniques
NT2 Agglutination tests
NT2 ELISA
NT2 Enzyme immunoassay
NT2 Immunoassay
NT2 Immunochemical analysis
NT2 Immunodiffusion
NT2 Immunoelectrophoresis
NT2 Immunofluorescence
NT2 Immunomagnetic separation
NT2 Radioimmunoassay
NT2 Serological tests
NT2 Serology
NT2 Serotyping
NT1 Impedance
NT1 Interferometry
NT1 Iodometry
NT1 Kjeldahl
NT1 Laser light scattering
NT1 Liquid phase microextraction
NT1 Machine vision
NT1 Manometry
NT1 Mapping
NT1 Matrix solid-phase dispersion
NT1 Metabolomics
NT1 Microarrays
NT1 Microscopy
NT2 Atomic force microscopy
NT2 Electron microscopy
NT3 EM
NT3 SEM
NT3 TEM
NT2 Fluorescence microscopy
NT2 Microscopes
NT1 Nephelometry
NT1 Neutron activation analysis
NT2 NAA
NT1 Penetrometry
NT1 Photodensitometry
NT1 Photography
NT1 Photometry
NT2 Flame photometry
NT1 Polarimetry
NT1 Polarography
NT1 Potentiometry
NT1 Proteomics
NT1 Pycnometry
NT1 Pyrolysis
NT1 Radiometry
NT1 Refractometry
NT1 Response surface methodology
NT1 Sensory analysis
NT2 Consumer panels
NT2 Flavour thresholds
NT2 Olfactometry
NT2 Panellists
NT2 Quantitative descriptive analysis
NT2 Sensory scores
NT2 Sensory thresholds
NT2 Taste panels
NT2 Texture profile analysis
NT2 Time intensity
NT1 Sequencing

NT1 Simultaneous distillation-extraction
NT1 Solid phase extraction
NT1 Solid phase microextraction
NT1 Spectroscopy
NT2 Atomic absorption spectroscopy
NT3 AAS
NT2 Atomic emission spectroscopy
NT3 ICP-AES
NT2 Circular dichroism
NT2 Electron paramagnetic resonance
NT2 Electron spin resonance
NT2 FTIR spectroscopy
NT2 ICP-OES
NT2 IR spectroscopy
NT3 IR analysis
NT3 IR spectra
NT2 Mass spectroscopy
NT3 Electrospray ionization MS
NT3 GC-MS
NT3 ICP-MS
NT3 LC-MS
NT3 MALDI-TOF-MS
NT3 MS
NT2 NIR spectroscopy
NT2 Nuclear magnetic resonance
NT3 Magnetic resonance imaging
NT3 NMR
NT3 Proton magnetic resonance
NT3 Proton resonance
NT2 Raman spectroscopy
NT2 Spectra
NT2 Spectrofluorometry
NT2 Spectrophotofluorometry
NT2 UV spectroscopy
NT2 X-ray fluorescence spectroscopy
NT1 Stable isotope techniques
NT1 Surface plasmon resonance
NT1 Telemetry
NT1 Tensiometry
NT1 Titration
NT2 Titrimetry
NT2 Volumetric analysis
NT1 Tomography
NT1 Turbidimetry
NT1 Video image analysis
NT1 Viscometry
NT1 Voltammetry
NT1 X-ray absorptiometry
RT Food reference materials
RT Quality control
RT Reference materials
RT Sampling
UF Analytical methods

Anaphylaxis
BT1 Allergies
BT2 Diseases

Anardana
BT1 Additives

Anasazi
BT1 Common beans
BT2 Legumes
BT3 Vegetables specific
BT4 Vegetables
BT5 Crops
BT6 Plants
BT5 Plant foods
BT6 Foods

Anatoxins
BT1 Neurotoxins
BT2 Toxins
BT3 Residues
RT *Anabaena*

Anchovies
HN used up to vol. 29 (1997)
USE **Anchovy**

Anchovy
BT1 Marine fish
BT2 Fish
BT3 Animals
BT3 Sea foods
BT4 Aquatic foods
BT5 Animal foods
BT6 Foods
BT1 Oily fish
BT2 Fish
BT3 Animals
BT3 Sea foods
BT4 Aquatic foods
BT5 Animal foods
BT6 Foods
NT1 Anchovy pastes
NT1 Budu
NT1 *Engraulis encrasicholus*
UF Anchovies

Anchovy oils
BT1 Fish oils
BT2 Oils fish
BT3 Fish products
BT4 Sea foods
BT5 Aquatic foods
BT6 Animal foods
BT7 Foods
BT3 Marine oils
BT4 Oils
BT5 Lipids
BT6 Nutrients

Anchovy pastes
BT1 Anchovy
BT2 Marine fish
BT3 Fish
BT4 Animals
BT4 Sea foods
BT5 Aquatic foods
BT6 Animal foods
BT7 Foods
BT2 Oily fish
BT3 Fish
BT4 Animals
BT4 Sea foods
BT5 Aquatic foods
BT6 Animal foods
BT7 Foods
BT1 Fish pastes
BT2 Fish products
BT3 Sea foods
BT4 Aquatic foods
BT5 Animal foods
BT6 Foods
BT2 Pastes
BT3 Processed foods
BT4 Foods

Andorra
BT1 Europe

Androgens
HN introduced from vol. 41, issue 1 (2009)
BT1 Hormones
BT2 Residues
NT1 Testosterone

Androlla
HN introduced from vol. 37, issue 5 (2005)
BT1 Sausages
BT2 Meat products
BT3 Animal foods
BT4 Foods

Androstenone
BT1 Hormones
BT2 Residues
RT Taints

Anencephaly
USE **Neural tube defects**

Anethole
HN also under Flavourings up to vol. 42 (2010)
BT1 Aroma compounds
BT2 Flavour compounds
BT2 Volatile compounds
BT1 Aromatic compounds
BT2 Organic compounds

Aneurin
USE **Thiamin**

Aneurine
USE **Thiamin**

Angel cakes
BT1 Cakes
BT2 Bakery products
BT3 Cereal products
BT4 Plant foods
BT5 Foods

Angelica
HN under Spices up to vol. 42 (2010)
BT1 Herbs
BT2 Spices
BT3 Flavourings
BT4 Additives

Angelica keiskei
BT1 Plants

Angiogenesis
HN introduced from vol. 39, issue 1 (2007)
BT1 Human physiology
BT2 Physiology

BT3 Science
RT Cancer

Angiogenin
HN introduced from vol. 39, issue 1 (2007)
BT1 Proteins
BT2 Nutrients
BT1 Ribonucleases
BT2 Nucleases
BT3 Esterases
BT4 Hydrolases
BT5 Enzymes

Angiotensin I-converting enzymes
USE **Peptidyl-dipeptidase A**

Angkak
SN pigment produced by Monascus species and used as a colorant
BT1 Colorants
BT2 Additives
UF Red rice

Angola
BT1 Southern Africa
BT2 Africa

Anhydrous milk fats
BT1 Milk fats
BT2 Fats milk
BT3 Fats animal
BT4 Animal foods
BT5 Foods
BT4 Fats
BT5 Lipids
BT6 Nutrients

Anilazine
BT1 Fungicides
BT2 Pesticides
BT3 Biocides
BT3 Residues

Aniline
BT1 Amines
BT2 Organic nitrogen compounds
BT1 Heterocyclic compounds

Animal carcasses
BT1 Carcasses
BT2 Meat
BT3 Animal foods
BT4 Foods

Animal diseases
SN index heading is Diseases animal
BT1 Diseases animal
BT2 Diseases
NT1 Avian flu
NT1 Brucellosis
NT1 Coccidiosis
NT1 Cysticercosis
NT1 Foot and mouth disease
NT1 Malignant hyperthermia
NT1 Mastitis
NT1 Swine fever
RT Prion diseases
RT Zoonoses

Animal fats
SN index heading is Fats animal
BT1 Fats animal
BT2 Animal foods
BT3 Foods
BT2 Fats
BT3 Lipids
BT4 Nutrients
NT1 Adipose tissues
NT1 Backfat
NT1 Belly fat
NT1 Blubber
NT2 Seal blubber
NT1 Dripping
NT1 Fatness
NT1 Intramuscular fat
NT1 Lard
NT1 Marbling
NT1 Subcutaneous fat
NT1 Suet
NT1 Tallow
RT Fish oils
RT Oils fish

Animal foods
HN heading from vol. 25 (1993); under Animals up to vol. 24 (1992)
SN general use only
BT1 Foods
NT1 Aquatic foods
NT1 Birds nests
NT1 Bone marrow
NT1 Cloned animal foods
NT1 Dairy products
NT1 Earthworms
NT1 Egg products
NT1 Eggs
NT1 Fats animal
NT1 Insect foods
NT1 Meat
NT1 Meat products
NT1 Offal
RT Animals
UF Animal products

Animal models
RT Health
RT Human physiology

Animal nutrition
USE **Feeds**

Animal products
USE **Animal foods**

Animal proteins
SN index heading is Proteins animal
BT1 Proteins animal
BT2 Proteins
BT3 Nutrients
NT1 Actins
NT2 F-actin
NT1 Actomyosin
NT1 Blood proteins
NT1 Bovine serum albumin
NT1 Collagen
NT2 Collagen sausage casings
NT1 Connectin
NT1 Desmin
NT1 Egg proteins
NT2 Avidin
NT2 Conalbumin
NT2 Ovalbumins
NT2 Ovomucins
NT2 Ovomucoid
NT2 Ovotransferrin
NT2 Phosvitin
NT1 Elastin
NT1 Fibrin
NT1 Fibrinogen
NT1 Fish proteins
NT1 Gelatin
NT2 Isinglass
NT1 Globins
NT1 γ-Globulins
NT1 Haemoglobin
NT1 Haemoproteins
NT1 Immunoglobulins
NT2 Immunoglobulin A
NT2 Immunoglobulin E
NT2 Immunoglobulin G
NT2 Immunoglobulin Y
NT1 Keratin
NT1 Lactoferrin
NT1 Mucins
NT1 Myofibrillar proteins
NT1 Myoglobin
NT2 Deoxymyoglobin
NT2 Metmyoglobin
NT2 Nitrosylmyoglobin
NT2 Oxymyoglobin
NT1 Myosin
NT2 Myosin heavy chains
NT2 Myosin light chains
NT1 Protamine
NT1 Proteins milk
NT2 Milk proteins
NT3 Butyrophilin
NT3 Casein
NT4 Acid casein
NT4 α_s-Casein
NT4 α_{s1}-Casein
NT4 α_{s2}-Casein
NT4 β-Casein
NT4 γ-Casein
NT4 κ-Casein
NT4 Casein micelles
NT3 β-Casomorphins
NT3 Lactalbumins
NT4 α-Lactalbumin
NT3 Lactoglobulins
NT4 β-Lactoglobulin
NT3 Milk protein concentrates
NT3 Proteose peptones
NT3 Whey proteins
NT4 Whey protein concentrates
NT1 Sarcoplasmic proteins
NT1 Titin
NT1 Transferrins
NT1 Tropomyosin
NT1 Troponin

Animal rennets
BT1 Rennets
BT2 Milk clotting enzymes
BT3 Enzymes milk clotting
BT4 Proteinases

BT5 Hydrolases
BT6 Enzymes

Animals
HN used for specific animals as well as animals in general from vol. 25 (1993)
NT1 Animal stress
NT1 Antelope meat
NT1 Antelopes
NT1 Ass milk
NT1 Bears
NT1 Beluga whales
NT1 Bison
NT1 Buffaloes
NT1 Camels
NT1 Capybaras
NT1 Caribou
NT1 Cattle
NT1 Cetacea
NT1 Cloned animals
NT1 Coypu
NT1 Crocodiles
NT1 Deer
NT1 Dolphins
NT1 Elks
NT1 Fish
NT1 Frogs
NT1 Game
NT1 Gazelles
NT1 Goats
NT1 Hares
NT1 Horses
NT1 Impala
NT1 Kangaroos
NT1 Lambs
NT1 Moose
NT1 Moufflon
NT1 Porpoises
NT1 Rabbits
NT1 Reindeer
NT1 Ruminants
NT1 Seals
NT1 Sheep
NT1 Shellfish
NT1 Slaughter animals
NT1 Snakes
NT1 Swine
NT1 Transgenic animals
NT1 Turtles
NT1 Walruses
NT1 Whale meat
NT1 Whales
NT1 Yaks
RT Animal foods
RT Birds
RT Eukaryotes
RT Pets
UF Animals specific
UF Livestock

Animal science
BT1 Science
NT1 Poultry science
RT Dairy science

Animals specific
HN heading up to vol. 24 (1992); under Animals from vol. 25 (1993)
USE **Animals**

Animal stress
HN introduced from vol. 39, issue 1 (2007)
BT1 Animals
BT1 Stress
RT Animal welfare
RT Dark cutting defect
RT DFD defect
RT PSE defect
RT Slaughter

Animal tissues
USE **Meat**

Animal welfare
RT Animal stress

Anion exchange
BT1 Ion exchange

Anions
BT1 Ions

Anisakiasis
SN syn. anisakidosis
BT1 Diseases
BT1 Poisoning
NT1 Anisakidosis
RT *Anisakis*
RT *Pseudoterranova*

Anisakidosis
SN syn. anisakiasis
BT1 Anisakiasis
BT2 Diseases
BT2 Poisoning
RT *Anisakis*
RT Fish

Anisakis
BT1 Parasites
BT2 Pests
NT1 *Anisakis simplex*
RT Anisakiasis
RT Anisakidosis

Anisakis simplex
HN introduced from vol. 39, issue 1 (2007)
BT1 *Anisakis*
BT2 Parasites
BT3 Pests

Anisaldehyde
HN also under Flavour compounds up to vol. 42 (2010)
BT1 Aldehydes
BT2 Carbonyl compounds
BT3 Organic compounds
BT1 Aroma compounds
BT2 Flavour compounds
BT2 Volatile compounds
BT1 Aromatic compounds
BT2 Organic compounds

Anise
USE **Aniseed**

Aniseed
BT1 Spices
BT2 Flavourings
BT3 Additives
UF Anise

Anisette
BT1 Liqueurs
BT2 Alcoholic beverages
BT3 Beverages alcoholic
BT4 Beverages

Anisidine
BT1 Amines
BT2 Organic nitrogen compounds

Anisole
HN under Flavour compounds and Aromatic compounds up to vol. 42 (2010)
BT1 Aroma compounds
BT2 Flavour compounds
BT2 Volatile compounds
BT1 Phenols
BT2 Alcohols
BT2 Aromatic compounds
BT3 Organic compounds

Ann
BT1 Bean jams
BT2 Vegetable products
BT3 Plant foods
BT4 Foods
UF An

Annatto
BT1 Colorants
BT2 Additives
RT Bixin

Annealing
BT1 Heating
BT2 Thermal processing
BT3 Processing thermal
BT4 Processing
BT5 Technology

Anserine
BT1 Peptides
BT2 Proteins
BT3 Nutrients

Antarctica

Antelope carcasses
BT1 Antelope meat
BT2 Animals
BT2 Meat specific
BT3 Meat
BT4 Animal foods
BT5 Foods
BT1 Carcasses
BT2 Meat
BT3 Animal foods
BT4 Foods

Antelope meat
BT1 Animals
BT1 Meat specific
BT2 Meat
BT3 Animal foods
BT4 Foods
NT1 Antelope carcasses

Antelopes
BT1 Animals

Anthelmintics
BT1 Drugs
BT2 Residues
NT1 Albendazole
NT1 Fasciolicides
NT1 Fenbendazole
NT1 Ivermectin
NT1 Levamisoles
NT1 Moxidectin
NT1 Nitroxynil

Anthio
USE **Formothion**

Anthocyanidins
BT1 Flavonoids
BT2 Aromatic compounds
BT3 Organic compounds
BT2 Pigments
NT1 Cyanidin
NT1 Delphinidin
NT1 Leucoanthocyanidins
NT2 Leucocyanidin
NT1 Malvidin
NT1 Pelargonidin
NT1 Peonidin
NT1 Petunidin
NT1 Proanthocyanidins
NT2 Procyanidins
RT Anthocyanins
RT Glycosides

Anthocyanins
BT1 Flavonoids
BT2 Aromatic compounds
BT3 Organic compounds
BT2 Pigments
NT1 Leucoanthocyanins
NT2 Anthocyanogens
NT1 Oenocyanins
NT1 Pyranoanthocyanins
RT Anthocyanidins
RT Glycosides

Anthocyanogens
BT1 Leucoanthocyanins
BT2 Anthocyanins
BT3 Flavonoids
BT4 Aromatic compounds
BT5 Organic compounds
BT4 Pigments

Anthracene
BT1 Hydrocarbons
BT2 Organic compounds

Anthracnose
BT1 Plant diseases
BT2 Diseases plant
BT3 Diseases
RT *Colletotrichum gloeosporioides*

Anthranilic acid
BT1 Heterocyclic compounds
BT1 Organic acids
BT2 Acids
BT1 Organic nitrogen compounds
RT Avenanthramides

Anthraquinones
BT1 Pigments
NT1 Emodin

Anthrax
HN introduced from vol. 39, issue 1 (2007)
BT1 Diseases
RT *Bacillus anthracis*

Anthropological groups
BT1 Population groups
NT1 Cultural groups
NT1 Ethnic groups
NT1 Religious groups

Anthropometric parameters
HN introduced from vol. 38, issue 8 (2006); heading
BT1 Health
NT1 Body composition
NT1 Body wt.
NT2 Birth wt.
NT2 Body mass index
NT2 Overweight
NT2 Wt. loss diet
NT1 Growth (human)
RT Obesity

Anti-ageing activity
HN introduced from vol. 42, issue 1 (2010)
BT1 Health

Antiallergic activity
HN introduced from vol. 40, issue 1 (2008)
BT1 Health
RT Allergies

Antiatherogenic activity
BT1 Health

Antibacterial activity
BT1 Antimicrobial activity
BT2 Inhibition
BT2 Microorganisms
BT1 Bacteria
BT2 Microorganisms

Antibacterial compounds
BT1 Antibiotics
BT2 Drugs
BT3 Residues

Antibiotics
BT1 Drugs
BT2 Residues
NT1 Actinomycin
NT1 Aminoglycoside antibiotics
NT2 Dihydrostreptomycin
NT2 Gentamicin
NT2 Hygromycins
NT2 Kanamycin
NT2 Neomycin
NT2 Spectinomycin
NT2 Streptomycin
NT1 Antibacterial compounds
NT1 Antibiotics resistance
NT1 Antimicrobial compounds
NT1 Avoparcin
NT1 Bacitracin
NT1 Bacteriocins
NT2 Acidocins
NT2 Amylovorins
NT2 Bacteriocins resistance
NT2 Bavaricins
NT2 Divercins
NT2 Enterocins
NT2 Epidermin
NT2 Gassericins
NT2 Lactacins
NT2 Lacticins
NT2 Lactocins
NT2 Lactococcins
NT2 Lantibiotics
NT2 Leucocins
NT2 Mesentericins
NT2 Nisin
NT2 Pediocins
NT2 Piscicolins
NT2 Plantaricins
NT2 Propionicins
NT2 Sakacins
NT2 Subtilins
NT1 Blasticidin S
NT1 Cerulenin
NT1 Chloramphenicol
NT1 Cycloheximide
NT1 Cycloserine
NT1 Flavomycin
NT1 Florfenicol
NT1 Gliotoxin
NT1 Griseofulvin
NT1 3-Hydroxypropionaldehyde
NT1 Isoniazid
NT1 β-Lactam antibiotics
NT2 Cephalosporins
NT3 Ceftazidime
NT3 Ceftiofur
NT3 Cephapirin
NT2 Penicillins
NT3 Amoxicillin
NT3 Ampicillin
NT3 Benzylpenicillin
NT3 Cloxacillin
NT3 Dicloxacillin
NT3 Oxacillin
NT3 Penicillin G
NT1 Lasalocids
NT1 Lincomycin
NT1 Macrolide antibiotics
NT2 Erythromycin
NT2 Nystatin
NT2 Oleandomycin
NT2 Spiramycin
NT2 Tilmicosin
NT2 Tylosin
NT1 Metronidazole
NT1 Monensin
NT1 Nitrofurans
NT2 Furazolidone
NT2 Nitrofurazone
NT2 Nitrovin
NT1 Novobiocin
NT1 Penicillic acid
NT1 Polymyxins
NT1 Quinolones

NT2 Ciprofloxacin
NT2 Enrofloxacin
NT2 Flumequine
NT2 Nalidixic acid
NT2 Oxolinic acid
NT1 Reuterin
NT1 Salinomycin
NT1 Sulfonamides
NT2 Chloramine T
NT2 Sulfadiazine
NT2 Sulfamethazine
NT3 Sulfadimidine
NT2 Sulfanilamide
NT2 Sulfathiazole
NT1 Surfactin
NT1 Tetracyclines
NT2 Chlortetracycline
NT2 Doxycycline
NT2 Oxytetracycline
NT1 Thiamphenicol
NT1 Tiamulin
NT1 Trimethoprim
NT1 Vancomycin
NT1 Virginiamycin
RT Bactericides
RT Biocides
RT Fungicides
RT Inhibition
RT Microbicidal compounds
RT Preservatives
UF β-Lactam antibiotics

Antibiotics resistance
BT1 Antibiotics
BT2 Drugs
BT3 Residues

Antibodies
BT1 Immunology
RT Immunoglobulins

Anticaking agents
BT1 Additives

Anticarcinogenicity
BT1 Health
RT Anticarcinogens
RT Nutrition

Anticarcinogens
BT1 Health
RT Anticarcinogenicity
RT Nutrition

Antifoaming agents
BT1 Additives
NT1 Dimethylpolysiloxane

Antifreeze proteins
HN proteins antifreeze also used in the index up to vol. 29 (1997)
BT1 Proteins
BT2 Nutrients
RT Stress

Antifungal activity
BT1 Antimicrobial activity
BT2 Inhibition
BT2 Microorganisms
BT1 Fungi
BT2 Microorganisms

Antifungal agents
USE **Fungicides**

Antifungal compounds
BT1 Fungicides
BT2 Pesticides
BT3 Biocides
BT3 Residues

Antigenicity
BT1 Immunology
RT Immunogenicity

Antigenotoxicity
BT1 Health
RT Antimutagenicity
RT Genotoxicity

Antigens
BT1 Immunology

Antigua and Barbuda
BT1 West Indies
BT2 America

Antihypertensive activity
BT1 Health
RT ACE inhibitors

Anti-inflammatory activity
BT1 Health
RT Inflammation

Antimicrobial activity
BT1 Inhibition
BT1 Microorganisms
NT1 Antibacterial activity
NT1 Antifungal activity
NT1 Antiviral activity

Antimicrobial compounds
BT1 Antibiotics
BT2 Drugs
BT3 Residues

Antimicrobial packaging films
BT1 Packaging films
BT2 Packaging materials
RT Active packaging

Antimony
USE **Sb**

Antimutagenicity
BT1 Health
RT Antigenotoxicity
RT Antimutagens
RT Cancer
RT Carcinogenicity
RT Diet
RT Mutagenicity
RT Nutrition

Antimutagens
BT1 Health
RT Antimutagenicity
RT Carcinogens
RT Diet
RT Mutagens
RT Nutrition

Antimycotics
USE **Fungicides**

Antinutritional factors
HN heading from vol. 25 (1993); under Nutrition up to vol. 24 (1992)
BT1 Nutritional values
NT1 Amylases inhibitors
NT2 α-Amylases inhibitors
NT1 Inositol
NT2 Inositol phosphates
NT2 Phytates
NT2 Phytic acid
NT1 Proteinases inhibitors
NT2 Calpastatins
NT2 Chymotrypsin inhibitors
NT2 Cystatins
NT2 Trypsin inhibitors
NT1 Vitamin antagonists
RT Malnutrition
RT Nutrients
RT Nutrition
RT Raffinose
RT Vicine

Antioxidant compounds
SN natural substances found in foods with antioxidative activity
RT Antioxidants

Antioxidants
BT1 Additives
NT1 *N*-Acetyl-L-cysteine
NT1 Alkylresorcinols
NT1 Ascorbates
NT2 Sodium ascorbate
NT1 Ascorbic acid
NT2 Dehydroascorbic acid
NT2 Vitamin C
NT1 Ascorbyl palmitate
NT1 BHA
NT1 BHT
NT1 Chalcones
NT2 Dihydrochalcones
NT3 Neohesperidin dihydrochalcone
NT3 Phloretin
NT2 Xanthohumol
NT1 Citric acid
NT1 Dihydroquercetin
NT1 Erythorbic acid
NT1 Ethoxyquin
NT1 Food antioxidants
NT1 Gallic acid
NT1 Isoascorbic acid
NT1 Nordihydroguaiaretic acid
NT2 NDGA
NT1 Octyl gallate
NT1 Oryzanols
NT1 Propyl gallate
NT1 Sesamol
NT1 TBHQ
NT1 Tenox
NT1 Thioredoxin
NT1 Vitamin E
NT2 Tocols
NT3 Tocopherols
NT4 α-Tocopherol
NT4 Tocotrienol

NT4 Vitamin E acetate
RT Antioxidant compounds

Antioxidant status
HN introduced from vol. 41, issue 1 (2009)
BT1 Nutritional status
BT2 Nutrition

Antioxidative activity
BT1 Oxidation
UF Antioxidative properties

Antioxidative properties
USE **Antioxidative activity**

Antiproliferative activity
HN introduced from vol. 39, issue 1 (2007)
BT1 Health
RT Apoptosis

Antisense technology
BT1 Gene silencing
BT2 Genetic techniques
BT3 Genetics
BT1 Technology

Antiseptics
BT1 Disinfectants
BT2 Disinfection
BT3 Hygiene
RT Germicides
RT Inhibition
RT Surfactants

Antisera
BT1 Immunology
RT Immunological techniques

Antisprouting agents
BT1 Plant growth regulators
BT2 Cultivation
BT3 Agriculture
NT1 Maleic hydrazide
UF Sprouting inhibitors

Antithrombotic activity
BT1 Health

Antithyroid agents
BT1 Drugs
BT2 Residues
NT1 Methimazole
NT1 Methylthiouracil
NT1 Thiouracil

Antitranspirants
BT1 Plant growth regulators
BT2 Cultivation
BT3 Agriculture

Antitumorigenicity
BT1 Health
RT Antitumour activity

Antitumour activity
BT1 Health
RT Antitumorigenicity

Antiviral activity
BT1 Antimicrobial activity
BT2 Inhibition
BT2 Microorganisms
BT1 Viruses
BT2 Microorganisms

Antivitamins
USE **Vitamin antagonists**

Ants
BT1 Insects
BT2 Pests

Anu
BT1 Vegetables specific
BT2 Vegetables
BT3 Crops
BT4 Plants
BT3 Plant foods
BT4 Foods
UF Mashua

AOAC
UF Association of Official Analytical Chemists

Aonla
USE **Amla**

Aperitifs
BT1 Alcoholic beverages
BT2 Beverages alcoholic
BT3 Beverages

Aphids
BT1 Insects
BT2 Pests

Apiculture
HN introduced from vol. 41, issue 1 (2009)
BT1 Agriculture
RT Bees
RT Honeys
RT Propolis
RT Royal jelly

Apigenin
BT1 Flavones
BT2 Flavonoids
BT3 Aromatic compounds
BT4 Organic compounds
BT3 Pigments

Apocarotenal
BT1 Carotenoids
BT2 Pigments
BT2 Terpenoids
BT3 Lipids
BT4 Nutrients

Apoproteins
BT1 Proteins
BT2 Nutrients

Apoptosis
BT1 Cell cycle
BT2 Physiology
BT3 Science
RT Antiproliferative activity

Apparatus
SN general term for machinery used in analytical procedures
BT1 Technology
NT1 Alveographs
NT1 Amylographs
NT1 Analysers
NT1 Butyrometers
NT1 Cameras
NT1 Detectors
NT1 Electrodes
NT2 Ion selective electrodes
NT1 Electronic noses
NT1 Electronic tongues
NT1 Extensographs
NT1 Farinographs
NT1 Finometers
NT1 Friabilimeters
NT1 Instruments
NT1 Lasers
NT1 Meters
NT1 Microchip technology
NT1 Micrometers
NT1 Mixographs
NT1 Penetrometers
NT1 Reflectometers
NT1 Sensors
NT1 Transducers

Apparent density
BT1 Density
BT2 Physical properties

Appearance
BT1 Sensory properties

Appenzeller cheese
BT1 Cheese varieties
BT2 Cheese
BT3 Dairy products
BT4 Animal foods
BT5 Foods

Appetite
BT1 Human physiology
BT2 Physiology
BT3 Science

Apple brandy
BT1 Fruit brandies
BT2 Brandies
BT3 Spirits
BT4 Alcoholic beverages
BT5 Beverages alcoholic
BT6 Beverages
NT1 Calvados

Apple cider
SN use for unfermented apple juices; for alcoholic beverages manufactured using fermented apple juices see Cider
BT1 Apple juices
BT2 Fruit juices
BT3 Fruit products
BT4 Plant foods
BT5 Foods
BT3 Soft drinks
BT4 Beverages

Apple juice concentrates
BT1 Apple juices
BT2 Fruit juices
BT3 Fruit products
BT4 Plant foods
BT5 Foods
BT3 Soft drinks
BT4 Beverages
BT1 Fruit juice concentrates
BT2 Concentrates
BT3 Processed foods
BT4 Foods
BT2 Fruit juices
BT3 Fruit products
BT4 Plant foods
BT5 Foods
BT3 Soft drinks
BT4 Beverages

Apple juices
BT1 Fruit juices
BT2 Fruit products
BT3 Plant foods
BT4 Foods
BT2 Soft drinks
BT3 Beverages
NT1 Apple cider
NT1 Apple juice concentrates
RT Apples
RT Cider

Apple musts
BT1 Apples
BT2 Fruits specific
BT3 Fruits
BT4 Crops
BT5 Plants
BT4 Plant foods
BT5 Foods
BT1 Musts
BT2 Fruit juices
BT3 Fruit products
BT4 Plant foods
BT5 Foods
BT3 Soft drinks
BT4 Beverages

Apple pectins
BT1 Apples
BT2 Fruits specific
BT3 Fruits
BT4 Crops
BT5 Plants
BT4 Plant foods
BT5 Foods
BT1 Pectins
BT2 Pectic substances
BT3 Polysaccharides
BT4 Carbohydrates
BT5 Nutrients
BT5 Organic compounds

Apple peel
BT1 Apples
BT2 Fruits specific
BT3 Fruits
BT4 Crops
BT5 Plants
BT4 Plant foods
BT5 Foods
BT1 Peel
RT Fruit peel

Apple pomaces
BT1 Apples
BT2 Fruits specific
BT3 Fruits
BT4 Crops
BT5 Plants
BT4 Plant foods
BT5 Foods
BT1 Pomaces
BT2 Wastes

Apple pulps
BT1 Apples
BT2 Fruits specific
BT3 Fruits
BT4 Crops
BT5 Plants
BT4 Plant foods
BT5 Foods
BT1 Fruit pulps
BT2 Fruit products
BT3 Plant foods
BT4 Foods
BT2 Pulps
BT3 Processed foods
BT4 Foods

Apple purees
BT1 Apples
BT2 Fruits specific
BT3 Fruits
BT4 Crops
BT5 Plants
BT4 Plant foods
BT5 Foods
BT1 Fruit purees
BT2 Fruit products
BT3 Plant foods
BT4 Foods
BT2 Purees
BT3 Pulps
BT4 Processed foods
BT5 Foods

Apples
BT1 Fruits specific
BT2 Fruits
BT3 Crops
BT4 Plants
BT3 Plant foods
BT4 Foods
NT1 Apple musts
NT1 Apple pectins
NT1 Apple peel
NT1 Apple pomaces
NT1 Apple pulps
NT1 Apple purees
NT1 Apple sauces
NT1 Cider apples
RT Apple juices
RT Bitter pit

Apple sauces
BT1 Apples
BT2 Fruits specific
BT3 Fruits
BT4 Crops
BT5 Plants
BT4 Plant foods
BT5 Foods
BT1 Sauces
BT2 Condiments
BT3 Flavourings
BT4 Additives

Apple vinegar
BT1 Fruit vinegars
BT2 Vinegar
BT3 Condiments
BT4 Flavourings
BT5 Additives
BT3 Fermented foods
BT4 Processed foods
BT5 Foods

Apple wines
BT1 Fruit wines
BT2 Alcoholic beverages
BT3 Beverages alcoholic
BT4 Beverages
RT Cider

Apricot jams
BT1 Apricots
BT2 Fruits specific
BT3 Fruits
BT4 Crops
BT5 Plants
BT4 Plant foods
BT5 Foods
BT1 Jams
BT2 Fruit preserves
BT3 Fruit products
BT4 Plant foods
BT5 Foods
BT3 Preserves
BT4 Processed foods
BT5 Foods

Apricot juices
BT1 Fruit juices
BT2 Fruit products
BT3 Plant foods
BT4 Foods
BT2 Soft drinks
BT3 Beverages
RT Apricot nectars
RT Apricots

Apricot kernels
BT1 Apricots
BT2 Fruits specific
BT3 Fruits
BT4 Crops
BT5 Plants
BT4 Plant foods
BT5 Foods

Apricot nectars
BT1 Fruit nectars
BT2 Fruit juices
BT3 Fruit products
BT4 Plant foods
BT5 Foods
BT3 Soft drinks
BT4 Beverages

RT Apricot juices
RT Apricots

Apricot pulps
BT1 Apricots
BT2 Fruits specific
BT3 Fruits
BT4 Crops
BT5 Plants
BT4 Plant foods
BT5 Foods
BT1 Fruit pulps
BT2 Fruit products
BT3 Plant foods
BT4 Foods
BT2 Pulps
BT3 Processed foods
BT4 Foods

Apricot purees
BT1 Apricots
BT2 Fruits specific
BT3 Fruits
BT4 Crops
BT5 Plants
BT4 Plant foods
BT5 Foods
BT1 Fruit purees
BT2 Fruit products
BT3 Plant foods
BT4 Foods
BT2 Purees
BT3 Pulps
BT4 Processed foods
BT5 Foods

Apricots
BT1 Fruits specific
BT2 Fruits
BT3 Crops
BT4 Plants
BT3 Plant foods
BT4 Foods
NT1 Apricot jams
NT1 Apricot kernels
NT1 Apricot pulps
NT1 Apricot purees
NT1 Apricot seeds
RT Apricot juices
RT Apricot nectars

Apricot seeds
BT1 Apricots
BT2 Fruits specific
BT3 Fruits
BT4 Crops
BT5 Plants
BT4 Plant foods
BT5 Foods
BT1 Seeds
BT2 Plant foods
BT3 Foods

Apricot wines
BT1 Fruit wines
BT2 Alcoholic beverages
BT3 Beverages alcoholic
BT4 Beverages

Apthovirus
HN introduced from vol. 43, issue 1 (2011)
BT1 Viruses
BT2 Microorganisms
NT1 Foot and mouth disease virus

Aquaculture
HN heading from vol. 25 (1993)
NT1 Fish farming
NT1 Stocking density (aquaculture)
RT Algae
RT Aquaculture products
RT Farmed fish
RT Farmed shellfish
RT Fish
RT Shellfish

Aquaculture products
BT1 Aquatic foods
BT2 Animal foods
BT3 Foods
RT Aquaculture
RT Sea foods

Aqualysins
BT1 Proteinases
BT2 Hydrolases
BT3 Enzymes

Aquatic foods
BT1 Animal foods
BT2 Foods
NT1 Aquaculture products
NT1 Sea foods
NT2 Ascidians
NT3 Sea squirts
NT2 Dried sea foods
NT3 Dried fish
NT2 Echinoderms
NT2 Fish
NT3 Bass
NT3 Char
NT4 Arctic char
NT3 Dried fish
NT3 Farmed fish
NT3 Finfish
NT3 Fish bones
NT3 Fish factories
NT3 Fish fillets
NT3 Fish industry
NT3 Fish livers
NT4 Cod livers
NT3 Fish mince
NT3 Fish skin
NT3 Freshwater fish
NT4 Ayu
NT4 Bream
NT4 Burbot
NT4 Carp
NT5 Bighead carp
NT6 *Aristichthys nobilis*
NT5 Crucian carp
NT5 *Cyprinus carpio*
NT5 Grass carp
NT6 White amur
NT5 Rohu
NT6 *Labeo rohita*
NT5 Silver carp
NT4 Catfish
NT5 Channel catfish
NT6 *Ictalurus punctatus*
NT5 *Silurus asotus*
NT4 Chub
NT5 *Leuciscus cephalus*
NT4 *Colossoma macropomum*
NT4 Eels
NT4 Nile perch
NT4 Pacu
NT4 Perch
NT5 *Perca fluviatilis*
NT5 Yellow perch
NT4 Pike
NT4 River fish
NT4 Roach
NT4 Snakehead
NT4 Sunfish
NT4 Tench
NT4 Tilapia
NT5 Nile tilapia
NT6 Bolti
NT6 *Oreochromis niloticus*
NT6 *Tilapia nilotica*
NT5 *Oreochromis*
NT6 *Oreochromis niloticus*
NT4 Vendace
NT5 Coregonus albula
NT4 Walleye
NT3 Lamprey
NT3 Marine fish
NT4 Alaska pollock
NT5 Alaska pollack
NT5 *Theragra chalcogramma*
NT5 Walleye pollack
NT4 Alewife
NT4 Anchovy
NT5 Anchovy pastes
NT5 Budu
NT5 *Engraulis encrasicholus*
NT4 Barracuda
NT4 Barramundi
NT4 Bigeye snapper
NT5 *Priacanthus macracanthus*
NT4 Bluefish
NT4 Blue whiting
NT5 *Micromesistius poutassou*
NT4 Bombay duck
NT4 Capelin
NT4 Coalfish
NT4 Cod
NT5 Cod livers
NT5 *Gadus morhua*
NT5 Rock cod
NT4 Conger eels
NT4 Croakers
NT4 Cutlassfish
NT4 Dogfish
NT4 Dolphinfish
NT5 Mahimahi
NT4 Drum
NT4 Filefish
NT4 Flatfish
NT5 Arrowtooth flounder

NT5 Bastard halibut
NT6 *Paralichthys olivaceus*
NT5 Dab
NT5 Flounders
NT6 Japanese flounders
NT7 *Paralichthys olivaceus*
NT6 *Platichthys flesus*
NT5 Halibut
NT6 Atlantic halibut
NT6 Greenland halibut
NT6 *Reinhardtius hippoglossoides*
NT5 Megrim
NT6 *Lepidorhombus boscii*
NT5 Plaice
NT6 *Pleuronectes platessa*
NT5 Sole
NT5 Turbot
NT4 Flying fish
NT4 Grenadier
NT4 Groundfish
NT4 Grouper
NT5 *Epinephelus guaza*
NT4 Gurnard
NT4 Haddock
NT4 Hagfish
NT4 Hairtail
NT4 Hake
NT5 *Merluccius australis*
NT5 *Merluccius hubbsi*
NT5 *Merluccius merluccius*
NT5 Pacific hake
NT6 *Merluccius productus*
NT6 Pacific whiting
NT5 Red hake
NT4 Herring
NT5 *Clupea harengus*
NT5 Kippers
NT5 Matjes
NT5 Rollmops
NT4 Hilsa
NT4 Hoki
NT4 Kilka
NT4 Kingklip
NT4 Lanternfish
NT4 Ling
NT5 *Molva molva*
NT4 Ling cod
NT5 *Ophiodon elongatus*
NT4 Lizardfish
NT4 Lumpfish
NT5 *Cyclopterus lumpus*
NT4 Mackerel
NT5 Atlantic mackerel
NT6 *Scomber scombrus*
NT5 Chub mackerel
NT6 *Scomber japonicus*
NT5 Frigate mackerel
NT5 Horse mackerel
NT5 Indian mackerel
NT5 Jack mackerel
NT6 *Trachurus japonicus*
NT6 *Trachurus murphyi*
NT5 Pacific mackerel
NT5 Scad
NT5 Seer fish
NT5 Smoked mackerel
NT5 Spanish mackerel
NT4 Marlins
NT4 Menhaden
NT5 *Brevoortia tyrannus*
NT4 Milkfish
NT5 *Chanos chanos*
NT4 Monkfish
NT4 Morwong
NT4 Mullet
NT5 *Mugil cephalus*
NT4 Orange roughy
NT4 Paddlefish
NT5 *Polyodon spathula*
NT4 Pilchards
NT4 Pollack
NT4 Pollock
NT4 Pomfret
NT5 Butterfish
NT4 *Priacanthus tayenus*
NT4 Pufferfish
NT4 Rabbitfish
NT4 Ray
NT4 Redfish
NT4 Redspot emperor
NT5 *Lethrinus lentjan*
NT4 Rockfish
NT4 Sablefish
NT4 Sailfish
NT4 Saithe
NT4 Sand lance
NT4 Sardine
NT5 Monterey sardine
NT5 *Sardina pilchardus*
NT4 *Sardinella*
NT4 Saury
NT4 Sculpin
NT4 Sea bass
NT5 Striped bass
NT6 *Morone saxatilis*
NT4 Sea bream
NT5 Bogue
NT6 *Boops boops*
NT5 Red sea bream
NT6 *Pagrus major*
NT5 *Sparus aurata*
NT4 Sea fish
NT4 Sea perch
NT4 Shad
NT5 Indian shad
NT4 Sharks
NT5 Shark fins
NT4 Sheatfish
NT4 Skate
NT4 Snapper
NT4 Sprat
NT4 Swordfish
NT4 Threadfin bream
NT4 Tuna
NT5 Bigeye tuna
NT5 Bonito
NT5 Skipjack tuna
NT6 Katsuobushi
NT5 White tuna
NT6 Albacore
NT5 Yellowfin tuna
NT4 Whitebait
NT4 White fish
NT4 Whiting
NT4 Wreckfish
NT5 *Polyprion americanus*
NT4 Yellowfin
NT4 Yellowtail
NT3 Oily fish
NT4 Anchovy
NT5 Anchovy pastes
NT5 Budu
NT5 *Engraulis encrasicholus*
NT4 Carp
NT5 Bighead carp
NT6 *Aristichthys nobilis*
NT5 Crucian carp
NT5 *Cyprinus carpio*
NT5 Grass carp
NT6 White amur
NT5 Rohu
NT6 *Labeo rohita*
NT5 Silver carp
NT4 Eels
NT4 Herring
NT5 *Clupea harengus*
NT5 Kippers
NT5 Matjes
NT5 Rollmops
NT4 Hilsa
NT4 Mackerel
NT5 Atlantic mackerel
NT6 *Scomber scombrus*
NT5 Chub mackerel
NT6 *Scomber japonicus*
NT5 Frigate mackerel
NT5 Horse mackerel
NT5 Indian mackerel
NT5 Jack mackerel
NT6 *Trachurus japonicus*
NT6 *Trachurus murphyi*
NT5 Pacific mackerel
NT5 Scad
NT5 Seer fish
NT5 Smoked mackerel
NT5 Spanish mackerel
NT4 Orange roughy
NT4 Pilchards
NT4 Salmon
NT5 Atlantic salmon
NT6 *Salmo salar*
NT5 Pacific salmon
NT6 Cherry salmon
NT7 Masu salmon
NT6 Chinook salmon
NT7 King salmon
NT6 Chum salmon
NT7 Keta salmon
NT7 *Oncorhynchus keta*
NT6 Coho salmon
NT6 Pink salmon
NT6 Sockeye salmon
NT7 Red salmon
NT5 Smoked salmon
NT4 Sardine
NT5 Monterey sardine
NT5 *Sardina pilchardus*
NT4 Sprat
NT4 Swordfish
NT4 Trout
NT5 Brook trout
NT5 Brown trout
NT5 Rainbow trout
NT6 *Oncorhynchus mykiss*
NT5 Sea trout

NT5 Smoked trout
NT4 Tuna
NT5 Bigeye tuna
NT5 Bonito
NT5 Skipjack tuna
NT6 Katsuobushi
NT5 White tuna
NT6 Albacore
NT5 Yellowfin tuna
NT4 Whitebait
NT3 Sturgeon
NT4 Beluga
NT3 Whitefish
NT4 *Coregonus lavaretus*
NT2 Fish products
NT3 Ceviche
NT3 Fish balls
NT3 Fishburgers
NT3 Fish cakes
NT3 Fish crackers
NT3 Fish fingers
NT3 Fish hydrolysates
NT3 Fish in marinades
NT3 Fish in oils
NT3 Fish in sauces
NT3 Fish meal
NT3 Fish noodles
NT3 Fish pastes
NT4 Anchovy pastes
NT3 Fish pates
NT3 Fish preserves
NT3 Fish sauces
NT4 Budu
NT4 Ishiru
NT4 Nuoc-mam
NT4 Patis
NT3 Fish sausages
NT3 Fish soups
NT3 Kamaboko
NT3 Katsuobushi
NT3 Kusaya
NT3 Matjes
NT3 Momoni
NT3 Nukazuke
NT3 Oils fish
NT4 Fish oils
NT5 Anchovy oils
NT5 Cod liver oils
NT5 Fish liver oils
NT5 Menhaden oils
NT5 Salmon oils
NT5 Sardine oils
NT5 Tuna oils
NT3 Pates
NT4 Fish pates
NT4 Liver pates
NT4 Terrines
NT3 Restructured fish products
NT3 Roes
NT4 Caviar
NT4 Caviar substitutes
NT4 Milt
NT3 Rollmops
NT3 Salted fish
NT3 Sashimi
NT3 Smoked fish
NT4 Kippers
NT4 Smoked mackerel
NT4 Smoked salmon
NT4 Smoked trout
NT3 Surimi
NT3 Sushi
NT2 Jellyfish
NT2 Jeotgal
NT2 Plankton
NT2 Sea cucumbers
NT2 Sea food products
NT2 Sea foods industry
NT2 Sea urchins
NT3 Sea urchin gonads
NT2 Seaweeds
NT3 *Caulerpa*
NT3 *Chondrus*
NT4 *Chondrus crispus*
NT3 *Cystoseira*
NT3 Dulse
NT4 *Palmaria palmata*
NT3 *Ecklonia*
NT3 *Eucheuma*
NT3 *Fucus*
NT3 *Furcellaria*
NT3 *Gigartina*
NT3 *Gracilaria*
NT3 *Hizikia*
NT3 *Iridaea*
NT3 *Laminaria*
NT4 Kombu
NT3 Laver
NT3 *Macrocystis*
NT3 Onigusa
NT3 *Phyllophora*
NT3 *Porphyra*
NT4 Nori
NT4 *Porphyra yezoensis*
NT3 *Sargassum*
NT3 *Ulva*
NT4 Sea lettuces
NT4 *Ulva lactuca*
NT3 *Undaria*
NT4 *Undaria pinnatifida*
NT4 Wakame
NT2 Shellfish
NT3 Crustacea
NT4 Crabs
NT5 Blue crabs
NT6 *Callinectes sapidus*
NT5 Crab meat
NT6 Crab legs
NT5 Mud crabs
NT5 Red crabs
NT5 Snow crabs
NT4 Crawfish
NT4 Crayfish
NT4 Krill
NT4 Lobsters
NT5 American lobsters
NT4 Norway lobsters
NT5 Langoustines
NT5 Scampi
NT4 Prawns
NT5 Kuruma prawns
NT5 Prawn crackers
NT4 Shrimps
NT5 *Crangon crangon*
NT5 *Pandalus borealis*
NT5 Tiger shrimps
NT3 Farmed shellfish
NT3 Molluscs
NT4 Bivalves
NT5 Arkshells
NT5 Carpet shells
NT5 Clams
NT6 Freshwater clams
NT6 *Pseudocardium sachalinensis*
NT6 *Tapes philippinarum*
NT5 Cockles
NT5 Mussels
NT6 Blue mussels
NT6 Green mussels
NT6 *Mytilus edulis*
NT6 *Mytilus galloprovincialis*
NT6 *Mytilus trossulus*
NT5 Oysters
NT6 *Crassostrea gigas*
NT6 *Crassostrea virginica*
NT6 Oyster sauces
NT5 Razor shells
NT5 Scallops
NT6 *Patinopecten yessoensis*
NT4 Cephalopods
NT5 Cuttlefish
NT5 Octopus
NT5 Squid
NT6 Ika shiokara
NT6 *Illex argentinus*
NT6 *Ommastrephes bartrami*
NT4 Gastropods
NT5 Abalones
NT5 Limpets
NT5 Periwinkles
NT5 Snails
NT6 Land snails
NT6 Snail meat
NT5 Top shells
NT5 Trumpet shells
NT5 Turban shells
NT5 Whelks
NT2 Shiokara
NT3 Ika shiokara

Aquavit
BT1 Spirits
BT2 Alcoholic beverages
BT3 Beverages alcoholic
BT4 Beverages

Aqueous two phase systems
HN introduced from vol. 39, issue 1 (2007)
BT1 Solvents
RT Extraction
RT Separation
RT Water

Ar
HN under Minerals up to vol. 42 (2010)
BT1 Elements
BT2 Minerals
BT3 Nutrients
BT1 Gases
BT2 Physical phases
BT3 Chemistry
BT4 Science
UF Argon

Arabans
USE **Arabinans**

Arabic bread
BT1 Bread
BT2 Bakery products
BT3 Cereal products
BT4 Plant foods
BT5 Foods

Arabidopsis
BT1 Plants
NT1 *Arabidopsis thaliana*

Arabidopsis thaliana
BT1 *Arabidopsis*
BT2 Plants

Arabinans
HN introduced from vol. 39, issue 1 (2007)
BT1 Pentosans
BT2 Polysaccharides
BT3 Carbohydrates
BT4 Nutrients
BT4 Organic compounds
UF Arabans

α-*N*-Arabinofuranosidases
SN EC 3.2.1.55
BT1 Glycosidases
BT2 Hydrolases
BT3 Enzymes
UF Arabinosidases

Arabinogalactans
BT1 Polysaccharides
BT2 Carbohydrates
BT3 Nutrients
BT3 Organic compounds

Arabinose
HN under Sugars up to vol. 42 (2010)
BT1 Monosaccharides
BT2 Sugars
BT3 Carbohydrates
BT4 Nutrients
BT4 Organic compounds
BT3 Plant foods
BT4 Foods

Arabinose isomerases
HN introduced from vol. 39, issue 1 (2007)
BT1 Isomerases
BT2 Enzymes

Arabinosidases
USE **α-*N*-Arabinofuranosidases**

Arabinoxylans
BT1 Pentosans
BT2 Polysaccharides
BT3 Carbohydrates
BT4 Nutrients
BT4 Organic compounds

Arabitol
BT1 Polyols
BT2 Alcohols
BT2 Carbohydrates
BT3 Nutrients
BT3 Organic compounds

Arachidic acid
BT1 Saturated fatty acids
BT2 Fatty acids
BT3 Lipids
BT4 Nutrients
BT3 Organic acids
BT4 Acids

Arachidonic acid
BT1 Eicosatetraenoic acid
BT2 PUFA
BT3 Unsaturated fatty acids
BT4 Fatty acids
BT5 Lipids
BT6 Nutrients
BT5 Organic acids
BT6 Acids
BT1 ω-6 Fatty acids
BT2 PUFA
BT3 Unsaturated fatty acids
BT4 Fatty acids
BT5 Lipids
BT6 Nutrients
BT5 Organic acids
BT6 Acids

Arachin
BT1 Globulins
BT2 Proteins
BT3 Nutrients
BT1 Vegetable proteins
BT2 Proteins vegetable
BT3 Proteins
BT4 Nutrients
BT3 Vegetable products
BT4 Plant foods
BT5 Foods
RT Peanut proteins
RT Peanuts

Arachis oils
USE **Groundnut oils**

Arak
BT1 Spirits
BT2 Alcoholic beverages
BT3 Beverages alcoholic
BT4 Beverages
UF Arrack

Arare
BT1 Rice
BT2 Cereals
BT3 Crops
BT4 Plants
BT3 Seeds
BT4 Plant foods
BT5 Foods

Arbutin
HN introduced from vol. 39, issue 1 (2007)
BT1 Glycosides
BT2 Carbohydrates
BT3 Nutrients
BT3 Organic compounds
BT1 Phenols
BT2 Alcohols
BT2 Aromatic compounds
BT3 Organic compounds

Arbutus berries
HN used up to vol. 39 (2007)
USE **Strawberry tree fruits**

Archaea
HN introduced from vol. 41, issue 1 (2009); heading
BT1 Microorganisms
NT1 *Pyrococcus*
NT2 *Pyrococcus furiosus*
NT1 *Sulfolobus*
NT2 *Sulfolobus solfataricus*
NT1 *Thermococcus*
NT2 *Thermococcus kodakaraensis*

Arcobacter
BT1 Bacteria
BT2 Microorganisms
NT1 *Arcobacter butzleri*

Arcobacter butzleri
BT1 *Arcobacter*
BT2 Bacteria
BT3 Microorganisms

Arctic char
BT1 Char
BT2 Fish
BT3 Animals
BT3 Sea foods
BT4 Aquatic foods
BT5 Animal foods
BT6 Foods

Areca
BT1 Palms
BT2 Plants
NT1 *Areca catechu*
RT Betel nuts

Areca catechu
BT1 *Areca*
BT2 Palms
BT3 Plants

Areca nuts
USE **Betel nuts**

Arenga
BT1 Palms
BT2 Plants

Arepas
BT1 Bakery products
BT2 Cereal products
BT3 Plant foods
BT4 Foods

Argemone oils
BT1 Vegetable oils
BT2 Oils vegetable
BT3 Oils
BT4 Lipids
BT5 Nutrients
BT3 Vegetable products
BT4 Plant foods
BT5 Foods

Argentina
HN heading up to vol. 24 (1992)
BT1 South America
BT2 America

Arginine
HN heading from vol. 25 (1993); under Amino acids up to vol. 24 (1992)
BT1 Amino acids
BT2 Nutrients
BT2 Organic acids
BT3 Acids
BT2 Organic nitrogen compounds

Argon
USE **Ar**

Aristichthys nobilis
BT1 Bighead carp
BT2 Carp
BT3 Freshwater fish
BT4 Fish
BT5 Animals
BT5 Sea foods
BT6 Aquatic foods
BT7 Animal foods
BT8 Foods
BT3 Oily fish
BT4 Fish
BT5 Animals
BT5 Sea foods
BT6 Aquatic foods
BT7 Animal foods
BT8 Foods

Arkshells
BT1 Bivalves
BT2 Molluscs
BT3 Shellfish
BT4 Animals
BT4 Sea foods
BT5 Aquatic foods
BT6 Animal foods
BT7 Foods

Armagnac
BT1 Brandies
BT2 Spirits
BT3 Alcoholic beverages
BT4 Beverages alcoholic
BT5 Beverages

Armenia
BT1 Asia
BT1 Europe

Armillaria
BT1 Edible fungi
BT2 Fungi edible
BT3 Vegetables specific
BT4 Vegetables
BT5 Crops
BT6 Plants
BT5 Plant foods
BT6 Foods
NT1 *Armillaria mellea*
UF *Armillariella*

Armillaria mellea
BT1 *Armillaria*
BT2 Edible fungi
BT3 Fungi edible
BT4 Vegetables specific
BT5 Vegetables
BT6 Crops
BT7 Plants
BT6 Plant foods
BT7 Foods

Armillariella
SN former name for the fungal genus Armillaria
USE ***Armillaria***

Army rations
BT1 Meals
BT2 Processed foods
BT3 Foods
RT Military rations

Arochlor
BT1 Polychlorinated biphenyls
BT2 Chlorinated hydrocarbons
BT3 Organic halogen compounds

Aroma
BT1 Sensory properties
NT1 Aromatization
NT1 Bouquet
NT1 Odour activity values
NT1 Odour threshold values
NT1 Pungency
RT Aroma compounds
RT Flavour
RT Flavour compounds
RT Off odour
UF Odour
UF Smell

Aroma compounds
BT1 Flavour compounds
BT1 Volatile compounds
NT1 Acetaldehyde
NT2 Ethanal
NT1 Acetals
NT1 Acetoin
NT2 Acetylmethylcarbinol
NT2 3-Hydroxy-2-butanone
NT1 α-Acetolactate
NT1 Acetophenone
NT1 Allicin
NT1 Alliin
NT1 Allyl isothiocyanate
NT1 Allyl sulfides
NT2 Diallyl disulfide
NT1 Amyl alcohol
NT2 Pentanol
NT1 Anethole
NT1 Anisaldehyde
NT1 Anisole
NT1 Benzaldehyde
NT1 Benzothiazole
NT1 Benzyl alcohol
NT1 Benzyl isothiocyanate
NT1 Borneol
NT1 Butanoic acid
NT2 Butyric acid
NT1 Butanol
NT2 Butyl alcohol
NT1 Butanone
NT1 Butyl acetate
NT1 Camphene
NT1 Camphor
NT1 Carvacrol
NT1 Carveol
NT1 Carvone
NT1 Caryophyllene
NT1 Cineole
NT2 Eucalyptol
NT1 Cinnamaldehyde
NT1 Cinnamic acid
NT1 Citral
NT2 Geranial
NT2 Neral
NT1 Citronellal
NT1 Citronellol
NT1 Cuminaldehyde
NT1 Cymene
NT1 Cysteine sulfoxides
NT1 γ-Decalactone
NT1 Decanal
NT1 Decanoic acid
NT2 Capric acid
NT1 Decanol
NT1 Diacetyl
NT2 2,3-Butanedione
NT1 Dill ether
NT1 Dimethyl disulfide
NT1 Dimethyl trisulfide
NT1 Dodecanoic acid
NT2 Lauric acid
NT1 Ethyl acetate
NT1 Ethyl butyrate
NT1 Ethyl caprylate
NT1 Ethyl decanoate
NT1 Ethyl formate
NT1 Ethyl hexanoate
NT2 Ethyl caproate
NT1 Ethyl octanoate
NT1 Ethyl vanillin
NT1 Eugenol
NT1 Farnesene
NT1 Farnesol
NT1 Filbertone
NT1 Furanones
NT2 Furaneol
NT3 2,5-Dimethyl-4-hydroxy-3(2*H*)-furanone
NT2 Sotolon
NT1 Geraniol
NT1 Geranyl acetate
NT1 Gingerols
NT1 Heptanoic acid
NT1 2-Heptanone
NT1 Heptenal
NT1 Hexanal
NT1 Hexanoic acid
NT2 Caproic acid
NT1 Hexanol
NT1 Hexenal
NT1 Hexyl acetate
NT1 Hotrienol
NT1 Humulene
NT1 Isoamyl acetate
NT1 Isoamyl alcohol
NT2 Isopentyl alcohol
NT2 Methyl butanol
NT1 Isobutanol

NT2 Isobutyl alcohol
NT2 Methyl propanol
NT1 Isobutyraldehyde
NT2 2-Methylpropanal
NT1 Isobutyric acid
NT1 Isocaproic acid
NT1 Isovaleric acid
NT1 Lenthionine
NT1 Limonene
NT1 Linalool
NT1 Linalyl acetate
NT1 Maltol
NT1 Menthol
NT1 Menthone
NT1 Methanethiol
NT2 Methyl mercaptan
NT1 Methional
NT1 Methionol
NT1 Methyl benzoate
NT1 3-Methylbutanal
NT2 Isovaleraldehyde
NT1 Myrcene
NT1 Myristicin
NT1 Nerol
NT1 Nonanal
NT1 Nonanone
NT1 Nonenal
NT1 Nootkatone
NT1 Norisoprenoids
NT2 β-Damascenone
NT2 Ionones
NT1 Octanal
NT1 Octanoic acid
NT2 Caprylic acid
NT1 Octanone
NT1 1-Octen-3-ol
NT1 Pentanal
NT2 Valeraldehyde
NT1 Pentanedione
NT2 Acetylacetone
NT1 Pentanoic acid
NT2 Valeric acid
NT1 Phenylacetaldehyde
NT1 Phenylethanol
NT2 Phenethyl alcohol
NT1 Pinenes
NT1 Piperidine
NT1 Piperine
NT1 Propanal
NT2 Propionaldehyde
NT1 Pyrazines
NT1 Safranal
NT1 Safrole
NT1 Terpinene
NT1 Terpineol
NT1 Terpinyl acetate
NT1 Thiazoles
NT1 Thioesters
NT1 Thujone
NT1 Thymol
NT1 Undecanone
NT1 Zingerone
RT Alcohols
RT Aldehydes
RT Aroma
RT Aroma concentrates
RT Aromatization
RT Benzophenone
RT Decenoic acid
RT Dimethyl sulfide
RT Esters
RT Flavour
RT Flavour compounds
RT Flavourings
RT Glyoxal
RT Guaiacol
RT Ketones
RT Lactones
RT Off odour
RT Organic sulfur compounds
RT Phenylacetic acid
RT Pyrones
RT Pyrroles
RT Terpenes
RT Terpenoids
RT Thiophenes
RT Trimethylamine
RT Volatile fatty acids
RT Volatile sulfur compounds
UF Aroma volatiles
UF Odorant

Aroma concentrates
HN heading from vol. 25 (1993)
BT1 Additives
BT1 Concentrates
BT2 Processed foods
BT3 Foods
RT Aroma compounds
RT Flavourings

Aromatic compounds
BT1 Organic compounds
NT1 Acetophenone
NT1 Anethole
NT1 Anisaldehyde
NT1 Benzaldehyde
NT1 Benzene
NT1 Benzidine
NT1 Benzophenone
NT1 Benzoyl compounds
NT1 Benzyl alcohol
NT1 Cinnamaldehyde
NT1 Cuminaldehyde
NT1 Cymene
NT1 Ethyl vanillin
NT1 Flavonoids
NT2 Anthocyanidins
NT3 Cyanidin
NT3 Delphinidin
NT3 Leucoanthocyanidins
NT4 Leucocyanidin
NT3 Malvidin
NT3 Pelargonidin
NT3 Peonidin
NT3 Petunidin
NT3 Proanthocyanidins
NT4 Procyanidins
NT2 Anthocyanins
NT3 Leucoanthocyanins
NT4 Anthocyanogens
NT3 Oenocyanins
NT3 Pyranoanthocyanins
NT2 Bioflavonoids
NT2 Chalcones
NT3 Dihydrochalcones
NT4 Neohesperidin dihydrochalcone
NT4 Phloretin
NT3 Xanthohumol
NT2 Flavanols
NT3 Catechols
NT4 Catechin
NT4 Epicatechin
NT4 Epicatechin gallate
NT4 Epicatechol
NT4 Epigallocatechin
NT4 Epigallocatechin gallate
NT4 Gallocatechin gallate
NT4 Pyrocatechol
NT2 Flavanones
NT3 Hesperetin
NT3 Hesperidin
NT3 Naringenin
NT3 Naringin
NT3 Narirutin
NT3 Neohesperidin
NT2 Flavones
NT3 Apigenin
NT3 Chrysin
NT3 Luteolin
NT2 Flavonols
NT3 Dihydroquercetin
NT3 Fisetin
NT3 Isorhamnetin
NT3 Kaempferol
NT3 Morin
NT3 Myricetin
NT3 Quercetin
NT3 Quercitrin
NT3 Rutin
NT2 Isoflavonoids
NT3 Coumestrol
NT3 Isoflavones
NT4 Daidzein
NT4 Equol
NT4 Genistein
NT4 Glycitein
NT4 Puerarin
NT2 Theaflavins
NT2 Thearubigins
NT1 Fluoranthene
NT1 Fluorene
NT1 Heterocyclic aromatic amines
NT1 Myristicin
NT1 Naphthalene
NT1 Oryzanols
NT1 Perylene
NT1 Phenanthrene
NT1 Phenols
NT2 Alkylphenols
NT2 Alkylresorcinols
NT2 Anisole
NT2 Arbutin
NT2 Avenanthramides
NT2 Bisphenol A
NT2 Bisphenol A diglycidyl ether
NT2 Bisphenol F diglycidyl ether
NT2 Bromophenols
NT2 Caffeic acid
NT2 Carvacrol
NT2 Catechols
NT3 Catechin
NT3 Epicatechin
NT3 Epicatechin gallate
NT3 Epicatechol
NT3 Epigallocatechin

NT3 Epigallocatechin gallate
NT3 Gallocatechin gallate
NT3 Pyrocatechol
NT2 Chlorogenic acid
NT3 Caffeoylquinic acid
NT2 Chlorophenol
NT2 Cinnamic acid
NT2 Coumarins
NT3 Coumarin
NT3 Coumestrol
NT3 Esculetin
NT3 Furocoumarins
NT4 Bergapten
NT4 Psoralens
NT4 Xanthotoxin
NT3 Scopoletin
NT2 Cresols
NT2 Curcuminoids
NT3 Curcumin
NT2 Ellagic acid
NT2 Ellagitannins
NT2 Estragole
NT2 Eugenol
NT2 Ferulic acid
NT2 Feruloylquinic acid
NT2 Gingerols
NT2 Guaiacol
NT2 4-Hexylresorcinol
NT2 Hydroquinone
NT2 Hydroxycinnamic acid
NT3 Coumaric acid
NT2 Hydroxytyrosol
NT2 Isochlorogenic acid
NT2 Isoeugenol
NT2 Lignans
NT3 Sesamin
NT3 Sesamolin
NT2 Naphthol
NT2 Nordihydroguaiaretic acid
NT3 NDGA
NT2 Oleuropein
NT2 Phenylpropanoids
NT2 Phloroglucinol
NT2 Polyphenols
NT2 Protocatechuic acid
NT2 Pyrogallol
NT2 Resorcinol
NT2 Rosmarinic acid
NT2 Sesamol
NT2 Stilbenes
NT3 Piceatannol
NT3 Piceid
NT3 Resveratrol
NT2 Syringic acid
NT2 Thymol
NT2 Tyrosol
NT2 Vanillic acid
NT2 Vanillin
NT2 Zingerone
NT1 Phenylacetic acid
NT1 Phthalic acid
NT1 Pyrene
NT1 Quinones
NT2 Coenzyme Q
NT1 Safrole
NT1 Tannins
NT2 Ellagitannins
NT2 Proanthocyanidins
NT3 Procyanidins
NT2 Tannic acid
NT1 Toluene
NT1 Xylene
RT Heterocyclic compounds
RT Hydrocarbons
RT Styrene

Aromatization
BT1 Aroma
BT2 Sensory properties
RT Aroma compounds

Aromatized wines
BT1 Wines
BT2 Alcoholic beverages
BT3 Beverages alcoholic
BT4 Beverages
NT1 Retsina
NT1 Sangria
NT1 Vermouths
NT1 Wine coolers

Aromatizing agents
USE **Flavourings**

Aroma volatiles
USE **Aroma compounds**

Aronia
BT1 Fruits specific
BT2 Fruits
BT3 Crops
BT4 Plants
BT3 Plant foods
BT4 Foods

Arracacha
BT1 Vegetables specific
BT2 Vegetables
BT3 Crops
BT4 Plants
BT3 Plant foods
BT4 Foods
UF Peruvian carrots
UF Peruvian parsnips

Arrack
USE **Arak**

Arrowhead
BT1 Vegetables specific
BT2 Vegetables
BT3 Crops
BT4 Plants
BT3 Plant foods
BT4 Foods

Arrowroot
BT1 Starch
BT2 Glucans
BT3 Polysaccharides
BT4 Carbohydrates
BT5 Nutrients
BT5 Organic compounds
BT2 Thickeners
BT3 Additives

Arrowtooth flounder
BT1 Flatfish
BT2 Marine fish
BT3 Fish
BT4 Animals
BT4 Sea foods
BT5 Aquatic foods
BT6 Animal foods
BT7 Foods

Arsenates
BT1 Salts

Arsenic
SN symbol As is also used in the index
BT1 Contaminants
BT2 Contamination
BT1 Elements
BT2 Minerals
BT3 Nutrients
NT1 Arsenicals
NT2 Arsenobetaine
NT2 Dimethylarsinic acid
NT2 Methylarsonic acid
NT1 As

Arsenicals
HN introduced from vol. 39, issue 1 (2007)
BT1 Arsenic
BT2 Contaminants
BT3 Contamination
BT2 Elements
BT3 Minerals
BT4 Nutrients
NT1 Arsenobetaine
NT1 Dimethylarsinic acid
NT1 Methylarsonic acid

Arsenobetaine
HN introduced from vol. 39, issue 1 (2007)
BT1 Arsenicals
BT2 Arsenic
BT3 Contaminants
BT4 Contamination
BT3 Elements
BT4 Minerals
BT5 Nutrients

Artemisia
HN under Spices up to vol. 42 (2010)
BT1 Herbs
BT2 Spices
BT3 Flavourings
BT4 Additives

Artemisia vulgaris
HN under Spices up to vol. 42 (2010)
BT1 Mugwort
BT2 Herbs
BT3 Spices
BT4 Flavourings
BT5 Additives

Arthritis
BT1 Diseases

Arthrobacter
BT1 Bacteria
BT2 Microorganisms
NT1 *Arthrobacter globiformis*
NT1 *Arthrobacter protophormiae*

Arthrobacter globiformis
BT1 *Arthrobacter*
BT2 Bacteria
BT3 Microorganisms

Arthrobacter protophormiae
BT1 *Arthrobacter*
BT2 Bacteria
BT3 Microorganisms

Artichokes
BT1 Vegetables specific
BT2 Vegetables
BT3 Crops
BT4 Plants
BT3 Plant foods
BT4 Foods
RT Globe artichokes
RT Jerusalem artichokes

Artificial colorants
HN colorants artificial also used in the index up to vol. 29 (1997)
BT1 Colorants
BT2 Additives

Artificial flavourings
HN flavourings artificial also used in the index up to vol. 29 (1997)
BT1 Flavourings
BT2 Additives

Artificial foods
BT1 Simulated foods
BT2 Processed foods
BT3 Foods

Artificial neural networks
BT1 Information technology
BT2 Technology
BT1 Modelling
RT Fuzzy control
RT Fuzzy logic process control
UF Neural networks

Artificial sweeteners
HN sweeteners artificial also used in the index up to vol. 29 (1997)
BT1 Sweeteners
BT2 Additives

Arxula
HN introduced from vol. 43, issue 1 (2011)
BT1 Yeasts
BT2 Fungi
BT3 Microorganisms
NT1 *Arxula adeninivorans*

Arxula adeninivorans
BT1 *Arxula*
BT2 Yeasts
BT3 Fungi
BT4 Microorganisms

Aryl-alcohol oxidases
SN EC 1.1.3.7
BT1 Alcohol oxidases
BT2 Oxidases
BT3 Oxidoreductases
BT4 Enzymes

Arzua cheese
BT1 Cheese varieties
BT2 Cheese
BT3 Dairy products
BT4 Animal foods
BT5 Foods

As
SN index heading is Arsenic
BT1 Arsenic
BT2 Contaminants
BT3 Contamination
BT2 Elements
BT3 Minerals
BT4 Nutrients

Asafoetida
BT1 Spices
BT2 Flavourings
BT3 Additives

Asbestos
BT1 Minerals
BT2 Nutrients
RT Carcinogens
RT Filtration

Ascidians
SN syn. sea squirts
BT1 Sea foods
BT2 Aquatic foods
BT3 Animal foods
BT4 Foods
NT1 Sea squirts

Ascomycetes
BT1 Fungi
BT2 Microorganisms

Ascorbases
USE **L-Ascorbate oxidases**

Ascorbate oxidases
USE **L-Ascorbate oxidases**

L-Ascorbate oxidases
SN EC 1.10.3.3
BT1 Oxidases
BT2 Oxidoreductases
BT3 Enzymes
UF Ascorbases
UF Ascorbate oxidases

Ascorbates
BT1 Antioxidants
BT2 Additives
BT1 Bakery additives
BT2 Additives
BT1 Salts
NT1 Sodium ascorbate
RT Ascorbic acid

Ascorbic acid
BT1 Antioxidants
BT2 Additives
BT1 Bakery additives
BT2 Additives
BT1 Vitamins
BT2 Nutrients
NT1 Dehydroascorbic acid
NT1 Vitamin C
RT Ascorbates

Ascorbyl palmitate
BT1 Antioxidants
BT2 Additives
BT1 Fatty acid esters
BT2 Esters
BT3 Organic compounds

Ascospores
USE **Fungal spores**

Aseptic packaging
SN index heading is Packaging aseptic
BT1 Packaging aseptic
BT2 Packaging
BT3 Technology

Aseptic processing
HN processing aseptic used in the index up to vol. 29 (1997)
BT1 Processing
BT2 Technology

Ash
BT1 Minerals
BT2 Nutrients

Ashbya
HN introduced from vol. 43, issue 1 (2011)
SN synonymous with Eremothecium
BT1 Yeasts
BT2 Fungi
BT3 Microorganisms
NT1 *Ashbya gossypii*

Ashbya gossypii
HN introduced from vol. 39, issue 1 (2007); under Fungi up to vol. 42 (2010)
BT1 *Ashbya*
BT2 Yeasts
BT3 Fungi
BT4 Microorganisms

Asia
HN heading up to vol. 24 (1992)
NT1 Afghanistan
NT1 Armenia
NT1 Azerbaijan
NT1 Bangladesh
NT1 Bhutan
NT1 Brunei
NT1 Cambodia
NT1 China
NT2 Hong Kong
NT2 Tibet
NT1 East Timor
NT1 Georgia
NT1 India
NT1 Indonesia
NT1 Iran
NT1 Iraq
NT1 Israel
NT1 Japan
NT1 Jordan
NT1 Kazakhstan
NT1 Korea
NT1 Kuwait
NT1 Kyrgyzstan

NT1 Laos
NT1 Lebanon
NT1 Malaysia
NT1 Mongolia
NT1 Myanmar
NT1 Nepal
NT1 North Korea
NT1 Oman
NT1 Pakistan
NT1 Philippines
NT1 Qatar
NT1 Russia
NT1 Sabah
NT1 Sarawak
NT1 Saudi Arabia
NT1 Singapore
NT1 South Korea
NT1 Sri Lanka
NT1 Taiwan
NT1 Tajikistan
NT1 Thailand
NT1 Turkey
NT1 Turkmenistan
NT1 United Arab Emirates
NT1 Uzbekistan
NT1 Vietnam
NT1 Yemen
RT Middle East

Asiago cheese
BT1 Cheese varieties
BT2 Cheese
BT3 Dairy products
BT4 Animal foods
BT5 Foods

Asiago Pressato cheese
BT1 Cheese varieties
BT2 Cheese
BT3 Dairy products
BT4 Animal foods
BT5 Foods

Asian pears
SN syn. Japanese pears
BT1 Pears
BT2 Fruits specific
BT3 Fruits
BT4 Crops
BT5 Plants
BT4 Plant foods
BT5 Foods

Asparaginases
HN introduced from vol. 41, issue 1 (2009)
SN EC 3.5.1.1
BT1 Hydrolases
BT2 Enzymes

Asparagine
BT1 Amino acids
BT2 Nutrients
BT2 Organic acids
BT3 Acids
BT2 Organic nitrogen compounds

Asparagus
HN heading from vol. 25 (1993); under Vegetables specific up to vol. 24 (1992)
BT1 Vegetables specific
BT2 Vegetables
BT3 Crops
BT4 Plants
BT3 Plant foods
BT4 Foods

Asparagus beans
BT1 Legumes
BT2 Vegetables specific
BT3 Vegetables
BT4 Crops
BT5 Plants
BT4 Plant foods
BT5 Foods
UF Sitao
UF Yard-long beans

Asparagus peas
BT1 Legumes
BT2 Vegetables specific
BT3 Vegetables
BT4 Crops
BT5 Plants
BT4 Plant foods
BT5 Foods

Aspartame
HN heading from vol. 25 (1993); under Sweeteners up to vol. 24 (1992)
BT1 Sweeteners
BT2 Additives
NT1 NutraSweet
RT Neotame
UF Aspartyl phenylalanine methyl ester

Aspartate aminotransferases
USE **Aspartate transaminases**

Aspartate kinases
SN EC 2.7.2.4
BT1 Kinases
BT2 Phosphotransferases
BT3 Transferases
BT4 Enzymes

Aspartate transaminases
HN introduced from vol. 39, issue 1 (2007)
SN EC 2.6.1.1
BT1 Transaminases
BT2 Transferases
BT3 Enzymes
UF Aspartate aminotransferases

Aspartic acid
HN heading from vol. 25 (1993); under Amino acids up to vol. 24 (1992)
BT1 Amino acids
BT2 Nutrients
BT2 Organic acids
BT3 Acids
BT2 Organic nitrogen compounds

Aspartyl phenylalanine methyl ester
USE **Aspartame**

Aspergillus
BT1 Fungi
BT2 Microorganisms
NT1 *Aspergillus aculeatus*
NT1 *Aspergillus awamori*
NT1 *Aspergillus candidus*
NT1 *Aspergillus carbonarius*
NT1 *Aspergillus clavatus*
NT1 *Aspergillus ficuum*
NT1 *Aspergillus flavus*
NT1 *Aspergillus foetidus*
NT1 *Aspergillus fumigatus*
NT1 *Aspergillus japonicus*
NT1 *Aspergillus kawachii*
NT1 *Aspergillus melleus*
NT1 *Aspergillus nidulans*
NT1 *Aspergillus niger*
NT1 *Aspergillus ochraceus*
NT1 *Aspergillus oryzae*
NT1 *Aspergillus parasiticus*
NT1 *Aspergillus phoenicis*
NT2 *Aspergillus saitoi*
NT1 *Aspergillus repens*
NT1 *Aspergillus sojae*
NT1 *Aspergillus terreus*
NT1 *Aspergillus tubingensis*
NT1 *Aspergillus ustus*
NT1 *Aspergillus versicolor*
RT Aflatoxicosis
RT Aflatoxins

Aspergillus aculeatus
BT1 *Aspergillus*
BT2 Fungi
BT3 Microorganisms

Aspergillus awamori
BT1 *Aspergillus*
BT2 Fungi
BT3 Microorganisms

Aspergillus candidus
BT1 *Aspergillus*
BT2 Fungi
BT3 Microorganisms

Aspergillus carbonarius
BT1 *Aspergillus*
BT2 Fungi
BT3 Microorganisms

Aspergillus clavatus
HN introduced from vol. 39, issue 1 (2007)
BT1 *Aspergillus*
BT2 Fungi
BT3 Microorganisms

Aspergillus ficuum
BT1 *Aspergillus*
BT2 Fungi
BT3 Microorganisms

Aspergillus flavus
BT1 *Aspergillus*
BT2 Fungi
BT3 Microorganisms

Aspergillus foetidus
HN introduced from vol. 39, issue 1 (2007)
BT1 _Aspergillus_
BT2 Fungi
BT3 Microorganisms

Aspergillus fumigatus
BT1 _Aspergillus_
BT2 Fungi
BT3 Microorganisms

Aspergillus japonicus
BT1 _Aspergillus_
BT2 Fungi
BT3 Microorganisms

Aspergillus kawachii
BT1 _Aspergillus_
BT2 Fungi
BT3 Microorganisms

Aspergillus melleus
BT1 _Aspergillus_
BT2 Fungi
BT3 Microorganisms

Aspergillus nidulans
SN synonymous with Emericella nidulans
BT1 _Aspergillus_
BT2 Fungi
BT3 Microorganisms

Aspergillus niger
BT1 _Aspergillus_
BT2 Fungi
BT3 Microorganisms

Aspergillus ochraceus
BT1 _Aspergillus_
BT2 Fungi
BT3 Microorganisms

Aspergillus oryzae
BT1 _Aspergillus_
BT2 Fungi
BT3 Microorganisms

Aspergillus parasiticus
BT1 _Aspergillus_
BT2 Fungi
BT3 Microorganisms

Aspergillus phoenicis
SN synonymous with Aspergilllus saitoi
BT1 _Aspergillus_
BT2 Fungi
BT3 Microorganisms
NT1 _Aspergillus saitoi_

Aspergillus repens
BT1 _Aspergillus_
BT2 Fungi
BT3 Microorganisms

Aspergillus saitoi
HN introduced from vol. 39, issue 1 (2007)
SN synonymous with Aspergillus phoenicis
BT1 _Aspergillus phoenicis_
BT2 _Aspergillus_
BT3 Fungi
BT4 Microorganisms

Aspergillus sojae
BT1 _Aspergillus_
BT2 Fungi
BT3 Microorganisms

Aspergillus terreus
BT1 _Aspergillus_
BT2 Fungi
BT3 Microorganisms

Aspergillus tubingensis
BT1 _Aspergillus_
BT2 Fungi
BT3 Microorganisms

Aspergillus ustus
BT1 _Aspergillus_
BT2 Fungi
BT3 Microorganisms

Aspergillus versicolor
HN introduced from vol. 39, issue 1 (2007)
BT1 _Aspergillus_
BT2 Fungi
BT3 Microorganisms

Aspic
BT1 Gels
BT2 Physical phases
BT3 Chemistry
BT4 Science

Aspirators
BT1 Equipment
BT2 Technology

Assay
BT1 Analytical techniques

Ass milk
BT1 Animals
BT1 Milk
BT2 Dairy products
BT3 Animal foods
BT4 Foods

Association of Official Analytical Chemists
HN heading up to vol. 10 (1978)
USE **AOAC**

Astacene
BT1 Carotenoids
BT2 Pigments
BT2 Terpenoids
BT3 Lipids
BT4 Nutrients

Astaxanthin
BT1 Xanthophylls
BT2 Carotenoids
BT3 Pigments
BT3 Terpenoids
BT4 Lipids
BT5 Nutrients

Asthma
BT1 Diseases

Astringency
BT1 Flavour
BT2 Sensory properties

Astrocaryum
BT1 Palms
BT2 Plants

Astroviruses
HN introduced from vol. 42, issue 1 (2010); under Enteric viruses up to vol. 42 (2010)
SN for descriptive use only
BT1 Viruses
BT2 Microorganisms
NT1 Mamastrovirus
NT2 Human astrovirus

Asulam
BT1 Carbamate pesticides
BT2 Pesticides
BT3 Biocides
BT3 Residues
BT1 Herbicides
BT2 Pesticides
BT3 Biocides
BT3 Residues

Atherosclerosis
BT1 Diseases

Athletes
HN introduced from vol. 38, issue 8 (2006)
BT1 Population groups

Atlantic halibut
HN introduced from vol. 39, issue 1 (2007)
BT1 Halibut
BT2 Flatfish
BT3 Marine fish
BT4 Fish
BT5 Animals
BT5 Sea foods
BT6 Aquatic foods
BT7 Animal foods
BT8 Foods

Atlantic mackerel
BT1 Mackerel
BT2 Marine fish
BT3 Fish
BT4 Animals
BT4 Sea foods
BT5 Aquatic foods
BT6 Animal foods
BT7 Foods
BT2 Oily fish
BT3 Fish
BT4 Animals
BT4 Sea foods
BT5 Aquatic foods
BT6 Animal foods
BT7 Foods
NT1 _Scomber scombrus_

Atlantic salmon
BT1 Salmon
BT2 Oily fish
BT3 Fish
BT4 Animals
BT4 Sea foods
BT5 Aquatic foods
BT6 Animal foods
BT7 Foods
NT1 *Salmo salar*

Atm
HN used as abbrev. for atmosphere up to vol. 24 (1992)
USE **Atmosphere**

Atmosphere
HN abbrev. atm used up to vol. 24 (1992)
BT1 Air
BT2 Gases
BT3 Physical phases
BT4 Chemistry
BT5 Science
UF Atm

Atomic absorption spectrophotometry
USE **AAS**

Atomic absorption spectroscopy
SN abbrev. AAS is also used in the index
BT1 Spectroscopy
BT2 Analytical techniques
NT1 AAS

Atomic emission spectroscopy
BT1 Spectroscopy
BT2 Analytical techniques
NT1 ICP-AES

Atomic force microscopy
BT1 Microscopy
BT2 Analytical techniques

Atomizers
BT1 Dispensers
BT2 Equipment
BT3 Technology

ATP
BT1 Nucleotides
UF Adenosine triphosphate

ATPases
SN EC 3.6.1.3 and members of EC 3.6.3 and EC 3.6.4
BT1 Hydrolases
BT2 Enzymes
UF Adenosinetriphosphatases

Atractylodes lancea
BT1 Plants

Atrazine
BT1 Triazine herbicides
BT2 Herbicides
BT3 Pesticides
BT4 Biocides
BT4 Residues

Atta
BT1 Cereal flours
BT2 Flours cereal
BT3 Cereal products
BT4 Plant foods
BT5 Foods
BT1 Wheat
BT2 Cereals
BT3 Crops
BT4 Plants
BT3 Seeds
BT4 Plant foods
BT5 Foods

Attieke
BT1 Cassava
BT2 Vegetables specific
BT3 Vegetables
BT4 Crops
BT5 Plants
BT4 Plant foods
BT5 Foods
BT1 Fermented foods
BT2 Processed foods
BT3 Foods

Au
HN under Minerals up to vol. 42 (2010)
BT1 Metals
BT2 Elements
BT3 Minerals
BT4 Nutrients
UF Gold

Aubergines
HN heading from vol. 30 (1998); under Vegetables specific up to vol. 29 (1997)
BT1 Vegetables specific
BT2 Vegetables
BT3 Crops
BT4 Plants
BT3 Plant foods
BT4 Foods
UF Brinjal
UF Egg plants

Aureobasidium
BT1 Fungi
BT2 Microorganisms
NT1 *Aureobasidium pullulans*

Aureobasidium pullulans
BT1 *Aureobasidium*
BT2 Fungi
BT3 Microorganisms
RT Pullulan

Aureomycin
USE **Chlortetracycline**

Auricularia
BT1 Edible fungi
BT2 Fungi edible
BT3 Vegetables specific
BT4 Vegetables
BT5 Crops
BT6 Plants
BT5 Plant foods
BT6 Foods
NT1 *Auricularia auricula*
NT1 *Auricularia polytricha*

Auricularia auricula
HN introduced from vol. 39, issue 1 (2007)
BT1 *Auricularia*
BT2 Edible fungi
BT3 Fungi edible
BT4 Vegetables specific
BT5 Vegetables
BT6 Crops
BT7 Plants
BT6 Plant foods
BT7 Foods

Auricularia polytricha
HN introduced from vol. 39, issue 1 (2007)
BT1 *Auricularia*
BT2 Edible fungi
BT3 Fungi edible
BT4 Vegetables specific
BT5 Vegetables
BT6 Crops
BT7 Plants
BT6 Plant foods
BT7 Foods

Australasia
HN heading up to vol. 24 (1992)
BT1 Oceania
NT1 New Caledonia

Australia
HN heading up to vol. 24 (1992)
BT1 Oceania
RT Organization for Economic Cooperation and Development

Australian chestnuts
BT1 Nuts
BT2 Fruits
BT3 Crops
BT4 Plants
BT3 Plant foods
BT4 Foods
BT2 Oilseeds
BT3 Seeds
BT4 Plant foods
BT5 Foods

Austria
HN heading up to vol. 24 (1992)
BT1 Europe
BT1 European Union
RT Organization for Economic Cooperation and Development

Authenticity
BT1 Purity

Autoclaves
BT1 Equipment
BT2 Technology
BT1 Sterilization
BT2 Thermal processing

BT3 Processing thermal
BT4 Processing
BT5 Technology

Autofluorescence
HN introduced from vol. 39, issue 1 (2007)
BT1 Fluorescence
BT2 Analytical techniques
BT2 Optical properties
BT3 Physical properties

Autolysins
SN EC 3.4.24.38
BT1 Lysins
BT2 Proteinases
BT3 Hydrolases
BT4 Enzymes

Autolysis
BT1 Lysis
BT2 Decomposition

Automation
HN heading from vol. 25 (1993); under Mechanization up to vol. 24 (1992)
BT1 Technology
NT1 Robotics
RT Mechanization

Autoxidation
BT1 Oxidation

Auxins
BT1 Plant growth regulators
BT2 Cultivation
BT3 Agriculture
NT1 Indole acetic acid
NT2 Indol-3-ylacetic acid
NT1 Naphthaleneacetic acid
NT2 2-(1-Naphthyl)acetic acid
NT2 (2-Naphthyloxy)acetic acid

Availability
BT1 Bioavailability
BT2 Nutritional values

Avena fatua
BT1 Oats
BT2 Cereals
BT3 Crops
BT4 Plants
BT3 Seeds
BT4 Plant foods
BT5 Foods

Avenanthramides
HN introduced from vol. 39, issue 1 (2007)
BT1 Amides
BT2 Organic nitrogen compounds
BT1 Phenols
BT2 Alcohols
BT2 Aromatic compounds
BT3 Organic compounds
RT Anthranilic acid
RT Oats

Avenasterol
BT1 Sterols
BT2 Alcohols
BT2 Steroids
BT3 Lipids
BT4 Nutrients

Avenins
BT1 Cereal proteins
BT2 Proteins cereal
BT3 Vegetable proteins
BT4 Proteins vegetable
BT5 Proteins
BT6 Nutrients
BT5 Vegetable products
BT6 Plant foods
BT7 Foods

Avermectins
BT1 Insecticides
BT2 Pesticides
BT3 Biocides
BT3 Residues
NT1 Emamectin

Avian flu
HN introduced from vol. 40, issue 1 (2008)
BT1 Animal diseases
BT2 Diseases animal
BT3 Diseases

Avidin
BT1 Egg proteins
BT2 Animal proteins
BT3 Proteins animal
BT4 Proteins
BT5 Nutrients
BT1 Glycoproteins
BT2 Proteins
BT3 Nutrients

Avocado oils
BT1 Vegetable oils
BT2 Oils vegetable
BT3 Oils
BT4 Lipids
BT5 Nutrients
BT3 Vegetable products
BT4 Plant foods
BT5 Foods

Avocados
BT1 Vegetables specific
BT2 Vegetables
BT3 Crops
BT4 Plants
BT3 Plant foods
BT4 Foods
NT1 Guacamole
UF Alligator pears

Avoparcin
BT1 Antibiotics
BT2 Drugs
BT3 Residues

a_w
SN index heading is Water activity
BT1 Water activity
RT Humidity
RT Moisture content

Awamori
BT1 Spirits
BT2 Alcoholic beverages
BT3 Beverages alcoholic
BT4 Beverages

Ayu
BT1 Freshwater fish
BT2 Fish
BT3 Animals
BT3 Sea foods
BT4 Aquatic foods
BT5 Animal foods
BT6 Foods

Azaperone
BT1 Drugs
BT2 Residues
UF Stresnil

Azaspiracids
BT1 Toxins
BT2 Residues

Azerbaijan
BT1 Asia
BT1 Europe

Azinphos-methyl
BT1 Acaricides
BT2 Pesticides
BT3 Biocides
BT3 Residues
BT1 Organophosphorus insecticides
BT2 Insecticides
BT3 Pesticides
BT4 Biocides
BT4 Residues
BT2 Organophosphorus pesticides
BT3 Pesticides
BT4 Biocides
BT4 Residues
UF Guthion

Azodicarbonamide
BT1 Amides
BT2 Organic nitrogen compounds
BT1 Bakery additives
BT2 Additives

Azodrin
USE **Monocrotophos**

Azo dyes
BT1 Colorants
BT2 Additives

Azotobacter
BT1 Bacteria
BT2 Microorganisms
NT1 *Azotobacter chroococcum*
NT1 *Azotobacter vinelandii*

Azotobacter chroococcum
BT1 *Azotobacter*
BT2 Bacteria
BT3 Microorganisms

Azotobacter vinelandii
BT1 *Azotobacter*
BT2 Bacteria
BT3 Microorganisms

Azoxystrobin
BT1 Fungicides
BT2 Pesticides
BT3 Biocides
BT3 Residues

B

B
HN under Minerals up to vol. 42 (2010)
BT1 Elements
BT2 Minerals
BT3 Nutrients
UF Boron

Ba
HN under Minerals up to vol. 42 (2010)
BT1 Metals
BT2 Elements
BT3 Minerals
BT4 Nutrients
UF Barium

Babaco
BT1 Fruits specific
BT2 Fruits
BT3 Crops
BT4 Plants
BT3 Plant foods
BT4 Foods

Babassu oils
BT1 Palm oils
BT2 Palms
BT3 Plants
BT2 Vegetable oils
BT3 Oils vegetable
BT4 Oils
BT5 Lipids
BT6 Nutrients
BT4 Vegetable products
BT5 Plant foods
BT6 Foods

Babassu palm kernels
BT1 Oilseeds
BT2 Seeds
BT3 Plant foods
BT4 Foods
BT1 Palms
BT2 Plants

Babies
USE **Infants**

Baby corn
BT1 Corn
BT2 Cereals
BT3 Crops
BT4 Plants
BT3 Seeds
BT4 Plant foods
BT5 Foods

Baby foods
USE **Infant foods**

Bacilli
BT1 Bacteria
BT2 Microorganisms

Bacillus
BT1 Bacteria
BT2 Microorganisms
NT1 *Bacillus acidopullulyticus*
NT1 *Bacillus agaradhaerens*
NT1 *Bacillus alcalophilus*
NT1 *Bacillus amyloliquefaciens*
NT1 *Bacillus anthracis*
NT1 *Bacillus brevis*
NT1 *Bacillus cereus*
NT1 *Bacillus circulans*
NT1 *Bacillus coagulans*
NT1 *Bacillus firmus*
NT1 *Bacillus halodurans*
NT1 *Bacillus lentus*
NT1 *Bacillus licheniformis*
NT1 *Bacillus macerans*
NT1 *Bacillus megaterium*
NT1 *Bacillus mojavensis*
NT1 *Bacillus polymyxa*
NT1 *Bacillus pumilus*
NT1 *Bacillus sphaericus*
NT1 *Bacillus sporothermodurans*
NT1 *Bacillus stearothermophilus*
NT1 *Bacillus subtilis*
NT2 *Bacillus natto*
NT1 *Bacillus thermoleovorans*
NT1 *Bacillus thermoproteolyticus*
NT1 *Bacillus thuringiensis*

Bacillus acidopullulyticus
HN introduced from vol. 39, issue 1 (2007)
BT1 *Bacillus*
BT2 Bacteria
BT3 Microorganisms

Bacillus agaradhaerens
BT1 *Bacillus*
BT2 Bacteria
BT3 Microorganisms

Bacillus alcalophilus
BT1 *Bacillus*
BT2 Bacteria
BT3 Microorganisms

Bacillus amyloliquefaciens
BT1 *Bacillus*
BT2 Bacteria
BT3 Microorganisms

Bacillus anthracis
BT1 *Bacillus*
BT2 Bacteria
BT3 Microorganisms
RT Anthrax

Bacillus brevis
SN synonymous with Brevibacillus brevis
BT1 *Bacillus*
BT2 Bacteria
BT3 Microorganisms

Bacillus cereus
BT1 *Bacillus*
BT2 Bacteria
BT3 Microorganisms
RT Cereulide

Bacillus circulans
BT1 *Bacillus*
BT2 Bacteria
BT3 Microorganisms

Bacillus coagulans
BT1 *Bacillus*
BT2 Bacteria
BT3 Microorganisms

Bacillus firmus
HN introduced from vol. 39, issue 1 (2007)
BT1 *Bacillus*
BT2 Bacteria
BT3 Microorganisms

Bacillus halodurans
BT1 *Bacillus*
BT2 Bacteria
BT3 Microorganisms

Bacillus lentus
HN introduced from vol. 39, issue 1 (2007)
BT1 *Bacillus*
BT2 Bacteria
BT3 Microorganisms

Bacillus licheniformis
BT1 *Bacillus*
BT2 Bacteria
BT3 Microorganisms

Bacillus macerans
SN synonymous with Paenibacillus macerans
BT1 *Bacillus*
BT2 Bacteria
BT3 Microorganisms

Bacillus megaterium
BT1 *Bacillus*
BT2 Bacteria
BT3 Microorganisms

Bacillus mojavensis
BT1 *Bacillus*
BT2 Bacteria
BT3 Microorganisms

Bacillus natto
SN current name is Bacillus subtilis subsp. natto
BT1 *Bacillus subtilis*
BT2 *Bacillus*
BT3 Bacteria
BT4 Microorganisms

Bacillus polymyxa
SN synonymous with Paenibacillus polymyxa
BT1 *Bacillus*
BT2 Bacteria
BT3 Microorganisms

Bacillus pumilus
BT1 *Bacillus*
BT2 Bacteria
BT3 Microorganisms

Bacillus sphaericus
SN synonymous with Lysinibacillus sphaericus
BT1 *Bacillus*
BT2 Bacteria
BT3 Microorganisms

Bacillus sporothermodurans
HN introduced from vol. 39, issue 1 (2007)
BT1 *Bacillus*
BT2 Bacteria
BT3 Microorganisms

Bacillus stearothermophilus
SN synonymous with Geobacillus stearothermophilus
BT1 *Bacillus*
BT2 Bacteria
BT3 Microorganisms

Bacillus subtilis
BT1 *Bacillus*
BT2 Bacteria
BT3 Microorganisms
NT1 *Bacillus natto*
RT Subtilins

Bacillus thermoleovorans
SN synonymous with Geobacillus thermoleovorans
BT1 *Bacillus*
BT2 Bacteria
BT3 Microorganisms

Bacillus thermoproteolyticus
BT1 *Bacillus*
BT2 Bacteria
BT3 Microorganisms

Bacillus thuringiensis
BT1 *Bacillus*
BT2 Bacteria
BT3 Microorganisms

Bacitracin
BT1 Antibiotics
BT2 Drugs
BT3 Residues

Backfat
BT1 Animal fats
BT2 Fats animal
BT3 Animal foods
BT4 Foods
BT3 Fats
BT4 Lipids
BT5 Nutrients

Bacon
BT1 Meat products
BT2 Animal foods
BT3 Foods
NT1 Baconburgers
RT Ham
RT Pork
RT Swine

Baconburgers
BT1 Bacon
BT2 Meat products
BT3 Animal foods
BT4 Foods
BT1 Burgers
BT2 Meat products
BT3 Animal foods
BT4 Foods

Bacteria
HN Eubacteria also used in the index up to vol. 42 (2010)
BT1 Microorganisms
NT1 Acetic acid bacteria
NT1 *Acetobacter*
NT2 *Acetobacter aceti*
NT2 *Acetobacter diazotrophicus*
NT2 *Acetobacter pasteurianus*
NT2 *Acetobacter suboxydans*
NT2 *Acetobacter xylinum*
NT1 *Achromobacter*
NT1 *Acinetobacter*
NT2 *Acinetobacter calcoaceticus*
NT2 *Acinetobacter haemolyticus*
NT2 *Acinetobacter radioresistens*
NT1 *Actinobacillus*
NT1 *Actinobacteria*
NT2 Actinomycetes
NT1 *Actinomyces*
NT1 Actinomycetales
NT1 *Actinoplanes*
NT1 *Aerococcus*
NT1 *Aeromonas*
NT2 *Aeromonas caviae*
NT2 *Aeromonas hydrophila*
NT1 *Agrobacterium*
NT2 *Agrobacterium tumefaciens*
NT3 *Agrobacterium radiobacter*
NT1 *Alcaligenes*
NT2 *Alcaligenes eutrophus*
NT2 *Alcaligenes faecalis*
NT2 *Alcaligenes xylosoxydans*
NT1 *Alicyclobacillus*
NT2 *Alicyclobacillus acidocaldarius*
NT2 *Alicyclobacillus acidoterrestris*
NT1 *Alteromonas*
NT1 *Amycolatopsis*
NT1 Antibacterial activity
NT1 *Arcobacter*
NT2 *Arcobacter butzleri*
NT1 *Arthrobacter*
NT2 *Arthrobacter globiformis*
NT2 *Arthrobacter protophormiae*
NT1 *Azotobacter*
NT2 *Azotobacter chroococcum*
NT2 *Azotobacter vinelandii*
NT1 Bacilli
NT1 *Bacillus*
NT2 *Bacillus acidopullulyticus*
NT2 *Bacillus agaradhaerens*
NT2 *Bacillus alcalophilus*
NT2 *Bacillus amyloliquefaciens*
NT2 *Bacillus anthracis*
NT2 *Bacillus brevis*
NT2 *Bacillus cereus*
NT2 *Bacillus circulans*
NT2 *Bacillus coagulans*
NT2 *Bacillus firmus*
NT2 *Bacillus halodurans*
NT2 *Bacillus lentus*
NT2 *Bacillus licheniformis*
NT2 *Bacillus macerans*
NT2 *Bacillus megaterium*
NT2 *Bacillus mojavensis*
NT2 *Bacillus polymyxa*
NT2 *Bacillus pumilus*
NT2 *Bacillus sphaericus*
NT2 *Bacillus sporothermodurans*
NT2 *Bacillus stearothermophilus*
NT2 *Bacillus subtilis*
NT3 *Bacillus natto*
NT2 *Bacillus thermoleovorans*
NT2 *Bacillus thermoproteolyticus*
NT2 *Bacillus thuringiensis*
NT1 Bacterial biomass
NT1 Bacterial contamination
NT1 *Bacteroides*
NT1 *Bdellovibrio*
NT1 *Beijerinckia*
NT1 *Bifidobacterium*
NT2 *Bifidobacterium adolescentis*
NT2 *Bifidobacterium animalis*
NT2 *Bifidobacterium bifidum*
NT2 *Bifidobacterium breve*
NT2 *Bifidobacterium infantis*
NT2 *Bifidobacterium lactis*
NT2 *Bifidobacterium longum*
NT2 *Bifidobacterium pseudolongum*
NT2 *Bifidobacterium thermophilum*
NT1 *Brevibacillus*
NT1 *Brevibacterium*
NT2 *Brevibacterium flavum*
NT2 *Brevibacterium helvolum*
NT2 *Brevibacterium lactofermentum*
NT2 *Brevibacterium linens*
NT1 *Brochothrix*
NT2 *Brochothrix thermosphacta*
NT1 *Brucella*
NT1 *Burkholderia*
NT2 *Burkholderia cepacia*
NT2 *Burkholderia gladioli*
NT1 *Butyrivibrio*
NT2 *Butyrivibrio fibrisolvens*
NT1 *Campylobacter*
NT2 *Campylobacter coli*
NT2 *Campylobacter fetus*
NT2 *Campylobacter jejuni*
NT2 *Campylobacter lari*
NT1 *Carnobacterium*
NT2 *Carnobacterium divergens*
NT2 *Carnobacterium maltaromaticum*

NT3 *Carnobacterium piscicola*
NT1 *Cellulomonas*
NT2 *Cellulomonas fimi*
NT2 *Cellulomonas flavigena*
NT1 *Cellvibrio*
NT1 *Chromobacterium*
NT2 *Chromobacterium violaceum*
NT2 *Chromobacterium viscosum*
NT1 *Chryseobacterium*
NT1 *Citrobacter*
NT2 *Citrobacter freundii*
NT1 *Clostridium*
NT2 *Clostridium absonum*
NT2 *Clostridium acetobutylicum*
NT2 *Clostridium beijerinckii*
NT2 *Clostridium botulinum*
NT2 *Clostridium butyricum*
NT2 *Clostridium cellulolyticum*
NT2 *Clostridium difficile*
NT2 *Clostridium josui*
NT2 *Clostridium lentocellum*
NT2 *Clostridium perfringens*
NT2 *Clostridium sporogenes*
NT2 *Clostridium stercorarium*
NT3 *Clostridium thermolacticum*
NT2 *Clostridium thermoaceticum*
NT2 *Clostridium thermocellum*
NT2 *Clostridium thermosuccinogenes*
NT2 *Clostridium thermosulfurogenes*
NT2 *Clostridium tyrobutyricum*
NT1 Cocci
NT1 Coliforms
NT1 *Comamonas*
NT1 Corynebacteriaceae
NT1 *Corynebacterium*
NT2 *Corynebacterium casei*
NT2 *Corynebacterium glutamicum*
NT1 *Coxiella*
NT1 Cyanobacteria
NT2 *Anabaena*
NT2 Blue green algae
NT2 *Microcystis*
NT2 *Nostoc*
NT2 *Spirulina*
NT3 *Spirulina maxima*
NT3 *Spirulina platensis*
NT2 *Synechococcus*
NT2 *Synechocystis*
NT1 *Cytophaga*
NT1 *Desulfovibrio*
NT1 *Edwardsiella*
NT1 *Enterobacter*
NT2 *Enterobacter aerogenes*
NT2 *Enterobacter cloacae*
NT2 *Enterobacter sakazakii*
NT1 Enterobacteria
NT1 Enterobacteriaceae
NT1 *Enterococcus*
NT2 *Enterococcus casseliflavus*
NT2 *Enterococcus faecalis*
NT2 *Enterococcus faecium*
NT2 *Enterococcus gallinarum*
NT1 *Erwinia*
NT2 *Erwinia carotovora*
NT2 *Erwinia chrysanthemi*
NT2 *Erwinia herbicola*
NT1 *Erysipelothrix*
NT1 *Escherichia*
NT2 *Escherichia coli*
NT1 *Fibrobacter*
NT1 *Flavimonas oryzihabitans*
NT1 *Flavobacterium*
NT2 *Flavobacterium aurantiacum*
NT2 *Flavobacterium meningosepticum*
NT1 *Francisella*
NT2 *Francisella tularensis*
NT1 *Geobacillus*
NT2 *Geobacillus stearothermophilus*
NT2 *Geobacillus thermoleovorans*
NT1 *Gluconacetobacter*
NT1 *Gluconobacter*
NT2 *Acetomonas*
NT2 *Gluconobacter frateurii*
NT2 *Gluconobacter oxydans*
NT1 Gram negative bacteria
NT1 Gram positive bacteria
NT1 *Hafnia*
NT2 *Hafnia alvei*
NT1 *Halomonas*
NT1 *Helicobacter*
NT2 *Helicobacter canadensis*
NT2 *Helicobacter pylori*
NT1 Hiochi bacteria
NT1 *Klebsiella*
NT2 *Klebsiella aerogenes*
NT2 *Klebsiella oxytoca*
NT2 *Klebsiella pneumoniae*
NT2 *Klebsiella terrigena*
NT1 *Kocuria*
NT2 *Kocuria varians*
NT1 *Kurthia*
NT1 Lactic acid bacteria
NT1 Lactobacillaceae
NT1 *Lactobacillus*
NT2 *Lactobacillus acidophilus*
NT2 *Lactobacillus alimentarius*
NT2 *Lactobacillus amylophilus*
NT2 *Lactobacillus amylovorus*
NT2 *Lactobacillus brevis*
NT2 *Lactobacillus buchneri*
NT2 *Lactobacillus casei*
NT2 *Lactobacillus collinoides*
NT2 *Lactobacillus crispatus*
NT2 *Lactobacillus curvatus*
NT2 *Lactobacillus delbrueckii*
NT3 *Lactobacillus bulgaricus*
NT3 *Lactobacillus lactis*
NT2 *Lactobacillus fermentum*
NT2 *Lactobacillus fructivorans*
NT2 *Lactobacillus gasseri*
NT2 *Lactobacillus helveticus*
NT2 *Lactobacillus hilgardii*
NT2 *Lactobacillus johnsonii*
NT2 *Lactobacillus kefiranofaciens*
NT2 *Lactobacillus kefiri*
NT2 *Lactobacillus leichmannii*
NT2 *Lactobacillus lindneri*
NT2 *Lactobacillus paracasei*
NT2 *Lactobacillus paraplantarum*
NT2 *Lactobacillus pentosus*
NT2 *Lactobacillus plantarum*
NT2 *Lactobacillus pontis*
NT2 *Lactobacillus reuteri*
NT2 *Lactobacillus rhamnosus*
NT2 *Lactobacillus sakei*
NT2 *Lactobacillus salivarius*
NT2 *Lactobacillus sanfranciscensis*
NT2 *Lactobacillus viridescens*
NT1 *Lactococcus*
NT2 *Lactococcus lactis*
NT2 *Lactococcus raffinolactis*
NT1 *Legionella*
NT2 *Legionella pneumophila*
NT1 *Leptospira*
NT1 *Leuconostoc*
NT2 *Leuconostoc carnosum*
NT2 *Leuconostoc citreum*
NT2 *Leuconostoc mesenteroides*
NT2 *Leuconostoc oenos*
NT1 *Listeria*
NT2 *Listeria innocua*
NT2 *Listeria ivanovii*
NT2 *Listeria monocytogenes*
NT2 *Listeria seeligeri*
NT2 *Listeria welshimeri*
NT1 *Macrococcus*
NT2 *Macrococcus caseolyticus*
NT1 *Megasphaera*
NT1 *Methylobacillus*
NT1 *Methylococcus*
NT1 *Methylomonas*
NT1 *Microbacterium*
NT1 Micrococcaceae
NT1 *Micrococcus*
NT2 *Micrococcus luteus*
NT1 *Micromonospora*
NT1 *Moraxella*
NT1 *Morganella*
NT2 *Morganella morganii*
NT1 *Mycobacterium*
NT2 *Mycobacterium avium*
NT3 *Mycobacterium paratuberculosis*
NT2 *Mycobacterium bovis*
NT2 *Mycobacterium tuberculosis*
NT1 *Mycoplasma*
NT1 *Nitrosomonas*
NT1 *Nocardia*
NT1 *Nocardiopsis*
NT1 *Obesumbacterium*
NT1 *Oenococcus*
NT2 *Oenococcus oeni*
NT1 *Paenibacillus*
NT2 *Paenibacillus amylolyticus*
NT2 *Paenibacillus polymyxa*
NT1 *Pantoea*
NT2 *Pantoea agglomerans*
NT1 *Paracoccus*
NT1 *Pasteurella*
NT1 *Pectinatus*
NT2 *Pectinatus frisingensis*
NT1 *Pediococcus*
NT2 *Pediococcus acidilactici*
NT2 *Pediococcus damnosus*

NT2 *Pediococcus pentosaceus*
NT1 *Peptococcus*
NT1 *Photobacterium*
NT2 *Photobacterium phosphoreum*
NT1 *Plesiomonas*
NT2 *Plesiomonas shigelloides*
NT1 Probiotic bacteria
NT1 Propionibacteriaceae
NT1 *Propionibacterium*
NT2 *Propionibacterium acidipropionici*
NT3 *Propionibacterium acidi-propionici*
NT2 *Propionibacterium freudenreichii*
NT3 *Propionibacterium shermanii*
NT2 *Propionibacterium jensenii*
NT2 *Propionibacterium thoenii*
NT1 Propionic acid bacteria
NT1 Proteobacteria
NT1 *Proteus*
NT2 *Proteus mirabilis*
NT2 *Proteus vulgaris*
NT1 *Providencia*
NT1 *Pseudoalteromonas*
NT1 Pseudomonadaceae
NT1 *Pseudomonas*
NT2 *Pseudomonas aeruginosa*
NT2 *Pseudomonas cellulosa*
NT2 *Pseudomonas cepacia*
NT2 *Pseudomonas fluorescens*
NT2 *Pseudomonas fragi*
NT2 *Pseudomonas marginalis*
NT2 *Pseudomonas pseudoalcaligenes*
NT2 *Pseudomonas putida*
NT2 *Pseudomonas stutzeri*
NT2 *Pseudomonas syringae*
NT1 *Psychrobacter*
NT2 *Psychrobacter immobilis*
NT1 *Rahnella*
NT2 *Rahnella aquatilis*
NT1 *Rhizobium*
NT1 *Rhodobacter*
NT1 *Rhodococcus*
NT2 *Rhodococcus equi*
NT2 *Rhodococcus erythropolis*
NT2 *Rhodococcus opacus*
NT1 *Rhodothermus*
NT2 *Rhodothermus marinus*
NT1 *Rickettsia*
NT1 Ropy bacteria
NT1 *Ruminococcus*
NT1 *Salmonella*
NT2 *Salmonella* Agona
NT2 *Salmonella* Blockley
NT2 *Salmonella* Bredeney
NT2 *Salmonella* Choleraesuis
NT2 *Salmonella* Cubana
NT2 *Salmonella* Derby
NT2 *Salmonella* Diarizonae
NT2 *Salmonella* Dublin
NT2 Salmonellae
NT2 *Salmonella enterica*
NT2 *Salmonella* Enteritidis
NT2 *Salmonella* Gallinarum
NT2 *Salmonella* Heidelberg
NT2 *Salmonella* Indiana
NT2 *Salmonella* Infantis
NT2 *Salmonella* Java
NT2 *Salmonella* Kottbus
NT2 *Salmonella* Mbandaka
NT2 *Salmonella* Montevideo
NT2 *Salmonella* Muenchen
NT2 *Salmonella* Muenster
NT2 *Salmonella* Newport
NT2 *Salmonella* Ohio
NT2 *Salmonella* Oranienburg
NT2 *Salmonella* Panama
NT2 *Salmonella* Paratyphi
NT2 *Salmonella* Poona
NT2 *Salmonella* Pullorum
NT2 *Salmonella* Senftenberg
NT2 *Salmonella* Stanley
NT2 *Salmonella* Thompson
NT2 *Salmonella* Typhi
NT2 *Salmonella* Typhimurium
NT2 *Salmonella* Virchow
NT1 *Sarcina*
NT1 *Serratia*
NT2 *Serratia liquefaciens*
NT2 *Serratia marcescens*
NT1 *Shewanella*
NT2 *Shewanella putrefaciens*
NT1 *Shigella*
NT2 *Shigella boydii*
NT2 *Shigella dysenteriae*
NT2 *Shigella flexneri*
NT2 *Shigella sonnei*
NT1 Slime bacteria
NT1 *Sphingomonas*
NT2 *Sphingomonas paucimobilis*
NT1 Spoilage bacteria
NT1 *Staphylococcus*
NT2 *Staphylococcus aureus*
NT2 *Staphylococcus carnosus*
NT2 *Staphylococcus epidermidis*
NT2 *Staphylococcus equorum*
NT2 *Staphylococcus intermedius*
NT2 *Staphylococcus saprophyticus*
NT2 *Staphylococcus sciuri*
NT2 *Staphylococcus simulans*
NT2 *Staphylococcus xylosus*
NT1 Starters
NT2 Adjunct cultures
NT2 Butter starters
NT2 Cheese starters
NT2 Dairy starters
NT2 Lactic starters
NT2 Nuruk
NT2 Yoghurt starters
NT1 *Stenotrophomonas*
NT2 *Stenotrophomonas maltophilia*
NT1 *Streptococcus*
NT2 Lactic streptococci
NT2 *Streptococcus bovis*
NT2 *Streptococcus faecalis*
NT2 *Streptococcus faecium*
NT2 *Streptococcus macedonicus*
NT2 *Streptococcus mutans*
NT2 *Streptococcus pyogenes*
NT2 *Streptococcus salivarius*
NT2 *Streptococcus suis*
NT2 *Streptococcus thermophilus*
NT2 *Streptococcus uberis*
NT1 *Streptomyces*
NT2 *Streptomyces albulus*
NT2 *Streptomyces coelicolor*
NT2 *Streptomyces diastaticus*
NT2 *Streptomyces globisporus*
NT2 *Streptomyces griseus*
NT2 *Streptomyces lividans*
NT2 *Streptomyces murinus*
NT2 *Streptomyces olivaceoviridis*
NT2 *Streptomyces thermoviolaceus*
NT1 *Streptoverticillium*
NT2 *Streptoverticillium mobaraense*
NT1 *Tetragenococcus*
NT2 *Tetragenococcus halophilus*
NT1 *Thermoactinomyces*
NT2 *Thermoactinomyces vulgaris*
NT1 *Thermoanaerobacter*
NT2 *Thermoanaerobacter brockii*
NT2 *Thermoanaerobacter ethanolicus*
NT1 *Thermoanaerobacterium*
NT2 *Thermoanaerobacterium thermosulfurigenes*
NT1 *Thermobifida*
NT2 *Thermobifida fusca*
NT1 *Thermomonospora*
NT2 *Thermomonospora fusca*
NT1 *Thermotoga*
NT2 *Thermotoga maritima*
NT1 *Thermus*
NT2 *Thermus aquaticus*
NT2 *Thermus nonproteolyticus*
NT2 *Thermus thermophilus*
NT1 *Thiobacillus thiooxidans*
NT1 *Veillonella*
NT1 *Vibrio*
NT2 *Vibrio alginolyticus*
NT2 *Vibrio cholerae*
NT2 *Vibrio fischeri*
NT2 *Vibrio lentus*
NT2 *Vibrio metschnikovii*
NT2 *Vibrio mimicus*
NT2 *Vibrio parahaemolyticus*
NT2 *Vibrio vulnificus*
NT1 *Weissella*
NT2 *Weissella confusa*
NT2 *Weissella kimchii*
NT2 *Weissella paramesenteroides*
NT2 *Weissella viridescens*
NT1 *Xanthomonas*
NT2 *Xanthomonas campestris*
NT1 *Yersinia*
NT2 *Yersinia enterocolitica*
NT2 *Yersinia pseudotuberculosis*
NT2 *Yersinia ruckeri*
NT1 *Zymomonas*
NT2 *Zymomonas mobilis*
RT Bacteriology
RT Prokaryotes

RT Quorum sensing
UF Eubacteria

Bacterial biomass
BT1 Bacteria
BT2 Microorganisms
BT1 Microbial biomass
BT2 Biomass
BT3 Fermentation products
BT4 Biotechnology
BT5 Technology
BT2 Microorganisms

Bacterial contamination
BT1 Bacteria
BT2 Microorganisms
BT1 Microbial contamination
BT2 Contamination
BT2 Microorganisms
RT Microbial spoilage
RT Poisoning

Bacterial counts
BT1 Microbiological techniques
RT Plate counts

Bacterial spoilage
HN spoilage bacterial also used in the index up to vol. 29 (1997)
BT1 Spoilage
RT Spoilage bacteria

Bacterial spores
HN heading from vol. 25 (1993); under Spores up to vol. 24 (1992)
BT1 Microbial spores
BT2 Spores
RT Dipicolinic acid
RT Sporulation

Bactericides
BT1 Biocides
RT Antibiotics
RT Inhibition

Bacteriocins
HN heading from vol. 28 (1996)
BT1 Antibiotics
BT2 Drugs
BT3 Residues
NT1 Acidocins
NT1 Amylovorins
NT1 Bacteriocins resistance
NT1 Bavaricins
NT1 Divercins
NT1 Enterocins
NT1 Epidermin
NT1 Gassericins
NT1 Lactacins
NT1 Lacticins
NT1 Lactocins
NT1 Lactococcins
NT1 Lantibiotics
NT1 Leucocins
NT1 Mesentericins
NT1 Nisin
NT1 Pediocins
NT1 Piscicolins
NT1 Plantaricins
NT1 Propionicins
NT1 Sakacins
NT1 Subtilins

Bacteriocins resistance
HN introduced from vol. 39, issue 1 (2007)
BT1 Bacteriocins
BT2 Antibiotics
BT3 Drugs
BT4 Residues
RT Stress resistance

Bacteriological quality
BT1 Microbiological quality
RT Food safety

Bacteriology
BT1 Microbiology
NT1 Bacteriostats
RT Bacteria
RT Resazurin

Bacteriophages
BT1 Viruses
BT2 Microorganisms
NT1 Bacteriophages resistance
NT1 Coliphages
RT Cloning vectors
UF Phages

Bacteriophages resistance
BT1 Bacteriophages
BT2 Viruses
BT3 Microorganisms

Bacteriostats
BT1 Bacteriology
BT2 Microbiology
RT Inhibition

Bacteroides
BT1 Bacteria
BT2 Microorganisms

Bactofugation
BT1 Centrifugation
BT2 Separation
BT3 Processing
BT4 Technology

Bactris
BT1 Palms
BT2 Plants

Bacuri
BT1 Fruits specific
BT2 Fruits
BT3 Crops
BT4 Plants
BT3 Plant foods
BT4 Foods

Bael fruit
BT1 Fruits specific
BT2 Fruits
BT3 Crops
BT4 Plants
BT3 Plant foods
BT4 Foods
UF Bengal quinces

Bagasse
BT1 Cane sugar
BT2 Sugar
BT3 Plant foods
BT4 Foods
BT1 Wastes
NT1 Sugar cane bagasse

Bagels
BT1 Bakery products
BT2 Cereal products
BT3 Plant foods
BT4 Foods

Bagging
BT1 Bags
BT2 Containers

Bag in box packaging
HN packaging bag in box also used in the index up to vol. 29 (1997)
BT1 Bags
BT2 Containers
BT1 Packaging
BT2 Technology
UF Packaging bag in box

Bags
BT1 Containers
NT1 Bagging
NT1 Bag in box packaging
NT1 Plastics bags
NT1 Polyethylene bags
NT1 Sacks

Baguettes
BT1 Bread
BT2 Bakery products
BT3 Cereal products
BT4 Plant foods
BT5 Foods

Bahamas
BT1 West Indies
BT2 America

Bahrain
BT1 Middle East

Bajra
BT1 Millet
BT2 Cereals
BT3 Crops
BT4 Plants
BT3 Seeds
BT4 Plant foods
BT5 Foods

Baked beans
BT1 Haricot beans
BT2 Common beans
BT3 Legumes
BT4 Vegetables specific
BT5 Vegetables
BT6 Crops
BT7 Plants
BT6 Plant foods
BT7 Foods

Bakeries
BT1 Baking

BT2 Cooking
BT3 Thermal processing
BT4 Processing thermal
BT5 Processing
BT6 Technology

Bakers confectionery
BT1 Bakery products
BT2 Cereal products
BT3 Plant foods
BT4 Foods
RT Cakes

Bakers yeasts
SN index heading is Yeasts bakers
BT1 Yeasts bakers
BT2 *Saccharomyces*
BT3 Yeasts
BT4 Fungi
BT5 Microorganisms
RT Breadmaking

Bakery additives
BT1 Additives
NT1 Ascorbates
NT2 Sodium ascorbate
NT1 Ascorbic acid
NT2 Dehydroascorbic acid
NT2 Vitamin C
NT1 Azodicarbonamide
NT1 Baking powders
NT1 Bromates
NT2 Potassium bromate
NT1 Dough conditioners
NT1 Flour improvers
NT1 Persulfates
NT1 Raising agents
NT1 Sodium bicarbonate
RT Baking

Bakery fillings
BT1 Fillings

Bakery industry
USE **Baking industry**

Bakery product mixes
BT1 Bakery products
BT2 Cereal products
BT3 Plant foods
BT4 Foods
BT1 Mixes
BT2 Dried foods
BT3 Processed foods
BT4 Foods
BT2 Instant foods
BT3 Processed foods
BT4 Foods
RT Cake mixes

Bakery products
BT1 Cereal products
BT2 Plant foods
BT3 Foods
NT1 Arepas
NT1 Bagels
NT1 Bakers confectionery
NT1 Bakery product mixes
NT1 Batters
NT1 Biscuits
NT2 Biscuit dough
NT2 Biscuit factories
NT2 Cookies
NT2 Crackers
NT2 Saltine crackers
NT2 Shortbread
NT1 Bread
NT2 Arabic bread
NT2 Baguettes
NT2 Balady
NT2 Bread crumb
NT2 Breadcrumbs
NT2 Bread crust
NT2 Bread dough
NT2 Breadmaking
NT3 Breadmaking properties
NT4 Loaf vol.
NT3 Wheat breadmaking
NT2 Bread rolls
NT2 Chapattis
NT2 Corn bread
NT2 Crispbreads
NT2 Flat bread
NT2 French bread
NT2 Fruit bread
NT2 Gluten low bread
NT2 Injera
NT2 Kisra
NT2 Nan
NT2 Parottas
NT2 Pita bread
NT2 Poori
NT2 Pumpernickel
NT2 Rice bread
NT2 Rolls
NT2 Roti
NT2 Rye bread
NT2 Sangak
NT2 Soda bread
NT2 Sourdough bread
NT2 Steamed bread
NT2 Tanoor
NT2 Toast
NT2 Toast bread
NT2 Wheat bread
NT1 Brioches
NT1 Brownies
NT1 Buns
NT1 Cakes
NT2 Angel cakes
NT2 Baumkuchen
NT2 Cake batters
NT2 Cake mixes
NT2 Christstollen
NT2 Gateaux
NT2 Muffins
NT2 Sponge cakes
NT2 Stollen
NT2 Swiss rolls
NT2 Torten
NT1 Confectionery
NT2 Confectionery bars
NT3 Chocolate bars
NT2 Confectionery industry
NT2 Confectionery products
NT2 Confections
NT2 Frozen confectionery
NT1 Crepes
NT1 Croissants
NT1 Croutons
NT1 Crumpets
NT1 Crust
NT1 Dough
NT2 Biscuit dough
NT2 Bread dough
NT2 Frozen dough
NT2 Pizza dough
NT2 Sourdough
NT2 Sponge
NT2 Wheat dough
NT1 Doughnuts
NT1 Dumplings
NT1 English muffins
NT1 Flans
NT2 Flan cases
NT2 Torten
NT1 Florentines
NT1 Gingerbread
NT1 Ice cream cones
NT1 Kocho
NT1 Macaroons
NT1 Morning goods
NT1 Muffins
NT1 Pancakes
NT1 Panettone
NT1 Papads
NT1 Parathas
NT1 Pastries
NT2 Cream puffs
NT2 Danish pastries
NT2 Eclairs
NT2 Strudels
NT1 Pastry
NT2 Puff pastry
NT1 Patisserie products
NT1 Pelmeni
NT1 Pies
NT2 Fruit pies
NT2 Meat pies
NT3 Cornish pasties
NT2 Pie fillings
NT2 Quiches
NT2 Tarts
NT1 Pizzas
NT2 Pizza dough
NT2 Pizza fillings
NT1 Pretzels
NT1 Rusks
NT1 Scones
NT1 Tacos
NT1 Taco shells
NT1 Tamales
NT1 Tortillas
NT1 Wafers
NT2 Ice cream wafers
NT1 Waffles
NT1 Yakifu
NT1 Zwieback

Baking
BT1 Cooking
BT2 Thermal processing
BT3 Processing thermal
BT4 Processing
BT5 Technology
NT1 Bakeries
NT1 Baking industry
NT1 Baking properties
NT1 Baking quality

NT1 Proofers
NT1 Proofing
RT Bakery additives
RT Baking ovens
RT Breadmaking

Baking industry
BT1 Baking
BT2 Cooking
BT3 Thermal processing
BT4 Processing thermal
BT5 Processing
BT6 Technology
BT1 Food industry
BT2 Industries
UF Bakery industry

Baking ovens
BT1 Ovens
BT2 Equipment
BT3 Technology
RT Baking

Baking powders
BT1 Bakery additives
BT2 Additives

Baking properties
BT1 Baking
BT2 Cooking
BT3 Thermal processing
BT4 Processing thermal
BT5 Processing
BT6 Technology

Baking quality
BT1 Baking
BT2 Cooking
BT3 Thermal processing
BT4 Processing thermal
BT5 Processing
BT6 Technology

Balady
BT1 Bread
BT2 Bakery products
BT3 Cereal products
BT4 Plant foods
BT5 Foods

Balenine
BT1 Peptides
BT2 Proteins
BT3 Nutrients

Balsamic vinegar
BT1 Vinegar
BT2 Condiments
BT3 Flavourings
BT4 Additives
BT2 Fermented foods
BT3 Processed foods
BT4 Foods

Balsam pears
USE **Bitter gourds**

Bambara beans
USE **Bambara groundnuts**

Bambara groundnuts
BT1 Legumes
BT2 Vegetables specific
BT3 Vegetables
BT4 Crops
BT5 Plants
BT4 Plant foods
BT5 Foods
UF Bambara beans

Bamboo
BT1 Vegetables specific
BT2 Vegetables
BT3 Crops
BT4 Plants
BT3 Plant foods
BT4 Foods
NT1 Bamboo shoots

Bamboo shoots
BT1 Bamboo
BT2 Vegetables specific
BT3 Vegetables
BT4 Crops
BT5 Plants
BT4 Plant foods
BT5 Foods

Banaba
BT1 Plants
NT1 *Lagerstroemia speciosa*

Banana juices
BT1 Fruit juices
BT2 Fruit products
BT3 Plant foods
BT4 Foods
BT2 Soft drinks
BT3 Beverages
RT Bananas

Banana peel
BT1 Bananas
BT2 Fruits specific
BT3 Fruits
BT4 Crops
BT5 Plants
BT4 Plant foods
BT5 Foods
BT1 Peel
RT Fruit peel

Banana pulps
BT1 Bananas
BT2 Fruits specific
BT3 Fruits
BT4 Crops
BT5 Plants
BT4 Plant foods
BT5 Foods
BT1 Fruit pulps
BT2 Fruit products
BT3 Plant foods
BT4 Foods
BT2 Pulps
BT3 Processed foods
BT4 Foods

Banana purees
HN introduced from vol. 41, issue 1 (2009)
BT1 Bananas
BT2 Fruits specific
BT3 Fruits
BT4 Crops
BT5 Plants
BT4 Plant foods
BT5 Foods
BT1 Fruit purees
BT2 Fruit products
BT3 Plant foods
BT4 Foods
BT2 Purees
BT3 Pulps
BT4 Processed foods
BT5 Foods

Bananas
BT1 Fruits specific
BT2 Fruits
BT3 Crops
BT4 Plants
BT3 Plant foods
BT4 Foods
NT1 Banana peel
NT1 Banana pulps
NT1 Banana purees
NT1 *Musa cavendishii*
NT1 Plantains
RT Banana juices

Bangladesh
BT1 Asia

Banvel
USE **Dicamba**

Baobab
BT1 Vegetables specific
BT2 Vegetables
BT3 Crops
BT4 Plants
BT3 Plant foods
BT4 Foods

Baobab oils
BT1 Vegetable oils
BT2 Oils vegetable
BT3 Oils
BT4 Lipids
BT5 Nutrients
BT3 Vegetable products
BT4 Plant foods
BT5 Foods

Barbados
BT1 West Indies
BT2 America

Barbados cherries
BT1 Fruits specific
BT2 Fruits
BT3 Crops
BT4 Plants
BT3 Plant foods
BT4 Foods
RT Barbados cherry juices
UF Acerola

Barbados cherry juices
BT1 Fruit juices
BT2 Fruit products
BT3 Plant foods
BT4 Foods
BT2 Soft drinks
BT3 Beverages
RT Barbados cherries

Barbecued foods
BT1 Processed foods
BT2 Foods

Barberry figs
USE **Prickly pears**

Barbiturates
BT1 Drugs
BT2 Residues
NT1 Phenobarbital

Barbituric acid
BT1 Organic acids
BT2 Acids
BT1 Pyrimidines
BT2 Heterocyclic compounds
BT2 Organic nitrogen compounds

Bar codes
BT1 Labelling
BT2 Packaging
BT3 Technology

Barium
USE **Ba**

Barley
BT1 Cereals
BT2 Crops
BT3 Plants
BT2 Seeds
BT3 Plant foods
BT4 Foods
NT1 Barley fibre
NT1 Barley flour
NT1 Barley starch
NT1 Malting barley
NT1 Pearl barley
RT Hordein
RT Malt
RT Tritordeum

Barley fibre
HN introduced from vol. 41, issue 1 (2009)
BT1 Barley
BT2 Cereals
BT3 Crops
BT4 Plants
BT3 Seeds
BT4 Plant foods
BT5 Foods
BT1 Fibre

Barley flour
BT1 Barley
BT2 Cereals
BT3 Crops
BT4 Plants
BT3 Seeds
BT4 Plant foods
BT5 Foods
BT1 Cereal flours
BT2 Flours cereal
BT3 Cereal products
BT4 Plant foods
BT5 Foods

Barley malt
BT1 Malt
BT2 Cereal products
BT3 Plant foods
BT4 Foods

Barley starch
BT1 Barley
BT2 Cereals
BT3 Crops
BT4 Plants
BT3 Seeds
BT4 Plant foods
BT5 Foods
BT1 Starch
BT2 Glucans
BT3 Polysaccharides
BT4 Carbohydrates
BT5 Nutrients
BT5 Organic compounds
BT2 Thickeners
BT3 Additives

Barracuda
BT1 Marine fish
BT2 Fish
BT3 Animals
BT3 Sea foods
BT4 Aquatic foods
BT5 Animal foods
BT6 Foods

Barramundi
BT1 Marine fish
BT2 Fish
BT3 Animals
BT3 Sea foods
BT4 Aquatic foods
BT5 Animal foods
BT6 Foods

Barrels
BT1 Containers
NT1 Casks
NT1 Kegs

Barrier properties
HN introduced from vol. 39, issue 1 (2007)
BT1 Permeability

Basella
BT1 Indian spinach
BT2 Vegetables specific
BT3 Vegetables
BT4 Crops
BT5 Plants
BT4 Plant foods
BT5 Foods

Basidiomycetes
BT1 Fungi
BT2 Microorganisms

Basil
HN under Spices up to vol. 42 (2010)
BT1 Herbs
BT2 Spices
BT3 Flavourings
BT4 Additives
NT1 Sweet basil

Baskets
BT1 Containers

Basmati rice
BT1 Rice
BT2 Cereals
BT3 Crops
BT4 Plants
BT3 Seeds
BT4 Plant foods
BT5 Foods

Bass
BT1 Fish
BT2 Animals
BT2 Sea foods
BT3 Aquatic foods
BT4 Animal foods
BT5 Foods

Bastard halibut
BT1 Flatfish
BT2 Marine fish
BT3 Fish
BT4 Animals
BT4 Sea foods
BT5 Aquatic foods
BT6 Animal foods
BT7 Foods
NT1 *Paralichthys olivaceus*
RT Japanese flounders

Basting
HN introduced from vol. 39, issue 1 (2007)
BT1 Processing
BT2 Technology

Batters
SN for meat batters see Meat or specific type of meat
BT1 Bakery products
BT2 Cereal products
BT3 Plant foods
BT4 Foods
BT1 Coatings
RT Cake batters

Baumkuchen
BT1 Cakes
BT2 Bakery products
BT3 Cereal products
BT4 Plant foods
BT5 Foods

Bavaricins
BT1 Bacteriocins
BT2 Antibiotics
BT3 Drugs
BT4 Residues
RT *Lactobacillus*

Bavarois
BT1 Desserts
BT2 Processed foods
BT3 Foods

Bavistin
USE **Carbendazim**

Bay
HN under Spices up to vol. 42 (2010)
SN syn. laurel
BT1 Herbs
BT2 Spices
BT3 Flavourings
BT4 Additives
NT1 Bay leaves
NT1 Laurel

Bayberries
HN introduced from vol. 41, issue 1 (2009)
BT1 Berries
BT2 Fruits specific
BT3 Fruits
BT4 Crops
BT5 Plants
BT4 Plant foods
BT5 Foods

Bay leaves
HN under Spices up to vol. 42 (2010)
BT1 Bay
BT2 Herbs
BT3 Spices
BT4 Flavourings
BT5 Additives

Bayrusil
USE **Quinalphos**

Baytex
USE **Fenthion**

Bdellovibrio
BT1 Bacteria
BT2 Microorganisms

Be
HN under Minerals up to vol. 42 (2010)
BT1 Metals
BT2 Elements
BT3 Minerals
BT4 Nutrients
UF Beryllium

Beach peas
BT1 Legumes
BT2 Vegetables specific
BT3 Vegetables
BT4 Crops
BT5 Plants
BT4 Plant foods
BT5 Foods
NT1 *Lathyrus maritimus*

Beakers
BT1 Containers

Bean curd
BT1 Beans
BT2 Legumes
BT3 Vegetables specific
BT4 Vegetables
BT5 Crops
BT6 Plants
BT5 Plant foods
BT6 Foods

Bean jams
BT1 Vegetable products
BT2 Plant foods
BT3 Foods
NT1 Ann

Bean pastes
BT1 Beans
BT2 Legumes
BT3 Vegetables specific
BT4 Vegetables
BT5 Crops
BT6 Plants
BT5 Plant foods
BT6 Foods
BT1 Pastes
BT2 Processed foods
BT3 Foods

Beans
BT1 Legumes
BT2 Vegetables specific
BT3 Vegetables
BT4 Crops
BT5 Plants
BT4 Plant foods
BT5 Foods
NT1 Bean curd
NT1 Bean pastes

Bean sprouts
BT1 Legume sprouts
BT2 Legumes
BT3 Vegetables specific
BT4 Vegetables
BT5 Crops
BT6 Plants
BT5 Plant foods
BT6 Foods
BT2 Sprouts
BT3 Vegetables specific
BT4 Vegetables
BT5 Crops
BT6 Plants
BT5 Plant foods
BT6 Foods

Bearberries
HN introduced from vol. 37, issue 5 (2005)
BT1 Berries
BT2 Fruits specific
BT3 Fruits
BT4 Crops
BT5 Plants
BT4 Plant foods
BT5 Foods

Bear meat
BT1 Bears
BT2 Animals
BT1 Meat specific
BT2 Meat
BT3 Animal foods
BT4 Foods

Bears
BT1 Animals
NT1 Bear meat

Beating
BT1 Whipping
BT2 Processing
BT3 Technology

Beauty foods
HN introduced from vol. 41, issue 1 (2009)
BT1 Health foods
BT2 Processed foods
BT3 Foods
BT1 Novel foods
BT2 Foods

Beauveria
HN introduced from vol. 43, issue 1 (2011)
BT1 Fungi
BT2 Microorganisms
NT1 *Beauveria bassiana*

Beauveria bassiana
BT1 *Beauveria*
BT2 Fungi
BT3 Microorganisms

Beauvericin
BT1 Mycotoxins
BT2 Toxins
BT3 Residues

Beche de mer
USE **Sea cucumbers**

Beech nut oils
BT1 Nut oils
BT2 Vegetable oils
BT3 Oils vegetable
BT4 Oils
BT5 Lipids
BT6 Nutrients
BT4 Vegetable products
BT5 Plant foods
BT6 Foods

Beef
BT1 Meat specific
BT2 Meat
BT3 Animal foods
BT4 Foods
NT1 Beefburgers
NT1 Beef extracts
NT1 Beef loaf
NT1 Beef mince
NT1 Beef products
NT2 Beef patties
NT1 Beef roasts
NT1 Beef steaks
NT1 Calf carcasses
NT1 Cattle carcasses
NT1 Corned beef
NT1 Oxtail
RT Cattle
RT Pastrami

RT Veal
UF Beef muscles
UF Bovine muscles
UF Bull muscles
UF Calf meat
UF Calf muscles
UF Cattle muscles
UF Cattle tissues

Beefburgers
BT1 Beef
 BT2 Meat specific
  BT3 Meat
   BT4 Animal foods
    BT5 Foods
BT1 Burgers
 BT2 Meat products
  BT3 Animal foods
   BT4 Foods

Beef extracts
BT1 Beef
 BT2 Meat specific
  BT3 Meat
   BT4 Animal foods
    BT5 Foods
BT1 Extracts
 BT2 Flavourings
  BT3 Additives

Beef loaf
BT1 Beef
 BT2 Meat specific
  BT3 Meat
   BT4 Animal foods
    BT5 Foods
BT1 Meat products
 BT2 Animal foods
  BT3 Foods

Beef mince
BT1 Beef
 BT2 Meat specific
  BT3 Meat
   BT4 Animal foods
    BT5 Foods
UF Ground beef
UF Minced beef

Beef muscles
USE **Beef**

Beef patties
BT1 Beef products
 BT2 Beef
  BT3 Meat specific
   BT4 Meat
    BT5 Animal foods
     BT6 Foods
BT1 Meat patties
 BT2 Patties
  BT3 Meat products
   BT4 Animal foods
    BT5 Foods

Beef products
BT1 Beef
 BT2 Meat specific
  BT3 Meat
   BT4 Animal foods
    BT5 Foods
NT1 Beef patties

Beef roasts
BT1 Beef
 BT2 Meat specific
  BT3 Meat
   BT4 Animal foods
    BT5 Foods

Beef sausages
BT1 Sausages
 BT2 Meat products
  BT3 Animal foods
   BT4 Foods

Beef steaks
BT1 Beef
 BT2 Meat specific
  BT3 Meat
   BT4 Animal foods
    BT5 Foods
RT Steaks

Beer
BT1 Alcoholic beverages
 BT2 Beverages alcoholic
  BT3 Beverages
NT1 Alcohol low beer
NT1 Ale
NT1 Bouza
NT1 Draught beer
NT1 Happoshu
NT1 Lager
NT1 Lambic
NT1 Malt beverages
NT1 Merissa
NT1 Pito
NT1 Pombe
NT1 Shandy
NT1 Sorghum beer
NT1 Stout
NT1 Wheat beer
RT Brewers yeasts
RT Brewing
RT Hops
RT Malt
RT Worts
RT Yeasts brewers

Beermaking
USE **Brewing**

Beer manufacture
USE **Brewing**

Bees
BT1 Insects
 BT2 Pests
RT Apiculture

Beeswax
BT1 Waxes
 BT2 Fatty acid esters
  BT3 Esters
   BT4 Organic compounds

Beetles
BT1 Insects
 BT2 Pests
NT1 *Ahasverus advena*

Beet molasses
BT1 Molasses
 BT2 Sugar
  BT3 Plant foods
   BT4 Foods
RT Beet sugar
RT Sugar processes
UF Beet sugar molasses
UF Sugar beet molasses

Beetroot juices
BT1 Beetroots
 BT2 Beets
  BT3 Vegetables specific
   BT4 Vegetables
    BT5 Crops
     BT6 Plants
    BT5 Plant foods
     BT6 Foods
BT1 Colorants
 BT2 Additives

Beetroots
BT1 Beets
 BT2 Vegetables specific
  BT3 Vegetables
   BT4 Crops
    BT5 Plants
   BT4 Plant foods
    BT5 Foods
NT1 Beetroot juices

Beets
BT1 Vegetables specific
 BT2 Vegetables
  BT3 Crops
   BT4 Plants
  BT3 Plant foods
   BT4 Foods
NT1 Beetroots
 NT2 Beetroot juices
NT1 Red beets

Beet sugar
BT1 Sugar
 BT2 Plant foods
  BT3 Foods
NT1 Beet sugar factories
NT1 Beet sugar industry
NT1 Beet sugar products
RT Beet molasses
RT Sugar beets
RT Sugar processes

Beet sugar factories
BT1 Beet sugar
 BT2 Sugar
  BT3 Plant foods
   BT4 Foods
BT1 Food factories

Beet sugar industry
BT1 Beet sugar
 BT2 Sugar
  BT3 Plant foods
   BT4 Foods
BT1 Food industry
 BT2 Industries

Beet sugar juices
BT1 Sugar juices
BT2 Plant foods
BT3 Foods
RT Sugar processes
UF Sugar beet juices

Beet sugar molasses
USE **Beet molasses**

Beet sugar products
BT1 Beet sugar
BT2 Sugar
BT3 Plant foods
BT4 Foods

Beet sugar syrups
BT1 Sugar syrups
BT2 Plant foods
BT3 Foods

Behavioural effects
BT1 Human physiology
BT2 Physiology
BT3 Science
NT1 Cognitive performance
NT2 Cognitive development
NT2 Memory
NT1 Cravings
NT1 Mood
RT Diet
RT Psychophysiological effects

Behenic acid
BT1 Saturated fatty acids
BT2 Fatty acids
BT3 Lipids
BT4 Nutrients
BT3 Organic acids
BT4 Acids

Beijerinckia
HN introduced from vol. 41, issue 1 (2009)
BT1 Bacteria
BT2 Microorganisms

Belarus
BT1 Europe
UF Byelorussia

Belgium
HN heading up to vol. 24 (1992)
BT1 Europe
BT1 European Union
RT Organization for Economic Cooperation and Development

Belize
BT1 Central America
BT2 America
UF British Honduras

Bell peppers
BT1 Capsicums
BT2 Vegetables specific
BT3 Vegetables
BT4 Crops
BT5 Plants
BT4 Plant foods
BT5 Foods

Belly fat
HN introduced from vol. 39, issue 1 (2007)
BT1 Animal fats
BT2 Fats animal
BT3 Animal foods
BT4 Foods
BT3 Fats
BT4 Lipids
BT5 Nutrients

Belona
BT1 Cereal products
BT2 Plant foods
BT3 Foods

Beluga
BT1 Sturgeon
BT2 Fish
BT3 Animals
BT3 Sea foods
BT4 Aquatic foods
BT5 Animal foods
BT6 Foods

Beluga whales
BT1 Animals

Bengal gram
BT1 Chick peas
BT2 Legumes
BT3 Vegetables specific
BT4 Vegetables
BT5 Crops
BT6 Plants
BT5 Plant foods
BT6 Foods
NT1 Boondi

Bengal quinces
USE **Bael fruit**

Benin
BT1 West Africa
BT2 Africa
UF Dahomey

Benincasa hispida
BT1 Gourds
BT2 Vegetables specific
BT3 Vegetables
BT4 Crops
BT5 Plants
BT4 Plant foods
BT5 Foods

Benlate
USE **Benomyl**

Benomyl
BT1 Benzimidazole
BT2 Fungicides
BT3 Pesticides
BT4 Biocides
BT4 Residues
BT1 Carbamate pesticides
BT2 Pesticides
BT3 Biocides
BT3 Residues
UF Benlate

Bentazone
BT1 Herbicides
BT2 Pesticides
BT3 Biocides
BT3 Residues

Bentonite
HN heading up to vol. 24 (1992)
BT1 Filter aids
BT2 Filtration
BT3 Processing
BT4 Technology

Benzaldehyde
HN also under Flavour compounds up to vol. 42 (2010)
BT1 Aldehydes
BT2 Carbonyl compounds
BT3 Organic compounds
BT1 Aroma compounds
BT2 Flavour compounds
BT2 Volatile compounds
BT1 Aromatic compounds
BT2 Organic compounds

Benzene
BT1 Aromatic compounds
BT2 Organic compounds
BT1 Solvents
RT Carcinogens

Benzidine
BT1 Amines
BT2 Organic nitrogen compounds
BT1 Aromatic compounds
BT2 Organic compounds

Benzimidazole
BT1 Fungicides
BT2 Pesticides
BT3 Biocides
BT3 Residues
NT1 Benomyl
NT1 Carbendazim
NT1 Thiabendazole
NT1 Thiophanate
NT1 Thiophanate-methyl
UF Benzimidazole fungicides

Benzimidazole fungicides
USE **Benzimidazole**

Benzoates
SN for benzoic acid salts; see also specific esters
BT1 Preservatives
BT2 Additives
BT1 Salts
NT1 Sodium benzoate
RT Benzoic acid

Benzoic acid
BT1 Organic acids
BT2 Acids
BT1 Preservatives
BT2 Additives
RT Benzoates

Benzophenone
HN introduced from vol. 39, issue 1 (2007)
BT1 Aromatic compounds
BT2 Organic compounds
BT1 Contaminants
BT2 Contamination
BT1 Ketones
BT2 Carbonyl compounds
BT3 Organic compounds
RT Aroma compounds

Benzopyrene
HN heading up to vol. 24 (1992)
BT1 Carcinogens
BT2 Mutagens

Benzothiazole
HN also under Flavour compounds up to vol. 42 (2010)
BT1 Aroma compounds
BT2 Flavour compounds
BT2 Volatile compounds
BT1 Organic nitrogen compounds
BT1 Organic sulfur compounds

Benzoyl compounds
BT1 Aromatic compounds
BT2 Organic compounds

Benzoylprop-ethyl
BT1 Herbicides
BT2 Pesticides
BT3 Biocides
BT3 Residues
UF Suffix

Benzyladenine
SN syn. 6-benzylaminopurine
BT1 Cytokinins
BT2 Plant growth regulators
BT3 Cultivation
BT4 Agriculture
NT1 6-Benzylaminopurine

Benzyl alcohol
HN also under Flavour compounds up to vol. 42 (2010)
BT1 Alcohols
BT1 Aroma compounds
BT2 Flavour compounds
BT2 Volatile compounds
BT1 Aromatic compounds
BT2 Organic compounds

6-Benzylaminopurine
SN syn. benzyladenine
BT1 Benzyladenine
BT2 Cytokinins
BT3 Plant growth regulators
BT4 Cultivation
BT5 Agriculture

Benzyl isothiocyanate
BT1 Aroma compounds
BT2 Flavour compounds
BT2 Volatile compounds
BT1 Isothiocyanates
BT2 Organic nitrogen compounds
BT2 Organic sulfur compounds
BT2 Volatile sulfur compounds
BT3 Volatile compounds

Benzylpenicillin
SN syn. penicillin G
BT1 Penicillins
BT2 β-Lactam antibiotics
BT3 Antibiotics
BT4 Drugs
BT5 Residues

Berberries
BT1 Berries
BT2 Fruits specific
BT3 Fruits
BT4 Crops
BT5 Plants
BT4 Plant foods
BT5 Foods

Ber fruits
USE **Jujubes**

Bergamot essential oils
BT1 Citrus essential oils
BT2 Essential oils
BT3 Flavourings
BT4 Additives
BT3 Vegetable oils
BT4 Oils vegetable
BT5 Oils
BT6 Lipids
BT7 Nutrients
BT5 Vegetable products
BT6 Plant foods
BT7 Foods
NT1 Bergamot oils
RT Citrus fruits

Bergamot oils
BT1 Bergamot essential oils
BT2 Citrus essential oils
BT3 Essential oils
BT4 Flavourings
BT5 Additives
BT4 Vegetable oils
BT5 Oils vegetable
BT6 Oils
BT7 Lipids
BT8 Nutrients
BT6 Vegetable products
BT7 Plant foods
BT8 Foods
RT Citrus fruits

Bergapten
BT1 Furocoumarins
BT2 Coumarins
BT3 Lactones
BT4 Esters
BT5 Organic compounds
BT4 Heterocyclic compounds
BT3 Phenols
BT4 Alcohols
BT4 Aromatic compounds
BT5 Organic compounds

Bergkaese cheese
BT1 Cheese varieties
BT2 Cheese
BT3 Dairy products
BT4 Animal foods
BT5 Foods

Bermuda
BT1 North America
BT2 America

Berries
BT1 Fruits specific
BT2 Fruits
BT3 Crops
BT4 Plants
BT3 Plant foods
BT4 Foods
NT1 Bayberries
NT1 Bearberries
NT1 Berberries
NT1 Bilberries
NT1 Blackberries
NT1 Blackcurrants
NT1 Black nightshade
NT1 Blueberries
NT1 Boysenberries
NT1 Chokeberries
NT1 Cloudberries
NT1 Cranberries
NT1 Crowberries
NT1 Dewberries
NT1 Elderberries
NT1 Gooseberries
NT1 Grapes
NT2 Grape jams
NT2 Grape pomaces
NT2 Grape seeds
NT2 Grape skins
NT2 Muscadine grapes
NT2 Seedless grapes
NT2 Table grapes
NT2 *Vitis vinifera*
NT2 Winemaking grapes
NT1 Huckleberries
NT1 Lingonberries
NT2 Cowberries
NT1 Loganberries
NT1 Mulberries
NT1 Raspberries
NT1 Redcurrants
NT1 Rowanberries
NT1 Strawberries
NT2 Strawberry jams
NT2 Strawberry pulps
NT2 Strawberry purees
NT1 Strawberry tree fruits
NT1 Whitecurrants
NT1 Wolfberries
NT1 Youngberries
RT Berry juices

Berry juices
BT1 Fruit juices
BT2 Fruit products
BT3 Plant foods
BT4 Foods
BT2 Soft drinks
BT3 Beverages
NT1 Bilberry juices
NT1 Blackberry juices
NT1 Blackcurrant juices
NT1 Blueberry juices
NT1 Cranberry juices

NT1 Elderberry juices
NT1 Raspberry juices
NT1 Redcurrant juices
NT1 Strawberry juices
RT Berries

Beryllium
USE **Be**

Betacoccus
SN obsolete name for Leuconostoc
USE ***Leuconostoc***

Betacyanins
BT1 Betalains
BT2 Organic nitrogen compounds
BT2 Pigments
NT1 Betanin
NT1 Betanine

Betaine
BT1 Ammonium compounds
BT1 Organic nitrogen compounds

Betalaines
BT1 Betalains
BT2 Organic nitrogen compounds
BT2 Pigments

Betalains
BT1 Organic nitrogen compounds
BT1 Pigments
NT1 Betacyanins
NT2 Betanin
NT2 Betanine
NT1 Betalaines
NT1 Betaxanthin

Betanal
USE **Phenmedipham**

Betanin
BT1 Betacyanins
BT2 Betalains
BT3 Organic nitrogen compounds
BT3 Pigments

Betanine
BT1 Betacyanins
BT2 Betalains
BT3 Organic nitrogen compounds
BT3 Pigments

Betaxanthin
BT1 Betalains
BT2 Organic nitrogen compounds
BT2 Pigments

Betel leaves
BT1 Plants
RT Betel nuts

Betel nuts
BT1 Seeds
BT2 Plant foods
BT3 Foods
RT *Areca*
RT Betel leaves
UF Areca nuts

Beverage concentrates
BT1 Beverages
BT1 Concentrates
BT2 Processed foods
BT3 Foods

Beverage mixes
BT1 Beverages
BT1 Mixes
BT2 Dried foods
BT3 Processed foods
BT4 Foods
BT2 Instant foods
BT3 Processed foods
BT4 Foods

Beverage powders
BT1 Beverages
BT1 Powders
BT2 Dried foods
BT3 Processed foods
BT4 Foods
BT2 Instant foods
BT3 Processed foods
BT4 Foods

Beverages
NT1 Beverage concentrates
NT1 Beverage mixes
NT1 Beverage powders
NT1 Beverages alcoholic
NT2 Alcoholic beverages
NT3 Alcoholic soft drinks
NT3 Aperitifs
NT3 Beer
NT4 Alcohol low beer
NT4 Ale
NT4 Bouza
NT4 Draught beer
NT4 Happoshu
NT4 Lager
NT4 Lambic
NT4 Malt beverages
NT4 Merissa
NT4 Pito
NT4 Pombe
NT4 Shandy
NT4 Sorghum beer
NT4 Stout
NT4 Wheat beer
NT3 Boza
NT3 Cereal wines
NT4 Rice wines
NT5 Sake
NT6 Ginjoshu
NT6 Narazuke
NT5 Takju
NT5 Yakju
NT3 Cider
NT3 Cocktails
NT3 Egg nog
NT3 Fruit wines
NT4 Apple wines
NT4 Apricot wines
NT4 Orange wines
NT3 Kvass
NT3 Liqueurs
NT4 Anisette
NT4 Cordials
NT4 Cream liqueurs
NT4 Fruit liqueurs
NT5 Cassis
NT5 Cherry brandy
NT5 Limoncello
NT4 Pernod
NT3 Mead
NT3 Melomel
NT3 Perry
NT3 Pulque
NT3 Spirits
NT4 Absinthe
NT4 Aquavit
NT4 Arak
NT4 Awamori
NT4 Brandies
NT5 Armagnac
NT5 Brandy
NT5 Cognac
NT5 Eau de vie
NT5 Fruit brandies
NT6 Apple brandy
NT7 Calvados
NT6 Kirsch
NT6 Rakia
NT6 Slivovitz
NT5 Grappa
NT5 Pisco
NT4 Distillates
NT5 Wine distillates
NT4 Gin
NT4 Grape spirits
NT4 Lambanog
NT4 Mezcal
NT4 Ouzo
NT4 Raki
NT4 Rum
NT4 Schnapps
NT4 Shochu
NT4 Sugar cane spirits
NT5 Cachaca
NT4 Tequila
NT4 Vodka
NT4 Whiskies
NT5 Whiskey
NT6 Bourbon whiskey
NT5 Whisky
NT6 Scotch whisky
NT3 Wines
NT4 Alcohol low wines
NT4 Aromatized wines
NT5 Retsina
NT5 Sangria
NT5 Vermouths
NT5 Wine coolers
NT4 Dessert wines
NT4 Fortified wines
NT5 Madeira
NT5 Marsala
NT5 Port
NT5 Sherry
NT4 Ice wines
NT5 Eiswein
NT4 Red wines
NT4 Rose wines
NT4 White wines

NT4 Wines sparkling
NT5 Sparkling wines
NT6 Cavas
NT6 Champagne
NT6 Sekts
NT3 Wines palm
NT4 Palm wines
NT5 Coconut toddy
NT5 Toddy
NT5 Tuba
NT1 Beverages alcohol low
NT2 Alcohol low beverages
NT3 Alcohol free beverages
NT3 Alcohol low beer
NT3 Alcohol low wines
NT1 Beverages factories
NT1 Beverages industry
NT1 Calories low beverages
NT1 Chicory (beverages)
NT1 Chilled beverages
NT1 Chocolate beverages
NT2 Drinking chocolate
NT1 Cocoa
NT2 Cocoa beans
NT3 Cocoa nibs
NT2 Cocoa industry
NT1 Cocoa beverages
NT1 Coconut water
NT1 Coffee
NT2 Coffee bags
NT2 Coffee beans
NT2 Coffee grounds
NT2 Coffee industry
NT2 Coffee products
NT3 Coffee beverages
NT4 Cappuccino coffee
NT4 Espresso coffee
NT4 Iced coffee
NT3 Coffee extracts
NT3 Coffee powders
NT3 Instant coffee
NT4 Coffee granules
NT2 Decaffeinated coffee
NT2 Green coffee
NT2 Ground coffee
NT2 Roasted coffee
NT2 Roasting coffee
NT1 Dairy beverages
NT2 Lactic beverages
NT2 Milk beverages
NT2 Milkshakes
NT2 Whey beverages
NT2 Yoghurt beverages
NT3 Drinking yoghurt
NT1 Fermented beverages
NT1 Flavoured beverages
NT1 Frozen beverages
NT2 Soft frozen beverages
NT1 Functional beverages
NT1 Health beverages
NT2 Energy drinks
NT2 Ginseng beverages
NT2 Isotonic drinks
NT2 Sports drinks
NT1 Herbal beverages
NT1 Honey beverages
NT1 Horchata
NT1 Hot beverages
NT1 Instant beverages
NT2 Instant cocoa
NT2 Instant coffee
NT3 Coffee granules
NT2 Instant tea
NT1 Kava
NT1 Kunun zaki
NT1 Lite beverages
NT1 Mahewu
NT1 Organic beverages
NT1 Rice milk
NT1 Sikhe
NT1 Soft drinks
NT2 Carbonated beverages
NT2 Coca-cola
NT2 Cola beverages
NT2 Energy drinks
NT2 Fruit cordials
NT2 Fruit juice beverages
NT3 Citrus beverages
NT3 Fruit beverages
NT3 Orange juice beverages
NT2 Fruit juices
NT3 Apple juices
NT4 Apple cider
NT4 Apple juice concentrates
NT3 Apricot juices
NT3 Banana juices
NT3 Barbados cherry juices
NT3 Berry juices
NT4 Bilberry juices
NT4 Blackberry juices
NT4 Blackcurrant juices
NT4 Blueberry juices
NT4 Cranberry juices
NT4 Elderberry juices
NT4 Raspberry juices
NT4 Redcurrant juices
NT4 Strawberry juices
NT3 Cashew apple juices
NT3 Cherry juices
NT3 Citrus juices
NT4 Citrus juice concentrates
NT5 Orange juice concentrates
NT4 Grapefruit juices
NT4 Lemon juices
NT4 Lime juices
NT4 Orange juices
NT5 Mandarin juices
NT6 Tangerine juices
NT5 Orange juice concentrates
NT3 Fig juices
NT3 Fruit juice concentrates
NT4 Apple juice concentrates
NT4 Citrus juice concentrates
NT5 Orange juice concentrates
NT4 Grape juice concentrates
NT3 Fruit nectars
NT4 Apricot nectars
NT4 Mango nectars
NT4 Papaya nectars
NT4 Peach nectars
NT4 Pineapple nectars
NT3 Grape juices
NT4 Grape juice concentrates
NT3 Guava juices
NT3 Hawthorn juices
NT3 Kiwifruit juices
NT3 Mango juices
NT3 Melon juices
NT3 Musts
NT4 Apple musts
NT4 Grape musts
NT5 Concentrated rectified musts
NT3 Noni juices
NT3 Passion fruit juices
NT3 Peach juices
NT3 Pear juices
NT3 Persimmon juices
NT3 Pineapple juices
NT3 Plum juices
NT3 Pomegranate juices
NT3 Prune juices
NT3 Quince juices
NT3 Sea buckthorn juices
NT3 Tomato juices
NT3 Watermelon juices
NT2 Ginger ale
NT2 Ginger beer
NT2 Guarana
NT3 *Paullinia cupana*
NT2 Isotonic drinks
NT2 Lemonade
NT2 Mineral waters
NT3 Bottled mineral waters
NT3 Soda water
NT3 Spring waters
NT2 Orange beverages
NT2 Performance drinks
NT2 Smoothies
NT2 Sports drinks
NT2 Squash
NT2 Tonic waters
NT2 Vegetable juice beverages
NT2 Vegetable juices
NT3 Cabbage juices
NT3 Carrot juices
NT3 Vegetable juice concentrates
NT3 Vegetable nectars
NT1 Soy beverages
NT2 Soymilk
NT1 Teas
NT2 Fruit tea
NT2 Herb tea
NT3 Honeybush tea
NT3 Mate
NT4 Yerba mate
NT5 *Ilex paraguariensis*
NT3 Rooibos tea
NT3 Tochu tea
NT2 Instant tea
NT2 Tea
NT3 Black tea
NT3 Brick tea
NT3 Decaffeinated tea
NT3 Green tea
NT3 Oolong tea
NT3 Pouchong tea
NT3 Pu-erh tea
NT3 Tea extracts
NT3 Tea leaves
NT2 Tea bags
NT2 Tea beverages
NT3 Chai

NT3 Iced tea
NT3 Kombucha
NT3 Lemon tea
NT2 Tea granules
NT2 Tea powders
RT Chocolate
RT Clouding agents
RT Drinking habits
RT Drinking straws
RT Drinking water
UF Drinks

Beverages alcoholic
SN alcoholic beverages is also used in the index
BT1 Beverages
NT1 Alcoholic beverages
NT2 Alcoholic soft drinks
NT2 Aperitifs
NT2 Beer
NT3 Alcohol low beer
NT3 Ale
NT3 Bouza
NT3 Draught beer
NT3 Happoshu
NT3 Lager
NT3 Lambic
NT3 Malt beverages
NT3 Merissa
NT3 Pito
NT3 Pombe
NT3 Shandy
NT3 Sorghum beer
NT3 Stout
NT3 Wheat beer
NT2 Boza
NT2 Cereal wines
NT3 Rice wines
NT4 Sake
NT5 Ginjoshu
NT5 Narazuke
NT4 Takju
NT4 Yakju
NT2 Cider
NT2 Cocktails
NT2 Egg nog
NT2 Fruit wines
NT3 Apple wines
NT3 Apricot wines
NT3 Orange wines
NT2 Kvass
NT2 Liqueurs
NT3 Anisette
NT3 Cordials
NT3 Cream liqueurs
NT3 Fruit liqueurs
NT4 Cassis
NT4 Cherry brandy
NT4 Limoncello
NT3 Pernod
NT2 Mead
NT2 Melomel
NT2 Perry
NT2 Pulque
NT2 Spirits
NT3 Absinthe
NT3 Aquavit
NT3 Arak
NT3 Awamori
NT3 Brandies
NT4 Armagnac
NT4 Brandy
NT4 Cognac
NT4 Eau de vie
NT4 Fruit brandies
NT5 Apple brandy
NT6 Calvados
NT5 Kirsch
NT5 Rakia
NT5 Slivovitz
NT4 Grappa
NT4 Pisco
NT3 Distillates
NT4 Wine distillates
NT3 Gin
NT3 Grape spirits
NT3 Lambanog
NT3 Mezcal
NT3 Ouzo
NT3 Raki
NT3 Rum
NT3 Schnapps
NT3 Shochu
NT3 Sugar cane spirits
NT4 Cachaca
NT3 Tequila
NT3 Vodka
NT3 Whiskies
NT4 Whiskey
NT5 Bourbon whiskey
NT4 Whisky
NT5 Scotch whisky
NT2 Wines
NT3 Alcohol low wines
NT3 Aromatized wines
NT4 Retsina
NT4 Sangria
NT4 Vermouths
NT4 Wine coolers
NT3 Dessert wines
NT3 Fortified wines
NT4 Madeira
NT4 Marsala
NT4 Port
NT4 Sherry
NT3 Ice wines
NT4 Eiswein
NT3 Red wines
NT3 Rose wines
NT3 White wines
NT3 Wines sparkling
NT4 Sparkling wines
NT5 Cavas
NT5 Champagne
NT5 Sekts
NT2 Wines palm
NT3 Palm wines
NT4 Coconut toddy
NT4 Toddy
NT4 Tuba

Beverages alcohol low
HN heading from vol. 25 (1993)
SN alcohol low beverages is also used in the index
BT1 Beverages
NT1 Alcohol low beverages
NT2 Alcohol free beverages
NT2 Alcohol low beer
NT2 Alcohol low wines
RT Lite beverages

Beverages factories
BT1 Beverages
BT1 Food factories

Beverages industry
BT1 Beverages
BT1 Food industry
BT2 Industries

Beyaz cheese
BT1 Cheese varieties
BT2 Cheese
BT3 Dairy products
BT4 Animal foods
BT5 Foods

BHA
BT1 Antioxidants
BT2 Additives
UF Butylated hydroxyanisole

BHC
HN heading up to vol. 24 (1992)
USE **HCH**

BHT
BT1 Antioxidants
BT2 Additives
UF Butylated hydroxytoluene
UF Ionol

Bhutan
BT1 Asia

Bi
HN under Minerals up to vol. 42 (2010)
BT1 Metals
BT2 Elements
BT3 Minerals
BT4 Nutrients
UF Bismuth

Bibliographies
BT1 Books

Bicarbonates
BT1 Salts
NT1 Sodium bicarbonate

Bierschinken
BT1 Sausages
BT2 Meat products
BT3 Animal foods
BT4 Foods

Bierwurst
BT1 Sausages
BT2 Meat products
BT3 Animal foods
BT4 Foods

Bifenox
BT1 Herbicides
BT2 Pesticides
BT3 Biocides
BT3 Residues

Bifidobacterium
HN heading from vol. 25 (1993); under Lactobacillus up to vol. 24 (1992)
BT1 Bacteria
BT2 Microorganisms
NT1 *Bifidobacterium adolescentis*
NT1 *Bifidobacterium animalis*
NT1 *Bifidobacterium bifidum*
NT1 *Bifidobacterium breve*
NT1 *Bifidobacterium infantis*
NT1 *Bifidobacterium lactis*
NT1 *Bifidobacterium longum*
NT1 *Bifidobacterium pseudolongum*
NT1 *Bifidobacterium thermophilum*
RT Bifidus milk
RT Lactic acid bacteria
RT Probiotic bacteria

Bifidobacterium adolescentis
BT1 *Bifidobacterium*
BT2 Bacteria
BT3 Microorganisms

Bifidobacterium animalis
BT1 *Bifidobacterium*
BT2 Bacteria
BT3 Microorganisms

Bifidobacterium bifidum
BT1 *Bifidobacterium*
BT2 Bacteria
BT3 Microorganisms

Bifidobacterium breve
BT1 *Bifidobacterium*
BT2 Bacteria
BT3 Microorganisms

Bifidobacterium infantis
BT1 *Bifidobacterium*
BT2 Bacteria
BT3 Microorganisms

Bifidobacterium lactis
BT1 *Bifidobacterium*
BT2 Bacteria
BT3 Microorganisms

Bifidobacterium longum
BT1 *Bifidobacterium*
BT2 Bacteria
BT3 Microorganisms

Bifidobacterium pseudolongum
BT1 *Bifidobacterium*
BT2 Bacteria
BT3 Microorganisms

Bifidobacterium thermophilum
BT1 *Bifidobacterium*
BT2 Bacteria
BT3 Microorganisms

Bifidus factors
BT1 Carbohydrates
BT2 Nutrients
BT2 Organic compounds
BT1 Glycoproteins
BT2 Proteins
BT3 Nutrients

Bifidus milk
BT1 Fermented milk
BT2 Fermented dairy products
BT3 Dairy products
BT4 Animal foods
BT5 Foods
BT3 Fermented foods
BT4 Processed foods
BT5 Foods
BT2 Milk
BT3 Dairy products
BT4 Animal foods
BT5 Foods
RT *Bifidobacterium*

Bigeye snapper
BT1 Marine fish
BT2 Fish
BT3 Animals
BT3 Sea foods
BT4 Aquatic foods
BT5 Animal foods
BT6 Foods
NT1 *Priacanthus macracanthus*

Bigeye tuna
BT1 Tuna
BT2 Marine fish
BT3 Fish
BT4 Animals
BT4 Sea foods
BT5 Aquatic foods
BT6 Animal foods
BT7 Foods
BT2 Oily fish
BT3 Fish
BT4 Animals
BT4 Sea foods
BT5 Aquatic foods
BT6 Animal foods
BT7 Foods

Bighead carp
BT1 Carp
BT2 Freshwater fish
BT3 Fish
BT4 Animals
BT4 Sea foods
BT5 Aquatic foods
BT6 Animal foods
BT7 Foods
BT2 Oily fish
BT3 Fish
BT4 Animals
BT4 Sea foods
BT5 Aquatic foods
BT6 Animal foods
BT7 Foods
NT1 *Aristichthys nobilis*

Bilberries
BT1 Berries
BT2 Fruits specific
BT3 Fruits
BT4 Crops
BT5 Plants
BT4 Plant foods
BT5 Foods
RT Bilberry juices

Bilberry juices
BT1 Berry juices
BT2 Fruit juices
BT3 Fruit products
BT4 Plant foods
BT5 Foods
BT3 Soft drinks
BT4 Beverages
RT Bilberries

Bile acids
BT1 Acids
RT Bile salts

Bile salt hydrolases
USE **Choloylglycine hydrolases**

Bile salts
RT Bile acids

Biltong
BT1 Meat products
BT2 Animal foods
BT3 Foods

Binders
BT1 Additives

Binding
HN heading up to vol. 24 (1992); binding capacity under Functional properties from vol. 25 (1993)
RT Integrins

Binding agents
BT1 Additives

Binding capacity
BT1 Functional properties
BT2 Physical properties

Bins
BT1 Containers
NT1 Hoppers
RT Silos

Bioaccumulation
HN introduced from vol. 39, issue 1 (2007)
BT1 Metabolism
BT2 Physiology
BT3 Science
RT Residues

Bioactive compounds
NT1 Bioactive peptides

Bioactive peptides
BT1 Bioactive compounds
BT1 Peptides
BT2 Proteins
BT3 Nutrients

Bioassay
BT1 Analytical techniques
RT Biosensors

Bioavailability
HN heading from vol. 30 (1998); under Nutritional values up to vol. 29 (1997)
BT1 Nutritional values
NT1 Availability

Biocatalysts
HN heading for vol. 23 (1991) only
BT1 Biotechnology
BT2 Technology

Biochemical oxygen demand
USE **Biological oxygen demand**

Biochemistry
HN heading from vol. 25 (1993); under Chemistry up to vol. 24 (1992)
BT1 Science
RT Biology
RT Chemistry

Biocides
HN heading up to vol. 24 (1992)
NT1 Bactericides
NT1 Fumigants
NT1 Microbicidal compounds
NT1 Pesticides
RT Antibiotics
RT Disinfection
RT Germicides

Biocontrol
BT1 Disinfestation
BT2 Pests

Bioconversions
HN heading from vol. 24 (1992)
BT1 Fermentation products
BT2 Biotechnology
BT3 Technology
NT1 Biotransformations

Biodegradability
BT1 Decomposition

Biodegradation
BT1 Decomposition

Biodeterioration
BT1 Spoilage
RT Biotechnology
RT Wastes

Biofilms
BT1 Microorganisms

Bioflavonoids
HN also under Nutrients up to vol. 42 (2010)
BT1 Flavonoids
BT2 Aromatic compounds
BT3 Organic compounds
BT2 Pigments
UF Vitamin P

Biofuels
HN introduced from vol. 43, issue 1 (2011)
BT1 Biotechnology
BT2 Technology
RT Biogas

Biogarde
BT1 Fermented milk
BT2 Fermented dairy products
BT3 Dairy products
BT4 Animal foods
BT5 Foods
BT3 Fermented foods
BT4 Processed foods
BT5 Foods
BT2 Milk
BT3 Dairy products
BT4 Animal foods
BT5 Foods

Biogas
BT1 Gases
BT2 Physical phases
BT3 Chemistry
BT4 Science
BT1 Hydrocarbons
BT2 Organic compounds
RT Biofuels
RT Methane

Biogenic amines
BT1 Amines
BT2 Organic nitrogen compounds
NT1 Cadaverine
NT1 Catecholamines
NT2 Adrenaline
NT2 Noradrenaline
NT1 Choline
NT1 Dopamine
NT1 Histamine
NT1 Hordenine
NT1 5-Hydroxytryptamine
NT1 Putrescine
NT1 Serotonin
NT1 Skatole
NT1 Spermine
NT1 Tryptamine
NT1 Tyramine

Bioghurt
BT1 Fermented milk
BT2 Fermented dairy products
BT3 Dairy products
BT4 Animal foods
BT5 Foods
BT3 Fermented foods
BT4 Processed foods
BT5 Foods
BT2 Milk
BT3 Dairy products
BT4 Animal foods
BT5 Foods

Biohydrogenation
HN introduced from vol. 39, issue 1 (2007)
BT1 Metabolism
BT2 Physiology
BT3 Science

Bioko
BT1 Equatorial Guinea
BT2 West Africa
BT3 Africa
UF Fernando Po

Biological activity
RT Biomarkers

Biological membranes
NT1 Egg shell membranes
RT Membranes

Biological oxygen demand
HN abbrev. BOD used in the index up to vol. 24 (1992)
RT Wastes
UF Biochemical oxygen demand
UF BOD

Biological values
BT1 Nutritional values

Biology
BT1 Science
RT Biochemistry

Bioluminescence
BT1 Fluorescence
BT2 Analytical techniques
BT2 Optical properties
BT3 Physical properties

Biomagnification
HN introduced from vol. 39, issue 1 (2007)
BT1 Metabolism
BT2 Physiology
BT3 Science
RT Residues

Biomarkers
RT Biological activity

Biomass
HN heading from vol. 22 (1990); under Single cell proteins up to vol. 21 (1989)
BT1 Fermentation products
BT2 Biotechnology
BT3 Technology
NT1 Microbial biomass
NT2 Bacterial biomass
NT2 Yeast biomass
NT1 Mycoprotein
NT2 Quorn
NT1 Single cell proteins

Biomycin
USE **Chlortetracycline**

Biopolymers
NT1 Cutin
NT1 Latex
NT1 Lignin
NT2 Lignocelluloses
NT1 Suberin
RT Carbohydrates
RT Polymers

Bioreactors
HN heading from vol. 24 (1992)
BT1 Fermentation technology
BT2 Biotechnology
BT3 Technology
BT2 Process control
BT3 Technology
NT1 Chemostats

NT1 Membrane bioreactors
NT1 Packed bed bioreactors
NT1 Stirred tank bioreactors
NT1 UASB bioreactors
RT Immobilized cells

Bioremediation
HN heading from vol. 30 (1998); under Biotechnology up to vol. 29 (1997)
BT1 Biotechnology
BT2 Technology
NT1 Anaerobic digestion
NT1 Composting
NT1 Dechlorination
RT *Coriolus*

Biosecurity
HN introduced from vol. 42, issue 1 (2010)
BT1 Food safety
RT Contamination

Biosensors
HN heading from vol. 24 (1992)
BT1 Biotechnology
BT2 Technology
NT1 Enzyme electrodes
RT Bioassay
RT Electrodes

Biosurfactants
BT1 Surfactants

Biotechnologically derived foods
BT1 Biotechnology
BT2 Technology
BT1 Novel foods
BT2 Foods
RT Genetically engineered foods
RT GM foods

Biotechnology
HN heading from vol. 22 (1990); under Product technology up to vol. 21 (1989)
BT1 Technology
NT1 Biocatalysts
NT1 Biofuels
NT1 Bioremediation
NT2 Anaerobic digestion
NT2 Composting
NT2 Dechlorination
NT1 Biosensors
NT2 Enzyme electrodes
NT1 Biotechnologically derived foods
NT1 Fermentation products
NT2 Bioconversions
NT3 Biotransformations
NT2 Biomass
NT3 Microbial biomass
NT4 Bacterial biomass
NT4 Yeast biomass
NT3 Mycoprotein
NT4 Quorn
NT3 Single cell proteins
NT1 Fermentation technology
NT2 Bioreactors
NT3 Chemostats
NT3 Membrane bioreactors
NT3 Packed bed bioreactors
NT3 Stirred tank bioreactors
NT3 UASB bioreactors
NT2 Cofermentation
NT2 Downstream processing
NT2 Extractive fermentation
NT2 Fermenters
NT2 Simultaneous saccharification and fermentation
NT2 Solid state fermentation
NT2 Submerged fermentation
NT1 Immobilization
NT1 Immobilized cells
NT1 Immobilized enzymes
RT Biodeterioration

Biotechnology products
HN heading from vol. 24 (1992) to vol. 27 (1995). Used up to vol. 39 (2007)
USE **Fermentation products**

Bioterrorism
HN introduced from vol. 39, issue 1 (2007)
BT1 Food safety
RT Contamination

Biotin
BT1 Vitamin B group
BT2 Vitamins
BT3 Nutrients
UF Vitamin H

Biotransformations
BT1 Bioconversions
BT2 Fermentation products
BT3 Biotechnology
BT4 Technology

Biphenyl
BT1 Fungicides
BT2 Pesticides
BT3 Biocides
BT3 Residues
UF Diphenyl

Bird foods
HN introduced from vol. 39, issue 1 (2007)
SN use for foods for domestic pet birds but not feeds for birds reared for meat
BT1 Pet foods
RT Pet birds

Bird rape
BT1 Rapeseeds
BT2 Oilseeds
BT3 Seeds
BT4 Plant foods
BT5 Foods

Birds
NT1 Partridges
NT2 Partridge meat
NT3 Partridge carcasses
NT1 Pheasants
NT2 Pheasant meat
NT3 Pheasant carcasses
NT1 Pigeons
NT2 Pigeon meat
NT3 Pigeon carcasses
NT1 Poultry
NT2 Chickens
NT3 Chicken bones
NT3 Chicken gizzard pickles
NT3 Chicken livers
NT3 Chicken meat
NT4 Chicken carcasses
NT4 Chicken drumsticks
NT4 Chicken mince
NT4 Chicken nuggets
NT4 Chicken products
NT5 Chicken patties
NT3 Chicken skin
NT2 Chukars
NT2 Ducks
NT3 Duck eggs
NT4 Pidan
NT3 Duck livers
NT3 Duck meat
NT4 Duck carcasses
NT2 Emus
NT3 Emu meat
NT4 Emu carcasses
NT2 Fowl
NT2 Geese
NT3 Goose eggs
NT3 Goose livers
NT3 Goose meat
NT4 Goose carcasses
NT2 Guinea fowl
NT2 Ostriches
NT3 Ostrich meat
NT4 Ostrich carcasses
NT2 Quails
NT3 Quail carcasses
NT3 Quail eggs
NT3 Quail meat
NT4 Quail carcasses
NT2 Rheas
NT3 Rhea meat
NT4 Rhea carcasses
NT2 Turkeys
NT3 Turkey meat
NT4 Turkey carcasses
NT4 Turkey mince
NT4 Turkey products
NT5 Turkey ham
NT5 Turkey patties
NT2 Waterfowl
NT1 Ptarmigans
NT1 Woodcock
NT1 Wood pigeons
RT Animals
RT Pets

Birds nests
BT1 Animal foods
BT2 Foods

Birefringence
BT1 Optical properties
BT2 Physical properties

Birth wt.
HN introduced from vol. 41, issue 1 (2009)
BT1 Body wt.

BT2 Anthropometric parameters
BT3 Health

Biscuit dough
BT1 Biscuits
BT2 Bakery products
BT3 Cereal products
BT4 Plant foods
BT5 Foods
BT1 Dough
BT2 Bakery products
BT3 Cereal products
BT4 Plant foods
BT5 Foods

Biscuit factories
BT1 Biscuits
BT2 Bakery products
BT3 Cereal products
BT4 Plant foods
BT5 Foods
BT1 Food factories

Biscuits
BT1 Bakery products
BT2 Cereal products
BT3 Plant foods
BT4 Foods
NT1 Biscuit dough
NT1 Biscuit factories
NT1 Cookies
NT1 Crackers
NT1 Saltine crackers
NT1 Shortbread

Bismuth
USE **Bi**

Bison
BT1 Animals
NT1 Bison meat
NT2 Bison carcasses
RT Buffaloes

Bison carcasses
BT1 Bison meat
BT2 Bison
BT3 Animals
BT2 Meat specific
BT3 Meat
BT4 Animal foods
BT5 Foods
BT1 Carcasses
BT2 Meat
BT3 Animal foods
BT4 Foods

Bison meat
BT1 Bison
BT2 Animals
BT1 Meat specific
BT2 Meat
BT3 Animal foods
BT4 Foods
NT1 Bison carcasses
RT Buffalo meat

Bisphenol A
BT1 Phenols
BT2 Alcohols
BT2 Aromatic compounds
BT3 Organic compounds
RT Polycarbonates

Bisphenol A diglycidyl ether
BT1 Ethers
BT2 Organic compounds
BT1 Phenols
BT2 Alcohols
BT2 Aromatic compounds
BT3 Organic compounds

Bisphenol F diglycidyl ether
HN introduced from vol. 41, issue 1 (2009)
BT1 Ethers
BT2 Organic compounds
BT1 Phenols
BT2 Alcohols
BT2 Aromatic compounds
BT3 Organic compounds

Bisulfites
BT1 Sulfites
BT2 Salts
UF Bisulphites

Bisulphites
HN used for bisulfites up to vol. 35, issue 6 (2003)
USE **Bisulfites**

Bitter acids
SN use for hop bitter compounds
BT1 Bitter compounds
BT2 Flavour compounds
BT1 Organic acids
BT2 Acids
NT1 α-Acids
NT2 Humulones
NT3 Adhumulone
NT3 Cohumulone
NT3 Humulinic acid
NT1 β-Acids
NT2 Hulupones
NT2 Lupulones
NT3 Colupulone
NT1 Iso-α-acids
NT2 Isohumulones
NT1 Lupulin
RT Bitterness
RT Bitter principles
RT Hops

Bitter almond oils
BT1 Essential oils
BT2 Flavourings
BT3 Additives
BT2 Vegetable oils
BT3 Oils vegetable
BT4 Oils
BT5 Lipids
BT6 Nutrients
BT4 Vegetable products
BT5 Plant foods
BT6 Foods
RT Bitter almonds

Bitter almonds
BT1 Flavourings
BT2 Additives
RT Bitter almond oils

Bitter compounds
HN heading from vol. 25 (1993); under Bitter principles up to vol. 24 (1992)
BT1 Flavour compounds
NT1 Bitter acids
NT2 α-Acids
NT3 Humulones
NT4 Adhumulone
NT4 Cohumulone
NT4 Humulinic acid
NT2 β-Acids
NT3 Hulupones
NT3 Lupulones
NT4 Colupulone
NT2 Iso-α-acids
NT3 Isohumulones
NT2 Lupulin
NT1 Bitter peptides
NT1 Bitter principles
NT1 Cucurbitacins
NT1 Diketopiperazines
NT1 Ipomeamarone
NT1 Limonoids
NT2 Limonin
NT2 Limonoid glucosides
NT2 Nomilin
NT1 Naringin
NT1 Oleuropein
NT1 Progoitrin
NT1 Propylthiouracil
NT1 Quassin
NT1 Quinine
RT Bitterness

Bitter gourds
BT1 Gourds
BT2 Vegetables specific
BT3 Vegetables
BT4 Crops
BT5 Plants
BT4 Plant foods
BT5 Foods
UF Balsam pears

Bitterness
BT1 Flavour
BT2 Sensory properties
RT Bitter acids
RT Bitter compounds
RT Debittering
RT Naringin

Bitter orange essential oils
HN introduced from vol. 39, issue 1 (2007)
BT1 Citrus essential oils
BT2 Essential oils
BT3 Flavourings
BT4 Additives
BT3 Vegetable oils
BT4 Oils vegetable
BT5 Oils
BT6 Lipids
BT7 Nutrients
BT5 Vegetable products
BT6 Plant foods
BT7 Foods
RT Bitter oranges

Bitter oranges
HN introduced from vol. 39, issue 1 (2007)
BT1 Citrus fruits
BT2 Fruits specific
BT3 Fruits
BT4 Crops
BT5 Plants
BT4 Plant foods
BT5 Foods
RT Bitter orange essential oils

Bitter peptides
BT1 Bitter compounds
BT2 Flavour compounds
BT1 Peptides
BT2 Proteins
BT3 Nutrients

Bitter pit
BT1 Plant disorders
BT2 Diseases plant
BT3 Diseases
RT Apples

Bitter principles
HN heading up to vol. 24 (1992)
BT1 Bitter compounds
BT2 Flavour compounds
RT Bitter acids

Bitto cheese
BT1 Cheese varieties
BT2 Cheese
BT3 Dairy products
BT4 Animal foods
BT5 Foods

Bivalves
BT1 Molluscs
BT2 Shellfish
BT3 Animals
BT3 Sea foods
BT4 Aquatic foods
BT5 Animal foods
BT6 Foods
NT1 Arkshells
NT1 Carpet shells
NT1 Clams
NT2 Freshwater clams
NT2 *Pseudocardium sachalinensis*
NT2 *Tapes philippinarum*
NT1 Cockles
NT1 Mussels
NT2 Blue mussels
NT2 Green mussels
NT2 *Mytilus edulis*
NT2 *Mytilus galloprovincialis*
NT2 *Mytilus trossulus*
NT1 Oysters
NT2 *Crassostrea gigas*
NT2 *Crassostrea virginica*
NT2 Oyster sauces
NT1 Razor shells
NT1 Scallops
NT2 *Patinopecten yessoensis*

Bixin
BT1 Carotenoids
BT2 Pigments
BT2 Terpenoids
BT3 Lipids
BT4 Nutrients
BT1 Colorants
BT2 Additives
RT Annatto

Black beans
BT1 Common beans
BT2 Legumes
BT3 Vegetables specific
BT4 Vegetables
BT5 Crops
BT6 Plants
BT5 Plant foods
BT6 Foods

Blackberries
BT1 Berries
BT2 Fruits specific
BT3 Fruits
BT4 Crops
BT5 Plants
BT4 Plant foods
BT5 Foods
RT Blackberry juices

Blackberry juices
HN introduced from vol. 39, issue 1 (2007)
BT1 Berry juices
BT2 Fruit juices
BT3 Fruit products
BT4 Plant foods
BT5 Foods
BT3 Soft drinks
BT4 Beverages
RT Blackberries

Black cumin
BT1 Spices
BT2 Flavourings
BT3 Additives

Blackcurrant juices
BT1 Berry juices
BT2 Fruit juices
BT3 Fruit products
BT4 Plant foods
BT5 Foods
BT3 Soft drinks
BT4 Beverages
RT Blackcurrants

Blackcurrants
BT1 Berries
BT2 Fruits specific
BT3 Fruits
BT4 Crops
BT5 Plants
BT4 Plant foods
BT5 Foods
RT Blackcurrant juices

Blackeyed peas
BT1 Cowpeas
BT2 Legumes
BT3 Vegetables specific
BT4 Vegetables
BT5 Crops
BT6 Plants
BT5 Plant foods
BT6 Foods

Black gram
BT1 Legumes
BT2 Vegetables specific
BT3 Vegetables
BT4 Crops
BT5 Plants
BT4 Plant foods
BT5 Foods
NT1 Dosai
UF Munggo
UF Urd beans

Black nightshade
BT1 Berries
BT2 Fruits specific
BT3 Fruits
BT4 Crops
BT5 Plants
BT4 Plant foods
BT5 Foods

Black olives
BT1 Olives
BT2 Fruits specific
BT3 Fruits
BT4 Crops
BT5 Plants
BT4 Plant foods
BT5 Foods
BT2 Oilseeds
BT3 Seeds
BT4 Plant foods
BT5 Foods

Black pepper
BT1 Pepper
BT2 Spices
BT3 Flavourings
BT4 Additives

Black puddings
BT1 Blood sausages
BT2 Sausages
BT3 Meat products
BT4 Animal foods
BT5 Foods

Black rice
BT1 Rice
BT2 Cereals
BT3 Crops
BT4 Plants
BT3 Seeds
BT4 Plant foods
BT5 Foods

Black salsify
BT1 Vegetables specific
BT2 Vegetables
BT3 Crops
BT4 Plants
BT3 Plant foods
BT4 Foods

Black sea sprat
USE **Kilka**

Black soybeans
BT1 Soybeans
BT2 Legumes
BT3 Vegetables specific
BT4 Vegetables
BT5 Crops
BT6 Plants
BT5 Plant foods
BT6 Foods
BT2 Oilseeds
BT3 Seeds
BT4 Plant foods
BT5 Foods

Black spot
USE **Blackspot**

Blackspot
BT1 Defects
BT1 Discoloration
RT Melanosis
UF Black spot

Black tea
BT1 Tea
BT2 Teas
BT3 Beverages
BT3 Crops
BT4 Plants
BT3 Plant foods
BT4 Foods

Black truffles
BT1 *Tuber*
BT2 Edible fungi
BT3 Fungi edible
BT4 Vegetables specific
BT5 Vegetables
BT6 Crops
BT7 Plants
BT6 Plant foods
BT7 Foods

Bladders
BT1 Offal
BT2 Animal foods
BT3 Foods

Blakeslea
BT1 Fungi
BT2 Microorganisms
NT1 *Blakeslea trispora*

Blakeslea trispora
BT1 *Blakeslea*
BT2 Fungi
BT3 Microorganisms

Blanching
BT1 Cooking
BT2 Thermal processing
BT3 Processing thermal
BT4 Processing
BT5 Technology

Blancmanges
BT1 Desserts
BT2 Processed foods
BT3 Foods

Blasticidin S
BT1 Antibiotics
BT2 Drugs
BT3 Residues

Bleaching
BT1 Processing
BT2 Technology
NT1 Bleaching agents
RT Decoloration

Bleaching agents
BT1 Bleaching
BT2 Processing
BT3 Technology

Bleeding
BT1 Blood

Blending
BT1 Mixing
BT2 Processing
BT3 Technology

Blights
BT1 Plant diseases
BT2 Diseases plant
BT3 Diseases

Blood
NT1 Bleeding
NT1 Blood proteins
UF Plasma
UF Serum

Blood pressure
BT1 Cardiovascular physiology
BT2 Human physiology
BT3 Physiology
BT4 Science

Blood proteins
BT1 Animal proteins
BT2 Proteins animal
BT3 Proteins
BT4 Nutrients
BT1 Blood

Blood sausages
BT1 Sausages
BT2 Meat products
BT3 Animal foods
BT4 Foods
NT1 Black puddings
UF Blutwurst

Bloom
BT1 Spoilage
RT Chocolate

Blossom end rot
BT1 Plant disorders
BT2 Diseases plant
BT3 Diseases

Blotting
BT1 Hybridization
BT2 Genetic techniques
BT3 Genetics
NT1 Northern blotting
NT1 Southern blotting
NT1 Western blotting

Blowing
BT1 Spoilage

Blubber
BT1 Animal fats
BT2 Fats animal
BT3 Animal foods
BT4 Foods
BT3 Fats
BT4 Lipids
BT5 Nutrients
NT1 Seal blubber

Blueberries
BT1 Berries
BT2 Fruits specific
BT3 Fruits
BT4 Crops
BT5 Plants
BT4 Plant foods
BT5 Foods
RT Blueberry juices

Blueberry juices
HN introduced from vol. 39, issue 1 (2007)
BT1 Berry juices
BT2 Fruit juices
BT3 Fruit products
BT4 Plant foods
BT5 Foods
BT3 Soft drinks
BT4 Beverages
RT Blueberries

Blue cheese
BT1 Cheese varieties
BT2 Cheese
BT3 Dairy products
BT4 Animal foods
BT5 Foods

Blue crabs
BT1 Crabs
BT2 Crustacea
BT3 Shellfish
BT4 Animals
BT4 Sea foods
BT5 Aquatic foods
BT6 Animal foods
BT7 Foods
NT1 *Callinectes sapidus*

Bluefish
HN introduced from vol. 37, issue 5 (2005)
BT1 Marine fish
BT2 Fish
BT3 Animals
BT3 Sea foods
BT4 Aquatic foods
BT5 Animal foods
BT6 Foods

Blue green algae
SN older name for cyanobacteria
BT1 Cyanobacteria
BT2 Bacteria

BT3 Microorganisms
RT Algae

Blue mussels
BT1 Mussels
BT2 Bivalves
BT3 Molluscs
BT4 Shellfish
BT5 Animals
BT5 Sea foods
BT6 Aquatic foods
BT7 Animal foods
BT8 Foods

Blue whiting
BT1 Marine fish
BT2 Fish
BT3 Animals
BT3 Sea foods
BT4 Aquatic foods
BT5 Animal foods
BT6 Foods
NT1 *Micromesistius poutassou*

Blutwurst
USE **Blood sausages**

Boar carcasses
USE **Swine carcasses**

Board
BT1 Packaging materials
NT1 Cardboard
NT1 Cartonboard
NT1 Fibreboard
NT1 Paperboard
NT1 Pulpboard

Boar meat
BT1 Pork
BT2 Meat specific
BT3 Meat
BT4 Animal foods
BT5 Foods

Boars
HN types of swine not specified in the index from vol. 25 (1993)
USE **Swine**

Boar taint
BT1 Taints
BT2 Flavour
BT3 Sensory properties

Bockwurst
BT1 Sausages
BT2 Meat products
BT3 Animal foods
BT4 Foods

BOD
HN used as abbrev. for biological oxygen demand up to vol. 24 (1992)
USE **Biological oxygen demand**

Body
BT1 Texture
BT2 Sensory properties

Body composition
HN introduced from vol. 40, issue 1 (2008)
BT1 Anthropometric parameters
BT2 Health
RT Obesity

Body fats
HN introduced from vol. 42, issue 1 (2010)
BT1 Human physiology
BT2 Physiology
BT3 Science
RT Adipose tissues

Bodying agents
BT1 Additives

Body mass index
BT1 Body wt.
BT2 Anthropometric parameters
BT3 Health

Body wt.
HN introduced from vol. 38, issue 8 (2006)
BT1 Anthropometric parameters
BT2 Health
NT1 Birth wt.
NT1 Body mass index
NT1 Overweight
NT1 Wt. loss diet
RT Obesity

Bogue
BT1 Sea bream
BT2 Marine fish
BT3 Fish
BT4 Animals
BT4 Sea foods
BT5 Aquatic foods
BT6 Animal foods
BT7 Foods
NT1 *Boops boops*

Boiled ham
BT1 Ham
BT2 Meat products
BT3 Animal foods
BT4 Foods

Boiled sausages
BT1 Sausages
BT2 Meat products
BT3 Animal foods
BT4 Foods

Boiled sweets
BT1 Sugar confectionery
BT2 Plant foods
BT3 Foods

Boilers
BT1 Boiling
BT2 Cooking
BT3 Thermal processing
BT4 Processing thermal
BT5 Processing
BT6 Technology
BT1 Equipment
BT2 Technology

Boiling
BT1 Cooking
BT2 Thermal processing
BT3 Processing thermal
BT4 Processing
BT5 Technology
NT1 Boilers
NT1 Parboiling

Boiling point
USE **b.p.**

Boletus
BT1 Edible fungi
BT2 Fungi edible
BT3 Vegetables specific
BT4 Vegetables
BT5 Crops
BT6 Plants
BT5 Plant foods
BT6 Foods
NT1 *Boletus edulis*

Boletus edulis
BT1 *Boletus*
BT2 Edible fungi
BT3 Fungi edible
BT4 Vegetables specific
BT5 Vegetables
BT6 Crops
BT7 Plants
BT6 Plant foods
BT7 Foods

Bolivia
BT1 South America
BT2 America

Bologna
BT1 Sausages
BT2 Meat products
BT3 Animal foods
BT4 Foods

Bolti
BT1 Nile tilapia
BT2 Tilapia
BT3 Freshwater fish
BT4 Fish
BT5 Animals
BT5 Sea foods
BT6 Aquatic foods
BT7 Animal foods
BT8 Foods

Bombay duck
BT1 Marine fish
BT2 Fish
BT3 Animals
BT3 Sea foods
BT4 Aquatic foods
BT5 Animal foods
BT6 Foods

Bonbons
BT1 Sugar confectionery
BT2 Plant foods
BT3 Foods

Bone health
HN introduced from vol. 38, issue 8 (2006)
BT1 Health

Bone marrow
HN under Fats animal up to vol. 42 (2010)
BT1 Animal foods
BT2 Foods
BT1 Connective tissues
RT Bones

Bone mineral density
BT1 Health

Bones
HN heading from vol. 25 (1993); under Boning up to vol. 24 (1992)
SN use for properties or use of bones
NT1 Chicken bones
NT1 Fish bones
RT Bone marrow
RT Boning

Bongkrek
BT1 Coconuts
BT2 Nuts
BT3 Fruits
BT4 Crops
BT5 Plants
BT4 Plant foods
BT5 Foods
BT3 Oilseeds
BT4 Seeds
BT5 Plant foods
BT6 Foods
BT1 Fermented foods
BT2 Processed foods
BT3 Foods

Boning
SN use for separation of bone from other tissues
BT1 Processing
BT2 Technology
NT1 Cold boning
NT1 Hot boning
NT1 Mechanical boning
RT Bones
RT Slaughter
UF Deboning

Bonito
HN under Fish up to vol. 42 (2010)
BT1 Tuna
BT2 Marine fish
BT3 Fish
BT4 Animals
BT4 Sea foods
BT5 Aquatic foods
BT6 Animal foods
BT7 Foods
BT2 Oily fish
BT3 Fish
BT4 Animals
BT4 Sea foods
BT5 Aquatic foods
BT6 Animal foods
BT7 Foods
UF Bonitos
UF Sarda

Bonitos
HN used up to vol. 29 (1997)
USE **Bonito**

Books
NT1 Bibliographies
NT1 Dictionaries
NT1 Directories
NT1 Encyclopaedias
NT1 Guides
RT Conference proceedings
RT Proceedings

Boondi
BT1 Bengal gram
BT2 Chick peas
BT3 Legumes
BT4 Vegetables specific
BT5 Vegetables
BT6 Crops
BT7 Plants
BT6 Plant foods
BT7 Foods

Boops boops
BT1 Bogue
BT2 Sea bream
BT3 Marine fish
BT4 Fish
BT5 Animals
BT5 Sea foods
BT6 Aquatic foods
BT7 Animal foods
BT8 Foods

Borage
HN under Spices up to vol. 42 (2010)
BT1 Herbs
BT2 Spices
BT3 Flavourings
BT4 Additives
BT1 Plants
BT1 Vegetables specific
BT2 Vegetables
BT3 Crops
BT4 Plants
BT3 Plant foods
BT4 Foods

Borage oils
BT1 Vegetable oils
BT2 Oils vegetable
BT3 Oils
BT4 Lipids
BT5 Nutrients
BT3 Vegetable products
BT4 Plant foods
BT5 Foods

Borassus
BT1 Palms
BT2 Plants

Bordeaux mixture
BT1 Fungicides
BT2 Pesticides
BT3 Biocides
BT3 Residues

Boric acid
BT1 Acids

Borneol
HN also under Volatile compounds up to vol. 42 (2010)
BT1 Aroma compounds
BT2 Flavour compounds
BT2 Volatile compounds
BT1 Monoterpenoids
BT2 Terpenoids
BT3 Lipids
BT4 Nutrients

Borneo tallow
BT1 Vegetable fats
BT2 Fats vegetable
BT3 Fats
BT4 Lipids
BT5 Nutrients
BT3 Vegetable products
BT4 Plant foods
BT5 Foods

Boron
USE **B**

Boronia
BT1 Plants
NT1 *Boronia megastigma*

Boronia megastigma
BT1 *Boronia*
BT2 Plants

Borshch
BT1 Soups
BT2 Processed foods
BT3 Foods

Bosnia and Herzegovina
BT1 Europe

Botanical origin
BT1 Origin

Botrytis
BT1 Fungi
BT2 Microorganisms
NT1 *Botrytis cinerea*
RT Diseases plant

Botrytis cinerea
SN anamorph of Botryotinia fuckeliana
BT1 *Botrytis*
BT2 Fungi
BT3 Microorganisms

Botswana
BT1 Southern Africa
BT2 Africa

Bottled mineral waters
BT1 Mineral waters
BT2 Soft drinks
BT3 Beverages
BT2 Water

Bottled water
BT1 Drinking water
BT2 Water

Bottles
BT1 Containers
NT1 Glass bottles
NT1 Plastics bottles
RT Bottling

Bottling
BT1 Packaging
BT2 Technology
BT1 Preservation
BT2 Technology
RT Bottles

Bottom fermenting yeasts
BT1 Brewers yeasts
BT2 Yeasts brewers
BT3 *Saccharomyces*
BT4 Yeasts
BT5 Fungi
BT6 Microorganisms
RT Brewing

Botulism
BT1 Diseases
BT1 Poisoning
RT Botulotoxins
RT *Clostridium*

Botulotoxins
BT1 Toxins
BT2 Residues
RT Botulism
RT *Clostridium*

Bouillon
BT1 Soups
BT2 Processed foods
BT3 Foods

Bouquet
BT1 Aroma
BT2 Sensory properties

Bourbon whiskey
HN under Spirits up to vol. 42 (2010)
BT1 Whiskey
BT2 Whiskies
BT3 Spirits
BT4 Alcoholic beverages
BT5 Beverages alcoholic
BT6 Beverages

Bouza
BT1 Beer
BT2 Alcoholic beverages
BT3 Beverages alcoholic
BT4 Beverages

Bovine
USE **Cattle**

Bovine immunodeficiency virus
HN introduced from vol. 43, issue 1 (2011); bovine immunodeficiency viruses also used in the index up to vol. 42 (2010)
BT1 Lentivirus
BT2 Viruses
BT3 Microorganisms
UF Bovine immunodeficiency viruses

Bovine immunodeficiency viruses
HN Bovine immunodeficiency virus used in the index from vol. 43 (2011)
USE **Bovine immunodeficiency virus**

Bovine muscles
USE **Beef**

Bovine serum albumin
BT1 Albumins
BT2 Proteins
BT3 Nutrients
BT1 Animal proteins
BT2 Proteins animal
BT3 Proteins
BT4 Nutrients

Bovine somatotropin
BT1 Somatotropin
BT2 Hormones
BT3 Residues

Bovine spongiform encephalopathy
USE **BSE**

Bowels
BT1 Offal
BT2 Animal foods
BT3 Foods

Bowls
BT1 Containers

Boxes
BT1 Containers
NT1 Cases

Boxthorn
BT1 Vegetables specific
BT2 Vegetables
BT3 Crops
BT4 Plants
BT3 Plant foods
BT4 Foods

Boysenberries
BT1 Berries
BT2 Fruits specific
BT3 Fruits
BT4 Crops
BT5 Plants
BT4 Plant foods
BT5 Foods

Boza
BT1 Alcoholic beverages
BT2 Beverages alcoholic
BT3 Beverages

b.p.
BT1 Thermophysical properties
BT2 Physical properties
UF Boiling point

Br
BT1 Halogens
BT2 Elements
BT3 Minerals
BT4 Nutrients
RT Bromides
RT Organobromine compounds
UF Bromine

Bracken
BT1 Ferns

Brains
BT1 Central nervous system tissues
BT2 Wastes
BT1 Offal
BT2 Animal foods
BT3 Foods

Braising
BT1 Cooking
BT2 Thermal processing
BT3 Processing thermal
BT4 Processing
BT5 Technology

Bran
BT1 Cereal products
BT2 Plant foods
BT3 Foods
NT1 Cereal bran
NT1 Corn bran
NT1 Oat bran
NT1 Rice bran
NT1 Rye bran
NT1 Wheat bran
RT Debranning
RT Fibre

Branched chain fatty acids
HN introduced from vol. 39, issue 1 (2007)
BT1 Fatty acids
BT2 Lipids
BT3 Nutrients
BT2 Organic acids
BT3 Acids
NT1 Isobutyric acid
NT1 Isocaproic acid
NT1 Isovaleric acid

Branching enzymes
USE **1,4-α-Glucan branching enzymes**

Brandies
HN heading from vol. 25 (1993); under Brandy up to vol. 24 (1992)
BT1 Spirits
BT2 Alcoholic beverages
BT3 Beverages alcoholic
BT4 Beverages
NT1 Armagnac
NT1 Brandy
NT1 Cognac
NT1 Eau de vie
NT1 Fruit brandies
NT2 Apple brandy
NT3 Calvados
NT2 Kirsch

  NT2 Rakia
  NT2 Slivovitz
 NT1 Grappa
 NT1 Pisco
 RT Wine distillates

Branding
 BT1 Labelling
  BT2 Packaging
   BT3 Technology
 RT Private labels

Brands
 BT1 Labelling
  BT2 Packaging
   BT3 Technology

Brandy
HN heading up to vol. 24 (1992); under Brandies from vol. 25 (1993)
 BT1 Brandies
  BT2 Spirits
   BT3 Alcoholic beverages
    BT4 Beverages alcoholic
     BT5 Beverages

Brassica
 BT1 Vegetables specific
  BT2 Vegetables
   BT3 Crops
    BT4 Plants
   BT3 Plant foods
    BT4 Foods
 NT1 *Brassica carinata*
 NT1 *Brassica napus*
 NT1 *Brassica oleracea*

Brassica carinata
 BT1 *Brassica*
  BT2 Vegetables specific
   BT3 Vegetables
    BT4 Crops
     BT5 Plants
    BT4 Plant foods
     BT5 Foods
 BT1 Ethiopian mustard
  BT2 Mustard greens
   BT3 Vegetables specific
    BT4 Vegetables
     BT5 Crops
      BT6 Plants
     BT5 Plant foods
      BT6 Foods
  BT2 Mustard seeds
   BT3 Oilseeds
    BT4 Seeds
     BT5 Plant foods
      BT6 Foods
   BT3 Spices
    BT4 Flavourings
     BT5 Additives

Brassica napus
 BT1 *Brassica*
  BT2 Vegetables specific
   BT3 Vegetables
    BT4 Crops
     BT5 Plants
    BT4 Plant foods
     BT5 Foods
 BT1 Rapeseeds
  BT2 Oilseeds
   BT3 Seeds
    BT4 Plant foods
     BT5 Foods

Brassica oleracea
 BT1 *Brassica*
  BT2 Vegetables specific
   BT3 Vegetables
    BT4 Crops
     BT5 Plants
    BT4 Plant foods
     BT5 Foods

***Brassica* seeds**
 BT1 Oilseeds
  BT2 Seeds
   BT3 Plant foods
    BT4 Foods

Brassicasterol
 BT1 Sterols
  BT2 Alcohols
  BT2 Steroids
   BT3 Lipids
    BT4 Nutrients

Brassinosteroids
 BT1 Steroids
  BT2 Lipids
   BT3 Nutrients

Bratwurst
 BT1 Sausages
  BT2 Meat products
   BT3 Animal foods
    BT4 Foods

Brawn
 BT1 Meat products
  BT2 Animal foods
   BT3 Foods

Brazil
HN heading up to vol. 24 (1992)
 BT1 South America
  BT2 America

Brazil nut oils
 BT1 Nut oils
  BT2 Vegetable oils
   BT3 Oils vegetable
    BT4 Oils
     BT5 Lipids
      BT6 Nutrients
    BT4 Vegetable products
     BT5 Plant foods
      BT6 Foods

Brazil nuts
 BT1 Nuts
  BT2 Fruits
   BT3 Crops
    BT4 Plants
   BT3 Plant foods
    BT4 Foods
  BT2 Oilseeds
   BT3 Seeds
    BT4 Plant foods
     BT5 Foods

Brazzein
 BT1 Sweet proteins
  BT2 Proteins
   BT3 Nutrients
  BT2 Sweeteners
   BT3 Additives

Bread
 BT1 Bakery products
  BT2 Cereal products
   BT3 Plant foods
    BT4 Foods
 NT1 Arabic bread
 NT1 Baguettes
 NT1 Balady
 NT1 Bread crumb
 NT1 Breadcrumbs
 NT1 Bread crust
 NT1 Bread dough
 NT1 Breadmaking
  NT2 Breadmaking properties
   NT3 Loaf vol.
  NT2 Wheat breadmaking
 NT1 Bread rolls
 NT1 Chapattis
 NT1 Corn bread
 NT1 Crispbreads
 NT1 Flat bread
 NT1 French bread
 NT1 Fruit bread
 NT1 Gluten low bread
 NT1 Injera
 NT1 Kisra
 NT1 Nan
 NT1 Parottas
 NT1 Pita bread
 NT1 Poori
 NT1 Pumpernickel
 NT1 Rice bread
 NT1 Rolls
 NT1 Roti
 NT1 Rye bread
 NT1 Sangak
 NT1 Soda bread
 NT1 Sourdough bread
 NT1 Steamed bread
 NT1 Tanoor
 NT1 Toast
 NT1 Toast bread
 NT1 Wheat bread

Bread crumb
 BT1 Bread
  BT2 Bakery products
   BT3 Cereal products
    BT4 Plant foods
     BT5 Foods

Breadcrumbs
 BT1 Bread
  BT2 Bakery products
   BT3 Cereal products
    BT4 Plant foods
     BT5 Foods
 BT1 Coatings

Bread crust
 BT1 Bread
  BT2 Bakery products
   BT3 Cereal products

BT4 Plant foods
BT5 Foods

Bread dough
BT1 Bread
BT2 Bakery products
BT3 Cereal products
BT4 Plant foods
BT5 Foods
BT1 Dough
BT2 Bakery products
BT3 Cereal products
BT4 Plant foods
BT5 Foods

Breadfruit
BT1 Fruits specific
BT2 Fruits
BT3 Crops
BT4 Plants
BT3 Plant foods
BT4 Foods

Breading
BT1 Coating
BT2 Processing
BT3 Technology

Breadings
BT1 Coatings

Breadmaking
BT1 Bread
BT2 Bakery products
BT3 Cereal products
BT4 Plant foods
BT5 Foods
BT1 Processing
BT2 Technology
NT1 Breadmaking properties
NT2 Loaf vol.
NT1 Wheat breadmaking
RT Bakers yeasts
RT Baking
RT Kneading
RT Yeasts bakers
UF Bread manufacture

Breadmaking properties
BT1 Breadmaking
BT2 Bread
BT3 Bakery products
BT4 Cereal products
BT5 Plant foods
BT6 Foods
BT2 Processing
BT3 Technology
NT1 Loaf vol.

Bread manufacture
USE **Breadmaking**

Bread rolls
BT1 Bread
BT2 Bakery products
BT3 Cereal products
BT4 Plant foods
BT5 Foods

Breakage
BT1 Damage

Breakdown
BT1 Decomposition

Breakfast
BT1 Meals
BT2 Processed foods
BT3 Foods
NT1 Breakfast foods
RT Morning goods

Breakfast cereals
BT1 Cereal products
BT2 Plant foods
BT3 Foods

Breakfast foods
BT1 Breakfast
BT2 Meals
BT3 Processed foods
BT4 Foods

Bream
BT1 Freshwater fish
BT2 Fish
BT3 Animals
BT3 Sea foods
BT4 Aquatic foods
BT5 Animal foods
BT6 Foods

Breast cancer
BT1 Cancer
BT2 Diseases

Breast feeding
BT1 Human physiology
BT2 Physiology
BT3 Science
RT Human lactation
RT Human milk
RT Weaning

Breast milk
USE **Human milk**

Breed
HN heading up to vol. 24 (1992)
RT Genetics
RT var

Breeding
RT Crossbreeding
RT Genetics

Bregott
BT1 Dairy products
BT2 Animal foods
BT3 Foods

Bresaola
BT1 Meat products
BT2 Animal foods
BT3 Foods

Brettanomyces
BT1 Yeasts
BT2 Fungi
BT3 Microorganisms
NT1 *Brettanomyces anomalus*
NT1 *Brettanomyces bruxellensis*
NT1 *Brettanomyces intermedius*

Brettanomyces anomalus
HN introduced from vol. 39, issue 1 (2007)
SN anamorph of Dekkera anomala
BT1 *Brettanomyces*
BT2 Yeasts
BT3 Fungi
BT4 Microorganisms

Brettanomyces bruxellensis
SN anamorph of Dekkera bruxellensis; synonymous with Brettanomyces custersii
BT1 *Brettanomyces*
BT2 Yeasts
BT3 Fungi
BT4 Microorganisms

Brettanomyces intermedius
HN introduced from vol. 39, issue 1 (2007)
BT1 *Brettanomyces*
BT2 Yeasts
BT3 Fungi
BT4 Microorganisms

Brevetoxins
BT1 Toxins
BT2 Residues
RT Paralytic shellfish poisoning
RT Paralytic shellfish toxins

Brevibacillus
HN introduced from vol. 39, issue 1 (2007)
BT1 Bacteria
BT2 Microorganisms

Brevibacterium
HN heading from vol. 30 (1998); under Bacteria up to vol. 29 (1997)
BT1 Bacteria
BT2 Microorganisms
NT1 *Brevibacterium flavum*
NT1 *Brevibacterium helvolum*
NT1 *Brevibacterium lactofermentum*
NT1 *Brevibacterium linens*

Brevibacterium flavum
BT1 *Brevibacterium*
BT2 Bacteria
BT3 Microorganisms

Brevibacterium helvolum
SN synonymous with Pseudoclavibacter helvolus
BT1 *Brevibacterium*
BT2 Bacteria
BT3 Microorganisms

Brevibacterium lactofermentum
SN synonymous with Corynebacterium glutamicum
BT1 *Brevibacterium*
BT2 Bacteria
BT3 Microorganisms

Brevibacterium linens
BT1 *Brevibacterium*

BT2 Bacteria
BT3 Microorganisms

Brevoortia tyrannus
BT1 Menhaden
BT2 Marine fish
BT3 Fish
BT4 Animals
BT4 Sea foods
BT5 Aquatic foods
BT6 Animal foods
BT7 Foods

Breweries
BT1 Brewing
BT2 Processing
BT3 Technology
NT1 Breweries effluents
NT1 Inn breweries
NT1 Microbreweries

Breweries effluents
BT1 Breweries
BT2 Brewing
BT3 Processing
BT4 Technology
BT1 Effluents
BT2 Waste water
BT3 Wastes
BT3 Water

Brewers grains
BT1 Brewing by-products
BT2 By-products
NT1 Brewers spent grains

Brewers spent grains
BT1 Brewers grains
BT2 Brewing by-products
BT3 By-products

Brewers yeasts
SN index heading is Yeasts brewers
BT1 Yeasts brewers
BT2 *Saccharomyces*
BT3 Yeasts
BT4 Fungi
BT5 Microorganisms
NT1 Bottom fermenting yeasts
NT1 Top fermenting yeasts
RT Beer
RT Brewing

Brewing
BT1 Processing
BT2 Technology
NT1 Breweries
NT2 Breweries effluents
NT2 Inn breweries
NT2 Microbreweries
NT1 Brewing adjuncts
NT1 Brewing industry
NT1 High gravity brewing
NT1 Hopping
RT Beer
RT Bottom fermenting yeasts
RT Brewers yeasts
RT Fermentation
RT Hops
RT Malting
RT Mashing
RT Stillage
RT Top fermenting yeasts
RT Worts
RT Yeasts brewers
UF Beermaking
UF Beer manufacture

Brewing adjuncts
BT1 Brewing
BT2 Processing
BT3 Technology

Brewing by-products
BT1 By-products
NT1 Brewers grains
NT2 Brewers spent grains

Brewing industry
BT1 Brewing
BT2 Processing
BT3 Technology
BT1 Food industry
BT2 Industries

Brick tea
HN under Teas up to vol. 42 (2010)
BT1 Tea
BT2 Teas
BT3 Beverages
BT3 Crops
BT4 Plants
BT3 Plant foods
BT4 Foods

Brie cheese
BT1 Cheese varieties
BT2 Cheese
BT3 Dairy products
BT4 Animal foods
BT5 Foods

Brightness
BT1 Optical properties
BT2 Physical properties

Brilliance
BT1 Optical properties
BT2 Physical properties

Brilliant Blue
BT1 Colorants
BT2 Additives

Brined cucumbers
USE **Cucumber pickles**

Brined meat
BT1 Meat products
BT2 Animal foods
BT3 Foods

Brines
BT1 Brining
BT2 Processing
BT3 Technology

Brining
BT1 Processing
BT2 Technology
NT1 Brines
NT1 Curing brines
RT Curing
RT Pickling
RT Salt
RT Salting

Brinjal
USE **Aubergines**

Brioches
BT1 Bakery products
BT2 Cereal products
BT3 Plant foods
BT4 Foods

Briquetting
BT1 Pressing
BT2 Processing
BT3 Technology

British Honduras
USE **Belize**

Brix values
BT1 Density
BT2 Physical properties
RT Solids

Broad beans
HN heading up to vol. 24 (1992); under Faba beans from vol. 25 (1993)
BT1 Faba beans
BT2 Legumes
BT3 Vegetables specific
BT4 Vegetables
BT5 Crops
BT6 Plants
BT5 Plant foods
BT6 Foods

Broccoli
HN heading from vol. 30 (1998); under Vegetables specific up to vol. 29 (1997)
BT1 Vegetables specific
BT2 Vegetables
BT3 Crops
BT4 Plants
BT3 Plant foods
BT4 Foods

Brochothrix
BT1 Bacteria
BT2 Microorganisms
NT1 *Brochothrix thermosphacta*

Brochothrix thermosphacta
BT1 *Brochothrix*
BT2 Bacteria
BT3 Microorganisms

Broiler carcasses
USE **Chicken carcasses**

Broiler meat
USE **Chicken meat**

Broiler muscles
USE **Chicken meat**

Broilers
HN types of chicken not specified in the index from vol. 25 (1993)

USE **Chickens**

Broiling
BT1 Cooking
BT2 Thermal processing
BT3 Processing thermal
BT4 Processing
BT5 Technology

Bromates
BT1 Bakery additives
BT2 Additives
BT1 Salts
NT1 Potassium bromate

Bromelains
SN EC 3.4.22.32; EC 3.4.22.33
BT1 Proteinases
BT2 Hydrolases
BT3 Enzymes

Bromides
BT1 Salts
RT Br

Bromine
USE **Br**

Bromocyclen
BT1 Acaricides
BT2 Pesticides
BT3 Biocides
BT3 Residues
BT1 Organochlorine insecticides
BT2 Insecticides
BT3 Pesticides
BT4 Biocides
BT4 Residues
BT2 Organochlorine pesticides
BT3 Pesticides
BT4 Biocides
BT4 Residues

Bromomethane
USE **Methyl bromide**

Bromophenols
HN introduced from vol. 39, issue 1 (2007)
BT1 Organobromine compounds
BT2 Organic halogen compounds
BT1 Phenols
BT2 Alcohols
BT2 Aromatic compounds
BT3 Organic compounds

Bromophos
BT1 Organophosphorus insecticides
BT2 Insecticides
BT3 Pesticides
BT4 Biocides
BT4 Residues
BT2 Organophosphorus pesticides
BT3 Pesticides
BT4 Biocides
BT4 Residues

Bromoxynil
BT1 Herbicides
BT2 Pesticides
BT3 Biocides
BT3 Residues

Brook trout
HN introduced from vol. 39, issue 1 (2007)
BT1 Trout
BT2 Oily fish
BT3 Fish
BT4 Animals
BT4 Sea foods
BT5 Aquatic foods
BT6 Animal foods
BT7 Foods

Broths
BT1 Soups
BT2 Processed foods
BT3 Foods

Brown heart
BT1 Plant disorders
BT2 Diseases plant
BT3 Diseases

Brownies
BT1 Bakery products
BT2 Cereal products
BT3 Plant foods
BT4 Foods

Browning
NT1 Browning agents
NT1 Browning inhibitors
NT2 4-Hexylresorcinol
NT2 Kojic acid
NT1 Enzymic browning
NT1 Nonenzymic browning
RT Discoloration
RT Furosine
RT Spoilage
UF Browning reactions

Browning agents
BT1 Browning

Browning inhibitors
BT1 Browning
NT1 4-Hexylresorcinol
NT1 Kojic acid

Browning reactions
USE **Browning**

Browning susceptors
USE **Microwave susceptors**

Brown rice
BT1 Rice
BT2 Cereals
BT3 Crops
BT4 Plants
BT3 Seeds
BT4 Plant foods
BT5 Foods

Brown rot
BT1 Rots
BT2 Plant diseases
BT3 Diseases plant
BT4 Diseases

Brown sugar
BT1 Sugar
BT2 Plant foods
BT3 Foods

Brown trout
BT1 Trout
BT2 Oily fish
BT3 Fish
BT4 Animals
BT4 Sea foods
BT5 Aquatic foods
BT6 Animal foods
BT7 Foods
RT Sea trout

Brucella
BT1 Bacteria
BT2 Microorganisms
RT Brucellosis

Brucellosis
BT1 Animal diseases
BT2 Diseases animal
BT3 Diseases
BT1 Diseases
RT *Brucella*

Bruehwurst
BT1 Sausages
BT2 Meat products
BT3 Animal foods
BT4 Foods

Bruising
BT1 Damage

Brunei
HN present as Brunei Darussalam up to vol. 39, issue 1 (2007)
BT1 Asia

Brussels sprouts
BT1 Vegetables specific
BT2 Vegetables
BT3 Crops
BT4 Plants
BT3 Plant foods
BT4 Foods

Bryndza cheese
BT1 Cheese varieties
BT2 Cheese
BT3 Dairy products
BT4 Animal foods
BT5 Foods

BSE
BT1 Prion diseases
BT2 Diseases
RT CJD
UF Bovine spongiform encephalopathy

Bubble gums
HN under Chewing gums up to vol. 29 (1997)

BT1 Gum confectionery
BT2 Sugar confectionery
BT3 Plant foods
BT4 Foods

Bubbles
RT Aeration
RT Carbonation
RT Gases

Buchu oils
BT1 Essential oils
BT2 Flavourings
BT3 Additives
BT2 Vegetable oils
BT3 Oils vegetable
BT4 Oils
BT5 Lipids
BT6 Nutrients
BT4 Vegetable products
BT5 Plant foods
BT6 Foods

Buckwheat
BT1 Pseudocereals
BT2 Seeds
BT3 Plant foods
BT4 Foods
NT1 Buckwheat flour
NT1 Buckwheat starch

Buckwheat flour
BT1 Buckwheat
BT2 Pseudocereals
BT3 Seeds
BT4 Plant foods
BT5 Foods
BT1 Cereal flours
BT2 Flours cereal
BT3 Cereal products
BT4 Plant foods
BT5 Foods

Buckwheat starch
HN introduced from vol. 39, issue 1 (2007)
BT1 Buckwheat
BT2 Pseudocereals
BT3 Seeds
BT4 Plant foods
BT5 Foods
BT1 Starch
BT2 Glucans
BT3 Polysaccharides
BT4 Carbohydrates
BT5 Nutrients
BT5 Organic compounds
BT2 Thickeners
BT3 Additives

Budu
BT1 Anchovy
BT2 Marine fish
BT3 Fish
BT4 Animals
BT4 Sea foods
BT5 Aquatic foods
BT6 Animal foods
BT7 Foods
BT2 Oily fish
BT3 Fish
BT4 Animals
BT4 Sea foods
BT5 Aquatic foods
BT6 Animal foods
BT7 Foods
BT1 Fermented foods
BT2 Processed foods
BT3 Foods
BT1 Fish sauces
BT2 Fish products
BT3 Sea foods
BT4 Aquatic foods
BT5 Animal foods
BT6 Foods
BT2 Sauces
BT3 Condiments
BT4 Flavourings
BT5 Additives

Buffalo butter
BT1 Buffaloes
BT2 Animals
BT1 Butter
BT2 Dairy products
BT3 Animal foods
BT4 Foods

Buffalo carcasses
BT1 Buffalo meat
BT2 Buffaloes
BT3 Animals
BT2 Meat specific
BT3 Meat
BT4 Animal foods
BT5 Foods
BT1 Carcasses
BT2 Meat
BT3 Animal foods
BT4 Foods

Buffalo cheese
BT1 Buffaloes
BT2 Animals
BT1 Cheese varieties
BT2 Cheese
BT3 Dairy products
BT4 Animal foods
BT5 Foods
NT1 Buffalo mozzarella cheese
UF Buffalo milk cheese

Buffaloes
BT1 Animals
NT1 Buffalo butter
NT1 Buffalo cheese
NT2 Buffalo mozzarella cheese
NT1 Buffalo meat
NT2 Buffalo carcasses
NT1 Buffalo milk
NT2 Shrikhand
NT1 Buffalo yoghurt
NT1 Carabao
RT Bison

Buffalo gourds
BT1 Gourds
BT2 Vegetables specific
BT3 Vegetables
BT4 Crops
BT5 Plants
BT4 Plant foods
BT5 Foods

Buffalo meat
BT1 Buffaloes
BT2 Animals
BT1 Meat specific
BT2 Meat
BT3 Animal foods
BT4 Foods
NT1 Buffalo carcasses
RT Bison meat

Buffalo milk
BT1 Buffaloes
BT2 Animals
BT1 Milk
BT2 Dairy products
BT3 Animal foods
BT4 Foods
NT1 Shrikhand

Buffalo milk cheese
USE **Buffalo cheese**

Buffalo mozzarella cheese
BT1 Buffalo cheese
BT2 Buffaloes
BT3 Animals
BT2 Cheese varieties
BT3 Cheese
BT4 Dairy products
BT5 Animal foods
BT6 Foods
BT1 Mozzarella cheese
BT2 Cheese varieties
BT3 Cheese
BT4 Dairy products
BT5 Animal foods
BT6 Foods

Buffalo yoghurt
BT1 Buffaloes
BT2 Animals
BT1 Yoghurt
BT2 Fermented milk
BT3 Fermented dairy products
BT4 Dairy products
BT5 Animal foods
BT6 Foods
BT4 Fermented foods
BT5 Processed foods
BT6 Foods
BT3 Milk
BT4 Dairy products
BT5 Animal foods
BT6 Foods

Buffering capacity
BT1 Functional properties
BT2 Physical properties

Bulgaria
HN heading up to vol. 24 (1992)
BT1 Europe

Bulgur
BT1 Wheat
BT2 Cereals
BT3 Crops

BT4 Plants
BT3 Seeds
BT4 Plant foods
BT5 Foods

Bulk density
BT1 Density
BT2 Physical properties

Bulking agents
BT1 Thickeners
BT2 Additives
NT1 Methylcellulose

Bull carcasses
USE **Cattle carcasses**

Bull muscles
USE **Beef**

Bulls
HN types of cattle not specified in the index from vol. 25 (1993)
USE **Cattle**

Buns
BT1 Bakery products
BT2 Cereal products
BT3 Plant foods
BT4 Foods

Bupirimate
BT1 Fungicides
BT2 Pesticides
BT3 Biocides
BT3 Residues

Burbot
BT1 Freshwater fish
BT2 Fish
BT3 Animals
BT3 Sea foods
BT4 Aquatic foods
BT5 Animal foods
BT6 Foods

Burdock
BT1 Vegetables specific
BT2 Vegetables
BT3 Crops
BT4 Plants
BT3 Plant foods
BT4 Foods

Burfee
BT1 Dairy products
BT2 Animal foods
BT3 Foods
UF Burfi

Burfi
USE **Burfee**

Burgers
BT1 Meat products
BT2 Animal foods
BT3 Foods
NT1 Baconburgers
NT1 Beefburgers
NT1 Cheeseburgers
NT1 Hamburgers

Burgos cheese
BT1 Cheese varieties
BT2 Cheese
BT3 Dairy products
BT4 Animal foods
BT5 Foods

Burkholderia
BT1 Bacteria
BT2 Microorganisms
NT1 *Burkholderia cepacia*
NT1 *Burkholderia gladioli*
RT *Pseudomonas*

Burkholderia cepacia
SN synonymous with Pseudomonas cepacia
BT1 *Burkholderia*
BT2 Bacteria
BT3 Microorganisms

Burkholderia gladioli
BT1 *Burkholderia*
BT2 Bacteria
BT3 Microorganisms

Burkina Faso
BT1 West Africa
BT2 Africa
UF Upper Volta

Burma
HN used up to vol. 29 (1997)
USE **Myanmar**

Burundi
BT1 Central Africa
BT2 Africa

Bush butter
BT1 Fruits specific
BT2 Fruits
BT3 Crops
BT4 Plants
BT3 Plant foods
BT4 Foods

Bush okra
USE **Ewedu**

Butanal
SN syn. butyraldehyde
BT1 Aldehydes
BT2 Carbonyl compounds
BT3 Organic compounds
BT1 Volatile compounds

Butane
BT1 Gases
BT2 Physical phases
BT3 Chemistry
BT4 Science
BT1 Hydrocarbons
BT2 Organic compounds

1,3-Butanediol
USE **1,3-Butylene glycol**

2,3-Butanediol
USE **2,3-Butylene glycol**

2,3-Butanedione
HN under Flavour compounds and Ketones up to vol. 42 (2010)
SN syn. diacetyl
BT1 Diacetyl
BT2 Aroma compounds
BT3 Flavour compounds
BT3 Volatile compounds
BT2 Diketones
BT3 Ketones
BT4 Carbonyl compounds
BT5 Organic compounds

Butanoic acid
HN under Butyric acid up to vol. 42 (2010)
SN syn. butyric acid
BT1 Aroma compounds
BT2 Flavour compounds
BT2 Volatile compounds
BT1 Saturated fatty acids
BT2 Fatty acids
BT3 Lipids
BT4 Nutrients
BT3 Organic acids
BT4 Acids
BT1 Short chain fatty acids
BT2 Volatile fatty acids
BT3 Fatty acids
BT4 Lipids
BT5 Nutrients
BT4 Organic acids
BT5 Acids
BT3 Volatile compounds
NT1 Butyric acid

Butanol
HN also under Flavour compounds up to vol. 42 (2010)
SN syn. butyl alcohol
BT1 Alcohols
BT1 Aroma compounds
BT2 Flavour compounds
BT2 Volatile compounds
NT1 Butyl alcohol

Butanone
HN also under Flavour compounds up to vol. 42 (2010)
BT1 Aroma compounds
BT2 Flavour compounds
BT2 Volatile compounds
BT1 Ketones
BT2 Carbonyl compounds
BT3 Organic compounds

Butcheries
BT1 Slaughterhouses

Butonate
BT1 Organophosphorus insecticides
BT2 Insecticides
BT3 Pesticides
BT4 Biocides
BT4 Residues
BT2 Organophosphorus pesticides
BT3 Pesticides
BT4 Biocides
BT4 Residues

Butralin
BT1 Herbicides
BT2 Pesticides
BT3 Biocides
BT3 Residues

Butter
BT1 Dairy products
BT2 Animal foods
BT3 Foods
NT1 Buffalo butter
NT1 Butter spreads
NT1 Samna
NT1 Smen
RT Buttermaking
RT Fats milk
RT Ghee
RT Milk fats

Butter beans
USE **Lima beans**

Butterbur
BT1 Vegetables specific
BT2 Vegetables
BT3 Crops
BT4 Plants
BT3 Plant foods
BT4 Foods

Butter factories
BT1 Buttermaking
BT2 Processing
BT3 Technology
BT1 Food factories

Butterfat
BT1 Milk fats
BT2 Fats milk
BT3 Fats animal
BT4 Animal foods
BT5 Foods
BT4 Fats
BT5 Lipids
BT6 Nutrients

Butterfish
SN syn. pomfret
BT1 Pomfret
BT2 Marine fish
BT3 Fish
BT4 Animals
BT4 Sea foods
BT5 Aquatic foods
BT6 Animal foods
BT7 Foods

Butterine
BT1 Spreads
BT2 Processed foods
BT3 Foods

Buttermaking
BT1 Processing
BT2 Technology
NT1 Butter factories
NT1 Churning
RT Butter
RT Buttermilk
RT Butter starters
RT Starters
UF Butter manufacture

Butter manufacture
USE **Buttermaking**

Buttermilk
BT1 Dairy products
BT2 Animal foods
BT3 Foods
NT1 Cultured buttermilk
NT1 Rabadi
RT Buttermaking
RT Fermented milk

Butternuts
BT1 Nuts
BT2 Fruits
BT3 Crops
BT4 Plants
BT3 Plant foods
BT4 Foods
BT2 Oilseeds
BT3 Seeds
BT4 Plant foods
BT5 Foods

Butter oils
BT1 Milk fats
BT2 Fats milk
BT3 Fats animal
BT4 Animal foods
BT5 Foods
BT4 Fats
BT5 Lipids
BT6 Nutrients

Butterscotch
BT1 Sugar confectionery
BT2 Plant foods
BT3 Foods

Butter spreads
BT1 Butter
BT2 Dairy products
BT3 Animal foods
BT4 Foods
BT1 Spreads
BT2 Processed foods
BT3 Foods

Butter starters
BT1 Starters
BT2 Bacteria
BT3 Microorganisms
RT Buttermaking

Butter substitutes
BT1 Simulated foods
BT2 Processed foods
BT3 Foods

Butyl acetate
HN introduced from vol. 41, issue 1 (2009)
BT1 Acetates
BT1 Aroma compounds
BT2 Flavour compounds
BT2 Volatile compounds
BT1 Esters
BT2 Organic compounds

Butyl alcohol
HN also under Flavour compounds up to vol. 42 (2010)
SN syn. butanol
BT1 Butanol
BT2 Alcohols
BT2 Aroma compounds
BT3 Flavour compounds
BT3 Volatile compounds

Butylamine
SN syn. 2-aminobutane
BT1 Fungicides
BT2 Pesticides
BT3 Biocides
BT3 Residues
UF Tutane

Butylated hydroxyanisole
USE **BHA**

Butylated hydroxytoluene
USE **BHT**

1,3-Butylene glycol
BT1 Glycols
BT2 Alcohols
UF 1,3-Butanediol

2,3-Butylene glycol
BT1 Glycols
BT2 Alcohols
UF 2,3-Butanediol

Butyltins
BT1 Organotin compounds
BT2 Contaminants
BT3 Contamination
BT2 Organic compounds
NT1 Tributyltin

Butyraldehyde
SN syn. butanal
BT1 Aldehydes
BT2 Carbonyl compounds
BT3 Organic compounds
BT1 Volatile compounds

Butyric acid
HN heading up to vol. 42 (2010)
SN syn. butanoic acid
BT1 Butanoic acid
BT2 Aroma compounds
BT3 Flavour compounds
BT3 Volatile compounds
BT2 Saturated fatty acids
BT3 Fatty acids
BT4 Lipids
BT5 Nutrients
BT4 Organic acids
BT5 Acids
BT2 Short chain fatty acids
BT3 Volatile fatty acids
BT4 Fatty acids
BT5 Lipids
BT6 Nutrients
BT5 Organic acids
BT6 Acids
BT4 Volatile compounds
RT Butyric fermentation

Butyric fermentation
BT1 Fermentation
RT Butyric acid

Butyrivibrio
HN introduced from vol. 43, issue 1 (2011)
BT1 Bacteria
BT2 Microorganisms
NT1 *Butyrivibrio fibrisolvens*

Butyrivibrio fibrisolvens
HN introduced from vol. 39, issue 1 (2007)
BT1 *Butyrivibrio*
BT2 Bacteria
BT3 Microorganisms

Butyrometers
BT1 Apparatus
BT2 Technology

Butyrophilin
BT1 Milk proteins
BT2 Proteins milk
BT3 Animal proteins
BT4 Proteins animal
BT5 Proteins
BT6 Nutrients

Buyers guides
RT Directories

Byelorussia
USE **Belarus**

By-products
NT1 Brewing by-products
NT2 Brewers grains
NT3 Brewers spent grains
NT1 Cereal by-products
NT1 Coffee grounds
NT1 Distillers grains
NT2 Distillers spent grains
NT1 Hides
NT1 Lees
NT1 Marc
NT2 Grape marc
RT Offal
RT Wastes

Byssochlamic acid
BT1 Mycotoxins
BT2 Toxins
BT3 Residues
RT *Byssochlamys*

Byssochlamys
BT1 Fungi
BT2 Microorganisms
NT1 *Byssochlamys fulva*
RT Byssochlamic acid
RT Patulin

Byssochlamys fulva
BT1 *Byssochlamys*
BT2 Fungi
BT3 Microorganisms

C

C
SN index heading is Carbon
BT1 Carbon
BT2 Elements
BT3 Minerals
BT4 Nutrients

Ca
SN index heading is Calcium
BT1 Calcium
BT2 Metals
BT3 Elements
BT4 Minerals
BT5 Nutrients

Cabbage juices
BT1 Vegetable juices
BT2 Soft drinks
BT3 Beverages
BT2 Vegetable products
BT3 Plant foods
BT4 Foods

Cabbages
BT1 Vegetables specific
BT2 Vegetables
BT3 Crops
BT4 Plants
BT3 Plant foods
BT4 Foods
NT1 Red cabbages
NT1 Sauerkraut
NT1 Savoy cabbages
NT1 White cabbages

Cabrales cheese
BT1 Cheese varieties
BT2 Cheese
BT3 Dairy products
BT4 Animal foods
BT5 Foods

Cacao
USE **Cocoa**

Cacao beans
USE **Cocoa beans**

Cachaca
HN introduced from vol. 39, issue 1 (2007)
BT1 Sugar cane spirits
BT2 Spirits
BT3 Alcoholic beverages
BT4 Beverages alcoholic
BT5 Beverages

Caciocavallo cheese
HN introduced from vol. 41, issue 1 (2009)
BT1 Cheese varieties
BT2 Cheese
BT3 Dairy products
BT4 Animal foods
BT5 Foods
NT1 Caciocavallo Palermitano cheese

Caciocavallo Palermitano cheese
BT1 Caciocavallo cheese
BT2 Cheese varieties
BT3 Cheese
BT4 Dairy products
BT5 Animal foods
BT6 Foods

Cacioricotta cheese
BT1 Cheese varieties
BT2 Cheese
BT3 Dairy products
BT4 Animal foods
BT5 Foods

Caciotta cheese
BT1 Cheese varieties
BT2 Cheese
BT3 Dairy products
BT4 Animal foods
BT5 Foods

$CaCl_2$
HN also under Calcium up to vol. 42 (2010)
BT1 Additives
BT1 Chlorides
BT2 Salts
UF Calcium chloride

Cacodylic acid
USE **Dimethylarsinic acid**

Cacti
BT1 Fruits specific
BT2 Fruits
BT3 Crops
BT4 Plants
BT3 Plant foods
BT4 Foods

Cactus fruits
USE **Cactus pears**

Cactus pears
SN syn. prickly pears
BT1 Fruits specific
BT2 Fruits
BT3 Crops
BT4 Plants
BT3 Plant foods
BT4 Foods
UF Cactus fruits

Cadaba farinosa
BT1 Plants

Cadaverine
BT1 Biogenic amines
BT2 Amines
BT3 Organic nitrogen compounds

Cadmium
SN symbol Cd is also used in the index
BT1 Metals
BT2 Elements
BT3 Minerals
BT4 Nutrients
NT1 Cd

Caesium
USE **Cs**

Cafestol
BT1 Alcohols
BT1 Diterpenoids
BT2 Terpenoids
BT3 Lipids
BT4 Nutrients

Cafeterias
BT1 Restaurants

Caffeic acid
BT1 Organic acids
BT2 Acids
BT1 Phenols
BT2 Alcohols
BT2 Aromatic compounds
BT3 Organic compounds

Caffeine
BT1 Alkaloids
BT2 Organic nitrogen compounds
BT1 Purines
BT2 Heterocyclic compounds
BT2 Organic nitrogen compounds
RT Coffee
RT Decaffeination
RT Tea

Caffeoylquinic acid
SN syn. chlorogenic acid
BT1 Chlorogenic acid
BT2 Organic acids
BT3 Acids
BT2 Phenols
BT3 Alcohols
BT3 Aromatic compounds
BT4 Organic compounds

Caja
BT1 Fruits specific
BT2 Fruits
BT3 Crops
BT4 Plants
BT3 Plant foods
BT4 Foods

Cake batters
BT1 Cakes
BT2 Bakery products
BT3 Cereal products
BT4 Plant foods
BT5 Foods
RT Batters

Cake mixes
BT1 Cakes
BT2 Bakery products
BT3 Cereal products
BT4 Plant foods
BT5 Foods
BT1 Mixes
BT2 Dried foods
BT3 Processed foods
BT4 Foods
BT2 Instant foods
BT3 Processed foods
BT4 Foods
RT Bakery product mixes

Cakes
BT1 Bakery products
BT2 Cereal products
BT3 Plant foods
BT4 Foods
NT1 Angel cakes
NT1 Baumkuchen
NT1 Cake batters
NT1 Cake mixes
NT1 Christstollen
NT1 Gateaux
NT1 Muffins
NT1 Sponge cakes
NT1 Stollen
NT1 Swiss rolls
NT1 Torten
RT Bakers confectionery

Caking
BT1 Solidification

Calamintha
HN under Spices up to vol. 42 (2010)
BT1 Herbs
BT2 Spices
BT3 Flavourings
BT4 Additives

Calamus
BT1 Flavourings
BT2 Additives
BT1 Plants
UF *Acorus calamus*

Calciferol
USE **Vitamin D_2**

Calcium
SN symbol Ca is also used in the index
BT1 Metals
BT2 Elements
BT3 Minerals
BT4 Nutrients
NT1 Ca

Calcium chloride
USE **$CaCl_2$**

Calcium hydroxide
USE **$Ca(OH)_2$**

Calcium lactate
HN introduced from vol. 39, issue 1 (2007)
BT1 Lactates
BT2 Preservatives
BT3 Additives
BT2 Salts

Calcium tartrate
BT1 Tartrates
BT2 Salts
RT Tartaric acid

Calendula officinalis
BT1 Plants

Calf carcasses
BT1 Beef
BT2 Meat specific
BT3 Meat
BT4 Animal foods
BT5 Foods
BT1 Carcasses
BT2 Meat
BT3 Animal foods
BT4 Foods

Calf meat
USE **Beef**

Calf muscles
USE **Beef**

Calf rennets
BT1 Rennets
BT2 Milk clotting enzymes
BT3 Enzymes milk clotting
BT4 Proteinases
BT5 Hydrolases
BT6 Enzymes

Caliciviruses
SN for descriptive use only
BT1 Viruses
BT2 Microorganisms
NT1 Noroviruses
NT2 Norovirus
NT3 Norwalk virus
NT4 Norwalk-like virus
NT4 Small round structured virus
NT1 Sapoviruses
NT2 Sapovirus
NT3 Sapporo virus

Callinectes sapidus
BT1 Blue crabs
BT2 Crabs
BT3 Crustacea
BT4 Shellfish
BT5 Animals
BT5 Sea foods
BT6 Aquatic foods
BT7 Animal foods
BT8 Foods

Callipyge phenotype
BT1 Genetic disorders

Callus culture
BT1 Cell culture

Calmodulin
BT1 Proteins
BT2 Nutrients

Calocybe
BT1 Edible fungi
BT2 Fungi edible
BT3 Vegetables specific
BT4 Vegetables
BT5 Crops
BT6 Plants
BT5 Plant foods
BT6 Foods

Calories
BT1 Nutrition
NT1 Calories high foods

NT1 Calories low beverages
NT1 Calories low diet
NT1 Calories low foods
NT2 Calories low spreads
RT Calorific values
RT Health foods
RT Nutritional values

Calories high foods
BT1 Calories
BT2 Nutrition
UF High calorie foods

Calories low beverages
HN introduced from vol. 41, issue 1 (2009)
BT1 Beverages
BT1 Calories
BT2 Nutrition
RT Lite beverages
UF Diet drinks
UF Low calorie beverages

Calories low diet
HN introduced from vol. 38, issue 8 (2006)
BT1 Calories
BT2 Nutrition
BT1 Diet therapy
BT2 Diet
BT3 Nutrition
BT2 Therapy
UF Low calorie diet

Calories low foods
BT1 Calories
BT2 Nutrition
NT1 Calories low spreads
RT Lite foods
UF Calories reduced foods
UF Low calorie foods

Calories low spreads
BT1 Calories low foods
BT2 Calories
BT3 Nutrition
BT1 Spreads
BT2 Processed foods
BT3 Foods
UF Low calorie spreads

Calories reduced foods
USE **Calories low foods**

Calorific values
BT1 Nutritional values
NT1 Energy density
RT Calories
UF Energy values

Calorimetry
BT1 Analytical techniques

Calpains
SN includes EC 3.4.22.52 and EC 3.4.22.53, formerly EC 3.4.22.17
BT1 Proteinases
BT2 Hydrolases
BT3 Enzymes
RT Calpastatins

Calpastatins
BT1 Proteinases inhibitors
BT2 Antinutritional factors
BT3 Nutritional values
BT2 Enzyme inhibitors
BT3 Enzymes
RT Calpains

Calvados
BT1 Apple brandy
BT2 Fruit brandies
BT3 Brandies
BT4 Spirits
BT5 Alcoholic beverages
BT6 Beverages alcoholic
BT7 Beverages

Calves
HN types of cattle not specified in the index from vol. 25 (1993)
USE **Cattle**

Cambodia
BT1 Asia
UF Kampuchea

Camel carcasses
BT1 Camel meat
BT2 Camels
BT3 Animals
BT2 Meat specific
BT3 Meat
BT4 Animal foods
BT5 Foods
BT1 Carcasses
BT2 Meat
BT3 Animal foods
BT4 Foods

Camelina oils
HN introduced from vol. 41, issue 1 (2009)
BT1 Vegetable oils
BT2 Oils vegetable
BT3 Oils
BT4 Lipids
BT5 Nutrients
BT3 Vegetable products
BT4 Plant foods
BT5 Foods

Camelina sativa
HN introduced from vol. 41, issue 1 (2009)
BT1 Oilseeds
BT2 Seeds
BT3 Plant foods
BT4 Foods
BT1 Plants

Camel meat
BT1 Camels
BT2 Animals
BT1 Meat specific
BT2 Meat
BT3 Animal foods
BT4 Foods
NT1 Camel carcasses

Camel milk
BT1 Camels
BT2 Animals
BT1 Milk
BT2 Dairy products
BT3 Animal foods
BT4 Foods
NT1 Shubat

Camels
HN heading from vol. 25 (1993); under Animals specific up to vol. 24 (1992)
BT1 Animals
NT1 Camel meat
NT2 Camel carcasses
NT1 Camel milk
NT2 Shubat

Camembert cheese
BT1 Cheese varieties
BT2 Cheese
BT3 Dairy products
BT4 Animal foods
BT5 Foods

Cameras
HN introduced from vol. 41, issue 1 (2009)
BT1 Apparatus
BT2 Technology
RT Imaging
RT Photography

Cameroon
BT1 West Africa
BT2 Africa

Cameros cheese
BT1 Cheese varieties
BT2 Cheese
BT3 Dairy products
BT4 Animal foods
BT5 Foods

Camomile
HN under Spices up to vol. 42 (2010)
SN syn. chamomile
BT1 Chamomile
BT2 Herbs
BT3 Spices
BT4 Flavourings
BT5 Additives

cAMP
BT1 Nucleotides

Campesterol
BT1 Sterols
BT2 Alcohols
BT2 Steroids
BT3 Lipids
BT4 Nutrients

Camphechlor
BT1 Acaricides
BT2 Pesticides
BT3 Biocides
BT3 Residues
BT1 Organochlorine insecticides
BT2 Insecticides
BT3 Pesticides
BT4 Biocides
BT4 Residues

BT2 Organochlorine pesticides
BT3 Pesticides
BT4 Biocides
BT4 Residues
UF Toxaphene

Camphene
BT1 Aroma compounds
BT2 Flavour compounds
BT2 Volatile compounds
BT1 Monoterpenes
BT2 Hydrocarbons
BT3 Organic compounds
BT2 Monoterpenoids
BT3 Terpenoids
BT4 Lipids
BT5 Nutrients

Camphor
BT1 Aroma compounds
BT2 Flavour compounds
BT2 Volatile compounds
BT1 Ketones
BT2 Carbonyl compounds
BT3 Organic compounds
BT1 Monoterpenoids
BT2 Terpenoids
BT3 Lipids
BT4 Nutrients

Campylobacter
HN heading from vol. 25 (1993); under Vibrio up to vol. 24 (1992)
BT1 Bacteria
BT2 Microorganisms
NT1 *Campylobacter coli*
NT1 *Campylobacter fetus*
NT1 *Campylobacter jejuni*
NT1 *Campylobacter lari*
RT Campylobacteriosis

Campylobacter coli
BT1 *Campylobacter*
BT2 Bacteria
BT3 Microorganisms

Campylobacter fetus
BT1 *Campylobacter*
BT2 Bacteria
BT3 Microorganisms

Campylobacteriosis
BT1 Diseases
BT1 Poisoning
RT *Campylobacter*

Campylobacter jejuni
BT1 *Campylobacter*
BT2 Bacteria
BT3 Microorganisms

Campylobacter lari
HN introduced from vol. 39, issue 1 (2007)
BT1 *Campylobacter*
BT2 Bacteria
BT3 Microorganisms

Camu-camu
BT1 Fruits specific
BT2 Fruits
BT3 Crops
BT4 Plants
BT3 Plant foods
BT4 Foods

Canada
HN heading up to vol. 24 (1992)
BT1 North America
BT2 America
RT Organization for Economic Cooperation and Development

Canapes
BT1 Snack foods
BT2 Processed foods
BT3 Foods

Canary grass
BT1 Pseudocereals
BT2 Seeds
BT3 Plant foods
BT4 Foods

Canary Islands
BT1 Spain
BT2 Europe
BT2 European Union

Canavalia ensiformis
BT1 Jack beans
BT2 Legumes
BT3 Vegetables specific
BT4 Vegetables
BT5 Crops
BT6 Plants
BT5 Plant foods
BT6 Foods

Canavalia gladiata
BT1 Sword beans
BT2 Legumes
BT3 Vegetables specific
BT4 Vegetables
BT5 Crops
BT6 Plants
BT5 Plant foods
BT6 Foods

Canavanine
BT1 Amino acids
BT2 Nutrients
BT2 Organic acids
BT3 Acids
BT2 Organic nitrogen compounds

Canbra oils
USE **Rapeseed oils**

Cancer
BT1 Diseases
NT1 Breast cancer
NT1 Colorectal cancer
NT1 Gastric cancer
NT1 Lung cancer
NT1 Ovarian cancer
NT1 Prostate cancer
RT Angiogenesis
RT Antimutagenicity
RT Carcinogenesis
RT Carcinogens
RT Mutagens
UF Tumours

Candida
SN formerly Monilia
BT1 Yeasts
BT2 Fungi
BT3 Microorganisms
NT1 *Candida albicans*
NT1 *Candida antarctica*
NT1 *Candida boidinii*
NT1 *Candida bombicola*
NT1 *Candida cylindracea*
NT1 *Candida famata*
NT1 *Candida glycerinogenes*
NT1 *Candida guilliermondii*
NT1 *Candida humilis*
NT2 *Candida milleri*
NT1 *Candida intermedia*
NT1 *Candida kefyr*
NT2 *Candida pseudotropicalis*
NT1 *Candida krusei*
NT1 *Candida lipolytica*
NT1 *Candida magnoliae*
NT1 *Candida maltosa*
NT1 *Candida mogii*
NT1 *Candida molischiana*
NT1 *Candida oleophila*
NT1 *Candida parapsilosis*
NT1 *Candida rugosa*
NT1 *Candida saitoana*
NT1 *Candida sake*
NT1 *Candida shehatae*
NT1 *Candida stellata*
NT1 *Candida tropicalis*
NT1 *Candida utilis*
NT1 *Candida valida*
NT1 *Candida versatilis*
NT1 *Candida wickerhamii*
NT1 *Candida zeylanoides*
NT1 Torula yeast

Candida albicans
BT1 *Candida*
BT2 Yeasts
BT3 Fungi
BT4 Microorganisms

Candida antarctica
BT1 *Candida*
BT2 Yeasts
BT3 Fungi
BT4 Microorganisms

Candida boidinii
BT1 *Candida*
BT2 Yeasts
BT3 Fungi
BT4 Microorganisms

Candida bombicola
BT1 *Candida*
BT2 Yeasts
BT3 Fungi
BT4 Microorganisms

Candida cylindracea
BT1 *Candida*
BT2 Yeasts

BT3 Fungi
BT4 Microorganisms

Candida famata
BT1 *Candida*
BT2 Yeasts
BT3 Fungi
BT4 Microorganisms

Candida glycerinogenes
BT1 *Candida*
BT2 Yeasts
BT3 Fungi
BT4 Microorganisms

Candida guilliermondii
SN anamorph of Pichia guilliermondii
BT1 *Candida*
BT2 Yeasts
BT3 Fungi
BT4 Microorganisms

Candida humilis
SN Genbank synonym is Candida milleri
BT1 *Candida*
BT2 Yeasts
BT3 Fungi
BT4 Microorganisms
NT1 *Candida milleri*

Candida intermedia
BT1 *Candida*
BT2 Yeasts
BT3 Fungi
BT4 Microorganisms

Candida kefyr
HN introduced from vol. 43, issue 1 (2011)
SN teleomorph is Kluyveromyces marxianus
BT1 *Candida*
BT2 Yeasts
BT3 Fungi
BT4 Microorganisms
NT1 *Candida pseudotropicalis*

Candida krusei
SN synonymous with Pichia kudriavzevii; teleomorph is Issatchenkia orientalis
BT1 *Candida*
BT2 Yeasts
BT3 Fungi
BT4 Microorganisms

Candida lipolytica
SN teleomorph is Yarrowia lipolytica
BT1 *Candida*
BT2 Yeasts
BT3 Fungi
BT4 Microorganisms

Candida magnoliae
BT1 *Candida*
BT2 Yeasts
BT3 Fungi
BT4 Microorganisms

Candida maltosa
HN introduced from vol. 39, issue 1 (2007)
BT1 *Candida*
BT2 Yeasts
BT3 Fungi
BT4 Microorganisms

Candida milleri
HN introduced from vol. 39, issue 1 (2007)
SN Genbank synonym of Candida humilis
BT1 *Candida humilis*
BT2 *Candida*
BT3 Yeasts
BT4 Fungi
BT5 Microorganisms

Candida mogii
BT1 *Candida*
BT2 Yeasts
BT3 Fungi
BT4 Microorganisms

Candida molischiana
HN introduced from vol. 39, issue 1 (2007)
BT1 *Candida*
BT2 Yeasts
BT3 Fungi
BT4 Microorganisms

Candida oleophila
HN introduced from vol. 39, issue 1 (2007)
BT1 *Candida*
BT2 Yeasts
BT3 Fungi
BT4 Microorganisms

Candida parapsilosis
BT1 *Candida*
BT2 Yeasts
BT3 Fungi
BT4 Microorganisms

Candida pseudotropicalis
SN anamorph is Candida kefyr; synonymous with Kluyveromyces marxianus
BT1 *Candida kefyr*
BT2 *Candida*
BT3 Yeasts
BT4 Fungi
BT5 Microorganisms

Candida rugosa
BT1 *Candida*
BT2 Yeasts
BT3 Fungi
BT4 Microorganisms

Candida saitoana
BT1 *Candida*
BT2 Yeasts
BT3 Fungi
BT4 Microorganisms

Candida sake
BT1 *Candida*
BT2 Yeasts
BT3 Fungi
BT4 Microorganisms

Candida shehatae
BT1 *Candida*
BT2 Yeasts
BT3 Fungi
BT4 Microorganisms

Candida stellata
BT1 *Candida*
BT2 Yeasts
BT3 Fungi
BT4 Microorganisms

Candida tropicalis
BT1 *Candida*
BT2 Yeasts
BT3 Fungi
BT4 Microorganisms

Candida utilis
SN anamorph of Pichia jadinii (common name Torula yeast)
BT1 *Candida*
BT2 Yeasts
BT3 Fungi
BT4 Microorganisms

Candida valida
SN Genbank anamorph of Pichia membranifaciens
BT1 *Candida*
BT2 Yeasts
BT3 Fungi
BT4 Microorganisms

Candida versatilis
BT1 *Candida*
BT2 Yeasts
BT3 Fungi
BT4 Microorganisms

Candida wickerhamii
BT1 *Candida*
BT2 Yeasts
BT3 Fungi
BT4 Microorganisms

Candida zeylanoides
BT1 *Candida*
BT2 Yeasts
BT3 Fungi
BT4 Microorganisms

Candied fruits
BT1 Fruit products
BT2 Plant foods
BT3 Foods

Candling
BT1 Analytical techniques

Candy
BT1 Sugar confectionery
BT2 Plant foods
BT3 Foods
NT1 Chewy candy

Candy floss
BT1 Sugar confectionery
BT2 Plant foods

BT3 Foods
RT Cotton candy

Cane molasses
BT1 Molasses
BT2 Sugar
BT3 Plant foods
BT4 Foods
RT Cane sugar
RT Sugar processes
UF Sugar cane molasses

Canestrato Pugliese cheese
BT1 Cheese varieties
BT2 Cheese
BT3 Dairy products
BT4 Animal foods
BT5 Foods

Cane sugar
BT1 Sugar
BT2 Plant foods
BT3 Foods
NT1 Bagasse
NT2 Sugar cane bagasse
NT1 Cane sugar factories
NT1 Cane sugar industry
NT1 Cane sugar products
NT1 Sugar cane bagasse
RT Cane molasses
RT Sugar cane
RT Sugar processes

Cane sugar factories
BT1 Cane sugar
BT2 Sugar
BT3 Plant foods
BT4 Foods
BT1 Food factories

Cane sugar industry
BT1 Cane sugar
BT2 Sugar
BT3 Plant foods
BT4 Foods
BT1 Food industry
BT2 Industries

Cane sugar juices
BT1 Sugar juices
BT2 Plant foods
BT3 Foods
RT Sugar processes
UF Sugar cane juices

Cane sugar products
BT1 Cane sugar
BT2 Sugar
BT3 Plant foods
BT4 Foods

Cane sugar syrups
BT1 Sugar syrups
BT2 Plant foods
BT3 Foods

Canisters
BT1 Containers

Canna
HN introduced from vol. 39, issue 1 (2007)
BT1 Vegetables specific
BT2 Vegetables
BT3 Crops
BT4 Plants
BT3 Plant foods
BT4 Foods
NT1 Canna starch

Canna starch
HN introduced from vol. 39, issue 1 (2007)
BT1 Canna
BT2 Vegetables specific
BT3 Vegetables
BT4 Crops
BT5 Plants
BT4 Plant foods
BT5 Foods
BT1 Starch
BT2 Glucans
BT3 Polysaccharides
BT4 Carbohydrates
BT5 Nutrients
BT5 Organic compounds
BT2 Thickeners
BT3 Additives

Canned foods
BT1 Processed foods
BT2 Foods
NT1 Canned pet foods
RT Canneries
RT Canning
RT Cans

Canned pet foods
HN introduced from vol. 39, issue 1 (2007)
BT1 Canned foods
BT2 Processed foods
BT3 Foods
BT1 Pet foods

Canneloni
BT1 Pasta
BT2 Cereal products
BT3 Plant foods
BT4 Foods

Canneries
BT1 Canning
BT2 Packaging
BT3 Technology
BT2 Preservation
BT3 Technology
RT Canned foods

Canning
BT1 Packaging
BT2 Technology
BT1 Preservation
BT2 Technology
NT1 Canneries
NT1 Canning equipment
NT1 Canning industry
NT1 Canning quality
RT Canned foods
RT Cans
RT Sterilization

Canning equipment
BT1 Canning
BT2 Packaging
BT3 Technology
BT2 Preservation
BT3 Technology

Canning industry
BT1 Canning
BT2 Packaging
BT3 Technology
BT2 Preservation
BT3 Technology
BT1 Food industry
BT2 Industries

Canning quality
BT1 Canning
BT2 Packaging
BT3 Technology
BT2 Preservation
BT3 Technology

Canola
USE **Rapeseeds**

Canola oils
USE **Rapeseed oils**

Canopy
BT1 Cultivation
BT2 Agriculture

Cans
BT1 Containers
RT Canned foods
RT Canning

Cantaloupes
BT1 Melons
BT2 Fruits specific
BT3 Fruits
BT4 Crops
BT5 Plants
BT4 Plant foods
BT5 Foods

Canteen meals
BT1 Meals
BT2 Processed foods
BT3 Foods
RT Canteens

Canteens
BT1 Restaurants
RT Canteen meals

Cantharellus
BT1 Edible fungi
BT2 Fungi edible
BT3 Vegetables specific
BT4 Vegetables
BT5 Crops
BT6 Plants
BT5 Plant foods
BT6 Foods
UF Chantarelles

Canthaxanthin
BT1 Xanthophylls
BT2 Carotenoids
BT3 Pigments
BT3 Terpenoids
BT4 Lipids
BT5 Nutrients

$Ca(OH)_2$
HN introduced from vol. 39, issue 1 (2007)
BT1 Alkalies
BT1 Hydroxides
BT2 Salts
UF Calcium hydroxide

CAP
BT1 Food policy
BT2 Economics
UF Common Agricultural Policy

Capacitance
BT1 Electrical properties
BT2 Physical properties

Cape gooseberries
SN syn. goldenberries
BT1 Fruits specific
BT2 Fruits
BT3 Crops
BT4 Plants
BT3 Plant foods
BT4 Foods
NT1 Goldenberries
UF Physalis

Capelin
BT1 Marine fish
BT2 Fish
BT3 Animals
BT3 Sea foods
BT4 Aquatic foods
BT5 Animal foods
BT6 Foods

Capers
BT1 Spices
BT2 Flavourings
BT3 Additives

Cape Verde
BT1 West Africa
BT2 Africa

Capillary electrochromatography
HN introduced from vol. 41, issue 1 (2009)
BT1 Chromatography
BT2 Analytical techniques

Capillary electrophoresis
HN electrophoresis capillary also used in the index up to vol. 29 (1997)
BT1 Electrophoresis
BT2 Analytical techniques

Capocollo
HN introduced from vol. 37, issue 5 (2005)
BT1 Sausages
BT2 Meat products
BT3 Animal foods
BT4 Foods

Capons
HN types of chicken not specified in the index from vol. 25 (1993)
USE **Chickens**

Capping devices
USE **Caps**

Cappuccino coffee
BT1 Coffee beverages
BT2 Coffee products
BT3 Coffee
BT4 Beverages
BT4 Crops
BT5 Plants
BT4 Plant foods
BT5 Foods

Caprenin
USE **Fat substitutes**

Capretto
HN introduced from vol. 37, issue 5 (2005)
BT1 Goat meat
BT2 Goats
BT3 Animals
BT2 Meat specific
BT3 Meat
BT4 Animal foods
BT5 Foods

Capric acid
HN under Flavour compounds and Fatty acids up to vol. 42 (2010)
SN syn. decanoic acid
BT1 Decanoic acid
BT2 Aroma compounds
BT3 Flavour compounds
BT3 Volatile compounds
BT2 Saturated fatty acids
BT3 Fatty acids
BT4 Lipids
BT5 Nutrients
BT4 Organic acids
BT5 Acids

Caprine
USE **Goats**

Caproic acid
HN under Flavour compounds and Fatty acids up to vol. 42 (2010)
SN syn. hexanoic acid
BT1 Hexanoic acid
BT2 Aroma compounds
BT3 Flavour compounds
BT3 Volatile compounds
BT2 Saturated fatty acids
BT3 Fatty acids
BT4 Lipids
BT5 Nutrients
BT4 Organic acids
BT5 Acids
BT2 Short chain fatty acids
BT3 Volatile fatty acids
BT4 Fatty acids
BT5 Lipids
BT6 Nutrients
BT5 Organic acids
BT6 Acids
BT4 Volatile compounds

Caprylic acid
HN under Flavour compounds and Fatty acids up to vol. 42 (2010)
SN syn. octanoic acid
BT1 Octanoic acid
BT2 Aroma compounds
BT3 Flavour compounds
BT3 Volatile compounds
BT2 Saturated fatty acids
BT3 Fatty acids
BT4 Lipids
BT5 Nutrients
BT4 Organic acids
BT5 Acids

Caps
BT1 Closures
BT2 Packaging
BT3 Technology
NT1 Screw caps
UF Capping devices

Capsaicin
BT1 Capsaicinoids
BT2 Amides
BT3 Organic nitrogen compounds
BT2 Pungent principles
BT3 Flavour compounds
RT Chilli
RT Chillies

Capsaicinoids
BT1 Amides
BT2 Organic nitrogen compounds
BT1 Pungent principles
BT2 Flavour compounds
NT1 Capsaicin
RT Chilli
RT Chillies

Capsanthin
BT1 Carotenoids
BT2 Pigments
BT2 Terpenoids
BT3 Lipids
BT4 Nutrients

Capsicum annuum
BT1 Capsicums
BT2 Vegetables specific
BT3 Vegetables
BT4 Crops
BT5 Plants
BT4 Plant foods
BT5 Foods

Capsicums
HN heading from vol. 25 (1993); under Peppers up to vol. 24 (1992)
BT1 Vegetables specific
BT2 Vegetables
BT3 Crops
BT4 Plants
BT3 Plant foods

BT4 Foods
NT1 Bell peppers
NT1 *Capsicum annuum*
NT1 Chillies
NT2 Jalapeno peppers
NT2 Red chillies
NT1 Green peppers
NT1 Hot peppers
NT1 Kochujang
NT1 Peppers
NT1 Pimento peppers
NT2 Pimiento peppers
NT1 Red peppers
NT1 Sweet peppers

Captafol
BT1 Dicarboximide fungicides
BT2 Fungicides
BT3 Pesticides
BT4 Biocides
BT4 Residues

Captan
BT1 Dicarboximide fungicides
BT2 Fungicides
BT3 Pesticides
BT4 Biocides
BT4 Residues
NT1 Tetrahydrophthalimide
UF Orthocide

Capybaras
BT1 Animals

Carabao
BT1 Buffaloes
BT2 Animals

Carambolas
SN syn. star fruit
BT1 Fruits specific
BT2 Fruits
BT3 Crops
BT4 Plants
BT3 Plant foods
BT4 Foods
NT1 Star fruit

Caramel
BT1 Flavourings
BT2 Additives

Caramel colorants
BT1 Colorants
BT2 Additives

Caramelization
HN introduced from vol. 41, issue 1 (2009)
RT Maillard reaction
RT Nonenzymic browning

Caramels
BT1 Sugar confectionery
BT2 Plant foods
BT3 Foods

Caraway
BT1 Spices
BT2 Flavourings
BT3 Additives

Carbadox
BT1 Drugs
BT2 Residues

Carbamate pesticides
BT1 Pesticides
BT2 Biocides
BT2 Residues
NT1 Asulam
NT1 Benomyl
NT1 Carbendazim
NT1 Carbetamide
NT1 Chlorpropham
NT1 Dimetilan
NT1 *N*-Methylcarbamate pesticides
NT2 *N*-Methylcarbamate insecticides
NT3 Aldicarb
NT3 Carbaryl
NT3 Carbofuran
NT3 Ethiofencarb
NT3 Methomyl
NT3 Oxamyl
NT3 Pirimicarb
NT3 Propoxur
NT1 Phenmedipham
NT1 Propham
NT1 Thiophanate
NT1 Thiophanate-methyl

Carbamide
SN syn. urea
BT1 Amides
BT2 Organic nitrogen compounds

Carbarsone
BT1 Drugs
BT2 Residues

Carbaryl
HN heading up to vol. 18 (1986)
BT1 Acaricides
BT2 Pesticides
BT3 Biocides
BT3 Residues
BT1 *N*-Methylcarbamate insecticides
BT2 Insecticides
BT3 Pesticides
BT4 Biocides
BT4 Residues
BT2 *N*-Methylcarbamate pesticides
BT3 Carbamate pesticides
BT4 Pesticides
BT5 Biocides
BT5 Residues
BT1 Nematocides
BT2 Pesticides
BT3 Biocides
BT3 Residues
RT Naphthol
UF Naphthylmethylcarbamate
UF Sevin
UF Vioxan

Carbendazim
BT1 Benzimidazole
BT2 Fungicides
BT3 Pesticides
BT4 Biocides
BT4 Residues
BT1 Carbamate pesticides
BT2 Pesticides
BT3 Biocides
BT3 Residues
UF Bavistin
UF Carbendazole

Carbendazole
USE **Carbendazim**

Carbetamide
BT1 Carbamate pesticides
BT2 Pesticides
BT3 Biocides
BT3 Residues
BT1 Herbicides
BT2 Pesticides
BT3 Biocides
BT3 Residues
UF Legurame

Carbofos
USE **Malathion**

Carbofuran
BT1 Acaricides
BT2 Pesticides
BT3 Biocides
BT3 Residues
BT1 *N*-Methylcarbamate insecticides
BT2 Insecticides
BT3 Pesticides
BT4 Biocides
BT4 Residues
BT2 *N*-Methylcarbamate pesticides
BT3 Carbamate pesticides
BT4 Pesticides
BT5 Biocides
BT5 Residues
BT1 Nematocides
BT2 Pesticides
BT3 Biocides
BT3 Residues

Carbohydrases
HN heading up to vol. 24 (1992)
BT1 Glycosidases
BT2 Hydrolases
BT3 Enzymes

Carbohydrates
BT1 Nutrients
BT1 Organic compounds
NT1 Bifidus factors
NT1 Carbohydrates low diet
NT1 Carbohydrates low foods
NT1 Glycosides
NT2 Aglycones
NT2 Amygdalin
NT2 Arbutin
NT2 Convicine
NT2 Cyanogenic glycosides
NT2 Digitonin
NT2 Diglucosides

NT2 Dihydrochalcones
NT3 Neohesperidin dihydrochalcone
NT3 Phloretin
NT2 Galactosides
NT2 Glucides
NT2 Glucosides
NT3 Geniposide
NT3 Limonoid glucosides
NT3 Piceid
NT3 Puerarin
NT2 Glucosinolates
NT3 Glucobrassicin
NT3 Glucoraphanin
NT3 Progoitrin
NT3 Sinigrin
NT2 Glycyrrhizic acid
NT2 Glycyrrhizin
NT2 Gymnemic acid
NT2 Hesperidin
NT2 Linamarin
NT2 Naringenin
NT2 Naringin
NT2 Neohesperidin
NT2 Oleuropein
NT2 Prunasin
NT2 Quercitrin
NT2 Rebaudiosides
NT2 Rutin
NT2 Saponins
NT3 Digitonin
NT3 Ginsenosides
NT3 Quillaja saponins
NT2 Simmondsin
NT2 Stevioside
NT2 Tannins
NT3 Ellagitannins
NT3 Proanthocyanidins
NT4 Procyanidins
NT3 Tannic acid
NT2 Thioglycosides
NT2 Vicine
NT1 Polyols
NT2 Alditols
NT2 Arabitol
NT2 Dulcitol
NT2 Erythritol
NT2 Galactitol
NT2 Glycerol
NT3 Glycerin
NT3 Glycerine
NT2 Inositol
NT3 Inositol phosphates
NT3 Phytates
NT3 Phytic acid
NT2 Lactitol
NT2 Maltitol
NT2 Mannitol
NT2 Sorbitol
NT2 Sugar alcohols
NT2 Xylitol
NT1 Polysaccharides
NT2 Agar
NT3 Agar gels
NT3 Agarose
NT2 Alginates
NT3 Alginate gels
NT3 Alginic acid
NT2 Arabinogalactans
NT2 Carrageenans
NT3 Carrageenan gels
NT2 Chitin
NT3 Chitosan
NT2 Exopolysaccharides
NT2 Fructans
NT3 Inulin
NT3 Levans
NT2 Fucoidans
NT2 Galactans
NT2 Gellan
NT3 Gellan gums
NT2 Glucans
NT3 Alternan
NT3 Celluloses
NT4 Carboxymethylcellulose
NT4 Cellulose acetate
NT4 Cellulose ether
NT4 Cellulose sausage casings
NT4 Hydroxypropylcellulose
NT4 Hydroxypropylmethylcellulose
NT4 Lignocelluloses
NT4 Methylcellulose
NT4 Microcrystalline celluloses
NT4 Regenerated cellulose
NT4 Tylose
NT3 Curdlan
NT3 Dextran
NT3 β-Glucans
NT3 Glycogen
NT3 Laminarin
NT3 Polydextrose
NT3 Pullulan
NT3 Starch
NT4 Amaranth starch
NT4 Amylopectins
NT4 Amyloses
NT4 Arrowroot
NT4 Barley starch
NT4 Buckwheat starch
NT4 Canna starch
NT4 Cassava starch
NT5 Tapioca
NT4 Corn starch
NT5 High amylose corn starch
NT4 Dextrins
NT5 Amylodextrins
NT5 Cyclodextrins
NT5 Maltodextrins
NT5 Pyrodextrins
NT4 Farina
NT4 Legume starch
NT4 Millet starch
NT4 Modified starches
NT4 Mung bean starch
NT4 Oat starch
NT4 Pea starch
NT4 Potato starch
NT4 Resistant starch
NT4 Rice starch
NT4 Rye starch
NT4 Sago
NT4 Sorghum starch
NT4 Starch granules
NT4 Sweet potato starch
NT4 Wheat starch
NT4 Yam starch
NT3 Xyloglucans
NT2 Glycosaminoglycans
NT3 Chondroitin
NT3 Hyaluronic acid
NT3 Mucopolysaccharides
NT2 Gums
NT3 Cassia gums
NT3 Furcellaran
NT3 Gellan gums
NT3 Guar gums
NT3 Gum arabic
NT4 Gum acacia
NT3 Gum ghatti
NT3 Gum kondagogu
NT3 Gum tragacanth
NT3 Karaya gums
NT3 Locust bean gums
NT4 Carob gums
NT3 Mesquite seed gums
NT3 Mucilage
NT3 Psyllium gums
NT3 Tara gums
NT3 Xanthan gums
NT2 Hemicelluloses
NT2 Kefiran
NT2 Lipopolysaccharides
NT2 Mannans
NT3 Galactomannans
NT3 Glucomannans
NT4 Konjac glucomannans
NT2 Nonstarch polysaccharides
NT2 Oligosaccharides
NT3 Chitooligosaccharides
NT3 Fructooligosaccharides
NT4 Kestose
NT4 Nystose
NT3 Galactooligosaccharides
NT3 Glucooligosaccharides
NT4 Isomaltooligosaccharides
NT4 Maltooligosaccharides
NT5 Maltohexaose
NT5 Maltotetraose
NT5 Maltotriose
NT4 Panose
NT3 Lactosucrose
NT3 Melezitose
NT3 Raffinose
NT3 Stachyose
NT3 Verbascose
NT3 Xylooligosaccharides
NT2 Pectic substances
NT3 Galacturonic acid
NT3 Pectins
NT4 Apple pectins
NT4 Citrus pectins
NT4 Sugar beet pectins
NT3 Polyuronides
NT3 Rhamnogalacturonans
NT2 Pentosans
NT3 Arabinans
NT3 Arabinoxylans
NT2 Proteoglycans
NT2 Xanthan
NT3 Xanthan gums
NT2 Xylan
NT1 Prebiotics

NT1 Sugars
NT2 Amino sugars
NT3 *N*-Acetylglucosamine
NT3 Furosine
NT3 Hexosamines
NT4 Galactosamine
NT4 Glucosamine
NT2 Disaccharides
NT3 Cellobiose
NT3 Difructose anhydride
NT3 Gentiobiose
NT3 Isomaltose
NT3 Isomaltulose
NT4 Palatinose
NT3 Lactose
NT4 Lactose low foods
NT3 Lactulose
NT3 Maltose
NT3 Melibiose
NT3 Nigerose
NT3 Sucrose
NT3 Trehalose
NT2 Monosaccharides
NT3 Aldoses
NT3 Arabinose
NT3 Fructose
NT3 Fucose
NT3 Galactose
NT3 Glucose
NT4 Glucose-6-phosphate
NT3 Hexoses
NT3 Ketoses
NT3 Mannose
NT3 Pentoses
NT3 Psicose
NT3 Rhamnose
NT3 Ribose
NT3 Sorbose
NT3 Tagatose
NT3 Xylose
NT3 Xylulose
NT2 Nonreducing sugars
NT2 Oligosaccharides
NT3 Chitooligosaccharides
NT3 Fructooligosaccharides
NT4 Kestose
NT4 Nystose
NT3 Galactooligosaccharides
NT3 Glucooligosaccharides
NT4 Isomaltooligosaccharides
NT4 Maltooligosaccharides
NT5 Maltohexaose
NT5 Maltotetraose
NT5 Maltotriose
NT4 Panose
NT3 Lactosucrose
NT3 Melezitose
NT3 Raffinose
NT3 Stachyose
NT3 Verbascose
NT3 Xylooligosaccharides
NT2 Reducing sugars
NT2 Saccharides
NT2 Uronic acids
NT3 Galacturonic acid
NT3 Glucuronic acid
NT3 Polyuronides
RT Biopolymers
RT Macronutrients

Carbohydrates low diet
HN introduced from vol. 38, issue 8 (2006)
BT1 Carbohydrates
BT2 Nutrients
BT2 Organic compounds
BT1 Diet therapy
BT2 Diet
BT3 Nutrition
BT2 Therapy

Carbohydrates low foods
HN introduced from vol. 39, issue 1 (2007)
BT1 Carbohydrates
BT2 Nutrients
BT2 Organic compounds

Carbolines
BT1 Alkaloids
BT2 Organic nitrogen compounds
RT Carcinogens
RT Harman
RT Norharman

Carbon
SN symbol C is also used in the index
BT1 Elements
BT2 Minerals
BT3 Nutrients
NT1 Activated C
NT2 Activated carbon
NT1 C
NT1 Charcoal

Carbonatation
BT1 Sugar processes
BT2 Processing
BT3 Technology

Carbonated beverages
BT1 Soft drinks
BT2 Beverages

Carbonates
BT1 Salts

Carbonation
BT1 Processing
BT2 Technology
RT Aeration
RT Bubbles
RT Carbon dioxide

Carbon dioxide
SN symbol CO2 is also used in the index
BT1 Gases
BT2 Physical phases
BT3 Chemistry
BT4 Science
BT1 Inorganic compounds
BT1 Oxides
BT1 Solvents
NT1 CO_2
NT1 Dry Ice
NT1 Supercritical CO_2 extraction
RT Carbonation
RT Flushing
RT Respiration

Carbon disulfide
BT1 Disulfides
BT2 Sulfides
BT3 Salts
BT1 Fumigants
BT2 Biocides
UF Carbon disulphide

Carbon disulphide
HN used for carbon disulfide up to vol. 35, issue 6 (2003)
USE **Carbon disulfide**

Carbonic acid
BT1 Acids
RT CO_2

Carbonic maceration
BT1 Maceration
BT2 Processing
BT3 Technology

Carbon monoxide
BT1 Gases
BT2 Physical phases
BT3 Chemistry
BT4 Science
BT1 Inorganic compounds
BT1 Oxides

Carbon tetrachloride
SN syn. tetrachloromethane
BT1 Chlorinated hydrocarbons
BT2 Organic halogen compounds
BT1 Fumigants
BT2 Biocides
BT1 Solvents

Carbonyl compounds
BT1 Organic compounds
NT1 Aldehydes
NT2 Acetaldehyde
NT3 Ethanal
NT2 Acetals
NT2 Acrolein
NT3 Propenal
NT2 Alkanals
NT2 Anisaldehyde
NT2 Benzaldehyde
NT2 Butanal
NT2 Butyraldehyde
NT2 Cinnamaldehyde
NT2 Citral
NT3 Geranial
NT3 Neral
NT2 Citronellal
NT2 Cuminaldehyde
NT2 Decanal
NT2 Formaldehyde
NT3 Formalin
NT3 Formol
NT3 Methanal
NT2 Fural
NT2 Furaldehyde
NT2 Furfural
NT2 Glutaraldehyde
NT2 Glyceraldehyde
NT2 Glycolaldehyde
NT2 Glyoxal

NT2 Heptenal
NT2 Hexanal
NT2 Hexenal
NT2 5-(Hydroxymethyl)-2-furaldehyde
NT2 Hydroxymethylfurfural
NT2 3-Hydroxypropionaldehyde
NT2 Isobutyraldehyde
NT3 2-Methylpropanal
NT2 Malonaldehyde
NT2 Malondialdehyde
NT2 Methional
NT2 3-Methylbutanal
NT3 Isovaleraldehyde
NT2 Methylglyoxal
NT2 Nonanal
NT2 Nonenal
NT2 Octanal
NT2 Paraformaldehyde
NT2 Pentanal
NT3 Valeraldehyde
NT2 Phenylacetaldehyde
NT2 Propanal
NT3 Propionaldehyde
NT2 Pyruvaldehyde
NT2 Reuterin
NT2 Safranal
NT1 Dinitrophenylhydrazones
NT1 Ketones
NT2 Acetoin
NT3 Acetylmethylcarbinol
NT3 3-Hydroxy-2-butanone
NT2 α-Acetolactate
NT2 Acetone
NT2 Acetophenone
NT2 Alkylcyclobutanones
NT2 Aloin
NT2 Benzophenone
NT2 Butanone
NT2 Camphor
NT2 Carvone
NT2 β-Damascenone
NT2 Dihydroxyacetone
NT2 Diketones
NT3 Diacetyl
NT4 2,3-Butanedione
NT2 Filbertone
NT2 Furanones
NT3 Furaneol
NT4 2,5-Dimethyl-4-hydroxy-3(2*H*)-furanone
NT3 Sotolon
NT2 2-Heptanone
NT2 Ionones
NT2 Keto acids
NT2 Nonanone
NT2 Nootkatone
NT2 Octanone
NT2 Pentanedione
NT3 Acetylacetone
NT2 Propanone
NT2 Thujone
NT2 Undecanone
NT2 Zingerone

Carbophenothion
BT1 Acaricides
BT2 Pesticides
BT3 Biocides
BT3 Residues
BT1 Organophosphorus insecticides
BT2 Insecticides
BT3 Pesticides
BT4 Biocides
BT4 Residues
BT2 Organophosphorus pesticides
BT3 Pesticides
BT4 Biocides
BT4 Residues
UF Trithion

Carboxin
BT1 Fungicides
BT2 Pesticides
BT3 Biocides
BT3 Residues
UF Vitavax

Carboxylesterases
SN EC 3.1.1.1
BT1 Esterases
BT2 Hydrolases
BT3 Enzymes

Carboxylic acids
BT1 Organic acids
BT2 Acids

Carboxymethylation
BT1 Modification

Carboxymethylcellulases
USE **Cellulases**

Carboxymethylcellulose
HN abbrev. CMC used in the index up to vol. 24 (1992)
BT1 Celluloses
BT2 Glucans
BT3 Polysaccharides
BT4 Carbohydrates
BT5 Nutrients
BT5 Organic compounds
UF CMC

Carboxypeptidases
SN EC 3.4.16 - 3.4.18
BT1 Proteinases
BT2 Hydrolases
BT3 Enzymes
UF Carboxypeptidase Y

Carboxypeptidase Y
USE **Carboxypeptidases**

Carcass by-products
USE **Offal**

Carcass condemnation
HN introduced from vol. 41, issue 1 (2009)
BT1 Carcasses
BT2 Meat
BT3 Animal foods
BT4 Foods
RT Inspection

Carcasses
BT1 Meat
BT2 Animal foods
BT3 Foods
NT1 Animal carcasses
NT1 Antelope carcasses
NT1 Bison carcasses
NT1 Buffalo carcasses
NT1 Calf carcasses
NT1 Camel carcasses
NT1 Carcass condemnation
NT1 Cattle carcasses
NT1 Chicken carcasses
NT1 Deer carcasses
NT1 Duck carcasses
NT1 Emu carcasses
NT1 Game carcasses
NT1 Gazelle carcasses
NT1 Goat carcasses
NT1 Goose carcasses
NT1 Hare carcasses
NT1 Horse carcasses
NT1 Lamb carcasses
NT1 Ostrich carcasses
NT1 Partridge carcasses
NT1 Pheasant carcasses
NT1 Pigeon carcasses
NT1 Poultry carcasses
NT1 Quail carcasses
NT1 Rabbit carcasses
NT1 Ram carcasses
NT1 Reindeer carcasses
NT1 Rhea carcasses
NT1 Seal carcasses
NT1 Sheep carcasses
NT1 Swine carcasses
NT1 Turkey carcasses
NT1 Veal calf carcasses
NT1 Whale carcasses
NT1 Wild boar carcasses
NT1 Yak carcasses
RT Fatness
RT Offal
RT Slaughter
UF Sides

Carcinogenesis
HN under Mutagenesis up to vol. 41 (2009)
BT1 Diseases
RT Cancer
RT Carcinogenicity
RT Carcinogenicity testing

Carcinogenicity
HN heading from vol. 25 (1993); under Carcinogens up to vol. 24 (1992)
RT Antimutagenicity
RT Carcinogenesis
RT Carcinogenicity testing
RT Carcinogens
RT Genetics
RT Mutagenicity
RT Mutagens
RT Mutants
RT Mutations

Carcinogenicity testing
RT Ames test
RT Carcinogenesis
RT Carcinogenicity

Carcinogens
BT1 Mutagens
NT1 Agaritine
NT1 Benzopyrene
NT1 Cycasin
NT1 Dioxane
NT1 Ethyl carbamate
NT1 Methyl carbamate
NT1 Urethane
RT Aflatoxins
RT Amines
RT Antimutagens
RT Asbestos
RT Benzene
RT Cancer
RT Carbolines
RT Carcinogenicity
RT Mutagenicity
RT Mutants
RT Mutations
RT Nitrosamines
RT Nitroso compounds
RT Norharman
RT Polybrominated biphenyls
RT Polychlorinated biphenyls
RT Teratogenesis
RT Toxins

Cardamom
BT1 Spices
BT2 Flavourings
BT3 Additives

Cardboard
BT1 Board
BT2 Packaging materials

Cardiovascular diseases
BT1 Diseases
NT1 Coronary heart diseases
NT2 Myocardial infarction
NT1 Stroke
RT Cardiovascular physiology

Cardiovascular physiology
HN introduced from vol. 41, issue 1 (2009)
SN includes cardiac function, and vascular and endothelial physiology
BT1 Human physiology
BT2 Physiology
BT3 Science
NT1 Blood pressure
RT Cardiovascular diseases

Cardoons
BT1 Vegetables specific
BT2 Vegetables
BT3 Crops
BT4 Plants
BT3 Plant foods
BT4 Foods
NT1 *Cynara cardunculus*

Caribbean
HN heading up to vol. 24 (1992)
USE **West Indies**

Caribou
BT1 Animals

Caries
USE **Dental caries**

Carmin
BT1 Vegetable proteins
BT2 Proteins vegetable
BT3 Proteins
BT4 Nutrients
BT3 Vegetable products
BT4 Plant foods
BT5 Foods

Carmine
BT1 Colorants
BT2 Additives

Carminic acid
BT1 Colorants
BT2 Additives
RT Cochineal

Carmoisine
BT1 Colorants
BT2 Additives

Carnauba wax
BT1 Coatings
BT1 Waxes
BT2 Fatty acid esters
BT3 Esters
BT4 Organic compounds

Carnitine
HN under Nutrients up to vol. 42 (2010)
BT1 Organic nitrogen compounds
RT Vitamin B group

Carnobacterium
BT1 Bacteria
BT2 Microorganisms
NT1 *Carnobacterium divergens*
NT1 *Carnobacterium maltaromaticum*
NT2 *Carnobacterium piscicola*

Carnobacterium divergens
BT1 *Carnobacterium*
BT2 Bacteria
BT3 Microorganisms
RT Divercins

Carnobacterium maltaromaticum
HN introduced from vol. 42, issue 1 (2010)
SN synonymous with Carnobacterium piscicola
BT1 *Carnobacterium*
BT2 Bacteria
BT3 Microorganisms
NT1 *Carnobacterium piscicola*

Carnobacterium piscicola
SN synonymous with Carnobacterium maltaromaticum
BT1 *Carnobacterium maltaromaticum*
BT2 *Carnobacterium*
BT3 Bacteria
BT4 Microorganisms
RT Piscicolins

Carnosic acid
HN introduced from vol. 39, issue 1 (2007)
BT1 Diterpenoids
BT2 Terpenoids
BT3 Lipids
BT4 Nutrients

Carnosine
BT1 Peptides
BT2 Proteins
BT3 Nutrients

Carnosol
HN introduced from vol. 39, issue 1 (2007)
BT1 Alcohols
BT1 Diterpenoids
BT2 Terpenoids
BT3 Lipids
BT4 Nutrients

Carob beans
BT1 Legumes
BT2 Vegetables specific
BT3 Vegetables
BT4 Crops
BT5 Plants
BT4 Plant foods
BT5 Foods
RT Carob gums
RT Locust bean gums
UF Locust beans

Carob gums
BT1 Locust bean gums
BT2 Gums
BT3 Polysaccharides
BT4 Carbohydrates
BT5 Nutrients
BT5 Organic compounds
BT3 Stabilizers
BT4 Additives
BT3 Thickeners
BT4 Additives
RT Carob beans

Carob pods
BT1 Legumes
BT2 Vegetables specific
BT3 Vegetables
BT4 Crops
BT5 Plants
BT4 Plant foods
BT5 Foods

α-Carotene
HN introduced from vol. 37, issue 5 (2005)
BT1 Carotenes
BT2 Carotenoids
BT3 Pigments
BT3 Terpenoids
BT4 Lipids
BT5 Nutrients

β-Carotene
BT1 Carotenes
BT2 Carotenoids
BT3 Pigments
BT3 Terpenoids

BT4 Lipids
BT5 Nutrients

Carotenes
BT1 Carotenoids
BT2 Pigments
BT2 Terpenoids
BT3 Lipids
BT4 Nutrients
NT1 α-Carotene
NT1 β-Carotene
NT1 Provitamin A

Carotenoids
BT1 Pigments
BT1 Terpenoids
BT2 Lipids
BT3 Nutrients
NT1 Apocarotenal
NT1 Astacene
NT1 Bixin
NT1 Capsanthin
NT1 Carotenes
NT2 α-Carotene
NT2 β-Carotene
NT2 Provitamin A
NT1 Crocin
NT2 Crocetin
NT1 Lycopene
NT1 Norisoprenoids
NT2 β-Damascenone
NT2 Ionones
NT1 Phytoene
NT1 Phytofluene
NT1 Xanthophylls
NT2 Astaxanthin
NT2 Canthaxanthin
NT2 Cryptoxanthin
NT2 Diatoxanthin
NT2 Fucoxanthin
NT2 Lutein
NT2 Neoxanthin
NT2 Tunaxanthin
NT2 Violaxanthin
NT2 Zeaxanthin
RT Retinoids
RT Riboflavin

Carp
HN heading from vol. 30 (1998); under Fishes up to vol. 29 (1997)
BT1 Freshwater fish
BT2 Fish
BT3 Animals
BT3 Sea foods
BT4 Aquatic foods
BT5 Animal foods
BT6 Foods
BT1 Oily fish
BT2 Fish
BT3 Animals
BT3 Sea foods
BT4 Aquatic foods
BT5 Animal foods
BT6 Foods
NT1 Bighead carp
NT2 *Aristichthys nobilis*
NT1 Crucian carp
NT1 *Cyprinus carpio*
NT1 Grass carp
NT2 White amur
NT1 Rohu
NT2 *Labeo rohita*
NT1 Silver carp

Carpet shells
BT1 Bivalves
BT2 Molluscs
BT3 Shellfish
BT4 Animals
BT4 Sea foods
BT5 Aquatic foods
BT6 Animal foods
BT7 Foods
UF Clovis

Carrageenan gels
BT1 Carrageenans
BT2 Emulsifiers
BT3 Additives
BT2 Polysaccharides
BT3 Carbohydrates
BT4 Nutrients
BT4 Organic compounds
BT2 Stabilizers
BT3 Additives
BT2 Thickeners
BT3 Additives
BT1 Gels
BT2 Physical phases
BT3 Chemistry
BT4 Science

Carrageenans
BT1 Emulsifiers
BT2 Additives
BT1 Polysaccharides
BT2 Carbohydrates
BT3 Nutrients
BT3 Organic compounds
BT1 Stabilizers
BT2 Additives
BT1 Thickeners
BT2 Additives
NT1 Carrageenan gels
RT Seaweeds

Carriers
BT1 Containers

Carrot chips
BT1 Carrots
BT2 Vegetables specific
BT3 Vegetables
BT4 Crops
BT5 Plants
BT4 Plant foods
BT5 Foods
BT1 Chips
BT2 Processed foods
BT3 Foods

Carrot juices
BT1 Vegetable juices
BT2 Soft drinks
BT3 Beverages
BT2 Vegetable products
BT3 Plant foods
BT4 Foods
RT Carrots

Carrot pulps
BT1 Carrots
BT2 Vegetables specific
BT3 Vegetables
BT4 Crops
BT5 Plants
BT4 Plant foods
BT5 Foods
BT1 Vegetable pulps
BT2 Pulps
BT3 Processed foods
BT4 Foods
BT2 Vegetable products
BT3 Plant foods
BT4 Foods

Carrots
BT1 Vegetables specific
BT2 Vegetables
BT3 Crops
BT4 Plants
BT3 Plant foods
BT4 Foods
NT1 Carrot chips
NT1 Carrot pulps
RT Carrot juices

Carthamin
BT1 Colorants
BT2 Additives
RT Saffron

Cartonboard
BT1 Board
BT2 Packaging materials

Cartoning
BT1 Cartons
BT2 Containers
BT1 Packaging
BT2 Technology

Cartons
BT1 Containers
NT1 Cartoning

Cartridges
HN introduced from vol. 41, issue 1 (2009)
BT1 Containers

Carvacrol
HN also under Flavour compounds up to vol. 42 (2010)
BT1 Aroma compounds
BT2 Flavour compounds
BT2 Volatile compounds
BT1 Monoterpenoids
BT2 Terpenoids
BT3 Lipids
BT4 Nutrients
BT1 Phenols
BT2 Alcohols
BT2 Aromatic compounds
BT3 Organic compounds

Carveol
BT1 Aroma compounds
BT2 Flavour compounds
BT2 Volatile compounds
BT1 Monoterpenoids

BT2 Terpenoids
BT3 Lipids
BT4 Nutrients

Carvone
HN also under Flavour compounds up to vol. 42 (2010)
BT1 Aroma compounds
BT2 Flavour compounds
BT2 Volatile compounds
BT1 Ketones
BT2 Carbonyl compounds
BT3 Organic compounds
BT1 Monoterpenoids
BT2 Terpenoids
BT3 Lipids
BT4 Nutrients

Carya
USE **Hickory nuts**

Caryophyllene
BT1 Aroma compounds
BT2 Flavour compounds
BT2 Volatile compounds
BT1 Sesquiterpenes
BT2 Hydrocarbons
BT3 Organic compounds
BT2 Sesquiterpenoids
BT3 Terpenoids
BT4 Lipids
BT5 Nutrients

Casein
BT1 Milk proteins
BT2 Proteins milk
BT3 Animal proteins
BT4 Proteins animal
BT5 Proteins
BT6 Nutrients
NT1 Acid casein
NT1 α_s-Casein
NT1 α_{s1}-Casein
NT1 α_{s2}-Casein
NT1 β-Casein
NT1 γ-Casein
NT1 κ-Casein
NT1 Casein micelles
RT Caseinates
RT Caseinomacropeptides

α_s-Casein
BT1 Casein
BT2 Milk proteins
BT3 Proteins milk
BT4 Animal proteins
BT5 Proteins animal
BT6 Proteins
BT7 Nutrients

α_{s1}-Casein
BT1 Casein
BT2 Milk proteins
BT3 Proteins milk
BT4 Animal proteins
BT5 Proteins animal
BT6 Proteins
BT7 Nutrients

α_{s2}-Casein
BT1 Casein
BT2 Milk proteins
BT3 Proteins milk
BT4 Animal proteins
BT5 Proteins animal
BT6 Proteins
BT7 Nutrients

β-Casein
BT1 Casein
BT2 Milk proteins
BT3 Proteins milk
BT4 Animal proteins
BT5 Proteins animal
BT6 Proteins
BT7 Nutrients

γ-Casein
BT1 Casein
BT2 Milk proteins
BT3 Proteins milk
BT4 Animal proteins
BT5 Proteins animal
BT6 Proteins
BT7 Nutrients

κ-Casein
BT1 Casein
BT2 Milk proteins
BT3 Proteins milk
BT4 Animal proteins
BT5 Proteins animal
BT6 Proteins
BT7 Nutrients

Caseinates
BT1 Protein products
NT1 Sodium caseinate
RT Casein

Casein curd
BT1 Curd
BT2 Dairy products
BT3 Animal foods
BT4 Foods

Casein micelles
BT1 Casein
BT2 Milk proteins
BT3 Proteins milk
BT4 Animal proteins
BT5 Proteins animal
BT6 Proteins
BT7 Nutrients

Caseinomacropeptides
BT1 Peptides
BT2 Proteins
BT3 Nutrients
RT Casein

Casein whey
BT1 Whey
BT2 Dairy products
BT3 Animal foods
BT4 Foods

Cases
BT1 Boxes
BT2 Containers

Cashew apple juices
HN introduced from vol. 39, issue 1 (2007)
BT1 Fruit juices
BT2 Fruit products
BT3 Plant foods
BT4 Foods
BT2 Soft drinks
BT3 Beverages
RT Cashew apples

Cashew apples
BT1 Fruits specific
BT2 Fruits
BT3 Crops
BT4 Plants
BT3 Plant foods
BT4 Foods
RT Cashew apple juices

Cashew nuts
BT1 Nuts
BT2 Fruits
BT3 Crops
BT4 Plants
BT3 Plant foods
BT4 Foods
BT2 Oilseeds
BT3 Seeds
BT4 Plant foods
BT5 Foods

Casings
NT1 Sausage casings
NT2 Cellulose sausage casings
NT2 Collagen sausage casings

Casks
BT1 Barrels
BT2 Containers

β-Casomorphins
BT1 Milk proteins
BT2 Proteins milk
BT3 Animal proteins
BT4 Proteins animal
BT5 Proteins
BT6 Nutrients

Casoron
USE **Dichlobenil**

Caspases
HN introduced from vol. 42, issue 1 (2010)
SN EC 3.4.22; includes caspase-1 to caspase-11
BT1 Proteinases
BT2 Hydrolases
BT3 Enzymes

Cassava
BT1 Vegetables specific
BT2 Vegetables
BT3 Crops
BT4 Plants
BT3 Plant foods

BT4 Foods
NT1 Attieke
NT1 Cassava chips
NT1 Cassava meal
NT1 Cassava starch
NT2 Tapioca
NT1 Gari
NT1 Koko
NT1 Manioc
NT1 Tape
NT2 Tape ketan
NT1 Uji

Cassava chips
BT1 Cassava
BT2 Vegetables specific
BT3 Vegetables
BT4 Crops
BT5 Plants
BT4 Plant foods
BT5 Foods

Cassava meal
HN introduced from vol. 41, issue 1 (2009)
BT1 Cassava
BT2 Vegetables specific
BT3 Vegetables
BT4 Crops
BT5 Plants
BT4 Plant foods
BT5 Foods
BT1 Flours
BT2 Plant foods
BT3 Foods

Cassava starch
SN syn. tapioca
BT1 Cassava
BT2 Vegetables specific
BT3 Vegetables
BT4 Crops
BT5 Plants
BT4 Plant foods
BT5 Foods
BT1 Starch
BT2 Glucans
BT3 Polysaccharides
BT4 Carbohydrates
BT5 Nutrients
BT5 Organic compounds
BT2 Thickeners
BT3 Additives
NT1 Tapioca

Casseroles
BT1 Meals
BT2 Processed foods
BT3 Foods

Cassia
BT1 Spices
BT2 Flavourings
BT3 Additives
RT Cinnamon

Cassia gums
BT1 Gums
BT2 Polysaccharides
BT3 Carbohydrates
BT4 Nutrients
BT4 Organic compounds
BT2 Stabilizers
BT3 Additives
BT2 Thickeners
BT3 Additives
RT *Cassia* seeds

***Cassia* seeds**
BT1 Legumes
BT2 Vegetables specific
BT3 Vegetables
BT4 Crops
BT5 Plants
BT4 Plant foods
BT5 Foods
RT Cassia gums

Cassis
BT1 Fruit liqueurs
BT2 Liqueurs
BT3 Alcoholic beverages
BT4 Beverages alcoholic
BT5 Beverages

Castor beans
BT1 Oilseeds
BT2 Seeds
BT3 Plant foods
BT4 Foods

Castor oils
BT1 Vegetable oils
BT2 Oils vegetable
BT3 Oils
BT4 Lipids
BT5 Nutrients
BT3 Vegetable products
BT4 Plant foods
BT5 Foods

Castration
RT Sex

Catalases
SN EC 1.11.1.6
BT1 Peroxidases
BT2 Oxidoreductases
BT3 Enzymes

Catalysts
RT Enzymes

Catechin
BT1 Catechols
BT2 Flavanols
BT3 Flavonoids
BT4 Aromatic compounds
BT5 Organic compounds
BT4 Pigments
BT2 Phenols
BT3 Alcohols
BT3 Aromatic compounds
BT4 Organic compounds

Catechins
USE **Catechols**

Catecholamines
BT1 Biogenic amines
BT2 Amines
BT3 Organic nitrogen compounds
BT1 Hormones
BT2 Residues
NT1 Adrenaline
NT1 Noradrenaline

Catechol oxidases
SN EC 1.10.3.1; also catalyses the reaction of monophenol monooxygenase (EC 1.14.18.1) under certain conditions
BT1 Phenolases
BT2 Oxidoreductases
BT3 Enzymes
UF Diphenol oxidases
UF Polyphenol oxidases

Catechols
BT1 Flavanols
BT2 Flavonoids
BT3 Aromatic compounds
BT4 Organic compounds
BT3 Pigments
BT1 Phenols
BT2 Alcohols
BT2 Aromatic compounds
BT3 Organic compounds
NT1 Catechin
NT1 Epicatechin
NT1 Epicatechin gallate
NT1 Epicatechol
NT1 Epigallocatechin
NT1 Epigallocatechin gallate
NT1 Gallocatechin gallate
NT1 Pyrocatechol
UF Catechins

Catering
NT1 Catering establishments
NT1 Catering industry
NT1 Foods service
NT1 Hotels
NT1 Kitchens
RT Meals
RT Menus
RT Restaurants

Catering establishments
BT1 Catering

Catering industry
BT1 Catering
BT1 Food industry
BT2 Industries

Catfish
HN heading from vol. 30 (1998); under Fishes up to vol. 29 (1997)
BT1 Freshwater fish
BT2 Fish
BT3 Animals
BT3 Sea foods
BT4 Aquatic foods
BT5 Animal foods
BT6 Foods
NT1 Channel catfish
NT2 *Ictalurus punctatus*
NT1 *Silurus asotus*

Cat foods
HN introduced from vol. 39, issue 1 (2007)
BT1 Pet foods
NT1 Cat milks
NT2 Kitten milks
NT1 Kitten foods
RT Cats

Catharanthus roseus
BT1 Plants

Cathepsins
BT1 Proteinases
BT2 Hydrolases
BT3 Enzymes

Cations
BT1 Ions

Cat milks
HN introduced from vol. 39, issue 1 (2007)
BT1 Cat foods
BT2 Pet foods
NT1 Kitten milks
RT Cats

Catmint
HN under Spices up to vol. 42 (2010)
BT1 Herbs
BT2 Spices
BT3 Flavourings
BT4 Additives

Cats
HN introduced from vol. 39, issue 1 (2007)
BT1 Pets
RT Cat foods
RT Cat milks
RT Kitten foods
RT Kitten milks

Catsups
SN syn. ketchups
BT1 Ketchups
BT2 Sauces
BT3 Condiments
BT4 Flavourings
BT5 Additives
NT1 Tomato catsups

Cattle
BT1 Animals
NT1 Cattle kidneys
NT1 Cattle livers
RT Beef
RT Veal
UF Bovine
UF Bulls
UF Calves
UF Cows
UF Heifers
UF Oxen
UF Steers

Cattle carcasses
BT1 Beef
BT2 Meat specific
BT3 Meat
BT4 Animal foods
BT5 Foods
BT1 Carcasses
BT2 Meat
BT3 Animal foods
BT4 Foods
UF Bull carcasses

Cattle kidneys
BT1 Cattle
BT2 Animals
BT1 Kidneys
BT2 Offal
BT3 Animal foods
BT4 Foods

Cattle livers
BT1 Cattle
BT2 Animals
BT1 Livers
BT2 Offal
BT3 Animal foods
BT4 Foods

Cattle muscles
USE **Beef**

Cattle tissues
USE **Beef**

Caucas
USE **Wild garlic**

Caulerpa
BT1 Seaweeds
BT2 Algae
BT3 Microorganisms
BT2 Sea foods
BT3 Aquatic foods
BT4 Animal foods
BT5 Foods

Cauliflowers
HN heading from vol. 30 (1998); under Vegetables specific up to vol. 29 (1997)
BT1 Vegetables specific
BT2 Vegetables
BT3 Crops
BT4 Plants
BT3 Plant foods
BT4 Foods

Cavas
HN introduced from vol. 39, issue 1 (2007)
BT1 Sparkling wines
BT2 Wines sparkling
BT3 Wines
BT4 Alcoholic beverages
BT5 Beverages alcoholic
BT6 Beverages

Caviar
BT1 Roes
BT2 Fish products
BT3 Sea foods
BT4 Aquatic foods
BT5 Animal foods
BT6 Foods
UF Caviare

Caviare
USE **Caviar**

Caviar substitutes
BT1 Roes
BT2 Fish products
BT3 Sea foods
BT4 Aquatic foods
BT5 Animal foods
BT6 Foods

Cayenne pepper
BT1 Spices
BT2 Flavourings
BT3 Additives

Cayman Islands
BT1 West Indies
BT2 America

CCC
USE **Chlormequat**

Cd
SN index heading is Cadmium
BT1 Cadmium
BT2 Metals
BT3 Elements
BT4 Minerals
BT5 Nutrients

cDNA
BT1 DNA
BT2 Nucleic acids
BT3 Organic acids
BT4 Acids

CD-ROMs
HN introduced from vol. 41, issue 1 (2009)
SN used for publications only available in this format
RT Electronic publications

Ce
HN under Minerals up to vol. 42 (2010)
BT1 Metals
BT2 Elements
BT3 Minerals
BT4 Nutrients
UF Cerium

Cebreiro cheese
BT1 Cheese varieties
BT2 Cheese
BT3 Dairy products
BT4 Animal foods
BT5 Foods

Cedar nuts
BT1 Nuts
BT2 Fruits
BT3 Crops
BT4 Plants
BT3 Plant foods
BT4 Foods
BT2 Oilseeds
BT3 Seeds
BT4 Plant foods
BT5 Foods

Ceftazidime
BT1 Cephalosporins
BT2 β-Lactam antibiotics
BT3 Antibiotics
BT4 Drugs
BT5 Residues

Ceftiofur
BT1 Cephalosporins
BT2 β-Lactam antibiotics
BT3 Antibiotics
BT4 Drugs
BT5 Residues

Celeriac
BT1 Vegetables specific
BT2 Vegetables
BT3 Crops
BT4 Plants
BT3 Plant foods
BT4 Foods
UF Turnip rooted celery

Celery
HN heading from vol. 30 (1998); under Vegetables specific up to vol. 29 (1997)
BT1 Vegetables specific
BT2 Vegetables
BT3 Crops
BT4 Plants
BT3 Plant foods
BT4 Foods

Celery seeds
BT1 Spices
BT2 Flavourings
BT3 Additives

Cell counts
BT1 Microbiological techniques
RT Plate counts

Cell culture
HN heading from vol. 22 (1990)
NT1 Callus culture
NT1 Cell lines
NT1 Culture
NT1 Regeneration
NT1 Suspension cultures
RT Incubation
RT Media
RT Microbiological techniques

Cell cycle
HN introduced from vol. 39, issue 1 (2007)
BT1 Physiology
BT2 Science
NT1 Apoptosis
NT1 Mitosis
RT Cells

Cell lines
BT1 Cell culture

Cellobiases
USE **β-Glucosidases**

Cellobiohydrolases
USE **Cellulose 1,4-β-cellobiosidases**

Cellobiose
HN under Sugars up to vol. 42 (2010)
BT1 Disaccharides
BT2 Sugars
BT3 Carbohydrates
BT4 Nutrients
BT4 Organic compounds
BT3 Plant foods
BT4 Foods

Cellophane
HN heading up to vol. 24 (1992)
BT1 Cellulose films
BT2 Plastics films
BT3 Plastics
BT4 Packaging materials
RT Regenerated cellulose

Cells
NT1 Adipocytes
NT1 Cell walls
NT1 Chromoplasts
NT1 Erythrocytes
NT2 Haemolysis
NT1 Fimbriae
NT1 Flagella
NT1 Immobilized cells
NT1 Leukocytes
NT1 Mitochondria
NT1 Pili
NT1 Platelets
NT1 Protoplasts
NT1 Somatic cells
NT1 Somatic cells counts
RT Cell cycle

Cells somatic
HN used in addition to somatic cells up to vol. 29 (1997)
USE **Somatic cells**

Cellulases
SN EC 3.2.1.4
BT1 Glycosidases
BT2 Hydrolases
BT3 Enzymes
UF Carboxymethylcellulases

Cellulolytic enzymes
BT1 Glycosidases
BT2 Hydrolases
BT3 Enzymes

Cellulomonas
BT1 Bacteria
BT2 Microorganisms
NT1 *Cellulomonas fimi*
NT1 *Cellulomonas flavigena*

Cellulomonas fimi
BT1 *Cellulomonas*
BT2 Bacteria
BT3 Microorganisms

Cellulomonas flavigena
BT1 *Cellulomonas*
BT2 Bacteria
BT3 Microorganisms

Cellulose acetate
HN under Cellulose films up to vol. 42 (2010)
BT1 Acetates
BT1 Celluloses
BT2 Glucans
BT3 Polysaccharides
BT4 Carbohydrates
BT5 Nutrients
BT5 Organic compounds
RT Cellulose films

Cellulose 1,4-β-cellobiosidases
SN EC 3.2.1.91
BT1 Glycosidases
BT2 Hydrolases
BT3 Enzymes
UF Cellobiohydrolases

Cellulose ether
BT1 Celluloses
BT2 Glucans
BT3 Polysaccharides
BT4 Carbohydrates
BT5 Nutrients
BT5 Organic compounds

Cellulose films
HN heading from vol. 25 (1993)
BT1 Plastics films
BT2 Plastics
BT3 Packaging materials
NT1 Cellophane
RT Cellulose acetate

Celluloses
BT1 Glucans
BT2 Polysaccharides
BT3 Carbohydrates
BT4 Nutrients
BT4 Organic compounds
NT1 Carboxymethylcellulose
NT1 Cellulose acetate
NT1 Cellulose ether
NT1 Cellulose sausage casings
NT1 Hydroxypropylcellulose
NT1 Hydroxypropylmethylcellulose
NT1 Lignocelluloses
NT1 Methylcellulose
NT1 Microcrystalline celluloses
NT1 Regenerated cellulose
NT1 Tylose
RT Lignin
RT Stabilizers
RT Thickeners

Cellulose sausage casings
HN sausage casings cellulose also used in the index up to vol. 29 (1997)
BT1 Celluloses
BT2 Glucans
BT3 Polysaccharides
BT4 Carbohydrates
BT5 Nutrients
BT5 Organic compounds

BT1 Sausage casings
BT2 Casings

Cellulosomes
BT1 Glycosidases
BT2 Hydrolases
BT3 Enzymes

Cellvibrio
BT1 Bacteria
BT2 Microorganisms

Cell walls
BT1 Cells

Central Africa
BT1 Africa
NT1 Burundi
NT1 Central African Republic
NT1 Chad
NT1 Democratic Republic of the Congo
NT1 Gabon
NT1 Rwanda
NT1 Zaire

Central African Republic
BT1 Central Africa
BT2 Africa

Central America
HN heading up to vol. 24 (1992)
BT1 America
NT1 Belize
NT1 Costa Rica
NT1 El Salvador
NT1 Guatemala
NT1 Honduras
NT1 Mexico
NT1 Nicaragua
NT1 Panama

Central nervous system tissues
BT1 Wastes
NT1 Brains
NT1 Spinal cord tissues

Centres
BT1 Fillings

Centrifugal separators
BT1 Centrifuges
BT2 Centrifugation
BT3 Separation
BT4 Processing
BT5 Technology
BT2 Equipment
BT3 Technology
BT1 Separators
BT2 Equipment
BT3 Technology
BT2 Separation
BT3 Processing
BT4 Technology

Centrifugation
BT1 Separation
BT2 Processing
BT3 Technology
NT1 Bactofugation
NT1 Centrifuges
NT2 Centrifugal separators
NT1 Ultracentrifugation

Centrifuges
BT1 Centrifugation
BT2 Separation
BT3 Processing
BT4 Technology
BT1 Equipment
BT2 Technology
NT1 Centrifugal separators

Cephalins
BT1 Phospholipids
BT2 Lipids
BT3 Nutrients

Cephalopods
HN heading from vol. 30 (1998); under Molluscs up to vol. 29 (1997)
BT1 Molluscs
BT2 Shellfish
BT3 Animals
BT3 Sea foods
BT4 Aquatic foods
BT5 Animal foods
BT6 Foods
NT1 Cuttlefish
NT1 Octopus
NT1 Squid
NT2 Ika shiokara
NT2 *Illex argentinus*
NT2 *Ommastrephes bartrami*

Cephalosporins
BT1 β-Lactam antibiotics
BT2 Antibiotics
BT3 Drugs
BT4 Residues
NT1 Ceftazidime
NT1 Ceftiofur
NT1 Cephapirin

Cephalosporium
SN obsolete synonym for Acremonium
BT1 *Acremonium*
BT2 Fungi
BT3 Microorganisms

Cephapirin
BT1 Cephalosporins
BT2 β-Lactam antibiotics
BT3 Antibiotics
BT4 Drugs
BT5 Residues

Ceramic membranes
BT1 Membranes

Ceramics
BT1 Surfaces
BT1 Utensils
BT2 Equipment
BT3 Technology

Ceramides
BT1 Phospholipids
BT2 Lipids
BT3 Nutrients

Ceratocystis
BT1 Fungi
BT2 Microorganisms
NT1 *Ceratocystis fimbriata*

Ceratocystis fimbriata
HN introduced from vol. 39, issue 1 (2007)
BT1 *Ceratocystis*
BT2 Fungi
BT3 Microorganisms

Cereal bars
BT1 Food bars
BT2 Snack foods
BT3 Processed foods
BT4 Foods
NT1 Muesli bars

Cereal bran
BT1 Bran
BT2 Cereal products
BT3 Plant foods
BT4 Foods

Cereal by-products
BT1 By-products

Cereal flours
SN index heading is Flours cereal
BT1 Flours cereal
BT2 Cereal products
BT3 Plant foods
BT4 Foods
NT1 Amaranth flour
NT1 Atta
NT1 Barley flour
NT1 Buckwheat flour
NT1 Composite flours
NT1 Corn flour
NT1 Flour
NT1 Maida
NT1 Millet flour
NT1 Oat flour
NT1 Oatmeal
NT1 Quinoa flour
NT1 Rice flour
NT1 Rye flour
NT1 Sorghum flour
NT1 Triticale flour
NT1 Wheat flour
NT1 Wholemeal
RT Semolina

Cereal products
BT1 Plant foods
BT2 Foods
NT1 Bakery products
NT2 Arepas
NT2 Bagels
NT2 Bakers confectionery
NT2 Bakery product mixes
NT2 Batters
NT2 Biscuits
NT3 Biscuit dough
NT3 Biscuit factories
NT3 Cookies
NT3 Crackers
NT3 Saltine crackers
NT3 Shortbread

NT2 Bread
NT3 Arabic bread
NT3 Baguettes
NT3 Balady
NT3 Bread crumb
NT3 Breadcrumbs
NT3 Bread crust
NT3 Bread dough
NT3 Breadmaking
NT4 Breadmaking properties
NT5 Loaf vol.
NT4 Wheat breadmaking
NT3 Bread rolls
NT3 Chapattis
NT3 Corn bread
NT3 Crispbreads
NT3 Flat bread
NT3 French bread
NT3 Fruit bread
NT3 Gluten low bread
NT3 Injera
NT3 Kisra
NT3 Nan
NT3 Parottas
NT3 Pita bread
NT3 Poori
NT3 Pumpernickel
NT3 Rice bread
NT3 Rolls
NT3 Roti
NT3 Rye bread
NT3 Sangak
NT3 Soda bread
NT3 Sourdough bread
NT3 Steamed bread
NT3 Tanoor
NT3 Toast
NT3 Toast bread
NT3 Wheat bread
NT2 Brioches
NT2 Brownies
NT2 Buns
NT2 Cakes
NT3 Angel cakes
NT3 Baumkuchen
NT3 Cake batters
NT3 Cake mixes
NT3 Christstollen
NT3 Gateaux
NT3 Muffins
NT3 Sponge cakes
NT3 Stollen
NT3 Swiss rolls
NT3 Torten
NT2 Confectionery
NT3 Confectionery bars
NT4 Chocolate bars
NT3 Confectionery industry
NT3 Confectionery products
NT3 Confections
NT3 Frozen confectionery
NT2 Crepes
NT2 Croissants
NT2 Croutons
NT2 Crumpets
NT2 Crust
NT2 Dough
NT3 Biscuit dough
NT3 Bread dough
NT3 Frozen dough
NT3 Pizza dough
NT3 Sourdough
NT3 Sponge
NT3 Wheat dough
NT2 Doughnuts
NT2 Dumplings
NT2 English muffins
NT2 Flans
NT3 Flan cases
NT3 Torten
NT2 Florentines
NT2 Gingerbread
NT2 Ice cream cones
NT2 Kocho
NT2 Macaroons
NT2 Morning goods
NT2 Muffins
NT2 Pancakes
NT2 Panettone
NT2 Papads
NT2 Parathas
NT2 Pastries
NT3 Cream puffs
NT3 Danish pastries
NT3 Eclairs
NT3 Strudels
NT2 Pastry
NT3 Puff pastry
NT2 Patisserie products
NT2 Pelmeni
NT2 Pies
NT3 Fruit pies
NT3 Meat pies
NT4 Cornish pasties
NT3 Pie fillings
NT3 Quiches
NT3 Tarts
NT2 Pizzas
NT3 Pizza dough
NT3 Pizza fillings
NT2 Pretzels
NT2 Rusks
NT2 Scones
NT2 Tacos
NT2 Taco shells
NT2 Tamales
NT2 Tortillas
NT2 Wafers
NT3 Ice cream wafers
NT2 Waffles
NT2 Yakifu
NT2 Zwieback
NT1 Belona
NT1 Bran
NT2 Cereal bran
NT2 Corn bran
NT2 Oat bran
NT2 Rice bran
NT2 Rye bran
NT2 Wheat bran
NT1 Breakfast cereals
NT1 Cornflakes
NT1 Couscous
NT1 Flours cereal
NT2 Cereal flours
NT3 Amaranth flour
NT3 Atta
NT3 Barley flour
NT3 Buckwheat flour
NT3 Composite flours
NT3 Corn flour
NT3 Flour
NT3 Maida
NT3 Millet flour
NT3 Oat flour
NT3 Oatmeal
NT3 Quinoa flour
NT3 Rice flour
NT3 Rye flour
NT3 Sorghum flour
NT3 Triticale flour
NT3 Wheat flour
NT3 Wholemeal
NT1 Germ
NT2 Wheat germ
NT1 Gofio
NT1 Granola
NT1 Grits
NT1 Groats
NT1 Hominy
NT1 Kishk
NT1 Koji
NT2 Rice koji
NT1 Malt
NT2 Barley malt
NT2 Rye malt
NT2 Sorghum malt
NT2 Wheat malt
NT1 Muesli
NT1 Ogi
NT1 Paps
NT1 Pasta
NT2 Alimentary pastes
NT2 Canneloni
NT2 Egg pasta
NT2 Lasagne
NT2 Macaroni
NT2 Noodles
NT3 Instant noodles
NT2 Ravioli
NT2 Somen
NT2 Spaghetti
NT2 Tagliatelli
NT2 Tortellini
NT2 Udon
NT2 Vermicelli
NT1 Porridges
NT2 Dalia
NT2 Gruel
NT2 Koko
NT2 Mawe
NT2 Polenta
NT2 Porridge
NT2 Uji
NT1 Rabadi
NT1 Rice noodles
NT1 Semolina
NT1 Tarhana
NT1 Trahanas
NT1 Wholegrain foods
RT Cereals

Cereal proteins
SN index heading is Proteins cereal
BT1 Proteins cereal
BT2 Vegetable proteins
BT3 Proteins vegetable
BT4 Proteins

BT5 Nutrients
BT4 Vegetable products
BT5 Plant foods
BT6 Foods
NT1 Avenins
NT1 Friabilins
NT1 Gliadins
NT1 Glutelins
NT1 Gluten
NT2 Gluten low foods
NT3 Gluten low bread
NT2 Vital gluten
NT2 Wheat gluten
NT1 Glutenin
NT1 Hordein
NT1 Hordothionins
NT1 Kafirins
NT1 Opaque 2
NT1 Oryzenin
NT1 Prolamins
NT1 Puroindolines
NT1 Purothionin
NT1 Secalins
NT1 Thionins
NT1 Zein

Cereals
BT1 Crops
BT2 Plants
BT1 Seeds
BT2 Plant foods
BT3 Foods
NT1 Acha
NT1 Barley
NT2 Barley fibre
NT2 Barley flour
NT2 Barley starch
NT2 Malting barley
NT2 Pearl barley
NT1 Corn
NT2 Baby corn
NT2 Corn bran
NT2 Corn bread
NT2 Corn chips
NT2 Corn cobs
NT2 Cornflakes
NT2 Corn flour
NT2 Corn masa
NT2 Corn starch
NT3 High amylose corn starch
NT2 Kenkey
NT2 Kwoka
NT2 Popcorn
NT3 Microwave popcorn
NT2 Pozol
NT2 Sweetcorn
NT1 Jobs tears
NT1 Millet
NT2 Bajra
NT2 Common millet
NT2 Finger millet
NT2 Fonio
NT2 Foxtail millet
NT2 Millet flour
NT2 Millet starch
NT2 Pearl millet
NT2 Ragi
NT2 Teff
NT1 Oats
NT2 *Avena fatua*
NT2 Oat bran
NT2 Oat fibre
NT2 Oat flakes
NT2 Oat flour
NT2 Oatmeal
NT2 Oat starch
NT2 Porridge
NT1 Rice
NT2 Arare
NT2 Basmati rice
NT2 Black rice
NT2 Brown rice
NT2 Dosai
NT2 Idli
NT2 Lao-chao
NT2 Paddy
NT2 Puffed rice
NT2 Puto
NT2 Rice bran
NT2 Rice bread
NT2 Rice cakes
NT2 Rice crackers
NT2 Rice flour
NT2 Rice koji
NT2 Rice milk
NT2 Rice noodles
NT2 Rice powders
NT2 Rice starch
NT2 Sikhe
NT2 Tape
NT3 Tape ketan
NT2 Yukwa
NT1 Rye
NT2 Rye bran
NT2 Rye bread
NT2 Rye flour
NT2 Rye starch
NT1 Sorghum
NT2 Jowar
NT2 Milo
NT2 Sorghum flour
NT2 Sorghum starch
NT1 Triticale
NT2 Triticale flour
NT1 Tritordeum
NT1 Wheat
NT2 Atta
NT2 Bulgur
NT2 Durum wheat
NT2 Einkorn
NT2 Emmer
NT2 Maida
NT2 Spelt
NT3 Spelt wheat
NT2 Wheat bran
NT2 Wheat bread
NT2 Wheat breadmaking
NT2 Wheat dough
NT2 Wheat fibre
NT2 Wheat flour
NT2 Wheat germ
NT2 Wheat gluten
NT2 Wheat starch
NT1 Wild rice
RT Aleurone
RT Cereal products
RT Falling number
RT Micronization
RT Pelshenke values
RT Winnowers
RT Zeleny values

Cereal wines
BT1 Alcoholic beverages
BT2 Beverages alcoholic
BT3 Beverages
NT1 Rice wines
NT2 Sake
NT3 Ginjoshu
NT3 Narazuke
NT2 Takju
NT2 Yakju

Cerebrosides
BT1 Glycolipids
BT2 Lipids
BT3 Nutrients
RT Galactolipids

Cereulide
HN introduced from vol. 39, issue 1 (2007)
BT1 Toxins
BT2 Residues
RT *Bacillus cereus*

Cerium
USE **Ce**

Certification
RT Accreditation
RT Standards

Cerulenin
BT1 Antibiotics
BT2 Drugs
BT3 Residues

Cervelat
BT1 Sausages
BT2 Meat products
BT3 Animal foods
BT4 Foods

Cestodes
BT1 Parasites
BT2 Pests

Cetacea
BT1 Animals
RT Dolphins
RT Porpoises
RT Whales

Cetavlon
SN syn. cetyltrimethylammonium bromide
BT1 Surfactants

Cetylpyridinium chloride
BT1 Disinfectants
BT2 Disinfection
BT3 Hygiene
BT1 Heterocyclic compounds
BT1 Organic nitrogen compounds

Cetyltrimethylammonium bromide
SN syn. cetavlon
BT1 Surfactants

Cevapcici
BT1 Meat products
BT2 Animal foods
BT3 Foods

Ceviche
BT1 Fish products
BT2 Sea foods
BT3 Aquatic foods
BT4 Animal foods
BT5 Foods

Ceylon
USE **Sri Lanka**

Ceylon spinach
BT1 Vegetables specific
BT2 Vegetables
BT3 Crops
BT4 Plants
BT3 Plant foods
BT4 Foods
UF Malabar nightshade

Chaconine
BT1 Glycoalkaloids
BT2 Alkaloids
BT3 Organic nitrogen compounds
RT Potatoes

Chad
BT1 Central Africa
BT2 Africa

Chaetomium
BT1 Fungi
BT2 Microorganisms

Chai
HN introduced from vol. 37, issue 5 (2005)
BT1 Tea beverages
BT2 Teas
BT3 Beverages
BT3 Crops
BT4 Plants
BT3 Plant foods
BT4 Foods

Chakka
BT1 Dairy products
BT2 Animal foods
BT3 Foods

Chalcones
BT1 Antioxidants
BT2 Additives
BT1 Flavonoids
BT2 Aromatic compounds
BT3 Organic compounds
BT2 Pigments
NT1 Dihydrochalcones
NT2 Neohesperidin dihydrochalcone
NT2 Phloretin
NT1 Xanthohumol

Chalkiness
HN introduced from vol. 39, issue 1 (2007)
BT1 Optical properties
BT2 Physical properties
BT1 Sensory properties

Chalva
USE **Halva**

Chamomile
HN under Spices up to vol. 42 (2010)
SN syn. camomile
BT1 Herbs
BT2 Spices
BT3 Flavourings
BT4 Additives
NT1 Camomile

Champagne
BT1 Sparkling wines
BT2 Wines sparkling
BT3 Wines
BT4 Alcoholic beverages
BT5 Beverages alcoholic
BT6 Beverages

Champagnization
BT1 Sparkling winemaking
BT2 Winemaking
BT3 Processing
BT4 Technology

Champignons
BT1 Edible fungi
BT2 Fungi edible
BT3 Vegetables specific
BT4 Vegetables
BT5 Crops
BT6 Plants
BT5 Plant foods
BT6 Foods

Channel catfish
BT1 Catfish
BT2 Freshwater fish
BT3 Fish
BT4 Animals
BT4 Sea foods
BT5 Aquatic foods
BT6 Animal foods
BT7 Foods
NT1 *Ictalurus punctatus*

Channel Islands
BT1 Europe

Chanos chanos
BT1 Milkfish
BT2 Marine fish
BT3 Fish
BT4 Animals
BT4 Sea foods
BT5 Aquatic foods
BT6 Animal foods
BT7 Foods

Chantarelles
USE ***Cantharellus***

Chapattis
BT1 Bread
BT2 Bakery products
BT3 Cereal products
BT4 Plant foods
BT5 Foods

Chaperones
BT1 Proteins
BT2 Nutrients

Chaptalization
BT1 Winemaking
BT2 Processing
BT3 Technology

Char
BT1 Fish
BT2 Animals
BT2 Sea foods
BT3 Aquatic foods
BT4 Animal foods
BT5 Foods
NT1 Arctic char

Charcoal
BT1 Carbon
BT2 Elements
BT3 Minerals
BT4 Nutrients
RT Activated C
RT Activated carbon

Charcuterie products
BT1 Pork products
BT2 Pork
BT3 Meat specific
BT4 Meat
BT5 Animal foods
BT6 Foods

Chard
USE **Swiss chard**

Charqui
BT1 Meat products
BT2 Animal foods
BT3 Foods

Chayote
BT1 Vegetables specific
BT2 Vegetables
BT3 Crops
BT4 Plants
BT3 Plant foods
BT4 Foods
UF Mirliton

Cheddar cheese
BT1 Cheese varieties
BT2 Cheese
BT3 Dairy products
BT4 Animal foods
BT5 Foods

Cheddaring
BT1 Cheesemaking
BT2 Cheese
BT3 Dairy products
BT4 Animal foods
BT5 Foods
BT2 Processing
BT3 Technology

Cheese
SN unspecified types of cows milk cheese; use Cheese varieties for specific types and cheeses of different species
BT1 Dairy products
BT2 Animal foods
BT3 Foods
NT1 Cheese factories
NT1 Cheesemaking
NT2 Cheddaring
NT1 Cheese rind
NT1 Cheese sauces
NT1 Cheese slices
NT1 Cheese spreads
NT1 Cheese varieties
NT2 Abondance cheese
NT2 Acid curd cheese
NT2 Afuega'l Pitu cheese
NT2 Appenzeller cheese
NT2 Arzua cheese
NT2 Asiago cheese
NT2 Asiago Pressato cheese
NT2 Bergkaese cheese
NT2 Beyaz cheese
NT2 Bitto cheese
NT2 Blue cheese
NT2 Brie cheese
NT2 Bryndza cheese
NT2 Buffalo cheese
NT3 Buffalo mozzarella cheese
NT2 Burgos cheese
NT2 Cabrales cheese
NT2 Caciocavallo cheese
NT3 Caciocavallo Palermitano cheese
NT2 Cacioricotta cheese
NT2 Caciotta cheese
NT2 Camembert cheese
NT2 Cameros cheese
NT2 Canestrato Pugliese cheese
NT2 Cebreiro cheese
NT2 Cheddar cheese
NT2 Chihuahua cheese
NT2 Colby cheese
NT2 Comte cheese
NT2 Cottage cheese
NT2 Cream cheese
NT2 Cremoso Argentino cheese
NT2 Crescenza cheese
NT2 Cuartirolo argentino cheese
NT2 Curd cheese
NT2 Danbo cheese
NT2 Domiati cheese
NT2 Edam cheese
NT2 Emmental cheese
NT2 Ewe cheese
NT2 Feta cheese
NT2 Fior di Latte cheese
NT2 Fiore Sardo cheese
NT2 Fontina cheese
NT2 Fossa cheese
NT2 Fresh cheese
NT2 Fynbo cheese
NT2 Goat cheese
NT2 Gorgonzola cheese
NT2 Gouda cheese
NT2 Grana cheese
NT2 Grana Padano cheese
NT2 Gruyere cheese
NT2 Halloumi cheese
NT2 Hard cheese
NT2 Havarti cheese
NT2 Herrgard cheese
NT2 Hispanico cheese
NT2 Idiazabal cheese
NT2 Jarlsberg cheese
NT2 Kachkaval cheese
NT2 Kajmak cheese
NT2 Kareish cheese
NT2 Kashar cheese
NT2 Kasseri cheese
NT2 Kefalograviera cheese
NT2 Kefalotyri cheese
NT2 Kostroma cheese
NT2 La Serena cheese
NT2 Limburg cheese
NT2 Los Pedroches cheese
NT2 Lymeswold cheese
NT2 Mahon cheese
NT2 Manchego cheese
NT2 Maribo cheese
NT2 Mascarpone cheese
NT2 Minas cheese
NT2 Minas Frescal cheese
NT2 Montasio cheese
NT2 Monterey Jack cheese
NT2 Mozzarella cheese
NT3 Buffalo mozzarella cheese
NT2 Muenster cheese
NT2 Munster cheese
NT2 Norvegia cheese
NT2 Ostiepok cheese
NT2 Parmesan cheese
NT2 Parmigiano Reggiano cheese
NT2 Pasta filata cheese
NT2 Patagras cheese
NT2 Pecorino cheese
NT2 Pecorino Sardo cheese
NT2 Penamellera cheese
NT2 Picante cheese
NT2 Pickled cheese
NT2 Pont-l'Eveque cheese
NT2 Port Salut cheese
NT2 Prato cheese
NT2 Processed cheese
NT2 Provolone cheese
NT2 Quarg
NT3 Tvaroh
NT3 Tvorog
NT3 Twarog
NT2 Quartirolo cheese
NT2 Queso Blanco cheese
NT2 Queso fresco cheese
NT2 Raclette cheese
NT2 Ragusano cheese
NT2 Ras cheese
NT2 Reggianito cheese
NT2 Ricotta cheese
NT2 Robiola cheese
NT2 Rokpol cheese
NT2 Romano cheese
NT2 Roncal cheese
NT2 Roquefort cheese
NT2 Rossiiskii cheese
NT2 Saint-Nectaire cheese
NT2 Saint-Paulin cheese
NT2 Salers cheese
NT2 Samso cheese
NT2 San Simon cheese
NT2 Serra cheese
NT2 Smear cheese
NT2 Soft cheese
NT2 Sovetskii cheese
NT2 Stilton cheese
NT2 Stracchino cheese
NT2 Suluguni cheese
NT2 Swiss cheese
NT2 Taleggio cheese
NT2 Teleme cheese
NT2 Tetilla cheese
NT2 Tilsit cheese
NT2 Toma cheese
NT2 Trappist cheese
NT2 Travnik cheese
NT2 Tulum cheese
NT2 Whey cheese
NT2 White cheese
NT2 White mould cheese
NT2 White pickled cheese
RT Curd
UF Cow cheese
UF Cow milk cheese

Cheese analogues
USE **Cheese substitutes**

Cheeseburgers
BT1 Burgers
BT2 Meat products
BT3 Animal foods
BT4 Foods

Cheesecakes
BT1 Desserts
BT2 Processed foods
BT3 Foods

Cheese curd
BT1 Curd
BT2 Dairy products
BT3 Animal foods
BT4 Foods

Cheese factories
HN under Cheesemaking up to vol. 29 (1997)
BT1 Cheese
BT2 Dairy products
BT3 Animal foods
BT4 Foods
BT1 Food factories
RT Cheesemaking

Cheesemaking
BT1 Cheese
BT2 Dairy products
BT3 Animal foods
BT4 Foods
BT1 Processing
BT2 Technology
NT1 Cheddaring
RT Adjunct cultures
RT Cheese factories
RT Cheesemaking milk
RT Cheese milk
RT Cheese starters

RT Enzymes milk clotting
RT Starters
RT Vats
UF Cheese manufacture

Cheesemaking milk
BT1 Milk
BT2 Dairy products
BT3 Animal foods
BT4 Foods
RT Cheesemaking

Cheese manufacture
USE **Cheesemaking**

Cheese milk
BT1 Milk
BT2 Dairy products
BT3 Animal foods
BT4 Foods
RT Cheesemaking

Cheese rind
HN introduced from vol. 41, issue 1 (2009)
BT1 Cheese
BT2 Dairy products
BT3 Animal foods
BT4 Foods
UF Rind

Cheese sauces
BT1 Cheese
BT2 Dairy products
BT3 Animal foods
BT4 Foods
BT1 Sauces
BT2 Condiments
BT3 Flavourings
BT4 Additives

Cheese slices
BT1 Cheese
BT2 Dairy products
BT3 Animal foods
BT4 Foods

Cheese spreads
BT1 Cheese
BT2 Dairy products
BT3 Animal foods
BT4 Foods
BT1 Spreads
BT2 Processed foods
BT3 Foods

Cheeses specific
HN used as a heading for specific cheeses up to vol. 24 (1992)
USE **Cheese varieties**

Cheese starters
BT1 Starters
BT2 Bacteria
BT3 Microorganisms
RT Cheesemaking

Cheese substitutes
BT1 Simulated foods
BT2 Processed foods
BT3 Foods
RT Imitation cheese
UF Cheese analogues

Cheese varieties
HN heading from vol. 25 (1993); under Cheeses specific up to vol. 24 (1992)
SN specific types of cheese and cheese from animals other than cows
BT1 Cheese
BT2 Dairy products
BT3 Animal foods
BT4 Foods
NT1 Abondance cheese
NT1 Acid curd cheese
NT1 Afuega'l Pitu cheese
NT1 Appenzeller cheese
NT1 Arzua cheese
NT1 Asiago cheese
NT1 Asiago Pressato cheese
NT1 Bergkaese cheese
NT1 Beyaz cheese
NT1 Bitto cheese
NT1 Blue cheese
NT1 Brie cheese
NT1 Bryndza cheese
NT1 Buffalo cheese
NT2 Buffalo mozzarella cheese
NT1 Burgos cheese
NT1 Cabrales cheese
NT1 Caciocavallo cheese
NT2 Caciocavallo Palermitano cheese
NT1 Cacioricotta cheese
NT1 Caciotta cheese
NT1 Camembert cheese
NT1 Cameros cheese
NT1 Canestrato Pugliese cheese
NT1 Cebreiro cheese
NT1 Cheddar cheese
NT1 Chihuahua cheese
NT1 Colby cheese
NT1 Comte cheese
NT1 Cottage cheese
NT1 Cream cheese
NT1 Cremoso Argentino cheese
NT1 Crescenza cheese
NT1 Cuartirolo argentino cheese
NT1 Curd cheese
NT1 Danbo cheese
NT1 Domiati cheese
NT1 Edam cheese
NT1 Emmental cheese
NT1 Ewe cheese
NT1 Feta cheese
NT1 Fior di Latte cheese
NT1 Fiore Sardo cheese
NT1 Fontina cheese
NT1 Fossa cheese
NT1 Fresh cheese
NT1 Fynbo cheese
NT1 Goat cheese
NT1 Gorgonzola cheese
NT1 Gouda cheese
NT1 Grana cheese
NT1 Grana Padano cheese
NT1 Gruyere cheese
NT1 Halloumi cheese
NT1 Hard cheese
NT1 Havarti cheese
NT1 Herrgard cheese
NT1 Hispanico cheese
NT1 Idiazabal cheese
NT1 Jarlsberg cheese
NT1 Kachkaval cheese
NT1 Kajmak cheese
NT1 Kareish cheese
NT1 Kashar cheese
NT1 Kasseri cheese
NT1 Kefalograviera cheese
NT1 Kefalotyri cheese
NT1 Kostroma cheese
NT1 La Serena cheese
NT1 Limburg cheese
NT1 Los Pedroches cheese
NT1 Lymeswold cheese
NT1 Mahon cheese
NT1 Manchego cheese
NT1 Maribo cheese
NT1 Mascarpone cheese
NT1 Minas cheese
NT1 Minas Frescal cheese
NT1 Montasio cheese
NT1 Monterey Jack cheese
NT1 Mozzarella cheese
NT2 Buffalo mozzarella cheese
NT1 Muenster cheese
NT1 Munster cheese
NT1 Norvegia cheese
NT1 Ostiepok cheese
NT1 Parmesan cheese
NT1 Parmigiano Reggiano cheese
NT1 Pasta filata cheese
NT1 Patagras cheese
NT1 Pecorino cheese
NT1 Pecorino Sardo cheese
NT1 Penamellera cheese
NT1 Picante cheese
NT1 Pickled cheese
NT1 Pont-l'Eveque cheese
NT1 Port Salut cheese
NT1 Prato cheese
NT1 Processed cheese
NT1 Provolone cheese
NT1 Quarg
NT2 Tvaroh
NT2 Tvorog
NT2 Twarog
NT1 Quartirolo cheese
NT1 Queso Blanco cheese
NT1 Queso fresco cheese
NT1 Raclette cheese
NT1 Ragusano cheese
NT1 Ras cheese
NT1 Reggianito cheese
NT1 Ricotta cheese
NT1 Robiola cheese
NT1 Rokpol cheese
NT1 Romano cheese
NT1 Roncal cheese
NT1 Roquefort cheese
NT1 Rossiiskii cheese
NT1 Saint-Nectaire cheese
NT1 Saint-Paulin cheese
NT1 Salers cheese
NT1 Samso cheese
NT1 San Simon cheese
NT1 Serra cheese

NT1 Smear cheese
NT1 Soft cheese
NT1 Sovetskii cheese
NT1 Stilton cheese
NT1 Stracchino cheese
NT1 Suluguni cheese
NT1 Swiss cheese
NT1 Taleggio cheese
NT1 Teleme cheese
NT1 Tetilla cheese
NT1 Tilsit cheese
NT1 Toma cheese
NT1 Trappist cheese
NT1 Travnik cheese
NT1 Tulum cheese
NT1 Whey cheese
NT1 White cheese
NT1 White mould cheese
NT1 White pickled cheese
UF Cheeses specific

Cheese whey
BT1 Whey
BT2 Dairy products
BT3 Animal foods
BT4 Foods

Chelating agents
BT1 Additives
RT Sequestrants

Chemesthesis
BT1 Sensory properties

Chemical contamination
BT1 Contamination
RT Pollution

Chemical oxygen demand
RT Wastes

Chemicals
BT1 Residues

Chemiluminescence
BT1 Fluorescence
BT2 Analytical techniques
BT2 Optical properties
BT3 Physical properties

Chemistry
BT1 Science
NT1 Histochemistry
NT1 Physical phases
NT2 Colloids
NT3 Colloidal stability
NT3 Hydrocolloids
NT2 Crystals
NT2 Dispersions
NT3 Dispersion
NT2 Emulsions
NT3 Food emulsions
NT3 Microemulsions
NT2 Gases
NT3 Acetylene
NT3 Air
NT4 Airborne
NT4 Air conditioning
NT4 Air speed
NT4 Atmosphere
NT3 Ammonia
NT4 NH_3
NT3 Ar
NT3 Biogas
NT3 Butane
NT3 Carbon dioxide
NT4 CO_2
NT4 Dry Ice
NT4 Supercritical CO_2 extraction
NT3 Carbon monoxide
NT3 Chlorine dioxide
NT3 Ethane
NT3 Ethylene
NT4 ACC
NT4 Ethephon
NT3 H_2
NT3 He
NT3 H_2S
NT3 Methane
NT3 N_2
NT3 Nitric oxide
NT3 Nitrous oxide
NT3 NO_2
NT3 O_2
NT3 Ozone
NT3 Propane
NT3 Sulfur dioxide
NT4 SO_2
NT3 Vapours
NT4 Water vapour
NT3 Xe
NT2 Gels
NT3 Agar gels
NT3 Alginate gels
NT3 Aspic
NT3 Carrageenan gels
NT3 Silica gels
NT2 Ice
NT2 Liquids
NT3 Fluids
NT4 Supercritical fluids
NT3 Juices
NT4 Stocks
NT3 Liquid foods
NT2 Solids
NT3 SNF
NT3 Soluble solids
NT3 TS
NT3 TSS
NT2 Vapours
NT3 Water vapour
RT Biochemistry

Chemometrics
BT1 Statistical analysis
BT2 Mathematics
BT3 Science

Chemostats
BT1 Bioreactors
BT2 Fermentation technology
BT3 Biotechnology
BT4 Technology
BT3 Process control
BT4 Technology

Chemotaxis
HN introduced from vol. 39, issue 1 (2007)
BT1 Physiology
BT2 Science
BT1 Virulence factors
RT Motility

Cherimoya
BT1 Fruits specific
BT2 Fruits
BT3 Crops
BT4 Plants
BT3 Plant foods
BT4 Foods

Cherries
BT1 Fruits specific
BT2 Fruits
BT3 Crops
BT4 Plants
BT3 Plant foods
BT4 Foods
NT1 Morello cherries
NT1 Sour cherries
NT1 Sweet cherries
RT Cherry juices

Cherry brandy
SN use for the cherry liqueur; for the distilled spirit see Kirsch
BT1 Fruit liqueurs
BT2 Liqueurs
BT3 Alcoholic beverages
BT4 Beverages alcoholic
BT5 Beverages
RT Kirsch

Cherry juices
BT1 Fruit juices
BT2 Fruit products
BT3 Plant foods
BT4 Foods
BT2 Soft drinks
BT3 Beverages
RT Cherries

Cherry laurel
BT1 Fruits specific
BT2 Fruits
BT3 Crops
BT4 Plants
BT3 Plant foods
BT4 Foods

Cherry salmon
SN syn. masu salmon
BT1 Pacific salmon
BT2 Salmon
BT3 Oily fish
BT4 Fish
BT5 Animals
BT5 Sea foods
BT6 Aquatic foods
BT7 Animal foods
BT8 Foods
NT1 Masu salmon

Cherry tomatoes
BT1 Tomatoes
BT2 Fruits specific
BT3 Fruits
BT4 Crops
BT5 Plants

BT4 Plant foods
BT5 Foods

Chervil
HN under Spices up to vol. 42 (2010)
BT1 Herbs
BT2 Spices
BT3 Flavourings
BT4 Additives

Chestnuts
HN heading from vol. 30 (1998); under Nuts up to vol. 29 (1997)
BT1 Nuts
BT2 Fruits
BT3 Crops
BT4 Plants
BT3 Plant foods
BT4 Foods
BT2 Oilseeds
BT3 Seeds
BT4 Plant foods
BT5 Foods
NT1 Japanese chestnuts
NT1 Sweet chestnuts

Chevon
BT1 Goat meat
BT2 Goats
BT3 Animals
BT2 Meat specific
BT3 Meat
BT4 Animal foods
BT5 Foods

Chewiness
BT1 Texture
BT2 Sensory properties

Chewing gums
BT1 Gum confectionery
BT2 Sugar confectionery
BT3 Plant foods
BT4 Foods
NT1 Polyvinyl acetate
UF Chicle gums
UF Gum balls

Chewy candy
HN introduced from vol. 39, issue 1 (2007)
BT1 Candy
BT2 Sugar confectionery
BT3 Plant foods
BT4 Foods

Chhana
BT1 Dairy products
BT2 Animal foods
BT3 Foods

Chicken bones
BT1 Bones
BT1 Chickens
BT2 Poultry
BT3 Birds

Chicken carcasses
BT1 Carcasses
BT2 Meat
BT3 Animal foods
BT4 Foods
BT1 Chicken meat
BT2 Chickens
BT3 Poultry
BT4 Birds
BT2 Poultry meat
BT3 Meat specific
BT4 Meat
BT5 Animal foods
BT6 Foods
UF Broiler carcasses

Chicken drumsticks
BT1 Chicken meat
BT2 Chickens
BT3 Poultry
BT4 Birds
BT2 Poultry meat
BT3 Meat specific
BT4 Meat
BT5 Animal foods
BT6 Foods

Chicken gizzard pickles
BT1 Chickens
BT2 Poultry
BT3 Birds
BT1 Offal
BT2 Animal foods
BT3 Foods
BT1 Pickles
BT2 Fermented foods
BT3 Processed foods
BT4 Foods

Chicken livers
BT1 Chickens
BT2 Poultry
BT3 Birds
BT1 Livers
BT2 Offal
BT3 Animal foods
BT4 Foods

Chicken meat
HN heading from vol. 30 (1998); under Chickens and Poultry meat up to vol. 29 (1997)
BT1 Chickens
BT2 Poultry
BT3 Birds
BT1 Poultry meat
BT2 Meat specific
BT3 Meat
BT4 Animal foods
BT5 Foods
NT1 Chicken carcasses
NT1 Chicken drumsticks
NT1 Chicken mince
NT1 Chicken nuggets
NT1 Chicken products
NT2 Chicken patties
UF Broiler meat
UF Broiler muscles
UF Hen meat

Chicken mince
BT1 Chicken meat
BT2 Chickens
BT3 Poultry
BT4 Birds
BT2 Poultry meat
BT3 Meat specific
BT4 Meat
BT5 Animal foods
BT6 Foods
UF Ground chicken

Chicken nuggets
BT1 Chicken meat
BT2 Chickens
BT3 Poultry
BT4 Birds
BT2 Poultry meat
BT3 Meat specific
BT4 Meat
BT5 Animal foods
BT6 Foods
BT1 Meat products
BT2 Animal foods
BT3 Foods

Chicken patties
BT1 Chicken products
BT2 Chicken meat
BT3 Chickens
BT4 Poultry
BT5 Birds
BT3 Poultry meat
BT4 Meat specific
BT5 Meat
BT6 Animal foods
BT7 Foods
BT1 Meat patties
BT2 Patties
BT3 Meat products
BT4 Animal foods
BT5 Foods

Chicken products
BT1 Chicken meat
BT2 Chickens
BT3 Poultry
BT4 Birds
BT2 Poultry meat
BT3 Meat specific
BT4 Meat
BT5 Animal foods
BT6 Foods
NT1 Chicken patties

Chickens
BT1 Poultry
BT2 Birds
NT1 Chicken bones
NT1 Chicken gizzard pickles
NT1 Chicken livers
NT1 Chicken meat
NT2 Chicken carcasses
NT2 Chicken drumsticks
NT2 Chicken mince
NT2 Chicken nuggets
NT2 Chicken products
NT3 Chicken patties
NT1 Chicken skin
RT Poultry meat
UF Broilers
UF Capons
UF Hens

Chicken sausages
BT1 Sausages
BT2 Meat products
BT3 Animal foods
BT4 Foods
RT Poultry sausages

Chicken skin
BT1 Chickens
BT2 Poultry
BT3 Birds
BT1 Skin

Chick peas
HN heading from vol. 25 (1993); under Legumes up to vol. 24 (1992)
BT1 Legumes
BT2 Vegetables specific
BT3 Vegetables
BT4 Crops
BT5 Plants
BT4 Plant foods
BT5 Foods
NT1 Bengal gram
NT2 Boondi
NT1 Humous
UF Garbanzo beans

Chicle gums
USE **Chewing gums**

Chicory
HN heading from vol. 43 (2011); under Beverages and Vegetables specific up to vol. 42 (2010)
BT1 Crops
BT2 Plants
NT1 Chicory (beverages)
NT1 Chicory (vegetables)
UF Witloof

Chicory (beverages)
HN introduced from vol. 43, issue 1 (2011)
BT1 Beverages
BT1 Chicory
BT2 Crops
BT3 Plants
RT Coffee

Chicory (vegetables)
HN introduced from vol. 43, issue 1 (2011)
BT1 Chicory
BT2 Crops
BT3 Plants
BT1 Vegetables specific
BT2 Vegetables
BT3 Crops
BT4 Plants
BT3 Plant foods
BT4 Foods

Chihuahua cheese
BT1 Cheese varieties
BT2 Cheese
BT3 Dairy products
BT4 Animal foods
BT5 Foods

Children
SN generally <13 years of age
BT1 Population groups

Chile
BT1 South America
BT2 America

Chilean hazelnuts
HN introduced from vol. 37, issue 5 (2005)
BT1 Nuts
BT2 Fruits
BT3 Crops
BT4 Plants
BT3 Plant foods
BT4 Foods
BT2 Oilseeds
BT3 Seeds
BT4 Plant foods
BT5 Foods

Chilled beverages
HN introduced from vol. 39, issue 1 (2007)
SN general use only; see also other specified chilled beverages
BT1 Beverages
RT Chilled foods

Chilled foods
BT1 Processed foods
BT2 Foods
NT1 Refrigerated foods
RT Chilled beverages
RT Salads

Chillers
BT1 Chilling
BT2 Cooling
BT3 Thermal processing
BT4 Processing thermal
BT5 Processing
BT6 Technology
BT1 Equipment
BT2 Technology
RT Refrigerators

Chilli
BT1 Spices
BT2 Flavourings
BT3 Additives
RT Capsaicin
RT Capsaicinoids

Chillies
BT1 Capsicums
BT2 Vegetables specific
BT3 Vegetables
BT4 Crops
BT5 Plants
BT4 Plant foods
BT5 Foods
NT1 Jalapeno peppers
NT1 Red chillies
RT Capsaicin
RT Capsaicinoids

Chilling
BT1 Cooling
BT2 Thermal processing
BT3 Processing thermal
BT4 Processing
BT5 Technology
NT1 Chillers

Chilling injury
BT1 Spoilage

China
BT1 Asia
NT1 Hong Kong
NT1 Tibet

Chinese cabbages
HN heading from vol. 30 (1998); under Vegetables specific up to vol. 29 (1997)
BT1 Vegetables specific
BT2 Vegetables
BT3 Crops
BT4 Plants
BT3 Plant foods
BT4 Foods
NT1 Pak choi

Chinese chives
BT1 Vegetables specific
BT2 Vegetables
BT3 Crops
BT4 Plants
BT3 Plant foods
BT4 Foods

Chinese dates
USE **Jujubes**

Chinese gooseberries
USE **Kiwifruit**

Chinese pears
BT1 Pears
BT2 Fruits specific
BT3 Fruits
BT4 Crops
BT5 Plants
BT4 Plant foods
BT5 Foods

Chinese sausages
BT1 Sausages
BT2 Meat products
BT3 Animal foods
BT4 Foods

Chinese water chestnuts
BT1 Vegetables specific
BT2 Vegetables
BT3 Crops
BT4 Plants
BT3 Plant foods
BT4 Foods
RT Water chestnuts

Chinook salmon
SN syn. king salmon
BT1 Pacific salmon
BT2 Salmon
BT3 Oily fish
BT4 Fish
BT5 Animals
BT5 Sea foods

BT6 Aquatic foods
BT7 Animal foods
BT8 Foods
NT1 King salmon

Chipping properties
BT1 Functional properties
BT2 Physical properties

Chips
BT1 Processed foods
BT2 Foods
NT1 Carrot chips
NT1 Corn chips
NT1 Crisps
NT1 French fries
NT1 Pommes frites
NT1 Potato chips
NT1 Potato crisps
NT1 Tortilla chips
RT Fried foods

Chistorra
BT1 Sausages
BT2 Meat products
BT3 Animal foods
BT4 Foods

Chitin
HN chitins used in the index up to vol. 29 (1997)
BT1 Polysaccharides
BT2 Carbohydrates
BT3 Nutrients
BT3 Organic compounds
NT1 Chitosan
RT Chitooligosaccharides
UF Chitins

Chitinases
SN EC 3.2.1.14
BT1 Glycosidases
BT2 Hydrolases
BT3 Enzymes

Chitin deacetylases
BT1 Hydrolases
BT2 Enzymes

Chitins
HN chitin used in the index from vol. 30 (1998)
USE **Chitin**

Chitooligosaccharides
HN introduced from vol. 43, issue 1 (2011)
BT1 Oligosaccharides
BT2 Polysaccharides
BT3 Carbohydrates
BT4 Nutrients
BT4 Organic compounds
BT2 Sugars
BT3 Carbohydrates
BT4 Nutrients
BT4 Organic compounds
BT3 Plant foods
BT4 Foods
RT Chitin

Chitosan
HN chitosans used in the index up to vol. 29 (1997)
BT1 Chitin
BT2 Polysaccharides
BT3 Carbohydrates
BT4 Nutrients
BT4 Organic compounds
UF Chitosans

Chitosanases
SN EC 3.2.1.132
BT1 Glycosidases
BT2 Hydrolases
BT3 Enzymes

Chitosans
HN chitosan used in the index from vol. 30 (1998)
USE **Chitosan**

Chitterlings
BT1 Offal
BT2 Animal foods
BT3 Foods
RT Intestines

Chives
HN under Spices up to vol. 42 (2010)
BT1 Herbs
BT2 Spices
BT3 Flavourings
BT4 Additives

Chlamydomonas
BT1 Microalgae
BT2 Algae
BT3 Microorganisms

Chloral hydrate
BT1 Drugs
BT2 Residues

Chloramben
BT1 Herbicides
BT2 Pesticides
BT3 Biocides
BT3 Residues
UF Amiben

Chloramines
HN introduced from vol. 39, issue 1 (2007)
BT1 Amines
BT2 Organic nitrogen compounds
BT1 Chlorides
BT2 Salts
BT1 Disinfectants
BT2 Disinfection
BT3 Hygiene
NT1 Monochloramine

Chloramine T
BT1 Sulfonamides
BT2 Antibiotics
BT3 Drugs
BT4 Residues

Chloramphenicol
BT1 Antibiotics
BT2 Drugs
BT3 Residues
UF Chloromycetin

Chlorate
BT1 Herbicides
BT2 Pesticides
BT3 Biocides
BT3 Residues

Chlorates
BT1 Disinfectants
BT2 Disinfection
BT3 Hygiene
RT Perchlorates

Chlordane
BT1 Organochlorine insecticides
BT2 Insecticides
BT3 Pesticides
BT4 Biocides
BT4 Residues
BT2 Organochlorine pesticides
BT3 Pesticides
BT4 Biocides
BT4 Residues
NT1 Nonachlor

Chlordecone
BT1 Organochlorine insecticides
BT2 Insecticides
BT3 Pesticides
BT4 Biocides
BT4 Residues
BT2 Organochlorine pesticides
BT3 Pesticides
BT4 Biocides
BT4 Residues
UF Kepone

Chlordimeform
BT1 Acaricides
BT2 Pesticides
BT3 Biocides
BT3 Residues
BT1 Insecticides
BT2 Pesticides
BT3 Biocides
BT3 Residues

Chlorella
BT1 Microalgae
BT2 Algae
BT3 Microorganisms
NT1 *Chlorella vulgaris*

Chlorella vulgaris
BT1 *Chlorella*
BT2 Microalgae
BT3 Algae
BT4 Microorganisms

Chlorfenvinphos
BT1 Acaricides
BT2 Pesticides
BT3 Biocides
BT3 Residues
BT1 Organophosphorus insecticides
BT2 Insecticides
BT3 Pesticides
BT4 Biocides

BT4 Residues
BT2 Organophosphorus pesticides
BT3 Pesticides
BT4 Biocides
BT4 Residues

Chlorflurecol
BT1 Herbicides
BT2 Pesticides
BT3 Biocides
BT3 Residues
UF Chlorflurenol

Chlorflurenol
USE **Chlorflurecol**

Chloridazon
BT1 Herbicides
BT2 Pesticides
BT3 Biocides
BT3 Residues
UF Pyramin
UF Pyrazon

Chlorides
BT1 Salts
NT1 $CaCl_2$
NT1 Chloramines
NT2 Monochloramine
NT1 KCl
NT1 $MgCl_2$
NT1 NaCl
RT Chlorine

Chlorinated hydrocarbons
BT1 Organic halogen compounds
NT1 Carbon tetrachloride
NT1 Chloroform
NT1 Dichloroacetic acid
NT1 Dichloromethane
NT1 Epichlorohydrin
NT1 Hexachlorobutadiene
NT1 Methylene chloride
NT1 Polychlorinated biphenyls
NT2 Arochlor
NT2 Hexachlorobiphenyl
NT2 PCB
NT1 Tetrachloromethane
NT1 Trichloromethane
RT Chlorine
RT Organochlorine compounds

Chlorination
BT1 Disinfection
BT2 Hygiene

Chlorine
SN symbol Cl is also used in the index
BT1 Halogens
BT2 Elements
BT3 Minerals
BT4 Nutrients
NT1 Cl
RT Chlorides
RT Chlorinated hydrocarbons
RT Chlorine dioxide
RT Disinfection
RT Organochlorine compounds

Chlorine dioxide
BT1 Gases
BT2 Physical phases
BT3 Chemistry
BT4 Science
BT1 Inorganic compounds
BT1 Oxides
BT1 Oxidizing agents
BT2 Additives
RT Chlorine

Chlorites
BT1 Disinfectants
BT2 Disinfection
BT3 Hygiene

Chlormequat
BT1 Herbicides
BT2 Pesticides
BT3 Biocides
BT3 Residues
BT1 Plant growth regulators
BT2 Cultivation
BT3 Agriculture
UF CCC
UF Chlorocholine chloride
UF Cycocel

Chloroanisoles
USE **Haloanisoles**

Chlorobenzilate
HN under Insecticides up to vol. 42 (2010)
BT1 Acaricides
BT2 Pesticides
BT3 Biocides
BT3 Residues
BT1 Organochlorine pesticides
BT2 Pesticides
BT3 Biocides
BT3 Residues

Chlorocholine chloride
USE **Chlormequat**

Chlorococcum
BT1 Microalgae
BT2 Algae
BT3 Microorganisms

Chloroethylphosphonic acid
USE **Ethephon**

(2-Chloroethyl)phosphonic acid
USE **Ethephon**

Chlorofluorocarbons
BT1 Refrigerants
BT2 Refrigeration
BT3 Thermal processing
BT4 Processing thermal
BT5 Processing
BT6 Technology

Chloroform
SN syn. trichloromethane
BT1 Chlorinated hydrocarbons
BT2 Organic halogen compounds
BT1 Fumigants
BT2 Biocides
BT1 Solvents

Chlorogenic acid
SN syn. caffeoylquinic acid
BT1 Organic acids
BT2 Acids
BT1 Phenols
BT2 Alcohols
BT2 Aromatic compounds
BT3 Organic compounds
NT1 Caffeoylquinic acid

Chloromycetin
USE **Chloramphenicol**

Chlorophenol
BT1 Organic halogen compounds
BT1 Phenols
BT2 Alcohols
BT2 Aromatic compounds
BT3 Organic compounds

Chlorophenoxyacetic acid
BT1 Phenoxy herbicides
BT2 Herbicides
BT3 Pesticides
BT4 Biocides
BT4 Residues

Chlorophos
USE **Trichlorfon**

Chlorophyllases
SN EC 3.1.1.14
BT1 Esterases
BT2 Hydrolases
BT3 Enzymes

Chlorophylls
BT1 Porphyrins
BT2 Heterocyclic compounds
BT2 Organic nitrogen compounds
BT2 Pigments

Chloropicrin
BT1 Fumigants
BT2 Biocides

Chloropropanols
HN introduced from vol. 39, issue 1 (2007)
BT1 Contaminants
BT2 Contamination
BT1 Organochlorine compounds
BT2 Organic halogen compounds
BT1 Propanol
BT2 Alcohols
BT2 Solvents

Chlorothalonil
BT1 Fungicides
BT2 Pesticides
BT3 Biocides
BT3 Residues
UF Daconil
UF Tetrachloroisophthalonitrile

Chloroxuron
BT1 Herbicides
BT2 Pesticides
BT3 Biocides
BT3 Residues
UF Tenoran

Chlorphoxim
BT1 Organophosphorus insecticides
BT2 Insecticides
BT3 Pesticides
BT4 Biocides
BT4 Residues
BT2 Organophosphorus pesticides
BT3 Pesticides
BT4 Biocides
BT4 Residues

Chlorpropham
BT1 Carbamate pesticides
BT2 Pesticides
BT3 Biocides
BT3 Residues
BT1 Herbicides
BT2 Pesticides
BT3 Biocides
BT3 Residues
UF CIPC

Chlorpyrifos
BT1 Acaricides
BT2 Pesticides
BT3 Biocides
BT3 Residues
BT1 Nematocides
BT2 Pesticides
BT3 Biocides
BT3 Residues
BT1 Organophosphorus insecticides
BT2 Insecticides
BT3 Pesticides
BT4 Biocides
BT4 Residues
BT2 Organophosphorus pesticides
BT3 Pesticides
BT4 Biocides
BT4 Residues
UF Dursban

Chlorpyrifos-methyl
BT1 Acaricides
BT2 Pesticides
BT3 Biocides
BT3 Residues
BT1 Organophosphorus insecticides
BT2 Insecticides
BT3 Pesticides
BT4 Biocides
BT4 Residues
BT2 Organophosphorus pesticides
BT3 Pesticides
BT4 Biocides
BT4 Residues

Chlortetracycline
BT1 Tetracyclines
BT2 Antibiotics
BT3 Drugs
BT4 Residues
UF Aureomycin
UF Biomycin

Chocolate
BT1 Sugar confectionery
BT2 Plant foods
BT3 Foods
NT1 Chocolate crumb
NT1 Chocolate factories
NT1 Chocolate industry
NT1 Chocolate liquor
NT1 Chocolate mass
NT1 Chocolate products
NT2 Chocolate bars
NT2 Chocolate beverages
NT3 Drinking chocolate
NT2 Chocolate chips
NT2 Chocolate coatings
NT2 Chocolate confectionery
NT2 Chocolate couverture
NT2 Chocolate desserts
NT2 Chocolate dragees
NT2 Chocolate milk
NT2 Chocolate powders
NT2 Chocolates
NT2 Chocolate truffles
NT2 Dark chocolate
NT2 Milk chocolate
NT2 White chocolate
RT Beverages
RT Bloom
RT Cocoa
RT Cocoa butter
RT Cocoa products
RT Cupuacu
RT Panning
RT Tempering

Chocolate bars
BT1 Chocolate products
BT2 Chocolate
BT3 Sugar confectionery
BT4 Plant foods
BT5 Foods
BT1 Confectionery bars
BT2 Confectionery
BT3 Bakery products
BT4 Cereal products
BT5 Plant foods
BT6 Foods
BT3 Sugar confectionery
BT4 Plant foods
BT5 Foods
BT2 Food bars
BT3 Snack foods
BT4 Processed foods
BT5 Foods

Chocolate beverages
BT1 Beverages
BT1 Chocolate products
BT2 Chocolate
BT3 Sugar confectionery
BT4 Plant foods
BT5 Foods
NT1 Drinking chocolate

Chocolate chips
BT1 Chocolate products
BT2 Chocolate
BT3 Sugar confectionery
BT4 Plant foods
BT5 Foods

Chocolate coatings
BT1 Chocolate products
BT2 Chocolate
BT3 Sugar confectionery
BT4 Plant foods
BT5 Foods
BT1 Coatings

Chocolate confectionery
BT1 Chocolate products
BT2 Chocolate
BT3 Sugar confectionery
BT4 Plant foods
BT5 Foods

Chocolate couverture
BT1 Chocolate products
BT2 Chocolate
BT3 Sugar confectionery
BT4 Plant foods
BT5 Foods

Chocolate crumb
BT1 Chocolate
BT2 Sugar confectionery
BT3 Plant foods
BT4 Foods

Chocolate desserts
BT1 Chocolate products
BT2 Chocolate
BT3 Sugar confectionery
BT4 Plant foods
BT5 Foods
BT1 Desserts
BT2 Processed foods
BT3 Foods

Chocolate dragees
BT1 Chocolate products
BT2 Chocolate
BT3 Sugar confectionery
BT4 Plant foods
BT5 Foods

Chocolate factories
BT1 Chocolate
BT2 Sugar confectionery
BT3 Plant foods
BT4 Foods
BT1 Food factories

Chocolate fillings
BT1 Confectionery fillings
BT2 Fillings

Chocolate industry
BT1 Chocolate
BT2 Sugar confectionery
BT3 Plant foods
BT4 Foods

BT1 Food industry
BT2 Industries

Chocolate liquor
BT1 Chocolate
BT2 Sugar confectionery
BT3 Plant foods
BT4 Foods

Chocolate mass
BT1 Chocolate
BT2 Sugar confectionery
BT3 Plant foods
BT4 Foods

Chocolate milk
BT1 Chocolate products
BT2 Chocolate
BT3 Sugar confectionery
BT4 Plant foods
BT5 Foods
BT1 Milk
BT2 Dairy products
BT3 Animal foods
BT4 Foods

Chocolate powders
BT1 Chocolate products
BT2 Chocolate
BT3 Sugar confectionery
BT4 Plant foods
BT5 Foods
BT1 Powders
BT2 Dried foods
BT3 Processed foods
BT4 Foods
BT2 Instant foods
BT3 Processed foods
BT4 Foods

Chocolate products
HN heading from vol. 25 (1993); under Chocolate up tovol. 24 (1992)
BT1 Chocolate
BT2 Sugar confectionery
BT3 Plant foods
BT4 Foods
NT1 Chocolate bars
NT1 Chocolate beverages
NT2 Drinking chocolate
NT1 Chocolate chips
NT1 Chocolate coatings
NT1 Chocolate confectionery
NT1 Chocolate couverture
NT1 Chocolate desserts
NT1 Chocolate dragees
NT1 Chocolate milk
NT1 Chocolate powders
NT1 Chocolates
NT1 Chocolate truffles
NT1 Dark chocolate
NT1 Milk chocolate
NT1 White chocolate

Chocolates
BT1 Chocolate products
BT2 Chocolate
BT3 Sugar confectionery
BT4 Plant foods
BT5 Foods

Chocolate truffles
BT1 Chocolate products
BT2 Chocolate
BT3 Sugar confectionery
BT4 Plant foods
BT5 Foods

Chokeberries
HN introduced from vol. 37, issue 5 (2005)
BT1 Berries
BT2 Fruits specific
BT3 Fruits
BT4 Crops
BT5 Plants
BT4 Plant foods
BT5 Foods

Cholecalciferol
SN syn. vitamin D3; syn. calciol
BT1 Vitamins
BT2 Nutrients
NT1 Vitamin D_3

Cholera
BT1 Diseases
RT Cholera toxin
RT *Vibrio*

Cholera toxin
BT1 Enterotoxins
BT2 Toxins
BT3 Residues
RT Cholera

Cholesterol
BT1 Sterols
BT2 Alcohols
BT2 Steroids
BT3 Lipids
BT4 Nutrients
NT1 Cholesterol low foods
NT1 Cholesterol oxidation products
NT2 Cholesterol oxides
RT Nutrition

Cholesterol low foods
HN introduced from vol. 42, issue 1 (2010)
BT1 Cholesterol
BT2 Sterols
BT3 Alcohols
BT3 Steroids
BT4 Lipids
BT5 Nutrients
UF Low cholesterol foods

Cholesterol oxidases
SN EC 1.1.3.6
BT1 Oxidases
BT2 Oxidoreductases
BT3 Enzymes

Cholesterol oxidation products
BT1 Cholesterol
BT2 Sterols
BT3 Alcohols
BT3 Steroids
BT4 Lipids
BT5 Nutrients
NT1 Cholesterol oxides
UF Oxysterols

Cholesterol oxides
BT1 Cholesterol oxidation products
BT2 Cholesterol
BT3 Sterols
BT4 Alcohols
BT4 Steroids
BT5 Lipids
BT6 Nutrients

Choline
HN also under Nutrients up to vol. 42 (2010)
BT1 Biogenic amines
BT2 Amines
BT3 Organic nitrogen compounds

Cholinesterases
SN EC 3.1.1.8
BT1 Esterases
BT2 Hydrolases
BT3 Enzymes

Choloylglycine hydrolases
SN EC 3.5.1.24
BT1 Hydrolases
BT2 Enzymes
UF Bile salt hydrolases

Chondroitin
HN introduced from vol. 39, issue 1 (2007)
BT1 Glycosaminoglycans
BT2 Polysaccharides
BT3 Carbohydrates
BT4 Nutrients
BT4 Organic compounds
RT Connective tissues

Chondrus
BT1 Seaweeds
BT2 Algae
BT3 Microorganisms
BT2 Sea foods
BT3 Aquatic foods
BT4 Animal foods
BT5 Foods
NT1 *Chondrus crispus*

Chondrus crispus
BT1 *Chondrus*
BT2 Seaweeds
BT3 Algae
BT4 Microorganisms
BT3 Sea foods
BT4 Aquatic foods
BT5 Animal foods
BT6 Foods

Chopi
HN introduced from vol. 37, issue 5 (2005)
BT1 Spices
BT2 Flavourings
BT3 Additives

Chopping
BT1 Cutting
BT2 Processing
BT3 Technology
NT1 Chopping boards
RT Comminution

Chopping boards
BT1 Chopping
BT2 Cutting
BT3 Processing
BT4 Technology

Chorizo
BT1 Sausages
BT2 Meat products
BT3 Animal foods
BT4 Foods

Christstollen
BT1 Cakes
BT2 Bakery products
BT3 Cereal products
BT4 Plant foods
BT5 Foods

Chromatography
BT1 Analytical techniques
NT1 Affinity chromatography
NT1 Capillary electrochromatography
NT1 Column chromatography
NT1 Countercurrent chromatography
NT1 Gas chromatography
NT2 Gas solid chromatography
NT2 GC
NT2 GC-MS
NT2 GLC
NT1 Gel filtration
NT1 Gel permeation chromatography
NT1 High performance liquid chromatography
NT2 HPLC
NT2 LC
NT2 LC-MS
NT2 Supercritical HPLC
NT2 UPLC
NT1 Immunoaffinity chromatography
NT1 Ion chromatography
NT1 Ion exchange chromatography
NT1 Micellar electrokinetic chromatography
NT1 Paper chromatography
NT1 Size exclusion chromatography
NT1 Supercritical fluid chromatography
NT1 Thin layer chromatography
NT2 HPTLC
NT2 TLC
RT Electrophoresis

Chromista
HN introduced from vol. 43, issue 1 (2011)
BT1 Microorganisms
NT1 *Phytophthora*
NT1 *Schizochytrium*
NT1 *Thraustochytrium*

Chromium
USE **Cr**

Chromobacterium
BT1 Bacteria
BT2 Microorganisms
NT1 *Chromobacterium violaceum*
NT1 *Chromobacterium viscosum*

Chromobacterium violaceum
BT1 *Chromobacterium*
BT2 Bacteria
BT3 Microorganisms

Chromobacterium viscosum
BT1 *Chromobacterium*
BT2 Bacteria
BT3 Microorganisms

Chromoplasts
BT1 Cells

Chromosomes
BT1 Genetics
NT1 Genes
NT2 Alleles
NT2 Gene-nutrient interactions
NT2 Genotype
NT2 Introns
NT2 Marker genes
NT2 QTL
NT2 Reporter genes
NT2 Transgenes
RT Clastogenicity
RT DNA
RT Genomes

Chrysanthemum
BT1 Plants
NT1 *Chrysanthemum coronarium*

Chrysanthemum coronarium
BT1 *Chrysanthemum*
BT2 Plants

Chrysene
BT1 Hydrocarbons
BT2 Organic compounds

Chryseobacterium
HN introduced from vol. 39, issue 1 (2007)
BT1 Bacteria
BT2 Microorganisms

Chrysin
HN introduced from vol. 39, issue 1 (2007)
BT1 Flavones
BT2 Flavonoids
BT3 Aromatic compounds
BT4 Organic compounds
BT3 Pigments

Chrysosporium
BT1 Fungi
BT2 Microorganisms

Chub
BT1 Freshwater fish
BT2 Fish
BT3 Animals
BT3 Sea foods
BT4 Aquatic foods
BT5 Animal foods
BT6 Foods
NT1 *Leuciscus cephalus*

Chub mackerel
SN syn. Pacific mackerel; Spanish mackerel
BT1 Mackerel
BT2 Marine fish
BT3 Fish
BT4 Animals
BT4 Sea foods
BT5 Aquatic foods
BT6 Animal foods
BT7 Foods
BT2 Oily fish
BT3 Fish
BT4 Animals
BT4 Sea foods
BT5 Aquatic foods
BT6 Animal foods
BT7 Foods
NT1 *Scomber japonicus*

Chufa nuts
SN syn. tigernuts
BT1 Vegetables specific
BT2 Vegetables
BT3 Crops
BT4 Plants
BT3 Plant foods
BT4 Foods
NT1 Tigernuts
NT2 *Cyperus esculentus*

Chukars
BT1 Poultry
BT2 Birds

Chum salmon
SN syn. keta salmon
BT1 Pacific salmon
BT2 Salmon
BT3 Oily fish
BT4 Fish
BT5 Animals
BT5 Sea foods
BT6 Aquatic foods
BT7 Animal foods
BT8 Foods
NT1 Keta salmon
NT1 *Oncorhynchus keta*

Chungkook-jang
BT1 Fermented foods
BT2 Processed foods
BT3 Foods
BT1 Soy products
BT2 Vegetable products
BT3 Plant foods
BT4 Foods

Churning
BT1 Buttermaking

BT2 Processing
BT3 Technology

Chutneys
BT1 Pickles
BT2 Fermented foods
BT3 Processed foods
BT4 Foods

Chymosin
HN heading up to vol. 24 (1992)
SN EC 3.4.23.4
BT1 Milk clotting enzymes
BT2 Enzymes milk clotting
BT3 Proteinases
BT4 Hydrolases
BT5 Enzymes
UF Rennin

Chymotrypsin
SN EC 3.4.21.1
BT1 Proteinases
BT2 Hydrolases
BT3 Enzymes

Chymotrypsin inhibitors
BT1 Proteinases inhibitors
BT2 Antinutritional factors
BT3 Nutritional values
BT2 Enzyme inhibitors
BT3 Enzymes

Cider
BT1 Alcoholic beverages
BT2 Beverages alcoholic
BT3 Beverages
RT Apple juices
RT Apple wines
RT Perry

Cider apples
BT1 Apples
BT2 Fruits specific
BT3 Fruits
BT4 Crops
BT5 Plants
BT4 Plant foods
BT5 Foods

Cider vinegar
BT1 Vinegar
BT2 Condiments
BT3 Flavourings
BT4 Additives
BT2 Fermented foods
BT3 Processed foods
BT4 Foods

Cider yeasts
BT1 Yeasts
BT2 Fungi
BT3 Microorganisms

Cigarette smoking
HN introduced from vol. 39, issue 1 (2007)
RT Diseases
RT Nicotine

Ciguatera
SN syn. paralytic shellfish poisoning
BT1 Poisoning
RT Ciguatoxin

Ciguatoxin
BT1 Toxins
BT2 Residues
RT Ciguatera

Cilantro
USE **Coriander**

Cimaterol
BT1 β-Adrenergic agonists
BT2 Drugs
BT3 Residues
RT Clenbuterol

Cineole
HN also under Flavour compounds up to vol. 42 (2010)
BT1 Aroma compounds
BT2 Flavour compounds
BT2 Volatile compounds
BT1 Monoterpenoids
BT2 Terpenoids
BT3 Lipids
BT4 Nutrients
NT1 Eucalyptol

Cinnamaldehyde
BT1 Aldehydes
BT2 Carbonyl compounds
BT3 Organic compounds
BT1 Aroma compounds
BT2 Flavour compounds
BT2 Volatile compounds
BT1 Aromatic compounds
BT2 Organic compounds
RT Cinnamon

Cinnamic acid
BT1 Aroma compounds
BT2 Flavour compounds
BT2 Volatile compounds
BT1 Organic acids
BT2 Acids
BT1 Phenols
BT2 Alcohols
BT2 Aromatic compounds
BT3 Organic compounds

Cinnamomum zeylanicum
BT1 Cinnamon
BT2 Spices
BT3 Flavourings
BT4 Additives

Cinnamon
BT1 Spices
BT2 Flavourings
BT3 Additives
NT1 *Cinnamomum zeylanicum*
RT *Cassia*
RT Cinnamaldehyde
RT Cinnamon oils

Cinnamon oils
BT1 Essential oils
BT2 Flavourings
BT3 Additives
BT2 Vegetable oils
BT3 Oils vegetable
BT4 Oils
BT5 Lipids
BT6 Nutrients
BT4 Vegetable products
BT5 Plant foods
BT6 Foods
RT Cinnamon

Ciodrin
USE **Crotoxyphos**

CIPC
USE **Chlorpropham**

Ciprofloxacin
BT1 Quinolones
BT2 Antibiotics
BT3 Drugs
BT4 Residues

Circular dichroism
BT1 Spectroscopy
BT2 Analytical techniques

Citral
BT1 Aldehydes
BT2 Carbonyl compounds
BT3 Organic compounds
BT1 Aroma compounds
BT2 Flavour compounds
BT2 Volatile compounds
BT1 Monoterpenoids
BT2 Terpenoids
BT3 Lipids
BT4 Nutrients
NT1 Geranial
NT1 Neral

Citramalic acid
BT1 Organic acids
BT2 Acids

Citrates
BT1 Salts
RT Citric acid

Citrate synthases
SN includes EC 2.3.3.1 (formerly EC 4.1.3.7) and EC 2.3.3.3 (formerly EC 4.1.3.28)
BT1 Transferases
BT2 Enzymes

Citreoviridin
BT1 Mycotoxins
BT2 Toxins
BT3 Residues

Citric acid
BT1 Antioxidants
BT2 Additives
BT1 Organic acids
BT2 Acids
RT Citrates
RT Citric fermentation
RT Isocitric acid

Citric fermentation
BT1 Fermentation
RT Citric acid

Citrinin
BT1 Mycotoxins
BT2 Toxins
BT3 Residues

Citrobacter
HN under Enterobacteriaceae up to vol. 24 (1992)
BT1 Bacteria
BT2 Microorganisms
NT1 *Citrobacter freundii*

Citrobacter freundii
BT1 *Citrobacter*
BT2 Bacteria
BT3 Microorganisms

Citronella
BT1 Plants
RT Citronella essential oils

Citronella essential oils
BT1 Essential oils
BT2 Flavourings
BT3 Additives
BT2 Vegetable oils
BT3 Oils vegetable
BT4 Oils
BT5 Lipids
BT6 Nutrients
BT4 Vegetable products
BT5 Plant foods
BT6 Foods
RT Citronella

Citronellal
HN also under Flavour compounds up to vol. 42 (2010)
BT1 Aldehydes
BT2 Carbonyl compounds
BT3 Organic compounds
BT1 Aroma compounds
BT2 Flavour compounds
BT2 Volatile compounds
BT1 Monoterpenoids
BT2 Terpenoids
BT3 Lipids
BT4 Nutrients

Citronellol
HN also under Flavour compounds up to vol. 42 (2010)
BT1 Alcohols
BT1 Aroma compounds
BT2 Flavour compounds
BT2 Volatile compounds
BT1 Monoterpenoids
BT2 Terpenoids
BT3 Lipids
BT4 Nutrients

Citrons
BT1 Citrus fruits
BT2 Fruits specific
BT3 Fruits
BT4 Crops
BT5 Plants
BT4 Plant foods
BT5 Foods

Citrulline
BT1 Amino acids
BT2 Nutrients
BT2 Organic acids
BT3 Acids
BT2 Organic nitrogen compounds

Citrus beverages
BT1 Fruit juice beverages
BT2 Soft drinks
BT3 Beverages
RT Citrus fruits
RT Citrus juices

Citrus essential oils
BT1 Essential oils
BT2 Flavourings
BT3 Additives
BT2 Vegetable oils
BT3 Oils vegetable
BT4 Oils
BT5 Lipids
BT6 Nutrients
BT4 Vegetable products
BT5 Plant foods
BT6 Foods
NT1 Bergamot essential oils
NT2 Bergamot oils
NT1 Bitter orange essential oils
NT1 Citrus oils
NT1 Lemon essential oils
NT1 Lime essential oils
NT1 Neroli oils
NT1 Orange essential oils
RT Citrus fruits

Citrus fruits
BT1 Fruits specific
BT2 Fruits
BT3 Crops
BT4 Plants
BT3 Plant foods
BT4 Foods
NT1 Bitter oranges
NT1 Citrons
NT1 Citrus pectins
NT1 Citrus peel
NT1 *Citrus tamurana*
NT1 Galgals
NT1 Grapefruit
NT2 Grapefruit peel
NT1 Ki-mikan
NT1 Kumquats
NT1 Lemons
NT2 Lemon peel
NT1 Limes
NT1 Oranges
NT2 Mandarins
NT3 Clementines
NT3 Kinnow mandarins
NT3 Ponkans
NT3 Satsuma mandarins
NT3 Satsumas
NT3 Tangerines
NT2 Orange peel
NT1 Ortanique
NT1 Pomelos
NT2 *Citrus grandis*
NT2 Pummelos
NT2 Shaddocks
NT1 Sweet limes
NT1 Tangelo
NT1 Tangor
NT1 Yuzu
RT Bergamot essential oils
RT Bergamot oils
RT Citrus beverages
RT Citrus essential oils
RT Citrus juice concentrates
RT Citrus juices
RT Citrus oils
RT Naringin
RT Neroli oils

Citrus grandis
BT1 Pomelos
BT2 Citrus fruits
BT3 Fruits specific
BT4 Fruits
BT5 Crops
BT6 Plants
BT5 Plant foods
BT6 Foods

Citrus juice concentrates
BT1 Citrus juices
BT2 Fruit juices
BT3 Fruit products
BT4 Plant foods
BT5 Foods
BT3 Soft drinks
BT4 Beverages
BT1 Fruit juice concentrates
BT2 Concentrates
BT3 Processed foods
BT4 Foods
BT2 Fruit juices
BT3 Fruit products
BT4 Plant foods
BT5 Foods
BT3 Soft drinks
BT4 Beverages
NT1 Orange juice concentrates
RT Citrus fruits

Citrus juices
BT1 Fruit juices
BT2 Fruit products
BT3 Plant foods
BT4 Foods
BT2 Soft drinks
BT3 Beverages
NT1 Citrus juice concentrates
NT2 Orange juice concentrates
NT1 Grapefruit juices
NT1 Lemon juices
NT1 Lime juices
NT1 Orange juices
NT2 Mandarin juices
NT3 Tangerine juices
NT2 Orange juice concentrates
RT Citrus beverages
RT Citrus fruits

Citrus oils
BT1 Citrus essential oils
BT2 Essential oils
BT3 Flavourings
BT4 Additives

BT3 Vegetable oils
BT4 Oils vegetable
BT5 Oils
BT6 Lipids
BT7 Nutrients
BT5 Vegetable products
BT6 Plant foods
BT7 Foods
RT Citrus fruits

Citrus pectins
BT1 Citrus fruits
BT2 Fruits specific
BT3 Fruits
BT4 Crops
BT5 Plants
BT4 Plant foods
BT5 Foods
BT1 Pectins
BT2 Pectic substances
BT3 Polysaccharides
BT4 Carbohydrates
BT5 Nutrients
BT5 Organic compounds

Citrus peel
BT1 Citrus fruits
BT2 Fruits specific
BT3 Fruits
BT4 Crops
BT5 Plants
BT4 Plant foods
BT5 Foods
BT1 Peel
RT Fruit peel

Citrus red
BT1 Colorants
BT2 Additives

Citrus tamurana
BT1 Citrus fruits
BT2 Fruits specific
BT3 Fruits
BT4 Crops
BT5 Plants
BT4 Plant foods
BT5 Foods

CJD
HN Creutzfeldt-Jakob disease used in the index up to vol. 35, issue 6 (2003)
BT1 Prion diseases
BT2 Diseases
RT BSE
UF Creutzfeldt-Jakob disease

Cl
SN index heading is Chlorine
BT1 Chlorine
BT2 Halogens
BT3 Elements
BT4 Minerals
BT5 Nutrients

CLA
HN conjugated linoleic acid used in the index up to vol. 35, issue 6 (2003)
BT1 Conjugated fatty acids
BT2 PUFA
BT3 Unsaturated fatty acids
BT4 Fatty acids
BT5 Lipids
BT6 Nutrients
BT5 Organic acids
BT6 Acids
BT1 Linoleic acid
BT2 ω-6 Fatty acids
BT3 PUFA
BT4 Unsaturated fatty acids
BT5 Fatty acids
BT6 Lipids
BT7 Nutrients
BT6 Organic acids
BT7 Acids
UF Conjugated linoleic acid

Cladosporium
BT1 Fungi
BT2 Microorganisms

Clams
BT1 Bivalves
BT2 Molluscs
BT3 Shellfish
BT4 Animals
BT4 Sea foods
BT5 Aquatic foods
BT6 Animal foods
BT7 Foods
NT1 Freshwater clams
NT1 *Pseudocardium sachalinensis*
NT1 *Tapes philippinarum*

Clarification
BT1 Processing
BT2 Technology
NT1 Clarifiers
NT1 Fining
NT2 Fining agents
NT1 Winterization
RT Filter aids

Clarifiers
BT1 Clarification
BT2 Processing
BT3 Technology
BT1 Equipment
BT2 Technology

Clarity
BT1 Optical properties
BT2 Physical properties

Clary sage essential oils
HN introduced from vol. 39, issue 1 (2007)
BT1 Essential oils
BT2 Flavourings
BT3 Additives
BT2 Vegetable oils
BT3 Oils vegetable
BT4 Oils
BT5 Lipids
BT6 Nutrients
BT4 Vegetable products
BT5 Plant foods
BT6 Foods

Classification
RT Grading

Clastogenicity
HN introduced from vol. 41, issue 1 (2009)
BT1 Mutagenicity
RT Chromosomes

Claviceps
BT1 Fungi
BT2 Microorganisms
NT1 *Claviceps purpurea*

Claviceps purpurea
BT1 *Claviceps*
BT2 Fungi
BT3 Microorganisms

Clays
BT1 Filter aids
BT2 Filtration
BT3 Processing
BT4 Technology

Cleaning
BT1 Hygiene
BT1 Processing
BT2 Technology
NT1 Cleaning agents
NT1 Cleaning in place
NT1 Depuration
NT1 Descaling
NT1 Dishwashers
NT1 Rinsing
NT1 Washing
RT Disinfection
RT Pigging
RT Surfactants

Cleaning agents
BT1 Cleaning
BT2 Hygiene
BT2 Processing
BT3 Technology

Cleaning in place
BT1 Cleaning
BT2 Hygiene
BT2 Processing
BT3 Technology
UF Clean in place

Clean in place
USE **Cleaning in place**

Clean room technology
BT1 Hygiene
BT1 Technology

Clementines
BT1 Mandarins
BT2 Oranges
BT3 Citrus fruits
BT4 Fruits specific
BT5 Fruits
BT6 Crops
BT7 Plants
BT6 Plant foods
BT7 Foods

Clenbuterol
BT1 β-Adrenergic agonists
BT2 Drugs
BT3 Residues
RT Cimaterol

Climate
RT Environment
RT Season
RT Weather

Clinical techniques
HN introduced from vol. 39, issue 1 (2007); heading
NT1 Diagnosis
NT1 Oral food challenges
NT1 Skin prick testing
RT Dietary study techniques
RT Diseases
RT Therapy

Clipping
BT1 Processing
BT2 Technology

Cloned animal foods
HN introduced from vol. 41, issue 1 (2009)
BT1 Animal foods
BT2 Foods
BT1 Novel foods
BT2 Foods
RT Cloned animals

Cloned animals
HN introduced from vol. 41, issue 1 (2009)
SN animals genetically identical to a single parent
BT1 Animals
BT1 Genetics
RT Cloned animal foods
RT Transgenic animals

Cloning technology
HN heading for vol. 22 and vol. 23 (1990-1991)
BT1 Gene cloning
BT2 Genetic techniques
BT3 Genetics
BT1 Technology
NT1 Marker genes
NT1 Marker proteins
NT2 Green fluorescent protein
NT1 Reporter genes

Cloning vectors
HN heading from vol. 24 (1992)
BT1 Genetic techniques
BT2 Genetics
NT1 Shuttle vectors
NT1 Vectors
NT2 Expression vectors
RT Bacteriophages
RT Plasmids

Clonorchis sinensis
BT1 Parasites
BT2 Pests

Clopidol
BT1 Coccidiostats
BT2 Drugs
BT3 Residues

Clostridium
BT1 Bacteria
BT2 Microorganisms
NT1 *Clostridium absonum*
NT1 *Clostridium acetobutylicum*
NT1 *Clostridium beijerinckii*
NT1 *Clostridium botulinum*
NT1 *Clostridium butyricum*
NT1 *Clostridium cellulolyticum*
NT1 *Clostridium difficile*
NT1 *Clostridium josui*
NT1 *Clostridium lentocellum*
NT1 *Clostridium perfringens*
NT1 *Clostridium sporogenes*
NT1 *Clostridium stercorarium*
NT2 *Clostridium thermolacticum*
NT1 *Clostridium thermoaceticum*
NT1 *Clostridium thermocellum*
NT1 *Clostridium thermosuccinogenes*
NT1 *Clostridium thermosulfurogenes*
NT1 *Clostridium tyrobutyricum*
RT Botulism
RT Botulotoxins

Clostridium absonum
SN synonymous with Clostridium sardiniense
BT1 *Clostridium*
BT2 Bacteria
BT3 Microorganisms

Clostridium acetobutylicum
BT1 *Clostridium*
BT2 Bacteria
BT3 Microorganisms

Clostridium beijerinckii
BT1 *Clostridium*
BT2 Bacteria
BT3 Microorganisms

Clostridium botulinum
BT1 *Clostridium*
BT2 Bacteria
BT3 Microorganisms

Clostridium butyricum
BT1 *Clostridium*
BT2 Bacteria
BT3 Microorganisms

Clostridium cellulolyticum
BT1 *Clostridium*
BT2 Bacteria
BT3 Microorganisms

Clostridium difficile
BT1 *Clostridium*
BT2 Bacteria
BT3 Microorganisms

Clostridium josui
BT1 *Clostridium*
BT2 Bacteria
BT3 Microorganisms

Clostridium lentocellum
BT1 *Clostridium*
BT2 Bacteria
BT3 Microorganisms

Clostridium perfringens
BT1 *Clostridium*
BT2 Bacteria
BT3 Microorganisms

Clostridium sporogenes
BT1 *Clostridium*
BT2 Bacteria
BT3 Microorganisms

Clostridium stercorarium
BT1 *Clostridium*
BT2 Bacteria
BT3 Microorganisms
NT1 *Clostridium thermolacticum*

Clostridium thermoaceticum
SN synonymous with Moorella thermoacetica
BT1 *Clostridium*
BT2 Bacteria
BT3 Microorganisms

Clostridium thermocellum
BT1 *Clostridium*
BT2 Bacteria
BT3 Microorganisms

Clostridium thermolacticum
SN current name is Clostridium stercorarium subsp. thermolacticum
BT1 *Clostridium stercorarium*
BT2 *Clostridium*
BT3 Bacteria
BT4 Microorganisms

Clostridium thermosuccinogenes
BT1 *Clostridium*
BT2 Bacteria
BT3 Microorganisms

Clostridium thermosulfurogenes
HN introduced from vol. 39, issue 1 (2007)
SN synonymous with Thermoanaerobacterium thermosulfurigenes
BT1 *Clostridium*
BT2 Bacteria
BT3 Microorganisms

Clostridium tyrobutyricum
BT1 *Clostridium*
BT2 Bacteria
BT3 Microorganisms

Closures
BT1 Packaging
BT2 Technology
NT1 Caps
NT2 Screw caps
NT1 Corks
NT1 Crown corks
NT1 Lids

NT1 Stoppers
NT1 Tamper evident closures
RT Openings
RT Sealing

Clotting
BT1 Coagulation
BT2 Processing
BT3 Technology
NT1 Milk clotting

Cloud
BT1 Turbidity
BT2 Optical properties
BT3 Physical properties
NT1 Clouding agents
RT Cloudiness

Cloudberries
BT1 Berries
BT2 Fruits specific
BT3 Fruits
BT4 Crops
BT5 Plants
BT4 Plant foods
BT5 Foods

Cloudiness
BT1 Turbidity
BT2 Optical properties
BT3 Physical properties
RT Cloud

Clouding agents
BT1 Additives
BT1 Cloud
BT2 Turbidity
BT3 Optical properties
BT4 Physical properties
RT Beverages

Clove oils
HN introduced from vol. 39, issue 1 (2007)
BT1 Essential oils
BT2 Flavourings
BT3 Additives
BT2 Vegetable oils
BT3 Oils vegetable
BT4 Oils
BT5 Lipids
BT6 Nutrients
BT4 Vegetable products
BT5 Plant foods
BT6 Foods
RT Cloves

Cloves
BT1 Spices
BT2 Flavourings
BT3 Additives
RT Clove oils

Clovis
USE **Carpet shells**

Cloxacillin
BT1 Penicillins
BT2 β-Lactam antibiotics
BT3 Antibiotics
BT4 Drugs
BT5 Residues

Clupea harengus
BT1 Herring
BT2 Marine fish
BT3 Fish
BT4 Animals
BT4 Sea foods
BT5 Aquatic foods
BT6 Animal foods
BT7 Foods
BT2 Oily fish
BT3 Fish
BT4 Animals
BT4 Sea foods
BT5 Aquatic foods
BT6 Animal foods
BT7 Foods

Cluster beans
SN syn. guar beans
BT1 Guar beans
BT2 Legumes
BT3 Vegetables specific
BT4 Vegetables
BT5 Crops
BT6 Plants
BT5 Plant foods
BT6 Foods

CMC
HN used as abbrev. for carboxymethylcellulose up to vol. 24 (1992)
USE **Carboxymethylcellulose**

Co
SN index heading is Cobalt
BT1 Cobalt
BT2 Metals
BT3 Elements
BT4 Minerals
BT5 Nutrients

CO_2
SN index heading is Carbon dioxide
BT1 Carbon dioxide
BT2 Gases
BT3 Physical phases
BT4 Chemistry
BT5 Science
BT2 Inorganic compounds
BT2 Oxides
BT2 Solvents
RT Carbonic acid
RT Decarbonation

Coagulants
BT1 Coagulation
BT2 Processing
BT3 Technology

Coagulation
BT1 Processing
BT2 Technology
NT1 Clotting
NT2 Milk clotting
NT1 Coagulants
NT1 Rennetability
RT Enzymes milk clotting

Coagulum
BT1 Curd
BT2 Dairy products
BT3 Animal foods
BT4 Foods

Coalfish
BT1 Marine fish
BT2 Fish
BT3 Animals
BT3 Sea foods
BT4 Aquatic foods
BT5 Animal foods
BT6 Foods

Coal tar dyes
BT1 Colorants
BT2 Additives

Coating
BT1 Processing
BT2 Technology
NT1 Breading
NT1 Enrobing
NT1 Glazing
NT1 Panning
RT Encapsulation

Coatings
NT1 Batters
NT1 Breadcrumbs
NT1 Breadings
NT1 Carnauba wax
NT1 Chocolate coatings
NT1 Glazes
NT1 Polyvinyl acetate
NT1 Shellac
NT1 Wax coatings
RT Films
RT Waxes

Cobalamins
BT1 Vitamin B group
BT2 Vitamins
BT3 Nutrients
RT Vitamin B_{12}

Cobalt
SN symbol Co is also used in index
BT1 Metals
BT2 Elements
BT3 Minerals
BT4 Nutrients
NT1 Co

Cobnuts
USE **Hazelnuts**

Coca-cola
BT1 Soft drinks
BT2 Beverages

Cocci
BT1 Bacteria
BT2 Microorganisms

Coccidiosis
BT1 Animal diseases
BT2 Diseases animal
BT3 Diseases
RT Coccidiostats

Coccidiostats
BT1 Drugs
 BT2 Residues
NT1 Amprolium
NT1 Clopidol
NT1 Decoquinate
NT1 Dimetridazole
NT1 Dinitolmide
NT1 Ethopabate
NT1 Lasalocids
NT1 Monensin
NT1 Nicarbazin
NT1 Pyrimethamine
NT1 Salinomycin
RT Coccidiosis

Cochineal
BT1 Colorants
 BT2 Additives
RT Carminic acid

Cockles
BT1 Bivalves
 BT2 Molluscs
  BT3 Shellfish
   BT4 Animals
   BT4 Sea foods
    BT5 Aquatic foods
     BT6 Animal foods
      BT7 Foods

Cockroaches
BT1 Insects
 BT2 Pests

Cocktails
BT1 Alcoholic beverages
 BT2 Beverages alcoholic
  BT3 Beverages

Cocoa
BT1 Beverages
BT1 Crops
 BT2 Plants
BT1 Plant foods
 BT2 Foods
NT1 Cocoa beans
 NT2 Cocoa nibs
NT1 Cocoa industry
RT Chocolate
RT Cocoa butter
RT Cocoa products
RT Theobromine
UF Cacao

Cocoa beans
HN heading from vol. 25 (1993); under Cocoa up to vol. 24 (1992)
BT1 Cocoa
 BT2 Beverages
 BT2 Crops
  BT3 Plants
 BT2 Plant foods
  BT3 Foods
NT1 Cocoa nibs
UF Cacao beans

Cocoa beverages
BT1 Beverages
BT1 Cocoa products
 BT2 Plant foods
  BT3 Foods

Cocoa butter
BT1 Vegetable fats
 BT2 Fats vegetable
  BT3 Fats
   BT4 Lipids
    BT5 Nutrients
  BT3 Vegetable products
   BT4 Plant foods
    BT5 Foods
NT1 Cocoa butter equivalents
NT1 Cocoa butter extenders
NT1 Cocoa butter substitutes
RT Chocolate
RT Cocoa

Cocoa butter equivalents
BT1 Cocoa butter
 BT2 Vegetable fats
  BT3 Fats vegetable
   BT4 Fats
    BT5 Lipids
     BT6 Nutrients
   BT4 Vegetable products
    BT5 Plant foods
     BT6 Foods

Cocoa butter extenders
BT1 Cocoa butter
 BT2 Vegetable fats
  BT3 Fats vegetable
   BT4 Fats
    BT5 Lipids
     BT6 Nutrients
   BT4 Vegetable products
    BT5 Plant foods
     BT6 Foods

Cocoa butter replacers
USE **Cocoa butter substitutes**

Cocoa butter substitutes
BT1 Cocoa butter
 BT2 Vegetable fats
  BT3 Fats vegetable
   BT4 Fats
    BT5 Lipids
     BT6 Nutrients
   BT4 Vegetable products
    BT5 Plant foods
     BT6 Foods
BT1 Simulated foods
 BT2 Processed foods
  BT3 Foods
UF Cocoa butter replacers

Cocoa industry
BT1 Cocoa
 BT2 Beverages
 BT2 Crops
  BT3 Plants
 BT2 Plant foods
  BT3 Foods
BT1 Food industry
 BT2 Industries

Cocoa liquor
HN introduced from vol. 39, issue 1 (2007)
BT1 Cocoa products
 BT2 Plant foods
  BT3 Foods

Cocoa mass
BT1 Cocoa products
 BT2 Plant foods
  BT3 Foods

Cocoa nibs
HN introduced from vol. 41, issue 1 (2009)
BT1 Cocoa beans
 BT2 Cocoa
  BT3 Beverages
  BT3 Crops
   BT4 Plants
  BT3 Plant foods
   BT4 Foods

Cocoa powders
BT1 Cocoa products
 BT2 Plant foods
  BT3 Foods
BT1 Powders
 BT2 Dried foods
  BT3 Processed foods
   BT4 Foods
 BT2 Instant foods
  BT3 Processed foods
   BT4 Foods

Cocoa products
HN heading from vol. 25 (1993); under Cocoa up to vol. 24 (1992)
BT1 Plant foods
 BT2 Foods
NT1 Cocoa beverages
NT1 Cocoa liquor
NT1 Cocoa mass
NT1 Cocoa powders
NT1 Instant cocoa
RT Chocolate
RT Cocoa

Cocona
BT1 Fruits specific
 BT2 Fruits
  BT3 Crops
   BT4 Plants
  BT3 Plant foods
   BT4 Foods

Coconut butter
BT1 Vegetable fats
 BT2 Fats vegetable
  BT3 Fats
   BT4 Lipids
    BT5 Nutrients
  BT3 Vegetable products
   BT4 Plant foods
    BT5 Foods

Coconut cream
BT1 Coconuts
 BT2 Nuts
  BT3 Fruits
   BT4 Crops
    BT5 Plants
   BT4 Plant foods
    BT5 Foods

BT3 Oilseeds
BT4 Seeds
BT5 Plant foods
BT6 Foods

Coconut milk
BT1 Coconuts
BT2 Nuts
BT3 Fruits
BT4 Crops
BT5 Plants
BT4 Plant foods
BT5 Foods
BT3 Oilseeds
BT4 Seeds
BT5 Plant foods
BT6 Foods

Coconut oils
BT1 Nut oils
BT2 Vegetable oils
BT3 Oils vegetable
BT4 Oils
BT5 Lipids
BT6 Nutrients
BT4 Vegetable products
BT5 Plant foods
BT6 Foods
UF Copra oils

Coconuts
BT1 Nuts
BT2 Fruits
BT3 Crops
BT4 Plants
BT3 Plant foods
BT4 Foods
BT2 Oilseeds
BT3 Seeds
BT4 Plant foods
BT5 Foods
NT1 Bongkrek
NT1 Coconut cream
NT1 Coconut milk
NT1 Coconut water
NT1 Copra
NT1 Desiccated coconut
NT1 Nata

Coconut toddy
BT1 Palm wines
BT2 Wines palm
BT3 Alcoholic beverages
BT4 Beverages alcoholic
BT5 Beverages
BT3 Palms
BT4 Plants

Coconut water
BT1 Beverages
BT1 Coconuts
BT2 Nuts
BT3 Fruits
BT4 Crops
BT5 Plants
BT4 Plant foods
BT5 Foods
BT3 Oilseeds
BT4 Seeds
BT5 Plant foods
BT6 Foods

Cocoyams
BT1 Vegetables specific
BT2 Vegetables
BT3 Crops
BT4 Plants
BT3 Plant foods
BT4 Foods

Cod
HN heading up to vol. 24 (1992) and from vol. 30 (1998)
BT1 Marine fish
BT2 Fish
BT3 Animals
BT3 Sea foods
BT4 Aquatic foods
BT5 Animal foods
BT6 Foods
NT1 Cod livers
NT1 *Gadus morhua*
NT1 Rock cod

Codex Alimentarius
HN heading up to vol. 24 (1992)

Cod liver oils
BT1 Fish oils
BT2 Oils fish
BT3 Fish products
BT4 Sea foods
BT5 Aquatic foods
BT6 Animal foods
BT7 Foods
BT3 Marine oils
BT4 Oils
BT5 Lipids
BT6 Nutrients

Cod livers
BT1 Cod
BT2 Marine fish
BT3 Fish
BT4 Animals
BT4 Sea foods
BT5 Aquatic foods
BT6 Animal foods
BT7 Foods
BT1 Fish livers
BT2 Fish
BT3 Animals
BT3 Sea foods
BT4 Aquatic foods
BT5 Animal foods
BT6 Foods
BT2 Livers
BT3 Offal
BT4 Animal foods
BT5 Foods

Coeliac disease
BT1 Diseases

Coenzyme Q
HN introduced from vol. 39, issue 1 (2007)
BT1 Coenzymes
BT2 Enzymes
BT1 Quinones
BT2 Aromatic compounds
BT3 Organic compounds
UF Ubiquinone

Coenzymes
BT1 Enzymes
NT1 *S*-Adenosyl-L-methionine
NT1 Coenzyme Q

Coertuek
BT1 Spices
BT2 Flavourings
BT3 Additives
NT1 *Echinophora tenuifolia*

Coextrusion
BT1 Extrusion
BT2 Processing
BT3 Technology

Cofermentation
BT1 Fermentation
BT1 Fermentation technology
BT2 Biotechnology
BT3 Technology
BT2 Process control
BT3 Technology

Coffee
BT1 Beverages
BT1 Crops
BT2 Plants
BT1 Plant foods
BT2 Foods
NT1 Coffee bags
NT1 Coffee beans
NT1 Coffee grounds
NT1 Coffee industry
NT1 Coffee products
NT2 Coffee beverages
NT3 Cappuccino coffee
NT3 Espresso coffee
NT3 Iced coffee
NT2 Coffee extracts
NT2 Coffee powders
NT2 Instant coffee
NT3 Coffee granules
NT1 Decaffeinated coffee
NT1 Green coffee
NT1 Ground coffee
NT1 Roasted coffee
NT1 Roasting coffee
RT Alkaloids
RT Caffeine
RT Chicory (beverages)

Coffee bags
BT1 Coffee
BT2 Beverages
BT2 Crops
BT3 Plants
BT2 Plant foods
BT3 Foods

Coffee bars
BT1 Restaurants

Coffee beans
BT1 Coffee
BT2 Beverages
BT2 Crops

BT3 Plants
BT2 Plant foods
BT3 Foods

Coffee beverages
BT1 Coffee products
BT2 Coffee
BT3 Beverages
BT3 Crops
BT4 Plants
BT3 Plant foods
BT4 Foods
NT1 Cappuccino coffee
NT1 Espresso coffee
NT1 Iced coffee

Coffee cream
BT1 Cream
BT2 Dairy products
BT3 Animal foods
BT4 Foods

Coffee extracts
BT1 Coffee products
BT2 Coffee
BT3 Beverages
BT3 Crops
BT4 Plants
BT3 Plant foods
BT4 Foods
BT1 Extracts
BT2 Flavourings
BT3 Additives

Coffee granules
BT1 Instant coffee
BT2 Coffee products
BT3 Coffee
BT4 Beverages
BT4 Crops
BT5 Plants
BT4 Plant foods
BT5 Foods
BT2 Instant beverages
BT3 Beverages
BT3 Instant foods
BT4 Processed foods
BT5 Foods

Coffee grounds
BT1 By-products
BT1 Coffee
BT2 Beverages
BT2 Crops
BT3 Plants
BT2 Plant foods
BT3 Foods

Coffee industry
BT1 Coffee
BT2 Beverages
BT2 Crops
BT3 Plants
BT2 Plant foods
BT3 Foods
BT1 Food industry
BT2 Industries

Coffee oils
BT1 Vegetable oils
BT2 Oils vegetable
BT3 Oils
BT4 Lipids
BT5 Nutrients
BT3 Vegetable products
BT4 Plant foods
BT5 Foods

Coffee powders
BT1 Coffee products
BT2 Coffee
BT3 Beverages
BT3 Crops
BT4 Plants
BT3 Plant foods
BT4 Foods
BT1 Powders
BT2 Dried foods
BT3 Processed foods
BT4 Foods
BT2 Instant foods
BT3 Processed foods
BT4 Foods
RT Instant coffee

Coffee products
BT1 Coffee
BT2 Beverages
BT2 Crops
BT3 Plants
BT2 Plant foods
BT3 Foods
NT1 Coffee beverages
NT2 Cappuccino coffee
NT2 Espresso coffee
NT2 Iced coffee
NT1 Coffee extracts
NT1 Coffee powders
NT1 Instant coffee
NT2 Coffee granules

Coffee substitutes
BT1 Simulated foods
BT2 Processed foods
BT3 Foods

Coffee whiteners
BT1 Whiteners
BT2 Additives

Cogeneration
HN introduced from vol. 39, issue 1 (2007)
BT1 Electricity
BT2 Energy

Cognac
BT1 Brandies
BT2 Spirits
BT3 Alcoholic beverages
BT4 Beverages alcoholic
BT5 Beverages

Cognitive development
HN introduced from vol. 39, issue 1 (2007)
BT1 Cognitive performance
BT2 Behavioural effects
BT3 Human physiology
BT4 Physiology
BT5 Science

Cognitive performance
BT1 Behavioural effects
BT2 Human physiology
BT3 Physiology
BT4 Science
NT1 Cognitive development
NT1 Memory
RT Performance drinks

Coho salmon
BT1 Pacific salmon
BT2 Salmon
BT3 Oily fish
BT4 Fish
BT5 Animals
BT5 Sea foods
BT6 Aquatic foods
BT7 Animal foods
BT8 Foods

Cohumulone
BT1 Humulones
BT2 α-Acids
BT3 Bitter acids
BT4 Bitter compounds
BT5 Flavour compounds
BT4 Organic acids
BT5 Acids

Cola beverages
BT1 Soft drinks
BT2 Beverages

Cola nitida
BT1 Cola nuts
BT2 Nuts
BT3 Fruits
BT4 Crops
BT5 Plants
BT4 Plant foods
BT5 Foods
BT3 Oilseeds
BT4 Seeds
BT5 Plant foods
BT6 Foods

Cola nuts
BT1 Nuts
BT2 Fruits
BT3 Crops
BT4 Plants
BT3 Plant foods
BT4 Foods
BT2 Oilseeds
BT3 Seeds
BT4 Plant foods
BT5 Foods
NT1 *Cola nitida*

Colby cheese
BT1 Cheese varieties
BT2 Cheese
BT3 Dairy products
BT4 Animal foods
BT5 Foods

Cold boning
HN boning cold also used in the index up to vol. 29 (1997)
BT1 Boning

BT2 Processing
BT3 Technology

Cold shock proteins
BT1 Stress proteins
BT2 Proteins
BT3 Nutrients
BT2 Stress

Cold shortening
BT1 Contraction

Cold storage
BT1 Storage cold
BT2 Storage
NT1 Cold stores

Cold stores
BT1 Cold storage
BT2 Storage cold
BT3 Storage

Coleslaw
BT1 Vegetable products
BT2 Plant foods
BT3 Foods

Colicins
BT1 Toxins
BT2 Residues

Coliforms
BT1 Bacteria
BT2 Microorganisms

Coliphages
BT1 Bacteriophages
BT2 Viruses
BT3 Microorganisms

Colitis
BT1 Diseases
RT Ulcerative colitis

Collagen
BT1 Animal proteins
BT2 Proteins animal
BT3 Proteins
BT4 Nutrients
NT1 Collagen sausage casings
RT Connective tissues

Collagenases
BT1 Proteinases
BT2 Hydrolases
BT3 Enzymes

Collagen sausage casings
HN sausage casings collagen also used in the index upto vol. 29 (1997)
BT1 Collagen
BT2 Animal proteins
BT3 Proteins animal
BT4 Proteins
BT5 Nutrients
BT1 Sausage casings
BT2 Casings

Collards
USE **Kale**

Colletotrichum
BT1 Fungi
BT2 Microorganisms
NT1 *Colletotrichum acutatum*
NT1 *Colletotrichum gloeosporioides*
RT Diseases plant

Colletotrichum acutatum
BT1 *Colletotrichum*
BT2 Fungi
BT3 Microorganisms

Colletotrichum gloeosporioides
HN introduced from vol. 39, issue 1 (2007)
BT1 *Colletotrichum*
BT2 Fungi
BT3 Microorganisms
RT Anthracnose

Colloidal stability
HN stability colloidal also used in the index up to vol. 29 (1997)
BT1 Colloids
BT2 Physical phases
BT3 Chemistry
BT4 Science
BT1 Stability
BT2 Physical properties

Colloids
BT1 Physical phases
BT2 Chemistry
BT3 Science
NT1 Colloidal stability
NT1 Hydrocolloids
RT Dispersions
RT Emulsions
RT Gels
RT Thickeners

Collybia
USE ***Flammulina***

Colombia
BT1 South America
BT2 America

Colonization
BT1 Virulence factors
NT1 Colonization factors
RT Adherence

Colonization factors
HN introduced from vol. 39, issue 1 (2007)
BT1 Colonization
BT2 Virulence factors
RT Adherence

Colony counting
BT1 Microbiological techniques

Colony counts
BT1 Microbiological techniques

Colorants
BT1 Additives
NT1 Allura Red
NT1 Amaranth
NT1 Angkak
NT1 Annatto
NT1 Artificial colorants
NT1 Azo dyes
NT1 Beetroot juices
NT1 Bixin
NT1 Brilliant Blue
NT1 Caramel colorants
NT1 Carmine
NT1 Carminic acid
NT1 Carmoisine
NT1 Carthamin
NT1 Citrus red
NT1 Coal tar dyes
NT1 Cochineal
NT1 Dyes
NT1 Edible inks
NT1 Erythrosine
NT1 FDC blue
NT1 FDC red
NT1 FDC yellow
NT1 Food colorants
NT1 Indigo carmine
NT1 Indigotine
NT1 Metanil yellow
NT1 Natural colorants
NT1 Norbixin
NT1 Phloxine
NT1 Ponceau
NT1 Rose Bengal
NT1 Roselle
NT1 Saffron
NT1 Sudan dyes
NT1 Sunset Yellow
NT1 Tartrazine
NT1 Xanthene dyes
RT *Gardenia*
RT *Monascus*
RT Pigments

Colorectal cancer
BT1 Cancer
BT2 Diseases

Colorimeters
BT1 Colorimetry
BT2 Analytical techniques

Colorimetry
BT1 Analytical techniques
NT1 Colorimeters
NT1 Photocolorimetry

Colossoma macropomum
BT1 Freshwater fish
BT2 Fish
BT3 Animals
BT3 Sea foods
BT4 Aquatic foods
BT5 Animal foods
BT6 Foods

Colostrum
BT1 Milk
BT2 Dairy products
BT3 Animal foods
BT4 Foods

Colour
BT1 Optical properties
BT2 Physical properties
RT Discoloration
RT Gloss
RT Pigmentation
RT Pigments
RT Sensory properties

Column chromatography
BT1 Chromatography
BT2 Analytical techniques

Colupulone
BT1 Lupulones
BT2 β-Acids
BT3 Bitter acids
BT4 Bitter compounds
BT5 Flavour compounds
BT4 Organic acids
BT5 Acids

Colza oils
USE **Rapeseed oils**

Comamonas
HN introduced from vol. 37, issue 5 (2005)
BT1 Bacteria
BT2 Microorganisms

Combustion
HN heading up to vol. 24 (1992)

Comet assay
HN introduced from vol. 39, issue 1 (2007)
BT1 Genetic techniques
BT2 Genetics

Comfrey
HN under Spices up to vol. 42 (2010)
BT1 Herbs
BT2 Spices
BT3 Flavourings
BT4 Additives

Comminution
BT1 Processing
BT2 Technology
NT1 Crumbling
NT1 Crushing
NT1 Flaking
NT1 Grating
NT1 Grinding
NT1 Mincing
NT2 Mincers
NT1 Pulverization
NT1 Shredding
RT Chopping
RT Cutting
RT Maceration
RT Milling
RT Pulping

Common Agricultural Policy
USE **CAP**

Common beans
HN heading from vol. 25 (1993); under Kidney beans up to vol. 24 (1992)
BT1 Legumes
BT2 Vegetables specific
BT3 Vegetables
BT4 Crops
BT5 Plants
BT4 Plant foods
BT5 Foods
NT1 Anasazi
NT1 Black beans
NT1 Dry beans
NT1 French beans
NT1 Green beans
NT1 Haricot beans
NT2 Baked beans
NT1 Kidney beans
NT1 Navy beans
NT1 Pea beans
NT1 Pinto beans
NT1 Pole beans
NT1 Snap beans
NT1 String beans
NT1 Wax beans
NT1 White beans
RT Phaseolins

Common millet
BT1 Millet
BT2 Cereals
BT3 Crops
BT4 Plants
BT3 Seeds
BT4 Plant foods
BT5 Foods
UF Proso millet

Comoros
BT1 Southern Africa
BT2 Africa

Companies
BT1 Food business
BT2 Economics
NT1 Food companies

Complexometry
BT1 Analytical techniques

Composite flours
SN may contain non-cereal ingredients
BT1 Cereal flours
BT2 Flours cereal
BT3 Cereal products
BT4 Plant foods
BT5 Foods

Composition

Composting
HN introduced from vol. 39, issue 1 (2007)
BT1 Bioremediation
BT2 Biotechnology
BT3 Technology

Compotes
BT1 Fruit products
BT2 Plant foods
BT3 Foods

Compressibility
BT1 Rheological properties
BT2 Mechanical properties
BT3 Physical properties
RT Texture

Compression
BT1 Pressing
BT2 Processing
BT3 Technology

Computerized data processing
BT1 Information technology
BT2 Technology

Computers
BT1 Equipment
BT2 Technology
NT1 Microprocessors
RT Computer software
RT Information technology
RT Modelling

Computer software
BT1 Information technology
BT2 Technology
RT Computers
UF Software

Comte cheese
BT1 Cheese varieties
BT2 Cheese
BT3 Dairy products
BT4 Animal foods
BT5 Foods

Conalbumin
BT1 Albumins
BT2 Proteins
BT3 Nutrients
BT1 Egg proteins
BT2 Animal proteins
BT3 Proteins animal
BT4 Proteins
BT5 Nutrients

Conarachin
BT1 Vegetable proteins
BT2 Proteins vegetable
BT3 Proteins
BT4 Nutrients
BT3 Vegetable products
BT4 Plant foods
BT5 Foods
RT Peanut proteins

Concanavalin A
BT1 Lectins
BT2 Glycoproteins
BT3 Proteins
BT4 Nutrients
BT2 Vegetable proteins
BT3 Proteins vegetable
BT4 Proteins
BT5 Nutrients
BT4 Vegetable products
BT5 Plant foods
BT6 Foods

Concentrated milk
BT1 Milk
BT2 Dairy products
BT3 Animal foods

BT4 Foods
RT Condensed milk
RT Evaporated milk

Concentrated rectified musts
BT1 Grape musts
BT2 Musts
BT3 Fruit juices
BT4 Fruit products
BT5 Plant foods
BT6 Foods
BT4 Soft drinks
BT5 Beverages

Concentrates
HN heading from vol. 25 (1993)
BT1 Processed foods
BT2 Foods
NT1 Aroma concentrates
NT1 Beverage concentrates
NT1 Fibre concentrates
NT1 Fruit concentrates
NT1 Fruit juice concentrates
NT2 Apple juice concentrates
NT2 Citrus juice concentrates
NT3 Orange juice concentrates
NT2 Grape juice concentrates
NT1 Protein concentrates
NT2 FPC
NT2 Milk protein concentrates
NT2 Pea protein concentrates
NT2 Soy protein concentrates
NT2 Whey protein concentrates
NT1 Tomato concentrates
NT1 Vegetable juice concentrates
NT1 Whey concentrates
RT Concentration
RT Extracts

Concentration
BT1 Processing
BT2 Technology
NT1 Freeze concentration
RT Concentrates
RT Condensation
RT Evaporation
RT Ultrafiltration

Conching
BT1 Mixing
BT2 Processing
BT3 Technology

Condensation
BT1 Processing
BT2 Technology
RT Concentration

Condensed milk
BT1 Milk
BT2 Dairy products
BT3 Animal foods
BT4 Foods
NT1 Mawa
RT Concentrated milk
RT Evaporated milk

Condiments
BT1 Flavourings
BT2 Additives
NT1 Mayonnaise
NT1 Mirin
NT1 Mustard
NT1 Relishes
NT1 Salad dressings
NT2 Dressings
NT2 French dressing
NT2 Salad cream
NT2 Salad oils
NT1 Salt
NT2 Desalination
NT2 Desalting
NT2 Iodized salt
NT2 NaCl
NT2 Salinity
NT2 Salt substitutes
NT1 Sauces
NT2 Apple sauces
NT2 Cheese sauces
NT2 Fish sauces
NT3 Budu
NT3 Ishiru
NT3 Nuoc-mam
NT3 Patis
NT2 Fondues
NT2 Gravy
NT3 Gravy powders
NT2 Hollandaise sauces
NT2 Ketchups
NT3 Catsups
NT4 Tomato catsups
NT3 Tomato ketchups
NT4 Tomato catsups
NT2 Meat sauces
NT2 Oyster sauces
NT2 Pasta sauces
NT3 Pesto
NT2 Roux
NT2 Salsa
NT2 Sauce mixes
NT2 Soy sauces
NT3 Kanjang
NT3 Kecap
NT3 Shoyu
NT2 Tomato sauces
NT2 Worcestershire sauces
NT1 Seasonings
NT1 Vinegar
NT2 Balsamic vinegar
NT2 Cider vinegar
NT2 Fruit vinegars
NT3 Apple vinegar
NT2 Malt vinegar
NT2 Rice vinegar
NT2 Wine vinegar

Conductimetry
BT1 Analytical techniques

Conductivity
HN heading up to vol. 24 (1992)
USE **Electrical conductivity**
USE **Thermal conductivity**

Confectionery
BT1 Bakery products
BT2 Cereal products
BT3 Plant foods
BT4 Foods
BT1 Sugar confectionery
BT2 Plant foods
BT3 Foods
NT1 Confectionery bars
NT2 Chocolate bars
NT1 Confectionery industry
NT1 Confectionery products
NT1 Confections
NT1 Frozen confectionery

Confectionery bars
BT1 Confectionery
BT2 Bakery products
BT3 Cereal products
BT4 Plant foods
BT5 Foods
BT2 Sugar confectionery
BT3 Plant foods
BT4 Foods
BT1 Food bars
BT2 Snack foods
BT3 Processed foods
BT4 Foods
NT1 Chocolate bars

Confectionery cream
BT1 Fillings

Confectionery fillings
BT1 Fillings
NT1 Chocolate fillings

Confectionery industry
BT1 Confectionery
BT2 Bakery products
BT3 Cereal products
BT4 Plant foods
BT5 Foods
BT2 Sugar confectionery
BT3 Plant foods
BT4 Foods
BT1 Food industry
BT2 Industries

Confectionery pastes
BT1 Pastes
BT2 Processed foods
BT3 Foods
BT1 Sugar confectionery
BT2 Plant foods
BT3 Foods
RT Nut pastes
RT Tahini
RT Tehineh

Confectionery products
BT1 Confectionery
BT2 Bakery products
BT3 Cereal products
BT4 Plant foods
BT5 Foods
BT2 Sugar confectionery
BT3 Plant foods
BT4 Foods

Confections
BT1 Confectionery
BT2 Bakery products
BT3 Cereal products
BT4 Plant foods
BT5 Foods
BT2 Sugar confectionery

BT3 Plant foods
BT4 Foods

Conference proceedings
RT Books
RT Proceedings
UF Conferences

Conferences
USE **Conference proceedings**

Conformation
RT Structure

Conger eels
BT1 Marine fish
BT2 Fish
BT3 Animals
BT3 Sea foods
BT4 Aquatic foods
BT5 Animal foods
BT6 Foods

Conglycinin
BT1 Soy proteins
BT2 Vegetable proteins
BT3 Proteins vegetable
BT4 Proteins
BT5 Nutrients
BT4 Vegetable products
BT5 Plant foods
BT6 Foods
RT Glycinin

β-Conglycinin
BT1 Soy proteins
BT2 Vegetable proteins
BT3 Proteins vegetable
BT4 Proteins
BT5 Nutrients
BT4 Vegetable products
BT5 Plant foods
BT6 Foods
RT Soy 7S globulins

Congo, Democratic Republic of the
USE **Democratic Republic of the Congo**

Congo, Republic of the
USE **Republic of the Congo**

Conidia
USE **Fungal spores**

Conjugases
USE **γ-Glutamyl hydrolases**

Conjugated fatty acids
HN introduced from vol. 41, issue 1 (2009)
BT1 PUFA
BT2 Unsaturated fatty acids
BT3 Fatty acids
BT4 Lipids
BT5 Nutrients
BT4 Organic acids
BT5 Acids
NT1 CLA
NT1 Eleostearic acid

Conjugated linoleic acid
HN CLA used in the index from vol. 35, issue 6 (2003)
USE **CLA**

Connectin
BT1 Animal proteins
BT2 Proteins animal
BT3 Proteins
BT4 Nutrients
RT Titin

Connective tissues
NT1 Bone marrow
RT Chondroitin
RT Collagen
RT Glycosaminoglycans
RT Meat

Conophor nuts
BT1 Nuts
BT2 Fruits
BT3 Crops
BT4 Plants
BT3 Plant foods
BT4 Foods
BT2 Oilseeds
BT3 Seeds
BT4 Plant foods
BT5 Foods

Consistency
BT1 Texture
BT2 Sensory properties
NT1 Consistometers
NT1 Creaminess
NT1 Graininess
NT1 Lumpiness
NT1 Pastiness
NT1 Plasticity
NT1 Smoothness
RT Rheological properties
RT Viscosity

Consistometers
BT1 Consistency
BT2 Texture
BT3 Sensory properties

Consommes
BT1 Soups
BT2 Processed foods
BT3 Foods

Constipation
BT1 Diseases

Consumer acceptability
BT1 Acceptability
BT2 Consumer response

Consumer acceptance
BT1 Acceptance
BT2 Consumer response

Consumer attitudes
BT1 Consumer response
RT Industry attitudes

Consumer awareness
BT1 Consumer response

Consumer behaviour
HN introduced from vol. 43, issue 1 (2011)
BT1 Consumer response
NT1 Drinking habits
NT1 Eating habits
NT2 Fasting
NT2 Food portions
NT3 Portion sizes
NT2 Healthy eating
NT2 Snacking
NT1 Purchasing behaviour

Consumer choice
BT1 Consumer response

Consumer complaints
BT1 Consumer response

Consumer concerns
BT1 Consumer response

Consumer demand
BT1 Demand
BT2 Consumer response

Consumer education
BT1 Education

Consumer expectations
BT1 Consumer response

Consumer information
BT1 Information
NT1 Health promotion
RT Nutritional labelling

Consumer liking
BT1 Consumer response

Consumer opinions
BT1 Consumer response

Consumer panels
BT1 Sensory analysis
BT2 Analytical techniques

Consumer perception
BT1 Consumer response

Consumer preference
BT1 Preference
BT2 Consumer response

Consumer protection
BT1 Economics
RT Product recalls

Consumer research
BT1 Marketing
BT2 Economics
RT Market research

Consumer response
NT1 Acceptability
NT2 Consumer acceptability
NT1 Acceptance
NT2 Consumer acceptance
NT1 Consumer attitudes
NT1 Consumer awareness
NT1 Consumer behaviour
NT2 Drinking habits

NT2 Eating habits
NT3 Fasting
NT3 Food portions
NT4 Portion sizes
NT3 Healthy eating
NT3 Snacking
NT2 Purchasing behaviour
NT1 Consumer choice
NT1 Consumer complaints
NT1 Consumer concerns
NT1 Consumer expectations
NT1 Consumer liking
NT1 Consumer opinions
NT1 Consumer perception
NT1 Consumer satisfaction
NT1 Demand
NT2 Consumer demand
NT1 Parental response
NT1 Preference
NT2 Consumer preference

Consumer satisfaction
BT1 Consumer response

Consumer spending
BT1 Marketing
BT2 Economics

Consumer surveys
BT1 Marketing
BT2 Economics

Consumption
BT1 Economics
RT Marketing
RT Sales
RT Sustainability

Contact Materials
RT Packaging materials
RT Surfaces

Containers
NT1 Bags
NT2 Bagging
NT2 Bag in box packaging
NT2 Plastics bags
NT2 Polyethylene bags
NT2 Sacks
NT1 Barrels
NT2 Casks
NT2 Kegs
NT1 Baskets
NT1 Beakers
NT1 Bins
NT2 Hoppers
NT1 Bottles
NT2 Glass bottles
NT2 Plastics bottles
NT1 Bowls
NT1 Boxes
NT2 Cases
NT1 Canisters
NT1 Cans
NT1 Carriers
NT1 Cartons
NT2 Cartoning
NT1 Cartridges
NT1 Crates
NT1 Drums
NT1 Edible containers
NT1 Glass containers
NT1 Jars
NT1 Microwaveable containers
NT1 Packs
NT2 Aerosol packs
NT2 Edible packs
NT2 Flexible packs
NT2 Multipacks
NT2 Nettings
NT2 Portion packs
NT2 Punnets
NT1 Pots
NT1 Pouches
NT2 Retort pouches
NT2 Sachets
NT1 Scoops
NT1 Silos
NT1 Tanks
NT1 Trays
NT1 Tubes
NT1 Tubs
NT1 Vessels
RT Packaging
RT Packaging materials

Contaminants
BT1 Contamination
NT1 Arsenic
NT2 Arsenicals
NT3 Arsenobetaine
NT3 Dimethylarsinic acid
NT3 Methylarsonic acid
NT2 As
NT1 Benzophenone
NT1 Chloropropanols
NT1 Dioxins
NT1 Dust
NT1 Filth
NT1 Hexachlorobutadiene
NT1 Impurities
NT1 Organotin compounds
NT2 Butyltins
NT3 Tributyltin
NT1 Perchlorates
NT1 Phthalic acid esters
NT1 Polychlorinated dibenzodioxins
NT1 Polychlorinated dibenzofurans
NT1 Polychlorinated dibenzo-*p*-dioxins
NT2 Tetrachlorodibenzo-*p*-dioxins
NT1 Semicarbazide
UF Foreign bodies

Contamination
NT1 Chemical contamination
NT1 Contaminants
NT2 Arsenic
NT3 Arsenicals
NT4 Arsenobetaine
NT4 Dimethylarsinic acid
NT4 Methylarsonic acid
NT3 As
NT2 Benzophenone
NT2 Chloropropanols
NT2 Dioxins
NT2 Dust
NT2 Filth
NT2 Hexachlorobutadiene
NT2 Impurities
NT2 Organotin compounds
NT3 Butyltins
NT4 Tributyltin
NT2 Perchlorates
NT2 Phthalic acid esters
NT2 Polychlorinated dibenzodioxins
NT2 Polychlorinated dibenzofurans
NT2 Polychlorinated dibenzo-*p*-dioxins
NT3 Tetrachlorodibenzo-*p*-dioxins
NT2 Semicarbazide
NT1 Cross-contamination
NT1 Decontamination
NT1 Endocrine disrupters
NT1 Environmental contamination
NT1 Faecal contamination
NT1 Microbial contamination
NT2 Bacterial contamination
NT1 Pollution
NT2 Environmental pollution
NT3 Air pollution
NT4 Air pollutants
NT5 Exhaust gases
NT5 Factory fumes
NT3 Water pollution
NT2 Pollutants
NT3 Air pollutants
NT4 Exhaust gases
NT4 Factory fumes
NT1 Radioactive contamination
NT2 Fallout
RT Adulteration
RT Biosecurity
RT Bioterrorism
RT Hygiene
RT Migration
RT Poisoning
RT Purity
RT Residues
RT Spoilage
RT Toxins
RT Wild yeasts

Continuous processing
HN processing continuous used in the index up to vol.31 (1999)
BT1 Processing
BT2 Technology
UF Processing continuous

Contraction
NT1 Cold shortening
NT1 Shortening

Controlled atmosphere packaging
HN packaging controlled atm used in the index up to vol. 24 (1992) and packaging controlled atmosphere up to vol. 31 (1999)
BT1 Packaging
BT2 Technology
RT Modified atmosphere packaging

UF Packaging controlled atm
UF Packaging controlled atmosphere

Controlled atmosphere storage
BT1 Storage controlled atmosphere
BT2 Storage

Control systems
BT1 Process control
BT2 Technology

Convenience foods
BT1 Processed foods
BT2 Foods

Conveying
BT1 Conveyors
BT2 Equipment
BT3 Technology

Conveyors
BT1 Equipment
BT2 Technology
NT1 Conveying
NT1 Pneumatic conveyors
RT Handling

Conveyors pneumatic
HN used for pneumatic conveyors up to vol. 31 (1999)
USE **Pneumatic conveyors**

Convicine
BT1 Glycosides
BT2 Carbohydrates
BT3 Nutrients
BT3 Organic compounds
RT Vicine

Cook chill foods
BT1 Processed foods
BT2 Foods

Cook chill processing
HN processing cook chill also used in the index up to vol. 29 (1997)
BT1 Thermal processing
BT2 Processing thermal
BT3 Processing
BT4 Technology

Cookers
BT1 Cooking
BT2 Thermal processing
BT3 Processing thermal
BT4 Processing
BT5 Technology
BT1 Equipment
BT2 Technology

Cookies
BT1 Biscuits
BT2 Bakery products
BT3 Cereal products
BT4 Plant foods
BT5 Foods

Cooking
BT1 Thermal processing
BT2 Processing thermal
BT3 Processing
BT4 Technology
NT1 Baking
NT2 Bakeries
NT2 Baking industry
NT2 Baking properties
NT2 Baking quality
NT2 Proofers
NT2 Proofing
NT1 Blanching
NT1 Boiling
NT2 Boilers
NT2 Parboiling
NT1 Braising
NT1 Broiling
NT1 Cookers
NT1 Cooking properties
NT2 Cooking loss
NT1 Frying
NT2 Deep frying
NT2 Frying properties
NT2 Stir frying
NT1 Grilling
NT1 Hard to cook defect
NT1 Microwave cooking
NT1 Roasting
NT1 Sauteing
NT1 Simmering
NT1 Slow cooking
NT1 Sous vide
NT1 Steaming
NT2 Steam
NT1 Stewing
NT1 Toasting
RT Endpoint temp. indicators
RT Heating

Cooking fats
BT1 Fats
BT2 Lipids
BT3 Nutrients
RT Frying fats

Cooking loss
HN introduced from vol. 39, issue 1 (2007)
BT1 Cooking properties
BT2 Cooking
BT3 Thermal processing
BT4 Processing thermal
BT5 Processing
BT6 Technology

Cooking oils
BT1 Oils
BT2 Lipids
BT3 Nutrients
RT Frying oils

Cooking properties
BT1 Cooking
BT2 Thermal processing
BT3 Processing thermal
BT4 Processing
BT5 Technology
NT1 Cooking loss

Coolers
BT1 Cooling
BT2 Thermal processing
BT3 Processing thermal
BT4 Processing
BT5 Technology
BT1 Equipment
BT2 Technology

Cooling
BT1 Thermal processing
BT2 Processing thermal
BT3 Processing
BT4 Technology
NT1 Air cooling
NT1 Chilling
NT2 Chillers
NT1 Coolers
NT1 Hydrocooling
NT1 Supercooling
NT1 Vacuum cooling
RT Refrigeration

Cooperatives
BT1 Marketing
BT2 Economics

Coppas
BT1 Sausages
BT2 Meat products
BT3 Animal foods
BT4 Foods

Copper
SN symbol Cu is also used in the index
BT1 Metals
BT2 Elements
BT3 Minerals
BT4 Nutrients
NT1 Cu

Copra
BT1 Coconuts
BT2 Nuts
BT3 Fruits
BT4 Crops
BT5 Plants
BT4 Plant foods
BT5 Foods
BT3 Oilseeds
BT4 Seeds
BT5 Plant foods
BT6 Foods

Copra oils
USE **Coconut oils**

Coprinus
BT1 Edible fungi
BT2 Fungi edible
BT3 Vegetables specific
BT4 Vegetables
BT5 Crops
BT6 Plants
BT5 Plant foods
BT6 Foods
NT1 *Coprinus comatus*

Coprinus comatus
BT1 *Coprinus*
BT2 Edible fungi

BT3 Fungi edible
BT4 Vegetables specific
BT5 Vegetables
BT6 Crops
BT7 Plants
BT6 Plant foods
BT7 Foods

Corchorus olitorius
BT1 Vegetables specific
BT2 Vegetables
BT3 Crops
BT4 Plants
BT3 Plant foods
BT4 Foods

Cordials
BT1 Liqueurs
BT2 Alcoholic beverages
BT3 Beverages alcoholic
BT4 Beverages

Cordyceps
HN introduced from vol. 39, issue 1 (2007)
BT1 Edible fungi
BT2 Fungi edible
BT3 Vegetables specific
BT4 Vegetables
BT5 Crops
BT6 Plants
BT5 Plant foods
BT6 Foods
NT1 *Cordyceps militaris*
NT1 *Cordyceps sinensis*

Cordyceps militaris
BT1 *Cordyceps*
BT2 Edible fungi
BT3 Fungi edible
BT4 Vegetables specific
BT5 Vegetables
BT6 Crops
BT7 Plants
BT6 Plant foods
BT7 Foods

Cordyceps sinensis
HN introduced from vol. 41, issue 1 (2009)
BT1 *Cordyceps*
BT2 Edible fungi
BT3 Fungi edible
BT4 Vegetables specific
BT5 Vegetables
BT6 Crops
BT7 Plants
BT6 Plant foods
BT7 Foods

Coregonus albula
BT1 Vendace
BT2 Freshwater fish
BT3 Fish
BT4 Animals
BT4 Sea foods
BT5 Aquatic foods
BT6 Animal foods
BT7 Foods

Coregonus lavaretus
BT1 Whitefish
BT2 Fish
BT3 Animals
BT3 Sea foods
BT4 Aquatic foods
BT5 Animal foods
BT6 Foods

Corers
BT1 Coring
BT2 Cutting
BT3 Processing
BT4 Technology
BT1 Equipment
BT2 Technology

Coriander
BT1 Spices
BT2 Flavourings
BT3 Additives
NT1 Coriander leaves
NT1 Coriander seeds
UF Cilantro

Coriander leaves
HN introduced from vol. 43, issue 1 (2011)
BT1 Coriander
BT2 Spices
BT3 Flavourings
BT4 Additives
BT1 Herbs
BT2 Spices
BT3 Flavourings
BT4 Additives

Coriander seeds
HN introduced from vol. 43, issue 1 (2011)
BT1 Coriander
BT2 Spices
BT3 Flavourings
BT4 Additives

Coring
BT1 Cutting
BT2 Processing
BT3 Technology
NT1 Corers

Coriolus
SN obsolete genus; now called Trametes
USE ***Trametes***

Coriolus hirsutus
USE ***Trametes hirsuta***

Coriolus versicolor
USE ***Trametes versicolor***

Corks
HN heading from vol. 30 (1998); under Closures up to vol. 29 (1997)
BT1 Closures
BT2 Packaging
BT3 Technology

Cork spots
BT1 Plant disorders
BT2 Diseases plant
BT3 Diseases

Cork taint
BT1 Taints
BT2 Flavour
BT3 Sensory properties

Corn
BT1 Cereals
BT2 Crops
BT3 Plants
BT2 Seeds
BT3 Plant foods
BT4 Foods
NT1 Baby corn
NT1 Corn bran
NT1 Corn bread
NT1 Corn chips
NT1 Corn cobs
NT1 Cornflakes
NT1 Corn flour
NT1 Corn masa
NT1 Corn starch
NT2 High amylose corn starch
NT1 Kenkey
NT1 Kwoka
NT1 Popcorn
NT2 Microwave popcorn
NT1 Pozol
NT1 Sweetcorn
RT Nixtamalization
UF Maize

Corn bran
BT1 Bran
BT2 Cereal products
BT3 Plant foods
BT4 Foods
BT1 Corn
BT2 Cereals
BT3 Crops
BT4 Plants
BT3 Seeds
BT4 Plant foods
BT5 Foods

Corn bread
BT1 Bread
BT2 Bakery products
BT3 Cereal products
BT4 Plant foods
BT5 Foods
BT1 Corn
BT2 Cereals
BT3 Crops
BT4 Plants
BT3 Seeds
BT4 Plant foods
BT5 Foods

Corn chips
BT1 Chips
BT2 Processed foods
BT3 Foods
BT1 Corn
BT2 Cereals
BT3 Crops
BT4 Plants
BT3 Seeds

BT4 Plant foods
BT5 Foods

Corn cobs
BT1 Corn
BT2 Cereals
BT3 Crops
BT4 Plants
BT3 Seeds
BT4 Plant foods
BT5 Foods

Corn dogs
BT1 Sausages
BT2 Meat products
BT3 Animal foods
BT4 Foods

Corned beef
BT1 Beef
BT2 Meat specific
BT3 Meat
BT4 Animal foods
BT5 Foods
BT1 Meat products
BT2 Animal foods
BT3 Foods

Cornelian cherries
BT1 Fruits specific
BT2 Fruits
BT3 Crops
BT4 Plants
BT3 Plant foods
BT4 Foods

Corn fibre oils
BT1 Corn oils
BT2 Vegetable oils
BT3 Oils vegetable
BT4 Oils
BT5 Lipids
BT6 Nutrients
BT4 Vegetable products
BT5 Plant foods
BT6 Foods

Cornflakes
BT1 Cereal products
BT2 Plant foods
BT3 Foods
BT1 Corn
BT2 Cereals
BT3 Crops
BT4 Plants
BT3 Seeds
BT4 Plant foods
BT5 Foods

Corn flour
SN dry-milled product; distinct from cornflour
BT1 Cereal flours
BT2 Flours cereal
BT3 Cereal products
BT4 Plant foods
BT5 Foods
BT1 Corn
BT2 Cereals
BT3 Crops
BT4 Plants
BT3 Seeds
BT4 Plant foods
BT5 Foods
UF Maize meal

Cornflour
USE **Corn starch**

Cornish pasties
BT1 Meat pies
BT2 Meat products
BT3 Animal foods
BT4 Foods
BT2 Pies
BT3 Bakery products
BT4 Cereal products
BT5 Plant foods
BT6 Foods
BT1 Meat products
BT2 Animal foods
BT3 Foods

Corn masa
BT1 Corn
BT2 Cereals
BT3 Crops
BT4 Plants
BT3 Seeds
BT4 Plant foods
BT5 Foods
RT Snack foods

Corn oils
BT1 Vegetable oils
BT2 Oils vegetable
BT3 Oils
BT4 Lipids
BT5 Nutrients
BT3 Vegetable products
BT4 Plant foods
BT5 Foods
NT1 Corn fibre oils
UF Maize oils

Corn starch
BT1 Corn
BT2 Cereals
BT3 Crops
BT4 Plants
BT3 Seeds
BT4 Plant foods
BT5 Foods
BT1 Starch
BT2 Glucans
BT3 Polysaccharides
BT4 Carbohydrates
BT5 Nutrients
BT5 Organic compounds
BT2 Thickeners
BT3 Additives
NT1 High amylose corn starch
UF Cornflour

Corn steep liquor
BT1 Distillation
BT2 Processing
BT3 Technology

Corn syrups
BT1 Sugar syrups
BT2 Plant foods
BT3 Foods
NT1 Fructose high corn syrups
NT1 Isoglucose
NT1 Isosyrups
RT Glucose syrups

Coronary heart diseases
BT1 Cardiovascular diseases
BT2 Diseases
NT1 Myocardial infarction

Coronavirus
HN introduced from vol. 43, issue 1 (2011)
BT1 Viruses
BT2 Microorganisms

Corrinoids
BT1 Vitamin B group
BT2 Vitamins
BT3 Nutrients
NT1 Cyanocobalamin
NT2 Vitamin B_{12}

Corrosion
NT1 Rust

Cortisol
HN under Drugs up to vol. 43 (2011)
BT1 Glucocorticoids
BT2 Hormones
BT3 Residues
BT1 Steroids
BT2 Lipids
BT3 Nutrients

Corynebacteriaceae
HN heading up to vol. 24 (1992)
BT1 Bacteria
BT2 Microorganisms

Corynebacterium
HN heading from vol. 30 (1998); under Bacteria up to vol. 29 (1997)
BT1 Bacteria
BT2 Microorganisms
NT1 *Corynebacterium casei*
NT1 *Corynebacterium glutamicum*

Corynebacterium casei
HN introduced from vol. 41, issue 1 (2009)
BT1 *Corynebacterium*
BT2 Bacteria
BT3 Microorganisms

Corynebacterium glutamicum
SN synonymous with Brevibacterium lactofermentum
BT1 *Corynebacterium*
BT2 Bacteria
BT3 Microorganisms

Costa Rica
BT1 Central America
BT2 America

Costmary
HN under Spices up to vol. 42 (2010)
BT1 Herbs
BT2 Spices

BT3 Flavourings
BT4 Additives

Costs
BT1 Economics

Costus
USE **Kuth**

Cote d'Ivoire
BT1 West Africa
BT2 Africa
UF Ivory Coast

Cottage cheese
BT1 Cheese varieties
BT2 Cheese
BT3 Dairy products
BT4 Animal foods
BT5 Foods

Cotton candy
BT1 Sugar confectionery
BT2 Plant foods
BT3 Foods
RT Candy floss

Cottonseed meal
BT1 Cottonseeds
BT2 Oilseeds
BT3 Seeds
BT4 Plant foods
BT5 Foods
BT1 Flours
BT2 Plant foods
BT3 Foods

Cottonseed oils
BT1 Vegetable oils
BT2 Oils vegetable
BT3 Oils
BT4 Lipids
BT5 Nutrients
BT3 Vegetable products
BT4 Plant foods
BT5 Foods

Cottonseed proteins
BT1 Cottonseeds
BT2 Oilseeds
BT3 Seeds
BT4 Plant foods
BT5 Foods
BT1 Vegetable proteins
BT2 Proteins vegetable
BT3 Proteins
BT4 Nutrients
BT3 Vegetable products
BT4 Plant foods
BT5 Foods

Cottonseeds
BT1 Oilseeds
BT2 Seeds
BT3 Plant foods
BT4 Foods
NT1 Cottonseed meal
NT1 Cottonseed proteins
NT1 Gossypol

Cough drops
BT1 Sugar confectionery
BT2 Plant foods
BT3 Foods

Coulometry
BT1 Analytical techniques

Coumaphos
BT1 Acaricides
BT2 Pesticides
BT3 Biocides
BT3 Residues
BT1 Organophosphorus insecticides
BT2 Insecticides
BT3 Pesticides
BT4 Biocides
BT4 Residues
BT2 Organophosphorus pesticides
BT3 Pesticides
BT4 Biocides
BT4 Residues

Coumaric acid
SN syn. hydroxycinnamic acid
BT1 Hydroxycinnamic acid
BT2 Organic acids
BT3 Acids
BT2 Phenols
BT3 Alcohols
BT3 Aromatic compounds
BT4 Organic compounds

Coumarin
HN heading up to vol. 24 (1992)
BT1 Coumarins
BT2 Lactones
BT3 Esters
BT4 Organic compounds
BT3 Heterocyclic compounds
BT2 Phenols
BT3 Alcohols
BT3 Aromatic compounds
BT4 Organic compounds

Coumarins
HN introduced from vol. 39, issue 1 (2007)
BT1 Lactones
BT2 Esters
BT3 Organic compounds
BT2 Heterocyclic compounds
BT1 Phenols
BT2 Alcohols
BT2 Aromatic compounds
BT3 Organic compounds
NT1 Coumarin
NT1 Coumestrol
NT1 Esculetin
NT1 Furocoumarins
NT2 Bergapten
NT2 Psoralens
NT2 Xanthotoxin
NT1 Scopoletin

Coumestrol
BT1 Coumarins
BT2 Lactones
BT3 Esters
BT4 Organic compounds
BT3 Heterocyclic compounds
BT2 Phenols
BT3 Alcohols
BT3 Aromatic compounds
BT4 Organic compounds
BT1 Isoflavonoids
BT2 Flavonoids
BT3 Aromatic compounds
BT4 Organic compounds
BT3 Pigments

Countercurrent chromatography
BT1 Chromatography
BT2 Analytical techniques

Counters
BT1 Radioactivity

Countries
RT International
RT World

Couplers
BT1 Equipment
BT2 Technology

Courgettes
BT1 Vegetables specific
BT2 Vegetables
BT3 Crops
BT4 Plants
BT3 Plant foods
BT4 Foods
UF Zucchini
UF Zucchini squashes

Couscous
BT1 Cereal products
BT2 Plant foods
BT3 Foods

Cowberries
SN syn. lingonberries
BT1 Lingonberries
BT2 Berries
BT3 Fruits specific
BT4 Fruits
BT5 Crops
BT6 Plants
BT5 Plant foods
BT6 Foods

Cow cheese
USE **Cheese**

Cow milk
USE **Milk**

Cow milk cheese
USE **Cheese**

Cowpea meal
BT1 Cowpeas
BT2 Legumes
BT3 Vegetables specific
BT4 Vegetables
BT5 Crops
BT6 Plants
BT5 Plant foods

BT6 Foods
BT1 Flours
BT2 Plant foods
BT3 Foods

Cowpeas
HN heading from vol. 25 (1993); under Legumes up to vol. 24 (1992)
BT1 Legumes
BT2 Vegetables specific
BT3 Vegetables
BT4 Crops
BT5 Plants
BT4 Plant foods
BT5 Foods
NT1 Akara
NT1 Blackeyed peas
NT1 Cowpea meal
NT1 Moinmoin
NT1 Southern peas

Cows
USE **Cattle**

Coxiella
BT1 Bacteria
BT2 Microorganisms

Coxsackieviruses
HN introduced from vol. 39, issue 1 (2007); under Enteric viruses up to vol. 42 (2010)
SN for descriptive use only
BT1 Viruses
BT2 Microorganisms
RT Enterovirus

Coypu
SN syn. nutria
BT1 Animals
NT1 Nutria

CPTA
BT1 Plant growth regulators
BT2 Cultivation
BT3 Agriculture

Cr
HN under Minerals up to vol. 42 (2010)
BT1 Metals
BT2 Elements
BT3 Minerals
BT4 Nutrients
UF Chromium

Crab legs
BT1 Crab meat
BT2 Crabs
BT3 Crustacea
BT4 Shellfish
BT5 Animals
BT5 Sea foods
BT6 Aquatic foods
BT7 Animal foods
BT8 Foods

Crab meat
BT1 Crabs
BT2 Crustacea
BT3 Shellfish
BT4 Animals
BT4 Sea foods
BT5 Aquatic foods
BT6 Animal foods
BT7 Foods
NT1 Crab legs

Crabs
BT1 Crustacea
BT2 Shellfish
BT3 Animals
BT3 Sea foods
BT4 Aquatic foods
BT5 Animal foods
BT6 Foods
NT1 Blue crabs
NT2 *Callinectes sapidus*
NT1 Crab meat
NT2 Crab legs
NT1 Mud crabs
NT1 Red crabs
NT1 Snow crabs

Crackers
BT1 Biscuits
BT2 Bakery products
BT3 Cereal products
BT4 Plant foods
BT5 Foods

Cracking
SN used for cracking of eggs, damage to fruits or freeze cracking of foods
BT1 Damage
BT1 Processing
BT2 Technology
RT Egg shells
RT Shells

Crambe abyssinica
BT1 Crambe seeds
BT2 Oilseeds
BT3 Seeds
BT4 Plant foods
BT5 Foods

Crambe seeds
BT1 Oilseeds
BT2 Seeds
BT3 Plant foods
BT4 Foods
NT1 *Crambe abyssinica*

Cranberries
BT1 Berries
BT2 Fruits specific
BT3 Fruits
BT4 Crops
BT5 Plants
BT4 Plant foods
BT5 Foods
RT Cranberry juices

Cranberry juices
BT1 Berry juices
BT2 Fruit juices
BT3 Fruit products
BT4 Plant foods
BT5 Foods
BT3 Soft drinks
BT4 Beverages
RT Cranberries

Crangon crangon
BT1 Shrimps
BT2 Crustacea
BT3 Shellfish
BT4 Animals
BT4 Sea foods
BT5 Aquatic foods
BT6 Animal foods
BT7 Foods

Crassostrea gigas
BT1 Oysters
BT2 Bivalves
BT3 Molluscs
BT4 Shellfish
BT5 Animals
BT5 Sea foods
BT6 Aquatic foods
BT7 Animal foods
BT8 Foods

Crassostrea virginica
BT1 Oysters
BT2 Bivalves
BT3 Molluscs
BT4 Shellfish
BT5 Animals
BT5 Sea foods
BT6 Aquatic foods
BT7 Animal foods
BT8 Foods

Crates
BT1 Containers

Cravings
BT1 Behavioural effects
BT2 Human physiology
BT3 Physiology
BT4 Science

Crawfish
SN salt water species
BT1 Crustacea
BT2 Shellfish
BT3 Animals
BT3 Sea foods
BT4 Aquatic foods
BT5 Animal foods
BT6 Foods

Crayfish
SN freshwater species
BT1 Crustacea
BT2 Shellfish
BT3 Animals
BT3 Sea foods
BT4 Aquatic foods
BT5 Animal foods
BT6 Foods

Cream
BT1 Dairy products
BT2 Animal foods
BT3 Foods
NT1 Coffee cream
NT1 Creaming
NT1 Double cream
NT1 Fermented cream
NT2 Katyk

NT2 Ripened cream
NT2 Smetana
NT2 Sour cream
NT1 Half cream
NT1 Single cream
NT1 Sweet cream
NT1 UHT cream
NT1 Whipped cream
NT1 Whipping cream
RT Fats milk
RT Milk fats

Cream cheese
BT1 Cheese varieties
BT2 Cheese
BT3 Dairy products
BT4 Animal foods
BT5 Foods

Creameries
USE **Dairies**

Creaminess
BT1 Consistency
BT2 Texture
BT3 Sensory properties

Creaming
BT1 Cream
BT2 Dairy products
BT3 Animal foods
BT4 Foods

Cream liqueurs
BT1 Liqueurs
BT2 Alcoholic beverages
BT3 Beverages alcoholic
BT4 Beverages

Cream milk
BT1 Milk
BT2 Dairy products
BT3 Animal foods
BT4 Foods

Cream puffs
BT1 Pastries
BT2 Bakery products
BT3 Cereal products
BT4 Plant foods
BT5 Foods

Creatine
BT1 Organic nitrogen compounds

Creatinine
BT1 Organic nitrogen compounds

Creep
BT1 Rheological properties
BT2 Mechanical properties
BT3 Physical properties

Cremes
BT1 Fillings

Cremoso Argentino cheese
BT1 Cheese varieties
BT2 Cheese
BT3 Dairy products
BT4 Animal foods
BT5 Foods

Crepes
BT1 Bakery products
BT2 Cereal products
BT3 Plant foods
BT4 Foods

Crescenza cheese
BT1 Cheese varieties
BT2 Cheese
BT3 Dairy products
BT4 Animal foods
BT5 Foods

Cresols
BT1 Phenols
BT2 Alcohols
BT2 Aromatic compounds
BT3 Organic compounds

Cress
BT1 Vegetables specific
BT2 Vegetables
BT3 Crops
BT4 Plants
BT3 Plant foods
BT4 Foods

Creutzfeldt-Jakob disease
HN CJD used in the index from vol. 35, issue 6 (2003)
USE **CJD**

Crispbreads
BT1 Bread
BT2 Bakery products
BT3 Cereal products
BT4 Plant foods
BT5 Foods

Crispness
BT1 Texture
BT2 Sensory properties

Crisps
BT1 Chips
BT2 Processed foods
BT3 Foods

Crithmum maritimum
BT1 Sea fennel
BT2 Samphire
BT3 Herbs
BT4 Spices
BT5 Flavourings
BT6 Additives

Critical control points
BT1 Quality control
BT2 Technology
RT Food safety
RT HACCP

Croakers
BT1 Marine fish
BT2 Fish
BT3 Animals
BT3 Sea foods
BT4 Aquatic foods
BT5 Animal foods
BT6 Foods

Croatia
BT1 Europe

Crocetin
BT1 Crocin
BT2 Carotenoids
BT3 Pigments
BT3 Terpenoids
BT4 Lipids
BT5 Nutrients

Crocin
BT1 Carotenoids
BT2 Pigments
BT2 Terpenoids
BT3 Lipids
BT4 Nutrients
NT1 Crocetin

Crocodile meat
BT1 Crocodiles
BT2 Animals
BT1 Meat specific
BT2 Meat
BT3 Animal foods
BT4 Foods

Crocodiles
BT1 Animals
NT1 Crocodile meat

Crohns disease
BT1 Inflammatory bowel disease
BT2 Diseases

Croissants
BT1 Bakery products
BT2 Cereal products
BT3 Plant foods
BT4 Foods

Croneton
USE **Ethiofencarb**

Crops
HN heading from vol. 25 (1993); under Plants up to vol. 24 (1992)
BT1 Plants
NT1 Agricultural produce
NT1 Agricultural products
NT1 Cereals
NT1 Chicory
NT1 Cocoa
NT1 Coffee
NT1 Fruits
NT1 Horticultural products
NT1 Sugar beets
NT1 Sugar cane
NT1 Sugar crops
NT1 Sweet sorghum
NT1 Teas
NT1 Vanilla beans
NT1 Vegetables

Crops rotation
BT1 Cultivation
BT2 Agriculture

Croquant
BT1 Sugar confectionery
BT2 Plant foods
BT3 Foods
UF Krokant

Crossbreeding
RT Breeding
RT Genetics

Cross-contamination
HN introduced from vol. 39, issue 1 (2007)
BT1 Contamination

Cross-linking
HN introduced from vol. 39, issue 1 (2007)
BT1 Modification

Cross-reactivity
HN introduced from vol. 39, issue 1 (2007)
SN used only in immunological contexts
BT1 Immunology
RT Allergies
RT Immunological techniques

Crotoxyphos
BT1 Acaricides
BT2 Pesticides
BT3 Biocides
BT3 Residues
BT1 Organophosphorus insecticides
BT2 Insecticides
BT3 Pesticides
BT4 Biocides
BT4 Residues
BT2 Organophosphorus pesticides
BT3 Pesticides
BT4 Biocides
BT4 Residues
UF Ciodrin

Croutons
BT1 Bakery products
BT2 Cereal products
BT3 Plant foods
BT4 Foods

Crowberries
BT1 Berries
BT2 Fruits specific
BT3 Fruits
BT4 Crops
BT5 Plants
BT4 Plant foods
BT5 Foods

Crown corks
BT1 Closures
BT2 Packaging
BT3 Technology

Crucian carp
BT1 Carp
BT2 Freshwater fish
BT3 Fish
BT4 Animals
BT4 Sea foods
BT5 Aquatic foods
BT6 Animal foods
BT7 Foods
BT2 Oily fish
BT3 Fish
BT4 Animals
BT4 Sea foods
BT5 Aquatic foods
BT6 Animal foods
BT7 Foods

Cruciferae
SN see also cabbages
BT1 Vegetables specific
BT2 Vegetables
BT3 Crops
BT4 Plants
BT3 Plant foods
BT4 Foods

Cruciferins
BT1 Vegetable proteins
BT2 Proteins vegetable
BT3 Proteins
BT4 Nutrients
BT3 Vegetable products
BT4 Plant foods
BT5 Foods

Crude fibre
BT1 Fibre

Crumbliness
BT1 Texture
BT2 Sensory properties

Crumbling
BT1 Comminution
BT2 Processing
BT3 Technology

Crumpets
BT1 Bakery products
BT2 Cereal products
BT3 Plant foods
BT4 Foods

Crunchiness
BT1 Texture
BT2 Sensory properties

Crushing
BT1 Comminution
BT2 Processing
BT3 Technology

Crust
BT1 Bakery products
BT2 Cereal products
BT3 Plant foods
BT4 Foods

Crustacea
BT1 Shellfish
BT2 Animals
BT2 Sea foods
BT3 Aquatic foods
BT4 Animal foods
BT5 Foods
NT1 Crabs
NT2 Blue crabs
NT3 *Callinectes sapidus*
NT2 Crab meat
NT3 Crab legs
NT2 Mud crabs
NT2 Red crabs
NT2 Snow crabs
NT1 Crawfish
NT1 Crayfish
NT1 Krill
NT1 Lobsters
NT2 American lobsters
NT1 Norway lobsters
NT2 Langoustines
NT2 Scampi
NT1 Prawns
NT2 Kuruma prawns
NT2 Prawn crackers
NT1 Shrimps
NT2 *Crangon crangon*
NT2 *Pandalus borealis*
NT2 Tiger shrimps

Cryogenics
BT1 Freezing
BT2 Thermal processing
BT3 Processing thermal
BT4 Processing
BT5 Technology

Cryopreservation
BT1 Freezing
BT2 Thermal processing
BT3 Processing thermal
BT4 Processing
BT5 Technology

Cryoprotectants
BT1 Additives

Cryoscopes
BT1 Thermophysical properties
BT2 Physical properties

Cryoscopy
BT1 Analytical techniques
RT f.p.

Cryovac
BT1 Plastics
BT2 Packaging materials

Cryphonectria
HN introduced from vol. 43, issue 1 (2011)
BT1 Fungi
BT2 Microorganisms
NT1 *Cryphonectria parasitica*

Cryphonectria parasitica
HN introduced from vol. 39, issue 1 (2007)
BT1 *Cryphonectria*
BT2 Fungi
BT3 Microorganisms

Crypthecodinium
HN introduced from vol. 43, issue 1 (2011)
BT1 Microalgae
BT2 Algae

BT3 Microorganisms
NT1 *Crypthecodinium cohnii*

Crypthecodinium cohnii
BT1 *Crypthecodinium*
BT2 Microalgae
BT3 Algae
BT4 Microorganisms

Cryptococcus
BT1 Yeasts
BT2 Fungi
BT3 Microorganisms
NT1 *Cryptococcus albidus*
NT1 *Cryptococcus curvatus*
NT1 *Cryptococcus laurentii*
NT1 *Cryptococcus nodaensis*

Cryptococcus albidus
BT1 *Cryptococcus*
BT2 Yeasts
BT3 Fungi
BT4 Microorganisms

Cryptococcus curvatus
BT1 *Cryptococcus*
BT2 Yeasts
BT3 Fungi
BT4 Microorganisms

Cryptococcus laurentii
HN introduced from vol. 39, issue 1 (2007)
BT1 *Cryptococcus*
BT2 Yeasts
BT3 Fungi
BT4 Microorganisms

Cryptococcus nodaensis
SN synonymous with Cryptococcus flavescens
BT1 *Cryptococcus*
BT2 Yeasts
BT3 Fungi
BT4 Microorganisms

Cryptosporidiosis
BT1 Diseases
BT1 Poisoning
RT *Cryptosporidium*

Cryptosporidium
HN heading from vol. 30 (1998)
BT1 Parasites
BT2 Pests
NT1 *Cryptosporidium hominis*
NT1 *Cryptosporidium parvum*
RT Cryptosporidiosis

Cryptosporidium hominis
HN introduced from vol. 41, issue 1 (2009)
BT1 *Cryptosporidium*
BT2 Parasites
BT3 Pests

Cryptosporidium parvum
BT1 *Cryptosporidium*
BT2 Parasites
BT3 Pests

Cryptoxanthin
BT1 Xanthophylls
BT2 Carotenoids
BT3 Pigments
BT3 Terpenoids
BT4 Lipids
BT5 Nutrients

Crystallinity
HN introduced from vol. 39, issue 1 (2007)
BT1 Physical properties
RT Crystallization
RT Crystals

Crystallization
BT1 Processing
BT2 Technology
RT Crystallinity
RT Crystals
RT Precipitation
RT Retrogradation
RT Solidification

Crystallography
BT1 Analytical techniques
NT1 X-ray crystallography

Crystals
HN heading from vol. 25 (1993)
BT1 Physical phases
BT2 Chemistry
BT3 Science
RT Crystallinity
RT Crystallization

Cs
BT1 Radioelements
BT2 Isotopes
BT3 Elements
BT4 Minerals
BT5 Nutrients
BT2 Residues
UF Caesium

Cu
SN index heading is Copper
BT1 Copper
BT2 Metals
BT3 Elements
BT4 Minerals
BT5 Nutrients

Cuartirolo argentino cheese
BT1 Cheese varieties
BT2 Cheese
BT3 Dairy products
BT4 Animal foods
BT5 Foods

Cuba
BT1 West Indies
BT2 America

Cucumber pickles
BT1 Cucumbers
BT2 Vegetables specific
BT3 Vegetables
BT4 Crops
BT5 Plants
BT4 Plant foods
BT5 Foods
BT1 Vegetable pickles
BT2 Pickles
BT3 Fermented foods
BT4 Processed foods
BT5 Foods
BT2 Vegetable products
BT3 Plant foods
BT4 Foods
UF Brined cucumbers
UF Pickled cucumbers

Cucumbers
BT1 Vegetables specific
BT2 Vegetables
BT3 Crops
BT4 Plants
BT3 Plant foods
BT4 Foods
NT1 Cucumber pickles

Cucumber seeds
BT1 Oilseeds
BT2 Seeds
BT3 Plant foods
BT4 Foods

Cucumisins
BT1 Proteinases
BT2 Hydrolases
BT3 Enzymes

Cucurbitaceae
BT1 Vegetables specific
BT2 Vegetables
BT3 Crops
BT4 Plants
BT3 Plant foods
BT4 Foods

Cucurbitacins
BT1 Bitter compounds
BT2 Flavour compounds
BT1 Sterols
BT2 Alcohols
BT2 Steroids
BT3 Lipids
BT4 Nutrients
BT1 Triterpenoids
BT2 Terpenoids
BT3 Lipids
BT4 Nutrients

Cucurbita moschata
BT1 Squashes
BT2 Vegetables specific
BT3 Vegetables
BT4 Crops
BT5 Plants
BT4 Plant foods
BT5 Foods

Cultivar
USE **cv**

Cultivation
BT1 Agriculture
NT1 Canopy
NT1 Crops rotation
NT1 Defoliation
NT1 Fertilizers

NT2 Foliar sprays
NT1 Girdling
NT1 Hydroponics
NT1 Irrigation
NT2 Water stress
NT1 Mulching
NT1 Plant density
NT1 Plant growth regulators
NT2 Abscisic acid
NT2 Acetylene
NT2 Aminoethoxyvinylglycine
NT2 Antisprouting agents
NT3 Maleic hydrazide
NT2 Antitranspirants
NT2 Auxins
NT3 Indole acetic acid
NT4 Indol-3-ylacetic acid
NT3 Naphthaleneacetic acid
NT4 2-(1-Naphthyl)acetic acid
NT4 (2-Naphthyloxy)acetic acid
NT2 Chlormequat
NT2 CPTA
NT2 Cytokinins
NT3 Benzyladenine
NT4 6-Benzylaminopurine
NT3 Kinetin
NT3 Thidiazuron
NT3 Zeatin
NT2 Daminozide
NT2 Ethylene
NT3 ACC
NT3 Ethephon
NT2 Gibberellins
NT3 Gibberellic acid
NT2 Growth promoters (plant)
NT2 1-Methylcyclopropene
NT2 Methyl jasmonate
NT3 Jasmonic acid
NT2 Paclobutrazol
NT2 Phytohormones
NT2 Propylene
NT2 Triiodobenzoic acid
NT1 Planting
NT1 Pruning
NT1 Rootstocks
NT1 Shading
NT1 Soils
NT1 Sowing
NT1 Thinning
NT1 Viniculture
NT1 Viticulture
RT Horticulture
RT Pollination

Cultural groups
BT1 Anthropological groups
BT2 Population groups

Culture
HN heading up to vol. 21 (1989)
BT1 Cell culture

Cultured buttermilk
BT1 Buttermilk
BT2 Dairy products
BT3 Animal foods
BT4 Foods

Cultured cream
HN heading up to vol. 24
USE **Fermented cream**

Cultured dairy products
USE **Fermented dairy products**

Cultured foods
USE **Fermented foods**

Cultured milk beverages
USE **Fermented milk**

Cultured milk products
USE **Fermented dairy products**

Cultured milks
HN heading up to vol. 24
USE **Fermented milk**

Culture media
USE **Media**

Cumin
BT1 Spices
BT2 Flavourings
BT3 Additives
RT Cuminaldehyde

Cuminaldehyde
HN also under Flavour compounds up to vol. 42 (2010)
BT1 Aldehydes
BT2 Carbonyl compounds
BT3 Organic compounds
BT1 Aroma compounds
BT2 Flavour compounds
BT2 Volatile compounds
BT1 Aromatic compounds
BT2 Organic compounds
RT Cumin

Cunninghamella
BT1 Fungi
BT2 Microorganisms

Cuphea
BT1 Oilseeds
BT2 Seeds
BT3 Plant foods
BT4 Foods

Cupuacu
BT1 Fruits specific
BT2 Fruits
BT3 Crops
BT4 Plants
BT3 Plant foods
BT4 Foods
RT Chocolate

Curacao
BT1 West Indies
BT2 America

Curculigo latifolia
BT1 Fruits specific
BT2 Fruits
BT3 Crops
BT4 Plants
BT3 Plant foods
BT4 Foods
RT Curculin

Curculin
BT1 Sweet proteins
BT2 Proteins
BT3 Nutrients
BT2 Sweeteners
BT3 Additives
RT *Curculigo latifolia*

Curcuma
BT1 Vegetables specific
BT2 Vegetables
BT3 Crops
BT4 Plants
BT3 Plant foods
BT4 Foods

Curcuma zedoaria
BT1 Zedoary
BT2 Vegetables specific
BT3 Vegetables
BT4 Crops
BT5 Plants
BT4 Plant foods
BT5 Foods

Curcumin
BT1 Curcuminoids
BT2 Phenols
BT3 Alcohols
BT3 Aromatic compounds
BT4 Organic compounds
BT2 Pigments

Curcuminoids
HN introduced from vol. 41, issue 1 (2009)
BT1 Phenols
BT2 Alcohols
BT2 Aromatic compounds
BT3 Organic compounds
BT1 Pigments
NT1 Curcumin
RT Polyphenols

Curd
BT1 Dairy products
BT2 Animal foods
BT3 Foods
NT1 Casein curd
NT1 Cheese curd
NT1 Coagulum
NT1 Izvara
NT1 Paneer
RT Cheese
RT Quarg
RT Syneresis

Curd cheese
BT1 Cheese varieties
BT2 Cheese
BT3 Dairy products
BT4 Animal foods
BT5 Foods

Curdlan
HN under Polysaccharides up to vol. 42 (2010)
BT1 Glucans

BT2 Polysaccharides
BT3 Carbohydrates
BT4 Nutrients
BT4 Organic compounds
RT Exopolysaccharides

Cured meat
BT1 Meat products
BT2 Animal foods
BT3 Foods

Curing
BT1 Preservation
BT2 Technology
NT1 Curing agents
RT Brining
RT Nitrates
RT Nitrites
RT Pickling
RT Smoking

Curing agents
BT1 Curing
BT2 Preservation
BT3 Technology

Curing brines
BT1 Brining
BT2 Processing
BT3 Technology

Currants
BT1 Dried fruits
BT2 Fruits dried
BT3 Dried foods
BT4 Processed foods
BT5 Foods
BT3 Fruits
BT4 Crops
BT5 Plants
BT4 Plant foods
BT5 Foods

Curries
BT1 Meals
BT2 Processed foods
BT3 Foods

Curry leaves
HN under Spices up to vol. 42 (2010)
BT1 Herbs
BT2 Spices
BT3 Flavourings
BT4 Additives
NT1 *Murraya koenigii*

Curry powders
BT1 Spices
BT2 Flavourings
BT3 Additives

Curvularia
BT1 Fungi
BT2 Microorganisms

Custard apples
BT1 Fruits specific
BT2 Fruits
BT3 Crops
BT4 Plants
BT3 Plant foods
BT4 Foods

Custards
BT1 Desserts
BT2 Processed foods
BT3 Foods

Cutability
BT1 Cutting
BT2 Processing
BT3 Technology

Cutin
BT1 Biopolymers

Cutinases
SN EC 3.1.1.74
BT1 Esterases
BT2 Hydrolases
BT3 Enzymes

Cutlassfish
BT1 Marine fish
BT2 Fish
BT3 Animals
BT3 Sea foods
BT4 Aquatic foods
BT5 Animal foods
BT6 Foods

Cutting
BT1 Processing
BT2 Technology
NT1 Chopping
NT2 Chopping boards
NT1 Coring
NT2 Corers
NT1 Cutability
NT1 Dicing
NT1 Filleting
NT1 Jointing
NT1 Knives
NT1 Slicing
NT1 Splitting
NT1 Trimming
RT Comminution

Cuttlefish
BT1 Cephalopods
BT2 Molluscs
BT3 Shellfish
BT4 Animals
BT4 Sea foods
BT5 Aquatic foods
BT6 Animal foods
BT7 Foods

cv
RT Genetics
RT var
UF Cultivar

Cyanazine
BT1 Triazine herbicides
BT2 Herbicides
BT3 Pesticides
BT4 Biocides
BT4 Residues

Cyanides
BT1 Salts
NT1 Acetonitrile
NT1 Cyanogens
NT2 Cyanogenic glycosides
NT2 Prunasin
NT1 Hydrocyanic acid
NT1 Hydrogen cyanide

Cyanidin
BT1 Anthocyanidins
BT2 Flavonoids
BT3 Aromatic compounds
BT4 Organic compounds
BT3 Pigments

Cyanobacteria
SN also known as blue green algae (older terminology)
BT1 Bacteria
BT2 Microorganisms
NT1 *Anabaena*
NT1 Blue green algae
NT1 *Microcystis*
NT1 *Nostoc*
NT1 *Spirulina*
NT2 *Spirulina maxima*
NT2 *Spirulina platensis*
NT1 *Synechococcus*
NT1 *Synechocystis*
RT Algae

Cyanocobalamin
SN syn. vitamin B12
BT1 Corrinoids
BT2 Vitamin B group
BT3 Vitamins
BT4 Nutrients
NT1 Vitamin B_{12}

Cyanogenic glycosides
BT1 Cyanogens
BT2 Cyanides
BT3 Salts
BT1 Glycosides
BT2 Carbohydrates
BT3 Nutrients
BT3 Organic compounds

Cyanogens
BT1 Cyanides
BT2 Salts
NT1 Cyanogenic glycosides
NT1 Prunasin

Cycad seeds
BT1 Plants
BT1 Seeds
BT2 Plant foods
BT3 Foods

Cycasin
BT1 Carcinogens
BT2 Mutagens
BT1 Toxins
BT2 Residues

Cyclamates
BT1 Salts
BT1 Sweeteners
BT2 Additives

NT1 Sodium cyclamate
UF Sulfamates
UF Sulphamates

Cyclamic acid
BT1 Organic acids
BT2 Acids
BT1 Sweeteners
BT2 Additives
UF Cyclohexanesulfamic acid
UF Cyclohexanesulphamic acid

Cyclic fatty acids
HN introduced from vol. 39, issue 1 (2007)
BT1 Fatty acids
BT2 Lipids
BT3 Nutrients
BT2 Organic acids
BT3 Acids

Cyclochlorotine
BT1 Mycotoxins
BT2 Toxins
BT3 Residues

Cyclodextrin glucanotransferases
USE **Cyclomaltodextrin glucanotransferases**

Cyclodextrins
HN heading from vol. 43 (2011); under Dextrins up to vol. 42 (2010)
BT1 Dextrins
BT2 Starch
BT3 Glucans
BT4 Polysaccharides
BT5 Carbohydrates
BT6 Nutrients
BT6 Organic compounds
BT3 Thickeners
BT4 Additives
RT Oligosaccharides

Cyclohexanesulfamic acid
USE **Cyclamic acid**

Cyclohexanesulphamic acid
USE **Cyclamic acid**

Cycloheximide
BT1 Antibiotics
BT2 Drugs
BT3 Residues
UF Actidione

Cyclohexylamine
BT1 Amines
BT2 Organic nitrogen compounds

Cyclomaltodextrinases
SN EC 3.2.1.54
BT1 Glycosidases
BT2 Hydrolases
BT3 Enzymes

Cyclomaltodextrin glucanotransferases
SN EC 2.4.1.19
BT1 Glycosyltransferases
BT2 Transferases
BT3 Enzymes
UF Cyclodextrin glucanotransferases

Cyclones
HN under Sugar processes up to vol. 42 (2010)
BT1 Equipment
BT2 Technology

Cyclooxygenases
HN introduced from vol. 39, issue 1 (2007)
SN alternative name for prostaglandin-endoperoxide synthases
BT1 Oxidoreductases
BT2 Enzymes

Cyclopiazonic acid
BT1 Mycotoxins
BT2 Toxins
BT3 Residues

Cyclopterus lumpus
BT1 Lumpfish
BT2 Marine fish
BT3 Fish
BT4 Animals
BT4 Sea foods
BT5 Aquatic foods
BT6 Animal foods
BT7 Foods

Cycloserine
BT1 Antibiotics
BT2 Drugs
BT3 Residues

Cyclospora
BT1 Parasites
BT2 Pests
NT1 *Cyclospora cayetanensis*
RT Cyclosporiasis

Cyclospora cayetanensis
BT1 *Cyclospora*
BT2 Parasites
BT3 Pests

Cyclosporiasis
BT1 Diseases
BT1 Poisoning
RT *Cyclospora*

Cycocel
USE **Chlormequat**

Cyhexatin
HN under Insecticides up to vol. 42 (2010)
BT1 Acaricides
BT2 Pesticides
BT3 Biocides
BT3 Residues
UF Plictran
UF Tricyclohexyltin hydroxide

Cymene
HN also under Volatile compounds up to vol. 42 (2010)
BT1 Aroma compounds
BT2 Flavour compounds
BT2 Volatile compounds
BT1 Aromatic compounds
BT2 Organic compounds
BT1 Hydrocarbons
BT2 Organic compounds

Cynara cardunculus
BT1 Cardoons
BT2 Vegetables specific
BT3 Vegetables
BT4 Crops
BT5 Plants
BT4 Plant foods
BT5 Foods

Cynara humilis
BT1 Thistles
BT2 Plants

Cypermethrin
BT1 Acaricides
BT2 Pesticides
BT3 Biocides
BT3 Residues
BT1 Pyrethroid insecticides
BT2 Insecticides
BT3 Pesticides
BT4 Biocides
BT4 Residues

Cyperus esculentus
BT1 Tigernuts
BT2 Chufa nuts
BT3 Vegetables specific
BT4 Vegetables
BT5 Crops
BT6 Plants
BT5 Plant foods
BT6 Foods

Cyprex
USE **Dodine**

Cyprinus carpio
BT1 Carp
BT2 Freshwater fish
BT3 Fish
BT4 Animals
BT4 Sea foods
BT5 Aquatic foods
BT6 Animal foods
BT7 Foods
BT2 Oily fish
BT3 Fish
BT4 Animals
BT4 Sea foods
BT5 Aquatic foods
BT6 Animal foods
BT7 Foods

Cyprodinil
HN introduced from vol. 39, issue 1 (2007)
BT1 Fungicides
BT2 Pesticides
BT3 Biocides
BT3 Residues

Cyprus
BT1 European Union
BT1 Middle East

Cystatins
BT1 Proteinases inhibitors
BT2 Antinutritional factors
BT3 Nutritional values
BT2 Enzyme inhibitors
BT3 Enzymes

Cysteine
BT1 Amino acids
BT2 Nutrients
BT2 Organic acids
BT3 Acids
BT2 Organic nitrogen compounds
NT1 *N*-Acetyl-L-cysteine

Cysteine sulfoxides
HN also under Flavour compounds up to vol. 42 (2010)
BT1 Aroma compounds
BT2 Flavour compounds
BT2 Volatile compounds
BT1 Organic sulfur compounds
BT1 Oxides
UF Cysteine sulphoxides

Cysteine sulphoxides
HN used for cysteine sulfoxides up to vol. 35, issue 6 (2003)
USE **Cysteine sulfoxides**

Cysticercosis
BT1 Animal diseases
BT2 Diseases animal
BT3 Diseases
RT *Cysticercus*

Cysticercus
BT1 Parasites
BT2 Pests
RT Cysticercosis

Cystine
BT1 Amino acids
BT2 Nutrients
BT2 Organic acids
BT3 Acids
BT2 Organic nitrogen compounds

Cystoseira
BT1 Seaweeds
BT2 Algae
BT3 Microorganisms
BT2 Sea foods
BT3 Aquatic foods
BT4 Animal foods
BT5 Foods

Cytidine
BT1 Nucleosides

Cytochalasins
BT1 Mycotoxins
BT2 Toxins
BT3 Residues

Cytokines
BT1 Immunology

Cytokinins
BT1 Plant growth regulators
BT2 Cultivation
BT3 Agriculture
NT1 Benzyladenine
NT2 6-Benzylaminopurine
NT1 Kinetin
NT1 Thidiazuron
NT1 Zeatin

Cytolethal distending toxin
HN introduced from vol. 41, issue 1 (2009)
BT1 Toxins
BT2 Residues

Cytophaga
BT1 Bacteria
BT2 Microorganisms

Cytosine
BT1 Pyrimidines
BT2 Heterocyclic compounds
BT2 Organic nitrogen compounds

Cytotoxicity
BT1 Toxicity

Cytotoxins
BT1 Toxins
BT2 Residues

Czechoslovakia
HN heading up to vol. 24 (1992)
SN Czech Republic and Slovakia also present in index
BT1 Europe
RT Czech Republic
RT Slovakia

Czech Republic
BT1 Europe
BT1 European Union
RT Czechoslovakia
RT Organization for Economic Cooperation and Development

D

2,4-D
BT1 Phenoxy herbicides
BT2 Herbicides
BT3 Pesticides
BT4 Biocides
BT4 Residues
UF 2,4-Dichlorophenoxyacetic acid

Dab
BT1 Flatfish
BT2 Marine fish
BT3 Fish
BT4 Animals
BT4 Sea foods
BT5 Aquatic foods
BT6 Animal foods
BT7 Foods
UF Dabs

Dabs
HN used up to vol. 29 (1997)
USE **Dab**

Daconil
USE **Chlorothalonil**

Dahi
BT1 Fermented milk
BT2 Fermented dairy products
BT3 Dairy products
BT4 Animal foods
BT5 Foods
BT3 Fermented foods
BT4 Processed foods
BT5 Foods
BT2 Milk
BT3 Dairy products
BT4 Animal foods
BT5 Foods

Dahomey
USE **Benin**

Daidzein
BT1 Isoflavones
BT2 Isoflavonoids
BT3 Flavonoids
BT4 Aromatic compounds
BT5 Organic compounds
BT4 Pigments
RT Genistein
RT Puerarin

Dairies
BT1 Dairy products
BT2 Animal foods
BT3 Foods
NT1 Dairies wastes
NT2 Dairies effluents
NT1 Dairying
UF Creameries
UF Dairy factories

Dairies effluents
BT1 Dairies wastes
BT2 Dairies
BT3 Dairy products
BT4 Animal foods
BT5 Foods
BT2 Wastes
BT1 Effluents
BT2 Waste water
BT3 Wastes
BT3 Water

Dairies wastes
BT1 Dairies
BT2 Dairy products
BT3 Animal foods
BT4 Foods

BT1 Wastes
NT1 Dairies effluents

Dairy beverages
BT1 Beverages
BT1 Dairy products
BT2 Animal foods
BT3 Foods
NT1 Lactic beverages
NT1 Milk beverages
NT1 Milkshakes
NT1 Whey beverages
NT1 Yoghurt beverages
NT2 Drinking yoghurt

Dairy desserts
BT1 Dairy products
BT2 Animal foods
BT3 Foods
BT1 Desserts
BT2 Processed foods
BT3 Foods

Dairy factories
USE **Dairies**

Dairy industry
HN under Dairies up to vol. 24 (1992)
BT1 Dairy products
BT2 Animal foods
BT3 Foods
BT1 Food industry
BT2 Industries
RT International Dairy Federation

Dairying
BT1 Dairies
BT2 Dairy products
BT3 Animal foods
BT4 Foods

Dairy-lo
BT1 Fat substitutes
BT2 Fats
BT3 Lipids
BT4 Nutrients

Dairy products
BT1 Animal foods
BT2 Foods
NT1 Bregott
NT1 Burfee
NT1 Butter
NT2 Buffalo butter
NT2 Butter spreads
NT2 Samna
NT2 Smen
NT1 Buttermilk
NT2 Cultured buttermilk
NT2 Rabadi
NT1 Chakka
NT1 Cheese
NT2 Cheese factories
NT2 Cheesemaking
NT3 Cheddaring
NT2 Cheese rind
NT2 Cheese sauces
NT2 Cheese slices
NT2 Cheese spreads
NT2 Cheese varieties
NT3 Abondance cheese
NT3 Acid curd cheese
NT3 Afuega'l Pitu cheese
NT3 Appenzeller cheese
NT3 Arzua cheese
NT3 Asiago cheese
NT3 Asiago Pressato cheese
NT3 Bergkaese cheese
NT3 Beyaz cheese
NT3 Bitto cheese
NT3 Blue cheese
NT3 Brie cheese
NT3 Bryndza cheese
NT3 Buffalo cheese
NT4 Buffalo mozzarella cheese
NT3 Burgos cheese
NT3 Cabrales cheese
NT3 Caciocavallo cheese
NT4 Caciocavallo Palermitano cheese
NT3 Cacioricotta cheese
NT3 Caciotta cheese
NT3 Camembert cheese
NT3 Cameros cheese
NT3 Canestrato Pugliese cheese
NT3 Cebreiro cheese
NT3 Cheddar cheese
NT3 Chihuahua cheese
NT3 Colby cheese
NT3 Comte cheese
NT3 Cottage cheese
NT3 Cream cheese
NT3 Cremoso Argentino cheese
NT3 Crescenza cheese
NT3 Cuartirolo argentino cheese
NT3 Curd cheese
NT3 Danbo cheese
NT3 Domiati cheese
NT3 Edam cheese
NT3 Emmental cheese
NT3 Ewe cheese
NT3 Feta cheese
NT3 Fior di Latte cheese
NT3 Fiore Sardo cheese
NT3 Fontina cheese
NT3 Fossa cheese
NT3 Fresh cheese
NT3 Fynbo cheese
NT3 Goat cheese
NT3 Gorgonzola cheese
NT3 Gouda cheese
NT3 Grana cheese
NT3 Grana Padano cheese
NT3 Gruyere cheese
NT3 Halloumi cheese
NT3 Hard cheese
NT3 Havarti cheese
NT3 Herrgard cheese
NT3 Hispanico cheese
NT3 Idiazabal cheese
NT3 Jarlsberg cheese
NT3 Kachkaval cheese
NT3 Kajmak cheese
NT3 Kareish cheese
NT3 Kashar cheese
NT3 Kasseri cheese
NT3 Kefalograviera cheese
NT3 Kefalotyri cheese
NT3 Kostroma cheese
NT3 La Serena cheese
NT3 Limburg cheese
NT3 Los Pedroches cheese
NT3 Lymeswold cheese
NT3 Mahon cheese
NT3 Manchego cheese
NT3 Maribo cheese
NT3 Mascarpone cheese
NT3 Minas cheese
NT3 Minas Frescal cheese
NT3 Montasio cheese
NT3 Monterey Jack cheese
NT3 Mozzarella cheese
NT4 Buffalo mozzarella cheese
NT3 Muenster cheese
NT3 Munster cheese
NT3 Norvegia cheese
NT3 Ostiepok cheese
NT3 Parmesan cheese
NT3 Parmigiano Reggiano cheese
NT3 Pasta filata cheese
NT3 Patagras cheese
NT3 Pecorino cheese
NT3 Pecorino Sardo cheese
NT3 Penamellera cheese
NT3 Picante cheese
NT3 Pickled cheese
NT3 Pont-l'Eveque cheese
NT3 Port Salut cheese
NT3 Prato cheese
NT3 Processed cheese
NT3 Provolone cheese
NT3 Quarg
NT4 Tvaroh
NT4 Tvorog
NT4 Twarog
NT3 Quartirolo cheese
NT3 Queso Blanco cheese
NT3 Queso fresco cheese
NT3 Raclette cheese
NT3 Ragusano cheese
NT3 Ras cheese
NT3 Reggianito cheese
NT3 Ricotta cheese
NT3 Robiola cheese
NT3 Rokpol cheese
NT3 Romano cheese
NT3 Roncal cheese
NT3 Roquefort cheese
NT3 Rossiiskii cheese
NT3 Saint-Nectaire cheese
NT3 Saint-Paulin cheese
NT3 Salers cheese
NT3 Samso cheese
NT3 San Simon cheese
NT3 Serra cheese
NT3 Smear cheese
NT3 Soft cheese
NT3 Sovetskii cheese
NT3 Stilton cheese
NT3 Stracchino cheese
NT3 Suluguni cheese
NT3 Swiss cheese

NT3 Taleggio cheese
NT3 Teleme cheese
NT3 Tetilla cheese
NT3 Tilsit cheese
NT3 Toma cheese
NT3 Trappist cheese
NT3 Travnik cheese
NT3 Tulum cheese
NT3 Whey cheese
NT3 White cheese
NT3 White mould cheese
NT3 White pickled cheese
NT1 Chhana
NT1 Cream
NT2 Coffee cream
NT2 Creaming
NT2 Double cream
NT2 Fermented cream
NT3 Katyk
NT3 Ripened cream
NT3 Smetana
NT3 Sour cream
NT2 Half cream
NT2 Single cream
NT2 Sweet cream
NT2 UHT cream
NT2 Whipped cream
NT2 Whipping cream
NT1 Curd
NT2 Casein curd
NT2 Cheese curd
NT2 Coagulum
NT2 Izvara
NT2 Paneer
NT1 Dairies
NT2 Dairies wastes
NT3 Dairies effluents
NT2 Dairying
NT1 Dairy beverages
NT2 Lactic beverages
NT2 Milk beverages
NT2 Milkshakes
NT2 Whey beverages
NT2 Yoghurt beverages
NT3 Drinking yoghurt
NT1 Dairy desserts
NT1 Dairy industry
NT1 Dairy spreads
NT1 Dried dairy products
NT2 Dried milk
NT2 Dried skim milk
NT2 Dried whey
NT1 Dudh churpi
NT1 Dulce de leche
NT1 Fermented dairy products
NT2 Acidophilus pastes
NT2 Fermented cream
NT3 Katyk
NT3 Ripened cream
NT3 Smetana
NT3 Sour cream
NT2 Fermented milk
NT3 Acidophilin
NT3 Acidophilus milk
NT3 Amasi
NT3 Bifidus milk
NT3 Biogarde
NT3 Bioghurt
NT3 Dahi
NT3 Kefir
NT4 Kefir grains
NT3 Koumiss
NT3 Labneh
NT3 Lactic beverages
NT3 Lassi
NT3 Leben
NT3 Nono
NT3 Prostokvasha
NT3 Ryazhenka
NT3 Shrikhand
NT3 Shubat
NT3 Skyr
NT3 Snezhok
NT3 Sour milk
NT3 Tarag
NT3 Tykmaelk
NT3 Yakult
NT3 Ymer
NT3 Yoghurt
NT4 Buffalo yoghurt
NT4 Ewe yoghurt
NT4 Flavoured yoghurt
NT4 Frozen yoghurt
NT4 Fruit yoghurt
NT4 Goat yoghurt
NT4 Yoghurt beverages
NT5 Drinking yoghurt
NT3 Zabady
NT4 Zabadi
NT1 Fromage frais
NT1 Ghee
NT1 Gulabjamans
NT1 Ice cream
NT2 Ice cream bars
NT2 Ice cream factories
NT2 Ice cream mixes
NT2 Ice milk
NT2 Ices
NT2 Mellorine
NT2 Milk ice
NT1 Junket
NT1 Kalakand
NT1 Khoa
NT1 Kishk
NT1 Kulfi
NT1 Milk
NT2 Ass milk
NT2 Buffalo milk
NT3 Shrikhand
NT2 Camel milk
NT3 Shubat
NT2 Cheesemaking milk
NT2 Cheese milk
NT2 Chocolate milk
NT2 Colostrum
NT2 Concentrated milk
NT2 Condensed milk
NT3 Mawa
NT2 Cream milk
NT2 Dried milk
NT2 Evaporated milk
NT2 Ewe milk
NT2 Farm milk
NT2 Fermented milk
NT3 Acidophilin
NT3 Acidophilus milk
NT3 Amasi
NT3 Bifidus milk
NT3 Biogarde
NT3 Bioghurt
NT3 Dahi
NT3 Kefir
NT4 Kefir grains
NT3 Koumiss
NT3 Labneh
NT3 Lactic beverages
NT3 Lassi
NT3 Leben
NT3 Nono
NT3 Prostokvasha
NT3 Ryazhenka
NT3 Shrikhand
NT3 Shubat
NT3 Skyr
NT3 Snezhok
NT3 Sour milk
NT3 Tarag
NT3 Tykmaelk
NT3 Yakult
NT3 Ymer
NT3 Yoghurt
NT4 Buffalo yoghurt
NT4 Ewe yoghurt
NT4 Flavoured yoghurt
NT4 Frozen yoghurt
NT4 Fruit yoghurt
NT4 Goat yoghurt
NT4 Yoghurt beverages
NT5 Drinking yoghurt
NT3 Zabady
NT4 Zabadi
NT2 Flavoured milk
NT2 Goat milk
NT2 Half and half milk
NT2 Homogenized milk
NT2 Human milk
NT2 Jellied milk
NT2 Mare milk
NT3 Koumiss
NT2 Milk beverages
NT2 Milk powders
NT2 Milkshakes
NT2 Miltone
NT2 Pasteurized milk
NT2 Raw milk
NT2 Recombined milk
NT2 Semi skimmed milk
NT2 Skim milk
NT3 Dried skim milk
NT3 Skim milk powders
NT2 Sterilized milk
NT2 UHT milk
NT2 Whole milk
NT2 Yak milk
NT1 Peda
NT1 Pera
NT1 Rabri
NT1 Rasogolla
NT1 Sandesh
NT1 Tarhana
NT1 Trahanas
NT1 Vla
NT1 Whey
NT2 Acid whey
NT2 Casein whey
NT2 Cheese whey
NT2 Dried whey

NT2 Whey beverages
NT2 Whey concentrates
NT2 Whey proteins
NT3 Whey protein concentrates
RT Lactose
UF Milk products

Dairy science
BT1 Food science
BT2 Science
RT Animal science

Dairy spreads
BT1 Dairy products
BT2 Animal foods
BT3 Foods
BT1 Spreads
BT2 Processed foods
BT3 Foods

Dairy starters
BT1 Starters
BT2 Bacteria
BT3 Microorganisms

Dalapon
BT1 Herbicides
BT2 Pesticides
BT3 Biocides
BT3 Residues

Dalia
BT1 Porridges
BT2 Cereal products
BT3 Plant foods
BT4 Foods

Damage
NT1 Abrasion
NT1 Breakage
NT1 Bruising
NT1 Cracking
NT1 Injury
NT1 Scuffing
NT1 Splitting
NT1 Sunburn
NT1 Wounding
RT Spoilage

β-Damascenone
HN introduced from vol. 39, issue 1 (2007)
BT1 Ketones
BT2 Carbonyl compounds
BT3 Organic compounds
BT1 Norisoprenoids
BT2 Aroma compounds
BT3 Flavour compounds
BT3 Volatile compounds
BT2 Carotenoids
BT3 Pigments
BT3 Terpenoids
BT4 Lipids
BT5 Nutrients

Daminozide
BT1 Plant growth regulators
BT2 Cultivation
BT3 Agriculture
UF Alar
UF *N*-Dimethylaminosuccinamic acid
UF Kylar
UF SADH

Damsons
BT1 Plums
BT2 Fruits specific
BT3 Fruits
BT4 Crops
BT5 Plants
BT4 Plant foods
BT5 Foods

Danbo cheese
BT1 Cheese varieties
BT2 Cheese
BT3 Dairy products
BT4 Animal foods
BT5 Foods

Dandelions
BT1 Vegetables specific
BT2 Vegetables
BT3 Crops
BT4 Plants
BT3 Plant foods
BT4 Foods

Danish pastries
BT1 Pastries
BT2 Bakery products
BT3 Cereal products
BT4 Plant foods
BT5 Foods

Dark chocolate
HN introduced from vol. 39, issue 1 (2007)
BT1 Chocolate products
BT2 Chocolate
BT3 Sugar confectionery
BT4 Plant foods
BT5 Foods
UF Plain chocolate

Dark cutting defect
BT1 Genetic disorders
RT Animal stress
RT DFD defect

Darkening
BT1 Discoloration

Dark firm dry defect
USE **DFD defect**

Dasanit
USE **Fensulfothion**

Databanks
BT1 Information technology
BT2 Technology

Databases
BT1 Information technology
BT2 Technology

Data processing
BT1 Information technology
BT2 Technology

DATEM
BT1 Emulsifiers
BT2 Additives
UF Diacetyl tartaric acid esters of mono- and diglycerides

Date marking
BT1 Labelling
BT2 Packaging
BT3 Technology
RT Dating

Dates
BT1 Fruits specific
BT2 Fruits
BT3 Crops
BT4 Plants
BT3 Plant foods
BT4 Foods
RT *Phoenix*

Dating
BT1 Labelling
BT2 Packaging
BT3 Technology
RT Date marking

Davana
HN under Spices up to vol. 42 (2010)
BT1 Herbs
BT2 Spices
BT3 Flavourings
BT4 Additives

Dawadawa
BT1 African locust beans
BT2 Oilseeds
BT3 Seeds
BT4 Plant foods
BT5 Foods
BT1 Fermented foods
BT2 Processed foods
BT3 Foods
RT Iru

Day lilies
HN introduced from vol. 39, issue 1 (2007)
SN belonging to the genus Hemerocallis
BT1 Edible flowers
BT2 Plants
BT2 Vegetables specific
BT3 Vegetables
BT4 Crops
BT5 Plants
BT4 Plant foods
BT5 Foods

DDD
USE **TDE**

DDE
HN heading up to vol. 18 (1986); under Insecticides from vol. 19 (1987) up to vol. 42 (2010)
BT1 DDT
BT2 Acaricides
BT3 Pesticides
BT4 Biocides
BT4 Residues
BT2 Organochlorine insecticides

BT3 Insecticides
BT4 Pesticides
BT5 Biocides
BT5 Residues
BT3 Organochlorine pesticides
BT4 Pesticides
BT5 Biocides
BT5 Residues

DDT
BT1 Acaricides
BT2 Pesticides
BT3 Biocides
BT3 Residues
BT1 Organochlorine insecticides
BT2 Insecticides
BT3 Pesticides
BT4 Biocides
BT4 Residues
BT2 Organochlorine pesticides
BT3 Pesticides
BT4 Biocides
BT4 Residues
NT1 DDE
NT1 TDE

Deacetylation
BT1 Modification

Deacidification
BT1 Neutralization

Deaeration
BT1 Processing
BT2 Technology
UF Degassing

Deamidation
BT1 Modification

Deaminases
BT1 Hydrolases
BT2 Enzymes

Debaryomyces
SN synonymous with Schwanniomyces
BT1 Yeasts
BT2 Fungi
BT3 Microorganisms
NT1 *Debaryomyces hansenii*

Debaryomyces hansenii
BT1 *Debaryomyces*
BT2 Yeasts
BT3 Fungi
BT4 Microorganisms

Debittering
BT1 Processing
BT2 Technology
RT Bitterness

Deboning
USE **Boning**

Debranching enzymes
USE **Pullulanases**

Debranning
BT1 Processing
BT2 Technology
RT Bran

Decaffeinated coffee
BT1 Coffee
BT2 Beverages
BT2 Crops
BT3 Plants
BT2 Plant foods
BT3 Foods

Decaffeinated tea
BT1 Tea
BT2 Teas
BT3 Beverages
BT3 Crops
BT4 Plants
BT3 Plant foods
BT4 Foods

Decaffeination
BT1 Processing
BT2 Technology
RT Caffeine

γ-Decalactone
BT1 Aroma compounds
BT2 Flavour compounds
BT2 Volatile compounds
BT1 Lactones
BT2 Esters
BT3 Organic compounds
BT2 Heterocyclic compounds

Decalepis hamiltonii
BT1 Plants

Decanal
HN also under Flavour compounds up to vol. 42 (2010)
BT1 Aldehydes
BT2 Carbonyl compounds
BT3 Organic compounds
BT1 Aroma compounds
BT2 Flavour compounds
BT2 Volatile compounds

Decane
BT1 Hydrocarbons
BT2 Organic compounds
BT1 Solvents

Decanoic acid
HN under Flavour compounds and Fatty acids up to vol. 42 (2010)
SN syn. capric acid
BT1 Aroma compounds
BT2 Flavour compounds
BT2 Volatile compounds
BT1 Saturated fatty acids
BT2 Fatty acids
BT3 Lipids
BT4 Nutrients
BT3 Organic acids
BT4 Acids
NT1 Capric acid

Decanol
HN also under Flavour compounds up to vol. 42 (2010)
BT1 Alcohols
BT1 Aroma compounds
BT2 Flavour compounds
BT2 Volatile compounds
BT1 Solvents

Decanters
BT1 Dispensers
BT2 Equipment
BT3 Technology

Decarbonation
BT1 Processing
BT2 Technology
RT CO_2

Decarboxylases
SN members of subclass EC 4.1.1
BT1 Lyases
BT2 Enzymes
NT1 Acetolactate decarboxylases
NT1 Glutamate decarboxylases
NT1 Histidine decarboxylases

Decarboxylation
BT1 Modification

Decay
BT1 Microbial spoilage
BT2 Spoilage

Decenoic acid
HN introduced from vol. 39, issue 1 (2007)
BT1 Monounsaturated fatty acids
BT2 Unsaturated fatty acids
BT3 Fatty acids
BT4 Lipids
BT5 Nutrients
BT4 Organic acids
BT5 Acids
RT Aroma compounds

Dechlorination
BT1 Bioremediation
BT2 Biotechnology
BT3 Technology

Decoction
BT1 Mashing
BT2 Processing
BT3 Technology

Decoloration
BT1 Processing
BT2 Technology
RT Bleaching
UF Decolorization

Decolorization
USE **Decoloration**

Decomposition
NT1 Biodegradability
NT1 Biodegradation
NT1 Breakdown
NT1 Degradation
NT2 Modori
NT1 Lysis
NT2 Autolysis
NT2 Haemolysis

NT2 Photolysis
NT2 Pyrolysis

Decontamination
BT1 Contamination

Decoquinate
BT1 Coccidiostats
BT2 Drugs
BT3 Residues

Decoration
BT1 Processing
BT2 Technology

Decortication
HN introduced from vol. 39, issue 1 (2007)
BT1 Processing
BT2 Technology
RT Husking

Deep freezing
BT1 Freezing
BT2 Thermal processing
BT3 Processing thermal
BT4 Processing
BT5 Technology

Deep frying
BT1 Frying
BT2 Cooking
BT3 Thermal processing
BT4 Processing thermal
BT5 Processing
BT6 Technology

Deer
BT1 Animals
RT Venison

Deer carcasses
BT1 Carcasses
BT2 Meat
BT3 Animal foods
BT4 Foods
BT1 Venison
BT2 Meat specific
BT3 Meat
BT4 Animal foods
BT5 Foods

Deer meat
USE **Venison**

Defeathering
BT1 Processing
BT2 Technology
UF Plucking

Defecation
BT1 Purification
BT2 Processing
BT3 Technology

Defects
NT1 Blackspot
RT Spoilage

Deficiency diseases
BT1 Diseases
RT Nutritional status

Definitions
BT1 Nomenclature
RT Terminology

Defoaming agents
BT1 Additives

Defoliation
BT1 Cultivation
BT2 Agriculture

Deformation
HN heading up to vol. 24 (1992)
BT1 Rheological properties
BT2 Mechanical properties
BT3 Physical properties
RT Shear

Defrosting
BT1 Thawing
BT2 Thermal processing
BT3 Processing thermal
BT4 Processing
BT5 Technology

Degassing
USE **Deaeration**

Degradation
BT1 Decomposition
NT1 Modori

Degreening
BT1 Processing
BT2 Technology

Degumming
BT1 Processing
BT2 Technology

Degumming agents
BT1 Additives

Dehairing
BT1 Processing
BT2 Technology

Dehulling
BT1 Husking
BT2 Processing
BT3 Technology

Dehydrated foods
USE **Dried foods**

Dehydration
USE **Drying**

Dehydroacetic acid
BT1 Organic acids
BT2 Acids
BT1 Preservatives
BT2 Additives

Dehydroascorbic acid
BT1 Ascorbic acid
BT2 Antioxidants
BT3 Additives
BT2 Bakery additives
BT3 Additives
BT2 Vitamins
BT3 Nutrients

Dehydrogenases
HN heading from vol. 25 (1993); under Enzymes up to vol. 24 (1992)
BT1 Oxidoreductases
BT2 Enzymes
NT1 Alcohol dehydrogenases
NT1 Aldehyde dehydrogenases
NT1 Aldehyde reductases
NT1 Glutamate dehydrogenases
NT1 L-Iditol 2-dehydrogenases
NT1 Isocitrate dehydrogenases
NT1 Lactate dehydrogenases
NT1 D-Lactate dehydrogenases
NT1 L-Lactate dehydrogenases
NT1 Xanthine dehydrogenases
NT1 D-Xylulose reductases

Dekkera
BT1 Yeasts
BT2 Fungi
BT3 Microorganisms
NT1 *Dekkera anomala*
NT1 *Dekkera bruxellensis*

Dekkera anomala
SN anamorph is Brettanomyces anomalus
BT1 *Dekkera*
BT2 Yeasts
BT3 Fungi
BT4 Microorganisms

Dekkera bruxellensis
SN anamorph is Brettanomyces bruxellensis, and is synonymous with Brettanomyces custersii
BT1 *Dekkera*
BT2 Yeasts
BT3 Fungi
BT4 Microorganisms

Delicatessen foods
BT1 Processed foods
BT2 Foods
NT1 Delicatessen salads
RT Salads

Delicatessen salads
BT1 Delicatessen foods
BT2 Processed foods
BT3 Foods
BT1 Salads

Delphinidin
BT1 Anthocyanidins
BT2 Flavonoids
BT3 Aromatic compounds
BT4 Organic compounds
BT3 Pigments

Deltamethrin
BT1 Acaricides
BT2 Pesticides
BT3 Biocides
BT3 Residues
BT1 Pyrethroid insecticides
BT2 Insecticides
BT3 Pesticides
BT4 Biocides
BT4 Residues

Demand
BT1 Consumer response
NT1 Consumer demand

Dementia
USE **Neurodegenerative diseases**

Demeton
BT1 Acaricides
BT2 Pesticides
BT3 Biocides
BT3 Residues
BT1 Organophosphorus insecticides
BT2 Insecticides
BT3 Pesticides
BT4 Biocides
BT4 Residues
BT2 Organophosphorus pesticides
BT3 Pesticides
BT4 Biocides
BT4 Residues

Demeton-*S*-methyl
BT1 Acaricides
BT2 Pesticides
BT3 Biocides
BT3 Residues
BT1 Organophosphorus insecticides
BT2 Insecticides
BT3 Pesticides
BT4 Biocides
BT4 Residues
BT2 Organophosphorus pesticides
BT3 Pesticides
BT4 Biocides
BT4 Residues
UF Metasystox
UF Methylmercaptofos

Demineralization
BT1 Minerals
BT2 Nutrients

Democratic Republic of the Congo
HN introduced from vol. 39, issue 1 (2007)
BT1 Central Africa
BT2 Africa
RT Zaire
UF Congo, Democratic Republic of the

Denaturation
RT Proteins
RT Renaturation

Denitrification
BT1 Processing
BT2 Technology
RT Nitrates
RT Nitrification

Denmark
HN heading up to vol. 24
BT1 Europe
BT1 European Union
RT Organization for Economic Cooperation and Development

Densitometry
HN heading up to vol. 24 (1992)
BT1 Analytical techniques

Density
BT1 Physical properties
NT1 Apparent density
NT1 Brix values
NT1 Bulk density
NT1 Gravity
NT1 Original gravity
NT1 sp. gr.
NT2 Relative density
RT Weight

Dental caries
BT1 Diseases
RT Dental health
UF Caries
UF Tooth decay

Dental health
BT1 Health
RT Dental caries

Dentex
USE **Sea bream**

Deodorization
BT1 Purification
BT2 Processing
BT3 Technology

Deoxycholate
BT1 Surfactants
UF Desoxycholate

Deoxymyoglobin
HN introduced from vol. 39, issue 1 (2007)
BT1 Myoglobin
BT2 Animal proteins
BT3 Proteins animal
BT4 Proteins
BT5 Nutrients
BT2 Pigments

Deoxynivalenol
SN syn. vomitoxin
BT1 Trichothecenes
BT2 Mycotoxins
BT3 Toxins
BT4 Residues

Deoxyribonucleases
SN includes members of EC 3.1.11, 3.1.15, 3.1.16, 3.1.21, 3.1.22 and 3.1.25
BT1 Nucleases
BT2 Esterases
BT3 Hydrolases
BT4 Enzymes
UF DNases

Deoxyribonucleic acid
USE **DNA**

Depolymerization
HN introduced from vol. 39, issue 1 (2007)
BT1 Modification

Depositors
BT1 Equipment
BT2 Technology

Depuration
BT1 Cleaning
BT2 Hygiene
BT2 Processing
BT3 Technology

Dermatitis
BT1 Diseases
UF Eczema

Desalination
BT1 Salt
BT2 Condiments
BT3 Flavourings
BT4 Additives

Desalting
BT1 Salt
BT2 Condiments
BT3 Flavourings
BT4 Additives

Desaturases
SN includes EC 1.3.1.35 and members of subclass EC 1.14.99
BT1 Oxidoreductases
BT2 Enzymes

Desaturation
BT1 Modification

Descaling
SN removal of limescale from equipment; for removal of fish scales use scaling
BT1 Cleaning
BT2 Hygiene
BT2 Processing
BT3 Technology

Desiccated coconut
BT1 Coconuts
BT2 Nuts
BT3 Fruits
BT4 Crops
BT5 Plants
BT4 Plant foods
BT5 Foods
BT3 Oilseeds
BT4 Seeds
BT5 Plant foods
BT6 Foods
BT1 Dried foods
BT2 Processed foods
BT3 Foods

Desiccation
USE **Drying**

Designer foods
BT1 Novel foods
BT2 Foods

RT Functional foods
RT Nutraceutical foods

Desmetryn
BT1 Triazine herbicides
BT2 Herbicides
BT3 Pesticides
BT4 Biocides
BT4 Residues
UF Semeron

Desmin
HN introduced from vol. 39, issue 1 (2007)
BT1 Animal proteins
BT2 Proteins animal
BT3 Proteins
BT4 Nutrients

Desmosterol
BT1 Sterols
BT2 Alcohols
BT2 Steroids
BT3 Lipids
BT4 Nutrients

Desmutagenicity
BT1 Health

Desorption
BT1 Sorption

Desoxycholate
HN used up to vol. 39 (2007)
USE **Deoxycholate**

Dessert mixes
BT1 Desserts
BT2 Processed foods
BT3 Foods
BT1 Mixes
BT2 Dried foods
BT3 Processed foods
BT4 Foods
BT2 Instant foods
BT3 Processed foods
BT4 Foods

Desserts
BT1 Processed foods
BT2 Foods
NT1 Bavarois
NT1 Blancmanges
NT1 Cheesecakes
NT1 Chocolate desserts
NT1 Custards
NT1 Dairy desserts
NT1 Dessert mixes
NT1 Frozen desserts
NT1 Fruit desserts
NT1 Gateaux
NT1 Gulabjamans
NT1 Jelly
NT1 Junket
NT1 Kissel
NT1 Milk puddings
NT1 Mousses
NT1 Nata
NT1 Pera
NT1 Pudding mixes
NT1 Puddings
NT1 Rasogolla
NT1 Sorbets
NT1 Torten
NT1 Zefir

Dessert wines
BT1 Wines
BT2 Alcoholic beverages
BT3 Beverages alcoholic
BT4 Beverages
RT Fortified wines

Destun
USE **Perfluidone**

Desulfitation
BT1 Processing
BT2 Technology
RT Sulfites
UF Desulphitation

Desulfovibrio
BT1 Bacteria
BT2 Microorganisms

Desulphitation
HN used for desulfitation up to vol. 35, issue 6 (2003)
USE **Desulfitation**

Detarium microcarpum
BT1 Legumes
BT2 Vegetables specific
BT3 Vegetables
BT4 Crops
BT5 Plants
BT4 Plant foods
BT5 Foods

Detectors
BT1 Apparatus
BT2 Technology
BT1 Equipment
BT2 Technology

Detergents
BT1 Surfactants

Deterioration
BT1 Spoilage

Detoxification
BT1 Processing
BT2 Technology

Detoxification enzymes
HN introduced from vol. 39, issue 1 (2007)
BT1 Enzymes

Deuterium
HN under Minerals up to vol. 42 (2010)
BT1 Hydrogen
BT2 Elements
BT3 Minerals
BT4 Nutrients

Developing countries
HN heading up to vol. 24 (1992)

Developments
HN under Product development up to vol. 24 (1992)

Devices
USE **Equipment**

Dewatering
BT1 Processing
BT2 Technology

Dewaxing
BT1 Processing
BT2 Technology
RT Waxes

Dewberries
BT1 Berries
BT2 Fruits specific
BT3 Fruits
BT4 Crops
BT5 Plants
BT4 Plant foods
BT5 Foods

Dextran
HN heading from vol. 30 (1998); dextrans used in the index up to vol. 29 (1997)
BT1 Glucans
BT2 Polysaccharides
BT3 Carbohydrates
BT4 Nutrients
BT4 Organic compounds
UF Dextrans

Dextranases
SN EC 3.2.1.11
BT1 Glycosidases
BT2 Hydrolases
BT3 Enzymes

Dextrans
HN dextran used in the index from vol. 30 (1998)
USE **Dextran**

Dextransucrases
SN EC 2.4.1.5
BT1 Glycosyltransferases
BT2 Transferases
BT3 Enzymes

Dextrinases
BT1 Glycosidases
BT2 Hydrolases
BT3 Enzymes

α-Dextrin endo-1,6-α-glucosidases
USE **Pullulanases**

Dextrins
BT1 Starch
BT2 Glucans
BT3 Polysaccharides
BT4 Carbohydrates
BT5 Nutrients
BT5 Organic compounds
BT2 Thickeners
BT3 Additives

NT1 Amylodextrins
NT1 Cyclodextrins
NT1 Maltodextrins
NT1 Pyrodextrins

Dextrose
USE **Glucose**

Dextrose equivalent
HN introduced from vol. 39, issue 1 (2007)
RT Sugars

DFD defect
BT1 Genetic disorders
RT Animal stress
RT Dark cutting defect
UF Dark firm dry defect

Dhal
BT1 Legumes
BT2 Vegetables specific
BT3 Vegetables
BT4 Crops
BT5 Plants
BT4 Plant foods
BT5 Foods

Dhokla
BT1 Fermented foods
BT2 Processed foods
BT3 Foods
BT1 Legumes
BT2 Vegetables specific
BT3 Vegetables
BT4 Crops
BT5 Plants
BT4 Plant foods
BT5 Foods

Diabetes
BT1 Diseases
RT Diabetic diet
RT Insulin
RT Insulin resistance

Diabetic diet
HN introduced from vol. 38, issue 8 (2006)
BT1 Diet therapy
BT2 Diet
BT3 Nutrition
BT2 Therapy
RT Diabetes

Diabetic foods
BT1 Dietetic foods
BT2 Processed foods
BT3 Foods

Diacetoxyscirpenol
BT1 Trichothecenes
BT2 Mycotoxins
BT3 Toxins
BT4 Residues

Diacetyl
SN syn. 2,3-butanedione
BT1 Aroma compounds
BT2 Flavour compounds
BT2 Volatile compounds
BT1 Diketones
BT2 Ketones
BT3 Carbonyl compounds
BT4 Organic compounds
NT1 2,3-Butanedione

Diacetyl tartaric acid esters of mono- and diglycerides
USE **DATEM**

Diacylglycerols
SN syn. diglycerides
BT1 Diglycerides
BT2 Glycerides
BT3 Emulsifiers
BT4 Additives
BT3 Fatty acid esters
BT4 Esters
BT5 Organic compounds
BT3 Lipids
BT4 Nutrients

Diafiltration
BT1 Ultrafiltration
BT2 Filtration
BT3 Processing
BT4 Technology

Diagnosis
HN introduced from vol. 39, issue 1 (2007)
BT1 Clinical techniques

Dialifos
BT1 Acaricides
BT2 Pesticides
BT3 Biocides
BT3 Residues
BT1 Organophosphorus insecticides
BT2 Insecticides
BT3 Pesticides
BT4 Biocides
BT4 Residues
BT2 Organophosphorus pesticides
BT3 Pesticides
BT4 Biocides
BT4 Residues
UF Torak

Diallyl disulfide
HN also under Flavour compounds up to vol. 42 (2010)
BT1 Allyl sulfides
BT2 Aroma compounds
BT3 Flavour compounds
BT3 Volatile compounds
BT2 Organic sulfur compounds
BT2 Sulfides
BT3 Salts
BT1 Disulfides
BT2 Sulfides
BT3 Salts
RT Garlic
UF Diallyl disulphides

Diallyl disulphides
HN used for diallyl disulfide up to vol. 35, issue 6 (2003)
USE **Diallyl disulfide**

Dialysis
BT1 Processing
BT2 Technology
NT1 Electrodialysis
RT Filtration
RT Membranes
RT Reverse osmosis
RT Separation
RT Ultrafiltration

Diamine oxidases
USE **Amine oxidases**

Diarrhoea
BT1 Diseases
RT Gastroenteritis

Diarrhoetic shellfish poisoning
BT1 Diseases
BT1 Poisoning
RT Diarrhoetic shellfish toxins
RT Paralytic shellfish poisoning
RT Sea foods

Diarrhoetic shellfish toxins
BT1 Toxins
BT2 Residues
RT Diarrhoetic shellfish poisoning
RT Okadaic acid
RT Paralytic shellfish toxins

Diastases
USE **α-Amylases**

Diastatic activity
BT1 Amylases
BT2 Glycosidases
BT3 Hydrolases
BT4 Enzymes
RT Malt

Diatomaceous earths
BT1 Filter aids
BT2 Filtration
BT3 Processing
BT4 Technology

Diatoxanthin
BT1 Xanthophylls
BT2 Carotenoids
BT3 Pigments
BT3 Terpenoids
BT4 Lipids
BT5 Nutrients

Diazepam
BT1 Drugs
BT2 Residues

Diazinon
BT1 Acaricides
BT2 Pesticides
BT3 Biocides
BT3 Residues
BT1 Organophosphorus insecticides
BT2 Insecticides
BT3 Pesticides
BT4 Biocides
BT4 Residues

Dietary reference values
USE **DRV**

Dietary study techniques
HN introduced from vol. 38, issue 8 (2006)
BT1 Diet
BT2 Nutrition
NT1 Food frequency questionnaires
RT Clinical techniques
RT Nutritional assessment

Dietary supplements
USE **Food supplements**

Diet drinks
USE **Calories low beverages**

Dietetic foods
SN products intended for individuals with metabolic disorders or allergies
BT1 Processed foods
BT2 Foods
NT1 Diabetic foods
NT1 Gluten low foods
NT2 Gluten low bread
RT Diet
RT Diet therapy
RT Health foods
RT Nutrition

Diethylamine
BT1 Amines
BT2 Organic nitrogen compounds

Diethylene glycol
BT1 Glycols
BT2 Alcohols

Diethylnitrosamine
SN syn. N-nitrosodiethylamine
BT1 Nitrosamines
BT2 Amines
BT3 Organic nitrogen compounds
BT2 Nitroso compounds
BT3 Organic nitrogen compounds

Diethylpyrocarbonate
BT1 Esters
BT2 Organic compounds
BT1 Organic acids
BT2 Acids
BT1 Preservatives
BT2 Additives

Diethylstilboestrol
BT1 Drugs
BT2 Residues
RT Oestrogens

Diet therapy
HN introduced from vol. 38, issue 8 (2006)
BT1 Diet
BT2 Nutrition
BT1 Therapy
NT1 Calories low diet
NT1 Carbohydrates low diet
NT1 Diabetic diet
NT1 Fats low diet
NT1 Ketogenic diet
NT1 Sodium low diet
NT1 Wt. loss diet
RT Dietetic foods

Difenzoquat
BT1 Herbicides
BT2 Pesticides
BT3 Biocides
BT3 Residues

Differential scanning calorimetry
USE **DSC**

Differential thermal analysis
BT1 Analytical techniques

Diffraction
BT1 Optical properties
BT2 Physical properties

Diffusers
BT1 Equipment
BT2 Technology
RT Diffusion

Diffusion
NT1 Diffusivity
RT Diffusers
RT Osmosis
RT Permeability
RT Sorption

Diffusivity
BT1 Diffusion
RT Moisture transfer

Diflubenzuron
BT1 Insecticides
BT2 Pesticides
BT3 Biocides
BT3 Residues

Difructose anhydride
HN introduced from vol. 39, issue 1 (2007); under Sugars up to vol. 42 (2010)
BT1 Disaccharides
BT2 Sugars
BT3 Carbohydrates
BT4 Nutrients
BT4 Organic compounds
BT3 Plant foods
BT4 Foods
RT Prebiotics

Digestibility
BT1 Nutrition

Digestion
BT1 Human physiology
BT2 Physiology
BT3 Science

Digitonin
BT1 Glycosides
BT2 Carbohydrates
BT3 Nutrients
BT3 Organic compounds
BT1 Saponins
BT2 Glycosides
BT3 Carbohydrates
BT4 Nutrients
BT4 Organic compounds

Diglucosides
BT1 Glycosides
BT2 Carbohydrates
BT3 Nutrients
BT3 Organic compounds

Diglycerides
SN syn. diacylglycerols
BT1 Glycerides
BT2 Emulsifiers
BT3 Additives
BT2 Fatty acid esters
BT3 Esters
BT4 Organic compounds
BT2 Lipids
BT3 Nutrients
NT1 Diacylglycerols

Dihydrochalcones
BT1 Chalcones
BT2 Antioxidants
BT3 Additives
BT2 Flavonoids
BT3 Aromatic compounds
BT4 Organic compounds
BT3 Pigments
BT1 Glycosides
BT2 Carbohydrates
BT3 Nutrients
BT3 Organic compounds
NT1 Neohesperidin dihydrochalcone
NT1 Phloretin

Dihydroquercetin
BT1 Antioxidants
BT2 Additives
BT1 Flavonols
BT2 Alcohols
BT2 Flavonoids
BT3 Aromatic compounds
BT4 Organic compounds
BT3 Pigments

Dihydrostreptomycin
BT1 Aminoglycoside antibiotics
BT2 Antibiotics
BT3 Drugs
BT4 Residues

Dihydroxyacetone
BT1 Ketones
BT2 Carbonyl compounds
BT3 Organic compounds

3,4-Dihydroxyphenylalanine
USE **DOPA**

Dika nuts
SN syn. African mango seeds
BT1 African mango seeds
BT2 Oilseeds
BT3 Seeds
BT4 Plant foods
BT5 Foods

Diketones
BT1 Ketones
BT2 Carbonyl compounds
BT3 Organic compounds
NT1 Diacetyl
NT2 2,3-Butanedione

Diketopiperazines
HN introduced from vol. 39, issue 1 (2007)
BT1 Bitter compounds
BT2 Flavour compounds
BT1 Heterocyclic compounds

Dilatometry
BT1 Analytical techniques

Dill
BT1 Spices
BT2 Flavourings
BT3 Additives
NT1 Dill leaves
NT1 Dill seeds
RT Dill ether

Dill ether
BT1 Aroma compounds
BT2 Flavour compounds
BT2 Volatile compounds
BT1 Ethers
BT2 Organic compounds
BT1 Monoterpenoids
BT2 Terpenoids
BT3 Lipids
BT4 Nutrients
RT Dill

Dill leaves
HN introduced from vol. 43, issue 1 (2011)
BT1 Dill
BT2 Spices
BT3 Flavourings
BT4 Additives
BT1 Herbs
BT2 Spices
BT3 Flavourings
BT4 Additives

Dill seeds
HN introduced from vol. 43, issue 1 (2011)
BT1 Dill
BT2 Spices
BT3 Flavourings
BT4 Additives

Dilor
BT1 Organochlorine insecticides
BT2 Insecticides
BT3 Pesticides
BT4 Biocides
BT4 Residues
BT2 Organochlorine pesticides
BT3 Pesticides
BT4 Biocides
BT4 Residues

Dilution
BT1 Processing
BT2 Technology

Dimethoate
BT1 Acaricides
BT2 Pesticides
BT3 Biocides
BT3 Residues
BT1 Nematocides
BT2 Pesticides
BT3 Biocides
BT3 Residues
BT1 Organophosphorus insecticides
BT2 Insecticides
BT3 Pesticides
BT4 Biocides
BT4 Residues
BT2 Organophosphorus pesticides
BT3 Pesticides
BT4 Biocides
BT4 Residues
UF Phosphamide

Dimethylamine
BT1 Amines
BT2 Organic nitrogen compounds

N-Dimethylaminosuccinamic acid
USE **Daminozide**

Dimethylarsinic acid
BT1 Arsenicals
BT2 Arsenic
BT3 Contaminants
BT4 Contamination
BT3 Elements
BT4 Minerals
BT5 Nutrients
BT1 Herbicides
BT2 Pesticides
BT3 Biocides
BT3 Residues
UF Cacodylic acid

Dimethyl disulfide
BT1 Aroma compounds
BT2 Flavour compounds
BT2 Volatile compounds
BT1 Disulfides
BT2 Sulfides
BT3 Salts
BT1 Organic sulfur compounds
UF Dimethyl disulphide

Dimethyl disulphide
HN used for dimethyl disulfide up to vol. 35, issue 6 (2003)
USE **Dimethyl disulfide**

Dimethylformamide
BT1 Amides
BT2 Organic nitrogen compounds
BT1 Solvents

2,5-Dimethyl-4-hydroxy-3(2*H*)-furanone
SN syn. furaneol
BT1 Furaneol
BT2 Furanones
BT3 Aroma compounds
BT4 Flavour compounds
BT4 Volatile compounds
BT3 Furans
BT4 Heterocyclic compounds
BT3 Ketones
BT4 Carbonyl compounds
BT5 Organic compounds

Dimethylnitrosamine
BT1 Nitrosamines
BT2 Amines
BT3 Organic nitrogen compounds
BT2 Nitroso compounds
BT3 Organic nitrogen compounds

Dimethylpolysiloxane
BT1 Antifoaming agents
BT2 Additives

Dimethyl sulfide
SN syn. methyl sulfide
BT1 Organic sulfur compounds
BT1 Solvents
BT1 Sulfides
BT2 Salts
NT1 Methyl sulfide
RT Aroma compounds
RT Off odour
UF Dimethyl sulphide

Dimethyl sulfoxide
BT1 Organic sulfur compounds
BT1 Oxides
BT1 Solvents
UF Dimethyl sulphoxide

Dimethyl sulphide
HN used for dimethyl sulfide up to vol. 35, issue 6 (2003)
USE **Dimethyl sulfide**

Dimethyl sulphoxide
HN used for dimethyl sulfoxide up to vol. 32 (2000)
USE **Dimethyl sulfoxide**

Dimethyl trisulfide
HN introduced from vol. 41, issue 1 (2009)
BT1 Aroma compounds
BT2 Flavour compounds
BT2 Volatile compounds
BT1 Organic sulfur compounds
BT1 Sulfides
BT2 Salts

Dimetilan
BT1 Carbamate pesticides
BT2 Pesticides
BT3 Biocides
BT3 Residues
BT1 Insecticides
BT2 Pesticides
BT3 Biocides
BT3 Residues

Dimetridazole
BT1 Coccidiostats
BT2 Drugs
BT3 Residues

Dim sum
BT1 Snack foods
BT2 Processed foods
BT3 Foods

Dinitolmide
BT1 Coccidiostats
BT2 Drugs
BT3 Residues
UF Zoalene

Dinitramine
BT1 Herbicides
BT2 Pesticides
BT3 Biocides
BT3 Residues

Dinitrophenylhydrazones
BT1 Carbonyl compounds
BT2 Organic compounds

Dinners
BT1 Meals
BT2 Processed foods
BT3 Foods

Dinocap
BT1 Fungicides
BT2 Pesticides
BT3 Biocides
BT3 Residues
BT1 Insecticides
BT2 Pesticides
BT3 Biocides
BT3 Residues

Dinoflagellates
BT1 Microalgae
BT2 Algae
BT3 Microorganisms
NT1 *Alexandrium*
NT2 *Alexandrium catenella*
NT2 *Alexandrium minutum*
NT2 *Alexandrium tamarense*
RT Dinoflagellate toxins
RT Paralytic shellfish toxins

Dinoflagellate toxins
BT1 Toxins
BT2 Residues
RT Dinoflagellates
RT Paralytic shellfish poisoning
RT Saxitoxin

Dinoseb
BT1 Herbicides
BT2 Pesticides
BT3 Biocides
BT3 Residues
UF DNBP

Diols
BT1 Alcohols

Dioscorin
HN introduced from vol. 37, issue 5 (2005)
BT1 Vegetable proteins
BT2 Proteins vegetable
BT3 Proteins
BT4 Nutrients
BT3 Vegetable products
BT4 Plant foods
BT5 Foods

Dioxane
BT1 Carcinogens
BT2 Mutagens
BT1 Solvents

Dioxathion
BT1 Acaricides
BT2 Pesticides
BT3 Biocides
BT3 Residues
BT1 Organophosphorus insecticides
BT2 Insecticides
BT3 Pesticides
BT4 Biocides
BT4 Residues
BT2 Organophosphorus pesticides
BT3 Pesticides
BT4 Biocides
BT4 Residues

Dioxins
BT1 Contaminants
BT2 Contamination

Dioxygenases
SN includes members of EC 1.13.11 and EC 1.14
BT1 Oxidoreductases
BT2 Enzymes

Dipeptidases
SN EC 3.4.13 - 3.4.15
BT1 Proteinases
BT2 Hydrolases
BT3 Enzymes

Dipeptides
BT1 Peptides
BT2 Proteins
BT3 Nutrients
NT1 Dipeptide sweeteners

Dipeptide sweeteners
HN sweeteners dipeptide also used in the index up to vol. 29 (1997)
BT1 Dipeptides
BT2 Peptides
BT3 Proteins
BT4 Nutrients
BT1 Sweeteners
BT2 Additives

Diphenamid
BT1 Herbicides
BT2 Pesticides
BT3 Biocides
BT3 Residues

Diphenol oxidases
USE **Catechol oxidases**

Diphenyl
USE **Biphenyl**

Diphenylamine
BT1 Fungicides
BT2 Pesticides
BT3 Biocides
BT3 Residues
RT Scald

Diphyllobothrium
BT1 Parasites
BT2 Pests

Dipicolinic acid
BT1 Organic acids
BT2 Acids
RT Bacterial spores

Diplodia
BT1 Fungi
BT2 Microorganisms

Dipping
BT1 Processing
BT2 Technology

Dips
BT1 Processed foods
BT2 Foods

Diquat
BT1 Herbicides
BT2 Pesticides
BT3 Biocides
BT3 Residues

Directories
BT1 Books
RT Buyers guides

Disaccharides
HN heading from vol. 43 (2011); under Sugars up to vol. 42 (2010)
BT1 Sugars
BT2 Carbohydrates
BT3 Nutrients
BT3 Organic compounds
BT2 Plant foods
BT3 Foods
NT1 Cellobiose
NT1 Difructose anhydride
NT1 Gentiobiose
NT1 Isomaltose
NT1 Isomaltulose
NT2 Palatinose
NT1 Lactose
NT2 Lactose low foods
NT1 Lactulose
NT1 Maltose
NT1 Melibiose
NT1 Nigerose
NT1 Sucrose
NT1 Trehalose

Discoloration
NT1 Blackspot
NT1 Darkening

NT1 Melanosis
NT1 Mottling
NT1 Staining
RT Browning
RT Colour

Disease resistance
HN introduced from vol. 39, issue 1 (2007)
BT1 Plant diseases
 BT2 Diseases plant
  BT3 Diseases

Diseases
SN includes both diseases and disorders
NT1 AIDS
NT1 Alcohol-related disorders
NT1 Allergies
 NT2 Allergenicity
 NT2 Allergens
 NT2 Anaphylaxis
NT1 Amnesic shellfish poisoning
NT1 Amoebiasis
NT1 Anaemia
NT1 Anisakiasis
 NT2 Anisakidosis
NT1 Anthrax
NT1 Arthritis
NT1 Asthma
NT1 Atherosclerosis
NT1 Botulism
NT1 Brucellosis
NT1 Campylobacteriosis
NT1 Cancer
 NT2 Breast cancer
 NT2 Colorectal cancer
 NT2 Gastric cancer
 NT2 Lung cancer
 NT2 Ovarian cancer
 NT2 Prostate cancer
NT1 Carcinogenesis
NT1 Cardiovascular diseases
 NT2 Coronary heart diseases
  NT3 Myocardial infarction
 NT2 Stroke
NT1 Cholera
NT1 Coeliac disease
NT1 Colitis
NT1 Constipation
NT1 Cryptosporidiosis
NT1 Cyclosporiasis
NT1 Deficiency diseases
NT1 Dental caries
NT1 Dermatitis
NT1 Diabetes
NT1 Diarrhoea
NT1 Diarrhoetic shellfish poisoning
NT1 Diseases animal
 NT2 Animal diseases
  NT3 Avian flu
  NT3 Brucellosis
  NT3 Coccidiosis
  NT3 Cysticercosis
  NT3 Foot and mouth disease
  NT3 Malignant hyperthermia
  NT3 Mastitis
  NT3 Swine fever
NT1 Diseases plant
 NT2 Plant diseases
  NT3 Anthracnose
  NT3 Blights
  NT3 Disease resistance
  NT3 Ergot
  NT3 Fungal decay
  NT3 Rots
   NT4 Brown rot
  NT3 Rusts
  NT3 Scab
 NT2 Plant disorders
  NT3 Bitter pit
  NT3 Blossom end rot
  NT3 Brown heart
  NT3 Cork spots
  NT3 Pitting disorders
  NT3 Russeting
  NT3 Scald
  NT3 Skin spot
  NT3 Sunburn
  NT3 Tipburn
  NT3 Watercore
  NT3 Woolliness
NT1 Diverticulosis
NT1 Dracunculiasis
NT1 Epidemiology
NT1 Eye disorders
NT1 Fluorosis
NT1 Foodborne diseases
NT1 Gallstones
NT1 Gastritis
NT1 Gastroenteritis
NT1 Giardiasis
NT1 Goitre
NT1 Gout
NT1 Haemolytic uraemic syndrome
NT1 Hepatitis
NT1 Human genetic disorders
NT1 Hyperactivity
NT1 Hyperlipaemia
NT1 Hypertension
NT1 Infection
NT1 Inflammation
NT1 Inflammatory bowel disease
 NT2 Crohns disease
 NT2 Ulcerative colitis
NT1 Insulin resistance
NT1 Intolerance
 NT2 Food intolerance
  NT3 Lactose intolerance
NT1 Irritable bowel syndrome
NT1 Kidney stones
NT1 Legionellosis
NT1 Leptospirosis
NT1 Listeriosis
NT1 Malabsorption
NT1 Malnutrition
NT1 Metabolic disorders
NT1 Metabolic syndrome
NT1 Migraine
NT1 Mussel poisoning
NT1 Mycotoxicosis
 NT2 Aflatoxicosis
NT1 Neural tube defects
 NT2 Spina bifida
NT1 Neurodegenerative diseases
NT1 Neurological shellfish poisoning
NT1 Obesity
NT1 Oedema
NT1 Osteoporosis
NT1 Paralytic shellfish poisoning
 NT2 PSP
NT1 Paratyphoid
NT1 Pasteurellosis
NT1 PKU
NT1 Poliomyelitis
NT1 Prion diseases
 NT2 BSE
 NT2 CJD
 NT2 Scrapie
NT1 Psychiatric disorders
 NT2 Eating disorders
NT1 Salmonellosis
NT1 Scombroid poisoning
NT1 Shigellosis
NT1 Toxoplasmosis
NT1 Trichinosis
NT1 Tuberculosis
NT1 Typhoid
NT1 Urticaria
NT1 Yersiniosis
NT1 Yusho
NT1 Zoonoses
RT Cigarette smoking
RT Clinical techniques
RT Health
RT Pathogens
RT Poisoning
RT Risk factors
RT Therapy

Diseases animal
SN animal diseases is also used in the index; includes diseases and disorders
BT1 Diseases
NT1 Animal diseases
 NT2 Avian flu
 NT2 Brucellosis
 NT2 Coccidiosis
 NT2 Cysticercosis
 NT2 Foot and mouth disease
 NT2 Malignant hyperthermia
 NT2 Mastitis
 NT2 Swine fever

Diseases plant
SN plant diseases is also used in the index
BT1 Diseases
NT1 Plant diseases
 NT2 Anthracnose
 NT2 Blights
 NT2 Disease resistance
 NT2 Ergot
 NT2 Fungal decay
 NT2 Rots
  NT3 Brown rot
 NT2 Rusts
 NT2 Scab
NT1 Plant disorders
 NT2 Bitter pit
 NT2 Blossom end rot
 NT2 Brown heart
 NT2 Cork spots
 NT2 Pitting disorders
 NT2 Russeting

NT2 Scald
NT2 Skin spot
NT2 Sunburn
NT2 Tipburn
NT2 Watercore
NT2 Woolliness
RT *Botrytis*
RT *Colletotrichum*
RT *Rhizoctonia*
RT *Sclerotinia*
RT *Septoria*
RT Spoilage

Dishes
BT1 Meals
BT2 Processed foods
BT3 Foods
NT1 Meat dishes
NT1 Side dishes

Dishwashers
BT1 Cleaning
BT2 Hygiene
BT2 Processing
BT3 Technology
BT1 Equipment
BT2 Technology

Disinfectants
BT1 Disinfection
BT2 Hygiene
NT1 Antiseptics
NT1 Cetylpyridinium chloride
NT1 Chloramines
NT2 Monochloramine
NT1 Chlorates
NT1 Chlorites
NT1 Electrolysed water
NT1 Germicides
NT1 Hexachlorophene
NT1 Hypochlorites
NT1 Iodophors
NT1 Methyl iodide
NT1 Ozone
NT1 Perchlorates
NT1 Quaternary ammonium compounds
NT1 Sanitizers
RT Surfactants

Disinfection
BT1 Hygiene
NT1 Chlorination
NT1 Disinfectants
NT2 Antiseptics
NT2 Cetylpyridinium chloride
NT2 Chloramines
NT3 Monochloramine
NT2 Chlorates
NT2 Chlorites
NT2 Electrolysed water
NT2 Germicides
NT2 Hexachlorophene
NT2 Hypochlorites
NT2 Iodophors
NT2 Methyl iodide
NT2 Ozone
NT2 Perchlorates
NT2 Quaternary ammonium compounds
NT2 Sanitizers
NT1 Disinfection by-products
NT2 Dichloroacetic acid
NT2 Haloacetic acids
NT2 Trihalomethanes
NT1 Ozonation
NT1 Sanitation
RT Ammonium compounds
RT Biocides
RT Chlorine
RT Cleaning
RT Formaldehyde
RT Fumigation
RT Methanal

Disinfection by-products
BT1 Disinfection
BT2 Hygiene
NT1 Dichloroacetic acid
NT1 Haloacetic acids
NT1 Trihalomethanes

Disinfestation
BT1 Pests
NT1 Biocontrol
NT1 Entoleters
RT Fumigation

Dispensers
BT1 Equipment
BT2 Technology
NT1 Aerosols
NT1 Atomizers
NT1 Decanters
NT1 Dispensing
NT1 Taps

Dispensing
BT1 Dispensers
BT2 Equipment
BT3 Technology

Dispersibility
BT1 Functional properties
BT2 Physical properties

Dispersion
HN heading up to vol. 24 (1992)
BT1 Dispersions
BT2 Physical phases
BT3 Chemistry
BT4 Science

Dispersions
HN heading from vol. 25 (1993); was Dispersion up to vol. 24 (1992)
BT1 Physical phases
BT2 Chemistry
BT3 Science
NT1 Dispersion
RT Colloids
RT Emulsions
RT Foams
RT Gels

Display cabinets
BT1 Marketing
BT2 Economics
RT Retail display

Distillates
BT1 Spirits
BT2 Alcoholic beverages
BT3 Beverages alcoholic
BT4 Beverages
NT1 Wine distillates

Distillation
BT1 Processing
BT2 Technology
NT1 Corn steep liquor
NT1 Distilleries
NT2 Distilleries effluents
NT1 Distilling industry
NT1 Rectification
NT1 Vacuum distillation
RT Evaporation
RT Fractionation
RT Stillage

Distilleries
BT1 Distillation
BT2 Processing
BT3 Technology
NT1 Distilleries effluents

Distilleries effluents
BT1 Distilleries
BT2 Distillation
BT3 Processing
BT4 Technology
BT1 Effluents
BT2 Waste water
BT3 Wastes
BT3 Water

Distillers grains
BT1 By-products
NT1 Distillers spent grains

Distillers spent grains
BT1 Distillers grains
BT2 By-products

Distillers yeasts
HN yeasts distillers also used in the index up to vol. 29 (1997)
BT1 Yeasts
BT2 Fungi
BT3 Microorganisms

Distilling industry
BT1 Distillation
BT2 Processing
BT3 Technology
BT1 Food industry
BT2 Industries

Distribution
RT Logistics
RT Marketing
RT Transport

Disulfides
BT1 Sulfides
BT2 Salts
NT1 Carbon disulfide
NT1 Diallyl disulfide
NT1 Dimethyl disulfide
UF Disulphides

Disulfoton
BT1 Acaricides
BT2 Pesticides
BT3 Biocides
BT3 Residues
BT1 Organophosphorus insecticides
BT2 Insecticides
BT3 Pesticides
BT4 Biocides
BT4 Residues
BT2 Organophosphorus pesticides
BT3 Pesticides
BT4 Biocides
BT4 Residues
UF Disyston

Disulphides
HN used for disulfides up to vol. 35, issue 6 (2003)
USE **Disulfides**

Disyston
USE **Disulfoton**

Diterpenes
BT1 Diterpenoids
BT2 Terpenoids
BT3 Lipids
BT4 Nutrients
BT1 Hydrocarbons
BT2 Organic compounds

Diterpenoids
HN introduced from vol. 43, issue 1 (2011)
BT1 Terpenoids
BT2 Lipids
BT3 Nutrients
NT1 Cafestol
NT1 Carnosic acid
NT1 Carnosol
NT1 Diterpenes
NT1 Kahweol
NT1 Rebaudiosides
NT1 Steviol
NT1 Stevioside

Dithiocarbamate fungicides
HN introduced from vol. 43 (2011)
BT1 Fungicides
BT2 Pesticides
BT3 Biocides
BT3 Residues
NT1 Ethylenethiourea
NT1 Ferbam
NT1 Mancozeb
NT1 Maneb
NT1 Propineb
NT1 Thiram
NT1 Zineb
NT1 Ziram

Dithiothreitol
BT1 Thiols
BT2 Organic sulfur compounds

Dittany
HN under Spices up to vol. 42 (2010)
BT1 Herbs
BT2 Spices
BT3 Flavourings
BT4 Additives

Diuron
BT1 Herbicides
BT2 Pesticides
BT3 Biocides
BT3 Residues

Divercins
HN introduced from vol. 39, issue 1 (2007)
BT1 Bacteriocins
BT2 Antibiotics
BT3 Drugs
BT4 Residues
RT *Carnobacterium divergens*

Diverticulosis
BT1 Diseases

Djenkol beans
BT1 Legumes
BT2 Vegetables specific
BT3 Vegetables
BT4 Crops
BT5 Plants
BT4 Plant foods
BT5 Foods

Djibouti
BT1 East Africa
BT2 Africa

DM
SN index heading is Dry matter
BT1 Dry matter
RT Solids

DMDT
USE **Methoxychlor**

DNA
BT1 Nucleic acids
BT2 Organic acids
BT3 Acids
NT1 cDNA
NT1 Mitochondrial DNA
NT1 RAPD
RT Chromosomes
RT Genomes
UF Deoxyribonucleic acid

DNA-directed DNA polymerases
SN EC 2.7.7.7
BT1 Transferases
BT2 Enzymes
UF DNA polymerases

DNA-directed RNA polymerases
SN EC 2.7.7.6
BT1 Transferases
BT2 Enzymes
UF RNA polymerases

DNA fingerprinting
BT1 Genetic fingerprinting
BT2 Genetic techniques
BT3 Genetics
RT RFLP

DNA hybridization
BT1 Hybridization
BT2 Genetic techniques
BT3 Genetics

DNA microarrays
HN introduced from vol. 39, issue 1 (2007)
BT1 Genetic techniques
BT2 Genetics
RT Microarrays

DNA polymerases
USE **DNA-directed DNA polymerases**

DNA probes
BT1 Gene probes
BT2 Genetic techniques
BT3 Genetics
RT Oligonucleotides

DNases
USE **Deoxyribonucleases**

DNBP
USE **Dinoseb**

Docosahexaenoic acid
BT1 ω-3 Fatty acids
BT2 PUFA
BT3 Unsaturated fatty acids
BT4 Fatty acids
BT5 Lipids
BT6 Nutrients
BT5 Organic acids
BT6 Acids

Docosapentaenoic acid
BT1 ω-3 Fatty acids
BT2 PUFA
BT3 Unsaturated fatty acids
BT4 Fatty acids
BT5 Lipids
BT6 Nutrients
BT5 Organic acids
BT6 Acids

Docosenoic acid
BT1 Monounsaturated fatty acids
BT2 Unsaturated fatty acids
BT3 Fatty acids
BT4 Lipids
BT5 Nutrients
BT4 Organic acids
BT5 Acids
NT1 Erucic acid
RT Rapeseed oils

Dodecanoic acid
HN under Fatty acids up to vol. 42 (2010)
SN syn. lauric acid
BT1 Aroma compounds
BT2 Flavour compounds
BT2 Volatile compounds
BT1 Saturated fatty acids
BT2 Fatty acids

BT3 Lipids
BT4 Nutrients
BT3 Organic acids
BT4 Acids
NT1 Lauric acid

Dodine
BT1 Fungicides
BT2 Pesticides
BT3 Biocides
BT3 Residues
UF Cyprex

Doenjang
BT1 Fermented foods
BT2 Processed foods
BT3 Foods
BT1 Soy products
BT2 Vegetable products
BT3 Plant foods
BT4 Foods
UF Doenzang
UF Tenjan

Doenzang
USE **Doenjang**

Dog biscuits
HN introduced from vol. 39, issue 1 (2007)
BT1 Dog foods
BT2 Pet foods
RT Dogs

Dogfish
BT1 Marine fish
BT2 Fish
BT3 Animals
BT3 Sea foods
BT4 Aquatic foods
BT5 Animal foods
BT6 Foods

Dog foods
HN introduced from vol. 39, issue 1 (2007)
BT1 Pet foods
NT1 Dog biscuits
NT1 Puppy foods
RT Dogs

Dogs
HN introduced from vol. 39, issue 1 (2007)
SN use for domestic pets but not for animals reared for dog meat
BT1 Pets
RT Dog biscuits
RT Dog foods
RT Puppy foods

Dolphinfish
SN syn. mahimahi
BT1 Marine fish
BT2 Fish
BT3 Animals
BT3 Sea foods
BT4 Aquatic foods
BT5 Animal foods
BT6 Foods
NT1 Mahimahi

Dolphins
BT1 Animals
RT Cetacea

Domiati cheese
BT1 Cheese varieties
BT2 Cheese
BT3 Dairy products
BT4 Animal foods
BT5 Foods

Dominica
BT1 West Indies
BT2 America

Dominican Republic
BT1 West Indies
BT2 America

Domoic acid
BT1 Toxins
BT2 Residues

Doner kebabs
BT1 Meat products
BT2 Animal foods
BT3 Foods

Dongchimi
BT1 Fermented foods
BT2 Processed foods
BT3 Foods
BT1 Radishes
BT2 Vegetables specific
BT3 Vegetables
BT4 Crops
BT5 Plants
BT4 Plant foods
BT5 Foods

DOPA
BT1 Amino acids
BT2 Nutrients
BT2 Organic acids
BT3 Acids
BT2 Organic nitrogen compounds
UF 3,4-Dihydroxyphenylalanine

Dopamine
BT1 Biogenic amines
BT2 Amines
BT3 Organic nitrogen compounds

Dosa
USE **Dosai**

Dosai
HN under Cereal products up to vol. 42 (2010)
BT1 Black gram
BT2 Legumes
BT3 Vegetables specific
BT4 Vegetables
BT5 Crops
BT6 Plants
BT5 Plant foods
BT6 Foods
BT1 Fermented foods
BT2 Processed foods
BT3 Foods
BT1 Rice
BT2 Cereals
BT3 Crops
BT4 Plants
BT3 Seeds
BT4 Plant foods
BT5 Foods
UF Dosa

Dosimeters
BT1 Radioactivity

Double cream
BT1 Cream
BT2 Dairy products
BT3 Animal foods
BT4 Foods

Dough
BT1 Bakery products
BT2 Cereal products
BT3 Plant foods
BT4 Foods
NT1 Biscuit dough
NT1 Bread dough
NT1 Frozen dough
NT1 Pizza dough
NT1 Sourdough
NT1 Sponge
NT1 Wheat dough
RT Alveographs
RT Farinographs

Dough conditioners
BT1 Bakery additives
BT2 Additives

Doughnuts
BT1 Bakery products
BT2 Cereal products
BT3 Plant foods
BT4 Foods

Dowicide A
USE **2-Phenylphenol**

Downstream processing
HN heading from vol. 24 (1992)
BT1 Fermentation technology
BT2 Biotechnology
BT3 Technology
BT2 Process control
BT3 Technology
BT1 Purification
BT2 Processing
BT3 Technology

Doxycycline
BT1 Tetracyclines
BT2 Antibiotics
BT3 Drugs
BT4 Residues

Dracunculiasis
BT1 Diseases

Dragees
BT1 Sugar confectionery
BT2 Plant foods
BT3 Foods

Draught beer
BT1 Beer
BT2 Alcoholic beverages
BT3 Beverages alcoholic
BT4 Beverages

Dressing
BT1 Processing
BT2 Technology

Dressings
BT1 Salad dressings
BT2 Condiments
BT3 Flavourings
BT4 Additives

DRI
HN introduced from vol. 38, issue 8 (2006)
SN includes the estimated average requirement (EAR), tolerable upper intake (UL), adequate intake (AI) and recommended daily allowance (RDA)
BT1 Nutrient requirements
BT2 Nutrients
BT2 Nutrition
NT1 RDA
RT DRV
RT RDI
UF Dietary reference intakes

Dried dairy products
BT1 Dairy products
BT2 Animal foods
BT3 Foods
BT1 Powders
BT2 Dried foods
BT3 Processed foods
BT4 Foods
BT2 Instant foods
BT3 Processed foods
BT4 Foods
NT1 Dried milk
NT1 Dried skim milk
NT1 Dried whey

Dried egg products
BT1 Egg products
BT2 Animal foods
BT3 Foods
BT1 Powders
BT2 Dried foods
BT3 Processed foods
BT4 Foods
BT2 Instant foods
BT3 Processed foods
BT4 Foods
RT Dried eggs

Dried eggs
BT1 Eggs
BT2 Animal foods
BT3 Foods
BT1 Powders
BT2 Dried foods
BT3 Processed foods
BT4 Foods
BT2 Instant foods
BT3 Processed foods
BT4 Foods
RT Dried egg products
UF Egg powders

Dried figs
HN introduced from vol. 37, issue 5 (2005)
BT1 Dried fruits
BT2 Fruits dried
BT3 Dried foods
BT4 Processed foods
BT5 Foods
BT3 Fruits
BT4 Crops
BT5 Plants
BT4 Plant foods
BT5 Foods
BT1 Figs
BT2 Fruits specific
BT3 Fruits
BT4 Crops
BT5 Plants
BT4 Plant foods
BT5 Foods

Dried fish
BT1 Dried sea foods
BT2 Dried foods
BT3 Processed foods
BT4 Foods
BT2 Sea foods
BT3 Aquatic foods
BT4 Animal foods
BT5 Foods
BT1 Fish
BT2 Animals
BT2 Sea foods
BT3 Aquatic foods
BT4 Animal foods
BT5 Foods

Dried foods
BT1 Processed foods
BT2 Foods
NT1 Desiccated coconut
NT1 Dried meat
NT1 Dried meat products
NT1 Dried pet foods
NT1 Dried sea foods
NT2 Dried fish
NT1 Dried vegetables
NT2 Dried peas
NT1 Freeze dried foods
NT1 Fruits dried
NT2 Dried fruits
NT3 Currants
NT3 Dried figs
NT3 Prunes
NT3 Raisins
NT3 Sultanas
NT1 Meju
NT1 Mixes
NT2 Bakery product mixes
NT2 Beverage mixes
NT2 Cake mixes
NT2 Dessert mixes
NT2 Ice cream mixes
NT2 Soup mixes
NT1 Potato flakes
NT1 Powders
NT2 Beverage powders
NT2 Chocolate powders
NT2 Cocoa powders
NT2 Coffee powders
NT2 Dried dairy products
NT3 Dried milk
NT3 Dried skim milk
NT3 Dried whey
NT2 Dried egg products
NT2 Dried eggs
NT2 Milk powders
NT2 Rice powders
NT2 Skim milk powders
NT2 Tea powders
NT2 Tomato powders
NT1 Spray dried foods
RT Drying
RT Freeze drying
RT Granules
RT Instant foods
UF Dehydrated foods

Dried fruits
SN index heading is Fruits dried
BT1 Fruits dried
BT2 Dried foods
BT3 Processed foods
BT4 Foods
BT2 Fruits
BT3 Crops
BT4 Plants
BT3 Plant foods
BT4 Foods
NT1 Currants
NT1 Dried figs
NT1 Prunes
NT1 Raisins
NT1 Sultanas

Dried meat
BT1 Dried foods
BT2 Processed foods
BT3 Foods
BT1 Meat
BT2 Animal foods
BT3 Foods
RT Dried meat products

Dried meat products
BT1 Dried foods
BT2 Processed foods
BT3 Foods
BT1 Meat products
BT2 Animal foods
BT3 Foods
RT Dried meat

Dried milk
BT1 Dried dairy products
BT2 Dairy products
BT3 Animal foods
BT4 Foods
BT2 Powders
BT3 Dried foods
BT4 Processed foods
BT5 Foods
BT3 Instant foods
BT4 Processed foods
BT5 Foods
BT1 Milk
BT2 Dairy products

BT3 Animal foods
BT4 Foods
RT Dried skim milk
RT Milk powders
RT Skim milk powders

Dried peas
BT1 Dried vegetables
BT2 Dried foods
BT3 Processed foods
BT4 Foods
BT2 Vegetables
BT3 Crops
BT4 Plants
BT3 Plant foods
BT4 Foods
BT1 Peas
BT2 Legumes
BT3 Vegetables specific
BT4 Vegetables
BT5 Crops
BT6 Plants
BT5 Plant foods
BT6 Foods

Dried pet foods
HN introduced from vol. 39, issue 1 (2007)
BT1 Dried foods
BT2 Processed foods
BT3 Foods
BT1 Pet foods

Dried sea foods
HN introduced from vol. 41, issue 1 (2009)
BT1 Dried foods
BT2 Processed foods
BT3 Foods
BT1 Sea foods
BT2 Aquatic foods
BT3 Animal foods
BT4 Foods
NT1 Dried fish

Dried skim milk
BT1 Dried dairy products
BT2 Dairy products
BT3 Animal foods
BT4 Foods
BT2 Powders
BT3 Dried foods
BT4 Processed foods
BT5 Foods
BT3 Instant foods
BT4 Processed foods
BT5 Foods
BT1 Skim milk
BT2 Milk
BT3 Dairy products
BT4 Animal foods
BT5 Foods
RT Dried milk
RT Milk powders
RT Skim milk powders

Dried vegetables
BT1 Dried foods
BT2 Processed foods
BT3 Foods
BT1 Vegetables
BT2 Crops
BT3 Plants
BT2 Plant foods
BT3 Foods
NT1 Dried peas

Dried whey
BT1 Dried dairy products
BT2 Dairy products
BT3 Animal foods
BT4 Foods
BT2 Powders
BT3 Dried foods
BT4 Processed foods
BT5 Foods
BT3 Instant foods
BT4 Processed foods
BT5 Foods
BT1 Whey
BT2 Dairy products
BT3 Animal foods
BT4 Foods

Dried yeasts
HN yeasts dried also used in the index up to vol. 29 (1997)
BT1 Yeasts
BT2 Fungi
BT3 Microorganisms

Driers
BT1 Drying
BT2 Thermal processing
BT3 Processing thermal
BT4 Processing
BT5 Technology
BT1 Equipment
BT2 Technology
NT1 Freeze driers
NT1 Solar driers
NT1 Spray driers
UF Dryers

Drinking chocolate
BT1 Chocolate beverages
BT2 Beverages
BT2 Chocolate products
BT3 Chocolate
BT4 Sugar confectionery
BT5 Plant foods
BT6 Foods

Drinking habits
HN introduced from vol. 40, issue 4 (2008)
SN includes intake patterns for alcoholic and non-alcoholic beverages, problem drinking, abstinence from alcohol, etc.
BT1 Consumer behaviour
BT2 Consumer response
RT Beverages
RT Eating habits

Drinking straws
RT Beverages

Drinking water
BT1 Water
NT1 Bottled water
NT1 Potable water
NT1 Well water
RT Beverages
RT Mineral waters

Drinking yoghurt
BT1 Yoghurt beverages
BT2 Dairy beverages
BT3 Beverages
BT3 Dairy products
BT4 Animal foods
BT5 Foods
BT2 Yoghurt
BT3 Fermented milk
BT4 Fermented dairy products
BT5 Dairy products
BT6 Animal foods
BT7 Foods
BT5 Fermented foods
BT6 Processed foods
BT7 Foods
BT4 Milk
BT5 Dairy products
BT6 Animal foods
BT7 Foods

Drinks
USE **Beverages**

Drip
BT1 Thawing
BT2 Thermal processing
BT3 Processing thermal
BT4 Processing
BT5 Technology

Dripping
BT1 Animal fats
BT2 Fats animal
BT3 Animal foods
BT4 Foods
BT3 Fats
BT4 Lipids
BT5 Nutrients

Dropsy
USE **Oedema**

Drugs
BT1 Residues
NT1 β-Adrenergic agonists
NT2 Cimaterol
NT2 Clenbuterol
NT2 Propranolol
NT2 Ractopamine
NT2 Salbutamol
NT1 Anabolic agents
NT1 Anabolic steroids
NT2 Trenbolone acetate
NT1 Anthelmintics
NT2 Albendazole
NT2 Fasciolicides
NT2 Fenbendazole
NT2 Ivermectin
NT2 Levamisoles
NT2 Moxidectin
NT2 Nitroxynil
NT1 Antibiotics
NT2 Actinomycin

NT2 Aminoglycoside antibiotics
NT3 Dihydrostreptomycin
NT3 Gentamicin
NT3 Hygromycins
NT3 Kanamycin
NT3 Neomycin
NT3 Spectinomycin
NT3 Streptomycin
NT2 Antibacterial compounds
NT2 Antibiotics resistance
NT2 Antimicrobial compounds
NT2 Avoparcin
NT2 Bacitracin
NT2 Bacteriocins
NT3 Acidocins
NT3 Amylovorins
NT3 Bacteriocins resistance
NT3 Bavaricins
NT3 Divercins
NT3 Enterocins
NT3 Epidermin
NT3 Gassericins
NT3 Lactacins
NT3 Lacticins
NT3 Lactocins
NT3 Lactococcins
NT3 Lantibiotics
NT3 Leucocins
NT3 Mesentericins
NT3 Nisin
NT3 Pediocins
NT3 Piscicolins
NT3 Plantaricins
NT3 Propionicins
NT3 Sakacins
NT3 Subtilins
NT2 Blasticidin S
NT2 Cerulenin
NT2 Chloramphenicol
NT2 Cycloheximide
NT2 Cycloserine
NT2 Flavomycin
NT2 Florfenicol
NT2 Gliotoxin
NT2 Griseofulvin
NT2 3-Hydroxypropionaldehyde
NT2 Isoniazid
NT2 β-Lactam antibiotics
NT3 Cephalosporins
NT4 Ceftazidime
NT4 Ceftiofur
NT4 Cephapirin
NT3 Penicillins
NT4 Amoxicillin
NT4 Ampicillin
NT4 Benzylpenicillin
NT4 Cloxacillin
NT4 Dicloxacillin
NT4 Oxacillin
NT4 Penicillin G
NT2 Lasalocids
NT2 Lincomycin
NT2 Macrolide antibiotics
NT3 Erythromycin
NT3 Nystatin
NT3 Oleandomycin
NT3 Spiramycin
NT3 Tilmicosin
NT3 Tylosin
NT2 Metronidazole
NT2 Monensin
NT2 Nitrofurans
NT3 Furazolidone
NT3 Nitrofurazone
NT3 Nitrovin
NT2 Novobiocin
NT2 Penicillic acid
NT2 Polymyxins
NT2 Quinolones
NT3 Ciprofloxacin
NT3 Enrofloxacin
NT3 Flumequine
NT3 Nalidixic acid
NT3 Oxolinic acid
NT2 Reuterin
NT2 Salinomycin
NT2 Sulfonamides
NT3 Chloramine T
NT3 Sulfadiazine
NT3 Sulfamethazine
NT4 Sulfadimidine
NT3 Sulfanilamide
NT3 Sulfathiazole
NT2 Surfactin
NT2 Tetracyclines
NT3 Chlortetracycline
NT3 Doxycycline
NT3 Oxytetracycline
NT2 Thiamphenicol
NT2 Tiamulin
NT2 Trimethoprim
NT2 Vancomycin
NT2 Virginiamycin
NT1 Antithyroid agents
NT2 Methimazole
NT2 Methylthiouracil
NT2 Thiouracil
NT1 Azaperone
NT1 Barbiturates
NT2 Phenobarbital
NT1 Carbadox
NT1 Carbarsone
NT1 Chloral hydrate
NT1 Coccidiostats
NT2 Amprolium
NT2 Clopidol
NT2 Decoquinate
NT2 Dimetridazole
NT2 Dinitolmide
NT2 Ethopabate
NT2 Lasalocids
NT2 Monensin
NT2 Nicarbazin
NT2 Pyrimethamine
NT2 Salinomycin
NT1 Diazepam
NT1 Diethylstilboestrol
NT1 Halothane
NT1 Ipronidazole
NT1 Ormetoprim
NT1 Phenothiazine
NT1 Ronidazole
NT1 Roxarsone
NT1 Tranquilizers
NT1 Zeranol
RT Hormones
RT Pharmacological properties

Drum
BT1 Marine fish
BT2 Fish
BT3 Animals
BT3 Sea foods
BT4 Aquatic foods
BT5 Animal foods
BT6 Foods
UF *Pogonias*

Drum drying
HN drying drum also used in the index up to vol. 29 (1997)
BT1 Drying
BT2 Thermal processing
BT3 Processing thermal
BT4 Processing
BT5 Technology

Drums
BT1 Containers

DRV
BT1 Nutrient requirements
BT2 Nutrients
BT2 Nutrition
RT DRI
RT RDA
RT RDI
UF Dietary reference values

Dry beans
BT1 Common beans
BT2 Legumes
BT3 Vegetables specific
BT4 Vegetables
BT5 Crops
BT6 Plants
BT5 Plant foods
BT6 Foods

Dry cured ham
BT1 Ham
BT2 Meat products
BT3 Animal foods
BT4 Foods

Dryers
USE **Driers**

Dry ham
BT1 Ham
BT2 Meat products
BT3 Animal foods
BT4 Foods

Dry Ice
HN introduced from vol. 39, issue 1 (2007)
BT1 Carbon dioxide
BT2 Gases
BT3 Physical phases
BT4 Chemistry
BT5 Science
BT2 Inorganic compounds
BT2 Oxides
BT2 Solvents

Drying
BT1 Thermal processing
BT2 Processing thermal

BT3 Processing
BT4 Technology
NT1 Air drying
NT1 Driers
NT2 Freeze driers
NT2 Solar driers
NT2 Spray driers
NT1 Drum drying
NT1 Freeze drying
NT2 Freeze driers
NT1 Impingement drying
NT1 IR drying
NT1 Osmotic drying
NT1 Parching
NT1 Roller drying
NT1 Solar drying
NT2 Solar driers
NT1 Spray drying
NT2 Spray driers
NT1 Thin layer drying
NT1 Vacuum drying
NT1 Withering
RT Dried foods
RT Evaporation
RT Fluidized beds
UF Dehydration
UF Desiccation

Dry matter
SN abbrev. DM is also used in the index
NT1 DM
RT Solids

Dryness
BT1 Sensory properties

Dry sausages
BT1 Sausages
BT2 Meat products
BT3 Animal foods
BT4 Foods

DSC
BT1 Analytical techniques
UF Differential scanning calorimetry

Duck carcasses
BT1 Carcasses
BT2 Meat
BT3 Animal foods
BT4 Foods
BT1 Duck meat
BT2 Ducks
BT3 Poultry
BT4 Birds
BT2 Poultry meat
BT3 Meat specific
BT4 Meat
BT5 Animal foods
BT6 Foods

Duck eggs
BT1 Ducks
BT2 Poultry
BT3 Birds
BT1 Eggs
BT2 Animal foods
BT3 Foods
NT1 Pidan

Duck livers
BT1 Ducks
BT2 Poultry
BT3 Birds
BT1 Livers
BT2 Offal
BT3 Animal foods
BT4 Foods

Duck meat
BT1 Ducks
BT2 Poultry
BT3 Birds
BT1 Poultry meat
BT2 Meat specific
BT3 Meat
BT4 Animal foods
BT5 Foods
NT1 Duck carcasses

Ducks
HN heading from vol. 25 (1993); under Poultry up to vol. 24 (1992)
BT1 Poultry
BT2 Birds
NT1 Duck eggs
NT2 Pidan
NT1 Duck livers
NT1 Duck meat
NT2 Duck carcasses
UF Mallards

Dudh churpi
HN introduced from vol. 37, issue 5 (2005)
BT1 Dairy products
BT2 Animal foods
BT3 Foods

Dulce de leche
BT1 Dairy products
BT2 Animal foods
BT3 Foods
BT1 Sugar confectionery
BT2 Plant foods
BT3 Foods
UF Dulche de leche

Dulche de leche
USE **Dulce de leche**

Dulcin
BT1 Sweeteners
BT2 Additives

Dulcitol
SN syn. galactitol
BT1 Polyols
BT2 Alcohols
BT2 Carbohydrates
BT3 Nutrients
BT3 Organic compounds

Dulse
BT1 Seaweeds
BT2 Algae
BT3 Microorganisms
BT2 Sea foods
BT3 Aquatic foods
BT4 Animal foods
BT5 Foods
NT1 *Palmaria palmata*

Dumplings
BT1 Bakery products
BT2 Cereal products
BT3 Plant foods
BT4 Foods

Dunaliella
HN heading from vol. 25 (1993); under Algae up to vol. 24 (1992)
BT1 Microalgae
BT2 Algae
BT3 Microorganisms
NT1 *Dunaliella salina*

Dunaliella salina
BT1 *Dunaliella*
BT2 Microalgae
BT3 Algae
BT4 Microorganisms

Durian
BT1 Fruits specific
BT2 Fruits
BT3 Crops
BT4 Plants
BT3 Plant foods
BT4 Foods

Dursban
USE **Chlorpyrifos**

Durum wheat
BT1 Wheat
BT2 Cereals
BT3 Crops
BT4 Plants
BT3 Seeds
BT4 Plant foods
BT5 Foods

Dust
BT1 Contaminants
BT2 Contamination

Dust explosions
BT1 Explosions

Dutch Guiana
USE **Surinam**

Dye binding tests
BT1 Analytical techniques

Dyes
BT1 Colorants
BT2 Additives

Dyfonate
USE **Fonofos**

E

Earthworms
BT1 Animal foods
BT2 Foods

East Africa
BT1 Africa
NT1 Djibouti
NT1 Eritrea
NT1 Ethiopia
NT1 Kenya
NT1 Somalia
NT1 Sudan
NT1 Tanzania
NT1 Uganda

East Timor
HN introduced from vol. 39, issue 1 (2007)
BT1 Asia

Eating disorders
HN introduced from vol. 40, issue 1 (2008)
BT1 Psychiatric disorders
BT2 Diseases

Eating habits
HN heading from vol. 42 (2010); under Consumer response up to vol. 41 (2009)
BT1 Consumer behaviour
BT2 Consumer response
NT1 Fasting
NT1 Food portions
NT2 Portion sizes
NT1 Healthy eating
NT1 Snacking
RT Drinking habits

Eating quality
BT1 Sensory properties

Eau de vie
BT1 Brandies
BT2 Spirits
BT3 Alcoholic beverages
BT4 Beverages alcoholic
BT5 Beverages

EC
USE **European Community**

Echinacea
HN introduced from vol. 39, issue 1 (2007)
BT1 Plants
NT1 *Echinacea purpurea*

Echinacea purpurea
HN introduced from vol. 39, issue 1 (2007)
BT1 *Echinacea*
BT2 Plants

Echinococcus
BT1 Parasites
BT2 Pests

Echinoderms
BT1 Sea foods
BT2 Aquatic foods
BT3 Animal foods
BT4 Foods

Echinoids
USE **Sea urchins**

Echinophora tenuifolia
BT1 Coertuek
BT2 Spices
BT3 Flavourings
BT4 Additives

Echovirus
HN introduced from vol. 43, issue 1 (2011); echoviruses also used in the index up to vol. 42 (2010)
BT1 Enterovirus
BT2 Viruses
BT3 Microorganisms
UF Echoviruses

Echoviruses
HN introduced from vol. 39, issue 1 (2007); Echovirus used in the index from vol. 43 (2011)
USE **Echovirus**

Ecklonia
HN introduced from vol. 42, issue 1 (2010)
BT1 Seaweeds
BT2 Algae
BT3 Microorganisms
BT2 Sea foods
BT3 Aquatic foods
BT4 Animal foods
BT5 Foods

Eclairs
BT1 Pastries
BT2 Bakery products
BT3 Cereal products
BT4 Plant foods
BT5 Foods

Ecology
HN heading from vol. 25 (1993); under Environment up to vol. 24 (1992)
BT1 Science
NT1 Environmental protection
NT1 Environment friendly packaging materials
NT1 Environment friendly processes
NT1 Life cycle assessment
NT1 Recycling

E-commerce
BT1 Information technology
BT2 Technology
BT1 Marketing
BT2 Economics

Economics
NT1 Consumer protection
NT1 Consumption
NT1 Costs
NT1 Expenditure
NT1 Finance
NT1 Food business
NT2 Companies
NT3 Food companies
NT2 Franchising
NT2 Mergers
NT2 Suppliers
NT3 Supply chains
NT4 Efficient consumer response
NT1 Food policy
NT2 CAP
NT2 Food security
NT3 Food aid
NT4 Food stamps
NT2 Food Standards Agency
NT2 Policies
NT2 Policy
NT2 Pricing
NT3 Payment
NT3 Prices
NT2 Product liability
NT2 Taxation
NT1 Fraud
NT1 Globalization
NT1 Marketing
NT2 Advertising
NT2 Consumer research
NT2 Consumer spending
NT2 Consumer surveys
NT2 Cooperatives
NT2 Display cabinets
NT2 E-commerce
NT2 Grocery stores
NT2 Hypermarkets
NT2 Market research
NT2 Presentation
NT2 Retail
NT3 Product recalls
NT2 Shops
NT2 Supermarkets
NT2 Vending machines
NT2 Wholesale
NT1 Markets
NT2 Purchase
NT2 Single market
NT1 Poverty
NT1 Production
NT1 Profitability
NT1 Profits
NT1 Sales
NT1 Socioeconomic factors
NT1 Statistics
NT1 Subsidies
NT1 Supplies
NT2 Supply chains
NT3 Efficient consumer response
NT1 Trade
NT2 EFTA
NT2 Exports
NT2 Fair trade
NT2 Imports
NT2 Mercosur
NT2 Tariffs
NT2 Trade agreements
NT3 GATT
NT3 NAFTA
NT2 World Trade Organization

RT Management
RT Quality of life

Ecuador
BT1 South America
BT2 America

Eczema
USE **Dermatitis**

Edam cheese
BT1 Cheese varieties
BT2 Cheese
BT3 Dairy products
BT4 Animal foods
BT5 Foods

Edestin
BT1 Globulins
BT2 Proteins
BT3 Nutrients
BT1 Vegetable proteins
BT2 Proteins vegetable
BT3 Proteins
BT4 Nutrients
BT3 Vegetable products
BT4 Plant foods
BT5 Foods

Edible containers
BT1 Containers
RT Edible packs

Edible films
HN introduced from vol. 39, issue 1 (2007)
BT1 Films

Edible flowers
HN introduced from vol. 39, issue 1 (2007)
BT1 Plants
BT1 Vegetables specific
BT2 Vegetables
BT3 Crops
BT4 Plants
BT3 Plant foods
BT4 Foods
NT1 Day lilies
NT1 Marigolds

Edible fungi
SN index heading is Fungi edible
BT1 Fungi edible
BT2 Vegetables specific
BT3 Vegetables
BT4 Crops
BT5 Plants
BT4 Plant foods
BT5 Foods
NT1 *Agaricus*
NT2 *Agaricus bisporus*
NT2 *Agaricus blazei*
NT1 *Agrocybe*
NT1 *Amanita*
NT2 *Amanita phalloides*
NT1 *Armillaria*
NT2 *Armillaria mellea*
NT1 *Auricularia*
NT2 *Auricularia auricula*
NT2 *Auricularia polytricha*
NT1 *Boletus*
NT2 *Boletus edulis*
NT1 *Calocybe*
NT1 *Cantharellus*
NT1 Champignons
NT1 *Coprinus*
NT2 *Coprinus comatus*
NT1 *Cordyceps*
NT2 *Cordyceps militaris*
NT2 *Cordyceps sinensis*
NT1 *Flammulina*
NT2 *Flammulina velutipes*
NT1 *Ganoderma*
NT2 *Ganoderma applanatum*
NT2 *Ganoderma lucidum*
NT1 *Grifola frondosa*
NT1 *Gyromitra*
NT1 *Hericium erinaceus*
NT1 Huitlacoche
NT1 *Hydnum*
NT1 *Lactarius*
NT1 *Leccinum*
NT1 *Lentinula edodes*
NT1 *Lentinus*
NT1 *Lepista*
NT2 *Lepista nuda*
NT1 *Lycoperdon*
NT1 *Morchella*
NT2 *Morchella esculenta*
NT1 Mushrooms
NT2 Wild mushrooms
NT1 *Phellinus linteus*
NT1 *Pholiota*
NT1 *Pleurotus*
NT2 *Pleurotus citrinopileatus*
NT2 *Pleurotus eryngii*
NT2 *Pleurotus florida*
NT2 *Pleurotus ostreatus*
NT2 *Pleurotus sajor-caju*
NT2 *Pleurotus tuberregium*
NT1 *Poria cocos*
NT1 *Russula*
NT1 *Sarcodon aspratus*
NT1 *Sarcodon imbricatum*
NT1 *Schizophyllum*
NT2 *Schizophyllum commune*
NT1 Straw mushrooms
NT1 *Terfezia*
NT1 *Termitomyces*
NT1 *Tricholoma*
NT2 *Tricholoma matsutake*
NT1 *Tuber*
NT2 Black truffles
NT2 White truffles
NT1 *Volvariella*
NT2 *Volvariella volvacea*
NT1 *Xerocomus*
RT Fungi

Edible inks
HN introduced from vol. 42, issue 1 (2010)
BT1 Colorants
BT2 Additives
RT Inks

Edible oils
USE **Oils**

Edible packs
BT1 Packs
BT2 Containers
RT Edible containers

Edifenphos
BT1 Fungicides
BT2 Pesticides
BT3 Biocides
BT3 Residues
BT1 Organophosphorus pesticides
BT2 Pesticides
BT3 Biocides
BT3 Residues
UF Hinosan

EDTA
BT1 Additives
BT1 Organic acids
BT2 Acids
RT Trilon B

Education
NT1 Consumer education
NT1 Training
RT Information

Edwardsiella
BT1 Bacteria
BT2 Microorganisms

EEC
HN abbrev. used up to vol. 24 (1992)
USE **European Community**

Eels
BT1 Freshwater fish
BT2 Fish
BT3 Animals
BT3 Sea foods
BT4 Aquatic foods
BT5 Animal foods
BT6 Foods
BT1 Oily fish
BT2 Fish
BT3 Animals
BT3 Sea foods
BT4 Aquatic foods
BT5 Animal foods
BT6 Foods

Efficient consumer response
HN under Distribution up to vol. 42 (2010)
BT1 Supply chains
BT2 Suppliers
BT3 Food business
BT4 Economics
BT2 Supplies
BT3 Economics

Effluent
USE **Effluents**

Effluents
BT1 Waste water
BT2 Wastes
BT2 Water
NT1 Breweries effluents
NT1 Dairies effluents

NT1 Distilleries effluents
NT1 Food factories effluents
NT1 Olive oil mills effluents
NT1 Palm oil mills effluents
NT1 Stillage
NT1 Vinasse
UF Effluent

EFSA
USE **European Food Safety Authority**

EFTA
BT1 Trade
BT2 Economics

Egg nog
BT1 Alcoholic beverages
BT2 Beverages alcoholic
BT3 Beverages
BT1 Egg products
BT2 Animal foods
BT3 Foods

Egg pasta
BT1 Egg products
BT2 Animal foods
BT3 Foods
BT1 Pasta
BT2 Cereal products
BT3 Plant foods
BT4 Foods

Egg plants
USE **Aubergines**

Egg powders
USE **Dried eggs**

Egg products
BT1 Animal foods
BT2 Foods
NT1 Dried egg products
NT1 Egg nog
NT1 Egg pasta
NT1 Liquid egg
NT1 Liquid egg whites
NT1 Liquid egg yolks
NT1 Liquid whole egg
NT1 Meringues
NT1 Omelettes
NT1 Pickled eggs
NT1 Scrambled egg
NT1 Souffles
RT Eggs

Egg proteins
BT1 Animal proteins
BT2 Proteins animal
BT3 Proteins
BT4 Nutrients
NT1 Avidin
NT1 Conalbumin
NT1 Ovalbumins
NT1 Ovomucins
NT1 Ovomucoid
NT1 Ovotransferrin
NT1 Phosvitin

Eggs
SN hen eggs unless otherwise stated
BT1 Animal foods
BT2 Foods
NT1 Dried eggs
NT1 Duck eggs
NT2 Pidan
NT1 Egg shell membranes
NT1 Egg shells
NT1 Eggs lysozymes
NT1 Egg whites
NT2 Egg whites lysozymes
NT1 Egg yolks
NT1 Goose eggs
NT1 Haugh score
NT1 Quail eggs
RT Egg products
UF Hen eggs
UF Pullet eggs

Egg shell membranes
HN introduced from vol. 39, issue 1 (2007)
BT1 Biological membranes
BT1 Eggs
BT2 Animal foods
BT3 Foods

Egg shells
BT1 Eggs
BT2 Animal foods
BT3 Foods
RT Cracking

Eggs lysozymes
BT1 Eggs
BT2 Animal foods
BT3 Foods
BT1 Lysozymes
BT2 Glycosidases
BT3 Hydrolases
BT4 Enzymes

Egg whites
BT1 Eggs
BT2 Animal foods
BT3 Foods
NT1 Egg whites lysozymes
RT Liquid egg whites
RT Meringues
RT Ovomucins
RT Ovomucoid
RT Ovotransferrin
UF Albumen

Egg whites lysozymes
BT1 Egg whites
BT2 Eggs
BT3 Animal foods
BT4 Foods
BT1 Lysozymes
BT2 Glycosidases
BT3 Hydrolases
BT4 Enzymes

Egg yolks
BT1 Eggs
BT2 Animal foods
BT3 Foods
RT Liquid egg yolks
RT Phosvitin

Egusi
BT1 Oilseeds
BT2 Seeds
BT3 Plant foods
BT4 Foods
BT1 Watermelons
BT2 Fruits specific
BT3 Fruits
BT4 Crops
BT5 Plants
BT4 Plant foods
BT5 Foods

Egypt
BT1 Middle East
BT1 North Africa
BT2 Africa

Eicosanoids
HN introduced from vol. 41, issue 1 (2009)
BT1 Fatty acids
BT2 Lipids
BT3 Nutrients
BT2 Organic acids
BT3 Acids
NT1 Prostaglandins

Eicosapentaenoic acid
BT1 ω-3 Fatty acids
BT2 PUFA
BT3 Unsaturated fatty acids
BT4 Fatty acids
BT5 Lipids
BT6 Nutrients
BT5 Organic acids
BT6 Acids

Eicosatetraenoic acid
BT1 PUFA
BT2 Unsaturated fatty acids
BT3 Fatty acids
BT4 Lipids
BT5 Nutrients
BT4 Organic acids
BT5 Acids
NT1 Arachidonic acid

Eicosenoic acid
BT1 Monounsaturated fatty acids
BT2 Unsaturated fatty acids
BT3 Fatty acids
BT4 Lipids
BT5 Nutrients
BT4 Organic acids
BT5 Acids

Einkorn
BT1 Wheat
BT2 Cereals
BT3 Crops
BT4 Plants
BT3 Seeds
BT4 Plant foods
BT5 Foods
UF Einkorn wheat

Einkorn wheat
USE **Einkorn**

Eiswein
BT1 Ice wines
BT2 Wines
BT3 Alcoholic beverages
BT4 Beverages alcoholic
BT5 Beverages

Ekalux
USE **Quinalphos**

Elaeis
BT1 Palms
BT2 Plants
RT Palm oils

Elaeis oils
USE **Palm oils**

Elaidic acid
BT1 Octadecenoic acid
BT2 Monounsaturated fatty acids
BT3 Unsaturated fatty acids
BT4 Fatty acids
BT5 Lipids
BT6 Nutrients
BT5 Organic acids
BT6 Acids
BT1 *trans* Fatty acids
BT2 Unsaturated fatty acids
BT3 Fatty acids
BT4 Lipids
BT5 Nutrients
BT4 Organic acids
BT5 Acids

Elastase
HN introduced from vol. 39, issue 1 (2007)
BT1 Proteinases
BT2 Hydrolases
BT3 Enzymes

Elasticity
BT1 Rheological properties
BT2 Mechanical properties
BT3 Physical properties

Elastin
BT1 Animal proteins
BT2 Proteins animal
BT3 Proteins
BT4 Nutrients

Elderberries
BT1 Berries
BT2 Fruits specific
BT3 Fruits
BT4 Crops
BT5 Plants
BT4 Plant foods
BT5 Foods
RT Elderberry juices

Elderberry juices
BT1 Berry juices
BT2 Fruit juices
BT3 Fruit products
BT4 Plant foods
BT5 Foods
BT3 Soft drinks
BT4 Beverages
RT Elderberries

Elderflowers
BT1 Flowers
BT2 Plants

Elderly
BT1 Population groups

Electrical conductivity
HN under Conductivity up to vol. 24 (1992); conductivity electrical also used in the index up to vol. 29 (1997)
BT1 Electrical properties
BT2 Physical properties
RT Specific conductivity
UF Conductivity

Electrical properties
HN heading from vol. 25 (1993); under Electricity up to vol. 24 (1992)
BT1 Physical properties
NT1 Capacitance
NT1 Dielectric constant
NT1 Dielectric properties
NT1 Electrical conductivity
NT1 Electrical resistance
NT1 Electrostatic interactions
NT1 Impedance
NT1 Specific conductivity
RT Electricity

Electrical resistance
BT1 Electrical properties
BT2 Physical properties

Electrical stimulation
HN stimulation electrical also used in the index up to vol. 29 (1997)
BT1 Slaughter

Electrical stunning
HN stunning electrical also used in the index up to vol. 29 (1997)
BT1 Stunning
BT2 Slaughter

Electric fields
BT1 Electricity
BT2 Energy
NT1 Pulsed electric fields

Electricity
BT1 Energy
NT1 Cogeneration
NT1 Electric fields
NT2 Pulsed electric fields
RT Electrical properties

Electrocution
BT1 Slaughter

Electrodes
BT1 Apparatus
BT2 Technology
NT1 Ion selective electrodes
RT Biosensors

Electrodialysis
BT1 Dialysis
BT2 Processing
BT3 Technology

Electrolysed water
BT1 Disinfectants
BT2 Disinfection
BT3 Hygiene

Electrolytes
BT1 Salts
RT Ions

Electromagnetic fields
BT1 Energy
RT Magnetic fields

Electron beam irradiation
HN introduced from vol. 39, issue 1 (2007)
BT1 Irradiation
BT2 Processing
BT3 Technology

Electronic data processing
BT1 Information technology
BT2 Technology

Electronic noses
BT1 Apparatus
BT2 Technology
RT Electronic tongues
RT Sensory analysis

Electronic publications
HN introduced from vol. 41, issue 1 (2009)
SN used for publications only available in this format
RT CD-ROMs

Electronic tongues
BT1 Apparatus
BT2 Technology
RT Electronic noses

Electron microscopy
SN abbrev. EM is also used in the index
BT1 Microscopy
BT2 Analytical techniques
NT1 EM
NT1 SEM
NT1 TEM

Electron paramagnetic resonance
BT1 Spectroscopy
BT2 Analytical techniques

Electron spin resonance
BT1 Spectroscopy
BT2 Analytical techniques

Electrophoresis
BT1 Analytical techniques
NT1 Capillary electrophoresis
NT1 Gel electrophoresis
NT2 PFGE
NT1 IEF
NT1 Immunoelectrophoresis
NT1 Isotachophoresis
NT1 PAGE

NT1 SDS-PAGE
RT Chromatography

Electroporation
BT1 Gene transfer
BT2 Gene cloning
BT3 Genetic techniques
BT4 Genetics

Electrospray ionization MS
HN introduced from vol. 39, issue 1 (2007)
BT1 Mass spectroscopy
BT2 Spectroscopy
BT3 Analytical techniques

Electrostatic interactions
BT1 Electrical properties
BT2 Physical properties

Elements
HN heading from vol. 43 (2011); under Minerals up to vol. 42 (2010)
BT1 Minerals
BT2 Nutrients
NT1 Ar
NT1 Arsenic
NT2 Arsenicals
NT3 Arsenobetaine
NT3 Dimethylarsinic acid
NT3 Methylarsonic acid
NT2 As
NT1 B
NT1 Carbon
NT2 Activated C
NT3 Activated carbon
NT2 C
NT2 Charcoal
NT1 Ge
NT1 Halogens
NT2 Br
NT2 Chlorine
NT3 Cl
NT2 F
NT2 Iodine
NT3 I
NT3 Iodized salt
NT1 He
NT1 Hydrogen
NT2 Deuterium
NT2 H_2
NT2 Tritium
NT1 Isotopes
NT2 Radioelements
NT3 Cs
NT3 Po
NT3 Pu
NT3 Ra
NT3 Radionuclides
NT4 Radioisotopes
NT3 Rn
NT3 Sr
NT3 Tc
NT3 Tritium
NT3 U
NT1 Metals
NT2 Ag
NT2 Aluminium
NT3 Al
NT3 Al compounds
NT2 Au
NT2 Ba
NT2 Be
NT2 Bi
NT2 Cadmium
NT3 Cd
NT2 Calcium
NT3 Ca
NT2 Ce
NT2 Cobalt
NT3 Co
NT2 Copper
NT3 Cu
NT2 Cr
NT2 Ga
NT2 Heavy metals
NT2 Iron
NT3 Fe
NT3 Ferritin
NT2 Lanthanides
NT3 La
NT3 Yb
NT2 Lead
NT3 Pb
NT2 Li
NT2 Magnesium
NT3 Mg
NT2 Manganese
NT3 Mn
NT2 Mercury
NT3 Hg
NT3 Methylmercury
NT2 Mo
NT2 Nb
NT2 Ni
NT2 Os
NT2 Pd
NT2 Potassium
NT3 K
NT2 Pt
NT2 Rb
NT2 Re
NT2 Rhodium
NT2 Ru
NT2 Sc
NT2 Sodium
NT3 Na
NT3 Sodium low diet
NT3 Sodium low foods
NT2 Sr
NT2 Th
NT2 Ti
NT2 Tin
NT3 Sn
NT2 Tl
NT2 V
NT2 W
NT2 Y
NT2 Zinc
NT3 Zn
NT2 Zr
NT1 Nitrogen
NT2 Amino N
NT3 α-Amino N
NT2 Liquid nitrogen
NT2 N
NT2 N_2
NT2 Nitrogen compounds
NT3 N compounds
NT1 Oxygen
NT2 O_2
NT2 Oxygen absorbers
NT3 Oxygen scavengers
NT2 Ozone
NT1 Phosphorus
NT2 P
NT1 Sb
NT1 Selenium
NT2 Se
NT2 Selenites
NT2 Selenomethionine
NT2 Selenoproteins
NT1 Si
NT1 Sulfur
NT2 S
NT1 Te
NT1 Trace elements
NT1 Xe

Eleostearic acid
HN introduced from vol. 39, issue 1 (2007)
BT1 Conjugated fatty acids
BT2 PUFA
BT3 Unsaturated fatty acids
BT4 Fatty acids
BT5 Lipids
BT6 Nutrients
BT5 Organic acids
BT6 Acids
BT1 Linolenic acid
BT2 PUFA
BT3 Unsaturated fatty acids
BT4 Fatty acids
BT5 Lipids
BT6 Nutrients
BT5 Organic acids
BT6 Acids

Elephant yams
BT1 Vegetables specific
BT2 Vegetables
BT3 Crops
BT4 Plants
BT3 Plant foods
BT4 Foods
NT1 Konjac glucomannans
UF Konjac
UF Konnyaku

Eleusine coracana
USE **Finger millet**

Elicitation
HN introduced from vol. 39, issue 1 (2007)
RT Phytochemicals
RT Plant diseases
RT Plant disorders
RT Stress

ELISA
HN heading from vol. 30 (1998); under Immunological techniques up to vol. 29 (1997)
BT1 Immunological techniques
BT2 Analytical techniques

Elk meat
BT1 Elks

BT2 Animals
BT1 Meat specific
BT2 Meat
BT3 Animal foods
BT4 Foods

Elks
BT1 Animals
NT1 Elk meat

Ellagic acid
BT1 Organic acids
BT2 Acids
BT1 Phenols
BT2 Alcohols
BT2 Aromatic compounds
BT3 Organic compounds
RT Tannins

Ellagitannins
HN introduced from vol. 39, issue 1 (2007)
BT1 Phenols
BT2 Alcohols
BT2 Aromatic compounds
BT3 Organic compounds
BT1 Tannins
BT2 Aromatic compounds
BT3 Organic compounds
BT2 Glycosides
BT3 Carbohydrates
BT4 Nutrients
BT4 Organic compounds
BT2 Organic acids
BT3 Acids

El Salvador
BT1 Central America
BT2 America

EM
SN index heading is Electron microscopy
BT1 Electron microscopy
BT2 Microscopy
BT3 Analytical techniques

Emamectin
BT1 Avermectins
BT2 Insecticides
BT3 Pesticides
BT4 Biocides
BT4 Residues

Emmental cheese
BT1 Cheese varieties
BT2 Cheese
BT3 Dairy products
BT4 Animal foods
BT5 Foods

Emmer
HN introduced from vol. 39, issue 1 (2007)
BT1 Wheat
BT2 Cereals
BT3 Crops
BT4 Plants
BT3 Seeds
BT4 Plant foods
BT5 Foods

Emodin
HN under Drugs up to vol. 42 (2010)
BT1 Anthraquinones
BT2 Pigments

Emu carcasses
BT1 Carcasses
BT2 Meat
BT3 Animal foods
BT4 Foods
BT1 Emu meat
BT2 Emus
BT3 Poultry
BT4 Birds
BT2 Poultry meat
BT3 Meat specific
BT4 Meat
BT5 Animal foods
BT6 Foods

Emulsification
HN heading from vol. 25 (1993)
BT1 Processing
BT2 Technology
RT Emulsifiers
RT Emulsions
RT Mixing
RT Whipping

Emulsification properties
BT1 Functional properties
BT2 Physical properties

Emulsifiers
BT1 Additives
NT1 Carrageenans
NT2 Carrageenan gels
NT1 DATEM
NT1 Emulsifying agents
NT1 Food emulsifiers
NT1 Glycerides
NT2 Acylglycerols
NT2 Diglycerides
NT3 Diacylglycerols
NT2 Glycerol monostearate
NT2 Glyceryl monostearate
NT2 Monoglycerides
NT3 Monoacylglycerols
NT3 Monolaurin
NT2 Phosphoglycerides
NT2 Triglycerides
NT3 Olein
NT4 Palm olein
NT3 Stearin
NT4 Palm stearin
NT3 Triacetin
NT3 Triacylglycerols
NT3 Tricaprylin
NT3 Trilinolein
NT3 Triolein
NT3 Tripalmitin
NT3 Tristearin
NT1 Lactylates
NT2 Stearoyl lactylates
NT1 Lecithins
NT2 Lysolecithin
NT2 Soy lecithins
NT1 Polyglycerol fatty acid esters
NT1 Polyglycerol polyricinoleate
NT1 Polysorbate 60
NT1 Propylene glycol
NT1 Sorbitan
RT Emulsification

Emulsifying agents
BT1 Emulsifiers
BT2 Additives

Emulsifying capacity
BT1 Functional properties
BT2 Physical properties

Emulsions
BT1 Physical phases
BT2 Chemistry
BT3 Science
NT1 Food emulsions
NT1 Microemulsions
RT Colloids
RT Dispersions
RT Emulsification

Emu meat
BT1 Emus
BT2 Poultry
BT3 Birds
BT1 Poultry meat
BT2 Meat specific
BT3 Meat
BT4 Animal foods
BT5 Foods
NT1 Emu carcasses

Emus
BT1 Poultry
BT2 Birds
NT1 Emu meat
NT2 Emu carcasses

Enamels
BT1 Surfaces

Enantiomers
BT1 Isomers

Enantioselectivity
BT1 Isomers

Encapsulation
BT1 Technology
NT1 Microencapsulation
RT Coating

Encyclopaedias
BT1 Books

Endives
BT1 Vegetables specific
BT2 Vegetables
BT3 Crops
BT4 Plants
BT3 Plant foods
BT4 Foods
UF Escarole

Endocrine disrupters
HN introduced from vol. 39, issue 1 (2007)
BT1 Contamination
RT Alkylphenols
RT Endocrine system

Endocrine system
HN introduced from vol. 39, issue 1 (2007)
BT1 Physiology
BT2 Science
RT Endocrine disrupters

Endo-1,3(4)-β-glucanases
SN EC 3.2.1.6
BT1 Glycosidases
BT2 Hydrolases
BT3 Enzymes
UF Laminarinases

Endomyces
BT1 Fungi
BT2 Microorganisms

Endomycopsis
HN under Fungi up to vol. 42 (2010)
SN obsolete yeast genus; now called Guillermondella
BT1 Yeasts
BT2 Fungi
BT3 Microorganisms

Endonucleases
SN EC 3.1.21-3.1.31
BT1 Nucleases
BT2 Esterases
BT3 Hydrolases
BT4 Enzymes

Endopeptidases
SN includes subclasses EC 3.4.21-25 and 3.4.99
BT1 Proteinases
BT2 Hydrolases
BT3 Enzymes

Endopolygalacturonases
USE **Polygalacturonases**

Endosulfan
BT1 Acaricides
BT2 Pesticides
BT3 Biocides
BT3 Residues
BT1 Organochlorine insecticides
BT2 Insecticides
BT3 Pesticides
BT4 Biocides
BT4 Residues
BT2 Organochlorine pesticides
BT3 Pesticides
BT4 Biocides
BT4 Residues
UF Thiodan

Endothal
BT1 Herbicides
BT2 Pesticides
BT3 Biocides
BT3 Residues

Endothia
BT1 Fungi
BT2 Microorganisms

Endotoxins
BT1 Toxins
BT2 Residues
RT Virulence factors

Endo-1,3-β-xylanases
USE **Xylan endo-1,3-β-xylosidases**

Endo-1,4-β-xylanases
SN EC 3.2.1.8
BT1 Glycosidases
BT2 Hydrolases
BT3 Enzymes

Endpoint temp.
BT1 Temperature

Endpoint temp. indicators
BT1 Temperature
RT Cooking

Endrin
BT1 Organochlorine insecticides
BT2 Insecticides
BT3 Pesticides
BT4 Biocides
BT4 Residues
BT2 Organochlorine pesticides
BT3 Pesticides
BT4 Biocides
BT4 Residues
BT1 Rodenticides
BT2 Pesticides
BT3 Biocides
BT3 Residues

Energy
NT1 Electricity
NT2 Cogeneration
NT2 Electric fields
NT3 Pulsed electric fields
NT1 Electromagnetic fields
NT1 Energy conservation
NT1 Magnetic fields
NT1 Nuclear power
NT1 Power
NT1 Solar energy
NT1 Steam

Energy conservation
BT1 Energy

Energy density
HN introduced from vol. 39, issue 1 (2007)
BT1 Calorific values
BT2 Nutritional values

Energy drinks
BT1 Health beverages
BT2 Beverages
BT2 Health foods
BT3 Processed foods
BT4 Foods
BT1 Soft drinks
BT2 Beverages
RT Energy foods
RT Isotonic drinks

Energy foods
BT1 Health foods
BT2 Processed foods
BT3 Foods
RT Energy drinks

Energy values
USE **Calorific values**

Engineering
BT1 Science

England
BT1 United Kingdom
BT2 Europe
BT2 European Union

English muffins
BT1 Bakery products
BT2 Cereal products
BT3 Plant foods
BT4 Foods
RT Muffins

Engraulis encrasicholus
BT1 Anchovy
BT2 Marine fish
BT3 Fish
BT4 Animals
BT4 Sea foods
BT5 Aquatic foods
BT6 Animal foods
BT7 Foods
BT2 Oily fish
BT3 Fish
BT4 Animals
BT4 Sea foods
BT5 Aquatic foods
BT6 Animal foods
BT7 Foods

Enniatins
HN introduced from vol. 41, issue 1 (2009)
BT1 Mycotoxins
BT2 Toxins
BT3 Residues

Enokitake
USE ***Flammulina***

Enrichment
BT1 Food enrichment
RT Fortification

Enrichment techniques
BT1 Microbiological techniques

Enrobing
BT1 Coating
BT2 Processing
BT3 Technology

Enrofloxacin
BT1 Quinolones
BT2 Antibiotics
BT3 Drugs
BT4 Residues

Entamoeba
HN heading from vol. 30 (1998)
BT1 Parasites
BT2 Pests
NT1 *Entamoeba histolytica*

Entamoeba histolytica
BT1 *Entamoeba*
BT2 Parasites
BT3 Pests

Enteric viruses
HN heading from vol. 39, issue 1 (2007) up to vol. 42 (2010)
SN for descriptive use only
BT1 Viruses
BT2 Microorganisms

Enterobacter
HN under Enterobacteriaceae up to vol. 24 (1992); Aerobacter also used in the index up to vol. 42 (2010)
SN opportunist pathogens
BT1 Bacteria
BT2 Microorganisms
NT1 *Enterobacter aerogenes*
NT1 *Enterobacter cloacae*
NT1 *Enterobacter sakazakii*
UF *Aerobacter*

Enterobacter aerogenes
BT1 *Enterobacter*
BT2 Bacteria
BT3 Microorganisms

Enterobacter cloacae
BT1 *Enterobacter*
BT2 Bacteria
BT3 Microorganisms

Enterobacteria
BT1 Bacteria
BT2 Microorganisms
RT Enterobacteriaceae

Enterobacteriaceae
HN heading up to vol. 24 (1992)
BT1 Bacteria
BT2 Microorganisms
RT Enterobacteria

Enterobacter sakazakii
HN introduced from vol. 39, issue 1 (2007)
SN synonymous with Cronobacter sakazakii
BT1 *Enterobacter*
BT2 Bacteria
BT3 Microorganisms

Enterocins
BT1 Bacteriocins
BT2 Antibiotics
BT3 Drugs
BT4 Residues
RT *Enterococcus*

Enterococci
HN heading up to vol. 24 (1992)
USE ***Enterococcus***

Enterococcus
HN heading from vol. 30 (1998); under Bacteria up to vol. 29 (1997)
BT1 Bacteria
BT2 Microorganisms
NT1 *Enterococcus casseliflavus*
NT1 *Enterococcus faecalis*
NT1 *Enterococcus faecium*
NT1 *Enterococcus gallinarum*
RT Enterocins
UF Enterococci

Enterococcus casseliflavus
HN introduced from vol. 41, issue 1 (2009)
BT1 *Enterococcus*
BT2 Bacteria
BT3 Microorganisms

Enterococcus faecalis
SN synonymous with Streptococcus faecalis
BT1 *Enterococcus*
BT2 Bacteria
BT3 Microorganisms

Enterococcus faecium
SN synonymous with Streptococcus faecium
BT1 *Enterococcus*
BT2 Bacteria
BT3 Microorganisms

Enterococcus gallinarum
HN introduced from vol. 41, issue 1 (2009)
BT1 *Enterococcus*
BT2 Bacteria
BT3 Microorganisms

Enterotoxicity
BT1 Toxicity

Enterotoxins
BT1 Toxins
BT2 Residues
NT1 Cholera toxin

Enterovirus
HN introduced from vol. 43, issue 1 (2011); enteroviruses also used in the index up to vol. 42 (2010)
BT1 Viruses
BT2 Microorganisms
NT1 Echovirus
NT1 Human enterovirus
NT2 Human coxsackievirus
NT1 Poliovirus
RT Coxsackieviruses
UF Enteroviruses

Enteroviruses
HN Enterovirus used in the index from vol. 43 (2011)
USE **Enterovirus**

Enthalpy
BT1 Thermophysical properties
BT2 Physical properties

Entoleters
BT1 Disinfestation
BT2 Pests

Entrees
BT1 Meals
BT2 Processed foods
BT3 Foods

Entropy
HN introduced from vol. 39, issue 1 (2007)
BT1 Thermophysical properties
BT2 Physical properties

Environment
HN heading up to vol. 24 (1992)
RT Agriculture
RT Altitude
RT Climate
RT Season
RT Sustainability
RT Weather

Environmental contamination
BT1 Contamination
RT Environmental pollution

Environmental pollution
BT1 Pollution
BT2 Contamination
NT1 Air pollution
NT2 Air pollutants
NT3 Exhaust gases
NT3 Factory fumes
NT1 Water pollution
RT Environmental contamination

Environmental protection
BT1 Ecology
BT2 Science

Environment friendly packaging materials
BT1 Ecology
BT2 Science
BT1 Packaging materials

Environment friendly processes
BT1 Ecology
BT2 Science

Enzyme electrodes
BT1 Biosensors
BT2 Biotechnology
BT3 Technology

Enzyme immunoassay
BT1 Immunological techniques
BT2 Analytical techniques

Enzyme inhibitors
HN heading from vol. 30 (1998); under Antinutritional factors up to vol. 29 (1997)
BT1 Enzymes
NT1 ACE inhibitors
NT1 Amylases inhibitors
NT2 α-Amylases inhibitors
NT1 Esculetin
NT1 Proteinases inhibitors
NT2 Calpastatins
NT2 Chymotrypsin inhibitors
NT2 Cystatins
NT2 Trypsin inhibitors

Enzymes
NT1 Coenzymes
NT2 *S*-Adenosyl-L-methionine

NT2 Coenzyme Q
NT1 Detoxification enzymes
NT1 Enzyme inhibitors
NT2 ACE inhibitors
NT2 Amylases inhibitors
NT3 α-Amylases inhibitors
NT2 Esculetin
NT2 Proteinases inhibitors
NT3 Calpastatins
NT3 Chymotrypsin inhibitors
NT3 Cystatins
NT3 Trypsin inhibitors
NT1 Hydrolases
NT2 Amidases
NT2 Aminoacylases
NT2 Asparaginases
NT2 ATPases
NT2 Chitin deacetylases
NT2 Choloylglycine hydrolases
NT2 Deaminases
NT2 Esterases
NT3 Acetylcholinesterases
NT3 Carboxylesterases
NT3 Chlorophyllases
NT3 Cholinesterases
NT3 Cutinases
NT3 Feruloyl esterases
NT3 Lipases
NT4 Lecithinases
NT4 Lipoprotein lipases
NT4 Lysophospholipases
NT4 Phospholipases
NT4 Triacylglycerol lipases
NT3 Nucleases
NT4 Deoxyribonucleases
NT4 Endonucleases
NT4 Restriction endonucleases
NT4 Restriction enzymes
NT4 Ribonucleases
NT5 Angiogenin
NT3 Pectinesterases
NT3 Phosphatases
NT4 Acid phosphatases
NT4 Alkaline phosphatases
NT4 Nucleotidases
NT4 Phytases
NT5 3-Phytases
NT5 4-Phytases
NT3 Phosphodiesterases
NT3 Tannases
NT2 Glutaminases
NT2 Glycosidases
NT3 Acetylglucosaminidases
NT3 β-*N*-acetylhexosaminidases
NT3 Agarases
NT3 Amylases
NT4 α-Amylases
NT4 β-Amylases
NT4 Amylolytic enzymes
NT4 Diastatic activity
NT4 Glucan 1,4-α-glucosidases
NT4 Isoamylases
NT3 α-*N*-Arabinofuranosidases
NT3 Carbohydrases
NT3 Cellulases
NT3 Cellulolytic enzymes
NT3 Cellulose 1,4-β-cellobiosidases
NT3 Cellulosomes
NT3 Chitinases
NT3 Chitosanases
NT3 Cyclomaltodextrinases
NT3 Dextranases
NT3 Dextrinases
NT3 Endo-1,3(4)-β-glucanases
NT3 Endo-1,4-β-xylanases
NT3 β-Fructofuranosidases
NT3 Galactosidases
NT4 Galactanases
NT4 α-Galactosidases
NT4 β-Galactosidases
NT3 Glucanases
NT3 β-Glucanases
NT3 Glucan endo-1,3-β-D-glucosidases
NT3 α-Glucosidases
NT3 β-Glucosidases
NT3 α-Glucuronidases
NT3 β-Glucuronidases
NT3 Hemicellulases
NT3 Inulinases
NT3 Levanases
NT3 Licheninases
NT3 Limit dextrinases
NT3 Lysozymes
NT4 Eggs lysozymes
NT4 Egg whites lysozymes
NT3 Mannan endo-1,4-β-mannosidases
NT3 Mannosidases
NT3 α-Mannosidases
NT3 β-Mannosidases
NT3 Mutanolysins
NT3 Neopullulanases
NT3 Oligo-1,6-glucosidases
NT3 Pentosanases
NT3 Polygalacturonases
NT3 Pullulanases
NT3 α-L-rhamnosidases
NT3 Sucrose α-glucosidases
NT3 Thioglucosidases
NT3 α,α-Trehalases
NT3 Xylan degrading enzymes
NT3 Xylan endo-1,3-β-xylosidases
NT3 Xylan 1,4-β-xylosidases
NT2 β-Lactamases
NT2 Pancreatins
NT2 Proteinases
NT3 Actinidains
NT3 Aminopeptidases
NT3 Aqualysins
NT3 Bromelains
NT3 Calpains
NT3 Carboxypeptidases
NT3 Caspases
NT3 Cathepsins
NT3 Chymotrypsin
NT3 Collagenases
NT3 Cucumisins
NT3 Dipeptidases
NT3 Elastase
NT3 Endopeptidases
NT3 Enzymes milk clotting
NT4 Milk clotting enzymes
NT5 Chymosin
NT5 Rennets
NT6 Animal rennets
NT6 Calf rennets
NT6 Microbial rennets
NT6 Vegetable rennets
NT5 Rennet substitutes
NT3 Ficains
NT3 γ-Glutamyl hydrolases
NT3 Keratinases
NT3 Lysins
NT4 Autolysins
NT4 Thermolysins
NT3 Papain
NT3 Pepsins
NT3 Peptidases
NT3 Peptidyl-dipeptidase A
NT3 Plasmin
NT3 Plasminogen
NT3 Plasminogen activators
NT3 Pronase
NT3 Subtilisins
NT3 Trypsin
NT2 Pyrophosphatases
NT2 Ureases
NT1 Immobilized enzymes
NT1 Isoenzymes
NT1 Isomerases
NT2 Arabinose isomerases
NT2 Epimerases
NT3 Aldose 1-epimerases
NT2 Glucose isomerases
NT2 Phosphoglucomutases
NT2 Racemases
NT2 Xylose isomerases
NT1 Ligases
NT2 Acetyl-CoA carboxylases
NT2 Pyruvate carboxylases
NT1 Lyases
NT2 Alliin lyases
NT2 1-Aminocyclopropane-1-carboxylate synthases
NT2 Decarboxylases
NT3 Acetolactate decarboxylases
NT3 Glutamate decarboxylases
NT3 Histidine decarboxylases
NT2 Fructose-bisphosphate aldolases
NT2 Fumarate hydratases
NT2 Hydroperoxide lyases
NT2 Inulin fructotransferases (DFA-III-forming)
NT2 Isocitrate lyases
NT2 Pectate lyases
NT2 Pectin lyases
NT2 Phenylalanine ammonia-lyases
NT2 Phosphoenolpyruvate carboxylases
NT2 Poly(β-D-mannuronate) lyases
NT2 Pyruvate decarboxylases
NT1 Metalloenzymes
NT1 Naringinases
NT1 Oxidoreductases
NT2 Cyclooxygenases
NT2 Dehydrogenases
NT3 Alcohol dehydrogenases

NT3 Aldehyde dehydrogenases
NT3 Aldehyde reductases
NT3 Glutamate dehydrogenases
NT3 L-Iditol 2-dehydrogenases
NT3 Isocitrate dehydrogenases
NT3 Lactate dehydrogenases
NT3 D-Lactate dehydrogenases
NT3 L-Lactate dehydrogenases
NT3 Xanthine dehydrogenases
NT3 D-Xylulose reductases
NT2 Desaturases
NT2 Dioxygenases
NT2 Malate dehydrogenases
NT2 Monooxygenases
NT2 Oxidases
NT3 Alcohol oxidases
NT4 Aryl-alcohol oxidases
NT3 Amine oxidases
NT3 Amino acid oxidases
NT3 1-Aminocyclopropane-1-carboxylate oxidases
NT3 L-Ascorbate oxidases
NT3 Cholesterol oxidases
NT3 Glucose oxidases
NT3 L-Glutamate oxidases
NT3 Lactate 2-monooxygenases
NT3 Xanthine oxidases
NT2 Oxygenases
NT3 Lipoxygenases
NT2 Peroxidases
NT3 Catalases
NT3 Glutathione peroxidases
NT3 Lactoperoxidase systems
NT3 Ligninases
NT3 Lignin peroxidases
NT3 Manganese peroxidases
NT2 Phenolases
NT3 Catechol oxidases
NT3 Laccases
NT3 Monophenol monooxygenases
NT3 Tyrosinases
NT2 Prostaglandin-endoperoxide synthases
NT2 Reductases
NT3 Nitrate reductases
NT2 Superoxide dismutases
NT1 Pectic enzymes
NT2 Pectate lyases
NT2 Pectinesterases
NT2 Pectin lyases
NT2 Pectolytic enzymes
NT2 Polygalacturonases
NT1 Recombinant enzymes
NT1 Restriction modification systems
NT1 Synthases
NT1 Transferases
NT2 Acetolactate synthases
NT2 Acyltransferases
NT3 Acetyltransferases
NT3 Alcohol *O*-acetyltransferases
NT3 Fatty acid synthases
NT3 γ-Glutamyltransferases
NT3 Protein-glutamine γ-glutamyltransferases
NT2 Aminotransferases
NT2 Citrate synthases
NT2 DNA-directed DNA polymerases
NT2 DNA-directed RNA polymerases
NT2 Glucose-1-phosphate adenylyltransferases
NT2 Glutathione transferases
NT2 Glycosyltransferases
NT3 Alternansucrases
NT3 Cyclomaltodextrin glucanotransferases
NT3 Dextransucrases
NT3 Fructosyltransferases
NT3 1,4-α-Glucan branching enzymes
NT3 4-α-Glucanotransferases
NT3 Glucosyltransferases
NT3 Lactose synthases
NT3 Levansucrases
NT3 Starch synthases
NT3 Sucrose-phosphate synthases
NT3 Sucrose synthases
NT3 Transglucosylases
NT2 Methyltransferases
NT2 Phosphorylases
NT2 Phosphotransferases
NT3 Kinases
NT4 Aspartate kinases
NT4 Fructokinases
NT4 Glucokinases
NT4 Hexokinases
NT2 Transaminases
NT3 Aspartate transaminases
NT2 Transpeptidases
RT Active sites
RT Catalysts

Enzymes milk clotting
HN heading from vol. 25 (1993); see Chymosin, Rennets, Proteinases up to vol. 24 (1992)
SN milk clotting enzymes is also used in the index
BT1 Proteinases
BT2 Hydrolases
BT3 Enzymes
NT1 Milk clotting enzymes
NT2 Chymosin
NT2 Rennets
NT3 Animal rennets
NT3 Calf rennets
NT3 Microbial rennets
NT3 Vegetable rennets
NT2 Rennet substitutes
RT Cheesemaking
RT Coagulation

Enzymic browning
HN browning enzymic also used in the index up to vol. 29 (1997)
BT1 Browning

Enzymic techniques
BT1 Analytical techniques

Epicatechin
BT1 Catechols
BT2 Flavanols
BT3 Flavonoids
BT4 Aromatic compounds
BT5 Organic compounds
BT4 Pigments
BT2 Phenols
BT3 Alcohols
BT3 Aromatic compounds
BT4 Organic compounds

Epicatechin gallate
BT1 Catechols
BT2 Flavanols
BT3 Flavonoids
BT4 Aromatic compounds
BT5 Organic compounds
BT4 Pigments
BT2 Phenols
BT3 Alcohols
BT3 Aromatic compounds
BT4 Organic compounds

Epicatechol
BT1 Catechols
BT2 Flavanols
BT3 Flavonoids
BT4 Aromatic compounds
BT5 Organic compounds
BT4 Pigments
BT2 Phenols
BT3 Alcohols
BT3 Aromatic compounds
BT4 Organic compounds

Epichlorohydrin
BT1 Chlorinated hydrocarbons
BT2 Organic halogen compounds
BT1 Fumigants
BT2 Biocides

Epidemiology
BT1 Diseases

Epidermal growth factors
BT1 Hormones
BT2 Residues

Epidermin
SN lantibiotic produced by Staphylococcus epidermidis
BT1 Bacteriocins
BT2 Antibiotics
BT3 Drugs
BT4 Residues
RT *Staphylococcus epidermidis*

Epigallocatechin
BT1 Catechols
BT2 Flavanols
BT3 Flavonoids
BT4 Aromatic compounds
BT5 Organic compounds
BT4 Pigments
BT2 Phenols
BT3 Alcohols
BT3 Aromatic compounds
BT4 Organic compounds

Epigallocatechin gallate
BT1 Catechols
BT2 Flavanols

BT3 Flavonoids
BT4 Aromatic compounds
BT5 Organic compounds
BT4 Pigments
BT2 Phenols
BT3 Alcohols
BT3 Aromatic compounds
BT4 Organic compounds

Epimerases
SN includes members of subclass EC 5.1
BT1 Isomerases
BT2 Enzymes
NT1 Aldose 1-epimerases

Epinephelus guaza
BT1 Grouper
BT2 Marine fish
BT3 Fish
BT4 Animals
BT4 Sea foods
BT5 Aquatic foods
BT6 Animal foods
BT7 Foods

Epinephrine
USE **Adrenaline**

Epoxides
BT1 Plastics
BT2 Packaging materials

Eptam
USE **EPTC**

EPTC
BT1 Herbicides
BT2 Pesticides
BT3 Biocides
BT3 Residues
UF Eptam

Epuration
BT1 Purification
BT2 Processing
BT3 Technology

Equations
BT1 Mathematics
BT2 Science
RT Formulae

Equatorial Guinea
BT1 West Africa
BT2 Africa
NT1 Bioko

Equipment
SN general term for machinery used in food processing
BT1 Technology
NT1 Aspirators
NT1 Autoclaves
NT1 Boilers
NT1 Centrifuges
NT2 Centrifugal separators
NT1 Chillers
NT1 Clarifiers
NT1 Computers
NT2 Microprocessors
NT1 Conveyors
NT2 Conveying
NT2 Pneumatic conveyors
NT1 Cookers
NT1 Coolers
NT1 Corers
NT1 Couplers
NT1 Cyclones
NT1 Depositors
NT1 Detectors
NT1 Diffusers
NT1 Dishwashers
NT1 Dispensers
NT2 Aerosols
NT2 Atomizers
NT2 Decanters
NT2 Dispensing
NT2 Taps
NT1 Driers
NT2 Freeze driers
NT2 Solar driers
NT2 Spray driers
NT1 Evaporators
NT1 Extruders
NT1 Fans
NT1 Filters
NT1 Freezers
NT1 Gauges
NT1 Heaters
NT1 Heat exchangers
NT1 Holders
NT1 Homogenizers
NT1 Hydrocyclones
NT1 Impellers
NT1 Injectors
NT1 Kettles
NT1 Knives
NT1 Lasers
NT1 Lauter tuns
NT1 Metal detectors
NT1 Microchip technology
NT1 Milking machines
NT1 Mills
NT2 Flour mills
NT2 Roller mills
NT1 Mincers
NT1 Mixers
NT1 Oil expellers
NT1 Ovens
NT2 Baking ovens
NT2 Kilns
NT2 Microwave ovens
NT1 Pans
NT1 Pasteurizers
NT1 Pipes
NT1 Presses
NT1 Processing equipment
NT1 Processing lines
NT1 Pumps
NT1 Refrigerators
NT1 Sensors
NT1 Separators
NT2 Centrifugal separators
NT1 Sieves
NT1 Sifters
NT1 Strainers
NT1 Sugar pans
NT1 Utensils
NT2 Ceramics
NT2 Scoops
NT1 Vacuum pans
NT1 Valves
NT1 Vats
NT1 Winnowers
RT Lubricants
UF Devices
UF Machinery
UF Machines
UF Plant (machinery)

Equol
HN introduced from vol. 39, issue 1 (2007)
BT1 Isoflavones
BT2 Isoflavonoids
BT3 Flavonoids
BT4 Aromatic compounds
BT5 Organic compounds
BT4 Pigments

Eremofortin
BT1 Mycotoxins
BT2 Toxins
BT3 Residues

Eremothecium
HN under Fungi up to vol. 42 (2010)
SN synonymous with Ashbya
BT1 Yeasts
BT2 Fungi
BT3 Microorganisms

Ergocalciferol
SN syn. vitamin D2; syn. ercalciol
BT1 Vitamins
BT2 Nutrients

Ergosterol
SN converted to ergocalciferol (vitamin D2) by UV light
BT1 Sterols
BT2 Alcohols
BT2 Steroids
BT3 Lipids
BT4 Nutrients

Ergot
BT1 Plant diseases
BT2 Diseases plant
BT3 Diseases
RT Ergotamine

Ergotamine
BT1 Alkaloids
BT2 Organic nitrogen compounds
RT Ergot

Eritrea
BT1 East Africa
BT2 Africa

Eruca sativa
BT1 Vegetables specific
BT2 Vegetables
BT3 Crops
BT4 Plants
BT3 Plant foods
BT4 Foods

Erucic acid
BT1 Docosenoic acid
BT2 Monounsaturated fatty acids
BT3 Unsaturated fatty acids
BT4 Fatty acids
BT5 Lipids
BT6 Nutrients
BT5 Organic acids
BT6 Acids
RT Rapeseed oils

Erwinia
HN under Enterobacteriaceae up to vol. 24 (1992)
BT1 Bacteria
BT2 Microorganisms
NT1 *Erwinia carotovora*
NT1 *Erwinia chrysanthemi*
NT1 *Erwinia herbicola*

Erwinia carotovora
SN synonymous with Pectobacterium carotovorum
BT1 *Erwinia*
BT2 Bacteria
BT3 Microorganisms

Erwinia chrysanthemi
BT1 *Erwinia*
BT2 Bacteria
BT3 Microorganisms

Erwinia herbicola
SN synonymous with Pantoea agglomerans
BT1 *Erwinia*
BT2 Bacteria
BT3 Microorganisms

Erysipelothrix
BT1 Bacteria
BT2 Microorganisms

Erythorbic acid
SN syn. isoascorbic acid
BT1 Antioxidants
BT2 Additives
BT1 Organic acids
BT2 Acids

Erythritol
BT1 Polyols
BT2 Alcohols
BT2 Carbohydrates
BT3 Nutrients
BT3 Organic compounds

Erythrocytes
HN introduced from vol. 39, issue 1 (2007)
BT1 Cells
NT1 Haemolysis

Erythromycin
BT1 Macrolide antibiotics
BT2 Antibiotics
BT3 Drugs
BT4 Residues

Erythrosine
BT1 Colorants
BT2 Additives

Escarole
USE **Endives**

Escherichia
BT1 Bacteria
BT2 Microorganisms
NT1 *Escherichia coli*
RT Verotoxins

Escherichia coli
BT1 *Escherichia*
BT2 Bacteria
BT3 Microorganisms
RT Haemolytic uraemic syndrome

Esculetin
BT1 Coumarins
BT2 Lactones
BT3 Esters
BT4 Organic compounds
BT3 Heterocyclic compounds
BT2 Phenols
BT3 Alcohols
BT3 Aromatic compounds
BT4 Organic compounds
BT1 Enzyme inhibitors
BT2 Enzymes

Espresso coffee
BT1 Coffee beverages
BT2 Coffee products
BT3 Coffee
BT4 Beverages
BT4 Crops
BT5 Plants
BT4 Plant foods
BT5 Foods
UF Expresso coffee

Essences
BT1 Extracts
BT2 Flavourings
BT3 Additives

Essential fatty acids
HN introduced from vol. 43, issue 1 (2011)
SN general use only; see also specified essential fatty acids
BT1 Unsaturated fatty acids
BT2 Fatty acids
BT3 Lipids
BT4 Nutrients
BT3 Organic acids
BT4 Acids
RT Linoleic acid
RT α-Linolenic acid

Essential oils
BT1 Flavourings
BT2 Additives
BT1 Vegetable oils
BT2 Oils vegetable
BT3 Oils
BT4 Lipids
BT5 Nutrients
BT3 Vegetable products
BT4 Plant foods
BT5 Foods
NT1 Bitter almond oils
NT1 Buchu oils
NT1 Cinnamon oils
NT1 Citronella essential oils
NT1 Citrus essential oils
NT2 Bergamot essential oils
NT3 Bergamot oils
NT2 Bitter orange essential oils
NT2 Citrus oils
NT2 Lemon essential oils
NT2 Lime essential oils
NT2 Neroli oils
NT2 Orange essential oils
NT1 Clary sage essential oils
NT1 Clove oils
NT1 Garlic oils
NT1 Hop essential oils
NT1 Lemongrass oils
NT1 Mint oils
NT1 Nutmeg oils
NT1 Oleoresins
NT1 Oregano oils
NT1 Peppermint essential oils
NT1 Petitgrain oils
NT1 Rosemary essential oils
NT1 Sage essential oils
NT1 Tea tree oils
NT1 Thyme oils

Esterases
SN EC 3.1
BT1 Hydrolases
BT2 Enzymes
NT1 Acetylcholinesterases
NT1 Carboxylesterases
NT1 Chlorophyllases
NT1 Cholinesterases
NT1 Cutinases
NT1 Feruloyl esterases
NT1 Lipases
NT2 Lecithinases
NT2 Lipoprotein lipases
NT2 Lysophospholipases
NT2 Phospholipases
NT2 Triacylglycerol lipases
NT1 Nucleases
NT2 Deoxyribonucleases
NT2 Endonucleases
NT2 Restriction endonucleases
NT2 Restriction enzymes
NT2 Ribonucleases
NT3 Angiogenin
NT1 Pectinesterases
NT1 Phosphatases
NT2 Acid phosphatases
NT2 Alkaline phosphatases
NT2 Nucleotidases
NT2 Phytases
NT3 3-Phytases
NT3 4-Phytases
NT1 Phosphodiesterases
NT1 Tannases

Esterification
NT1 Acidolysis
NT1 Alcoholysis
NT2 Glycerolysis

NT2 Methanolysis
NT1 Interesterification
NT1 Transesterification
RT Esters
RT Modification

Esters
BT1 Organic compounds
NT1 Butyl acetate
NT1 Diethylpyrocarbonate
NT1 Ethyl acetate
NT1 Ethyl carbamate
NT1 Ethyl formate
NT1 Fatty acid esters
NT2 Ascorbyl palmitate
NT2 Ethyl butyrate
NT2 Ethyl caprylate
NT2 Ethyl decanoate
NT2 Ethyl hexanoate
NT3 Ethyl caproate
NT2 Ethyl octanoate
NT2 Ethyl oleate
NT2 Glycerides
NT3 Acylglycerols
NT3 Diglycerides
NT4 Diacylglycerols
NT3 Glycerol monostearate
NT3 Glyceryl monostearate
NT3 Monoglycerides
NT4 Monoacylglycerols
NT4 Monolaurin
NT3 Phosphoglycerides
NT3 Triglycerides
NT4 Olein
NT5 Palm olein
NT4 Stearin
NT5 Palm stearin
NT4 Triacetin
NT4 Triacylglycerols
NT4 Tricaprylin
NT4 Trilinolein
NT4 Triolein
NT4 Tripalmitin
NT4 Tristearin
NT2 Linoleates
NT3 Methyl linoleate
NT2 Polyglycerol fatty acid esters
NT2 Waxes
NT3 Beeswax
NT3 Carnauba wax
NT3 Wax coatings
NT3 Wax esters
NT1 Geranyl acetate
NT1 Hexyl acetate
NT1 Hydroxybenzoic acid esters
NT2 Parabens
NT3 Methylparaben
NT3 Propylparaben
NT1 Isoamyl acetate
NT1 Lactones
NT2 Coumarins
NT3 Coumarin
NT3 Coumestrol
NT3 Esculetin
NT3 Furocoumarins
NT4 Bergapten
NT4 Psoralens
NT4 Xanthotoxin
NT3 Scopoletin
NT2 γ-Decalactone
NT2 Glucono-δ-lactone
NT1 Linalyl acetate
NT1 Methyl benzoate
NT1 Methyl carbamate
NT1 Octyl gallate
NT1 Phthalic acid esters
NT1 Propyl gallate
NT1 Pyrocarbonic acid diethyl ester
NT1 Sinapine
NT1 Stanol esters
NT1 Sterol esters
NT1 Sucrose polyesters
NT2 Olestra
NT1 Terpinyl acetate
NT1 Thioesters
NT1 Urethane
NT1 Vitamin E acetate
RT Acetates
RT Aroma compounds
RT Esterification

Estonia
BT1 Europe
BT1 European Union

Estragole
BT1 Phenols
BT2 Alcohols
BT2 Aromatic compounds
BT3 Organic compounds

Ethanal
SN syn. acetaldehyde
BT1 Acetaldehyde
BT2 Aldehydes
BT3 Carbonyl compounds
BT4 Organic compounds
BT2 Aroma compounds
BT3 Flavour compounds
BT3 Volatile compounds

Ethane
BT1 Gases
BT2 Physical phases
BT3 Chemistry
BT4 Science
BT1 Hydrocarbons
BT2 Organic compounds

Ethanol
SN syn. alcohol
BT1 Alcohols
BT1 Solvents
NT1 Alcohol
NT1 Alcoholometers
UF Ethyl alcohol

Ethanolamine
BT1 Alcohols
BT1 Amines
BT2 Organic nitrogen compounds

Ethanolic fermentation
SN syn. alcoholic fermentation
BT1 Fermentation

Ethephon
HN heading from vol. 25 (1993) up to vol. 42 (2010); under Ethrel up to vol. 24 (1992)
BT1 Ethylene
BT2 Gases
BT3 Physical phases
BT4 Chemistry
BT5 Science
BT2 Hydrocarbons
BT3 Organic compounds
BT2 Plant growth regulators
BT3 Cultivation
BT4 Agriculture
UF Chloroethylphosphonic acid
UF (2-Chloroethyl)phosphonic acid
UF Ethrel

Etherification
HN introduced from vol. 41, issue 1 (2009)
BT1 Modification

Ethers
BT1 Organic compounds
NT1 Bisphenol A diglycidyl ether
NT1 Bisphenol F diglycidyl ether
NT1 Dill ether

Ethics

Ethiofencarb
BT1 *N*-Methylcarbamate insecticides
BT2 Insecticides
BT3 Pesticides
BT4 Biocides
BT4 Residues
BT2 *N*-Methylcarbamate pesticides
BT3 Carbamate pesticides
BT4 Pesticides
BT5 Biocides
BT5 Residues
UF Croneton

Ethion
BT1 Acaricides
BT2 Pesticides
BT3 Biocides
BT3 Residues
BT1 Organophosphorus insecticides
BT2 Insecticides
BT3 Pesticides
BT4 Biocides
BT4 Residues
BT2 Organophosphorus pesticides
BT3 Pesticides
BT4 Biocides
BT4 Residues

Ethiopia
BT1 East Africa
BT2 Africa

Ethiopian mustard
BT1 Mustard greens

BT2 Vegetables specific
BT3 Vegetables
BT4 Crops
BT5 Plants
BT4 Plant foods
BT5 Foods
BT1 Mustard seeds
BT2 Oilseeds
BT3 Seeds
BT4 Plant foods
BT5 Foods
BT2 Spices
BT3 Flavourings
BT4 Additives
NT1 *Brassica carinata*

Ethnic foods
BT1 Processed foods
BT2 Foods
RT Regional foods

Ethnic groups
BT1 Anthropological groups
BT2 Population groups

Ethopabate
BT1 Coccidiostats
BT2 Drugs
BT3 Residues

Ethoprop
USE **Ethoprophos**

Ethoprophos
BT1 Nematocides
BT2 Pesticides
BT3 Biocides
BT3 Residues
BT1 Organophosphorus insecticides
BT2 Insecticides
BT3 Pesticides
BT4 Biocides
BT4 Residues
BT2 Organophosphorus pesticides
BT3 Pesticides
BT4 Biocides
BT4 Residues
UF Ethoprop

Ethoxyquin
BT1 Antioxidants
BT2 Additives
UF Santoquin

Ethrel
HN heading up to vol. 24 (1992)
USE **Ethephon**

Ethyl acetate
HN also under Flavour compounds up to vol. 42 (2010)
BT1 Acetates
BT1 Aroma compounds
BT2 Flavour compounds
BT2 Volatile compounds
BT1 Esters
BT2 Organic compounds
BT1 Solvents

Ethyl alcohol
USE **Ethanol**

Ethylamine
BT1 Amines
BT2 Organic nitrogen compounds

Ethyl butyrate
HN also under Flavour compounds up to vol. 42 (2010)
BT1 Aroma compounds
BT2 Flavour compounds
BT2 Volatile compounds
BT1 Fatty acid esters
BT2 Esters
BT3 Organic compounds

Ethyl caproate
HN also under Flavour compounds up to vol. 42 (2010)
SN syn. ethyl hexanoate
BT1 Ethyl hexanoate
BT2 Aroma compounds
BT3 Flavour compounds
BT3 Volatile compounds
BT2 Fatty acid esters
BT3 Esters
BT4 Organic compounds

Ethyl caprylate
HN introduced from vol. 43, issue 1 (2011)
BT1 Aroma compounds
BT2 Flavour compounds
BT2 Volatile compounds
BT1 Fatty acid esters
BT2 Esters
BT3 Organic compounds

Ethyl carbamate
HN ethylcarbamate was used in the index up to vol. 24(1992)
SN syn. urethane
BT1 Carcinogens
BT2 Mutagens
BT1 Esters
BT2 Organic compounds
BT1 Organic nitrogen compounds
UF Ethylcarbamate

Ethylcarbamate
HN used in the index up to vol. 24 (1992)
USE **Ethyl carbamate**

Ethyl decanoate
HN introduced from vol. 41, issue 1 (2009)
BT1 Aroma compounds
BT2 Flavour compounds
BT2 Volatile compounds
BT1 Fatty acid esters
BT2 Esters
BT3 Organic compounds

Ethylene
BT1 Gases
BT2 Physical phases
BT3 Chemistry
BT4 Science
BT1 Hydrocarbons
BT2 Organic compounds
BT1 Plant growth regulators
BT2 Cultivation
BT3 Agriculture
NT1 ACC
NT1 Ethephon

Ethylenediamine
BT1 Amines
BT2 Organic nitrogen compounds

Ethylene dibromide
BT1 Fumigants
BT2 Biocides

Ethylene dichloride
BT1 Fumigants
BT2 Biocides

Ethylene glycol
BT1 Glycols
BT2 Alcohols

Ethylene oxide
BT1 Fumigants
BT2 Biocides
BT1 Oxides

Ethylenethiourea
BT1 Dithiocarbamate fungicides
BT2 Fungicides
BT3 Pesticides
BT4 Biocides
BT4 Residues

Ethyl formate
HN introduced from vol. 41, issue 1 (2009)
BT1 Aroma compounds
BT2 Flavour compounds
BT2 Volatile compounds
BT1 Esters
BT2 Organic compounds
BT1 Fumigants
BT2 Biocides

Ethyl hexanoate
HN introduced from vol. 39, issue 1 (2007); also under Flavour compounds up to vol. 42 (2010)
SN syn. ethyl caproate
BT1 Aroma compounds
BT2 Flavour compounds
BT2 Volatile compounds
BT1 Fatty acid esters
BT2 Esters
BT3 Organic compounds
NT1 Ethyl caproate

Ethyl octanoate
HN introduced from vol. 41, issue 1 (2009)
BT1 Aroma compounds
BT2 Flavour compounds
BT2 Volatile compounds
BT1 Fatty acid esters
BT2 Esters
BT3 Organic compounds

Ethyl oleate
HN introduced from vol. 39, issue 1 (2007)
BT1 Fatty acid esters
BT2 Esters
BT3 Organic compounds

Ethyl vanillin
HN under Flavourings up to vol. 42 (2010)
BT1 Aroma compounds
BT2 Flavour compounds
BT2 Volatile compounds
BT1 Aromatic compounds
BT2 Organic compounds

Etrimfos
BT1 Organophosphorus insecticides
BT2 Insecticides
BT3 Pesticides
BT4 Biocides
BT4 Residues
BT2 Organophosphorus pesticides
BT3 Pesticides
BT4 Biocides
BT4 Residues

EU
USE **European Union**

Eubacteria
USE **Bacteria**

Eucalyptol
HN also under Flavour compounds up to vol. 42 (2010)
BT1 Cineole
BT2 Aroma compounds
BT3 Flavour compounds
BT3 Volatile compounds
BT2 Monoterpenoids
BT3 Terpenoids
BT4 Lipids
BT5 Nutrients

Eucalyptus
BT1 Plants

Eucaryotes
USE **Eukaryotes**

Eucheuma
BT1 Seaweeds
BT2 Algae
BT3 Microorganisms
BT2 Sea foods
BT3 Aquatic foods
BT4 Animal foods
BT5 Foods

Eucommia ulmoides
BT1 Plants
RT Tochu tea

Eugenol
HN also under Flavour compounds up to vol. 42 (2010)
BT1 Aroma compounds
BT2 Flavour compounds
BT2 Volatile compounds
BT1 Phenols
BT2 Alcohols
BT2 Aromatic compounds
BT3 Organic compounds

Euglena
HN introduced from vol. 43, issue 1 (2011)
BT1 Microalgae
BT2 Algae
BT3 Microorganisms
NT1 *Euglena gracilis*

Euglena gracilis
BT1 *Euglena*
BT2 Microalgae
BT3 Algae
BT4 Microorganisms

Eukaryotes
RT Algae
RT Animals
RT Fungi
RT Oocysts
RT Plants
RT Protozoa
UF Eucaryotes

Euparen
USE **Dichlofluanid**

Euphorbia
BT1 Oilseeds
BT2 Seeds
BT3 Plant foods
BT4 Foods

Europe
HN heading up to vol. 24 (1992)
NT1 Albania
NT1 Andorra
NT1 Armenia
NT1 Austria
NT1 Azerbaijan
NT1 Belarus
NT1 Belgium
NT1 Bosnia and Herzegovina
NT1 Bulgaria
NT1 Channel Islands
NT1 Croatia
NT1 Czechoslovakia
NT1 Czech Republic
NT1 Denmark
NT1 Estonia
NT1 Finland
NT1 France
NT1 Georgia
NT1 Germany
NT1 Greece
NT1 Hungary
NT1 Iceland
NT1 Italy
NT1 Latvia
NT1 Liechtenstein
NT1 Lithuania
NT1 Luxembourg
NT1 Macedonia
NT1 Malta
NT1 Moldova
NT1 Monaco
NT1 Montenegro
NT1 Netherlands
NT1 Norway
NT1 Poland
NT1 Portugal
NT1 Republic of Ireland
NT1 Romania
NT1 Russia
NT1 San Marino
NT1 Scandinavia
NT1 Serbia
NT1 Slovakia
NT1 Slovenia
NT1 Spain
NT2 Canary Islands
NT1 Sweden
NT1 Switzerland
NT1 Turkey
NT1 Ukraine
NT1 United Kingdom
NT2 England
NT2 Northern Ireland
NT2 Scotland
NT2 St Helena
NT2 Wales
NT1 Yugoslavia
RT European Community
RT European Union
RT Middle East

European Community
SN European Union is also in index
RT Europe
RT European Union
UF EC
UF EEC
UF European Economic Community

European Economic Community
HN heading up to vol. 24
USE **European Community**

European Food Safety Authority
HN introduced from vol. 43, issue 1 (2011)
RT Food safety
UF EFSA

European Union
NT1 Austria
NT1 Belgium
NT1 Cyprus
NT1 Czech Republic
NT1 Denmark
NT1 Estonia
NT1 Finland
NT1 France
NT1 Germany
NT1 Greece
NT1 Hungary
NT1 Italy
NT1 Latvia
NT1 Lithuania
NT1 Luxembourg
NT1 Malta
NT1 Netherlands
NT1 Poland
NT1 Portugal
NT1 Republic of Ireland

NT1 Slovakia
NT1 Slovenia
NT1 Spain
NT2 Canary Islands
NT1 Sweden
NT1 United Kingdom
NT2 England
NT2 Northern Ireland
NT2 Scotland
NT2 St Helena
NT2 Wales
RT Europe
RT European Community
UF EU

Eurotium
BT1 Fungi
BT2 Microorganisms

Eurygaster
BT1 Insects
BT2 Pests

Evaluation
HN heading up to vol. 24 (1992)
BT1 Analytical techniques

Evaporated milk
BT1 Milk
BT2 Dairy products
BT3 Animal foods
BT4 Foods
RT Concentrated milk
RT Condensed milk

Evaporation
BT1 Thermal processing
BT2 Processing thermal
BT3 Processing
BT4 Technology
NT1 Evaporators
NT1 Vacuum evaporation
NT1 Vaporization
RT Concentration
RT Distillation
RT Drying

Evaporators
BT1 Equipment
BT2 Technology
BT1 Evaporation
BT2 Thermal processing
BT3 Processing thermal
BT4 Processing
BT5 Technology

Evening primrose oils
BT1 Vegetable oils
BT2 Oils vegetable
BT3 Oils
BT4 Lipids
BT5 Nutrients
BT3 Vegetable products
BT4 Plant foods
BT5 Foods

Evening primrose seeds
BT1 Oilseeds
BT2 Seeds
BT3 Plant foods
BT4 Foods

Evisceration
BT1 Processing
BT2 Technology
RT Gutting
RT Slaughter
RT Viscera

Ewe cheese
BT1 Cheese varieties
BT2 Cheese
BT3 Dairy products
BT4 Animal foods
BT5 Foods
BT1 Sheep
BT2 Animals
UF Ewe milk cheese
UF Sheep cheese
UF Sheep milk cheese

Ewedu
BT1 Vegetables specific
BT2 Vegetables
BT3 Crops
BT4 Plants
BT3 Plant foods
BT4 Foods
UF Bush okra

Ewe milk
BT1 Milk
BT2 Dairy products
BT3 Animal foods
BT4 Foods
BT1 Sheep
BT2 Animals
UF Sheep milk

Ewe milk cheese
USE **Ewe cheese**

Ewes
USE **Sheep**

Ewe yoghurt
HN introduced from vol. 39, issue 1 (2007)
BT1 Sheep
BT2 Animals
BT1 Yoghurt
BT2 Fermented milk
BT3 Fermented dairy products
BT4 Dairy products
BT5 Animal foods
BT6 Foods
BT4 Fermented foods
BT5 Processed foods
BT6 Foods
BT3 Milk
BT4 Dairy products
BT5 Animal foods
BT6 Foods

Exercise performance
HN introduced from vol. 39, issue 1 (2007)
BT1 Human physiology
BT2 Physiology
BT3 Science
BT1 Physical activity
BT2 Health
RT Performance drinks

Exhaust gases
BT1 Air pollutants
BT2 Air pollution
BT3 Environmental pollution
BT4 Pollution
BT5 Contamination
BT2 Pollutants
BT3 Pollution
BT4 Contamination

Exopolysaccharides
BT1 Polysaccharides
BT2 Carbohydrates
BT3 Nutrients
BT3 Organic compounds
RT Curdlan
RT Gellan
RT Kefiran
RT Pullulan
RT Xanthan

Exotic fruits
BT1 Fruits specific
BT2 Fruits
BT3 Crops
BT4 Plants
BT3 Plant foods
BT4 Foods

Exotic vegetables
BT1 Vegetables specific
BT2 Vegetables
BT3 Crops
BT4 Plants
BT3 Plant foods
BT4 Foods

Exotoxins
BT1 Toxins
BT2 Residues
RT Virulence factors

Exo-1,4-β-xylosidases
USE **Xylan 1,4-β-xylosidases**

Expansins
HN introduced from vol. 41, issue 1 (2009)
BT1 Vegetable proteins
BT2 Proteins vegetable
BT3 Proteins
BT4 Nutrients
BT3 Vegetable products
BT4 Plant foods
BT5 Foods

Expansion
HN introduced from vol. 39, issue 1 (2007)
BT1 Physical properties

Expenditure
BT1 Economics

Expert systems
BT1 Information technology
BT2 Technology

Explosions
NT1 Dust explosions
RT Safety

Exports
BT1 Trade
BT2 Economics

Expression vectors
HN introduced from vol. 39, issue 1 (2007)
BT1 Vectors
BT2 Cloning vectors
BT3 Genetic techniques
BT4 Genetics

Expresso coffee
USE **Espresso coffee**

Extensibility
BT1 Rheological properties
BT2 Mechanical properties
BT3 Physical properties

Extensographs
BT1 Apparatus
BT2 Technology

Extraction
BT1 Processing
BT2 Technology
NT1 Sonication
NT1 Supercritical CO_2 extraction
NT1 Supercritical fluid extraction
RT Aqueous two phase systems
RT Extracts
RT Mashing

Extractive fermentation
BT1 Fermentation technology
BT2 Biotechnology
BT3 Technology
BT2 Process control
BT3 Technology

Extracts
BT1 Flavourings
BT2 Additives
NT1 Beef extracts
NT1 Coffee extracts
NT1 Essences
NT1 Fruit extracts
NT1 Hop extracts
NT1 Infusions
NT1 Meat extracts
NT1 Tea extracts
NT1 Yeast extracts
RT Concentrates
RT Extraction

Extrudates
BT1 Extrusion
BT2 Processing
BT3 Technology
RT Extruded foods

Extruded foods
HN introduced from vol. 39, issue 1 (2007)
BT1 Processed foods
BT2 Foods
NT1 Extruded pet foods
RT Extrudates

Extruded pet foods
HN introduced from vol. 39, issue 1 (2007)
BT1 Extruded foods
BT2 Processed foods
BT3 Foods
BT1 Pet foods

Extruders
BT1 Equipment
BT2 Technology
BT1 Extrusion
BT2 Processing
BT3 Technology

Extrusion
BT1 Processing
BT2 Technology
NT1 Coextrusion
NT1 Extrudates
NT1 Extruders
NT1 Extrusion cooking
RT Texturization

Extrusion cooking
BT1 Extrusion
BT2 Processing
BT3 Technology

Eye disorders
HN introduced from vol. 39, issue 1 (2007)
SN includes cataracts, age-related macular degeneration, etc.
BT1 Diseases
RT Eye health
RT Vision

Eye health
HN introduced from vol. 42, issue 1 (2010)
BT1 Health
RT Eye disorders
RT Vision

F

F
BT1 Halogens
BT2 Elements
BT3 Minerals
BT4 Nutrients
RT Fluorides
UF Fluorine

Faba beans
HN heading from vol. 25 (1993); under Broad beans up to vol. 24 (1992)
BT1 Legumes
BT2 Vegetables specific
BT3 Vegetables
BT4 Crops
BT5 Plants
BT4 Plant foods
BT5 Foods
NT1 Broad beans
NT1 Field beans
NT1 Horse beans

σ Factors
BT1 Proteins
BT2 Nutrients
RT Stress
RT Transcription
UF Sigma factors

Factory fumes
BT1 Air pollutants
BT2 Air pollution
BT3 Environmental pollution
BT4 Pollution
BT5 Contamination
BT2 Pollutants
BT3 Pollution
BT4 Contamination

Faecal contamination
HN introduced from vol. 39, issue 1 (2007)
BT1 Contamination

Fair trade
HN introduced from vol. 39, issue 1 (2007)
BT1 Trade
BT2 Economics
RT Marketing
RT Markets

Falafel
BT1 Snack foods
BT2 Processed foods
BT3 Foods
BT1 Vegetable products
BT2 Plant foods
BT3 Foods

Falkland Islands
BT1 South America
BT2 America

Falling number
RT Cereals

Fallout
BT1 Radioactive contamination
BT2 Contamination
BT2 Radioactivity
RT Air pollution

Famophos
USE **Famphur**

Famphur
BT1 Organophosphorus insecticides
BT2 Insecticides
BT3 Pesticides
BT4 Biocides
BT4 Residues
BT2 Organophosphorus pesticides
BT3 Pesticides
BT4 Biocides
BT4 Residues
UF Famophos

Fans
HN introduced from vol. 39, issue 1 (2007)
BT1 Equipment
BT2 Technology

FAO
USE **Food and Agriculture Organization**

Farina
BT1 Starch
BT2 Glucans
BT3 Polysaccharides
BT4 Carbohydrates
BT5 Nutrients
BT5 Organic compounds
BT2 Thickeners
BT3 Additives

Farinographs
BT1 Apparatus
BT2 Technology
RT Dough

Farmed fish
BT1 Fish
BT2 Animals
BT2 Sea foods
BT3 Aquatic foods
BT4 Animal foods
BT5 Foods
RT Aquaculture

Farmed shellfish
HN introduced from vol. 37, issue 5 (2005)
BT1 Shellfish
BT2 Animals
BT2 Sea foods
BT3 Aquatic foods
BT4 Animal foods
BT5 Foods
RT Aquaculture

Farm milk
BT1 Milk
BT2 Dairy products
BT3 Animal foods
BT4 Foods

Farnesene
BT1 Aroma compounds
BT2 Flavour compounds
BT2 Volatile compounds
BT1 Sesquiterpenes
BT2 Hydrocarbons
BT3 Organic compounds
BT2 Sesquiterpenoids
BT3 Terpenoids
BT4 Lipids
BT5 Nutrients
RT Scald

Farnesol
BT1 Alcohols
BT1 Aroma compounds
BT2 Flavour compounds
BT2 Volatile compounds
BT1 Sesquiterpenoids
BT2 Terpenoids
BT3 Lipids
BT4 Nutrients

Fasciola
BT1 Parasites
BT2 Pests

Fasciolicides
BT1 Anthelmintics
BT2 Drugs
BT3 Residues

Fast foods
HN heading from vol. 25 (1993); under Meals up to vol. 24 (1992)
BT1 Processed foods
BT2 Foods
NT1 Street foods
NT1 Take away foods
RT Fried foods

Fasting
HN introduced from vol. 42, issue 1 (2010)
BT1 Eating habits
BT2 Consumer behaviour
BT3 Consumer response
RT Starvation

Fat mimetics
USE **Fat substitutes**

Fatness
HN introduced from vol. 39, issue 1 (2007)
BT1 Animal fats
BT2 Fats animal
BT3 Animal foods
BT4 Foods
BT3 Fats
BT4 Lipids
BT5 Nutrients
RT Carcasses

Fat replacers
USE **Fat substitutes**

Fats
BT1 Lipids
BT2 Nutrients
NT1 Cooking fats
NT1 Fats animal
NT2 Animal fats
NT3 Adipose tissues
NT3 Backfat
NT3 Belly fat
NT3 Blubber
NT4 Seal blubber
NT3 Dripping
NT3 Fatness
NT3 Intramuscular fat
NT3 Lard
NT3 Marbling
NT3 Subcutaneous fat
NT3 Suet
NT3 Tallow
NT2 Fats milk
NT3 Milk fats
NT4 Anhydrous milk fats
NT4 Butterfat
NT4 Butter oils
NT4 Milk fat globule membranes
NT4 Milk fat globules
NT1 Fats high diet
NT1 Fats low diet
NT1 Fats low foods
NT2 Fats low spreads
NT1 Fat substitutes
NT2 Dairy-lo
NT2 Litesse
NT2 Microcrystalline celluloses
NT2 Oatrim
NT2 Raftiline
NT2 Salatrim
NT2 Simplesse
NT2 Sucrose polyesters
NT3 Olestra
NT2 Z-Trim
NT1 Fats vegetable
NT2 Vegetable fats
NT3 Borneo tallow
NT3 Cocoa butter
NT4 Cocoa butter equivalents
NT4 Cocoa butter extenders
NT4 Cocoa butter substitutes
NT3 Coconut butter
NT3 Illipe butter
NT3 Kokum
NT3 Sal fats
NT3 Shea nut butter
NT3 Vanaspati
NT1 Frying fats
NT1 Hydrogenated fats
NT1 Margarines
NT2 Halvarine
NT1 Polyunsaturated fats
NT1 Saturated fats
NT1 Shortenings
NT1 Unsaturated fats
RT Hydrogenation
RT Iodine values
RT Oils

Fats animal
SN animal fats is also used in the index
BT1 Animal foods
BT2 Foods
BT1 Fats
BT2 Lipids
BT3 Nutrients
NT1 Animal fats
NT2 Adipose tissues
NT2 Backfat
NT2 Belly fat
NT2 Blubber
NT3 Seal blubber
NT2 Dripping
NT2 Fatness
NT2 Intramuscular fat
NT2 Lard
NT2 Marbling
NT2 Subcutaneous fat
NT2 Suet
NT2 Tallow
NT1 Fats milk
NT2 Milk fats
NT3 Anhydrous milk fats
NT3 Butterfat
NT3 Butter oils

NT3 Milk fat globule membranes
NT3 Milk fat globules

Fats high diet
HN introduced from vol. 41, issue 1 (2009)
BT1 Diet
BT2 Nutrition
BT1 Fats
BT2 Lipids
BT3 Nutrients
UF High fat diet

Fats low diet
HN introduced from vol. 38, issue 8 (2006)
BT1 Diet therapy
BT2 Diet
BT3 Nutrition
BT2 Therapy
BT1 Fats
BT2 Lipids
BT3 Nutrients
UF Low fat diet

Fats low foods
BT1 Fats
BT2 Lipids
BT3 Nutrients
NT1 Fats low spreads
RT Lite foods
UF Low fat foods

Fats low spreads
BT1 Fats low foods
BT2 Fats
BT3 Lipids
BT4 Nutrients
BT1 Spreads
BT2 Processed foods
BT3 Foods
UF Low fat spreads

Fats milk
SN milk fats is also used in the index
BT1 Fats animal
BT2 Animal foods
BT3 Foods
BT2 Fats
BT3 Lipids
BT4 Nutrients
NT1 Milk fats
NT2 Anhydrous milk fats
NT2 Butterfat
NT2 Butter oils
NT2 Milk fat globule membranes
NT2 Milk fat globules
RT Butter
RT Cream
RT Ghee

Fat substitutes
HN heading from vol. 30 (1998); under Fats up to vol.29 (1997)
BT1 Fats
BT2 Lipids
BT3 Nutrients
NT1 Dairy-lo
NT1 Litesse
NT1 Microcrystalline celluloses
NT1 Oatrim
NT1 Raftiline
NT1 Salatrim
NT1 Simplesse
NT1 Sucrose polyesters
NT2 Olestra
NT1 Z-Trim
UF Caprenin
UF Fat mimetics
UF Fat replacers

Fats vegetable
SN vegetable fats is also used in the index
BT1 Fats
BT2 Lipids
BT3 Nutrients
BT1 Vegetable products
BT2 Plant foods
BT3 Foods
NT1 Vegetable fats
NT2 Borneo tallow
NT2 Cocoa butter
NT3 Cocoa butter equivalents
NT3 Cocoa butter extenders
NT3 Cocoa butter substitutes
NT2 Coconut butter
NT2 Illipe butter
NT2 Kokum
NT2 Sal fats
NT2 Shea nut butter
NT2 Vanaspati
RT Oilseeds
RT Oils vegetable

Fattening
BT1 Feeds

Fatty acid esters
HN heading from vol. 25 (1993)
BT1 Esters
BT2 Organic compounds
NT1 Ascorbyl palmitate
NT1 Ethyl butyrate
NT1 Ethyl caprylate
NT1 Ethyl decanoate
NT1 Ethyl hexanoate
NT2 Ethyl caproate
NT1 Ethyl octanoate
NT1 Ethyl oleate
NT1 Glycerides
NT2 Acylglycerols
NT2 Diglycerides
NT3 Diacylglycerols
NT2 Glycerol monostearate
NT2 Glyceryl monostearate
NT2 Monoglycerides
NT3 Monoacylglycerols
NT3 Monolaurin
NT2 Phosphoglycerides
NT2 Triglycerides
NT3 Olein
NT4 Palm olein
NT3 Stearin
NT4 Palm stearin
NT3 Triacetin
NT3 Triacylglycerols
NT3 Tricaprylin
NT3 Trilinolein
NT3 Triolein
NT3 Tripalmitin
NT3 Tristearin
NT1 Linoleates
NT2 Methyl linoleate
NT1 Polyglycerol fatty acid esters
NT1 Waxes
NT2 Beeswax
NT2 Carnauba wax
NT2 Wax coatings
NT2 Wax esters
RT Fatty acids

Fatty acids
BT1 Lipids
BT2 Nutrients
BT1 Organic acids
BT2 Acids
NT1 Branched chain fatty acids
NT2 Isobutyric acid
NT2 Isocaproic acid
NT2 Isovaleric acid
NT1 Cyclic fatty acids
NT1 Eicosanoids
NT2 Prostaglandins
NT1 Malvalic acid
NT1 Saturated fatty acids
NT2 Arachidic acid
NT2 Behenic acid
NT2 Butanoic acid
NT3 Butyric acid
NT2 Decanoic acid
NT3 Capric acid
NT2 Dodecanoic acid
NT3 Lauric acid
NT2 Heptadecanoic acid
NT3 Margaric acid
NT2 Heptanoic acid
NT2 Hexadecanoic acid
NT3 Palmitic acid
NT2 Hexanoic acid
NT3 Caproic acid
NT2 Lignoceric acid
NT2 Myristic acid
NT2 Octadecanoic acid
NT3 Stearic acid
NT4 Hydroxystearic acid
NT2 Octanoic acid
NT3 Caprylic acid
NT2 Pentanoic acid
NT3 Valeric acid
NT1 Sterculic acid
NT1 Unsaturated fatty acids
NT2 Essential fatty acids
NT2 Monounsaturated fatty acids
NT3 Decenoic acid
NT3 Docosenoic acid
NT4 Erucic acid
NT3 Eicosenoic acid
NT3 Hexadecenoic acid
NT4 Palmitoleic acid
NT3 Octadecenoic acid
NT4 Elaidic acid
NT4 Oleic acid
NT4 Petroselinic acid
NT4 Vaccenic acid
NT3 Ricinoleic acid
NT2 PUFA
NT3 Conjugated fatty acids

NT4 CLA
NT4 Eleostearic acid
NT3 Eicosatetraenoic acid
NT4 Arachidonic acid
NT3 ω-3 Fatty acids
NT4 Docosahexaenoic acid
NT4 Docosapentaenoic acid
NT4 Eicosapentaenoic acid
NT4 α-Linolenic acid
NT4 Stearidonic acid
NT3 ω-6 Fatty acids
NT4 Arachidonic acid
NT4 Linoleic acid
NT5 CLA
NT4 γ-Linolenic acid
NT3 Linolenic acid
NT4 Eleostearic acid
NT4 α-Linolenic acid
NT4 γ-Linolenic acid
NT2 *trans* Fatty acids
NT3 Elaidic acid
NT3 Vaccenic acid
NT1 Volatile fatty acids
NT2 Short chain fatty acids
NT3 Butanoic acid
NT4 Butyric acid
NT3 Hexanoic acid
NT4 Caproic acid
NT3 Hydroxybutyric acid
NT3 Isobutyric acid
NT3 Isocaproic acid
NT3 Isovaleric acid
NT3 Pentanoic acid
NT4 Valeric acid
RT Acid values
RT Fatty acid esters
RT Lipolysis

ω-3 Fatty acids
BT1 PUFA
BT2 Unsaturated fatty acids
BT3 Fatty acids
BT4 Lipids
BT5 Nutrients
BT4 Organic acids
BT5 Acids
NT1 Docosahexaenoic acid
NT1 Docosapentaenoic acid
NT1 Eicosapentaenoic acid
NT1 α-Linolenic acid
NT1 Stearidonic acid
UF ω3 Fatty acids

ω-6 Fatty acids
HN introduced from vol. 37, issue 5 (2005)
BT1 PUFA
BT2 Unsaturated fatty acids
BT3 Fatty acids
BT4 Lipids
BT5 Nutrients
BT4 Organic acids
BT5 Acids
NT1 Arachidonic acid
NT1 Linoleic acid
NT2 CLA
NT1 γ-Linolenic acid

ω3 Fatty acids
HN used for <omega>-3 Fatty acids up to vol. 35, issue 6 (2003)
USE **ω-3 Fatty acids**

Fatty acid synthases
SN EC 2.3.1.85
BT1 Acyltransferases
BT2 Transferases
BT3 Enzymes

FDA
USE **Food and Drug Administration**

FDC blue
BT1 Colorants
BT2 Additives

FDC red
BT1 Colorants
BT2 Additives

FDC yellow
BT1 Colorants
BT2 Additives

Fe
SN index heading is Iron
BT1 Iron
BT2 Metals
BT3 Elements
BT4 Minerals
BT5 Nutrients

Feathers
BT1 Wastes

Federal Republic of Germany
HN Germany, Federal Republic of was heading up to vol. 24 (1992)
USE **Germany**

Feeding
BT1 Feeds

Feeds
NT1 Fattening
NT1 Feeding
NT1 Fodder
NT1 Pastures
NT1 Silage
RT Agriculture
UF Animal nutrition

Feijoa
BT1 Fruits specific
BT2 Fruits
BT3 Crops
BT4 Plants
BT3 Plant foods
BT4 Foods

Fenazaflor
BT1 Acaricides
BT2 Pesticides
BT3 Biocides
BT3 Residues
BT1 Insecticides
BT2 Pesticides
BT3 Biocides
BT3 Residues

Fenbendazole
BT1 Anthelmintics
BT2 Drugs
BT3 Residues

Fenchlorphos
BT1 Organophosphorus insecticides
BT2 Insecticides
BT3 Pesticides
BT4 Biocides
BT4 Residues
BT2 Organophosphorus pesticides
BT3 Pesticides
BT4 Biocides
BT4 Residues
UF Ronnel

Fenitrothion
BT1 Organophosphorus insecticides
BT2 Insecticides
BT3 Pesticides
BT4 Biocides
BT4 Residues
BT2 Organophosphorus pesticides
BT3 Pesticides
BT4 Biocides
BT4 Residues
UF Methylnitrophos

Fennel
BT1 Vegetables specific
BT2 Vegetables
BT3 Crops
BT4 Plants
BT3 Plant foods
BT4 Foods

Fennel seeds
BT1 Spices
BT2 Flavourings
BT3 Additives

Fenoprop
BT1 Phenoxy herbicides
BT2 Herbicides
BT3 Pesticides
BT4 Biocides
BT4 Residues
UF Silvex
UF 2,4,5-TP

Fensulfothion
BT1 Nematocides
BT2 Pesticides
BT3 Biocides
BT3 Residues
BT1 Organophosphorus insecticides
BT2 Insecticides
BT3 Pesticides
BT4 Biocides
BT4 Residues
BT2 Organophosphorus pesticides
BT3 Pesticides
BT4 Biocides

BT4 Residues
UF Dasanit

Fenthion
BT1 Acaricides
 BT2 Pesticides
  BT3 Biocides
  BT3 Residues
BT1 Organophosphorus insecticides
 BT2 Insecticides
  BT3 Pesticides
   BT4 Biocides
   BT4 Residues
 BT2 Organophosphorus pesticides
  BT3 Pesticides
   BT4 Biocides
   BT4 Residues
UF Baytex
UF Lebaycid
UF Mercaptophos

Fenugreek
BT1 Spices
 BT2 Flavourings
  BT3 Additives
BT1 Vegetables specific
 BT2 Vegetables
  BT3 Crops
   BT4 Plants
  BT3 Plant foods
   BT4 Foods

Fenuron
BT1 Herbicides
 BT2 Pesticides
  BT3 Biocides
  BT3 Residues

Fenvalerate
BT1 Acaricides
 BT2 Pesticides
  BT3 Biocides
  BT3 Residues
BT1 Pyrethroid insecticides
 BT2 Insecticides
  BT3 Pesticides
   BT4 Biocides
   BT4 Residues

Ferbam
BT1 Dithiocarbamate fungicides
 BT2 Fungicides
  BT3 Pesticides
   BT4 Biocides
   BT4 Residues

Fermentation
HN heading up to vol. 23 (1991) and from vol. 25 (1993)
NT1 Acetic fermentation
NT1 Alcoholic fermentation
NT1 Butyric fermentation
NT1 Citric fermentation
NT1 Cofermentation
NT1 Ethanolic fermentation
NT1 Lactic fermentation
NT1 Leavening
NT1 Malolactic fermentation
NT1 Propionic fermentation
RT Brewing
RT Starters
RT Winemaking
RT Worts
RT Yeasts

Fermentation products
HN heading from vol. 24 (1992)
BT1 Biotechnology
 BT2 Technology
NT1 Bioconversions
 NT2 Biotransformations
NT1 Biomass
 NT2 Microbial biomass
  NT3 Bacterial biomass
  NT3 Yeast biomass
 NT2 Mycoprotein
  NT3 Quorn
 NT2 Single cell proteins
UF Biotechnology products

Fermentation technology
HN heading from vol. 24 (1992)
BT1 Biotechnology
 BT2 Technology
BT1 Process control
 BT2 Technology
NT1 Bioreactors
 NT2 Chemostats
 NT2 Membrane bioreactors
 NT2 Packed bed bioreactors
 NT2 Stirred tank bioreactors
 NT2 UASB bioreactors
NT1 Cofermentation
NT1 Downstream processing
NT1 Extractive fermentation
NT1 Fermenters
NT1 Simultaneous saccharification and fermentation
NT1 Solid state fermentation
NT1 Submerged fermentation

Fermented beverages
SN general use only; see also other specified fermented beverages
BT1 Beverages
RT Fermented foods

Fermented cream
HN heading from vol. 25 (1993); under Cultured cream up to vol. 24 (1992)
BT1 Cream
 BT2 Dairy products
  BT3 Animal foods
   BT4 Foods
BT1 Fermented dairy products
 BT2 Dairy products
  BT3 Animal foods
   BT4 Foods
 BT2 Fermented foods
  BT3 Processed foods
   BT4 Foods
NT1 Katyk
NT1 Ripened cream
NT1 Smetana
NT1 Sour cream
UF Cultured cream

Fermented dairy products
HN heading from vol. 25 (1993); under Dairy products up to vol. 24 (1992)
BT1 Dairy products
 BT2 Animal foods
  BT3 Foods
BT1 Fermented foods
 BT2 Processed foods
  BT3 Foods
NT1 Acidophilus pastes
NT1 Fermented cream
 NT2 Katyk
 NT2 Ripened cream
 NT2 Smetana
 NT2 Sour cream
NT1 Fermented milk
 NT2 Acidophilin
 NT2 Acidophilus milk
 NT2 Amasi
 NT2 Bifidus milk
 NT2 Biogarde
 NT2 Bioghurt
 NT2 Dahi
 NT2 Kefir
  NT3 Kefir grains
 NT2 Koumiss
 NT2 Labneh
 NT2 Lactic beverages
 NT2 Lassi
 NT2 Leben
 NT2 Nono
 NT2 Prostokvasha
 NT2 Ryazhenka
 NT2 Shrikhand
 NT2 Shubat
 NT2 Skyr
 NT2 Snezhok
 NT2 Sour milk
 NT2 Tarag
 NT2 Tykmaelk
 NT2 Yakult
 NT2 Ymer
 NT2 Yoghurt
  NT3 Buffalo yoghurt
  NT3 Ewe yoghurt
  NT3 Flavoured yoghurt
  NT3 Frozen yoghurt
  NT3 Fruit yoghurt
  NT3 Goat yoghurt
  NT3 Yoghurt beverages
   NT4 Drinking yoghurt
 NT2 Zabady
  NT3 Zabadi
UF Cultured dairy products
UF Cultured milk products

Fermented foods
HN heading from vol. 25 (1993); under Fermented products up to vol. 23 (1991)
BT1 Processed foods
 BT2 Foods
NT1 Attieke
NT1 Bongkrek
NT1 Budu
NT1 Chungkook-jang
NT1 Dawadawa
NT1 Dhokla
NT1 Doenjang
NT1 Dongchimi

NT1 Dosai
NT1 Fermented dairy products
NT2 Acidophilus pastes
NT2 Fermented cream
NT3 Katyk
NT3 Ripened cream
NT3 Smetana
NT3 Sour cream
NT2 Fermented milk
NT3 Acidophilin
NT3 Acidophilus milk
NT3 Amasi
NT3 Bifidus milk
NT3 Biogarde
NT3 Bioghurt
NT3 Dahi
NT3 Kefir
NT4 Kefir grains
NT3 Koumiss
NT3 Labneh
NT3 Lactic beverages
NT3 Lassi
NT3 Leben
NT3 Nono
NT3 Prostokvasha
NT3 Ryazhenka
NT3 Shrikhand
NT3 Shubat
NT3 Skyr
NT3 Snezhok
NT3 Sour milk
NT3 Tarag
NT3 Tykmaelk
NT3 Yakult
NT3 Ymer
NT3 Yoghurt
NT4 Buffalo yoghurt
NT4 Ewe yoghurt
NT4 Flavoured yoghurt
NT4 Frozen yoghurt
NT4 Fruit yoghurt
NT4 Goat yoghurt
NT4 Yoghurt beverages
NT5 Drinking yoghurt
NT3 Zabady
NT4 Zabadi
NT1 Fermented sausages
NT1 Fufu
NT1 Gari
NT1 Idli
NT1 Iru
NT1 Ishiru
NT1 Jeotgal
NT1 Katsuobushi
NT1 Kawal
NT1 Kenkey
NT1 Kimchies
NT2 Kakdugi
NT1 Kinema
NT1 Kishk
NT1 Kochujang
NT1 Koji
NT2 Rice koji
NT1 Koko
NT1 Lao-chao
NT1 Meitauza
NT1 Miso
NT1 Momoni
NT1 Nata
NT1 Natto
NT1 Nukazuke
NT1 Nuoc-mam
NT1 Ogi
NT1 Ogiri
NT1 Ontjom
NT1 Patis
NT1 Pickles
NT2 Chicken gizzard pickles
NT2 Chutneys
NT2 Mango pickles
NT2 Vegetable pickles
NT3 Cucumber pickles
NT3 Narazuke
NT3 Pickled onions
NT1 Pidan
NT1 Poi
NT1 Pozol
NT1 Puto
NT1 Rabadi
NT1 Sauerkraut
NT1 Shiokara
NT2 Ika shiokara
NT1 Siljo
NT1 Soy sauces
NT2 Kanjang
NT2 Kecap
NT2 Shoyu
NT1 Sufu
NT1 Tape
NT2 Tape ketan
NT1 Tarhana
NT1 Tempeh
NT1 Trahanas
NT1 Ugba
NT1 Uji
NT1 Vinegar
NT2 Balsamic vinegar
NT2 Cider vinegar
NT2 Fruit vinegars
NT3 Apple vinegar
NT2 Malt vinegar
NT2 Rice vinegar
NT2 Wine vinegar
RT Fermented beverages
UF Cultured foods
UF Fermented products

Fermented milk
HN heading from vol. 25 (1993); under Cultured milks up to vol. 24 (1992)
BT1 Fermented dairy products
BT2 Dairy products
BT3 Animal foods
BT4 Foods
BT2 Fermented foods
BT3 Processed foods
BT4 Foods
BT1 Milk
BT2 Dairy products
BT3 Animal foods
BT4 Foods
NT1 Acidophilin
NT1 Acidophilus milk
NT1 Amasi
NT1 Bifidus milk
NT1 Biogarde
NT1 Bioghurt
NT1 Dahi
NT1 Kefir
NT2 Kefir grains
NT1 Koumiss
NT1 Labneh
NT1 Lactic beverages
NT1 Lassi
NT1 Leben
NT1 Nono
NT1 Prostokvasha
NT1 Ryazhenka
NT1 Shrikhand
NT1 Shubat
NT1 Skyr
NT1 Snezhok
NT1 Sour milk
NT1 Tarag
NT1 Tykmaelk
NT1 Yakult
NT1 Ymer
NT1 Yoghurt
NT2 Buffalo yoghurt
NT2 Ewe yoghurt
NT2 Flavoured yoghurt
NT2 Frozen yoghurt
NT2 Fruit yoghurt
NT2 Goat yoghurt
NT2 Yoghurt beverages
NT3 Drinking yoghurt
NT1 Zabady
NT2 Zabadi
RT Buttermilk
UF Cultured milk beverages
UF Cultured milks

Fermented products
HN heading up to vol. 23 (1991)
USE **Fermented foods**

Fermented sausages
SN general use only; see also other specified fermented sausages
BT1 Fermented foods
BT2 Processed foods
BT3 Foods
BT1 Sausages
BT2 Meat products
BT3 Animal foods
BT4 Foods

Fermenters
BT1 Fermentation technology
BT2 Biotechnology
BT3 Technology
BT2 Process control
BT3 Technology

Fernando Po
USE **Bioko**

Ferns
NT1 Bracken
NT1 Ostrich fern
RT Vegetables specific

Ferritin
HN introduced from vol. 39, issue 1 (2007)
BT1 Iron
BT2 Metals
BT3 Elements
BT4 Minerals
BT5 Nutrients

BT1 Proteins
BT2 Nutrients

Fertilizers
BT1 Cultivation
BT2 Agriculture
NT1 Foliar sprays

Ferulic acid
BT1 Organic acids
BT2 Acids
BT1 Phenols
BT2 Alcohols
BT2 Aromatic compounds
BT3 Organic compounds

Feruloyl esterases
HN introduced from vol. 39, issue 1 (2007)
SN EC 3.1.1.73
BT1 Esterases
BT2 Hydrolases
BT3 Enzymes

Feruloylquinic acid
BT1 Organic acids
BT2 Acids
BT1 Phenols
BT2 Alcohols
BT2 Aromatic compounds
BT3 Organic compounds

Feta cheese
BT1 Cheese varieties
BT2 Cheese
BT3 Dairy products
BT4 Animal foods
BT5 Foods

Fetal programming
USE **Prenatal nutrition**

Fetuses
BT1 Population groups
RT Prenatal nutrition

FIA
BT1 Analytical techniques
UF Flow injection analysis

Fibre
NT1 Barley fibre
NT1 Crude fibre
NT1 Dietary fibre
NT2 Insoluble fibre
NT2 Nonstarch polysaccharides
NT2 Soluble fibre
NT1 Fibre concentrates
NT1 Oat fibre
NT1 Roughage
NT1 Wheat fibre
RT Bran
RT Lignin

Fibreboard
BT1 Board
BT2 Packaging materials

Fibre concentrates
HN introduced from vol. 39, issue 1 (2007)
BT1 Concentrates
BT2 Processed foods
BT3 Foods
BT1 Fibre

Fibre optics
BT1 Analytical techniques

Fibrin
BT1 Animal proteins
BT2 Proteins animal
BT3 Proteins
BT4 Nutrients

Fibrinogen
BT1 Animal proteins
BT2 Proteins animal
BT3 Proteins
BT4 Nutrients

Fibrinolysin
USE **Plasmin**

Fibrobacter
BT1 Bacteria
BT2 Microorganisms

Ficains
SN EC 3.4.22.3
BT1 Proteinases
BT2 Hydrolases
BT3 Enzymes
UF Ficins

Ficins
USE **Ficains**

Ficus awkeotsang
BT1 Jelly figs
BT2 Fruits specific
BT3 Fruits
BT4 Crops
BT5 Plants
BT4 Plant foods
BT5 Foods

Field beans
BT1 Faba beans
BT2 Legumes
BT3 Vegetables specific
BT4 Vegetables
BT5 Crops
BT6 Plants
BT5 Plant foods
BT6 Foods

Field peas
BT1 Peas
BT2 Legumes
BT3 Vegetables specific
BT4 Vegetables
BT5 Crops
BT6 Plants
BT5 Plant foods
BT6 Foods

Fig juices
BT1 Fruit juices
BT2 Fruit products
BT3 Plant foods
BT4 Foods
BT2 Soft drinks
BT3 Beverages
RT Figs

Figs
HN heading from vol. 30 (1998); under Fruits specificup to vol. 29 (1997)
BT1 Fruits specific
BT2 Fruits
BT3 Crops
BT4 Plants
BT3 Plant foods
BT4 Foods
NT1 Dried figs
RT Fig juices

Fiji
BT1 Oceania

Filbertone
HN introduced from vol. 39, issue 1 (2007); also under Flavour compounds up to vol. 42 (2010)
BT1 Aroma compounds
BT2 Flavour compounds
BT2 Volatile compounds
BT1 Ketones
BT2 Carbonyl compounds
BT3 Organic compounds
RT Hazelnuts

Filberts
USE **Hazelnuts**

Filefish
BT1 Marine fish
BT2 Fish
BT3 Animals
BT3 Sea foods
BT4 Aquatic foods
BT5 Animal foods
BT6 Foods

Fillers
BT1 Filling
BT2 Packaging
BT3 Technology

Filleting
BT1 Cutting
BT2 Processing
BT3 Technology

Filling
BT1 Packaging
BT2 Technology
NT1 Fillers
NT1 Filling equipment

Filling equipment
BT1 Filling
BT2 Packaging
BT3 Technology

Fillings
NT1 Bakery fillings
NT1 Centres
NT1 Confectionery cream
NT1 Confectionery fillings
NT2 Chocolate fillings
NT1 Cremes
NT1 Forcemeat

NT1 Pie fillings
NT1 Pizza fillings
NT1 Stuffings

Films
SN used for food films not plastics films
NT1 Edible films
RT Coatings

Filter aids
HN heading from vol. 25 (1993)
BT1 Filtration
BT2 Processing
BT3 Technology
NT1 Bentonite
NT1 Clays
NT1 Diatomaceous earths
NT1 Kieselguhr
RT Clarification
RT Fining agents

Filters
BT1 Equipment
BT2 Technology
BT1 Filtration
BT2 Processing
BT3 Technology

Filth
BT1 Contaminants
BT2 Contamination

Filth tests
HN heading up to vol. 24 (1992)
BT1 Analytical techniques

Filtration
BT1 Processing
BT2 Technology
NT1 Filter aids
NT2 Bentonite
NT2 Clays
NT2 Diatomaceous earths
NT2 Kieselguhr
NT1 Filters
NT1 Microfiltration
NT1 Nanofiltration
NT1 Racking
NT1 Ultrafiltration
NT2 Diafiltration
RT Asbestos
RT Dialysis
RT Membranes

Fimbriae
BT1 Cells
BT1 Virulence factors
RT Adherence
RT Adhesins

Finance
BT1 Economics

Finfish
BT1 Fish
BT2 Animals
BT2 Sea foods
BT3 Aquatic foods
BT4 Animal foods
BT5 Foods

Finger millet
SN syn. ragi
BT1 Millet
BT2 Cereals
BT3 Crops
BT4 Plants
BT3 Seeds
BT4 Plant foods
BT5 Foods
UF *Eleusine coracana*
UF Kurakkan

Fining
BT1 Clarification
BT2 Processing
BT3 Technology
NT1 Fining agents

Fining agents
BT1 Fining
BT2 Clarification
BT3 Processing
BT4 Technology
RT Filter aids

Finland
HN heading up to vol. 24 (1992)
BT1 Europe
BT1 European Union
RT Organization for Economic Cooperation and Development

Finometers
BT1 Apparatus
BT2 Technology

Fior di Latte cheese
BT1 Cheese varieties
BT2 Cheese
BT3 Dairy products
BT4 Animal foods
BT5 Foods

Fiore Sardo cheese
HN introduced from vol. 39, issue 1 (2007)
BT1 Cheese varieties
BT2 Cheese
BT3 Dairy products
BT4 Animal foods
BT5 Foods

Firmness
BT1 Texture
BT2 Sensory properties
NT1 Penetrometers
NT1 *Rigor mortis*
NT1 Rigorometers
NT1 Softening
NT1 Softness
RT Rheological properties

Fisetin
HN introduced from vol. 39, issue 1 (2007)
BT1 Flavonols
BT2 Alcohols
BT2 Flavonoids
BT3 Aromatic compounds
BT4 Organic compounds
BT3 Pigments

Fish
HN used only for fish in general up to vol. 29 (1997)
BT1 Animals
BT1 Sea foods
BT2 Aquatic foods
BT3 Animal foods
BT4 Foods
NT1 Bass
NT1 Char
NT2 Arctic char
NT1 Dried fish
NT1 Farmed fish
NT1 Finfish
NT1 Fish bones
NT1 Fish factories
NT1 Fish fillets
NT1 Fish industry
NT1 Fish livers
NT2 Cod livers
NT1 Fish mince
NT1 Fish skin
NT1 Freshwater fish
NT2 Ayu
NT2 Bream
NT2 Burbot
NT2 Carp
NT3 Bighead carp
NT4 *Aristichthys nobilis*
NT3 Crucian carp
NT3 *Cyprinus carpio*
NT3 Grass carp
NT4 White amur
NT3 Rohu
NT4 *Labeo rohita*
NT3 Silver carp
NT2 Catfish
NT3 Channel catfish
NT4 *Ictalurus punctatus*
NT3 *Silurus asotus*
NT2 Chub
NT3 *Leuciscus cephalus*
NT2 *Colossoma macropomum*
NT2 Eels
NT2 Nile perch
NT2 Pacu
NT2 Perch
NT3 *Perca fluviatilis*
NT3 Yellow perch
NT2 Pike
NT2 River fish
NT2 Roach
NT2 Snakehead
NT2 Sunfish
NT2 Tench
NT2 Tilapia
NT3 Nile tilapia
NT4 Bolti
NT4 *Oreochromis niloticus*
NT4 *Tilapia nilotica*
NT3 *Oreochromis*
NT4 *Oreochromis niloticus*
NT2 Vendace
NT3 Coregonus albula
NT2 Walleye
NT1 Lamprey
NT1 Marine fish

NT2 Alaska pollock
NT3 Alaska pollack
NT3 *Theragra chalcogramma*
NT3 Walleye pollack
NT2 Alewife
NT2 Anchovy
NT3 Anchovy pastes
NT3 Budu
NT3 *Engraulis encrasicholus*
NT2 Barracuda
NT2 Barramundi
NT2 Bigeye snapper
NT3 *Priacanthus macracanthus*
NT2 Bluefish
NT2 Blue whiting
NT3 *Micromesistius poutassou*
NT2 Bombay duck
NT2 Capelin
NT2 Coalfish
NT2 Cod
NT3 Cod livers
NT3 *Gadus morhua*
NT3 Rock cod
NT2 Conger eels
NT2 Croakers
NT2 Cutlassfish
NT2 Dogfish
NT2 Dolphinfish
NT3 Mahimahi
NT2 Drum
NT2 Filefish
NT2 Flatfish
NT3 Arrowtooth flounder
NT3 Bastard halibut
NT4 *Paralichthys olivaceus*
NT3 Dab
NT3 Flounders
NT4 Japanese flounders
NT5 *Paralichthys olivaceus*
NT4 *Platichthys flesus*
NT3 Halibut
NT4 Atlantic halibut
NT4 Greenland halibut
NT4 *Reinhardtius hippoglossoides*
NT3 Megrim
NT4 *Lepidorhombus boscii*
NT3 Plaice
NT4 *Pleuronectes platessa*
NT3 Sole
NT3 Turbot
NT2 Flying fish
NT2 Grenadier
NT2 Groundfish
NT2 Grouper
NT3 *Epinephelus guaza*
NT2 Gurnard
NT2 Haddock
NT2 Hagfish
NT2 Hairtail
NT2 Hake
NT3 *Merluccius australis*
NT3 *Merluccius hubbsi*
NT3 *Merluccius merluccius*
NT3 Pacific hake
NT4 *Merluccius productus*
NT4 Pacific whiting
NT3 Red hake
NT2 Herring
NT3 *Clupea harengus*
NT3 Kippers
NT3 Matjes
NT3 Rollmops
NT2 Hilsa
NT2 Hoki
NT2 Kilka
NT2 Kingklip
NT2 Lanternfish
NT2 Ling
NT3 *Molva molva*
NT2 Ling cod
NT3 *Ophiodon elongatus*
NT2 Lizardfish
NT2 Lumpfish
NT3 *Cyclopterus lumpus*
NT2 Mackerel
NT3 Atlantic mackerel
NT4 *Scomber scombrus*
NT3 Chub mackerel
NT4 *Scomber japonicus*
NT3 Frigate mackerel
NT3 Horse mackerel
NT3 Indian mackerel
NT3 Jack mackerel
NT4 *Trachurus japonicus*
NT4 *Trachurus murphyi*
NT3 Pacific mackerel
NT3 Scad
NT3 Seer fish
NT3 Smoked mackerel
NT3 Spanish mackerel
NT2 Marlins
NT2 Menhaden
NT3 *Brevoortia tyrannus*
NT2 Milkfish
NT3 *Chanos chanos*
NT2 Monkfish
NT2 Morwong
NT2 Mullet
NT3 *Mugil cephalus*
NT2 Orange roughy
NT2 Paddlefish
NT3 *Polyodon spathula*
NT2 Pilchards
NT2 Pollack
NT2 Pollock
NT2 Pomfret
NT3 Butterfish
NT2 *Priacanthus tayenus*
NT2 Pufferfish
NT2 Rabbitfish
NT2 Ray
NT2 Redfish
NT2 Redspot emperor
NT3 *Lethrinus lentjan*
NT2 Rockfish
NT2 Sablefish
NT2 Sailfish
NT2 Saithe
NT2 Sand lance
NT2 Sardine
NT3 Monterey sardine
NT3 *Sardina pilchardus*
NT2 *Sardinella*
NT2 Saury
NT2 Sculpin
NT2 Sea bass
NT3 Striped bass
NT4 *Morone saxatilis*
NT2 Sea bream
NT3 Bogue
NT4 *Boops boops*
NT3 Red sea bream
NT4 *Pagrus major*
NT3 *Sparus aurata*
NT2 Sea fish
NT2 Sea perch
NT2 Shad
NT3 Indian shad
NT2 Sharks
NT3 Shark fins
NT2 Sheatfish
NT2 Skate
NT2 Snapper
NT2 Sprat
NT2 Swordfish
NT2 Threadfin bream
NT2 Tuna
NT3 Bigeye tuna
NT3 Bonito
NT3 Skipjack tuna
NT4 Katsuobushi
NT3 White tuna
NT4 Albacore
NT3 Yellowfin tuna
NT2 Whitebait
NT2 White fish
NT2 Whiting
NT2 Wreckfish
NT3 *Polyprion americanus*
NT2 Yellowfin
NT2 Yellowtail
NT1 Oily fish
NT2 Anchovy
NT3 Anchovy pastes
NT3 Budu
NT3 *Engraulis encrasicholus*
NT2 Carp
NT3 Bighead carp
NT4 *Aristichthys nobilis*
NT3 Crucian carp
NT3 *Cyprinus carpio*
NT3 Grass carp
NT4 White amur
NT3 Rohu
NT4 *Labeo rohita*
NT3 Silver carp
NT2 Eels
NT2 Herring
NT3 *Clupea harengus*
NT3 Kippers
NT3 Matjes
NT3 Rollmops
NT2 Hilsa
NT2 Mackerel
NT3 Atlantic mackerel
NT4 *Scomber scombrus*
NT3 Chub mackerel
NT4 *Scomber japonicus*
NT3 Frigate mackerel
NT3 Horse mackerel
NT3 Indian mackerel
NT3 Jack mackerel
NT4 *Trachurus japonicus*
NT4 *Trachurus murphyi*
NT3 Pacific mackerel
NT3 Scad

NT3 Seer fish
NT3 Smoked mackerel
NT3 Spanish mackerel
NT2 Orange roughy
NT2 Pilchards
NT2 Salmon
NT3 Atlantic salmon
NT4 *Salmo salar*
NT3 Pacific salmon
NT4 Cherry salmon
NT5 Masu salmon
NT4 Chinook salmon
NT5 King salmon
NT4 Chum salmon
NT5 Keta salmon
NT5 *Oncorhynchus keta*
NT4 Coho salmon
NT4 Pink salmon
NT4 Sockeye salmon
NT5 Red salmon
NT3 Smoked salmon
NT2 Sardine
NT3 Monterey sardine
NT3 *Sardina pilchardus*
NT2 Sprat
NT2 Swordfish
NT2 Trout
NT3 Brook trout
NT3 Brown trout
NT3 Rainbow trout
NT4 *Oncorhynchus mykiss*
NT3 Sea trout
NT3 Smoked trout
NT2 Tuna
NT3 Bigeye tuna
NT3 Bonito
NT3 Skipjack tuna
NT4 Katsuobushi
NT3 White tuna
NT4 Albacore
NT3 Yellowfin tuna
NT2 Whitebait
NT1 Sturgeon
NT2 Beluga
NT1 Whitefish
NT2 *Coregonus lavaretus*
RT Anisakidosis
RT Aquaculture
RT Fish products
UF Fishes

Fish balls
BT1 Fish products
BT2 Sea foods
BT3 Aquatic foods
BT4 Animal foods
BT5 Foods

Fish bones
BT1 Bones
BT1 Fish
BT2 Animals
BT2 Sea foods
BT3 Aquatic foods
BT4 Animal foods
BT5 Foods

Fishburgers
BT1 Fish products
BT2 Sea foods
BT3 Aquatic foods
BT4 Animal foods
BT5 Foods

Fish cakes
BT1 Fish products
BT2 Sea foods
BT3 Aquatic foods
BT4 Animal foods
BT5 Foods

Fish crackers
BT1 Fish products
BT2 Sea foods
BT3 Aquatic foods
BT4 Animal foods
BT5 Foods

Fishes
HN used for specific types of fish from vol. 25 (1993) to vol. 29 (1997); under Fish from vol. 30 (1998)
USE **Fish**

Fish factories
BT1 Fish
BT2 Animals
BT2 Sea foods
BT3 Aquatic foods
BT4 Animal foods
BT5 Foods

Fish farming
BT1 Aquaculture

Fish fillets
BT1 Fish
BT2 Animals
BT2 Sea foods
BT3 Aquatic foods
BT4 Animal foods
BT5 Foods

Fish fingers
BT1 Fish products
BT2 Sea foods
BT3 Aquatic foods
BT4 Animal foods
BT5 Foods

Fish foods
HN introduced from vol. 39, issue 1 (2007)
SN use for foods for domestic pet fish but not aquaculture feeds
BT1 Pet foods
RT Pet fish

Fish hydrolysates
BT1 Fish products
BT2 Sea foods
BT3 Aquatic foods
BT4 Animal foods
BT5 Foods

Fish industry
BT1 Fish
BT2 Animals
BT2 Sea foods
BT3 Aquatic foods
BT4 Animal foods
BT5 Foods
BT1 Food industry
BT2 Industries
RT Sea foods industry

Fish in marinades
BT1 Fish products
BT2 Sea foods
BT3 Aquatic foods
BT4 Animal foods
BT5 Foods

Fish in oils
BT1 Fish products
BT2 Sea foods
BT3 Aquatic foods
BT4 Animal foods
BT5 Foods

Fish in sauces
BT1 Fish products
BT2 Sea foods
BT3 Aquatic foods
BT4 Animal foods
BT5 Foods

Fish liver oils
BT1 Fish oils
BT2 Oils fish
BT3 Fish products
BT4 Sea foods
BT5 Aquatic foods
BT6 Animal foods
BT7 Foods
BT3 Marine oils
BT4 Oils
BT5 Lipids
BT6 Nutrients

Fish livers
BT1 Fish
BT2 Animals
BT2 Sea foods
BT3 Aquatic foods
BT4 Animal foods
BT5 Foods
BT1 Livers
BT2 Offal
BT3 Animal foods
BT4 Foods
NT1 Cod livers

Fish meal
BT1 Fish products
BT2 Sea foods
BT3 Aquatic foods
BT4 Animal foods
BT5 Foods

Fish mince
BT1 Fish
BT2 Animals
BT2 Sea foods
BT3 Aquatic foods
BT4 Animal foods
BT5 Foods

Fish noodles
BT1 Fish products
BT2 Sea foods
BT3 Aquatic foods

BT4 Animal foods
BT5 Foods

Fish oils
SN heading is Oils fish
BT1 Oils fish
BT2 Fish products
BT3 Sea foods
BT4 Aquatic foods
BT5 Animal foods
BT6 Foods
BT2 Marine oils
BT3 Oils
BT4 Lipids
BT5 Nutrients
NT1 Anchovy oils
NT1 Cod liver oils
NT1 Fish liver oils
NT1 Menhaden oils
NT1 Salmon oils
NT1 Sardine oils
NT1 Tuna oils
RT Animal fats

Fish pastes
BT1 Fish products
BT2 Sea foods
BT3 Aquatic foods
BT4 Animal foods
BT5 Foods
BT1 Pastes
BT2 Processed foods
BT3 Foods
NT1 Anchovy pastes

Fish pates
BT1 Fish products
BT2 Sea foods
BT3 Aquatic foods
BT4 Animal foods
BT5 Foods
BT1 Pates
BT2 Fish products
BT3 Sea foods
BT4 Aquatic foods
BT5 Animal foods
BT6 Foods
BT2 Meat products
BT3 Animal foods
BT4 Foods

Fish preserves
BT1 Fish products
BT2 Sea foods
BT3 Aquatic foods
BT4 Animal foods
BT5 Foods
BT1 Preserves
BT2 Processed foods
BT3 Foods

Fish products
BT1 Sea foods
BT2 Aquatic foods
BT3 Animal foods
BT4 Foods
NT1 Ceviche
NT1 Fish balls
NT1 Fishburgers
NT1 Fish cakes
NT1 Fish crackers
NT1 Fish fingers
NT1 Fish hydrolysates
NT1 Fish in marinades
NT1 Fish in oils
NT1 Fish in sauces
NT1 Fish meal
NT1 Fish noodles
NT1 Fish pastes
NT2 Anchovy pastes
NT1 Fish pates
NT1 Fish preserves
NT1 Fish sauces
NT2 Budu
NT2 Ishiru
NT2 Nuoc-mam
NT2 Patis
NT1 Fish sausages
NT1 Fish soups
NT1 Kamaboko
NT1 Katsuobushi
NT1 Kusaya
NT1 Matjes
NT1 Momoni
NT1 Nukazuke
NT1 Oils fish
NT2 Fish oils
NT3 Anchovy oils
NT3 Cod liver oils
NT3 Fish liver oils
NT3 Menhaden oils
NT3 Salmon oils
NT3 Sardine oils
NT3 Tuna oils
NT1 Pates
NT2 Fish pates
NT2 Liver pates
NT2 Terrines
NT1 Restructured fish products
NT1 Roes
NT2 Caviar
NT2 Caviar substitutes
NT2 Milt
NT1 Rollmops
NT1 Salted fish
NT1 Sashimi
NT1 Smoked fish
NT2 Kippers
NT2 Smoked mackerel
NT2 Smoked salmon
NT2 Smoked trout
NT1 Surimi
NT1 Sushi
RT Fish

Fish protein concentrates
HN heading up to vol. 24 (1992)
USE **FPC**

Fish proteins
BT1 Animal proteins
BT2 Proteins animal
BT3 Proteins
BT4 Nutrients

Fish sauces
BT1 Fish products
BT2 Sea foods
BT3 Aquatic foods
BT4 Animal foods
BT5 Foods
BT1 Sauces
BT2 Condiments
BT3 Flavourings
BT4 Additives
NT1 Budu
NT1 Ishiru
NT1 Nuoc-mam
NT1 Patis

Fish sausages
HN under Sausages up to vol. 24 (1992)
BT1 Fish products
BT2 Sea foods
BT3 Aquatic foods
BT4 Animal foods
BT5 Foods

Fish skin
HN introduced from vol. 39, issue 1 (2007)
BT1 Fish
BT2 Animals
BT2 Sea foods
BT3 Aquatic foods
BT4 Animal foods
BT5 Foods
BT1 Skin

Fish soups
BT1 Fish products
BT2 Sea foods
BT3 Aquatic foods
BT4 Animal foods
BT5 Foods
BT1 Soups
BT2 Processed foods
BT3 Foods

Flagella
HN introduced from vol. 39, issue 1 (2007)
BT1 Cells
BT1 Virulence factors
RT Flagellins
RT Motility

Flagellins
BT1 Microbial proteins
BT2 Microorganisms
BT2 Proteins
BT3 Nutrients
BT1 Virulence factors
RT Flagella

Flaking
BT1 Comminution
BT2 Processing
BT3 Technology

Flame photometry
BT1 Photometry
BT2 Analytical techniques

Flaming
BT1 Heating
BT2 Thermal processing
BT3 Processing thermal
BT4 Processing
BT5 Technology

Flammulina
BT1 Edible fungi
BT2 Fungi edible
BT3 Vegetables specific
BT4 Vegetables
BT5 Crops
BT6 Plants
BT5 Plant foods
BT6 Foods
NT1 *Flammulina velutipes*
UF *Collybia*
UF Enokitake

Flammulina velutipes
BT1 *Flammulina*
BT2 Edible fungi
BT3 Fungi edible
BT4 Vegetables specific
BT5 Vegetables
BT6 Crops
BT7 Plants
BT6 Plant foods
BT7 Foods

Flan cases
BT1 Flans
BT2 Bakery products
BT3 Cereal products
BT4 Plant foods
BT5 Foods

Flans
BT1 Bakery products
BT2 Cereal products
BT3 Plant foods
BT4 Foods
NT1 Flan cases
NT1 Torten

Flat bread
HN introduced from vol. 39, issue 1 (2007)
BT1 Bread
BT2 Bakery products
BT3 Cereal products
BT4 Plant foods
BT5 Foods

Flatfish
HN heading from vol. 30 (1998); under Fishes up to vol. 29 (1997)
BT1 Marine fish
BT2 Fish
BT3 Animals
BT3 Sea foods
BT4 Aquatic foods
BT5 Animal foods
BT6 Foods
NT1 Arrowtooth flounder
NT1 Bastard halibut
NT2 *Paralichthys olivaceus*
NT1 Dab
NT1 Flounders
NT2 Japanese flounders
NT3 *Paralichthys olivaceus*
NT2 *Platichthys flesus*
NT1 Halibut
NT2 Atlantic halibut
NT2 Greenland halibut
NT2 *Reinhardtius hippoglossoides*
NT1 Megrim
NT2 *Lepidorhombus boscii*
NT1 Plaice
NT2 *Pleuronectes platessa*
NT1 Sole
NT1 Turbot

Flatulence
HN introduced from vol. 39, issue 1 (2007)
BT1 Human physiology
BT2 Physiology
BT3 Science
NT1 Flatulence factors

Flatulence factors
HN introduced from vol. 39, issue 1 (2007)
BT1 Flatulence
BT2 Human physiology
BT3 Physiology
BT4 Science

Flavanols
HN heading up to vol. 24 (1992)
BT1 Flavonoids
BT2 Aromatic compounds
BT3 Organic compounds
BT2 Pigments
NT1 Catechols
NT2 Catechin
NT2 Epicatechin
NT2 Epicatechin gallate
NT2 Epicatechol
NT2 Epigallocatechin
NT2 Epigallocatechin gallate
NT2 Gallocatechin gallate
NT2 Pyrocatechol

Flavanones
BT1 Flavonoids
BT2 Aromatic compounds
BT3 Organic compounds
BT2 Pigments
NT1 Hesperetin
NT1 Hesperidin
NT1 Naringenin
NT1 Naringin
NT1 Narirutin
NT1 Neohesperidin

Flavimonas oryzihabitans
BT1 Bacteria
BT2 Microorganisms

Flavins
BT1 Pigments

Flavobacterium
BT1 Bacteria
BT2 Microorganisms
NT1 *Flavobacterium aurantiacum*
NT1 *Flavobacterium meningosepticum*

Flavobacterium aurantiacum
BT1 *Flavobacterium*
BT2 Bacteria
BT3 Microorganisms

Flavobacterium meningosepticum
BT1 *Flavobacterium*
BT2 Bacteria
BT3 Microorganisms

Flavomycin
BT1 Antibiotics
BT2 Drugs
BT3 Residues

Flavones
BT1 Flavonoids
BT2 Aromatic compounds
BT3 Organic compounds
BT2 Pigments
NT1 Apigenin
NT1 Chrysin
NT1 Luteolin

Flavonoids
BT1 Aromatic compounds
BT2 Organic compounds
BT1 Pigments
NT1 Anthocyanidins
NT2 Cyanidin
NT2 Delphinidin
NT2 Leucoanthocyanidins
NT3 Leucocyanidin
NT2 Malvidin
NT2 Pelargonidin
NT2 Peonidin
NT2 Petunidin
NT2 Proanthocyanidins
NT3 Procyanidins
NT1 Anthocyanins
NT2 Leucoanthocyanins
NT3 Anthocyanogens
NT2 Oenocyanins
NT2 Pyranoanthocyanins
NT1 Bioflavonoids
NT1 Chalcones
NT2 Dihydrochalcones
NT3 Neohesperidin dihydrochalcone
NT3 Phloretin
NT2 Xanthohumol
NT1 Flavanols
NT2 Catechols
NT3 Catechin
NT3 Epicatechin
NT3 Epicatechin gallate
NT3 Epicatechol
NT3 Epigallocatechin
NT3 Epigallocatechin gallate
NT3 Gallocatechin gallate
NT3 Pyrocatechol
NT1 Flavanones
NT2 Hesperetin
NT2 Hesperidin
NT2 Naringenin
NT2 Naringin
NT2 Narirutin
NT2 Neohesperidin
NT1 Flavones
NT2 Apigenin
NT2 Chrysin
NT2 Luteolin
NT1 Flavonols

NT2 Dihydroquercetin
NT2 Fisetin
NT2 Isorhamnetin
NT2 Kaempferol
NT2 Morin
NT2 Myricetin
NT2 Quercetin
NT2 Quercitrin
NT2 Rutin
NT1 Isoflavonoids
NT2 Coumestrol
NT2 Isoflavones
NT3 Daidzein
NT3 Equol
NT3 Genistein
NT3 Glycitein
NT3 Puerarin
NT1 Theaflavins
NT1 Thearubigins
RT Glycosides
RT Heterocyclic compounds
RT Polyphenols
RT Tannins

Flavonols
BT1 Alcohols
BT1 Flavonoids
BT2 Aromatic compounds
BT3 Organic compounds
BT2 Pigments
NT1 Dihydroquercetin
NT1 Fisetin
NT1 Isorhamnetin
NT1 Kaempferol
NT1 Morin
NT1 Myricetin
NT1 Quercetin
NT1 Quercitrin
NT1 Rutin

Flavour
BT1 Sensory properties
NT1 Aftertaste
NT1 Astringency
NT1 Bitterness
NT1 Fruitiness
NT1 Rancidity
NT1 Saltiness
NT1 Sharpness
NT1 Soapiness
NT1 Sourness
NT1 Sweetness
NT1 Taints
NT2 Boar taint
NT2 Cork taint
NT2 Off flavour
NT2 Off odour
NT2 Warmed over flavour
NT1 Umami
RT Aroma
RT Aroma compounds
RT Flavour compounds
RT Flavourings
RT Off flavour
UF Taste

Flavour compounds
NT1 Aroma compounds
NT2 Acetaldehyde
NT3 Ethanal
NT2 Acetals
NT2 Acetoin
NT3 Acetylmethylcarbinol
NT3 3-Hydroxy-2-butanone
NT2 α-Acetolactate
NT2 Acetophenone
NT2 Allicin
NT2 Alliin
NT2 Allyl isothiocyanate
NT2 Allyl sulfides
NT3 Diallyl disulfide
NT2 Amyl alcohol
NT3 Pentanol
NT2 Anethole
NT2 Anisaldehyde
NT2 Anisole
NT2 Benzaldehyde
NT2 Benzothiazole
NT2 Benzyl alcohol
NT2 Benzyl isothiocyanate
NT2 Borneol
NT2 Butanoic acid
NT3 Butyric acid
NT2 Butanol
NT3 Butyl alcohol
NT2 Butanone
NT2 Butyl acetate
NT2 Camphene
NT2 Camphor
NT2 Carvacrol
NT2 Carveol
NT2 Carvone
NT2 Caryophyllene
NT2 Cineole
NT3 Eucalyptol
NT2 Cinnamaldehyde
NT2 Cinnamic acid
NT2 Citral
NT3 Geranial
NT3 Neral
NT2 Citronellal
NT2 Citronellol
NT2 Cuminaldehyde
NT2 Cymene
NT2 Cysteine sulfoxides
NT2 γ-Decalactone
NT2 Decanal
NT2 Decanoic acid
NT3 Capric acid
NT2 Decanol
NT2 Diacetyl
NT3 2,3-Butanedione
NT2 Dill ether
NT2 Dimethyl disulfide
NT2 Dimethyl trisulfide
NT2 Dodecanoic acid
NT3 Lauric acid
NT2 Ethyl acetate
NT2 Ethyl butyrate
NT2 Ethyl caprylate
NT2 Ethyl decanoate
NT2 Ethyl formate
NT2 Ethyl hexanoate
NT3 Ethyl caproate
NT2 Ethyl octanoate
NT2 Ethyl vanillin
NT2 Eugenol
NT2 Farnesene
NT2 Farnesol
NT2 Filbertone
NT2 Furanones
NT3 Furaneol
NT4 2,5-Dimethyl-4-hydroxy-3(2*H*)-furanone
NT3 Sotolon
NT2 Geraniol
NT2 Geranyl acetate
NT2 Gingerols
NT2 Heptanoic acid
NT2 2-Heptanone
NT2 Heptenal
NT2 Hexanal
NT2 Hexanoic acid
NT3 Caproic acid
NT2 Hexanol
NT2 Hexenal
NT2 Hexyl acetate
NT2 Hotrienol
NT2 Humulene
NT2 Isoamyl acetate
NT2 Isoamyl alcohol
NT3 Isopentyl alcohol
NT3 Methyl butanol
NT2 Isobutanol
NT3 Isobutyl alcohol
NT3 Methyl propanol
NT2 Isobutyraldehyde
NT3 2-Methylpropanal
NT2 Isobutyric acid
NT2 Isocaproic acid
NT2 Isovaleric acid
NT2 Lenthionine
NT2 Limonene
NT2 Linalool
NT2 Linalyl acetate
NT2 Maltol
NT2 Menthol
NT2 Menthone
NT2 Methanethiol
NT3 Methyl mercaptan
NT2 Methional
NT2 Methionol
NT2 Methyl benzoate
NT2 3-Methylbutanal
NT3 Isovaleraldehyde
NT2 Myrcene
NT2 Myristicin
NT2 Nerol
NT2 Nonanal
NT2 Nonanone
NT2 Nonenal
NT2 Nootkatone
NT2 Norisoprenoids
NT3 β-Damascenone
NT3 Ionones
NT2 Octanal
NT2 Octanoic acid
NT3 Caprylic acid
NT2 Octanone
NT2 1-Octen-3-ol
NT2 Pentanal
NT3 Valeraldehyde
NT2 Pentanedione
NT3 Acetylacetone
NT2 Pentanoic acid
NT3 Valeric acid
NT2 Phenylacetaldehyde
NT2 Phenylethanol

NT3 Phenethyl alcohol
NT2 Pinenes
NT2 Piperidine
NT2 Piperine
NT2 Propanal
NT3 Propionaldehyde
NT2 Pyrazines
NT2 Safranal
NT2 Safrole
NT2 Terpinene
NT2 Terpineol
NT2 Terpinyl acetate
NT2 Thiazoles
NT2 Thioesters
NT2 Thujone
NT2 Thymol
NT2 Undecanone
NT2 Zingerone
NT1 Bitter compounds
NT2 Bitter acids
NT3 α-Acids
NT4 Humulones
NT5 Adhumulone
NT5 Cohumulone
NT5 Humulinic acid
NT3 β-Acids
NT4 Hulupones
NT4 Lupulones
NT5 Colupulone
NT3 Iso-α-acids
NT4 Isohumulones
NT3 Lupulin
NT2 Bitter peptides
NT2 Bitter principles
NT2 Cucurbitacins
NT2 Diketopiperazines
NT2 Ipomeamarone
NT2 Limonoids
NT3 Limonin
NT3 Limonoid glucosides
NT3 Nomilin
NT2 Naringin
NT2 Oleuropein
NT2 Progoitrin
NT2 Propylthiouracil
NT2 Quassin
NT2 Quinine
NT1 Glycyrrhizic acid
NT1 Glycyrrhizin
NT1 Pungent principles
NT2 Allicin
NT2 Allyl isothiocyanate
NT2 Capsaicinoids
NT3 Capsaicin
NT2 Gingerols
NT2 Piperine
NT2 Zingerone
RT Aroma
RT Aroma compounds
RT Flavour
RT Flavourings
RT Glutamates
RT Off flavour
RT Salt
RT Sugar
RT Sugars
RT Sweeteners
RT Sweet proteins
UF Tastant

Flavoured beverages
SN general use only; see also other specified flavoured beverages
BT1 Beverages
RT Flavoured milk

Flavoured milk
BT1 Milk
BT2 Dairy products
BT3 Animal foods
BT4 Foods
RT Flavoured beverages

Flavoured yoghurt
BT1 Yoghurt
BT2 Fermented milk
BT3 Fermented dairy products
BT4 Dairy products
BT5 Animal foods
BT6 Foods
BT4 Fermented foods
BT5 Processed foods
BT6 Foods
BT3 Milk
BT4 Dairy products
BT5 Animal foods
BT6 Foods

Flavour enhancers
BT1 Flavourings
BT2 Additives
RT Flavour modifiers
RT Glutamates
RT Glutamic acid
RT GMP
RT Monosodium glutamate

Flavour industry
USE **Flavourings industry**

Flavourings
BT1 Additives
NT1 Aconitic acid
NT1 Adipic acid
NT1 Artificial flavourings
NT1 Bitter almonds
NT1 Calamus
NT1 Caramel
NT1 Condiments
NT2 Mayonnaise
NT2 Mirin
NT2 Mustard
NT2 Relishes
NT2 Salad dressings
NT3 Dressings
NT3 French dressing
NT3 Salad cream
NT3 Salad oils
NT2 Salt
NT3 Desalination
NT3 Desalting
NT3 Iodized salt
NT3 NaCl
NT3 Salinity
NT3 Salt substitutes
NT2 Sauces
NT3 Apple sauces
NT3 Cheese sauces
NT3 Fish sauces
NT4 Budu
NT4 Ishiru
NT4 Nuoc-mam
NT4 Patis
NT3 Fondues
NT3 Gravy
NT4 Gravy powders
NT3 Hollandaise sauces
NT3 Ketchups
NT4 Catsups
NT5 Tomato catsups
NT4 Tomato ketchups
NT5 Tomato catsups
NT3 Meat sauces
NT3 Oyster sauces
NT3 Pasta sauces
NT4 Pesto
NT3 Roux
NT3 Salsa
NT3 Sauce mixes
NT3 Soy sauces
NT4 Kanjang
NT4 Kecap
NT4 Shoyu
NT3 Tomato sauces
NT3 Worcestershire sauces
NT2 Seasonings
NT2 Vinegar
NT3 Balsamic vinegar
NT3 Cider vinegar
NT3 Fruit vinegars
NT4 Apple vinegar
NT3 Malt vinegar
NT3 Rice vinegar
NT3 Wine vinegar
NT1 Essential oils
NT2 Bitter almond oils
NT2 Buchu oils
NT2 Cinnamon oils
NT2 Citronella essential oils
NT2 Citrus essential oils
NT3 Bergamot essential oils
NT4 Bergamot oils
NT3 Bitter orange essential oils
NT3 Citrus oils
NT3 Lemon essential oils
NT3 Lime essential oils
NT3 Neroli oils
NT3 Orange essential oils
NT2 Clary sage essential oils
NT2 Clove oils
NT2 Garlic oils
NT2 Hop essential oils
NT2 Lemongrass oils
NT2 Mint oils
NT2 Nutmeg oils
NT2 Oleoresins
NT2 Oregano oils
NT2 Peppermint essential oils
NT2 Petitgrain oils
NT2 Rosemary essential oils
NT2 Sage essential oils
NT2 Tea tree oils
NT2 Thyme oils
NT1 Extracts
NT2 Beef extracts
NT2 Coffee extracts
NT2 Essences
NT2 Fruit extracts
NT2 Hop extracts

NT2 Infusions
NT2 Meat extracts
NT2 Tea extracts
NT2 Yeast extracts
NT1 Flavour enhancers
NT1 Flavourings industry
NT1 Flavour modifiers
NT1 Food flavourings
NT1 Glutamates
NT2 Monosodium glutamate
NT1 Glutamic acid
NT2 Poly(γ-glutamic acid)
NT1 Hickory smoke
NT1 Hops
NT2 Hop extracts
NT2 Hop pellets
NT2 Hop substitutes
NT1 Jasmine
NT1 Liquid smoke
NT1 Liquorice
NT1 Myrrh
NT1 Natural flavourings
NT1 Smoke concentrates
NT1 Smoke flavourings
NT1 Spices
NT2 African nutmeg
NT2 *Afromomum danielli*
NT2 Ajowan
NT2 Allspice
NT2 Aniseed
NT2 Asafoetida
NT2 Black cumin
NT2 Capers
NT2 Caraway
NT2 Cardamom
NT2 *Cassia*
NT2 Cayenne pepper
NT2 Celery seeds
NT2 Chilli
NT2 Chopi
NT2 Cinnamon
NT3 *Cinnamomum zeylanicum*
NT2 Cloves
NT2 Coertuek
NT3 *Echinophora tenuifolia*
NT2 Coriander
NT3 Coriander leaves
NT3 Coriander seeds
NT2 Cumin
NT2 Curry powders
NT2 Dill
NT3 Dill leaves
NT3 Dill seeds
NT2 Fennel seeds
NT2 Fenugreek
NT2 Galangal
NT2 Garlic
NT2 Ginger
NT2 Herbs
NT3 *Agastache*
NT3 Angelica
NT3 *Artemisia*
NT3 Basil
NT4 Sweet basil
NT3 Bay
NT4 Bay leaves
NT4 Laurel
NT3 Borage
NT3 *Calamintha*
NT3 Catmint
NT3 Chamomile
NT4 Camomile
NT3 Chervil
NT3 Chives
NT3 Comfrey
NT3 Coriander leaves
NT3 Costmary
NT3 Curry leaves
NT4 *Murraya koenigii*
NT3 Davana
NT3 Dill leaves
NT3 Dittany
NT3 Hyssop
NT3 Lemon balm
NT3 Lemongrass
NT3 Marjoram
NT3 Mint
NT4 Peppermint
NT4 Spearmint
NT3 Mugwort
NT4 *Artemisia vulgaris*
NT3 Oregano
NT3 Palmarosa
NT3 Parsley
NT3 Rosemary
NT3 Rue
NT3 Sage
NT3 Samphire
NT4 Sea fennel
NT5 *Crithmum maritimum*
NT3 Savory
NT4 *Satureja*
NT3 Sorrel
NT3 Tansy
NT3 Tarragon
NT3 Thyme
NT3 Wormwood
NT2 Horseradish
NT2 Japanese pepper
NT2 Juniper
NT2 Kokum
NT2 Lovage
NT2 Mace
NT2 Mustard seeds
NT3 Ethiopian mustard
NT4 *Brassica carinata*
NT3 Indian mustard
NT2 Nutmeg
NT2 Paprika
NT2 Pepper
NT3 Black pepper
NT3 Peppercorns
NT3 *Piper longum*
NT3 White pepper
NT2 Poppy seeds
NT2 Saffron
NT2 Sarsaparilla
NT2 Star anise
NT2 Sumac
NT2 Turmeric
NT2 Wasabi
NT2 White mustard
NT2 Wild garlic
NT2 Yellow mustard
NT1 Vanilla
NT1 Vanillin
NT1 Wood smoke
RT Aroma compounds
RT Aroma concentrates
RT Flavour
RT Flavour compounds
RT Sweeteners
UF Aromatizing agents
UF Flavours

Flavourings industry
BT1 Flavourings
BT2 Additives
BT1 Food industry
BT2 Industries
UF Flavour industry

Flavour modifiers
BT1 Flavourings
BT2 Additives
RT Flavour enhancers

Flavours
USE **Flavourings**

Flavour thresholds
BT1 Sensory analysis
BT2 Analytical techniques
UF Taste thresholds

Flax seed oils
BT1 Vegetable oils
BT2 Oils vegetable
BT3 Oils
BT4 Lipids
BT5 Nutrients
BT3 Vegetable products
BT4 Plant foods
BT5 Foods
NT1 Linseed oils

Flax seeds
BT1 Oilseeds
BT2 Seeds
BT3 Plant foods
BT4 Foods
NT1 Linseeds

Fleischwurst
BT1 Sausages
BT2 Meat products
BT3 Animal foods
BT4 Foods

Flexible packs
HN packs flexible used up to vol. 31 (1999)
BT1 Packs
BT2 Containers
UF Packs flexible

Flies
BT1 Insects
BT2 Pests

Floc
BT1 Flocculation
BT2 Separation
BT3 Processing
BT4 Technology

Flocculants
BT1 Flocculation
BT2 Separation

BT3 Processing
BT4 Technology

Flocculation
HN heading up to vol. 24
BT1 Separation
BT2 Processing
BT3 Technology
NT1 Floc
NT1 Flocculants

Floors
HN introduced from vol. 39, issue 1 (2007)
BT1 Surfaces

Florentines
BT1 Bakery products
BT2 Cereal products
BT3 Plant foods
BT4 Foods

Florfenicol
HN introduced from vol. 37, issue 5 (2005)
BT1 Antibiotics
BT2 Drugs
BT3 Residues

Flotation
BT1 Separation
BT2 Processing
BT3 Technology

Flounders
BT1 Flatfish
BT2 Marine fish
BT3 Fish
BT4 Animals
BT4 Sea foods
BT5 Aquatic foods
BT6 Animal foods
BT7 Foods
NT1 Japanese flounders
NT2 *Paralichthys olivaceus*
NT1 *Platichthys flesus*

Flour
HN heading up to vol. 24 (1992)
SN use without further description to mean a cereal flour
BT1 Cereal flours
BT2 Flours cereal
BT3 Cereal products
BT4 Plant foods
BT5 Foods
RT Amylographs

Flour improvers
BT1 Bakery additives
BT2 Additives
RT Improvers

Flour mills
BT1 Mills
BT2 Equipment
BT3 Technology
BT2 Milling
BT3 Processing
BT4 Technology

Flours
HN heading from vol. 25 (1993) for non-cereal flours;under Meal up to vol. 24 (1992)
BT1 Plant foods
BT2 Foods
NT1 Cassava meal
NT1 Cottonseed meal
NT1 Cowpea meal
NT1 Legume meal
NT1 Lupin meal
NT1 Meal
NT1 Pea meal
NT1 Peanut meal
NT1 Potato meal
NT1 Rapeseed meal
NT1 Sesame seed meal
NT1 Soy meal
NT1 Sunflower meal
NT1 Yam meal

Flours cereal
HN heading from vol. 25 (1993)
SN cereal flours is also used in the index
BT1 Cereal products
BT2 Plant foods
BT3 Foods
NT1 Cereal flours
NT2 Amaranth flour
NT2 Atta
NT2 Barley flour
NT2 Buckwheat flour
NT2 Composite flours
NT2 Corn flour
NT2 Flour
NT2 Maida
NT2 Millet flour
NT2 Oat flour
NT2 Oatmeal
NT2 Quinoa flour
NT2 Rice flour
NT2 Rye flour
NT2 Sorghum flour
NT2 Triticale flour
NT2 Wheat flour
NT2 Wholemeal
RT Semolina
UF Flour specific

Flour specific
HN heading up to vol. 24 (1992) for flours of specified cereals
USE **Flours cereal**

Flow
BT1 Rheological properties
BT2 Mechanical properties
BT3 Physical properties
NT1 Flow meters
NT1 Gushing

Flow cytometry
BT1 Microbiological techniques

Flowers
BT1 Plants
NT1 Elderflowers
NT1 Safflowers

Flow injection analysis
USE **FIA**

Flow meters
BT1 Flow
BT2 Rheological properties
BT3 Mechanical properties
BT4 Physical properties

Fluchloralin
BT1 Herbicides
BT2 Pesticides
BT3 Biocides
BT3 Residues

Fludioxonil
HN introduced from vol. 39, issue 1 (2007)
BT1 Fungicides
BT2 Pesticides
BT3 Biocides
BT3 Residues

Fluidization
BT1 Processing
BT2 Technology
NT1 Fluidized beds
NT1 Microfluidization

Fluidized beds
BT1 Fluidization
BT2 Processing
BT3 Technology
RT Drying

Fluids
SN colloquial usage as synonym for liquids
BT1 Liquids
BT2 Physical phases
BT3 Chemistry
BT4 Science
NT1 Supercritical fluids
RT Microfluidic technology

Flukes
BT1 Parasites
BT2 Pests
NT1 Liver flukes

Flumequine
BT1 Quinolones
BT2 Antibiotics
BT3 Drugs
BT4 Residues

Fluometuron
BT1 Herbicides
BT2 Pesticides
BT3 Biocides
BT3 Residues

Fluoranthene
BT1 Aromatic compounds
BT2 Organic compounds
BT1 Hydrocarbons
BT2 Organic compounds

Fluorene
BT1 Aromatic compounds
BT2 Organic compounds

BT1 Hydrocarbons
BT2 Organic compounds

Fluorescence
BT1 Analytical techniques
BT1 Optical properties
BT2 Physical properties
NT1 Autofluorescence
NT1 Bioluminescence
NT1 Chemiluminescence
NT1 Green fluorescent protein
NT1 Luminescence
NT2 Phosphorescence
NT1 Thermoluminescence
RT Fluorometry
RT Radiation

Fluorescence *in situ* hybridization
HN introduced from vol. 39, issue 1 (2007)
BT1 Hybridization
BT2 Genetic techniques
BT3 Genetics

Fluorescence microscopy
BT1 Microscopy
BT2 Analytical techniques

Fluorescence spectroscopy
USE **Spectrofluorometry**

Fluorescent light
BT1 Light
BT2 Radiation

Fluoridation
BT1 Fluorides
BT2 Salts
RT Fluorosis

Fluorides
BT1 Salts
NT1 Fluoridation
RT F
RT Fluorosis

Fluorimetry
USE **Fluorometry**

Fluorine
USE **F**

Fluoroacetate
BT1 Rodenticides
BT2 Pesticides
BT3 Biocides
BT3 Residues

Fluorodensitometry
BT1 Analytical techniques

Fluorodifen
BT1 Herbicides
BT2 Pesticides
BT3 Biocides
BT3 Residues

Fluorometry
BT1 Analytical techniques
NT1 Spectrofluorometry
NT1 Spectrophotofluorometry
NT1 X-ray fluorescence spectroscopy
RT Fluorescence
RT Spectroscopy
UF Fluorimetry

Fluorosis
BT1 Diseases
RT Fluoridation
RT Fluorides

Fluridone
BT1 Herbicides
BT2 Pesticides
BT3 Biocides
BT3 Residues

Flushing
BT1 Processing
BT2 Technology
RT Carbon dioxide
RT Gases
RT Nitrogen

Fluted pumpkins
BT1 Pumpkins
BT2 Vegetables specific
BT3 Vegetables
BT4 Crops
BT5 Plants
BT4 Plant foods
BT5 Foods

Fluvalinate
BT1 Acaricides
BT2 Pesticides
BT3 Biocides
BT3 Residues
BT1 Pyrethroid insecticides
BT2 Insecticides
BT3 Pesticides
BT4 Biocides
BT4 Residues

Flying fish
BT1 Marine fish
BT2 Fish
BT3 Animals
BT3 Sea foods
BT4 Aquatic foods
BT5 Animal foods
BT6 Foods

Foamed plastics
BT1 Plastics
BT2 Packaging materials

Foam fractionation
HN introduced from vol. 39, issue 1 (2007)
BT1 Fractionation
BT2 Separation
BT3 Processing
BT4 Technology

Foaming
BT1 Functional properties
BT2 Physical properties
NT1 Foaming agents

Foaming agents
BT1 Foaming
BT2 Functional properties
BT3 Physical properties

Foaming capacity
BT1 Functional properties
BT2 Physical properties

Foaming properties
BT1 Functional properties
BT2 Physical properties

Foams
SN food foams
RT Dispersions
RT Frothing
RT Whipping

Fodder
BT1 Feeds

Foie gras
BT1 Livers
BT2 Offal
BT3 Animal foods
BT4 Foods

Foils
BT1 Packaging materials
NT1 Al foils

Folacin
BT1 Vitamin B group
BT2 Vitamins
BT3 Nutrients

Folate conjugases
USE **γ-Glutamyl hydrolases**

Folates
SN preferred syn. for pteroylglutamates
BT1 Vitamin B group
BT2 Vitamins
BT3 Nutrients
NT1 Tetrahydrofolate
RT Folic acid

Foliar sprays
BT1 Fertilizers
BT2 Cultivation
BT3 Agriculture

Folic acid
SN preferred syn. for pteroylglutamic acid
BT1 Vitamin B group
BT2 Vitamins
BT3 Nutrients
RT Folates

Folimat
USE **Omethoate**

Folpet
BT1 Dicarboximide fungicides
BT2 Fungicides
BT3 Pesticides
BT4 Biocides
BT4 Residues
UF Phaltan

Fomes
BT1 Fungi
BT2 Microorganisms

Fondants
BT1 Sugar confectionery
BT2 Plant foods
BT3 Foods

Fondues
BT1 Processed foods
BT2 Foods
BT1 Sauces
BT2 Condiments
BT3 Flavourings
BT4 Additives

Fonio
BT1 Millet
BT2 Cereals
BT3 Crops
BT4 Plants
BT3 Seeds
BT4 Plant foods
BT5 Foods

Fonofos
BT1 Organophosphorus insecticides
BT2 Insecticides
BT3 Pesticides
BT4 Biocides
BT4 Residues
BT2 Organophosphorus pesticides
BT3 Pesticides
BT4 Biocides
BT4 Residues
UF Dyfonate

Fontina cheese
BT1 Cheese varieties
BT2 Cheese
BT3 Dairy products
BT4 Animal foods
BT5 Foods

Food additives
BT1 Additives

Food aid
HN introduced from vol. 40, issue 1 (2008)
BT1 Food security
BT2 Food policy
BT3 Economics
NT1 Food stamps

Food and Agriculture Organization
HN heading up to vol. 24 (1992)
UF FAO

Food and Drug Administration
HN introduced from vol. 37, issue 5 (2005)
UF FDA

Food antioxidants
BT1 Antioxidants
BT2 Additives

Food bars
BT1 Snack foods
BT2 Processed foods
BT3 Foods
NT1 Cereal bars
NT2 Muesli bars
NT1 Confectionery bars
NT2 Chocolate bars
NT1 Ice cream bars

Foodborne diseases
SN includes diseases caused by foodborne and waterborne organisms
BT1 Diseases
RT Food poisoning

Food business
HN heading from vol. 24 (1992)
BT1 Economics
NT1 Companies
NT2 Food companies
NT1 Franchising
NT1 Mergers
NT1 Suppliers
NT2 Supply chains
NT3 Efficient consumer response
RT Planning

Food colorants
BT1 Colorants
BT2 Additives

Food companies
SN general use only; see specific commodity headings for individual company types
BT1 Companies
BT2 Food business
BT3 Economics

Food composition tables
HN introduced from vol. 39, issue 1 (2007)
BT1 Nutrition

Food emulsifiers
BT1 Emulsifiers
BT2 Additives

Food emulsions
BT1 Emulsions
BT2 Physical phases
BT3 Chemistry
BT4 Science

Food enrichment
HN heading from vol. 25 (1993); Foods enrichment up to vol. 24 (1992)
NT1 Enrichment
NT1 Fortification
NT2 Fortified foods
RT Nutritional values
UF Foods enrichment

Food factories
HN heading from vol. 25 (1993); Foods factories up to vol. 24 (1992)
NT1 Beet sugar factories
NT1 Beverages factories
NT1 Biscuit factories
NT1 Butter factories
NT1 Cane sugar factories
NT1 Cheese factories
NT1 Chocolate factories
NT1 Food factories wastes
NT2 Food factories effluents
NT1 Meat factories
NT1 Sugar factories
UF Foods factories

Food factories effluents
BT1 Effluents
BT2 Waste water
BT3 Wastes
BT3 Water
BT1 Food factories wastes
BT2 Food factories
BT2 Wastes

Food factories wastes
BT1 Food factories
BT1 Wastes
NT1 Food factories effluents

Food flavourings
BT1 Flavourings
BT2 Additives

Food frequency questionnaires
HN introduced from vol. 39, issue 1 (2007)
BT1 Dietary study techniques
BT2 Diet
BT3 Nutrition

Food guide pyramids
HN introduced from vol. 39, issue 1 (2007)
BT1 Nutrition

Food handlers
RT Handling

Food industry
HN heading from vol. 25 (1993)
BT1 Industries
NT1 Baking industry
NT1 Beet sugar industry
NT1 Beverages industry
NT1 Brewing industry
NT1 Cane sugar industry
NT1 Canning industry
NT1 Catering industry
NT1 Chocolate industry
NT1 Cocoa industry
NT1 Coffee industry
NT1 Confectionery industry
NT1 Dairy industry
NT1 Distilling industry
NT1 Fish industry
NT1 Flavourings industry
NT1 Fresh produce industry
NT1 Industry attitudes
NT1 Meat industry
NT1 Poultry meat industry
NT1 Sea foods industry
NT1 Sugar confectionery industry
NT1 Sugar industry
NT1 Wine industry
UF Foods industry

Food information
BT1 Information technology
BT2 Technology

Food intolerance
BT1 Intolerance
BT2 Diseases
NT1 Lactose intolerance
RT Allergies

Food poisoning
BT1 Poisoning
RT Foodborne diseases

Food policy
HN heading from vol. 24 (1992)
BT1 Economics
NT1 CAP
NT1 Food security
NT2 Food aid
NT3 Food stamps
NT1 Food Standards Agency
NT1 Policies
NT1 Policy
NT1 Pricing
NT2 Payment
NT2 Prices
NT1 Product liability
NT1 Taxation

Food portions
HN introduced from vol. 39, issue 1 (2007); under Cutting up to vol. 42 (2010)
BT1 Eating habits
BT2 Consumer behaviour
BT3 Consumer response
NT1 Portion sizes
RT Obesity
RT Portioning

Food powders
USE **Powders**

Food preservatives
BT1 Preservatives
BT2 Additives

Food products
USE **Foods**

Food reference materials
BT1 Reference materials
RT Analytical techniques

Foods
NT1 Animal foods
NT1 Fresh produce
NT1 Microwaveable foods
NT1 Natural foods
NT1 Novel foods
NT1 Organic foods
NT1 Perishable foods
NT1 Plant foods
NT1 Processed foods
NT1 Regional foods
UF Food products
UF Foodstuffs

Food safety
HN heading from vol. 24 (1992); under Health up to vol. 23 (1991)
SN general use only
NT1 Biosecurity
NT1 Bioterrorism
NT1 Food safety additives
NT1 Food safety animal foods
NT2 Food safety dairy products
NT1 Food safety beverages
NT1 Food safety pet foods
NT1 Food safety plant foods
NT1 GRAS status
NT1 GRAS substances
NT1 HACCP
RT Bacteriological quality
RT Critical control points
RT European Food Safety Authority
RT Hazards
RT Hazards analysis
RT Health
RT Health hazards
RT Hygiene
RT Microbiological quality
RT Parasites
RT Pathogens
RT Pests
RT Plasmids
RT Poisoning
RT Product recalls
RT Public health
RT Residues
RT Risk communication
RT Risks assessment
RT Risks management
RT Toxicology
RT Toxins

Food safety additives
HN heading from vol. 28 (1996)
BT1 Food safety
RT Migration
RT Plasticizers

Food safety animal foods
HN heading from vol. 28 (1996)
BT1 Food safety
NT1 Food safety dairy products

Food safety beverages
HN heading from vol. 28 (1996)
BT1 Food safety

Food safety dairy products
HN heading from vol. 28 (1996)
BT1 Food safety animal foods
BT2 Food safety

Food safety pet foods
HN introduced from vol. 39, issue 1 (2007); heading
BT1 Food safety

Food safety plant foods
HN heading from vol. 28 (1996)
BT1 Food safety

Food science
BT1 Science
NT1 Dairy science

Food security
HN heading from vol. 42 (2010); under Food policy up to vol. 41 (2009)
BT1 Food policy
BT2 Economics
NT1 Food aid
NT2 Food stamps
RT Poverty
RT Socioeconomic factors
RT Sustainability

Foods enrichment
HN heading up to vol. 24 (1992)
USE **Food enrichment**

Food service
USE **Foods service**

Foodservice
USE **Foods service**

Foods factories
HN heading up to vol. 24 (1992)
USE **Food factories**

Foods industry
USE **Food industry**

Foods service
BT1 Catering
UF Food service
UF Foodservice

Food stabilizers
BT1 Stabilizers
BT2 Additives

Food stamps
HN introduced from vol. 42, issue 1 (2010)
BT1 Food aid
BT2 Food security
BT3 Food policy
BT4 Economics

Food Standards Agency
BT1 Food policy
BT2 Economics

Foodstuffs
USE **Foods**

Food supplements
NT1 Sports supplements
RT Health foods
RT Nutrition
UF Dietary supplements

Food technology
BT1 Processing
BT2 Technology

Food thickeners
BT1 Thickeners
BT2 Additives

Foot and mouth disease
BT1 Animal diseases
BT2 Diseases animal
BT3 Diseases

Foot and mouth disease virus
HN introduced from vol. 43, issue 1 (2011)
BT1 Apthovirus
BT2 Viruses
BT3 Microorganisms

Forcemeat
BT1 Fillings

Foreign bodies
USE **Contaminants**

Formaldehyde
SN syn. methanal
BT1 Aldehydes
BT2 Carbonyl compounds
BT3 Organic compounds
BT1 Preservatives
BT2 Additives
NT1 Formalin
NT1 Formol
NT1 Methanal
RT Disinfection

Formalin
SN syn. formol
BT1 Formaldehyde
BT2 Aldehydes
BT3 Carbonyl compounds
BT4 Organic compounds
BT2 Preservatives
BT3 Additives

Formamide
BT1 Amides
BT2 Organic nitrogen compounds
BT1 Solvents

Formic acid
BT1 Organic acids
BT2 Acids
BT1 Preservatives
BT2 Additives

Formol
SN syn. formalin
BT1 Formaldehyde
BT2 Aldehydes
BT3 Carbonyl compounds
BT4 Organic compounds
BT2 Preservatives
BT3 Additives

Formosa
USE **Taiwan**

Formothion
BT1 Acaricides
BT2 Pesticides
BT3 Biocides
BT3 Residues
BT1 Organophosphorus insecticides
BT2 Insecticides
BT3 Pesticides
BT4 Biocides
BT4 Residues
BT2 Organophosphorus pesticides
BT3 Pesticides
BT4 Biocides
BT4 Residues
UF Anthio

Formulae
BT1 Mathematics
BT2 Science
RT Equations

Fortification
BT1 Food enrichment
NT1 Fortified foods
RT Enrichment

Fortified foods
HN introduced from vol. 39, issue 1 (2007)
BT1 Fortification
BT2 Food enrichment
BT1 Processed foods
BT2 Foods

Fortified wines
BT1 Wines
BT2 Alcoholic beverages
BT3 Beverages alcoholic
BT4 Beverages
NT1 Madeira
NT1 Marsala
NT1 Port
NT1 Sherry
RT Dessert wines

Fortunella
BT1 Fruits specific
BT2 Fruits
BT3 Crops
BT4 Plants
BT3 Plant foods
BT4 Foods

Fossa cheese
BT1 Cheese varieties
BT2 Cheese
BT3 Dairy products
BT4 Animal foods
BT5 Foods

Fouling
RT Membranes
RT Surfaces

Fourier transform IR spectroscopy
HN FTIR spectroscopy used in the index from vol. 35, issue 6 (2003)
USE **FTIR spectroscopy**

Fowl
BT1 Poultry
BT2 Birds

Foxtail millet
BT1 Millet
BT2 Cereals
BT3 Crops
BT4 Plants
BT3 Seeds
BT4 Plant foods
BT5 Foods

f.p.
BT1 Thermophysical properties
BT2 Physical properties
RT Cryoscopy
UF Freezing point

FPC
HN Fish protein concentrates was a heading up to vol. 24 (1992)
BT1 Protein concentrates
BT2 Concentrates
BT3 Processed foods
BT4 Foods
BT2 Protein products
UF Fish protein concentrates

Fractionation
BT1 Separation
BT2 Processing
BT3 Technology
NT1 Foam fractionation
RT Distillation

Fracture properties
BT1 Mechanical properties
BT2 Physical properties

France
HN heading up to vol. 24 (1992)
BT1 Europe
BT1 European Union
RT Organization for Economic Cooperation and Development

Franchising
BT1 Food business
BT2 Economics

Francisella
HN introduced from vol. 41, issue 1 (2009)
BT1 Bacteria
BT2 Microorganisms
NT1 *Francisella tularensis*

Francisella tularensis
HN introduced from vol. 41, issue 1 (2009)
BT1 *Francisella*
BT2 Bacteria
BT3 Microorganisms

Frankfurters
BT1 Sausages
BT2 Meat products
BT3 Animal foods
BT4 Foods
NT1 Hot dogs
NT1 Turkey frankfurters
NT1 Wieners

Frappe
BT1 Sugar confectionery
BT2 Plant foods
BT3 Foods

Fraud
BT1 Economics

Free radicals
BT1 Radicals

NT1 Reactive nitrogen species
NT2 Nitric oxide
NT2 Peroxynitrite
NT1 Reactive oxygen species
NT2 Peroxides
NT3 H_2O_2
NT3 Hydroperoxides
NT2 Superoxides
RT Health
RT Oxidation
RT Oxidative stress
RT Radical scavenging activity

Freeze concentration
BT1 Concentration
BT2 Processing
BT3 Technology

Freeze dried foods
BT1 Dried foods
BT2 Processed foods
BT3 Foods
RT Freeze drying

Freeze driers
BT1 Driers
BT2 Drying
BT3 Thermal processing
BT4 Processing thermal
BT5 Processing
BT6 Technology
BT2 Equipment
BT3 Technology
BT1 Freeze drying
BT2 Drying
BT3 Thermal processing
BT4 Processing thermal
BT5 Processing
BT6 Technology

Freeze drying
HN heading was Freeze-drying up to vol. 24 (1992)
BT1 Drying
BT2 Thermal processing
BT3 Processing thermal
BT4 Processing
BT5 Technology
NT1 Freeze driers
RT Dried foods
RT Freeze dried foods
UF Freeze-drying
UF Lyophilization

Freeze-drying
HN heading up to vol. 24 (1992)
USE **Freeze drying**

Freezers
BT1 Equipment
BT2 Technology
BT1 Freezing
BT2 Thermal processing
BT3 Processing thermal
BT4 Processing
BT5 Technology

Freeze-thaw stability
HN introduced from vol. 41, issue 1 (2009)
BT1 Freezing
BT2 Thermal processing
BT3 Processing thermal
BT4 Processing
BT5 Technology
BT1 Stability
BT2 Physical properties
BT1 Thawing
BT2 Thermal processing
BT3 Processing thermal
BT4 Processing
BT5 Technology

Freezing
BT1 Thermal processing
BT2 Processing thermal
BT3 Processing
BT4 Technology
NT1 Cryogenics
NT1 Cryopreservation
NT1 Deep freezing
NT1 Freezers
NT1 Freeze-thaw stability
NT1 Ice nucleation activity
NT1 Immersion freezing
NT1 Liquid nitrogen
NT1 Pressure shift freezing
RT Frozen foods
RT Refrigeration

Freezing point
USE **f.p.**

French beans
BT1 Common beans
BT2 Legumes
BT3 Vegetables specific
BT4 Vegetables
BT5 Crops
BT6 Plants
BT5 Plant foods
BT6 Foods

French bread
HN introduced from vol. 39, issue 1 (2007)
BT1 Bread
BT2 Bakery products
BT3 Cereal products
BT4 Plant foods
BT5 Foods

French dressing
BT1 Salad dressings
BT2 Condiments
BT3 Flavourings
BT4 Additives

French fries
BT1 Chips
BT2 Processed foods
BT3 Foods
BT1 Potato products
BT2 Potatoes
BT3 Vegetables specific
BT4 Vegetables
BT5 Crops
BT6 Plants
BT5 Plant foods
BT6 Foods

French Guiana
BT1 South America
BT2 America

Freons
HN heading up to vol. 24
BT1 Refrigerants
BT2 Refrigeration
BT3 Thermal processing
BT4 Processing thermal
BT5 Processing
BT6 Technology

Fresh cheese
BT1 Cheese varieties
BT2 Cheese
BT3 Dairy products
BT4 Animal foods
BT5 Foods

Freshness
BT1 Shelf life

Fresh produce
HN introduced from vol. 39, issue 1 (2007)
BT1 Foods
NT1 Fresh produce industry

Fresh produce industry
HN introduced from vol. 39, issue 1 (2007)
BT1 Food industry
BT2 Industries
BT1 Fresh produce
BT2 Foods

Freshwater clams
BT1 Clams
BT2 Bivalves
BT3 Molluscs
BT4 Shellfish
BT5 Animals
BT5 Sea foods
BT6 Aquatic foods
BT7 Animal foods
BT8 Foods

Freshwater fish
BT1 Fish
BT2 Animals
BT2 Sea foods
BT3 Aquatic foods
BT4 Animal foods
BT5 Foods
NT1 Ayu
NT1 Bream
NT1 Burbot
NT1 Carp
NT2 Bighead carp
NT3 *Aristichthys nobilis*
NT2 Crucian carp
NT2 *Cyprinus carpio*
NT2 Grass carp
NT3 White amur
NT2 Rohu
NT3 *Labeo rohita*
NT2 Silver carp
NT1 Catfish
NT2 Channel catfish
NT3 *Ictalurus punctatus*

NT2 *Silurus asotus*
NT1 Chub
NT2 *Leuciscus cephalus*
NT1 *Colossoma macropomum*
NT1 Eels
NT1 Nile perch
NT1 Pacu
NT1 Perch
NT2 *Perca fluviatilis*
NT2 Yellow perch
NT1 Pike
NT1 River fish
NT1 Roach
NT1 Snakehead
NT1 Sunfish
NT1 Tench
NT1 Tilapia
NT2 Nile tilapia
NT3 Bolti
NT3 *Oreochromis niloticus*
NT3 *Tilapia nilotica*
NT2 *Oreochromis*
NT3 *Oreochromis niloticus*
NT1 Vendace
NT2 Coregonus albula
NT1 Walleye

FRG
HN used as abbrev. for Federal Republic of Germany up to vol. 24 (1992)
USE **Germany**

Friabilimeters
BT1 Apparatus
BT2 Technology

Friabilins
BT1 Cereal proteins
BT2 Proteins cereal
BT3 Vegetable proteins
BT4 Proteins vegetable
BT5 Proteins
BT6 Nutrients
BT5 Vegetable products
BT6 Plant foods
BT7 Foods

Fricadelles
BT1 Meat products
BT2 Animal foods
BT3 Foods

Friction
HN introduced from vol. 39, issue 1 (2007)
BT1 Rheological properties
BT2 Mechanical properties
BT3 Physical properties

Fried foods
BT1 Processed foods
BT2 Foods
NT1 Fritters
NT1 Tempura
RT Chips
RT Fast foods
RT Frying

Frigate mackerel
HN introduced from vol. 37, issue 5 (2005)
BT1 Mackerel
BT2 Marine fish
BT3 Fish
BT4 Animals
BT4 Sea foods
BT5 Aquatic foods
BT6 Animal foods
BT7 Foods
BT2 Oily fish
BT3 Fish
BT4 Animals
BT4 Sea foods
BT5 Aquatic foods
BT6 Animal foods
BT7 Foods

Fritters
BT1 Fried foods
BT2 Processed foods
BT3 Foods

Frogs
BT1 Animals

Frogs legs
HN heading up to vol. 24
BT1 Meat products
BT2 Animal foods
BT3 Foods

Fromage frais
BT1 Dairy products
BT2 Animal foods
BT3 Foods

Frostings
BT1 Toppings

Frothing
BT1 Processing
BT2 Technology
RT Foams

Frozen beverages
BT1 Beverages
NT1 Soft frozen beverages

Frozen confectionery
HN introduced from vol. 39, issue 1 (2007)
BT1 Confectionery
BT2 Bakery products
BT3 Cereal products
BT4 Plant foods
BT5 Foods
BT2 Sugar confectionery
BT3 Plant foods
BT4 Foods
BT1 Frozen foods
BT2 Processed foods
BT3 Foods

Frozen desserts
BT1 Desserts
BT2 Processed foods
BT3 Foods
BT1 Frozen foods
BT2 Processed foods
BT3 Foods

Frozen dough
BT1 Dough
BT2 Bakery products
BT3 Cereal products
BT4 Plant foods
BT5 Foods
BT1 Frozen foods
BT2 Processed foods
BT3 Foods

Frozen foods
BT1 Processed foods
BT2 Foods
NT1 Frozen confectionery
NT1 Frozen desserts
NT1 Frozen dough
NT1 Frozen meals
NT1 Frozen pet foods
NT1 Frozen yoghurt
NT1 Ice cream
NT2 Ice cream bars
NT2 Ice cream factories
NT2 Ice cream mixes
NT2 Ice milk
NT2 Ices
NT2 Mellorine
NT2 Milk ice
NT1 Ice lollies
NT1 Water ices
RT Freezing

Frozen meals
BT1 Frozen foods
BT2 Processed foods
BT3 Foods
BT1 Meals
BT2 Processed foods
BT3 Foods

Frozen pet foods
HN introduced from vol. 39, issue 1 (2007)
BT1 Frozen foods
BT2 Processed foods
BT3 Foods
BT1 Pet foods

Frozen storage
BT1 Storage cold
BT2 Storage

Frozen yoghurt
BT1 Frozen foods
BT2 Processed foods
BT3 Foods
BT1 Yoghurt
BT2 Fermented milk
BT3 Fermented dairy products
BT4 Dairy products
BT5 Animal foods
BT6 Foods
BT4 Fermented foods
BT5 Processed foods
BT6 Foods
BT3 Milk
BT4 Dairy products
BT5 Animal foods

BT6 Foods
RT Ice cream

Fructans
BT1 Polysaccharides
BT2 Carbohydrates
BT3 Nutrients
BT3 Organic compounds
NT1 Inulin
NT1 Levans
RT Fructooligosaccharides

β-Fructofuranosidases
SN EC 3.2.1.26
BT1 Glycosidases
BT2 Hydrolases
BT3 Enzymes
UF Invertases
UF Saccharases

Fructokinases
SN EC 2.7.1.4
BT1 Kinases
BT2 Phosphotransferases
BT3 Transferases
BT4 Enzymes

Fructooligosaccharides
HN under Polysaccharides and Sugars up to vol. 42 (2010)
BT1 Oligosaccharides
BT2 Polysaccharides
BT3 Carbohydrates
BT4 Nutrients
BT4 Organic compounds
BT2 Sugars
BT3 Carbohydrates
BT4 Nutrients
BT4 Organic compounds
BT3 Plant foods
BT4 Foods
NT1 Kestose
NT1 Nystose
RT Fructans
UF Oligofructose

Fructose
HN under Sugars up to vol. 42 (2010)
BT1 Monosaccharides
BT2 Sugars
BT3 Carbohydrates
BT4 Nutrients
BT4 Organic compounds
BT3 Plant foods
BT4 Foods
UF Laevulose

Fructose-bisphosphate aldolases
SN EC 4.1.2.13
BT1 Lyases
BT2 Enzymes
UF Aldolases

Fructose high corn syrups
BT1 Corn syrups
BT2 Sugar syrups
BT3 Plant foods
BT4 Foods

Fructose syrups
BT1 Sugar syrups
BT2 Plant foods
BT3 Foods

Fructosyltransferases
SN includes members of EC 2.4.1
BT1 Glycosyltransferases
BT2 Transferases
BT3 Enzymes

Fruit beverages
BT1 Fruit juice beverages
BT2 Soft drinks
BT3 Beverages

Fruit brandies
HN under Spirits up to vol. 42 (2010)
BT1 Brandies
BT2 Spirits
BT3 Alcoholic beverages
BT4 Beverages alcoholic
BT5 Beverages
NT1 Apple brandy
NT2 Calvados
NT1 Kirsch
NT1 Rakia
NT1 Slivovitz

Fruit bread
BT1 Bread
BT2 Bakery products
BT3 Cereal products
BT4 Plant foods
BT5 Foods

Fruit compotes
BT1 Fruit products
BT2 Plant foods
BT3 Foods

Fruit concentrates
HN introduced from vol. 39, issue 1 (2007)
BT1 Concentrates
BT2 Processed foods
BT3 Foods
BT1 Fruit products
BT2 Plant foods
BT3 Foods

Fruit cordials
BT1 Soft drinks
BT2 Beverages
RT Squash

Fruit desserts
BT1 Desserts
BT2 Processed foods
BT3 Foods
BT1 Fruit products
BT2 Plant foods
BT3 Foods

Fruit extracts
BT1 Extracts
BT2 Flavourings
BT3 Additives
BT1 Fruit products
BT2 Plant foods
BT3 Foods

Fruit flies
BT1 Insects
BT2 Pests

Fruit gums
BT1 Jelly confectionery
BT2 Sugar confectionery
BT3 Plant foods
BT4 Foods

Fruitiness
BT1 Flavour
BT2 Sensory properties

Fruit jellies
BT1 Fruit products
BT2 Plant foods
BT3 Foods

Fruit juice beverages
HN heading from vol. 25 (1993)
BT1 Soft drinks
BT2 Beverages
NT1 Citrus beverages
NT1 Fruit beverages
NT1 Orange juice beverages
RT Fruit juices

Fruit juice concentrates
HN heading from vol. 30 (1998); under Fruit juices and Concentrates up to vol. 29 (1997)
BT1 Concentrates
BT2 Processed foods
BT3 Foods
BT1 Fruit juices
BT2 Fruit products
BT3 Plant foods
BT4 Foods
BT2 Soft drinks
BT3 Beverages
NT1 Apple juice concentrates
NT1 Citrus juice concentrates
NT2 Orange juice concentrates
NT1 Grape juice concentrates

Fruit juices
BT1 Fruit products
BT2 Plant foods
BT3 Foods
BT1 Soft drinks
BT2 Beverages
NT1 Apple juices
NT2 Apple cider
NT2 Apple juice concentrates
NT1 Apricot juices
NT1 Banana juices
NT1 Barbados cherry juices
NT1 Berry juices
NT2 Bilberry juices
NT2 Blackberry juices
NT2 Blackcurrant juices
NT2 Blueberry juices
NT2 Cranberry juices
NT2 Elderberry juices
NT2 Raspberry juices
NT2 Redcurrant juices
NT2 Strawberry juices
NT1 Cashew apple juices
NT1 Cherry juices
NT1 Citrus juices

NT2 Citrus juice concentrates
NT3 Orange juice concentrates
NT2 Grapefruit juices
NT2 Lemon juices
NT2 Lime juices
NT2 Orange juices
NT3 Mandarin juices
NT4 Tangerine juices
NT3 Orange juice concentrates
NT1 Fig juices
NT1 Fruit juice concentrates
NT2 Apple juice concentrates
NT2 Citrus juice concentrates
NT3 Orange juice concentrates
NT2 Grape juice concentrates
NT1 Fruit nectars
NT2 Apricot nectars
NT2 Mango nectars
NT2 Papaya nectars
NT2 Peach nectars
NT2 Pineapple nectars
NT1 Grape juices
NT2 Grape juice concentrates
NT1 Guava juices
NT1 Hawthorn juices
NT1 Kiwifruit juices
NT1 Mango juices
NT1 Melon juices
NT1 Musts
NT2 Apple musts
NT2 Grape musts
NT3 Concentrated rectified musts
NT1 Noni juices
NT1 Passion fruit juices
NT1 Peach juices
NT1 Pear juices
NT1 Persimmon juices
NT1 Pineapple juices
NT1 Plum juices
NT1 Pomegranate juices
NT1 Prune juices
NT1 Quince juices
NT1 Sea buckthorn juices
NT1 Tomato juices
NT1 Watermelon juices
RT Fruit juice beverages

Fruit leathers
BT1 Fruit products
BT2 Plant foods
BT3 Foods

Fruit liqueurs
BT1 Liqueurs
BT2 Alcoholic beverages
BT3 Beverages alcoholic
BT4 Beverages
NT1 Cassis
NT1 Cherry brandy
NT1 Limoncello

Fruit nectars
HN under Fruit products up to vol. 24 (1992)
BT1 Fruit juices
BT2 Fruit products
BT3 Plant foods
BT4 Foods
BT2 Soft drinks
BT3 Beverages
NT1 Apricot nectars
NT1 Mango nectars
NT1 Papaya nectars
NT1 Peach nectars
NT1 Pineapple nectars

Fruit pastes
HN introduced from vol. 41, issue 1 (2009)
BT1 Fruit products
BT2 Plant foods
BT3 Foods
BT1 Pastes
BT2 Processed foods
BT3 Foods

Fruit peel
BT1 Fruits
BT2 Crops
BT3 Plants
BT2 Plant foods
BT3 Foods
BT1 Peel
RT Apple peel
RT Banana peel
RT Citrus peel
RT Lemon peel
RT Orange peel

Fruit pies
BT1 Fruit products
BT2 Plant foods
BT3 Foods
BT1 Pies
BT2 Bakery products
BT3 Cereal products
BT4 Plant foods
BT5 Foods

Fruit preserves
HN heading from vol. 25 (1993); under Preserves up to vol. 24 (1992)
BT1 Fruit products
BT2 Plant foods
BT3 Foods
BT1 Preserves
BT2 Processed foods
BT3 Foods
NT1 Jams
NT2 Apricot jams
NT2 Grape jams
NT2 Jelly
NT2 Mango jams
NT2 Marmalades
NT2 Quince jams
NT2 Strawberry jams

Fruit products
BT1 Plant foods
BT2 Foods
NT1 Candied fruits
NT1 Compotes
NT1 Fruit compotes
NT1 Fruit concentrates
NT1 Fruit desserts
NT1 Fruit extracts
NT1 Fruit jellies
NT1 Fruit juices
NT2 Apple juices
NT3 Apple cider
NT3 Apple juice concentrates
NT2 Apricot juices
NT2 Banana juices
NT2 Barbados cherry juices
NT2 Berry juices
NT3 Bilberry juices
NT3 Blackberry juices
NT3 Blackcurrant juices
NT3 Blueberry juices
NT3 Cranberry juices
NT3 Elderberry juices
NT3 Raspberry juices
NT3 Redcurrant juices
NT3 Strawberry juices
NT2 Cashew apple juices
NT2 Cherry juices
NT2 Citrus juices
NT3 Citrus juice concentrates
NT4 Orange juice concentrates
NT3 Grapefruit juices
NT3 Lemon juices
NT3 Lime juices
NT3 Orange juices
NT4 Mandarin juices
NT5 Tangerine juices
NT4 Orange juice concentrates
NT2 Fig juices
NT2 Fruit juice concentrates
NT3 Apple juice concentrates
NT3 Citrus juice concentrates
NT4 Orange juice concentrates
NT3 Grape juice concentrates
NT2 Fruit nectars
NT3 Apricot nectars
NT3 Mango nectars
NT3 Papaya nectars
NT3 Peach nectars
NT3 Pineapple nectars
NT2 Grape juices
NT3 Grape juice concentrates
NT2 Guava juices
NT2 Hawthorn juices
NT2 Kiwifruit juices
NT2 Mango juices
NT2 Melon juices
NT2 Musts
NT3 Apple musts
NT3 Grape musts
NT4 Concentrated rectified musts
NT2 Noni juices
NT2 Passion fruit juices
NT2 Peach juices
NT2 Pear juices
NT2 Persimmon juices
NT2 Pineapple juices
NT2 Plum juices
NT2 Pomegranate juices
NT2 Prune juices
NT2 Quince juices
NT2 Sea buckthorn juices
NT2 Tomato juices
NT2 Watermelon juices
NT1 Fruit leathers
NT1 Fruit pastes

NT1 Fruit pies
NT1 Fruit preserves
NT2 Jams
NT3 Apricot jams
NT3 Grape jams
NT3 Jelly
NT3 Mango jams
NT3 Marmalades
NT3 Quince jams
NT3 Strawberry jams
NT1 Fruit pulps
NT2 Apple pulps
NT2 Apricot pulps
NT2 Banana pulps
NT2 Guava pulps
NT2 Mango pulps
NT2 Peach pulps
NT2 Strawberry pulps
NT2 Tomato pulps
NT1 Fruit purees
NT2 Apple purees
NT2 Apricot purees
NT2 Banana purees
NT2 Guava purees
NT2 Mango purees
NT2 Peach purees
NT2 Strawberry purees
NT2 Tomato purees
NT1 Fruit salads
NT1 Pekmez
RT Salads

Fruit pulps
BT1 Fruit products
BT2 Plant foods
BT3 Foods
BT1 Pulps
BT2 Processed foods
BT3 Foods
NT1 Apple pulps
NT1 Apricot pulps
NT1 Banana pulps
NT1 Guava pulps
NT1 Mango pulps
NT1 Peach pulps
NT1 Strawberry pulps
NT1 Tomato pulps

Fruit purees
BT1 Fruit products
BT2 Plant foods
BT3 Foods
BT1 Purees
BT2 Pulps
BT3 Processed foods
BT4 Foods
NT1 Apple purees
NT1 Apricot purees
NT1 Banana purees
NT1 Guava purees
NT1 Mango purees
NT1 Peach purees
NT1 Strawberry purees
NT1 Tomato purees

Fruits
SN use for fruits in general
BT1 Crops
BT2 Plants
BT1 Plant foods
BT2 Foods
NT1 Fruit peel
NT1 Fruits dried
NT2 Dried fruits
NT3 Currants
NT3 Dried figs
NT3 Prunes
NT3 Raisins
NT3 Sultanas
NT1 Fruits specific
NT2 Acai
NT2 Ackee
NT2 *Actinidia arguta*
NT2 Aiele fruits
NT2 Amla
NT2 Apples
NT3 Apple musts
NT3 Apple pectins
NT3 Apple peel
NT3 Apple pomaces
NT3 Apple pulps
NT3 Apple purees
NT3 Apple sauces
NT3 Cider apples
NT2 Apricots
NT3 Apricot jams
NT3 Apricot kernels
NT3 Apricot pulps
NT3 Apricot purees
NT3 Apricot seeds
NT2 *Aronia*
NT2 Babaco
NT2 Bacuri
NT2 Bael fruit
NT2 Bananas
NT3 Banana peel
NT3 Banana pulps
NT3 Banana purees
NT3 *Musa cavendishii*
NT3 Plantains
NT2 Barbados cherries
NT2 Berries
NT3 Bayberries
NT3 Bearberries
NT3 Berberries
NT3 Bilberries
NT3 Blackberries
NT3 Blackcurrants
NT3 Black nightshade
NT3 Blueberries
NT3 Boysenberries
NT3 Chokeberries
NT3 Cloudberries
NT3 Cranberries
NT3 Crowberries
NT3 Dewberries
NT3 Elderberries
NT3 Gooseberries
NT3 Grapes
NT4 Grape jams
NT4 Grape pomaces
NT4 Grape seeds
NT4 Grape skins
NT4 Muscadine grapes
NT4 Seedless grapes
NT4 Table grapes
NT4 *Vitis vinifera*
NT4 Winemaking grapes
NT3 Huckleberries
NT3 Lingonberries
NT4 Cowberries
NT3 Loganberries
NT3 Mulberries
NT3 Raspberries
NT3 Redcurrants
NT3 Rowanberries
NT3 Strawberries
NT4 Strawberry jams
NT4 Strawberry pulps
NT4 Strawberry purees
NT3 Strawberry tree fruits
NT3 Whitecurrants
NT3 Wolfberries
NT3 Youngberries
NT2 Breadfruit
NT2 Bush butter
NT2 Cacti
NT2 Cactus pears
NT2 Caja
NT2 Camu-camu
NT2 Cape gooseberries
NT3 Goldenberries
NT2 Carambolas
NT3 Star fruit
NT2 Cashew apples
NT2 Cherimoya
NT2 Cherries
NT3 Morello cherries
NT3 Sour cherries
NT3 Sweet cherries
NT2 Cherry laurel
NT2 Citrus fruits
NT3 Bitter oranges
NT3 Citrons
NT3 Citrus pectins
NT3 Citrus peel
NT3 *Citrus tamurana*
NT3 Galgals
NT3 Grapefruit
NT4 Grapefruit peel
NT3 Ki-mikan
NT3 Kumquats
NT3 Lemons
NT4 Lemon peel
NT3 Limes
NT3 Oranges
NT4 Mandarins
NT5 Clementines
NT5 Kinnow mandarins
NT5 Ponkans
NT5 Satsuma mandarins
NT5 Satsumas
NT5 Tangerines
NT4 Orange peel
NT3 Ortanique
NT3 Pomelos
NT4 *Citrus grandis*
NT4 Pummelos
NT4 Shaddocks
NT3 Sweet limes
NT3 Tangelo
NT3 Tangor
NT3 Yuzu
NT2 Cocona
NT2 Cornelian cherries
NT2 Cupuacu
NT2 *Curculigo latifolia*
NT2 Custard apples

NT2 Dates
NT2 Durian
NT2 Exotic fruits
NT2 Feijoa
NT2 Figs
 NT3 Dried figs
NT2 *Fortunella*
NT2 Guavas
 NT3 Guava pulps
 NT3 Guava purees
NT2 Hawthorn fruits
NT2 Jaboticaba
NT2 Jak fruits
NT2 Japanese apricots
 NT3 *Prunus mume*
NT2 Jelly figs
 NT3 *Ficus awkeotsang*
NT2 Jujubes
NT2 Kiwano
NT2 Kiwifruit
 NT3 *Actinidia chinensis*
 NT3 *Actinidia deliciosa*
 NT3 *Actinidia polygama*
NT2 Langsat
NT2 Litchis
NT2 Longans
NT2 Loquats
NT2 Malay apples
NT2 Mamey
NT2 Mangoes
 NT3 African mangoes
 NT3 Mango jams
 NT3 Mango kernels
 NT3 Mango pickles
 NT3 Mango pulps
 NT3 Mango purees
NT2 Mangosteens
NT2 Marula
 NT3 *Sclerocarya birrea*
NT2 Medlars
NT2 Melons
 NT3 Cantaloupes
 NT3 Honeydew melons
 NT3 Muskmelons
NT2 Myrobalans
NT2 Myrtle
NT2 Naranjilla
 NT3 Lulo
NT2 Noni
NT2 Olives
 NT3 Black olives
 NT3 Table olives
NT2 Omija
NT2 Papayas
 NT3 Pawpaws
NT2 Passion fruits
 NT3 *Passiflora edulis*
NT2 Peaches
 NT3 Nectarines
 NT3 Peach pulps
 NT3 Peach purees
NT2 Pears
 NT3 Asian pears
 NT3 Chinese pears
 NT3 Japanese pears
NT2 Pepino
NT2 Persimmons
NT2 Phalsa
NT2 Pineapples
NT2 Pitayos
NT2 Plums
 NT3 Damsons
 NT3 Greengages
 NT3 Japanese plums
NT2 Pome fruits
NT2 Pomegranates
NT2 Prickly pears
 NT3 *Opuntia ficus-indica*
NT2 Quinces
 NT3 Quince jams
NT2 Rambutan
NT2 Rose apples
NT2 Rosehips
NT2 Sapodillas
NT2 Saskatoon fruits
NT2 Sea buckthorn
NT2 Sloes
NT2 Soursop
NT2 *Spondias*
NT2 Star apples
NT2 Stone fruits
NT2 Sugar apples
NT2 Tamarillos
NT2 Tamarinds
NT2 Tomatillos
NT2 Tomatoes
 NT3 Cherry tomatoes
 NT3 Tomato products
  NT4 Tomato concentrates
  NT4 Tomato ketchups
   NT5 Tomato catsups
  NT4 Tomato pastes
  NT4 Tomato powders
  NT4 Tomato pulps
  NT4 Tomato purees
  NT4 Tomato sauces
 NT3 Tomato skins
NT2 Tropical fruits
NT2 Watermelons
 NT3 Egusi
NT1 Nuts
NT2 Acorns
NT2 Almonds
 NT3 Sweet almonds
NT2 Australian chestnuts
NT2 Brazil nuts
NT2 Butternuts
NT2 Cashew nuts
NT2 Cedar nuts
NT2 Chestnuts
 NT3 Japanese chestnuts
 NT3 Sweet chestnuts
NT2 Chilean hazelnuts
NT2 Coconuts
 NT3 Bongkrek
 NT3 Coconut cream
 NT3 Coconut milk
 NT3 Coconut water
 NT3 Copra
 NT3 Desiccated coconut
 NT3 Nata
NT2 Cola nuts
 NT3 *Cola nitida*
NT2 Conophor nuts
NT2 Ginkgo nuts
NT2 Gorgon nuts
NT2 Hazelnuts
NT2 Hickory nuts
NT2 Macadamia nuts
NT2 Nut pastes
 NT3 Peanut pastes
NT2 Nut products
NT2 Peanuts
 NT3 Ontjom
 NT3 Peanut butter
 NT3 Peanut meal
 NT3 Peanut milk
 NT3 Peanut pastes
 NT3 Peanut products
 NT3 Peanut proteins
 NT3 Roasted peanuts
NT2 Pecan nuts
NT2 Pine nuts
NT2 Pistachio nuts
NT2 Walnuts

Fruit salads
BT1 Fruit products
 BT2 Plant foods
  BT3 Foods
BT1 Salads

Fruits dried
SN dried fruits is also used in the index
BT1 Dried foods
 BT2 Processed foods
  BT3 Foods
BT1 Fruits
 BT2 Crops
  BT3 Plants
 BT2 Plant foods
  BT3 Foods
NT1 Dried fruits
 NT2 Currants
 NT2 Dried figs
 NT2 Prunes
 NT2 Raisins
 NT2 Sultanas

Fruits specific
SN use for specific types of fruit
BT1 Fruits
 BT2 Crops
  BT3 Plants
 BT2 Plant foods
  BT3 Foods
NT1 Acai
NT1 Ackee
NT1 *Actinidia arguta*
NT1 Aiele fruits
NT1 Amla
NT1 Apples
 NT2 Apple musts
 NT2 Apple pectins
 NT2 Apple peel
 NT2 Apple pomaces
 NT2 Apple pulps
 NT2 Apple purees
 NT2 Apple sauces
 NT2 Cider apples
NT1 Apricots
 NT2 Apricot jams
 NT2 Apricot kernels
 NT2 Apricot pulps
 NT2 Apricot purees
 NT2 Apricot seeds
NT1 *Aronia*
NT1 Babaco

NT1 Bacuri
NT1 Bael fruit
NT1 Bananas
NT2 Banana peel
NT2 Banana pulps
NT2 Banana purees
NT2 *Musa cavendishii*
NT2 Plantains
NT1 Barbados cherries
NT1 Berries
NT2 Bayberries
NT2 Bearberries
NT2 Berberries
NT2 Bilberries
NT2 Blackberries
NT2 Blackcurrants
NT2 Black nightshade
NT2 Blueberries
NT2 Boysenberries
NT2 Chokeberries
NT2 Cloudberries
NT2 Cranberries
NT2 Crowberries
NT2 Dewberries
NT2 Elderberries
NT2 Gooseberries
NT2 Grapes
NT3 Grape jams
NT3 Grape pomaces
NT3 Grape seeds
NT3 Grape skins
NT3 Muscadine grapes
NT3 Seedless grapes
NT3 Table grapes
NT3 *Vitis vinifera*
NT3 Winemaking grapes
NT2 Huckleberries
NT2 Lingonberries
NT3 Cowberries
NT2 Loganberries
NT2 Mulberries
NT2 Raspberries
NT2 Redcurrants
NT2 Rowanberries
NT2 Strawberries
NT3 Strawberry jams
NT3 Strawberry pulps
NT3 Strawberry purees
NT2 Strawberry tree fruits
NT2 Whitecurrants
NT2 Wolfberries
NT2 Youngberries
NT1 Breadfruit
NT1 Bush butter
NT1 Cacti
NT1 Cactus pears
NT1 Caja
NT1 Camu-camu
NT1 Cape gooseberries
NT2 Goldenberries
NT1 Carambolas
NT2 Star fruit
NT1 Cashew apples
NT1 Cherimoya
NT1 Cherries
NT2 Morello cherries
NT2 Sour cherries
NT2 Sweet cherries
NT1 Cherry laurel
NT1 Citrus fruits
NT2 Bitter oranges
NT2 Citrons
NT2 Citrus pectins
NT2 Citrus peel
NT2 *Citrus tamurana*
NT2 Galgals
NT2 Grapefruit
NT3 Grapefruit peel
NT2 Ki-mikan
NT2 Kumquats
NT2 Lemons
NT3 Lemon peel
NT2 Limes
NT2 Oranges
NT3 Mandarins
NT4 Clementines
NT4 Kinnow mandarins
NT4 Ponkans
NT4 Satsuma mandarins
NT4 Satsumas
NT4 Tangerines
NT3 Orange peel
NT2 Ortanique
NT2 Pomelos
NT3 *Citrus grandis*
NT3 Pummelos
NT3 Shaddocks
NT2 Sweet limes
NT2 Tangelo
NT2 Tangor
NT2 Yuzu
NT1 Cocona
NT1 Cornelian cherries
NT1 Cupuacu
NT1 *Curculigo latifolia*
NT1 Custard apples
NT1 Dates
NT1 Durian
NT1 Exotic fruits
NT1 Feijoa
NT1 Figs
NT2 Dried figs
NT1 *Fortunella*
NT1 Guavas
NT2 Guava pulps
NT2 Guava purees
NT1 Hawthorn fruits
NT1 Jaboticaba
NT1 Jak fruits
NT1 Japanese apricots
NT2 *Prunus mume*
NT1 Jelly figs
NT2 *Ficus awkeotsang*
NT1 Jujubes
NT1 Kiwano
NT1 Kiwifruit
NT2 *Actinidia chinensis*
NT2 *Actinidia deliciosa*
NT2 *Actinidia polygama*
NT1 Langsat
NT1 Litchis
NT1 Longans
NT1 Loquats
NT1 Malay apples
NT1 Mamey
NT1 Mangoes
NT2 African mangoes
NT2 Mango jams
NT2 Mango kernels
NT2 Mango pickles
NT2 Mango pulps
NT2 Mango purees
NT1 Mangosteens
NT1 Marula
NT2 *Sclerocarya birrea*
NT1 Medlars
NT1 Melons
NT2 Cantaloupes
NT2 Honeydew melons
NT2 Muskmelons
NT1 Myrobalans
NT1 Myrtle
NT1 Naranjilla
NT2 Lulo
NT1 Noni
NT1 Olives
NT2 Black olives
NT2 Table olives
NT1 Omija
NT1 Papayas
NT2 Pawpaws
NT1 Passion fruits
NT2 *Passiflora edulis*
NT1 Peaches
NT2 Nectarines
NT2 Peach pulps
NT2 Peach purees
NT1 Pears
NT2 Asian pears
NT2 Chinese pears
NT2 Japanese pears
NT1 Pepino
NT1 Persimmons
NT1 Phalsa
NT1 Pineapples
NT1 Pitayos
NT1 Plums
NT2 Damsons
NT2 Greengages
NT2 Japanese plums
NT1 Pome fruits
NT1 Pomegranates
NT1 Prickly pears
NT2 *Opuntia ficus-indica*
NT1 Quinces
NT2 Quince jams
NT1 Rambutan
NT1 Rose apples
NT1 Rosehips
NT1 Sapodillas
NT1 Saskatoon fruits
NT1 Sea buckthorn
NT1 Sloes
NT1 Soursop
NT1 *Spondias*
NT1 Star apples
NT1 Stone fruits
NT1 Sugar apples
NT1 Tamarillos
NT1 Tamarinds
NT1 Tomatillos
NT1 Tomatoes
NT2 Cherry tomatoes
NT2 Tomato products
NT3 Tomato concentrates
NT3 Tomato ketchups
NT4 Tomato catsups

NT3 Tomato pastes
NT3 Tomato powders
NT3 Tomato pulps
NT3 Tomato purees
NT3 Tomato sauces
NT2 Tomato skins
NT1 Tropical fruits
NT1 Watermelons
NT2 Egusi

Fruit syrups
BT1 Syrups
BT2 Sugar syrups
BT3 Plant foods
BT4 Foods

Fruit tea
BT1 Teas
BT2 Beverages
BT2 Crops
BT3 Plants
BT2 Plant foods
BT3 Foods

Fruit vinegars
HN introduced from vol. 42, issue 1 (2010)
BT1 Vinegar
BT2 Condiments
BT3 Flavourings
BT4 Additives
BT2 Fermented foods
BT3 Processed foods
BT4 Foods
NT1 Apple vinegar

Fruit wines
HN heading from vol. 30 (1998); under Wines up to vol. 29 (1997)
BT1 Alcoholic beverages
BT2 Beverages alcoholic
BT3 Beverages
NT1 Apple wines
NT1 Apricot wines
NT1 Orange wines
RT Wines

Fruit yoghurt
BT1 Yoghurt
BT2 Fermented milk
BT3 Fermented dairy products
BT4 Dairy products
BT5 Animal foods
BT6 Foods
BT4 Fermented foods
BT5 Processed foods
BT6 Foods
BT3 Milk
BT4 Dairy products
BT5 Animal foods
BT6 Foods

Frying
BT1 Cooking
BT2 Thermal processing
BT3 Processing thermal
BT4 Processing
BT5 Technology
NT1 Deep frying
NT1 Frying properties
NT1 Stir frying
RT Fried foods

Frying fats
BT1 Fats
BT2 Lipids
BT3 Nutrients
RT Cooking fats

Frying oils
BT1 Oils
BT2 Lipids
BT3 Nutrients
RT Cooking oils

Frying properties
BT1 Frying
BT2 Cooking
BT3 Thermal processing
BT4 Processing thermal
BT5 Processing
BT6 Technology

FTIR spectroscopy
HN Fourier transform IR spectroscopy used in the index up to vol. 35, issue 6 (2003)
BT1 Spectroscopy
BT2 Analytical techniques
UF Fourier transform IR spectroscopy

F2 toxin
SN syn. zearalenone
BT1 Mycotoxins
BT2 Toxins
BT3 Residues

Fucoidans
BT1 Polysaccharides
BT2 Carbohydrates
BT3 Nutrients
BT3 Organic compounds
RT Seaweeds

Fucose
HN under Sugars up to vol. 42 (2010)
BT1 Monosaccharides
BT2 Sugars
BT3 Carbohydrates
BT4 Nutrients
BT4 Organic compounds
BT3 Plant foods
BT4 Foods

Fucosylation
BT1 Modification

Fucoxanthin
HN introduced from vol. 39, issue 1 (2007)
BT1 Xanthophylls
BT2 Carotenoids
BT3 Pigments
BT3 Terpenoids
BT4 Lipids
BT5 Nutrients

Fucus
BT1 Seaweeds
BT2 Algae
BT3 Microorganisms
BT2 Sea foods
BT3 Aquatic foods
BT4 Animal foods
BT5 Foods

Fudges
BT1 Sugar confectionery
BT2 Plant foods
BT3 Foods

Fufu
BT1 Fermented foods
BT2 Processed foods
BT3 Foods
BT1 Vegetable products
BT2 Plant foods
BT3 Foods

Fumagillin
BT1 Mycotoxins
BT2 Toxins
BT3 Residues

Fumarases
USE **Fumarate hydratases**

Fumarate hydratases
SN EC 4.2.1.2
BT1 Lyases
BT2 Enzymes
UF Fumarases

Fumaric acid
BT1 Additives
BT1 Organic acids
BT2 Acids

Fumigants
HN heading from vol. 25 (1993); under Fumigation up to vol. 24 (1992)
BT1 Biocides
NT1 Acrylonitrile
NT1 Aluminium phosphide
NT1 Carbon disulfide
NT1 Carbon tetrachloride
NT1 Chloroform
NT1 Chloropicrin
NT1 1,2-Dichloropropane with 1,3-dichloropropene
NT1 Epichlorohydrin
NT1 Ethylene dibromide
NT1 Ethylene dichloride
NT1 Ethylene oxide
NT1 Ethyl formate
NT1 Methyl bromide
NT1 Paraformaldehyde
NT1 Phosphine
NT1 Phostoxin
NT1 Propylene oxide
NT1 Tetrachloromethane
NT1 Trichloroacetonitrile
NT1 Trichloroethylene
NT1 Trichloromethane
RT Fumigation
RT Hydrocyanic acid
RT Hydrogen cyanide
RT Pesticides

Fumigation
RT Disinfection
RT Disinfestation

RT Fumigants
RT Hygiene
RT Sterilization

Fumonisin B_1
BT1 Fumonisins
BT2 Mycotoxins
BT3 Toxins
BT4 Residues

Fumonisin B_2
BT1 Fumonisins
BT2 Mycotoxins
BT3 Toxins
BT4 Residues

Fumonisin B_3
BT1 Fumonisins
BT2 Mycotoxins
BT3 Toxins
BT4 Residues

Fumonisins
HN heading from vol. 30 (1998); under Mycotoxins up to vol. 29 (1997)
BT1 Mycotoxins
BT2 Toxins
BT3 Residues
NT1 Fumonisin B_1
NT1 Fumonisin B_2
NT1 Fumonisin B_3
RT *Fusarium*

Functional beverages
HN introduced from vol. 39, issue 1 (2007)
BT1 Beverages
BT1 Functional foods
BT2 Novel foods
BT3 Foods
RT Health beverages

Functional foods
HN heading from vol. 25 (1993)
SN syn. nutraceutical foods
BT1 Novel foods
BT2 Foods
NT1 Functional beverages
NT1 Nutraceutical foods
RT Designer foods
RT Health
RT Medical foods
RT Nutrition
RT Phytochemicals

Functional properties
HN heading from vol. 24 (1992)
BT1 Physical properties
NT1 Binding capacity
NT1 Buffering capacity
NT1 Chipping properties
NT1 Dispersibility
NT1 Emulsification properties
NT1 Emulsifying capacity
NT1 Foaming
NT2 Foaming agents
NT1 Foaming capacity
NT1 Foaming properties
NT1 Gelling capacity
NT1 Moisture retention
NT1 Oil absorption capacity
NT1 Pasting properties
NT1 Surface active properties
NT1 Swelling
NT1 Water binding capacity
NT1 Water holding capacity
NT1 Whipping properties
NT2 Whipping capacity

Fungal counts
BT1 Microbiological techniques
RT Plate counts
UF Mould counts

Fungal decay
BT1 Plant diseases
BT2 Diseases plant
BT3 Diseases

Fungal proteins
HN under Proteins up to vol. 42 (2010)
BT1 Fungi
BT2 Microorganisms
BT1 Microbial proteins
BT2 Microorganisms
BT2 Proteins
BT3 Nutrients
RT Mycoprotein
RT Quorn

Fungal spores
BT1 Microbial spores
BT2 Spores
RT Sporulation
UF Ascospores
UF Conidia

Fungi
BT1 Microorganisms
NT1 *Absidia*
NT2 *Absidia corymbifera*
NT1 *Acremonium*
NT2 *Acremonium cellulolyticus*
NT2 *Cephalosporium*
NT1 *Actinomucor*
NT2 *Actinomucor elegans*
NT1 *Alternaria*
NT2 *Alternaria alternata*
NT2 *Alternaria citri*
NT1 *Amylomyces*
NT2 *Amylomyces rouxii*
NT1 Antifungal activity
NT1 Ascomycetes
NT1 *Aspergillus*
NT2 *Aspergillus aculeatus*
NT2 *Aspergillus awamori*
NT2 *Aspergillus candidus*
NT2 *Aspergillus carbonarius*
NT2 *Aspergillus clavatus*
NT2 *Aspergillus ficuum*
NT2 *Aspergillus flavus*
NT2 *Aspergillus foetidus*
NT2 *Aspergillus fumigatus*
NT2 *Aspergillus japonicus*
NT2 *Aspergillus kawachii*
NT2 *Aspergillus melleus*
NT2 *Aspergillus nidulans*
NT2 *Aspergillus niger*
NT2 *Aspergillus ochraceus*
NT2 *Aspergillus oryzae*
NT2 *Aspergillus parasiticus*
NT2 *Aspergillus phoenicis*
NT3 *Aspergillus saitoi*
NT2 *Aspergillus repens*
NT2 *Aspergillus sojae*
NT2 *Aspergillus terreus*
NT2 *Aspergillus tubingensis*
NT2 *Aspergillus ustus*
NT2 *Aspergillus versicolor*
NT1 *Aureobasidium*
NT2 *Aureobasidium pullulans*
NT1 Basidiomycetes
NT1 *Beauveria*
NT2 *Beauveria bassiana*
NT1 *Blakeslea*
NT2 *Blakeslea trispora*
NT1 *Botrytis*
NT2 *Botrytis cinerea*
NT1 *Byssochlamys*
NT2 *Byssochlamys fulva*
NT1 *Ceratocystis*
NT2 *Ceratocystis fimbriata*
NT1 *Chaetomium*
NT1 *Chrysosporium*
NT1 *Cladosporium*
NT1 *Claviceps*
NT2 *Claviceps purpurea*
NT1 *Colletotrichum*
NT2 *Colletotrichum acutatum*
NT2 *Colletotrichum gloeosporioides*
NT1 *Cryphonectria*
NT2 *Cryphonectria parasitica*
NT1 *Cunninghamella*
NT1 *Curvularia*
NT1 *Diplodia*
NT1 *Endomyces*
NT1 *Endothia*
NT1 *Eurotium*
NT1 *Fomes*
NT1 Fungal proteins
NT1 *Fusarium*
NT2 *Fusarium avenaceum*
NT2 *Fusarium culmorum*
NT2 *Fusarium equiseti*
NT2 *Fusarium graminearum*
NT2 *Fusarium moniliforme*
NT2 *Fusarium oxysporum*
NT2 *Fusarium proliferatum*
NT2 *Fusarium sambucinum*
NT2 *Fusarium solani*
NT3 *Fusarium solani pisi*
NT2 *Fusarium sporotrichioides*
NT2 *Fusarium verticillioides*
NT1 *Fusidium*
NT1 *Geotrichum*
NT2 *Geotrichum candidum*
NT2 *Geotrichum klebahnii*
NT1 *Gibberella*
NT2 *Gibberella fujikuroi* complex
NT3 *Gibberella fujikuroi*
NT1 *Gliocladium*
NT1 *Helminthosporium*
NT1 *Humicola*
NT2 *Humicola grisea*
NT2 *Humicola insolens*
NT2 *Humicola lanuginosa*
NT1 *Irpex*
NT1 *Monascus*
NT2 *Monascus purpureus*

NT2 *Monascus ruber*
NT1 *Monilia*
NT1 *Monilinia*
NT2 *Monilinia fructicola*
NT2 *Monilinia fructigena*
NT2 *Monilinia laxa*
NT1 *Mortierella*
NT2 *Mortierella alliacea*
NT2 *Mortierella alpina*
NT2 *Mortierella isabellina*
NT1 *Mucor*
NT2 *Mucor circinelloides*
NT2 *Mucor miehei*
NT2 *Mucor rouxii*
NT1 *Myrothecium*
NT1 *Neocallimastix*
NT2 *Neocallimastix patriciarum*
NT1 *Neosartorya*
NT1 *Neurospora*
NT1 *Paecilomyces*
NT2 *Paecilomyces japonica*
NT2 *Paecilomyces sinclairii*
NT1 *Penicillium*
NT2 *Penicillium aurantiogriseum*
NT2 *Penicillium brasilianum*
NT2 *Penicillium camemberti*
NT2 *Penicillium canescens*
NT2 *Penicillium chrysogenum*
NT2 *Penicillium citrinum*
NT2 *Penicillium corylophilum*
NT2 *Penicillium crustosum*
NT2 *Penicillium decumbens*
NT2 *Penicillium digitatum*
NT2 *Penicillium expansum*
NT2 *Penicillium funiculosum*
NT2 *Penicillium glabrum*
NT2 *Penicillium griseoroseum*
NT2 *Penicillium italicum*
NT2 *Penicillium janthinellum*
NT2 *Penicillium nalgiovense*
NT2 *Penicillium olsonii*
NT2 *Penicillium oxalicum*
NT2 *Penicillium palitans*
NT2 *Penicillium purpurogenum*
NT2 *Penicillium restrictum*
NT2 *Penicillium roqueforti*
NT2 *Penicillium simplicissimum*
NT2 *Penicillium spinulosum*
NT2 *Penicillium verrucosum*
NT2 *Penicillium viridicatum*
NT1 *Phanerochaete*
NT2 *Phanerochaete chrysosporium*
NT1 *Phlebia*
NT2 *Phlebia radiata*
NT1 *Phoma*
NT1 *Pithomyces*
NT1 *Polyporus*
NT1 *Pycnoporus*
NT2 *Pycnoporus cinnabarinus*
NT1 *Rhizoctonia*
NT1 *Rhizomucor*
NT2 *Rhizomucor miehei*
NT1 *Rhizopus*
NT2 *Rhizopus arrhizus*
NT2 *Rhizopus chinensis*
NT2 *Rhizopus cohnii*
NT2 *Rhizopus delemar*
NT2 *Rhizopus japonicus*
NT2 *Rhizopus microsporus*
NT2 *Rhizopus niveus*
NT2 *Rhizopus oligosporus*
NT2 *Rhizopus oryzae*
NT2 *Rhizopus stolonifer*
NT3 *Rhizopus nigricans*
NT1 *Sclerotinia*
NT1 *Sclerotium*
NT1 *Scopulariopsis*
NT1 *Septoria*
NT1 Spoilage fungi
NT1 *Sporotrichum*
NT1 *Stachybotrys*
NT1 *Talaromyces*
NT2 *Talaromyces avellaneus*
NT2 *Talaromyces macrosporus*
NT1 *Thermoascus*
NT2 *Thermoascus aurantiacus*
NT1 *Thermomyces*
NT2 *Thermomyces lanuginosus*
NT1 *Thielaviopsis*
NT1 *Trametes*
NT2 *Trametes hirsuta*
NT2 *Trametes versicolor*
NT1 *Trichoderma*
NT2 *Trichoderma harzianum*
NT2 *Trichoderma koningii*
NT2 *Trichoderma longibrachiatum*
NT2 *Trichoderma reesei*
NT2 *Trichoderma viride*
NT1 *Trichophyton*
NT1 *Trichothecium*
NT1 *Verticillium*
NT1 *Wallemia*
NT2 *Wallemia sebi*
NT1 Yeasts
NT2 *Arxula*
NT3 *Arxula adeninivorans*
NT2 *Ashbya*
NT3 *Ashbya gossypii*
NT2 *Brettanomyces*
NT3 *Brettanomyces anomalus*
NT3 *Brettanomyces bruxellensis*
NT3 *Brettanomyces intermedius*
NT2 *Candida*
NT3 *Candida albicans*
NT3 *Candida antarctica*
NT3 *Candida boidinii*
NT3 *Candida bombicola*
NT3 *Candida cylindracea*
NT3 *Candida famata*
NT3 *Candida glycerinogenes*
NT3 *Candida guilliermondii*
NT3 *Candida humilis*
NT4 *Candida milleri*
NT3 *Candida intermedia*
NT3 *Candida kefyr*
NT4 *Candida pseudotropicalis*
NT3 *Candida krusei*
NT3 *Candida lipolytica*
NT3 *Candida magnoliae*
NT3 *Candida maltosa*
NT3 *Candida mogii*
NT3 *Candida molischiana*
NT3 *Candida oleophila*
NT3 *Candida parapsilosis*
NT3 *Candida rugosa*
NT3 *Candida saitoana*
NT3 *Candida sake*
NT3 *Candida shehatae*
NT3 *Candida stellata*
NT3 *Candida tropicalis*
NT3 *Candida utilis*
NT3 *Candida valida*
NT3 *Candida versatilis*
NT3 *Candida wickerhamii*
NT3 *Candida zeylanoides*
NT3 Torula yeast
NT2 Cider yeasts
NT2 *Cryptococcus*
NT3 *Cryptococcus albidus*
NT3 *Cryptococcus curvatus*
NT3 *Cryptococcus laurentii*
NT3 *Cryptococcus nodaensis*
NT2 *Debaryomyces*
NT3 *Debaryomyces hansenii*
NT2 *Dekkera*
NT3 *Dekkera anomala*
NT3 *Dekkera bruxellensis*
NT2 Distillers yeasts
NT2 Dried yeasts
NT2 *Endomycopsis*
NT2 *Eremothecium*
NT2 *Hanseniaspora*
NT3 *Hanseniaspora guilliermondii*
NT3 *Hanseniaspora osmophila*
NT3 *Hanseniaspora uvarum*
NT2 *Hansenula*
NT3 *Hansenula polymorpha*
NT2 *Issatchenkia*
NT3 *Issatchenkia orientalis*
NT2 Killer yeasts
NT2 *Kloeckera*
NT3 *Kloeckera apiculata*
NT2 *Kluyveromyces*
NT3 *Kluyveromyces bulgaricus*
NT3 *Kluyveromyces fragilis*
NT3 *Kluyveromyces lactis*
NT3 *Kluyveromyces marxianus*
NT3 *Kluyveromyces phaffii*
NT3 *Kluyveromyces thermotolerans*
NT2 *Metschnikowia*
NT3 *Metschnikowia pulcherrima*
NT2 *Pachysolen*
NT2 *Phaffia*
NT3 *Phaffia rhodozyma*
NT2 *Pichia*
NT3 *Pichia anomala*
NT3 *Pichia fermentans*
NT3 *Pichia guilliermondii*
NT3 *Pichia heedii*
NT3 *Pichia membranifaciens*
NT4 *Pichia membranefaciens*
NT3 *Pichia methanolica*
NT3 *Pichia pastoris*
NT3 *Pichia stipitis*
NT3 *Pichia subpelliculosa*
NT2 *Rhodosporidium*
NT3 *Rhodosporidium toruloides*
NT2 *Rhodotorula*
NT3 *Rhodotorula glutinis*
NT3 *Rhodotorula gracilis*

NT3 *Rhodotorula mucilaginosa*
NT4 *Rhodotorula rubra*
NT2 *Saccharomyces*
NT3 *Saccharomyces bayanus*
NT3 *Saccharomyces boulardii*
NT3 *Saccharomyces carlsbergensis*
NT3 *Saccharomyces cerevisiae*
NT3 *Saccharomyces diastaticus*
NT3 *Saccharomyces exiguus*
NT3 *Saccharomyces pastorianus*
NT3 *Saccharomyces uvarum*
NT3 Yeasts bakers
NT4 Bakers yeasts
NT3 Yeasts brewers
NT4 Brewers yeasts
NT5 Bottom fermenting yeasts
NT5 Top fermenting yeasts
NT3 Yeasts wine
NT4 Wine yeasts
NT5 Sake yeasts
NT2 *Saccharomycodes*
NT2 *Saccharomycopsis*
NT3 *Saccharomycopsis fibuligera*
NT2 *Schizosaccharomyces*
NT3 *Schizosaccharomyces pombe*
NT2 *Schwanniomyces*
NT2 Spoilage yeasts
NT2 *Sporobolomyces*
NT2 *Torulaspora*
NT3 *Torulaspora delbrueckii*
NT2 *Torulopsis*
NT3 *Torulopsis glabrata*
NT2 *Trichosporon*
NT3 *Trichosporon cutaneum*
NT3 *Trichosporon pullulans*
NT2 Wild yeasts
NT2 *Xanthophyllomyces*
NT3 *Xanthophyllomyces dendrorhous*
NT2 *Yarrowia*
NT3 *Yarrowia lipolytica*
NT2 Yeast biomass
NT2 Yeast extracts
NT2 Yeast proteins
NT2 *Zygosaccharomyces*
NT3 *Zygosaccharomyces bailii*
NT3 *Zygosaccharomyces rouxii*
RT Edible fungi
RT Eukaryotes
RT Fungi edible
RT Mycotoxicosis
RT Mycotoxins
RT Quorn
UF Moulds

Fungicides
BT1 Pesticides
BT2 Biocides
BT2 Residues
NT1 2-Aminobutane
NT1 Anilazine
NT1 Antifungal compounds
NT1 Azoxystrobin
NT1 Benzimidazole
NT2 Benomyl
NT2 Carbendazim
NT2 Thiabendazole
NT2 Thiophanate
NT2 Thiophanate-methyl
NT1 Biphenyl
NT1 Bordeaux mixture
NT1 Bupirimate
NT1 Butylamine
NT1 Carboxin
NT1 Chlorothalonil
NT1 Cyprodinil
NT1 Dicarboximide fungicides
NT2 Captafol
NT2 Captan
NT3 Tetrahydrophthalimide
NT2 Folpet
NT2 Iprodione
NT2 Procymidone
NT2 Vinclozolin
NT1 Dichlofluanid
NT1 Dichlozoline
NT1 Dinocap
NT1 Diphenylamine
NT1 Dithiocarbamate fungicides
NT2 Ethylenethiourea
NT2 Ferbam
NT2 Mancozeb
NT2 Maneb
NT2 Propineb
NT2 Thiram
NT2 Zineb
NT2 Ziram
NT1 Dodine
NT1 Edifenphos
NT1 Fludioxonil
NT1 Hexachlorobenzene
NT1 Imazalil
NT1 Malachite green
NT1 Metalaxyl
NT1 Natamycin
NT2 Pimaricin
NT1 Pentachlorobenzene
NT1 2-Phenylphenol
NT1 Pyrimethanil
NT1 Quinomethionate
NT1 Quintozene
NT1 Tebuconazole
NT1 Triadimefon
NT1 Triforine
RT Antibiotics
UF Antifungal agents
UF Antimycotics

Fungi edible
SN edible fungi is also used in the index
BT1 Vegetables specific
BT2 Vegetables
BT3 Crops
BT4 Plants
BT3 Plant foods
BT4 Foods
NT1 Edible fungi
NT2 *Agaricus*
NT3 *Agaricus bisporus*
NT3 *Agaricus blazei*
NT2 *Agrocybe*
NT2 *Amanita*
NT3 *Amanita phalloides*
NT2 *Armillaria*
NT3 *Armillaria mellea*
NT2 *Auricularia*
NT3 *Auricularia auricula*
NT3 *Auricularia polytricha*
NT2 *Boletus*
NT3 *Boletus edulis*
NT2 *Calocybe*
NT2 *Cantharellus*
NT2 Champignons
NT2 *Coprinus*
NT3 *Coprinus comatus*
NT2 *Cordyceps*
NT3 *Cordyceps militaris*
NT3 *Cordyceps sinensis*
NT2 *Flammulina*
NT3 *Flammulina velutipes*
NT2 *Ganoderma*
NT3 *Ganoderma applanatum*
NT3 *Ganoderma lucidum*
NT2 *Grifola frondosa*
NT2 *Gyromitra*
NT2 *Hericium erinaceus*
NT2 Huitlacoche
NT2 *Hydnum*
NT2 *Lactarius*
NT2 *Leccinum*
NT2 *Lentinula edodes*
NT2 *Lentinus*
NT2 *Lepista*
NT3 *Lepista nuda*
NT2 *Lycoperdon*
NT2 *Morchella*
NT3 *Morchella esculenta*
NT2 Mushrooms
NT3 Wild mushrooms
NT2 *Phellinus linteus*
NT2 *Pholiota*
NT2 *Pleurotus*
NT3 *Pleurotus citrinopileatus*
NT3 *Pleurotus eryngii*
NT3 *Pleurotus florida*
NT3 *Pleurotus ostreatus*
NT3 *Pleurotus sajor-caju*
NT3 *Pleurotus tuberregium*
NT2 *Poria cocos*
NT2 *Russula*
NT2 *Sarcodon aspratus*
NT2 *Sarcodon imbricatum*
NT2 *Schizophyllum*
NT3 *Schizophyllum commune*
NT2 Straw mushrooms
NT2 *Terfezia*
NT2 *Termitomyces*
NT2 *Tricholoma*
NT3 *Tricholoma matsutake*
NT2 *Tuber*
NT3 Black truffles
NT3 White truffles
NT2 *Volvariella*
NT3 *Volvariella volvacea*
NT2 *Xerocomus*
RT Fungi

Fural
SN syn. furfural
BT1 Aldehydes
BT2 Carbonyl compounds
BT3 Organic compounds

Furaldehyde
SN syn. furfural
BT1 Aldehydes
BT2 Carbonyl compounds
BT3 Organic compounds

Furaneol
SN syn. 2,5-dimethyl-4-hydroxy-3(2H)-furanone
BT1 Furanones
BT2 Aroma compounds
BT3 Flavour compounds
BT3 Volatile compounds
BT2 Furans
BT3 Heterocyclic compounds
BT2 Ketones
BT3 Carbonyl compounds
BT4 Organic compounds
NT1 2,5-Dimethyl-4-hydroxy-3(2*H*)-furanone

Furanones
BT1 Aroma compounds
BT2 Flavour compounds
BT2 Volatile compounds
BT1 Furans
BT2 Heterocyclic compounds
BT1 Ketones
BT2 Carbonyl compounds
BT3 Organic compounds
NT1 Furaneol
NT2 2,5-Dimethyl-4-hydroxy-3(2*H*)-furanone
NT1 Sotolon

Furans
BT1 Heterocyclic compounds
NT1 Furanones
NT2 Furaneol
NT3 2,5-Dimethyl-4-hydroxy-3(2*H*)-furanone
NT2 Sotolon
NT1 5-(Hydroxymethyl)-2-furaldehyde
NT1 Hydroxymethylfurfural

Furazolidone
BT1 Nitrofurans
BT2 Antibiotics
BT3 Drugs
BT4 Residues

Furcellaran
BT1 Gums
BT2 Polysaccharides
BT3 Carbohydrates
BT4 Nutrients
BT4 Organic compounds
BT2 Stabilizers
BT3 Additives
BT2 Thickeners
BT3 Additives
RT *Furcellaria*

Furcellaria
BT1 Seaweeds
BT2 Algae
BT3 Microorganisms
BT2 Sea foods
BT3 Aquatic foods
BT4 Animal foods
BT5 Foods
RT Furcellaran

Furfural
SN syn. fural; syn. furaldehyde
BT1 Aldehydes
BT2 Carbonyl compounds
BT3 Organic compounds

Furocoumarins
HN introduced from vol. 39, issue 1 (2007)
BT1 Coumarins
BT2 Lactones
BT3 Esters
BT4 Organic compounds
BT3 Heterocyclic compounds
BT2 Phenols
BT3 Alcohols
BT3 Aromatic compounds
BT4 Organic compounds
NT1 Bergapten
NT1 Psoralens
NT1 Xanthotoxin

Furosine
BT1 Amino sugars
BT2 Sugars
BT3 Carbohydrates
BT4 Nutrients
BT4 Organic compounds
BT3 Plant foods
BT4 Foods
RT Browning

Furylfuramide
BT1 Preservatives
BT2 Additives

Fusaproliferin
BT1 Mycotoxins
BT2 Toxins
BT3 Residues

Fusarenon X
BT1 Trichothecenes
BT2 Mycotoxins
BT3 Toxins
BT4 Residues

Fusarin C
BT1 Mycotoxins
BT2 Toxins
BT3 Residues
RT *Fusarium*

Fusarium
BT1 Fungi
BT2 Microorganisms
NT1 *Fusarium avenaceum*
NT1 *Fusarium culmorum*
NT1 *Fusarium equiseti*
NT1 *Fusarium graminearum*
NT1 *Fusarium moniliforme*
NT1 *Fusarium oxysporum*
NT1 *Fusarium proliferatum*
NT1 *Fusarium sambucinum*
NT1 *Fusarium solani*
NT2 *Fusarium solani pisi*
NT1 *Fusarium sporotrichioides*
NT1 *Fusarium verticillioides*
RT Fumonisins
RT Fusarin C
RT Mycotoxins

Fusarium avenaceum
BT1 *Fusarium*
BT2 Fungi
BT3 Microorganisms

Fusarium culmorum
BT1 *Fusarium*
BT2 Fungi
BT3 Microorganisms

Fusarium equiseti
HN introduced from vol. 39, issue 1 (2007)
BT1 *Fusarium*
BT2 Fungi
BT3 Microorganisms

Fusarium graminearum
SN genbank anamorph of Gibberella zeae
BT1 *Fusarium*
BT2 Fungi
BT3 Microorganisms

Fusarium moniliforme
SN synonymous with Fusarium verticillioides; teleomorph is Gibberella fujikuroi
BT1 *Fusarium*
BT2 Fungi
BT3 Microorganisms

Fusarium oxysporum
BT1 *Fusarium*
BT2 Fungi
BT3 Microorganisms

Fusarium proliferatum
BT1 *Fusarium*
BT2 Fungi
BT3 Microorganisms

Fusarium sambucinum
SN synonymous with Gibberella pulicaris
BT1 *Fusarium*
BT2 Fungi
BT3 Microorganisms

Fusarium solani
HN introduced from vol. 43, issue 1 (2011)
BT1 *Fusarium*
BT2 Fungi
BT3 Microorganisms
NT1 *Fusarium solani pisi*

Fusarium solani pisi
BT1 *Fusarium solani*
BT2 *Fusarium*
BT3 Fungi
BT4 Microorganisms

Fusarium sporotrichioides
BT1 *Fusarium*
BT2 Fungi
BT3 Microorganisms

Fusarium verticillioides
SN synonymous with Fusarium moniliforme
BT1 *Fusarium*
BT2 Fungi
BT3 Microorganisms

Fusel oils
BT1 Alcohols

Fusidium
SN obsolete genus; spp. reclassified into other genera, including Cylindrocarpon
BT1 Fungi
BT2 Microorganisms

Fusion proteins
BT1 Proteins
BT2 Nutrients

Fuzzy control
BT1 Process control
BT2 Technology
RT Artificial neural networks

Fuzzy logic process control
HN process control fuzzy logic also used in the index up to vol. 29 (1997)
BT1 Process control
BT2 Technology
RT Artificial neural networks

Fynbo cheese
BT1 Cheese varieties
BT2 Cheese
BT3 Dairy products
BT4 Animal foods
BT5 Foods

G

Ga
HN under Minerals up to vol. 42 (2010)
BT1 Metals
BT2 Elements
BT3 Minerals
BT4 Nutrients
UF Gallium

Gabon
BT1 Central Africa
BT2 Africa

Gadus morhua
BT1 Cod
BT2 Marine fish
BT3 Fish
BT4 Animals
BT4 Sea foods
BT5 Aquatic foods
BT6 Animal foods
BT7 Foods

Galactanases
BT1 Galactosidases
BT2 Glycosidases
BT3 Hydrolases
BT4 Enzymes

Galactans
BT1 Polysaccharides
BT2 Carbohydrates
BT3 Nutrients
BT3 Organic compounds

Galactitol
SN syn. dulcitol
BT1 Polyols
BT2 Alcohols
BT2 Carbohydrates
BT3 Nutrients
BT3 Organic compounds

Galactolipids
BT1 Glycolipids
BT2 Lipids
BT3 Nutrients
RT Cerebrosides

Galactomannans
BT1 Mannans
BT2 Polysaccharides
BT3 Carbohydrates
BT4 Nutrients
BT4 Organic compounds

Galactooligosaccharides
HN under Polysaccharides and Sugars up to vol. 42 (2010)
BT1 Oligosaccharides
BT2 Polysaccharides
BT3 Carbohydrates
BT4 Nutrients
BT4 Organic compounds
BT2 Sugars
BT3 Carbohydrates
BT4 Nutrients
BT4 Organic compounds
BT3 Plant foods
BT4 Foods
RT Galactosides

Galactosamine
BT1 Hexosamines
BT2 Amino sugars
BT3 Sugars
BT4 Carbohydrates
BT5 Nutrients
BT5 Organic compounds
BT4 Plant foods
BT5 Foods

Galactose
HN heading from vol. 25 (1993); under Sugars specific up to vol. 24 (1992)
BT1 Monosaccharides
BT2 Sugars
BT3 Carbohydrates
BT4 Nutrients
BT4 Organic compounds
BT3 Plant foods
BT4 Foods

Galactosidases
BT1 Glycosidases
BT2 Hydrolases
BT3 Enzymes
NT1 Galactanases
NT1 α-Galactosidases
NT1 β-Galactosidases

α-Galactosidases
SN EC 3.2.1.22
BT1 Galactosidases
BT2 Glycosidases
BT3 Hydrolases
BT4 Enzymes
UF Melibiases

β-Galactosidases
SN EC 3.2.1.23
BT1 Galactosidases
BT2 Glycosidases
BT3 Hydrolases
BT4 Enzymes
UF Lactases

Galactosides
BT1 Glycosides
BT2 Carbohydrates
BT3 Nutrients
BT3 Organic compounds
RT Galactooligosaccharides

Galacturonic acid
BT1 Pectic substances
BT2 Polysaccharides
BT3 Carbohydrates
BT4 Nutrients
BT4 Organic compounds
BT1 Uronic acids
BT2 Organic acids
BT3 Acids
BT2 Sugars
BT3 Carbohydrates
BT4 Nutrients
BT4 Organic compounds
BT3 Plant foods
BT4 Foods

Galangal
BT1 Spices
BT2 Flavourings
BT3 Additives

Galgals
BT1 Citrus fruits
BT2 Fruits specific
BT3 Fruits
BT4 Crops
BT5 Plants
BT4 Plant foods
BT5 Foods
RT Lemons

Gallic acid
BT1 Antioxidants
BT2 Additives
BT1 Organic acids
BT2 Acids

Gallium
USE **Ga**

Gallocatechin gallate
HN introduced from vol. 41, issue 1 (2009)
BT1 Catechols
BT2 Flavanols
BT3 Flavonoids
BT4 Aromatic compounds
BT5 Organic compounds
BT4 Pigments
BT2 Phenols
BT3 Alcohols
BT3 Aromatic compounds
BT4 Organic compounds

Gallstones
HN introduced from vol. 39, issue 1 (2007)
BT1 Diseases

Gambia
BT1 West Africa
BT2 Africa

Game
SN use only for game in general; individual species go under Animals or Birds
BT1 Animals
NT1 Game birds
NT1 Game meat
NT2 Game carcasses

Game birds
BT1 Game
BT2 Animals

Game carcasses
BT1 Carcasses
BT2 Meat
BT3 Animal foods
BT4 Foods
BT1 Game meat
BT2 Game
BT3 Animals
BT2 Meat specific
BT3 Meat
BT4 Animal foods
BT5 Foods

Game meat
BT1 Game
BT2 Animals
BT1 Meat specific
BT2 Meat
BT3 Animal foods
BT4 Foods
NT1 Game carcasses

Gamma irradiation
BT1 Irradiation
BT2 Processing
BT3 Technology

Gamma rays
HN heading up to vol. 24 (1992); under Irradiation from vol. 25 (1993)
BT1 Irradiation
BT2 Processing
BT3 Technology

Gammon
BT1 Ham
BT2 Meat products
BT3 Animal foods
BT4 Foods

Gangliosides
BT1 Glycolipids
BT2 Lipids
BT3 Nutrients

Ganoderma
BT1 Edible fungi
BT2 Fungi edible
BT3 Vegetables specific
BT4 Vegetables
BT5 Crops
BT6 Plants
BT5 Plant foods
BT6 Foods
NT1 *Ganoderma applanatum*
NT1 *Ganoderma lucidum*

Ganoderma applanatum
BT1 *Ganoderma*
BT2 Edible fungi
BT3 Fungi edible
BT4 Vegetables specific
BT5 Vegetables
BT6 Crops
BT7 Plants
BT6 Plant foods
BT7 Foods

Ganoderma lucidum
BT1 *Ganoderma*
BT2 Edible fungi
BT3 Fungi edible
BT4 Vegetables specific
BT5 Vegetables
BT6 Crops
BT7 Plants
BT6 Plant foods
BT7 Foods

Garbanzo beans
USE **Chick peas**

Gardenia
BT1 Plants
NT1 *Gardenia jasminoides*
RT Colorants
RT Geniposide

Gardenia jasminoides
BT1 *Gardenia*
BT2 Plants

Gardona
USE **Tetrachlorvinphos**

Gari
BT1 Cassava
BT2 Vegetables specific
BT3 Vegetables
BT4 Crops
BT5 Plants
BT4 Plant foods
BT5 Foods
BT1 Fermented foods
BT2 Processed foods
BT3 Foods

Garlic
HN heading from vol. 25 (1993); under Spices up to vol. 24 (1992)
BT1 Spices
BT2 Flavourings
BT3 Additives
RT Allicin
RT Alliin
RT Diallyl disulfide
RT Garlic oils
RT Wild garlic

Garlic oils
BT1 Essential oils
BT2 Flavourings
BT3 Additives
BT2 Vegetable oils
BT3 Oils vegetable
BT4 Oils
BT5 Lipids
BT6 Nutrients
BT4 Vegetable products
BT5 Plant foods
BT6 Foods
RT Garlic

Garnishes
HN introduced from vol. 37, issue 5 (2005)

Gas chromatography
HN heading from vol. 25 (1993); under Gas liquid chromatography up to vol. 24 (1992)
SN abbrev. GC is also used in the index
BT1 Chromatography
BT2 Analytical techniques
NT1 Gas solid chromatography
NT1 GC
NT1 GC-MS
NT1 GLC

Gases
BT1 Physical phases
BT2 Chemistry
BT3 Science
NT1 Acetylene
NT1 Air
NT2 Airborne
NT2 Air conditioning
NT2 Air speed
NT2 Atmosphere
NT1 Ammonia
NT2 NH_3
NT1 Ar
NT1 Biogas
NT1 Butane
NT1 Carbon dioxide
NT2 CO_2
NT2 Dry Ice
NT2 Supercritical CO_2 extraction
NT1 Carbon monoxide
NT1 Chlorine dioxide
NT1 Ethane
NT1 Ethylene
NT2 ACC
NT2 Ethephon
NT1 H_2

NT1 He
NT1 H_2S
NT1 Methane
NT1 N_2
NT1 Nitric oxide
NT1 Nitrous oxide
NT1 NO_2
NT1 O_2
NT1 Ozone
NT1 Propane
NT1 Sulfur dioxide
NT2 SO_2
NT1 Vapours
NT2 Water vapour
NT1 Xe
RT Bubbles
RT Flushing

Gas liquid chromatography
HN heading up to vol. 24 (1992)
USE **GLC**

Gassericins
BT1 Bacteriocins
BT2 Antibiotics
BT3 Drugs
BT4 Residues
RT *Lactobacillus gasseri*

Gas solid chromatography
BT1 Gas chromatography
BT2 Chromatography
BT3 Analytical techniques

Gastric cancer
HN introduced from vol. 41, issue 1 (2009)
BT1 Cancer
BT2 Diseases

Gastritis
BT1 Diseases
RT Gastroenteritis

Gastroenteritis
BT1 Diseases
RT Diarrhoea
RT Gastritis

Gastrointestinal tract
BT1 Human physiology
BT2 Physiology
BT3 Science
NT1 Malabsorption

Gastropods
BT1 Molluscs
BT2 Shellfish
BT3 Animals
BT3 Sea foods
BT4 Aquatic foods
BT5 Animal foods
BT6 Foods
NT1 Abalones
NT1 Limpets
NT1 Periwinkles
NT1 Snails
NT2 Land snails
NT2 Snail meat
NT1 Top shells
NT1 Trumpet shells
NT1 Turban shells
NT1 Whelks

Gateaux
BT1 Cakes
BT2 Bakery products
BT3 Cereal products
BT4 Plant foods
BT5 Foods
BT1 Desserts
BT2 Processed foods
BT3 Foods

GATT
BT1 Trade agreements
BT2 Trade
BT3 Economics
UF General Agreement on Trade and Tariffs

Gauges
BT1 Equipment
BT2 Technology

Gaza Strip
HN introduced from vol. 39, issue 1 (2007)
BT1 Middle East

Gazelle carcasses
BT1 Carcasses
BT2 Meat
BT3 Animal foods
BT4 Foods
BT1 Gazelle meat
BT2 Gazelles
BT3 Animals
BT2 Meat specific
BT3 Meat
BT4 Animal foods
BT5 Foods

Gazelle meat
BT1 Gazelles
BT2 Animals
BT1 Meat specific
BT2 Meat
BT3 Animal foods
BT4 Foods
NT1 Gazelle carcasses

Gazelles
BT1 Animals
NT1 Gazelle meat
NT2 Gazelle carcasses

GC
SN index heading is Gas chromatography
BT1 Gas chromatography
BT2 Chromatography
BT3 Analytical techniques

GC-MS
BT1 Gas chromatography
BT2 Chromatography
BT3 Analytical techniques
BT1 Mass spectroscopy
BT2 Spectroscopy
BT3 Analytical techniques

GDR
HN used as abbrev. for German Democratic Republic up to vol. 24 (1992)
USE **Germany**

Ge
HN under Minerals up to vol. 42 (2010)
BT1 Elements
BT2 Minerals
BT3 Nutrients
UF Germanium

Geese
HN heading from vol. 25 (1993); under Poultry up to vol. 24 (1992)
BT1 Poultry
BT2 Birds
NT1 Goose eggs
NT1 Goose livers
NT1 Goose meat
NT2 Goose carcasses

Gelatin
BT1 Animal proteins
BT2 Proteins animal
BT3 Proteins
BT4 Nutrients
NT1 Isinglass

Gelatinization
BT1 Gelation

Gelation
NT1 Gelatinization
NT1 Gelling agents
RT Gels
RT Solidification
UF Gelling

Gel electrophoresis
BT1 Electrophoresis
BT2 Analytical techniques
NT1 PFGE
RT PAGE

Gel filtration
BT1 Chromatography
BT2 Analytical techniques

Gelidium
USE **Onigusa**

Gellan
BT1 Polysaccharides
BT2 Carbohydrates
BT3 Nutrients
BT3 Organic compounds
NT1 Gellan gums
RT Exopolysaccharides

Gellan gums
BT1 Gellan
BT2 Polysaccharides
BT3 Carbohydrates
BT4 Nutrients
BT4 Organic compounds
BT1 Gums
BT2 Polysaccharides
BT3 Carbohydrates
BT4 Nutrients

BT4 Organic compounds
BT2 Stabilizers
BT3 Additives
BT2 Thickeners
BT3 Additives

Gelling
USE **Gelation**

Gelling agents
BT1 Gelation

Gelling capacity
BT1 Functional properties
BT2 Physical properties

Gel permeation chromatography
BT1 Chromatography
BT2 Analytical techniques

Gels
BT1 Physical phases
BT2 Chemistry
BT3 Science
NT1 Agar gels
NT1 Alginate gels
NT1 Aspic
NT1 Carrageenan gels
NT1 Silica gels
RT Colloids
RT Dispersions
RT Gelation
RT Syneresis

Gene cloning
HN heading from vol. 24 (1992)
BT1 Genetic techniques
BT2 Genetics
NT1 Cloning technology
NT2 Marker genes
NT2 Marker proteins
NT3 Green fluorescent protein
NT2 Reporter genes
NT1 Gene libraries
NT1 Gene transfer
NT2 Electroporation
NT2 Protoplast fusion
NT2 Transformation

Gene disruption
BT1 Genetic techniques
BT2 Genetics

Gene expression
HN heading from vol. 24 (1992)
BT1 Genetics
NT1 Transcription
NT2 Transcription factors
NT1 Translation
RT Marker genes
RT Operators
RT Operons
RT Promoters
RT Reporter genes
RT Structural genes

Gene libraries
HN heading from vol. 24 (1992) to vol. 29 (1997); under Gene cloning from vol. 30 (1998)
BT1 Gene cloning
BT2 Genetic techniques
BT3 Genetics

Gene-nutrient interactions
HN introduced from vol. 39, issue 1 (2007)
BT1 Genes
BT2 Chromosomes
BT3 Genetics
BT2 Genomes
BT3 Genetics
BT1 Nutrients
RT Nutrigenetics

Gene probes
HN heading from vol. 24 (1992)
BT1 Genetic techniques
BT2 Genetics
NT1 DNA probes
RT Hybridization
RT Oligonucleotides
UF Oligonucleotide probes

General Agreement on Trade and Tariffs
USE **GATT**

Genes
BT1 Chromosomes
BT2 Genetics
BT1 Genomes
BT2 Genetics
NT1 Alleles
NT1 Gene-nutrient interactions
NT1 Genotype
NT1 Introns
NT1 Marker genes
NT1 QTL
NT1 Reporter genes
NT1 Transgenes
RT Operators
RT Operons
RT Promoters
RT Sequencing
RT Structural genes

Gene silencing
HN introduced from vol. 39, issue 1 (2007)
BT1 Genetic techniques
BT2 Genetics
NT1 Antisense technology
NT1 RNA interference

Genetically engineered foods
BT1 Genetics
BT1 Novel foods
BT2 Foods
RT Biotechnologically derived foods
RT GM foods

Genetically modified foods
HN GM foods used in the index from vol. 35, issue 6 (2003)
USE **GM foods**

Genetically modified microorganisms
HN GM microorganisms used in the index from vol. 35, issue 6 (2003)
USE **GM microorganisms**

Genetically modified organisms
HN GM organisms/GMO used in the index from vol. 35, issue 6 (2003)
USE **GMO**

Genetic disorders
HN heading from vol. 30 (1998)
NT1 Callipyge phenotype
NT1 Dark cutting defect
NT1 DFD defect
NT1 Halothane sensitivity
NT1 Human genetic disorders
NT1 Malignant hyperthermia
NT1 PSE defect
NT1 Rendement Napole genes
NT1 RSE defect
RT Genetics

Genetic engineering
BT1 Genetic techniques
BT2 Genetics
RT Protein engineering

Genetic fingerprinting
BT1 Genetic techniques
BT2 Genetics
NT1 DNA fingerprinting
RT RFLP

Genetic mapping
BT1 Genetic techniques
BT2 Genetics

Genetic markers
HN introduced from vol. 42, issue 1 (2010)
BT1 Genetics

Genetics
NT1 Chromosomes
NT2 Genes
NT3 Alleles
NT3 Gene-nutrient interactions
NT3 Genotype
NT3 Introns
NT3 Marker genes
NT3 QTL
NT3 Reporter genes
NT3 Transgenes
NT1 Cloned animals
NT1 Gene expression
NT2 Transcription
NT3 Transcription factors
NT2 Translation
NT1 Genetically engineered foods
NT1 Genetic markers
NT1 Genetic techniques
NT2 AFLP
NT2 Cloning vectors
NT3 Shuttle vectors
NT3 Vectors
NT4 Expression vectors
NT2 Comet assay
NT2 DNA microarrays
NT2 Gene cloning

NT3 Cloning technology
NT4 Marker genes
NT4 Marker proteins
NT5 Green fluorescent protein
NT4 Reporter genes
NT3 Gene libraries
NT3 Gene transfer
NT4 Electroporation
NT4 Protoplast fusion
NT4 Transformation
NT2 Gene disruption
NT2 Gene probes
NT3 DNA probes
NT2 Gene silencing
NT3 Antisense technology
NT3 RNA interference
NT2 Genetic engineering
NT2 Genetic fingerprinting
NT3 DNA fingerprinting
NT2 Genetic mapping
NT2 Genotyping
NT2 Hybridization
NT3 Blotting
NT4 Northern blotting
NT4 Southern blotting
NT4 Western blotting
NT3 DNA hybridization
NT3 Fluorescence *in situ* hybridization
NT2 LAMP
NT2 Metabolic engineering
NT2 Microsatellite markers
NT2 Microsatellites
NT2 Mutagenesis
NT3 Site directed mutagenesis
NT2 PCR
NT2 Protein engineering
NT3 Site directed mutagenesis
NT2 RAPD
NT2 RFLP
NT2 Ribotyping
NT2 Typing
NT1 Genetic variants
NT1 Genomes
NT2 Genes
NT3 Alleles
NT3 Gene-nutrient interactions
NT3 Genotype
NT3 Introns
NT3 Marker genes
NT3 QTL
NT3 Reporter genes
NT3 Transgenes
NT1 Genomics
NT2 Nutrigenomics
NT1 GM foods
NT1 GM microorganisms
NT1 GMO
NT1 GM organisms
NT1 Heritability
NT1 Hybrids
NT1 Inheritance
NT1 Insertion sequences
NT1 Mutations
NT2 Mutants
NT1 Nucleotide sequences
NT1 Nutrigenetics
NT1 Operons
NT2 Operators
NT2 Promoters
NT2 Structural genes
NT1 Phenotype
NT1 Plasmids
NT1 Polymorphism
NT1 Recombinant microorganisms
NT1 Ribotype
NT1 Transgenic animals
NT1 Transgenic plants
NT1 Transposable elements
NT1 Transposition
NT1 Transposons
RT Breed
RT Breeding
RT Carcinogenicity
RT Crossbreeding
RT cv
RT Genetic disorders
RT Mutagenicity
RT Sex
RT var

Genetic techniques
HN heading from vol. 24 (1992)
BT1 Genetics
NT1 AFLP
NT1 Cloning vectors
NT2 Shuttle vectors
NT2 Vectors
NT3 Expression vectors
NT1 Comet assay
NT1 DNA microarrays
NT1 Gene cloning
NT2 Cloning technology
NT3 Marker genes
NT3 Marker proteins
NT4 Green fluorescent protein
NT3 Reporter genes
NT2 Gene libraries
NT2 Gene transfer
NT3 Electroporation
NT3 Protoplast fusion
NT3 Transformation
NT1 Gene disruption
NT1 Gene probes
NT2 DNA probes
NT1 Gene silencing
NT2 Antisense technology
NT2 RNA interference
NT1 Genetic engineering
NT1 Genetic fingerprinting
NT2 DNA fingerprinting
NT1 Genetic mapping
NT1 Genotyping
NT1 Hybridization
NT2 Blotting
NT3 Northern blotting
NT3 Southern blotting
NT3 Western blotting
NT2 DNA hybridization
NT2 Fluorescence *in situ* hybridization
NT1 LAMP
NT1 Metabolic engineering
NT1 Microsatellite markers
NT1 Microsatellites
NT1 Mutagenesis
NT2 Site directed mutagenesis
NT1 PCR
NT1 Protein engineering
NT2 Site directed mutagenesis
NT1 RAPD
NT1 RFLP
NT1 Ribotyping
NT1 Typing

Genetic variants
BT1 Genetics
RT Polymorphism

Gene transfer
HN heading for vol. 24 (1992) only
BT1 Gene cloning
BT2 Genetic techniques
BT3 Genetics
NT1 Electroporation
NT1 Protoplast fusion
NT1 Transformation

Geniposide
HN introduced from vol. 37, issue 5 (2005)
BT1 Glucosides
BT2 Glycosides
BT3 Carbohydrates
BT4 Nutrients
BT4 Organic compounds
RT *Gardenia*

Genistein
BT1 Isoflavones
BT2 Isoflavonoids
BT3 Flavonoids
BT4 Aromatic compounds
BT5 Organic compounds
BT4 Pigments
RT Daidzein

Genomes
BT1 Genetics
NT1 Genes
NT2 Alleles
NT2 Gene-nutrient interactions
NT2 Genotype
NT2 Introns
NT2 Marker genes
NT2 QTL
NT2 Reporter genes
NT2 Transgenes
RT Chromosomes
RT DNA
RT RNA

Genomics
BT1 Genetics
NT1 Nutrigenomics
RT Metabolomics
RT Proteomics

Genotoxicity
BT1 Mutagenicity
RT Antigenotoxicity

Genotype
BT1 Genes
BT2 Chromosomes
BT3 Genetics
BT2 Genomes

BT3 Genetics
RT Genotyping

Genotyping
BT1 Genetic techniques
BT2 Genetics
RT Genotype

Gentamicin
BT1 Aminoglycoside antibiotics
BT2 Antibiotics
BT3 Drugs
BT4 Residues

Gentians
HN introduced from vol. 39, issue 1 (2007)
BT1 Plants

Gentiobiose
HN under Sugars up to vol. 42 (2010)
BT1 Disaccharides
BT2 Sugars
BT3 Carbohydrates
BT4 Nutrients
BT4 Organic compounds
BT3 Plant foods
BT4 Foods

Geobacillus
HN introduced from vol. 37, issue 5 (2005)
BT1 Bacteria
BT2 Microorganisms
NT1 *Geobacillus stearothermophilus*
NT1 *Geobacillus thermoleovorans*

Geobacillus stearothermophilus
HN introduced from vol. 41, issue 1 (2009)
SN synonymous with Bacillus stearothermophilus
BT1 *Geobacillus*
BT2 Bacteria
BT3 Microorganisms

Geobacillus thermoleovorans
HN introduced from vol. 43, issue 1 (2011)
SN synonymous with Bacillus thermoleovorans
BT1 *Geobacillus*
BT2 Bacteria
BT3 Microorganisms

Geographical origin
BT1 Origin

Georgia
BT1 Asia
BT1 Europe

Geosmin
HN also under Heterocyclic compounds up to vol. 42 (2010)
BT1 Alcohols
BT1 Organic compounds
BT1 Volatile compounds
RT Taints

Geotrichum
HN heading up to vol. 24 (1992)
BT1 Fungi
BT2 Microorganisms
NT1 *Geotrichum candidum*
NT1 *Geotrichum klebahnii*

Geotrichum candidum
BT1 *Geotrichum*
BT2 Fungi
BT3 Microorganisms

Geotrichum klebahnii
BT1 *Geotrichum*
BT2 Fungi
BT3 Microorganisms

Geranial
HN also under Flavour compounds up to vol. 42 (2010)
BT1 Citral
BT2 Aldehydes
BT3 Carbonyl compounds
BT4 Organic compounds
BT2 Aroma compounds
BT3 Flavour compounds
BT3 Volatile compounds
BT2 Monoterpenoids
BT3 Terpenoids
BT4 Lipids
BT5 Nutrients
RT Neral

Geraniol
BT1 Alcohols
BT1 Aroma compounds
BT2 Flavour compounds
BT2 Volatile compounds
BT1 Monoterpenoids
BT2 Terpenoids
BT3 Lipids
BT4 Nutrients
RT Nerol

Geranyl acetate
HN also under Flavour compounds up to vol. 42 (2010)
BT1 Acetates
BT1 Aroma compounds
BT2 Flavour compounds
BT2 Volatile compounds
BT1 Esters
BT2 Organic compounds

Germ
BT1 Cereal products
BT2 Plant foods
BT3 Foods
NT1 Wheat germ

German Democratic Republic
HN heading up to vol. 24 (1992)
USE **Germany**

German Federal Republic
USE **Germany**

Germanium
USE **Ge**

Germany
BT1 Europe
BT1 European Union
RT Organization for Economic Cooperation and Development
UF Federal Republic of Germany
UF FRG
UF GDR
UF German Democratic Republic
UF German Federal Republic
UF Germany, East
UF Germany, Federal Republic of
UF Germany, West

Germany, East
USE **Germany**

Germany, Federal Republic of
HN heading up to vol. 24 (1992)
USE **Germany**

Germany, West
USE **Germany**

Germicides
BT1 Disinfectants
BT2 Disinfection
BT3 Hygiene
RT Antiseptics
RT Biocides

Germination
SN used in relation to seeds, e.g. cereals, legumes
NT1 Germination capacity
RT Malting

Germination capacity
BT1 Germination

Gesatop
USE **Simazine**

Gestagens
BT1 Hormones
BT2 Residues

Gevuina avellana
BT1 Plants

Ghana
BT1 West Africa
BT2 Africa

Ghee
BT1 Dairy products
BT2 Animal foods
BT3 Foods
RT Butter
RT Fats milk
RT Milk fats

Gherkins
BT1 Vegetables specific
BT2 Vegetables
BT3 Crops
BT4 Plants

BT3 Plant foods
BT4 Foods

Ghrelin
HN introduced from vol. 39, issue 1 (2007)
BT1 Hormones
BT2 Residues

Giardia
HN heading from vol. 30 (1998)
BT1 Parasites
BT2 Pests
NT1 *Giardia intestinalis*
NT1 *Giardia lamblia*
NT1 *Giardia muris*
RT Giardiasis

Giardia intestinalis
BT1 *Giardia*
BT2 Parasites
BT3 Pests

Giardia lamblia
BT1 *Giardia*
BT2 Parasites
BT3 Pests

Giardia muris
BT1 *Giardia*
BT2 Parasites
BT3 Pests

Giardiasis
BT1 Diseases
BT1 Poisoning
RT *Giardia*

Gibberella
HN introduced from vol. 43, issue 1 (2011)
BT1 Fungi
BT2 Microorganisms
NT1 *Gibberella fujikuroi* complex
NT2 *Gibberella fujikuroi*

Gibberella fujikuroi
HN introduced from vol. 41, issue 1 (2009)
SN teleomorph of Fusarium moniliforme
BT1 *Gibberella fujikuroi* complex
BT2 *Gibberella*
BT3 Fungi
BT4 Microorganisms

***Gibberella fujikuroi* complex**
HN introduced from vol. 43, issue 1 (2011)
BT1 *Gibberella*
BT2 Fungi
BT3 Microorganisms
NT1 *Gibberella fujikuroi*

Gibberellic acid
HN heading up to vol. 42 (2010)
BT1 Gibberellins
BT2 Plant growth regulators
BT3 Cultivation
BT4 Agriculture

Gibberellins
HN heading from vol. 43 (2011); under Gibberellic acid up to vol. 42 (2010)
BT1 Plant growth regulators
BT2 Cultivation
BT3 Agriculture
NT1 Gibberellic acid

Giblets
BT1 Offal
BT2 Animal foods
BT3 Foods

Gigartina
BT1 Seaweeds
BT2 Algae
BT3 Microorganisms
BT2 Sea foods
BT3 Aquatic foods
BT4 Animal foods
BT5 Foods

Gin
BT1 Spirits
BT2 Alcoholic beverages
BT3 Beverages alcoholic
BT4 Beverages

Gingelly oils
USE **Sesame oils**

Gingelly seeds
USE **Sesame seeds**

Ginger
HN heading from vol. 30 (1998); under Spices up to vol. 29 (1997)
BT1 Spices
BT2 Flavourings
BT3 Additives
RT Gingerols
RT Zingerone

Ginger ale
BT1 Soft drinks
BT2 Beverages

Ginger beer
BT1 Soft drinks
BT2 Beverages

Gingerbread
BT1 Bakery products
BT2 Cereal products
BT3 Plant foods
BT4 Foods

Gingerols
BT1 Aroma compounds
BT2 Flavour compounds
BT2 Volatile compounds
BT1 Phenols
BT2 Alcohols
BT2 Aromatic compounds
BT3 Organic compounds
BT1 Pungent principles
BT2 Flavour compounds
RT Ginger

Ginjoshu
BT1 Sake
BT2 Rice wines
BT3 Cereal wines
BT4 Alcoholic beverages
BT5 Beverages alcoholic
BT6 Beverages

Ginkgo biloba
BT1 Plants
RT Ginkgo nuts

Ginkgo nuts
BT1 Nuts
BT2 Fruits
BT3 Crops
BT4 Plants
BT3 Plant foods
BT4 Foods
BT2 Oilseeds
BT3 Seeds
BT4 Plant foods
BT5 Foods
RT *Ginkgo biloba*

Ginseng
HN heading from vol. 25 (1993)
BT1 Plants
NT1 *Panax notoginseng*
NT1 Red ginseng
RT Ginseng beverages
RT Ginsenosides

Ginseng beverages
HN introduced from vol. 39, issue 1 (2007)
BT1 Health beverages
BT2 Beverages
BT2 Health foods
BT3 Processed foods
BT4 Foods
RT Ginseng
RT Ginsenosides

Ginseng saponins
USE **Ginsenosides**

Ginsenosides
BT1 Saponins
BT2 Glycosides
BT3 Carbohydrates
BT4 Nutrients
BT4 Organic compounds
RT Ginseng
RT Ginseng beverages
UF Ginseng saponins

Girdling
BT1 Cultivation
BT2 Agriculture

Gizzards
BT1 Offal
BT2 Animal foods
BT3 Foods

Glass
BT1 Packaging materials
NT1 Glass bottles
NT1 Glass containers

Glass bottles
HN bottles glass used in the index up to vol. 31 (1999)
BT1 Bottles
BT2 Containers
BT1 Glass
BT2 Packaging materials

Glass containers
HN containers glass used up to vol. 29 (1997)
BT1 Containers
BT1 Glass
BT2 Packaging materials

Glassine
BT1 Paper
BT2 Packaging materials

Glassiness
BT1 Optical properties
BT2 Physical properties

Glass transition
BT1 Thermophysical properties
BT2 Physical properties

Glass transition temp.
BT1 Thermophysical properties
BT2 Physical properties

Glazes
BT1 Coatings

Glazing
BT1 Coating
BT2 Processing
BT3 Technology

GLC
BT1 Gas chromatography
BT2 Chromatography
BT3 Analytical techniques
UF Gas liquid chromatography

Gliadins
HN heading from vol. 30 (1998); under Proteins cereal up to vol. 29 (1997)
BT1 Cereal proteins
BT2 Proteins cereal
BT3 Vegetable proteins
BT4 Proteins vegetable
BT5 Proteins
BT6 Nutrients
BT5 Vegetable products
BT6 Plant foods
BT7 Foods

Gliocladium
BT1 Fungi
BT2 Microorganisms
RT Mycotoxins

Gliotoxin
BT1 Antibiotics
BT2 Drugs
BT3 Residues
BT1 Mycotoxins
BT2 Toxins
BT3 Residues

Globalization
HN introduced from vol. 39, issue 1 (2007)
BT1 Economics

Globe artichokes
BT1 Vegetables specific
BT2 Vegetables
BT3 Crops
BT4 Plants
BT3 Plant foods
BT4 Foods
RT Artichokes

Globins
BT1 Animal proteins
BT2 Proteins animal
BT3 Proteins
BT4 Nutrients

Globulins
BT1 Proteins
BT2 Nutrients
NT1 Actins
NT2 F-actin
NT1 Actomyosin
NT1 Arachin
NT1 Edestin
NT1 γ-Globulins
NT1 Immunoglobulins
NT2 Immunoglobulin A
NT2 Immunoglobulin E
NT2 Immunoglobulin G
NT2 Immunoglobulin Y
NT1 Lactoferrin
NT1 Lactoglobulins
NT2 β-Lactoglobulin
NT1 Legumin
NT1 Myosin
NT2 Myosin heavy chains
NT2 Myosin light chains
NT1 11S Globulins
NT1 7S Globulins
NT1 Vicilin

γ-Globulins
BT1 Animal proteins
BT2 Proteins animal
BT3 Proteins
BT4 Nutrients
BT1 Globulins
BT2 Proteins
BT3 Nutrients
RT Immunoglobulins

Gloss
BT1 Optical properties
BT2 Physical properties
RT Colour

Gloves
HN introduced from vol. 39, issue 1 (2007)
BT1 Handling

Glucagon
BT1 Hormones
BT2 Residues

Glucanases
BT1 Glycosidases
BT2 Hydrolases
BT3 Enzymes

β-Glucanases
BT1 Glycosidases
BT2 Hydrolases
BT3 Enzymes

1,4-α-Glucan branching enzymes
SN EC 2.4.1.18
BT1 Glycosyltransferases
BT2 Transferases
BT3 Enzymes
UF Branching enzymes

Glucan endo-1,3-β-D-glucosidases
SN EC 3.2.1.39
BT1 Glycosidases
BT2 Hydrolases
BT3 Enzymes
UF Laminarinases

Glucan 1,4-α-glucosidases
SN EC 3.2.1.3
BT1 Amylases
BT2 Glycosidases
BT3 Hydrolases
BT4 Enzymes
UF Amyloglucosidases
UF Glucoamylases

4-α-Glucanotransferases
SN EC 2.4.1.25
BT1 Glycosyltransferases
BT2 Transferases
BT3 Enzymes

Glucans
HN heading from vol. 25 (1993); under Polysaccharides up to vol. 24 (1992)
BT1 Polysaccharides
BT2 Carbohydrates
BT3 Nutrients
BT3 Organic compounds
NT1 Alternan
NT1 Celluloses
NT2 Carboxymethylcellulose
NT2 Cellulose acetate
NT2 Cellulose ether
NT2 Cellulose sausage casings
NT2 Hydroxypropylcellulose
NT2 Hydroxypropylmethylcellulose
NT2 Lignocelluloses
NT2 Methylcellulose
NT2 Microcrystalline celluloses
NT2 Regenerated cellulose
NT2 Tylose
NT1 Curdlan
NT1 Dextran
NT1 β-Glucans
NT1 Glycogen
NT1 Laminarin
NT1 Polydextrose
NT1 Pullulan
NT1 Starch
NT2 Amaranth starch

NT2 Amylopectins
NT2 Amyloses
NT2 Arrowroot
NT2 Barley starch
NT2 Buckwheat starch
NT2 Canna starch
NT2 Cassava starch
NT3 Tapioca
NT2 Corn starch
NT3 High amylose corn starch
NT2 Dextrins
NT3 Amylodextrins
NT3 Cyclodextrins
NT3 Maltodextrins
NT3 Pyrodextrins
NT2 Farina
NT2 Legume starch
NT2 Millet starch
NT2 Modified starches
NT2 Mung bean starch
NT2 Oat starch
NT2 Pea starch
NT2 Potato starch
NT2 Resistant starch
NT2 Rice starch
NT2 Rye starch
NT2 Sago
NT2 Sorghum starch
NT2 Starch granules
NT2 Sweet potato starch
NT2 Wheat starch
NT2 Yam starch
NT1 Xyloglucans

β-Glucans
SN general use only; see also other specified beta-glucans
BT1 Glucans
BT2 Polysaccharides
BT3 Carbohydrates
BT4 Nutrients
BT4 Organic compounds

Glucides
BT1 Glycosides
BT2 Carbohydrates
BT3 Nutrients
BT3 Organic compounds

Glucitol
USE **Sorbitol**

Glucoamylases
HN heading up to vol. 24 (1992)
USE **Glucan 1,4-α-glucosidases**

Glucobrassicin
BT1 Glucosinolates
BT2 Glycosides
BT3 Carbohydrates
BT4 Nutrients
BT4 Organic compounds
RT Indole-3-carbinol

Glucocorticoids
BT1 Hormones
BT2 Residues
NT1 Cortisol

Glucokinases
SN EC 2.7.1.2
BT1 Kinases
BT2 Phosphotransferases
BT3 Transferases
BT4 Enzymes

Glucomannans
BT1 Mannans
BT2 Polysaccharides
BT3 Carbohydrates
BT4 Nutrients
BT4 Organic compounds
NT1 Konjac glucomannans

Gluconacetobacter
HN introduced from vol. 39, issue 1 (2007)
BT1 Bacteria
BT2 Microorganisms

Gluconates
HN introduced from vol. 39, issue 1 (2007)
BT1 Salts
RT Gluconic acid

Gluconic acid
BT1 Organic acids
BT2 Acids
RT Gluconates

Gluconobacter
HN under Pseudomonadaceae up to vol. 24 (1992)
SN new name for obsolete genus Acetomonas
BT1 Bacteria
BT2 Microorganisms
NT1 *Acetomonas*
NT1 *Gluconobacter frateurii*
NT1 *Gluconobacter oxydans*
RT Acetic acid bacteria

Gluconobacter frateurii
BT1 *Gluconobacter*
BT2 Bacteria
BT3 Microorganisms

Gluconobacter oxydans
SN synonymous with Acetobacter diazotrophicus
BT1 *Gluconobacter*
BT2 Bacteria
BT3 Microorganisms

Glucono-δ-lactone
BT1 Additives
BT1 Lactones
BT2 Esters
BT3 Organic compounds
BT2 Heterocyclic compounds

Glucooligosaccharides
HN introduced from vol. 41, issue 1 (2009); under Polysaccharides and Sugars up to vol. 42 (2010)
BT1 Oligosaccharides
BT2 Polysaccharides
BT3 Carbohydrates
BT4 Nutrients
BT4 Organic compounds
BT2 Sugars
BT3 Carbohydrates
BT4 Nutrients
BT4 Organic compounds
BT3 Plant foods
BT4 Foods
NT1 Isomaltooligosaccharides
NT1 Maltooligosaccharides
NT2 Maltohexaose
NT2 Maltotetraose
NT2 Maltotriose
NT1 Panose

Glucoraphanin
HN introduced from vol. 39, issue 1 (2007)
BT1 Glucosinolates
BT2 Glycosides
BT3 Carbohydrates
BT4 Nutrients
BT4 Organic compounds
RT Sulforaphane

Glucosamine
BT1 Hexosamines
BT2 Amino sugars
BT3 Sugars
BT4 Carbohydrates
BT5 Nutrients
BT5 Organic compounds
BT4 Plant foods
BT5 Foods

Glucose
BT1 Monosaccharides
BT2 Sugars
BT3 Carbohydrates
BT4 Nutrients
BT4 Organic compounds
BT3 Plant foods
BT4 Foods
NT1 Glucose-6-phosphate
RT Glucose syrups
RT Glucose tolerance
RT Glycaemic load
RT Glycolysis
RT Hypoglycaemic activity
UF Dextrose

Glucose isomerases
SN EC entry for this enzyme has been deleted, activity now attributed to xylose isomerases (EC 5.3.1.5); term still widely used
BT1 Isomerases
BT2 Enzymes
RT Xylose isomerases

Glucose oxidases
SN EC 1.1.3.4
BT1 Oxidases
BT2 Oxidoreductases
BT3 Enzymes

Glucose-6-phosphate
BT1 Glucose
BT2 Monosaccharides
BT3 Sugars
BT4 Carbohydrates
BT5 Nutrients
BT5 Organic compounds
BT4 Plant foods
BT5 Foods

Glucose-1-phosphate adenylyltransferases
SN EC 2.7.7.27
BT1 Transferases
BT2 Enzymes
UF ADP-glucose pyrophosphorylases

Glucose syrups
BT1 Sugar syrups
BT2 Plant foods
BT3 Foods
RT Corn syrups
RT Glucose

Glucose tolerance
HN introduced from vol. 38, issue 8 (2006)
BT1 Human physiology
BT2 Physiology
BT3 Science
RT Glucose
RT Hypoglycaemic activity

Glucosidases
HN heading up to vol. 24 (1992)
USE **Glycosidases**

α-Glucosidases
SN EC 3.2.1.20
BT1 Glycosidases
BT2 Hydrolases
BT3 Enzymes
UF Maltases

β-Glucosidases
SN EC 3.2.1.21
BT1 Glycosidases
BT2 Hydrolases
BT3 Enzymes
UF Cellobiases
UF Linamarases

Glucosides
BT1 Glycosides
BT2 Carbohydrates
BT3 Nutrients
BT3 Organic compounds
NT1 Geniposide
NT1 Limonoid glucosides
NT1 Piceid
NT1 Puerarin

Glucosinolases
USE **Thioglucosidases**

Glucosinolates
BT1 Glycosides
BT2 Carbohydrates
BT3 Nutrients
BT3 Organic compounds
NT1 Glucobrassicin
NT1 Glucoraphanin
NT1 Progoitrin
NT1 Sinigrin
RT Poisoning

Glucosyltransferases
SN members of subclass EC 2.4.1; syn. transglucosylases
BT1 Glycosyltransferases
BT2 Transferases
BT3 Enzymes

Glucuronic acid
HN under Pectic substances up to vol. 42 (2010)
BT1 Uronic acids
BT2 Organic acids
BT3 Acids
BT2 Sugars
BT3 Carbohydrates
BT4 Nutrients
BT4 Organic compounds
BT3 Plant foods
BT4 Foods

α-Glucuronidases
SN EC 3.2.1.139
BT1 Glycosidases
BT2 Hydrolases
BT3 Enzymes

β-Glucuronidases
SN EC 3.2.1.31
BT1 Glycosidases
BT2 Hydrolases
BT3 Enzymes

Glutamate decarboxylases
SN EC 4.1.1.15
BT1 Decarboxylases
BT2 Lyases
BT3 Enzymes

Glutamate dehydrogenases
SN EC 1.4.1.2, 1.4.1.3 or 1.4.1.4 depending on acceptor molecule (NAD+, NAD(P)+ or NADP+, respectively)
BT1 Dehydrogenases
BT2 Oxidoreductases
BT3 Enzymes

Glutamate oxidases
USE **L-Glutamate oxidases**

L-Glutamate oxidases
SN EC 1.4.3.11
BT1 Oxidases
BT2 Oxidoreductases
BT3 Enzymes
UF Glutamate oxidases

Glutamates
BT1 Flavourings
BT2 Additives
BT1 Salts
NT1 Monosodium glutamate
RT Flavour compounds
RT Flavour enhancers
RT Glutamic acid

Glutamic acid
BT1 Amino acids
BT2 Nutrients
BT2 Organic acids
BT3 Acids
BT2 Organic nitrogen compounds
BT1 Flavourings
BT2 Additives
NT1 Poly(γ-glutamic acid)
RT Flavour enhancers
RT Glutamates

Glutaminases
SN EC 3.5.1.2
BT1 Hydrolases
BT2 Enzymes

Glutamine
BT1 Amino acids
BT2 Nutrients
BT2 Organic acids
BT3 Acids
BT2 Organic nitrogen compounds

γ-Glutamyl hydrolases
SN EC 3.4.19.9
BT1 Proteinases
BT2 Hydrolases
BT3 Enzymes
UF Conjugases
UF Folate conjugases

γ-Glutamyltransferases
SN EC 2.3.2.2
BT1 Acyltransferases
BT2 Transferases
BT3 Enzymes

Glutaraldehyde
BT1 Aldehydes
BT2 Carbonyl compounds
BT3 Organic compounds

Glutaric acid
BT1 Organic acids
BT2 Acids

Glutathione
BT1 Organic sulfur compounds
BT1 Peptides
BT2 Proteins
BT3 Nutrients

Glutathione peroxidases
HN introduced from vol. 42, issue 1 (2010)
SN EC 1.11.1.9
BT1 Peroxidases
BT2 Oxidoreductases
BT3 Enzymes

Glutathione transferases
HN introduced from vol. 39, issue 1 (2007)
SN EC 2.5.1.18
BT1 Transferases
BT2 Enzymes

Glutelins
BT1 Cereal proteins
BT2 Proteins cereal
BT3 Vegetable proteins
BT4 Proteins vegetable
BT5 Proteins
BT6 Nutrients
BT5 Vegetable products
BT6 Plant foods
BT7 Foods

Gluten
BT1 Cereal proteins
BT2 Proteins cereal
BT3 Vegetable proteins
BT4 Proteins vegetable
BT5 Proteins
BT6 Nutrients
BT5 Vegetable products
BT6 Plant foods
BT7 Foods
NT1 Gluten low foods
NT2 Gluten low bread
NT1 Vital gluten
NT1 Wheat gluten

Gluten free bread
USE **Gluten low bread**

Gluten free foods
USE **Gluten low foods**

Glutenin
BT1 Cereal proteins
BT2 Proteins cereal
BT3 Vegetable proteins
BT4 Proteins vegetable
BT5 Proteins
BT6 Nutrients
BT5 Vegetable products
BT6 Plant foods
BT7 Foods

Gluten low bread
BT1 Bread
BT2 Bakery products
BT3 Cereal products
BT4 Plant foods
BT5 Foods
BT1 Gluten low foods
BT2 Dietetic foods
BT3 Processed foods
BT4 Foods
BT2 Gluten
BT3 Cereal proteins
BT4 Proteins cereal
BT5 Vegetable proteins
BT6 Proteins vegetable
BT7 Proteins
BT8 Nutrients
BT7 Vegetable products
BT8 Plant foods
BT9 Foods
UF Gluten free bread

Gluten low foods
BT1 Dietetic foods
BT2 Processed foods
BT3 Foods
BT1 Gluten
BT2 Cereal proteins
BT3 Proteins cereal
BT4 Vegetable proteins
BT5 Proteins vegetable
BT6 Proteins
BT7 Nutrients
BT6 Vegetable products
BT7 Plant foods
BT8 Foods
NT1 Gluten low bread
UF Gluten free foods

Glycaemic index values
BT1 Nutritional values

Glycaemic load
HN introduced from vol. 39, issue 1 (2007)
BT1 Nutritional values
RT Glucose

Glycans
USE **Polysaccharides**

Glycation
HN introduced from vol. 37, issue 5 (2005)
BT1 Modification

Glyceraldehyde
BT1 Aldehydes
BT2 Carbonyl compounds
BT3 Organic compounds

Glycerides
SN syn. acylglycerols
BT1 Emulsifiers
BT2 Additives
BT1 Fatty acid esters
BT2 Esters
BT3 Organic compounds
BT1 Lipids
BT2 Nutrients
NT1 Acylglycerols
NT1 Diglycerides
NT2 Diacylglycerols
NT1 Glycerol monostearate
NT1 Glyceryl monostearate
NT1 Monoglycerides
NT2 Monoacylglycerols
NT2 Monolaurin
NT1 Phosphoglycerides
NT1 Triglycerides
NT2 Olein
NT3 Palm olein
NT2 Stearin
NT3 Palm stearin
NT2 Triacetin
NT2 Triacylglycerols
NT2 Tricaprylin
NT2 Trilinolein
NT2 Triolein
NT2 Tripalmitin
NT2 Tristearin

Glycerin
SN syn. glycerol
BT1 Glycerol
BT2 Polyols
BT3 Alcohols
BT3 Carbohydrates
BT4 Nutrients
BT4 Organic compounds

Glycerine
SN syn. glycerol
BT1 Glycerol
BT2 Polyols
BT3 Alcohols
BT3 Carbohydrates
BT4 Nutrients
BT4 Organic compounds

Glycerol
SN syn. glycerin; syn. glycerine
BT1 Polyols
BT2 Alcohols
BT2 Carbohydrates
BT3 Nutrients
BT3 Organic compounds
NT1 Glycerin
NT1 Glycerine
RT Polyglycerol fatty acid esters

Glycerolipids
USE **Glycolipids**

Glycerol monolaurate
USE **Monolaurin**

Glycerol monostearate
SN syn. glyceryl monostearate
BT1 Glycerides
BT2 Emulsifiers
BT3 Additives
BT2 Fatty acid esters
BT3 Esters
BT4 Organic compounds
BT2 Lipids
BT3 Nutrients

Glycerolysis
HN introduced from vol. 39, issue 1 (2007)
BT1 Alcoholysis
BT2 Esterification

Glyceryl monostearate
SN syn. glycerol monostearate
BT1 Glycerides
BT2 Emulsifiers
BT3 Additives
BT2 Fatty acid esters
BT3 Esters
BT4 Organic compounds
BT2 Lipids
BT3 Nutrients

Glycine
BT1 Amino acids
BT2 Nutrients
BT2 Organic acids
BT3 Acids
BT2 Organic nitrogen compounds

Glycine betaine
BT1 Ammonium compounds
BT1 Organic nitrogen compounds

Glycinin
BT1 Soy proteins
BT2 Vegetable proteins
BT3 Proteins vegetable
BT4 Proteins
BT5 Nutrients
BT4 Vegetable products
BT5 Plant foods
BT6 Foods
RT Conglycinin
RT Soy 11S globulins

Glycitein
HN introduced from vol. 41, issue 1 (2009)
BT1 Isoflavones
BT2 Isoflavonoids
BT3 Flavonoids
BT4 Aromatic compounds
BT5 Organic compounds
BT4 Pigments

Glycoalkaloids
BT1 Alkaloids
BT2 Organic nitrogen compounds
NT1 Chaconine
NT1 Solanine

Glycogen
HN heading up to vol. 24 (1992); under Starch from vol. 25 (1993) up to vol. 42 (2010)
BT1 Glucans
BT2 Polysaccharides
BT3 Carbohydrates
BT4 Nutrients
BT4 Organic compounds
RT Glycolysis

Glycolaldehyde
BT1 Aldehydes
BT2 Carbonyl compounds
BT3 Organic compounds

Glycolic acid
BT1 Organic acids
BT2 Acids

Glycolipids
BT1 Lipids
BT2 Nutrients
NT1 Cerebrosides
NT1 Galactolipids
NT1 Gangliosides
UF Glycerolipids

Glycols
BT1 Alcohols
NT1 1,3-Butylene glycol
NT1 2,3-Butylene glycol
NT1 Diethylene glycol
NT1 Ethylene glycol
NT1 Polyethylene glycol
NT1 1,2-Propanediol
NT1 Propylene glycol

Glycolysis
RT Glucose
RT Glycogen

Glycomacropeptides
BT1 Peptides
BT2 Proteins
BT3 Nutrients

Glycopeptides
BT1 Peptides
BT2 Proteins
BT3 Nutrients

Glycoproteins
BT1 Proteins
BT2 Nutrients
NT1 Avidin
NT1 Bifidus factors
NT1 Lectins
NT2 Concanavalin A
NT2 Haemagglutinins
NT2 Phytohaemagglutinins
NT2 Ricin
NT1 Mannoproteins
NT1 Miraculin
NT1 Mucins
NT1 Mucoids
NT1 Ovomucins
NT1 Ovomucoid
NT1 Ovotransferrin
NT1 Transferrins

Glycosaminoglycans
HN introduced from vol. 39, issue 1 (2007)
SN syn. mucopolysaccharides
BT1 Polysaccharides
BT2 Carbohydrates
BT3 Nutrients
BT3 Organic compounds
NT1 Chondroitin
NT1 Hyaluronic acid
NT1 Mucopolysaccharides
RT Connective tissues

Glycosidases
HN heading from vol. 25 (1993); under Carbohydrases or Glucosidases up to vol. 1992)
SN EC 3.2.1
BT1 Hydrolases
BT2 Enzymes
NT1 Acetylglucosaminidases
NT1 β-*N*-acetylhexosaminidases
NT1 Agarases
NT1 Amylases
NT2 α-Amylases
NT2 β-Amylases
NT2 Amylolytic enzymes
NT2 Diastatic activity
NT2 Glucan 1,4-α-glucosidases
NT2 Isoamylases
NT1 α-*N*-Arabinofuranosidases
NT1 Carbohydrases
NT1 Cellulases
NT1 Cellulolytic enzymes
NT1 Cellulose 1,4-β-cellobiosidases
NT1 Cellulosomes
NT1 Chitinases
NT1 Chitosanases
NT1 Cyclomaltodextrinases
NT1 Dextranases
NT1 Dextrinases
NT1 Endo-1,3(4)-β-glucanases
NT1 Endo-1,4-β-xylanases
NT1 β-Fructofuranosidases
NT1 Galactosidases
NT2 Galactanases
NT2 α-Galactosidases
NT2 β-Galactosidases
NT1 Glucanases
NT1 β-Glucanases
NT1 Glucan endo-1,3-β-D-glucosidases
NT1 α-Glucosidases
NT1 β-Glucosidases
NT1 α-Glucuronidases
NT1 β-Glucuronidases
NT1 Hemicellulases
NT1 Inulinases
NT1 Levanases
NT1 Licheninases
NT1 Limit dextrinases
NT1 Lysozymes
NT2 Eggs lysozymes
NT2 Egg whites lysozymes
NT1 Mannan endo-1,4-β-mannosidases
NT1 Mannosidases
NT1 α-Mannosidases
NT1 β-Mannosidases
NT1 Mutanolysins
NT1 Neopullulanases
NT1 Oligo-1,6-glucosidases
NT1 Pentosanases
NT1 Polygalacturonases
NT1 Pullulanases
NT1 α-L-rhamnosidases
NT1 Sucrose α-glucosidases
NT1 Thioglucosidases
NT1 α,α-Trehalases
NT1 Xylan degrading enzymes
NT1 Xylan endo-1,3-β-xylosidases
NT1 Xylan 1,4-β-xylosidases
UF Glucosidases

Glycosides
BT1 Carbohydrates
BT2 Nutrients
BT2 Organic compounds
NT1 Aglycones
NT1 Amygdalin
NT1 Arbutin
NT1 Convicine
NT1 Cyanogenic glycosides
NT1 Digitonin
NT1 Diglucosides
NT1 Dihydrochalcones
NT2 Neohesperidin dihydrochalcone
NT2 Phloretin
NT1 Galactosides
NT1 Glucides
NT1 Glucosides
NT2 Geniposide
NT2 Limonoid glucosides
NT2 Piceid
NT2 Puerarin
NT1 Glucosinolates
NT2 Glucobrassicin
NT2 Glucoraphanin
NT2 Progoitrin
NT2 Sinigrin
NT1 Glycyrrhizic acid
NT1 Glycyrrhizin
NT1 Gymnemic acid
NT1 Hesperidin
NT1 Linamarin
NT1 Naringenin
NT1 Naringin
NT1 Neohesperidin
NT1 Oleuropein

NT1 Prunasin
NT1 Quercitrin
NT1 Rebaudiosides
NT1 Rutin
NT1 Saponins
NT2 Digitonin
NT2 Ginsenosides
NT2 Quillaja saponins
NT1 Simmondsin
NT1 Stevioside
NT1 Tannins
NT2 Ellagitannins
NT2 Proanthocyanidins
NT3 Procyanidins
NT2 Tannic acid
NT1 Thioglycosides
NT1 Vicine
RT Alkaloids
RT Anthocyanidins
RT Anthocyanins
RT Flavonoids
RT Pigments
RT Sweeteners
RT Toxins

Glycosylation
BT1 Modification
NT1 Transglycosylation

Glycosyltransferases
HN heading from vol. 30 (1998); under Transferases up to vol. 29 (1997)
SN EC 2.4
BT1 Transferases
BT2 Enzymes
NT1 Alternansucrases
NT1 Cyclomaltodextrin glucanotransferases
NT1 Dextransucrases
NT1 Fructosyltransferases
NT1 1,4-α-Glucan branching enzymes
NT1 4-α-Glucanotransferases
NT1 Glucosyltransferases
NT1 Lactose synthases
NT1 Levansucrases
NT1 Starch synthases
NT1 Sucrose-phosphate synthases
NT1 Sucrose synthases
NT1 Transglucosylases

Glycyrrhizic acid
HN also under Organic acids up to vol. 42 (2010)
BT1 Flavour compounds
BT1 Glycosides
BT2 Carbohydrates
BT3 Nutrients
BT3 Organic compounds
BT1 Sweeteners
BT2 Additives
BT1 Triterpenoids
BT2 Terpenoids
BT3 Lipids
BT4 Nutrients
RT Liquorice

Glycyrrhizin
BT1 Flavour compounds
BT1 Glycosides
BT2 Carbohydrates
BT3 Nutrients
BT3 Organic compounds
BT1 Sweeteners
BT2 Additives
BT1 Triterpenoids
BT2 Terpenoids
BT3 Lipids
BT4 Nutrients
RT Liquorice

Glyoxal
BT1 Aldehydes
BT2 Carbonyl compounds
BT3 Organic compounds
RT Aroma compounds
RT Maillard reaction products

Glyphosate
BT1 Herbicides
BT2 Pesticides
BT3 Biocides
BT3 Residues
BT1 Organophosphorus pesticides
BT2 Pesticides
BT3 Biocides
BT3 Residues

GM foods
HN genetically modified foods used in the index up to vol. 35, issue 6 (2003)
BT1 Genetics
BT1 Novel foods
BT2 Foods
RT Biotechnologically derived foods
RT Genetically engineered foods
UF Genetically modified foods

GM microorganisms
HN genetically modified microorganisms used in the index up to vol. 35, issue 6 (2003)
BT1 Genetics
BT1 Microorganisms
RT GMO
RT GM organisms
UF Genetically modified microorganisms

GMO
HN genetically modified organisms used in the index up to vol. 35, issue 6 (2003)
BT1 Genetics
RT GM microorganisms
RT GM organisms
RT Transgenic animals
RT Transgenic plants
UF Genetically modified organisms

GM organisms
HN genetically modified organisms used in the index up to vol. 35, issue 6 (2003)
BT1 Genetics
RT GM microorganisms
RT GMO
RT Transgenic animals
RT Transgenic plants

GMP
BT1 Nucleotides
RT Flavour enhancers
RT Guanosine
UF Guanosine monophosphate
UF Guanylic acid

Gnocchi
BT1 Potato products
BT2 Potatoes
BT3 Vegetables specific
BT4 Vegetables
BT5 Crops
BT6 Plants
BT5 Plant foods
BT6 Foods

Goat carcasses
BT1 Carcasses
BT2 Meat
BT3 Animal foods
BT4 Foods
BT1 Goat meat
BT2 Goats
BT3 Animals
BT2 Meat specific
BT3 Meat
BT4 Animal foods
BT5 Foods

Goat cheese
BT1 Cheese varieties
BT2 Cheese
BT3 Dairy products
BT4 Animal foods
BT5 Foods
BT1 Goats
BT2 Animals
UF Goat milk cheese

Goat meat
HN heading from vol. 30 (1998); under Goats and Meat specific up to vol. 29 (1997)
BT1 Goats
BT2 Animals
BT1 Meat specific
BT2 Meat
BT3 Animal foods
BT4 Foods
NT1 Capretto
NT1 Chevon
NT1 Goat carcasses

Goat milk
BT1 Goats
BT2 Animals
BT1 Milk
BT2 Dairy products
BT3 Animal foods
BT4 Foods

Goat milk cheese
USE **Goat cheese**

Goats
BT1 Animals

NT1 Goat cheese
NT1 Goat meat
NT2 Capretto
NT2 Chevon
NT2 Goat carcasses
NT1 Goat milk
NT1 Goat yoghurt
UF Caprine
UF Kids

Goat yoghurt
HN introduced from vol. 39, issue 1 (2007)
BT1 Goats
BT2 Animals
BT1 Yoghurt
BT2 Fermented milk
BT3 Fermented dairy products
BT4 Dairy products
BT5 Animal foods
BT6 Foods
BT4 Fermented foods
BT5 Processed foods
BT6 Foods
BT3 Milk
BT4 Dairy products
BT5 Animal foods
BT6 Foods

Godulbaegi
BT1 Vegetables specific
BT2 Vegetables
BT3 Crops
BT4 Plants
BT3 Plant foods
BT4 Foods

Gofio
HN introduced from vol. 37, issue 5 (2005)
BT1 Cereal products
BT2 Plant foods
BT3 Foods

Goitre
HN introduced from vol. 40, issue 1 (2008)
BT1 Diseases
RT Goitrogens
RT Iodine

Goitrogens
BT1 Toxins
BT2 Residues
RT Goitre

Gold
USE **Au**

Goldenberries
HN introduced from vol. 37, issue 5 (2005)
SN syn. cape gooseberries
BT1 Cape gooseberries
BT2 Fruits specific
BT3 Fruits
BT4 Crops
BT5 Plants
BT4 Plant foods
BT5 Foods

Gonyautoxins
BT1 Toxins
BT2 Residues

Good Manufacturing Practice
BT1 Quality control
BT2 Technology

Gooseberries
BT1 Berries
BT2 Fruits specific
BT3 Fruits
BT4 Crops
BT5 Plants
BT4 Plant foods
BT5 Foods

Goose carcasses
BT1 Carcasses
BT2 Meat
BT3 Animal foods
BT4 Foods
BT1 Goose meat
BT2 Geese
BT3 Poultry
BT4 Birds
BT2 Poultry meat
BT3 Meat specific
BT4 Meat
BT5 Animal foods
BT6 Foods

Goose eggs
HN introduced from vol. 39, issue 1 (2007)
BT1 Eggs
BT2 Animal foods
BT3 Foods
BT1 Geese
BT2 Poultry
BT3 Birds

Goose livers
HN introduced from vol. 39, issue 1 (2007)
BT1 Geese
BT2 Poultry
BT3 Birds
BT1 Livers
BT2 Offal
BT3 Animal foods
BT4 Foods

Goose meat
BT1 Geese
BT2 Poultry
BT3 Birds
BT1 Poultry meat
BT2 Meat specific
BT3 Meat
BT4 Animal foods
BT5 Foods
NT1 Goose carcasses

Gorgon nuts
BT1 Nuts
BT2 Fruits
BT3 Crops
BT4 Plants
BT3 Plant foods
BT4 Foods
BT2 Oilseeds
BT3 Seeds
BT4 Plant foods
BT5 Foods
UF Makhana

Gorgonzola cheese
BT1 Cheese varieties
BT2 Cheese
BT3 Dairy products
BT4 Animal foods
BT5 Foods

Gossypol
BT1 Cottonseeds
BT2 Oilseeds
BT3 Seeds
BT4 Plant foods
BT5 Foods
BT1 Pigments
RT Poisoning

Gouda cheese
BT1 Cheese varieties
BT2 Cheese
BT3 Dairy products
BT4 Animal foods
BT5 Foods

Goulash
BT1 Meals
BT2 Processed foods
BT3 Foods

Gourds
BT1 Vegetables specific
BT2 Vegetables
BT3 Crops
BT4 Plants
BT3 Plant foods
BT4 Foods
NT1 *Benincasa hispida*
NT1 Bitter gourds
NT1 Buffalo gourds
NT1 Wax gourds

Gourd seeds
BT1 Oilseeds
BT2 Seeds
BT3 Plant foods
BT4 Foods

Gout
HN introduced from vol. 39, issue 1 (2007)
BT1 Diseases

Gouter
BT1 Meals
BT2 Processed foods
BT3 Foods

Gracilaria
BT1 Seaweeds
BT2 Algae
BT3 Microorganisms
BT2 Sea foods
BT3 Aquatic foods
BT4 Animal foods
BT5 Foods

Grading
NT1 Sorting
RT Classification

Grain
SN use for unspecified food grains
BT1 Seeds
BT2 Plant foods
BT3 Foods

Grain alcohols
USE **Spirits**

Grain amaranth
HN under Pseudocereals from vol. 25 (1993) to vol. 29(1997)
BT1 Amaranth grain
BT2 Pseudocereals
BT3 Seeds
BT4 Plant foods
BT5 Foods

Grain borers
HN introduced from vol. 41, issue 1 (2009)
BT1 Insects
BT2 Pests

Graininess
BT1 Consistency
BT2 Texture
BT3 Sensory properties

Gram negative bacteria
BT1 Bacteria
BT2 Microorganisms
RT Microbiological techniques

Gram positive bacteria
BT1 Bacteria
BT2 Microorganisms
RT Microbiological techniques

Grams
USE **Legumes**

Grana cheese
BT1 Cheese varieties
BT2 Cheese
BT3 Dairy products
BT4 Animal foods
BT5 Foods

Granadillas
USE **Passion fruits**

Grana Padano cheese
BT1 Cheese varieties
BT2 Cheese
BT3 Dairy products
BT4 Animal foods
BT5 Foods

Granola
BT1 Cereal products
BT2 Plant foods
BT3 Foods

Granulated sugar
BT1 Sugar
BT2 Plant foods
BT3 Foods

Granulation
BT1 Granules

Granules
NT1 Granulation
RT Agglomeration
RT Dried foods
RT Instant foods
RT Particles
RT Powders

Granulometry
BT1 Analytical techniques

Grapefruit
BT1 Citrus fruits
BT2 Fruits specific
BT3 Fruits
BT4 Crops
BT5 Plants
BT4 Plant foods
BT5 Foods
NT1 Grapefruit peel
RT Grapefruit juices

Grapefruit juices
BT1 Citrus juices
BT2 Fruit juices
BT3 Fruit products
BT4 Plant foods
BT5 Foods
BT3 Soft drinks
BT4 Beverages
RT Grapefruit

Grapefruit peel
BT1 Grapefruit
BT2 Citrus fruits
BT3 Fruits specific
BT4 Fruits
BT5 Crops
BT6 Plants
BT5 Plant foods
BT6 Foods
BT1 Peel

Grape jams
BT1 Grapes
BT2 Berries
BT3 Fruits specific
BT4 Fruits
BT5 Crops
BT6 Plants
BT5 Plant foods
BT6 Foods
BT1 Jams
BT2 Fruit preserves
BT3 Fruit products
BT4 Plant foods
BT5 Foods
BT3 Preserves
BT4 Processed foods
BT5 Foods

Grape juice concentrates
BT1 Fruit juice concentrates
BT2 Concentrates
BT3 Processed foods
BT4 Foods
BT2 Fruit juices
BT3 Fruit products
BT4 Plant foods
BT5 Foods
BT3 Soft drinks
BT4 Beverages
BT1 Grape juices
BT2 Fruit juices
BT3 Fruit products
BT4 Plant foods
BT5 Foods
BT3 Soft drinks
BT4 Beverages

Grape juices
BT1 Fruit juices
BT2 Fruit products
BT3 Plant foods
BT4 Foods
BT2 Soft drinks
BT3 Beverages
NT1 Grape juice concentrates
RT Grapes
RT Musts
RT Pekmez
RT Winemaking

Grape marc
BT1 Marc
BT2 By-products

Grape musts
BT1 Musts
BT2 Fruit juices
BT3 Fruit products
BT4 Plant foods
BT5 Foods
BT3 Soft drinks
BT4 Beverages
NT1 Concentrated rectified musts

Grape pomaces
BT1 Grapes
BT2 Berries
BT3 Fruits specific
BT4 Fruits
BT5 Crops
BT6 Plants
BT5 Plant foods
BT6 Foods
BT1 Pomaces
BT2 Wastes

Grapes
BT1 Berries
BT2 Fruits specific
BT3 Fruits
BT4 Crops
BT5 Plants
BT4 Plant foods
BT5 Foods
NT1 Grape jams
NT1 Grape pomaces
NT1 Grape seeds
NT1 Grape skins
NT1 Muscadine grapes
NT1 Seedless grapes
NT1 Table grapes
NT1 *Vitis vinifera*
NT1 Winemaking grapes
RT Grape juices

RT Vines
RT Winemaking

Grape seed oils
BT1 Vegetable oils
BT2 Oils vegetable
BT3 Oils
BT4 Lipids
BT5 Nutrients
BT3 Vegetable products
BT4 Plant foods
BT5 Foods

Grape seeds
BT1 Grapes
BT2 Berries
BT3 Fruits specific
BT4 Fruits
BT5 Crops
BT6 Plants
BT5 Plant foods
BT6 Foods
BT1 Seeds
BT2 Plant foods
BT3 Foods

Grape skins
BT1 Grapes
BT2 Berries
BT3 Fruits specific
BT4 Fruits
BT5 Crops
BT6 Plants
BT5 Plant foods
BT6 Foods
BT1 Peel

Grape spirits
BT1 Spirits
BT2 Alcoholic beverages
BT3 Beverages alcoholic
BT4 Beverages

Grappa
BT1 Brandies
BT2 Spirits
BT3 Alcoholic beverages
BT4 Beverages alcoholic
BT5 Beverages

Grass carp
SN syn. white amur
BT1 Carp
BT2 Freshwater fish
BT3 Fish
BT4 Animals
BT4 Sea foods
BT5 Aquatic foods
BT6 Animal foods
BT7 Foods
BT2 Oily fish
BT3 Fish
BT4 Animals
BT4 Sea foods
BT5 Aquatic foods
BT6 Animal foods
BT7 Foods
NT1 White amur

Grass peas
HN heading from vol. 30 (1998); under Legumes up to vol. 29 (1997)
BT1 Legumes
BT2 Vegetables specific
BT3 Vegetables
BT4 Crops
BT5 Plants
BT4 Plant foods
BT5 Foods
UF Kesari dhal

GRAS status
BT1 Food safety
RT GRAS substances

GRAS substances
BT1 Food safety
RT GRAS status

Grating
BT1 Comminution
BT2 Processing
BT3 Technology

Gravimetry
BT1 Analytical techniques
UF Thermogravimetric analysis

Gravity
BT1 Density
BT2 Physical properties
RT sp. gr.

Gravy
BT1 Meat products
BT2 Animal foods
BT3 Foods
BT1 Sauces
BT2 Condiments
BT3 Flavourings
BT4 Additives
NT1 Gravy powders

Gravy powders
BT1 Gravy
BT2 Meat products
BT3 Animal foods
BT4 Foods
BT2 Sauces
BT3 Condiments
BT4 Flavourings
BT5 Additives
BT1 Instant foods
BT2 Processed foods
BT3 Foods

Greasiness
BT1 Sensory properties

Great Britain
USE **United Kingdom**

Greece
BT1 Europe
BT1 European Union
RT Organization for Economic Cooperation and Development

Green beans
BT1 Common beans
BT2 Legumes
BT3 Vegetables specific
BT4 Vegetables
BT5 Crops
BT6 Plants
BT5 Plant foods
BT6 Foods

Green coffee
BT1 Coffee
BT2 Beverages
BT2 Crops
BT3 Plants
BT2 Plant foods
BT3 Foods

Green fluorescent protein
HN introduced from vol. 39, issue 1 (2007)
BT1 Fluorescence
BT2 Analytical techniques
BT2 Optical properties
BT3 Physical properties
BT1 Marker proteins
BT2 Cloning technology
BT3 Gene cloning
BT4 Genetic techniques
BT5 Genetics
BT3 Technology
BT2 Proteins
BT3 Nutrients

Greengages
BT1 Plums
BT2 Fruits specific
BT3 Fruits
BT4 Crops
BT5 Plants
BT4 Plant foods
BT5 Foods

Green gram
USE **Mung beans**

Greenland
HN heading from vol. 20 (1988) to vol. 24 (1992)
BT1 North America
BT2 America

Greenland halibut
HN introduced from vol. 37, issue 5 (2005)
BT1 Halibut
BT2 Flatfish
BT3 Marine fish
BT4 Fish
BT5 Animals
BT5 Sea foods
BT6 Aquatic foods
BT7 Animal foods
BT8 Foods

Green-lipped mussels
USE **Green mussels**

Green mussels
BT1 Mussels
BT2 Bivalves

BT3 Molluscs
BT4 Shellfish
BT5 Animals
BT5 Sea foods
BT6 Aquatic foods
BT7 Animal foods
BT8 Foods
UF Green-lipped mussels

Green peas
BT1 Peas
BT2 Legumes
BT3 Vegetables specific
BT4 Vegetables
BT5 Crops
BT6 Plants
BT5 Plant foods
BT6 Foods

Green peppers
BT1 Capsicums
BT2 Vegetables specific
BT3 Vegetables
BT4 Crops
BT5 Plants
BT4 Plant foods
BT5 Foods

Green tea
BT1 Tea
BT2 Teas
BT3 Beverages
BT3 Crops
BT4 Plants
BT3 Plant foods
BT4 Foods

Green vegetables
BT1 Vegetables specific
BT2 Vegetables
BT3 Crops
BT4 Plants
BT3 Plant foods
BT4 Foods

Grenada
BT1 West Indies
BT2 America

Grenadier
BT1 Marine fish
BT2 Fish
BT3 Animals
BT3 Sea foods
BT4 Aquatic foods
BT5 Animal foods
BT6 Foods
UF Grenadiers

Grenadiers
HN used up to vol. 29 (1997)
USE **Grenadier**

Grifola frondosa
BT1 Edible fungi
BT2 Fungi edible
BT3 Vegetables specific
BT4 Vegetables
BT5 Crops
BT6 Plants
BT5 Plant foods
BT6 Foods
UF Maitake

Grilling
BT1 Cooking
BT2 Thermal processing
BT3 Processing thermal
BT4 Processing
BT5 Technology

Grinding
BT1 Comminution
BT2 Processing
BT3 Technology

Griseofulvin
BT1 Antibiotics
BT2 Drugs
BT3 Residues
BT1 Mycotoxins
BT2 Toxins
BT3 Residues

Grits
BT1 Cereal products
BT2 Plant foods
BT3 Foods

Grittiness
BT1 Mouthfeel
BT2 Sensory properties

Groats
BT1 Cereal products
BT2 Plant foods
BT3 Foods

Grocery stores
BT1 Marketing
BT2 Economics

Groundbeans
BT1 Legumes
BT2 Vegetables specific
BT3 Vegetables
BT4 Crops
BT5 Plants
BT4 Plant foods
BT5 Foods

Ground beef
USE **Beef mince**

Ground chicken
USE **Chicken mince**

Ground coffee
BT1 Coffee
BT2 Beverages
BT2 Crops
BT3 Plants
BT2 Plant foods
BT3 Foods

Groundfish
BT1 Marine fish
BT2 Fish
BT3 Animals
BT3 Sea foods
BT4 Aquatic foods
BT5 Animal foods
BT6 Foods

Ground meat
USE **Meat mince**

Groundnut oils
BT1 Nut oils
BT2 Vegetable oils
BT3 Oils vegetable
BT4 Oils
BT5 Lipids
BT6 Nutrients
BT4 Vegetable products
BT5 Plant foods
BT6 Foods
UF Arachis oils
UF Peanut oils

Groundnuts
HN heading up to vol. 24 (1992)
USE **Peanuts**

Ground pork
USE **Pork mince**

Ground turkey
USE **Turkey mince**

Groundwater
BT1 Water

Grouper
BT1 Marine fish
BT2 Fish
BT3 Animals
BT3 Sea foods
BT4 Aquatic foods
BT5 Animal foods
BT6 Foods
NT1 *Epinephelus guaza*

Growth (human)
HN introduced from vol. 43, issue 1 (2011)
SN includes animal model studies
BT1 Anthropometric parameters
BT2 Health

Growth factors
HN introduced from vol. 37, issue 5 (2005)
BT1 Hormones
BT2 Residues
NT1 Myostatin

Growth hormone
USE **Somatotropin**

Growth promoters (animal)
BT1 Hormones
BT2 Residues
UF Growth stimulators

Growth promoters (microbial)
BT1 Microorganisms
UF Growth stimulators

Growth promoters (plant)
BT1 Plant growth regulators
BT2 Cultivation

BT3 Agriculture
UF Growth stimulators

Growth stimulators
USE **Growth promoters (animal)**
USE **Growth promoters (microbial)**
USE **Growth promoters (plant)**

Gruel
BT1 Porridges
BT2 Cereal products
BT3 Plant foods
BT4 Foods

Gruyere cheese
BT1 Cheese varieties
BT2 Cheese
BT3 Dairy products
BT4 Animal foods
BT5 Foods

Guacamole
BT1 Avocados
BT2 Vegetables specific
BT3 Vegetables
BT4 Crops
BT5 Plants
BT4 Plant foods
BT5 Foods

Guadeloupe
BT1 West Indies
BT2 America

Guaiacol
BT1 Phenols
BT2 Alcohols
BT2 Aromatic compounds
BT3 Organic compounds
RT Aroma compounds
RT Taints

Guam
BT1 Oceania

Guanidine
BT1 Organic nitrogen compounds

Guanosine
BT1 Nucleosides
RT GMP

Guanosine monophosphate
SN syn. guanylic acid
USE **GMP**

Guanylic acid
SN syn. guanosine monophosphate
USE **GMP**

Guarana
HN under Beverages up to vol. 42 (2010)
BT1 Soft drinks
BT2 Beverages
NT1 *Paullinia cupana*

Guar beans
SN syn. cluster beans
BT1 Legumes
BT2 Vegetables specific
BT3 Vegetables
BT4 Crops
BT5 Plants
BT4 Plant foods
BT5 Foods
NT1 Cluster beans
RT Guar gums

Guar gums
BT1 Gums
BT2 Polysaccharides
BT3 Carbohydrates
BT4 Nutrients
BT4 Organic compounds
BT2 Stabilizers
BT3 Additives
BT2 Thickeners
BT3 Additives
RT Guar beans

Guatemala
BT1 Central America
BT2 America

Guava juices
BT1 Fruit juices
BT2 Fruit products
BT3 Plant foods
BT4 Foods
BT2 Soft drinks
BT3 Beverages
RT Guavas

Guava pulps
BT1 Fruit pulps
BT2 Fruit products
BT3 Plant foods
BT4 Foods
BT2 Pulps
BT3 Processed foods
BT4 Foods
BT1 Guavas
BT2 Fruits specific
BT3 Fruits
BT4 Crops
BT5 Plants
BT4 Plant foods
BT5 Foods

Guava purees
BT1 Fruit purees
BT2 Fruit products
BT3 Plant foods
BT4 Foods
BT2 Purees
BT3 Pulps
BT4 Processed foods
BT5 Foods
BT1 Guavas
BT2 Fruits specific
BT3 Fruits
BT4 Crops
BT5 Plants
BT4 Plant foods
BT5 Foods

Guavas
HN heading from vol. 30 (1998); under Fruits specific up to vol. 29 (1997)
BT1 Fruits specific
BT2 Fruits
BT3 Crops
BT4 Plants
BT3 Plant foods
BT4 Foods
NT1 Guava pulps
NT1 Guava purees
RT Guava juices

Guidelines
RT Regulations

Guides
BT1 Books

Guinea
BT1 West Africa
BT2 Africa

Guinea-Bissau
BT1 West Africa
BT2 Africa

Guinea fowl
BT1 Poultry
BT2 Birds

Guizotia
BT1 Oilseeds
BT2 Seeds
BT3 Plant foods
BT4 Foods

Gulabjamans
BT1 Dairy products
BT2 Animal foods
BT3 Foods
BT1 Desserts
BT2 Processed foods
BT3 Foods

Gum acacia
SN syn. gum arabic
BT1 Gum arabic
BT2 Gums
BT3 Polysaccharides
BT4 Carbohydrates
BT5 Nutrients
BT5 Organic compounds
BT3 Stabilizers
BT4 Additives
BT3 Thickeners
BT4 Additives
RT *Acacia*

Gum arabic
SN syn. gum acacia
BT1 Gums
BT2 Polysaccharides
BT3 Carbohydrates
BT4 Nutrients
BT4 Organic compounds
BT2 Stabilizers
BT3 Additives
BT2 Thickeners
BT3 Additives
NT1 Gum acacia
RT *Acacia*

Gum balls
USE **Chewing gums**

Gum confectionery
BT1 Sugar confectionery
BT2 Plant foods
BT3 Foods
NT1 Bubble gums
NT1 Chewing gums
NT2 Polyvinyl acetate

Gum ghatti
BT1 Gums
BT2 Polysaccharides
BT3 Carbohydrates
BT4 Nutrients
BT4 Organic compounds
BT2 Stabilizers
BT3 Additives
BT2 Thickeners
BT3 Additives

Gum kondagogu
BT1 Gums
BT2 Polysaccharides
BT3 Carbohydrates
BT4 Nutrients
BT4 Organic compounds
BT2 Stabilizers
BT3 Additives
BT2 Thickeners
BT3 Additives

Gums
BT1 Polysaccharides
BT2 Carbohydrates
BT3 Nutrients
BT3 Organic compounds
BT1 Stabilizers
BT2 Additives
BT1 Thickeners
BT2 Additives
NT1 Cassia gums
NT1 Furcellaran
NT1 Gellan gums
NT1 Guar gums
NT1 Gum arabic
NT2 Gum acacia
NT1 Gum ghatti
NT1 Gum kondagogu
NT1 Gum tragacanth
NT1 Karaya gums
NT1 Locust bean gums
NT2 Carob gums
NT1 Mesquite seed gums
NT1 Mucilage
NT1 Psyllium gums
NT1 Tara gums
NT1 Xanthan gums
RT Hydrocolloids
RT Resins

Gum tragacanth
BT1 Gums
BT2 Polysaccharides
BT3 Carbohydrates
BT4 Nutrients
BT4 Organic compounds
BT2 Stabilizers
BT3 Additives
BT2 Thickeners
BT3 Additives

Gur
HN under Sugars up to vol. 42 (2010)
SN syn. jaggery
BT1 Jaggery
BT2 Sugar
BT3 Plant foods
BT4 Foods

Gurnard
BT1 Marine fish
BT2 Fish
BT3 Animals
BT3 Sea foods
BT4 Aquatic foods
BT5 Animal foods
BT6 Foods
UF Gurnards

Gurnards
HN used up to vol. 29 (1997)
USE **Gurnard**

Gushing
BT1 Flow
BT2 Rheological properties
BT3 Mechanical properties
BT4 Physical properties

Guthion
USE **Azinphos-methyl**

Gutting
BT1 Processing
BT2 Technology
RT Evisceration
RT Slaughter
RT Viscera

Guyana
BT1 South America
BT2 America

Gymnemic acid
BT1 Glycosides
BT2 Carbohydrates
BT3 Nutrients
BT3 Organic compounds

Gyromitra
BT1 Edible fungi
BT2 Fungi edible
BT3 Vegetables specific
BT4 Vegetables
BT5 Crops
BT6 Plants
BT5 Plant foods
BT6 Foods

Gyromitrin
BT1 Mycotoxins
BT2 Toxins
BT3 Residues

Gyros
BT1 Meat products
BT2 Animal foods
BT3 Foods

H

H_2
HN also under Minerals up to vol. 42 (2010)
SN use for gaseous form
BT1 Gases
BT2 Physical phases
BT3 Chemistry
BT4 Science
BT1 Hydrogen
BT2 Elements
BT3 Minerals
BT4 Nutrients

HACCP
HN heading from vol. 30 (1998); under Quality control up to vol. 29 (1997)
BT1 Food safety
BT1 Quality control
BT2 Technology
RT Critical control points
UF Hazard analysis critical control point

Haddock
BT1 Marine fish
BT2 Fish
BT3 Animals
BT3 Sea foods
BT4 Aquatic foods
BT5 Animal foods
BT6 Foods

Haem
BT1 Porphyrins
BT2 Heterocyclic compounds
BT2 Organic nitrogen compounds
BT2 Pigments

Haemagglutination
HN introduced from vol. 37, issue 5 (2005)
BT1 Agglutination
BT2 Aggregation
BT3 Agglomeration
RT Haemagglutinins

Haemagglutinins
BT1 Lectins
BT2 Glycoproteins
BT3 Proteins
BT4 Nutrients
BT2 Vegetable proteins
BT3 Proteins vegetable
BT4 Proteins
BT5 Nutrients
BT4 Vegetable products
BT5 Plant foods
BT6 Foods
RT Haemagglutination

Haematin
BT1 Porphyrins
BT2 Heterocyclic compounds
BT2 Organic nitrogen compounds
BT2 Pigments

Haematococcus
BT1 Microalgae
BT2 Algae
BT3 Microorganisms
NT1 *Haematococcus pluvialis*

Haematococcus pluvialis
BT1 *Haematococcus*
BT2 Microalgae
BT3 Algae
BT4 Microorganisms

Haemin
HN introduced from vol. 39, issue 1 (2007)
BT1 Porphyrins
BT2 Heterocyclic compounds
BT2 Organic nitrogen compounds
BT2 Pigments

Haemocyanin
BT1 Proteins
BT2 Nutrients

Haemoglobin
BT1 Animal proteins
BT2 Proteins animal
BT3 Proteins
BT4 Nutrients
BT1 Pigments

Haemolysins
BT1 Immunology

Haemolysis
HN introduced from vol. 41, issue 1 (2009)
BT1 Erythrocytes
BT2 Cells
BT1 Lysis
BT2 Decomposition

Haemolytic uraemic syndrome
HN introduced from vol. 42, issue 1 (2010)
BT1 Diseases
RT *Escherichia coli*
RT Shiga like toxins

Haemoproteins
BT1 Animal proteins
BT2 Proteins animal
BT3 Proteins
BT4 Nutrients
BT1 Pigments

Hafnia
HN under Enterobacteriaceae up to vol. 24 (1992)
BT1 Bacteria
BT2 Microorganisms
NT1 *Hafnia alvei*

Hafnia alvei
BT1 *Hafnia*
BT2 Bacteria
BT3 Microorganisms

Hagfish
BT1 Marine fish
BT2 Fish
BT3 Animals
BT3 Sea foods
BT4 Aquatic foods
BT5 Animal foods
BT6 Foods

Haggis
BT1 Meat products
BT2 Animal foods
BT3 Foods

Hairtail
HN introduced from vol. 37, issue 5 (2005)
BT1 Marine fish
BT2 Fish
BT3 Animals
BT3 Sea foods
BT4 Aquatic foods
BT5 Animal foods
BT6 Foods

Haiti
BT1 West Indies
BT2 America

Hake
HN heading up to vol. 24 (1992)
BT1 Marine fish
BT2 Fish
BT3 Animals
BT3 Sea foods
BT4 Aquatic foods
BT5 Animal foods
BT6 Foods
NT1 *Merluccius australis*
NT1 *Merluccius hubbsi*
NT1 *Merluccius merluccius*
NT1 Pacific hake
NT2 *Merluccius productus*
NT2 Pacific whiting
NT1 Red hake

Halal foods
BT1 Processed foods
BT2 Foods

Halawa
USE **Halva**

Half and half milk
BT1 Milk
BT2 Dairy products
BT3 Animal foods
BT4 Foods

Half cream
BT1 Cream
BT2 Dairy products
BT3 Animal foods
BT4 Foods

Halibut
BT1 Flatfish
BT2 Marine fish
BT3 Fish
BT4 Animals
BT4 Sea foods
BT5 Aquatic foods
BT6 Animal foods
BT7 Foods
NT1 Atlantic halibut
NT1 Greenland halibut
NT1 *Reinhardtius hippoglossoides*

Halides
BT1 Salts
RT Halogens

Halloumi cheese
BT1 Cheese varieties
BT2 Cheese
BT3 Dairy products
BT4 Animal foods
BT5 Foods

Haloacetic acids
HN introduced from vol. 39, issue 1 (2007)
BT1 Disinfection by-products
BT2 Disinfection
BT3 Hygiene
BT1 Organic halogen compounds

Haloanisoles
HN introduced from vol. 42, issue 1 (2010)
BT1 Organic halogen compounds
NT1 Trichloroanisole
UF Chloroanisoles

Halogenated compounds
HN heading up to vol. 24 (1992)
BT1 Organic halogen compounds

Halogens
BT1 Elements
BT2 Minerals
BT3 Nutrients
NT1 Br
NT1 Chlorine
NT2 Cl
NT1 F
NT1 Iodine
NT2 I
NT2 Iodized salt
RT Halides

Halomonas
BT1 Bacteria
BT2 Microorganisms

Halophiles
BT1 Microorganisms
UF Halophilic bacteria

Halophilic bacteria
USE **Halophiles**

Halothane
BT1 Drugs
BT2 Residues

Halothane sensitivity
BT1 Genetic disorders

Halva
BT1 Sesame seeds
BT2 Oilseeds
BT3 Seeds
BT4 Plant foods
BT5 Foods

BT1 Sugar confectionery
BT2 Plant foods
BT3 Foods
RT Tahini
RT Tehineh
UF Chalva
UF Halawa

Halvarine
BT1 Margarines
BT2 Fats
BT3 Lipids
BT4 Nutrients

Ham
BT1 Meat products
BT2 Animal foods
BT3 Foods
NT1 Boiled ham
NT1 Dry cured ham
NT1 Dry ham
NT1 Gammon
NT1 Iberian ham
NT1 Parma ham
NT1 Serrano ham
RT Bacon
RT Kasseler
RT Pork
RT Rendement Napole genes
RT Swine

Hamburgers
BT1 Burgers
BT2 Meat products
BT3 Animal foods
BT4 Foods

Handling
NT1 Gloves
NT1 Hot water dips
NT1 Stacking
RT Conveyors
RT Food handlers
RT Pallets
RT Transport

Hanseniaspora
HN under Fungi up to vol. 42 (2010)
BT1 Yeasts
BT2 Fungi
BT3 Microorganisms
NT1 *Hanseniaspora guilliermondii*
NT1 *Hanseniaspora osmophila*
NT1 *Hanseniaspora uvarum*

Hanseniaspora guilliermondii
HN introduced from vol. 41, issue 1 (2009); under Fungi up to vol. 42 (2010)
BT1 *Hanseniaspora*
BT2 Yeasts
BT3 Fungi
BT4 Microorganisms

Hanseniaspora osmophila
HN under Fungi up to vol. 42 (2010)
BT1 *Hanseniaspora*
BT2 Yeasts
BT3 Fungi
BT4 Microorganisms

Hanseniaspora uvarum
HN under Fungi up to vol. 42 (2010)
SN anamorph is Kloeckera apiculata
BT1 *Hanseniaspora*
BT2 Yeasts
BT3 Fungi
BT4 Microorganisms

Hansenula
SN obsolete genus name for Pichia spp.
BT1 Yeasts
BT2 Fungi
BT3 Microorganisms
NT1 *Hansenula polymorpha*

Hansenula polymorpha
SN synonymous with Pichia angusta
BT1 *Hansenula*
BT2 Yeasts
BT3 Fungi
BT4 Microorganisms

Happoshu
HN introduced from vol. 37, issue 5 (2005); under Beverages alcoholic up to vol. 42 (2010)
BT1 Beer
BT2 Alcoholic beverages
BT3 Beverages alcoholic
BT4 Beverages

Hard cheese
BT1 Cheese varieties
BT2 Cheese
BT3 Dairy products
BT4 Animal foods
BT5 Foods

Hardening
BT1 Hydrogenation
BT2 Processing
BT3 Technology

Hardness
BT1 Mechanical properties
BT2 Physical properties
RT Water hardness

Hard to cook defect
BT1 Cooking
BT2 Thermal processing
BT3 Processing thermal
BT4 Processing
BT5 Technology

Hare carcasses
BT1 Carcasses
BT2 Meat
BT3 Animal foods
BT4 Foods
BT1 Hare meat
BT2 Hares
BT3 Animals
BT2 Meat specific
BT3 Meat
BT4 Animal foods
BT5 Foods

Hare meat
BT1 Hares
BT2 Animals
BT1 Meat specific
BT2 Meat
BT3 Animal foods
BT4 Foods
NT1 Hare carcasses

Hares
BT1 Animals
NT1 Hare meat
NT2 Hare carcasses

Haricot beans
BT1 Common beans
BT2 Legumes
BT3 Vegetables specific
BT4 Vegetables
BT5 Crops
BT6 Plants
BT5 Plant foods
BT6 Foods
NT1 Baked beans

Harman
BT1 Alkaloids
BT2 Organic nitrogen compounds
RT Carbolines
RT Norharman

Harvesting
BT1 Agriculture
NT1 Mechanical harvesting
NT1 Picking
NT1 Threshers

Haugh score
BT1 Eggs
BT2 Animal foods
BT3 Foods

Havarti cheese
BT1 Cheese varieties
BT2 Cheese
BT3 Dairy products
BT4 Animal foods
BT5 Foods

Hawthorn fruits
BT1 Fruits specific
BT2 Fruits
BT3 Crops
BT4 Plants
BT3 Plant foods
BT4 Foods

Hawthorn juices
BT1 Fruit juices
BT2 Fruit products
BT3 Plant foods
BT4 Foods
BT2 Soft drinks
BT3 Beverages

Hazard analysis critical control point
USE **HACCP**

Hazards
RT Food safety
RT Health hazards
RT Risk communication

Hazards analysis
RT Food safety
RT Risks assessment

Haze
BT1 Turbidity
BT2 Optical properties
BT3 Physical properties

Hazelnut oils
BT1 Nut oils
BT2 Vegetable oils
BT3 Oils vegetable
BT4 Oils
BT5 Lipids
BT6 Nutrients
BT4 Vegetable products
BT5 Plant foods
BT6 Foods

Hazelnuts
HN heading from vol. 30 (1998); under Nuts up to vol. 29 (1997)
BT1 Nuts
BT2 Fruits
BT3 Crops
BT4 Plants
BT3 Plant foods
BT4 Foods
BT2 Oilseeds
BT3 Seeds
BT4 Plant foods
BT5 Foods
RT Filbertone
UF Cobnuts
UF Filberts

HCB
USE **Hexachlorobenzene**

HCH
BT1 Acaricides
BT2 Pesticides
BT3 Biocides
BT3 Residues
BT1 Organochlorine insecticides
BT2 Insecticides
BT3 Pesticides
BT4 Biocides
BT4 Residues
BT2 Organochlorine pesticides
BT3 Pesticides
BT4 Biocides
BT4 Residues
BT1 Rodenticides
BT2 Pesticides
BT3 Biocides
BT3 Residues
UF BHC
UF Hexachloran
UF Lindane

HCl
BT1 Acids
UF Hydrochloric acid

HDPE
BT1 Polyethylene
BT2 Plastics
BT3 Packaging materials
UF High density polyethylene

He
HN also under Minerals up to vol. 42 (2010)
BT1 Elements
BT2 Minerals
BT3 Nutrients
BT1 Gases
BT2 Physical phases
BT3 Chemistry
BT4 Science
UF Helium

Headspace analysis
BT1 Analytical techniques

Health
NT1 Anthropometric parameters
NT2 Body composition
NT2 Body wt.
NT3 Birth wt.
NT3 Body mass index
NT3 Overweight
NT3 Wt. loss diet
NT2 Growth (human)
NT1 Anti-ageing activity
NT1 Antiallergic activity
NT1 Antiatherogenic activity
NT1 Anticarcinogenicity
NT1 Anticarcinogens
NT1 Antigenotoxicity
NT1 Antihypertensive activity
NT1 Anti-inflammatory activity
NT1 Antimutagenicity
NT1 Antimutagens
NT1 Antiproliferative activity
NT1 Antithrombotic activity
NT1 Antitumorigenicity
NT1 Antitumour activity
NT1 Bone health
NT1 Bone mineral density
NT1 Dental health
NT1 Desmutagenicity
NT1 Eye health
NT1 Healthiness
NT1 Health promotion
NT1 Healthy eating
NT1 Hypoglycaemic activity
NT1 Hypolipaemic activity
NT1 Mental health
NT1 Oestrogenic activity
NT1 Physical activity
NT2 Exercise performance
NT1 Teratogenicity
RT Animal models
RT Diet
RT Diseases
RT Food safety
RT Free radicals
RT Functional foods
RT Health foods
RT Health hazards
RT Hygiene
RT Medicinal plants
RT Nutraceutical foods
RT Nutrition
RT Phytochemicals
RT Quality of life
RT Radicals
RT Residues
RT Safety
RT Toxicity

Health beverages
BT1 Beverages
BT1 Health foods
BT2 Processed foods
BT3 Foods
NT1 Energy drinks
NT1 Ginseng beverages
NT1 Isotonic drinks
NT1 Sports drinks
RT Functional beverages
RT Sports supplements

Health claims
BT1 Labelling
BT2 Packaging
BT3 Technology

Health foods
BT1 Processed foods
BT2 Foods
NT1 Beauty foods
NT1 Energy foods
NT1 Health beverages
NT2 Energy drinks
NT2 Ginseng beverages
NT2 Isotonic drinks
NT2 Sports drinks
NT1 Royal jelly
NT1 Sports foods
RT Calories
RT Diet
RT Dietetic foods
RT Food supplements
RT Health
RT Nutrition
RT Phytochemicals
RT Sports supplements

Health hazards
RT Food safety
RT Hazards
RT Health
RT Safety

Healthiness
HN introduced from vol. 40, issue 4 (2008)
SN includes healthiness of individuals, populations, foods, diets, lifestyles, etc.
BT1 Health

Health promotion
HN introduced from vol. 40, issue 4 (2008)
SN used for health promotion campaigns and programmes rather than health-promoting properties of foods
BT1 Consumer information
BT2 Information
BT1 Health
RT Policy

Healthy eating
HN introduced from vol. 40, issue 4 (2008)

BT1 Eating habits
BT2 Consumer behaviour
BT3 Consumer response
BT1 Health

Hearts
BT1 Offal
BT2 Animal foods
BT3 Foods

Heat
HN heading up to vol. 24 (1992)
BT1 Heating
BT2 Thermal processing
BT3 Processing thermal
BT4 Processing
BT5 Technology
RT Temperature

Heat distribution
BT1 Heating
BT2 Thermal processing
BT3 Processing thermal
BT4 Processing
BT5 Technology
RT Heat transfer

Heaters
BT1 Equipment
BT2 Technology
BT1 Heating
BT2 Thermal processing
BT3 Processing thermal
BT4 Processing
BT5 Technology

Heat exchangers
BT1 Equipment
BT2 Technology
RT Heating

Heating
BT1 Thermal processing
BT2 Processing thermal
BT3 Processing
BT4 Technology
NT1 Annealing
NT1 Dielectric heating
NT1 Flaming
NT1 Heat
NT1 Heat distribution
NT1 Heaters
NT1 Heat transfer
NT1 Induction heating
NT1 IR heating
NT1 Reheating
NT1 Thermization
NT1 Warming
RT Cooking
RT Heat exchangers
RT Pasteurization
RT Rendering
RT Scalding
UF Heat treatment

Heat resistance
BT1 Thermophysical properties
BT2 Physical properties
RT Heat stability
RT Stress resistance
RT Thermal stability

Heat shock proteins
BT1 Stress proteins
BT2 Proteins
BT3 Nutrients
BT2 Stress
UF Heat stress proteins

Heat stability
SN syn. thermal stability
BT1 Stability
BT2 Physical properties
BT1 Thermophysical properties
BT2 Physical properties
RT Heat resistance

Heat stress proteins
USE **Heat shock proteins**

Heat transfer
BT1 Heating
BT2 Thermal processing
BT3 Processing thermal
BT4 Processing
BT5 Technology
RT Heat distribution

Heat treatment
USE **Heating**

Heavy metals
HN under Minerals up to vol. 42 (2010)
BT1 Metals
BT2 Elements
BT3 Minerals
BT4 Nutrients

Heifers
HN type of cattle not specified in the index from vol. 25 (1993)
USE **Cattle**

Helianthinin
BT1 Vegetable proteins
BT2 Proteins vegetable
BT3 Proteins
BT4 Nutrients
BT3 Vegetable products
BT4 Plant foods
BT5 Foods

Helicobacter
HN heading from vol. 30 (1998); under Bacteria up to vol. 29 (1997)
BT1 Bacteria
BT2 Microorganisms
NT1 *Helicobacter canadensis*
NT1 *Helicobacter pylori*

Helicobacter canadensis
BT1 *Helicobacter*
BT2 Bacteria
BT3 Microorganisms

Helicobacter pylori
BT1 *Helicobacter*
BT2 Bacteria
BT3 Microorganisms

Helium
USE **He**

Helminthosporium
BT1 Fungi
BT2 Microorganisms

Helminths
BT1 Parasites
BT2 Pests

Hemicellulases
BT1 Glycosidases
BT2 Hydrolases
BT3 Enzymes

Hemicelluloses
HN under Celluloses up to vol. 42 (2010)
BT1 Polysaccharides
BT2 Carbohydrates
BT3 Nutrients
BT3 Organic compounds

Hemp
BT1 Plants

Hemp seeds
BT1 Oilseeds
BT2 Seeds
BT3 Plant foods
BT4 Foods

Hen eggs
USE **Eggs**

Hen meat
USE **Chicken meat**

Hens
USE **Chickens**

Hepatitis
BT1 Diseases
RT Hepatitis viruses

Hepatitis A virus
HN introduced from vol. 43, issue 1 (2011); hepatitis A viruses also used in the index up to vol. 42 (2010)
BT1 Hepatovirus
BT2 Hepatitis viruses
BT3 Viruses
BT4 Microorganisms
UF Hepatitis A viruses

Hepatitis A viruses
HN introduced from vol. 39, issue 1 (2007); Hepatitis A virus used in the index from vol. 43 (2011)
USE **Hepatitis A virus**

Hepatitis E virus
HN introduced from vol. 43, issue 1 (2011); hepatitis E viruses also used in the index up to vol. 42 (2010)
BT1 Hepevirus
BT2 Hepatitis viruses
BT3 Viruses
BT4 Microorganisms
UF Hepatitis E viruses

Hepatitis E viruses
HN introduced from vol. 39, issue 1 (2007); Hepatitis E virus used in the index from vol. 43 (2011)

USE **Hepatitis E virus**

Hepatitis viruses
HN under Enteric viruses up to vol. 42 (2010)
SN for descriptive use only
BT1 Viruses
BT2 Microorganisms
NT1 Hepatovirus
NT2 Hepatitis A virus
NT1 Hepevirus
NT2 Hepatitis E virus
RT Hepatitis

Hepatotoxicity
BT1 Toxicity

Hepatotoxins
BT1 Toxins
BT2 Residues
RT Aflatoxins

Hepatovirus
HN introduced from vol. 43, issue 1 (2011)
BT1 Hepatitis viruses
BT2 Viruses
BT3 Microorganisms
NT1 Hepatitis A virus

Hepevirus
HN introduced from vol. 43, issue 1 (2011)
BT1 Hepatitis viruses
BT2 Viruses
BT3 Microorganisms
NT1 Hepatitis E virus

Heptachlor
BT1 Organochlorine insecticides
BT2 Insecticides
BT3 Pesticides
BT4 Biocides
BT4 Residues
BT2 Organochlorine pesticides
BT3 Pesticides
BT4 Biocides
BT4 Residues
NT1 Heptachlor epoxide

Heptachlor epoxide
BT1 Heptachlor
BT2 Organochlorine insecticides
BT3 Insecticides
BT4 Pesticides
BT5 Biocides
BT5 Residues
BT3 Organochlorine pesticides
BT4 Pesticides
BT5 Biocides
BT5 Residues

Heptadecanoic acid
SN syn. margaric acid
BT1 Saturated fatty acids
BT2 Fatty acids
BT3 Lipids
BT4 Nutrients
BT3 Organic acids
BT4 Acids
NT1 Margaric acid

Heptane
BT1 Hydrocarbons
BT2 Organic compounds
BT1 Solvents

Heptanoic acid
HN under Fatty acids up to vol. 42 (2010)
BT1 Aroma compounds
BT2 Flavour compounds
BT2 Volatile compounds
BT1 Saturated fatty acids
BT2 Fatty acids
BT3 Lipids
BT4 Nutrients
BT3 Organic acids
BT4 Acids

2-Heptanone
BT1 Aroma compounds
BT2 Flavour compounds
BT2 Volatile compounds
BT1 Ketones
BT2 Carbonyl compounds
BT3 Organic compounds

Heptenal
BT1 Aldehydes
BT2 Carbonyl compounds
BT3 Organic compounds
BT1 Aroma compounds
BT2 Flavour compounds
BT2 Volatile compounds

Herbal beverages
BT1 Beverages
RT Herb tea

Herbal tea
USE **Herb tea**

Herbicides
BT1 Pesticides
BT2 Biocides
BT2 Residues
NT1 Alachlor
NT1 Amitrole
NT1 Asulam
NT1 Bentazone
NT1 Benzoylprop-ethyl
NT1 Bifenox
NT1 Bromoxynil
NT1 Butralin
NT1 Carbetamide
NT1 Chloramben
NT1 Chlorate
NT1 Chlorflurecol
NT1 Chloridazon
NT1 Chlormequat
NT1 Chloroxuron
NT1 Chlorpropham
NT1 Dalapon
NT1 Dicamba
NT1 Dichlobenil
NT1 Difenzoquat
NT1 Dimethylarsinic acid
NT1 Dinitramine
NT1 Dinoseb
NT1 Diphenamid
NT1 Diquat
NT1 Diuron
NT1 Endothal
NT1 EPTC
NT1 Fenuron
NT1 Fluchloralin
NT1 Fluometuron
NT1 Fluorodifen
NT1 Fluridone
NT1 Glyphosate
NT1 Lenacil
NT1 Linuron
NT1 Methabenzthiazuron
NT1 Methazole
NT1 Methylarsonic acid
NT1 Metolachlor
NT1 Metribuzin
NT1 Molinate
NT1 Monuron
NT1 Nitrofen
NT1 Norflurazon
NT1 Oryzalin
NT1 Oxadiazon
NT1 Paraquat
NT1 Perfluidone
NT1 Phenmedipham
NT1 Phenoxy herbicides
NT2 Chlorophenoxyacetic acid
NT2 2,4-D
NT2 Dichlorprop
NT2 Fenoprop
NT2 MCPA
NT2 2,4,5-T
NT1 Picloram
NT1 Propachlor
NT1 Propanil
NT1 Propham
NT1 Ronit
NT1 Terbacil
NT1 Tri-allate
NT1 Triazine herbicides
NT2 Atrazine
NT2 Cyanazine
NT2 Desmetryn
NT2 Prometryn
NT2 Propazine
NT2 Simazine
NT2 Terbuthylazine
NT1 Trifluralin
RT Plant growth regulators

Herbs
HN heading from vol. 43 (2011); under Spices up to vol. 42 (2010)
BT1 Spices
BT2 Flavourings
BT3 Additives
NT1 *Agastache*
NT1 Angelica
NT1 *Artemisia*
NT1 Basil
NT2 Sweet basil
NT1 Bay
NT2 Bay leaves
NT2 Laurel
NT1 Borage
NT1 *Calamintha*
NT1 Catmint
NT1 Chamomile
NT2 Camomile
NT1 Chervil

NT1 Chives
NT1 Comfrey
NT1 Coriander leaves
NT1 Costmary
NT1 Curry leaves
NT2 *Murraya koenigii*
NT1 Davana
NT1 Dill leaves
NT1 Dittany
NT1 Hyssop
NT1 Lemon balm
NT1 Lemongrass
NT1 Marjoram
NT1 Mint
NT2 Peppermint
NT2 Spearmint
NT1 Mugwort
NT2 *Artemisia vulgaris*
NT1 Oregano
NT1 Palmarosa
NT1 Parsley
NT1 Rosemary
NT1 Rue
NT1 Sage
NT1 Samphire
NT2 Sea fennel
NT3 *Crithmum maritimum*
NT1 Savory
NT2 *Satureja*
NT1 Sorrel
NT1 Tansy
NT1 Tarragon
NT1 Thyme
NT1 Wormwood

Herb tea
BT1 Teas
BT2 Beverages
BT2 Crops
BT3 Plants
BT2 Plant foods
BT3 Foods
NT1 Honeybush tea
NT1 Mate
NT2 Yerba mate
NT3 *Ilex paraguariensis*
NT1 Rooibos tea
NT1 Tochu tea
RT Herbal beverages
UF Herbal tea

Hericium erinaceus
BT1 Edible fungi
BT2 Fungi edible
BT3 Vegetables specific
BT4 Vegetables
BT5 Crops
BT6 Plants
BT5 Plant foods
BT6 Foods

Heritability
BT1 Genetics

Herpesviruses
HN under Enteric viruses up to vol. 42 (2010)
SN for descriptive use only
BT1 Viruses
BT2 Microorganisms

Herrgard cheese
HN introduced from vol. 37, issue 5 (2005)
BT1 Cheese varieties
BT2 Cheese
BT3 Dairy products
BT4 Animal foods
BT5 Foods

Herring
HN heading from vol. 30 (1998); under Fishes up to vol. 29 (1997)
BT1 Marine fish
BT2 Fish
BT3 Animals
BT3 Sea foods
BT4 Aquatic foods
BT5 Animal foods
BT6 Foods
BT1 Oily fish
BT2 Fish
BT3 Animals
BT3 Sea foods
BT4 Aquatic foods
BT5 Animal foods
BT6 Foods
NT1 *Clupea harengus*
NT1 Kippers
NT1 Matjes
NT1 Rollmops
UF Herrings

Herrings
HN heading up to vol. 24
USE **Herring**

Hesperetin
HN introduced from vol. 39, issue 1 (2007)
BT1 Flavanones
BT2 Flavonoids
BT3 Aromatic compounds
BT4 Organic compounds
BT3 Pigments

Hesperidin
BT1 Flavanones
BT2 Flavonoids
BT3 Aromatic compounds
BT4 Organic compounds
BT3 Pigments
BT1 Glycosides
BT2 Carbohydrates
BT3 Nutrients
BT3 Organic compounds

Heterocyclic amines
BT1 Amines
BT2 Organic nitrogen compounds
BT1 Heterocyclic compounds

Heterocyclic aromatic amines
BT1 Amines
BT2 Organic nitrogen compounds
BT1 Aromatic compounds
BT2 Organic compounds
BT1 Heterocyclic compounds

Heterocyclic compounds
NT1 Aniline
NT1 Anthranilic acid
NT1 Cetylpyridinium chloride
NT1 Diketopiperazines
NT1 Furans
NT2 Furanones
NT3 Furaneol
NT4 2,5-Dimethyl-4-hydroxy-3(2*H*)-furanone
NT3 Sotolon
NT2 5-(Hydroxymethyl)-2-furaldehyde
NT2 Hydroxymethylfurfural
NT1 Heterocyclic amines
NT1 Heterocyclic aromatic amines
NT1 Hypoxanthine
NT1 Imidazoles
NT2 Allantoin
NT1 Indoles
NT2 Indole-3-carbinol
NT1 Lactones
NT2 Coumarins
NT3 Coumarin
NT3 Coumestrol
NT3 Esculetin
NT3 Furocoumarins
NT4 Bergapten
NT4 Psoralens
NT4 Xanthotoxin
NT3 Scopoletin
NT2 γ-Decalactone
NT2 Glucono-δ-lactone
NT1 Lenthionine
NT1 Melamine
NT1 Melatonin
NT1 Morpholine
NT1 Pipecolic acid
NT1 Piperidine
NT1 Porphyrins
NT2 Chlorophylls
NT2 Haem
NT2 Haematin
NT2 Haemin
NT1 Purines
NT2 Adenine
NT2 Caffeine
NT2 Theobromine
NT2 Theophylline
NT2 Uric acid
NT1 Pyrazines
NT1 Pyridine
NT1 Pyrimidines
NT2 Barbituric acid
NT2 Cytosine
NT2 Propylthiouracil
NT2 Thymine
NT2 Uracil
NT1 Pyrones
NT2 Kojic acid
NT2 Maltol
NT1 Pyrroles
NT1 Resazurin
NT1 Safrole
NT1 Skatole
NT1 Tryptophol
NT1 Xanthones
NT2 Mangiferin

NT2 Sterigmatocystins
RT Aromatic compounds
RT Flavonoids
RT Organic compounds
RT Organic halogen compounds
RT Organic nitrogen compounds
RT Organic sulfur compounds
RT Toxins

Hexachloran
USE **HCH**

Hexachlorobenzene
BT1 Fungicides
BT2 Pesticides
BT3 Biocides
BT3 Residues
UF HCB

Hexachlorobiphenyl
BT1 Polychlorinated biphenyls
BT2 Chlorinated hydrocarbons
BT3 Organic halogen compounds
RT Poisoning

Hexachlorobutadiene
HN under Insecticides up to vol. 42 (2010)
BT1 Chlorinated hydrocarbons
BT2 Organic halogen compounds
BT1 Contaminants
BT2 Contamination

Hexachlorophene
BT1 Disinfectants
BT2 Disinfection
BT3 Hygiene

Hexadecanoic acid
SN syn. palmitic acid
BT1 Saturated fatty acids
BT2 Fatty acids
BT3 Lipids
BT4 Nutrients
BT3 Organic acids
BT4 Acids
NT1 Palmitic acid

Hexadecenoic acid
BT1 Monounsaturated fatty acids
BT2 Unsaturated fatty acids
BT3 Fatty acids
BT4 Lipids
BT5 Nutrients
BT4 Organic acids
BT5 Acids
NT1 Palmitoleic acid

Hexanal
BT1 Aldehydes
BT2 Carbonyl compounds
BT3 Organic compounds
BT1 Aroma compounds
BT2 Flavour compounds
BT2 Volatile compounds

Hexane
BT1 Hydrocarbons
BT2 Organic compounds
BT1 Solvents

Hexanoic acid
HN under Flavour compounds and Fatty acids up to vol. 42 (2010)
SN syn. caproic acid
BT1 Aroma compounds
BT2 Flavour compounds
BT2 Volatile compounds
BT1 Saturated fatty acids
BT2 Fatty acids
BT3 Lipids
BT4 Nutrients
BT3 Organic acids
BT4 Acids
BT1 Short chain fatty acids
BT2 Volatile fatty acids
BT3 Fatty acids
BT4 Lipids
BT5 Nutrients
BT4 Organic acids
BT5 Acids
BT3 Volatile compounds
NT1 Caproic acid

Hexanol
BT1 Alcohols
BT1 Aroma compounds
BT2 Flavour compounds
BT2 Volatile compounds

Hexenal
BT1 Aldehydes
BT2 Carbonyl compounds
BT3 Organic compounds
BT1 Aroma compounds
BT2 Flavour compounds
BT2 Volatile compounds

Hexokinases
SN EC 2.7.1.1
BT1 Kinases
BT2 Phosphotransferases
BT3 Transferases
BT4 Enzymes

Hexosamines
BT1 Amino sugars
BT2 Sugars
BT3 Carbohydrates
BT4 Nutrients
BT4 Organic compounds
BT3 Plant foods
BT4 Foods
NT1 Galactosamine
NT1 Glucosamine

Hexoses
HN under Sugars up to vol. 42 (2010)
BT1 Monosaccharides
BT2 Sugars
BT3 Carbohydrates
BT4 Nutrients
BT4 Organic compounds
BT3 Plant foods
BT4 Foods

Hexyl acetate
HN introduced from vol. 41, issue 1 (2009)
BT1 Acetates
BT1 Aroma compounds
BT2 Flavour compounds
BT2 Volatile compounds
BT1 Esters
BT2 Organic compounds

Hexylamine
BT1 Amines
BT2 Organic nitrogen compounds

4-Hexylresorcinol
BT1 Browning inhibitors
BT2 Browning
BT1 Phenols
BT2 Alcohols
BT2 Aromatic compounds
BT3 Organic compounds

Hg
SN index heading is Mercury
BT1 Mercury
BT2 Metals
BT3 Elements
BT4 Minerals
BT5 Nutrients

Hickory nuts
BT1 Nuts
BT2 Fruits
BT3 Crops
BT4 Plants
BT3 Plant foods
BT4 Foods
BT2 Oilseeds
BT3 Seeds
BT4 Plant foods
BT5 Foods
UF Carya

Hickory smoke
BT1 Flavourings
BT2 Additives
RT Smoking

Hides
BT1 By-products
RT Skin

High amylose corn starch
BT1 Corn starch
BT2 Corn
BT3 Cereals
BT4 Crops
BT5 Plants
BT4 Seeds
BT5 Plant foods
BT6 Foods
BT2 Starch
BT3 Glucans
BT4 Polysaccharides
BT5 Carbohydrates
BT6 Nutrients
BT6 Organic compounds
BT3 Thickeners
BT4 Additives

High calorie foods
USE **Calories high foods**

High density lipoproteins
HN introduced from vol. 39, issue 1 (2007)
BT1 Lipoproteins
BT2 Proteins
BT3 Nutrients

High density polyethylene
USE **HDPE**

High fat diet
USE **Fats high diet**

High gravity brewing
BT1 Brewing
BT2 Processing
BT3 Technology

High performance liquid chromatography
HN heading from vol. 18; under Chromatography up to vol. 17
SN abbrev. HPLC is also used in the index
BT1 Chromatography
BT2 Analytical techniques
NT1 HPLC
NT1 LC
NT1 LC-MS
NT1 Supercritical HPLC
NT1 UPLC

High pressure liquid chromatography
USE **HPLC**

High pressure processing
HN processing high pressure also used in the index up to vol. 29 (1997)
BT1 Pressure
BT1 Processing
BT2 Technology

High protein diet
USE **Proteins high diet**

High protein foods
USE **Proteins high foods**

Hilsa
BT1 Marine fish
BT2 Fish
BT3 Animals
BT3 Sea foods
BT4 Aquatic foods
BT5 Animal foods
BT6 Foods
BT1 Oily fish
BT2 Fish
BT3 Animals
BT3 Sea foods
BT4 Aquatic foods
BT5 Animal foods
BT6 Foods
UF Hilsah

Hilsah
USE **Hilsa**

Himegai
USE **Mussels**

Hinosan
USE **Edifenphos**

Hiochi bacteria
BT1 Bacteria
BT2 Microorganisms
RT *Lactobacillus*
RT Sake

Hippuric acid
BT1 Organic acids
BT2 Acids

Hispanico cheese
HN introduced from vol. 37, issue 5 (2005)
BT1 Cheese varieties
BT2 Cheese
BT3 Dairy products
BT4 Animal foods
BT5 Foods

Histamine
BT1 Biogenic amines
BT2 Amines
BT3 Organic nitrogen compounds
RT Scombroid poisoning

Histidine
BT1 Amino acids
BT2 Nutrients
BT2 Organic acids
BT3 Acids
BT2 Organic nitrogen compounds

Histidine decarboxylases
SN EC 4.1.1.22
BT1 Decarboxylases
BT2 Lyases
BT3 Enzymes

Histochemistry
BT1 Chemistry
BT2 Science

Histology
BT1 Science
NT1 Morphology

Histones
BT1 Proteins
BT2 Nutrients

Hizikia
HN present as Hijikia up to vol. 39, issue 1 (2007)
BT1 Seaweeds
BT2 Algae
BT3 Microorganisms
BT2 Sea foods
BT3 Aquatic foods
BT4 Animal foods
BT5 Foods

H_2O_2
HN under Hydrogen peroxide up to vol. 24 (1992)
BT1 Peroxides
BT2 Inorganic compounds
BT2 Oxides
BT2 Reactive oxygen species
BT3 Free radicals
BT4 Radicals
BT1 Preservatives
BT2 Additives
UF Hydrogen peroxide

Hogs
HN type of swine not specified in the index from vol.25
USE **Swine**

Hoki
BT1 Marine fish
BT2 Fish
BT3 Animals
BT3 Sea foods
BT4 Aquatic foods
BT5 Animal foods
BT6 Foods

Holders
BT1 Equipment
BT2 Technology

Holland
USE **Netherlands**

Hollandaise sauces
HN introduced from vol. 39, issue 1 (2007)
BT1 Sauces
BT2 Condiments
BT3 Flavourings
BT4 Additives

Hominy
BT1 Cereal products
BT2 Plant foods
BT3 Foods

Homocysteine
BT1 Amino acids
BT2 Nutrients
BT2 Organic acids
BT3 Acids
BT2 Organic nitrogen compounds
BT1 Organic sulfur compounds

Homogenization
BT1 Processing
BT2 Technology
NT1 Homogenizers
RT Mixing

Homogenized milk
BT1 Milk
BT2 Dairy products
BT3 Animal foods
BT4 Foods

Homogenizers
BT1 Equipment
BT2 Technology
BT1 Homogenization
BT2 Processing
BT3 Technology

Homoserine
BT1 Amino acids

BT2 Nutrients
BT2 Organic acids
BT3 Acids
BT2 Organic nitrogen compounds

Honduras
BT1 Central America
BT2 America

Honey beverages
BT1 Beverages
BT1 Honeys
BT2 Sugar
BT3 Plant foods
BT4 Foods
RT Mead
RT Melomel

Honeybush tea
BT1 Herb tea
BT2 Teas
BT3 Beverages
BT3 Crops
BT4 Plants
BT3 Plant foods
BT4 Foods

Honeycombs
BT1 Honeys
BT2 Sugar
BT3 Plant foods
BT4 Foods

Honeydew honey
BT1 Honeys
BT2 Sugar
BT3 Plant foods
BT4 Foods

Honeydew melons
BT1 Melons
BT2 Fruits specific
BT3 Fruits
BT4 Crops
BT5 Plants
BT4 Plant foods
BT5 Foods

Honeys
BT1 Sugar
BT2 Plant foods
BT3 Foods
NT1 Honey beverages
NT1 Honeycombs
NT1 Honeydew honey
NT1 Pollen
NT1 Propolis
RT Apiculture

Hong Kong
BT1 China
BT2 Asia

Hop essential oils
BT1 Essential oils
BT2 Flavourings
BT3 Additives
BT2 Vegetable oils
BT3 Oils vegetable
BT4 Oils
BT5 Lipids
BT6 Nutrients
BT4 Vegetable products
BT5 Plant foods
BT6 Foods
RT Hops

Hop extracts
BT1 Extracts
BT2 Flavourings
BT3 Additives
BT1 Hops
BT2 Flavourings
BT3 Additives

Hop pellets
BT1 Hops
BT2 Flavourings
BT3 Additives

Hoppers
BT1 Bins
BT2 Containers

Hopping
BT1 Brewing
BT2 Processing
BT3 Technology
RT Hops

Hops
BT1 Flavourings
BT2 Additives
NT1 Hop extracts
NT1 Hop pellets
NT1 Hop substitutes
RT Beer
RT Bitter acids
RT Brewing
RT Hop essential oils
RT Hopping
RT Humulene

Hop substitutes
BT1 Hops
BT2 Flavourings
BT3 Additives

Horchata
BT1 Beverages

Hordein
BT1 Cereal proteins
BT2 Proteins cereal
BT3 Vegetable proteins
BT4 Proteins vegetable
BT5 Proteins
BT6 Nutrients
BT5 Vegetable products
BT6 Plant foods
BT7 Foods
RT Barley

Hordenine
BT1 Biogenic amines
BT2 Amines
BT3 Organic nitrogen compounds

Hordeumin
HN introduced from vol. 37, issue 5 (2005)
BT1 Pigments

Hordothionins
BT1 Cereal proteins
BT2 Proteins cereal
BT3 Vegetable proteins
BT4 Proteins vegetable
BT5 Proteins
BT6 Nutrients
BT5 Vegetable products
BT6 Plant foods
BT7 Foods

Hormones
BT1 Residues
NT1 Adiponectin
NT1 Androgens
NT2 Testosterone
NT1 Androstenone
NT1 Catecholamines
NT2 Adrenaline
NT2 Noradrenaline
NT1 Epidermal growth factors
NT1 Gestagens
NT1 Ghrelin
NT1 Glucagon
NT1 Glucocorticoids
NT2 Cortisol
NT1 Growth factors
NT2 Myostatin
NT1 Growth promoters (animal)
NT1 Insulin
NT2 Insulin resistance
NT1 Insulin-like growth factors
NT1 Leptin
NT1 Melengestrol
NT1 Oestrogens
NT2 Oestradiol
NT2 Oestrogenic activity
NT2 Oestrone
NT1 Oxytocin
NT1 Progesterone
NT1 Prolactin
NT1 Somatotropin
NT2 Bovine somatotropin
NT2 Porcine somatotropin
NT1 Thyroxine
NT1 Triiodothyronine
RT Drugs
RT Pheromones

Horse beans
BT1 Faba beans
BT2 Legumes
BT3 Vegetables specific
BT4 Vegetables
BT5 Crops
BT6 Plants
BT5 Plant foods
BT6 Foods

Horse carcasses
BT1 Carcasses
BT2 Meat
BT3 Animal foods
BT4 Foods
BT1 Horse meat

Hulling
BT1 Husking
BT2 Processing
BT3 Technology

Hulls
BT1 Husking
BT2 Processing
BT3 Technology
BT1 Wastes
RT Seed coats

Hulupones
BT1 β-Acids
BT2 Bitter acids
BT3 Bitter compounds
BT4 Flavour compounds
BT3 Organic acids
BT4 Acids

Human adenovirus
HN introduced from vol. 43, issue 1 (2011)
BT1 Mastadenovirus
BT2 Adenoviruses
BT3 Viruses
BT4 Microorganisms

Human astrovirus
HN introduced from vol. 43, issue 1 (2011)
BT1 Mamastrovirus
BT2 Astroviruses
BT3 Viruses
BT4 Microorganisms

Human coxsackievirus
HN introduced from vol. 43, issue 1 (2011)
BT1 Human enterovirus
BT2 Enterovirus
BT3 Viruses
BT4 Microorganisms

Human enterovirus
HN introduced from vol. 43, issue 1 (2011)
BT1 Enterovirus
BT2 Viruses
BT3 Microorganisms
NT1 Human coxsackievirus

Human genetic disorders
HN introduced from vol. 39, issue 1 (2007)
SN includes animal model studies
BT1 Diseases
BT1 Genetic disorders

Human immunodeficiency virus
HN introduced from vol. 43, issue 1 (2011); human immunodeficiency viruses also used in the index up to vol. 42 (2010)
BT1 Lentivirus
BT2 Viruses
BT3 Microorganisms
UF Human immunodeficiency viruses

Human immunodeficiency viruses
HN Human immunodeficiency virus used in the index from vol. 43 (2011)
USE **Human immunodeficiency virus**

Humanized milk
BT1 Infant foods
BT2 Processed foods
BT3 Foods

Human lactation
SN includes animal model studies; for lactation in animals use lactation
BT1 Human physiology
BT2 Physiology
BT3 Science
RT Breast feeding
RT Human milk
RT Weaning

Human metabolism
HN introduced from vol. 38, issue 8 (2006)
SN includes animal model studies
BT1 Human physiology
BT2 Physiology
BT3 Science
RT Metabolism

Human milk
BT1 Milk
BT2 Dairy products
BT3 Animal foods
BT4 Foods
RT Breast feeding
RT Human lactation
UF Breast milk

Human milk substitutes
USE **Infant formulas**
USE **Milk infant formulas**

Human physiology
HN heading from vol. 32 (2000)
SN includes animal model studies
BT1 Physiology
BT2 Science
NT1 Angiogenesis
NT1 Appetite
NT1 Behavioural effects
NT2 Cognitive performance
NT3 Cognitive development
NT3 Memory
NT2 Cravings
NT2 Mood
NT1 Body fats
NT1 Breast feeding
NT1 Cardiovascular physiology
NT2 Blood pressure
NT1 Digestion
NT1 Exercise performance
NT1 Flatulence
NT2 Flatulence factors
NT1 Gastrointestinal tract
NT2 Malabsorption
NT1 Glucose tolerance
NT1 Human lactation
NT1 Human metabolism
NT1 Hunger
NT1 Lipaemic activity
NT1 Mastication
NT1 Physiological effects
NT1 Postprandial response
NT1 Psychophysiological effects
NT1 Reproduction
NT2 Menopause
NT2 Menstrual cycle
NT2 Pregnancy
NT1 Saliva
NT1 Satiety
NT1 Sensory perception
NT1 Sleep
NT1 Swallowing
NT1 Thermogenesis
NT1 Thirst
NT1 Vision
NT1 Weaning
RT Animal models
RT Nutritional status

Humectants
BT1 Additives

Humic acids
BT1 Organic acids
BT2 Acids

Humicola
HN heading from vol. 30 (1998); under Fungi up to vol. 29 (1997)
BT1 Fungi
BT2 Microorganisms
NT1 *Humicola grisea*
NT1 *Humicola insolens*
NT1 *Humicola lanuginosa*

Humicola grisea
BT1 *Humicola*
BT2 Fungi
BT3 Microorganisms

Humicola insolens
BT1 *Humicola*
BT2 Fungi
BT3 Microorganisms

Humicola lanuginosa
SN synonymous with Thermomyces lanuginosus
BT1 *Humicola*
BT2 Fungi
BT3 Microorganisms

Humidification
BT1 Humidity

Humidity
NT1 Humidification
NT1 Hygrometers
NT1 Moistness
NT1 RH
RT a_w
RT Moisture content
RT Sorption
RT Water
RT Water activity

Humous
BT1 Chick peas
BT2 Legumes

BT3 Vegetables specific
BT4 Vegetables
BT5 Crops
BT6 Plants
BT5 Plant foods
BT6 Foods

Humulene
BT1 Aroma compounds
BT2 Flavour compounds
BT2 Volatile compounds
BT1 Sesquiterpenes
BT2 Hydrocarbons
BT3 Organic compounds
BT2 Sesquiterpenoids
BT3 Terpenoids
BT4 Lipids
BT5 Nutrients
RT Hops

Humulinic acid
BT1 Humulones
BT2 α-Acids
BT3 Bitter acids
BT4 Bitter compounds
BT5 Flavour compounds
BT4 Organic acids
BT5 Acids

Humulones
BT1 α-Acids
BT2 Bitter acids
BT3 Bitter compounds
BT4 Flavour compounds
BT3 Organic acids
BT4 Acids
NT1 Adhumulone
NT1 Cohumulone
NT1 Humulinic acid

Hungary
HN heading up to vol. 24 (1992)
BT1 Europe
BT1 European Union
RT Organization for Economic Cooperation and Development

Hunger
BT1 Human physiology
BT2 Physiology
BT3 Science

Hurdle technology
BT1 Preservation
BT2 Technology

Husbandry
BT1 Agriculture
NT1 Milking
NT1 Stocking density (husbandry)
RT Rearing

Husking
BT1 Processing
BT2 Technology
NT1 Dehulling
NT1 Hulling
NT1 Hulls
NT1 Husks
RT Decortication
RT Winnowers

Husks
BT1 Husking
BT2 Processing
BT3 Technology
BT1 Wastes
RT Seed coats

Hyacinth beans
USE **Lablab beans**

Hyaluronic acid
HN introduced from vol. 39, issue 1 (2007)
BT1 Glycosaminoglycans
BT2 Polysaccharides
BT3 Carbohydrates
BT4 Nutrients
BT4 Organic compounds

Hybridization
BT1 Genetic techniques
BT2 Genetics
NT1 Blotting
NT2 Northern blotting
NT2 Southern blotting
NT2 Western blotting
NT1 DNA hybridization
NT1 Fluorescence *in situ* hybridization
RT Gene probes

Hybrids
BT1 Genetics

Hydnum
BT1 Edible fungi
BT2 Fungi edible
BT3 Vegetables specific
BT4 Vegetables
BT5 Crops
BT6 Plants
BT5 Plant foods
BT6 Foods

Hydration
BT1 Moisture content
RT Rehydration

Hydration status
HN introduced from vol. 41, issue 1 (2009)
BT1 Nutritional status
BT2 Nutrition

Hydrazine
BT1 Organic nitrogen compounds

Hydrocarbons
BT1 Organic compounds
NT1 Acetylene
NT1 Alkanes
NT1 Alkenes
NT1 Anthracene
NT1 Biogas
NT1 Butane
NT1 Chrysene
NT1 Cymene
NT1 Decane
NT1 Diterpenes
NT1 Ethane
NT1 Ethylene
NT2 ACC
NT2 Ethephon
NT1 Fluoranthene
NT1 Fluorene
NT1 Heptane
NT1 Hexane
NT1 Isoprene
NT1 Isoprenoids
NT1 Methane
NT1 Monoterpenes
NT2 Camphene
NT2 Limonene
NT2 Myrcene
NT2 Pinenes
NT2 Terpinene
NT1 Olefins
NT1 PAH
NT1 Paraffins
NT1 Pentane
NT1 Petroleum
NT1 Polyacetylenes
NT1 Polyhydroxyalkanoates
NT1 Pristane
NT1 Propane
NT1 Sesquiterpenes
NT2 Caryophyllene
NT2 Farnesene
NT2 Humulene
NT1 Terpenes
NT1 Triterpenes
NT2 Squalene
RT Aliphatic compounds
RT Aromatic compounds
RT Organic halogen compounds
RT Organic nitrogen compounds
RT Organic sulfur compounds
RT Styrene

Hydrochloric acid
USE **HCl**

Hydrocolloids
HN under Gums up to vol. 42 (2010)
BT1 Colloids
BT2 Physical phases
BT3 Chemistry
BT4 Science
RT Gums
RT Polysaccharides

Hydrocooling
BT1 Cooling
BT2 Thermal processing
BT3 Processing thermal
BT4 Processing
BT5 Technology

Hydrocyanic acid
SN syn. hydrogen cyanide
BT1 Cyanides
BT2 Salts
RT Fumigants

Hydrocyclones
HN under Sugar processes up to vol. 42 (2010)

BT1 Equipment
BT2 Technology

Hydrogen
HN introduced (as heading) from vol. 43, issue 1 (2011); H2 used previously
SN use generally for this element; use H2 for gaseous form
BT1 Elements
BT2 Minerals
BT3 Nutrients
NT1 Deuterium
NT1 H_2
NT1 Tritium

Hydrogenated fats
HN fats hydrogenated also used in the index up to vol. 29 (1997)
BT1 Fats
BT2 Lipids
BT3 Nutrients

Hydrogenation
BT1 Processing
BT2 Technology
NT1 Hardening
RT Fats
RT Oils
RT Reduction

Hydrogen cyanide
SN syn. hydrocyanic acid
BT1 Cyanides
BT2 Salts
RT Fumigants

Hydrogen ion concentration
USE **pH**

Hydrogen peroxide
HN heading up to vol. 24 (1992)
USE **H_2O_2**

Hydrogen sulfide
USE **H_2S**

Hydrogen sulphide
USE **H_2S**

Hydrolases
SN EC 3
BT1 Enzymes
NT1 Amidases
NT1 Aminoacylases
NT1 Asparaginases
NT1 ATPases
NT1 Chitin deacetylases
NT1 Choloylglycine hydrolases
NT1 Deaminases
NT1 Esterases
NT2 Acetylcholinesterases
NT2 Carboxylesterases
NT2 Chlorophyllases
NT2 Cholinesterases
NT2 Cutinases
NT2 Feruloyl esterases
NT2 Lipases
NT3 Lecithinases
NT3 Lipoprotein lipases
NT3 Lysophospholipases
NT3 Phospholipases
NT3 Triacylglycerol lipases
NT2 Nucleases
NT3 Deoxyribonucleases
NT3 Endonucleases
NT3 Restriction endonucleases
NT3 Restriction enzymes
NT3 Ribonucleases
NT4 Angiogenin
NT2 Pectinesterases
NT2 Phosphatases
NT3 Acid phosphatases
NT3 Alkaline phosphatases
NT3 Nucleotidases
NT3 Phytases
NT4 3-Phytases
NT4 4-Phytases
NT2 Phosphodiesterases
NT2 Tannases
NT1 Glutaminases
NT1 Glycosidases
NT2 Acetylglucosaminidases
NT2 β-*N*-acetylhexosaminidases
NT2 Agarases
NT2 Amylases
NT3 α-Amylases
NT3 β-Amylases
NT3 Amylolytic enzymes
NT3 Diastatic activity
NT3 Glucan 1,4-α-glucosidases
NT3 Isoamylases
NT2 α-*N*-Arabinofuranosidases
NT2 Carbohydrases
NT2 Cellulases
NT2 Cellulolytic enzymes
NT2 Cellulose 1,4-β-cellobiosidases
NT2 Cellulosomes
NT2 Chitinases
NT2 Chitosanases
NT2 Cyclomaltodextrinases
NT2 Dextranases
NT2 Dextrinases
NT2 Endo-1,3(4)-β-glucanases
NT2 Endo-1,4-β-xylanases
NT2 β-Fructofuranosidases
NT2 Galactosidases
NT3 Galactanases
NT3 α-Galactosidases
NT3 β-Galactosidases
NT2 Glucanases
NT2 β-Glucanases
NT2 Glucan endo-1,3-β-D-glucosidases
NT2 α-Glucosidases
NT2 β-Glucosidases
NT2 α-Glucuronidases
NT2 β-Glucuronidases
NT2 Hemicellulases
NT2 Inulinases
NT2 Levanases
NT2 Licheninases
NT2 Limit dextrinases
NT2 Lysozymes
NT3 Eggs lysozymes
NT3 Egg whites lysozymes
NT2 Mannan endo-1,4-β-mannosidases
NT2 Mannosidases
NT2 α-Mannosidases
NT2 β-Mannosidases
NT2 Mutanolysins
NT2 Neopullulanases
NT2 Oligo-1,6-glucosidases
NT2 Pentosanases
NT2 Polygalacturonases
NT2 Pullulanases
NT2 α-L-rhamnosidases
NT2 Sucrose α-glucosidases
NT2 Thioglucosidases
NT2 α,α-Trehalases
NT2 Xylan degrading enzymes
NT2 Xylan endo-1,3-β-xylosidases
NT2 Xylan 1,4-β-xylosidases
NT1 β-Lactamases
NT1 Pancreatins
NT1 Proteinases
NT2 Actinidains
NT2 Aminopeptidases
NT2 Aqualysins
NT2 Bromelains
NT2 Calpains
NT2 Carboxypeptidases
NT2 Caspases
NT2 Cathepsins
NT2 Chymotrypsin
NT2 Collagenases
NT2 Cucumisins
NT2 Dipeptidases
NT2 Elastase
NT2 Endopeptidases
NT2 Enzymes milk clotting
NT3 Milk clotting enzymes
NT4 Chymosin
NT4 Rennets
NT5 Animal rennets
NT5 Calf rennets
NT5 Microbial rennets
NT5 Vegetable rennets
NT4 Rennet substitutes
NT2 Ficains
NT2 γ-Glutamyl hydrolases
NT2 Keratinases
NT2 Lysins
NT3 Autolysins
NT3 Thermolysins
NT2 Papain
NT2 Pepsins
NT2 Peptidases
NT2 Peptidyl-dipeptidase A
NT2 Plasmin
NT2 Plasminogen
NT2 Plasminogen activators
NT2 Pronase
NT2 Subtilisins
NT2 Trypsin
NT1 Pyrophosphatases
NT1 Ureases

Hydrolysed lactose syrups
BT1 Sugar syrups
BT2 Plant foods
BT3 Foods

Hydrolysed starches
USE **Starch hydrolysates**

Hydrolysed starch syrups
BT1 Sugar syrups
BT2 Plant foods
BT3 Foods
NT1 Lycasin

Hydrolysis
HN heading up to vol. 24 (1992)
NT1 Lipolysis
NT1 Proteolysis
NT1 Saponification

Hydrometry
BT1 Analytical techniques

Hydroperoxide lyases
BT1 Lyases
BT2 Enzymes

Hydroperoxides
BT1 Peroxides
BT2 Inorganic compounds
BT2 Oxides
BT2 Reactive oxygen species
BT3 Free radicals
BT4 Radicals

Hydrophobicity
BT1 Physical properties

Hydroponics
BT1 Cultivation
BT2 Agriculture

Hydroquinone
BT1 Phenols
BT2 Alcohols
BT2 Aromatic compounds
BT3 Organic compounds

Hydrothermal processing
BT1 Thermal processing
BT2 Processing thermal
BT3 Processing
BT4 Technology

Hydroxides
HN introduced from vol. 39, issue 1 (2007)
BT1 Salts
NT1 $Ca(OH)_2$
NT1 KOH
NT1 NaOH
RT Alkalies

Hydroxybenzoic acid
HN introduced from vol. 37, issue 5 (2005)
BT1 Organic acids
BT2 Acids

Hydroxybenzoic acid esters
SN syn. parabens
BT1 Esters
BT2 Organic compounds
BT1 Preservatives
BT2 Additives
NT1 Parabens
NT2 Methylparaben
NT2 Propylparaben

3-Hydroxy-2-butanone
SN syn. acetoin
BT1 Acetoin
BT2 Aroma compounds
BT3 Flavour compounds
BT3 Volatile compounds
BT2 Ketones
BT3 Carbonyl compounds
BT4 Organic compounds

Hydroxybutyric acid
BT1 Short chain fatty acids
BT2 Volatile fatty acids
BT3 Fatty acids
BT4 Lipids
BT5 Nutrients
BT4 Organic acids
BT5 Acids
BT3 Volatile compounds

Hydroxycinnamic acid
SN syn. coumaric acid
BT1 Organic acids
BT2 Acids
BT1 Phenols
BT2 Alcohols
BT2 Aromatic compounds
BT3 Organic compounds
NT1 Coumaric acid

Hydroxycitric acid
HN introduced from vol. 39, issue 1 (2007)
BT1 Organic acids
BT2 Acids

Hydroxylamine
BT1 Amines
BT2 Organic nitrogen compounds

Hydroxylation
BT1 Modification

5-(Hydroxymethyl)-2-furaldehyde
SN syn. hydroxymethylfurfural
BT1 Aldehydes
BT2 Carbonyl compounds
BT3 Organic compounds
BT1 Furans
BT2 Heterocyclic compounds

Hydroxymethylfurfural
SN syn. 5-(hydroxymethyl)-2-furaldehyde
BT1 Aldehydes
BT2 Carbonyl compounds
BT3 Organic compounds
BT1 Furans
BT2 Heterocyclic compounds

Hydroxyproline
BT1 Amino acids
BT2 Nutrients
BT2 Organic acids
BT3 Acids
BT2 Organic nitrogen compounds

3-Hydroxypropionaldehyde
HN introduced from vol. 39, issue 1 (2007)
SN syn. reuterin
BT1 Aldehydes
BT2 Carbonyl compounds
BT3 Organic compounds
BT1 Antibiotics
BT2 Drugs
BT3 Residues

Hydroxypropylation
BT1 Modification

Hydroxypropylcellulose
BT1 Celluloses
BT2 Glucans
BT3 Polysaccharides
BT4 Carbohydrates
BT5 Nutrients
BT5 Organic compounds

Hydroxypropylmethylcellulose
HN introduced from vol. 39, issue 1 (2007)
BT1 Celluloses
BT2 Glucans
BT3 Polysaccharides
BT4 Carbohydrates
BT5 Nutrients
BT5 Organic compounds

Hydroxystearic acid
BT1 Stearic acid
BT2 Octadecanoic acid
BT3 Saturated fatty acids
BT4 Fatty acids
BT5 Lipids
BT6 Nutrients
BT5 Organic acids
BT6 Acids

5-Hydroxytryptamine
SN syn. serotonin
BT1 Biogenic amines
BT2 Amines
BT3 Organic nitrogen compounds

Hydroxytyrosol
HN introduced from vol. 39, issue 1 (2007)
BT1 Phenols
BT2 Alcohols
BT2 Aromatic compounds
BT3 Organic compounds

Hygiene
NT1 Cleaning
NT2 Cleaning agents
NT2 Cleaning in place
NT2 Depuration
NT2 Descaling
NT2 Dishwashers
NT2 Rinsing
NT2 Washing
NT1 Clean room technology
NT1 Disinfection
NT2 Chlorination
NT2 Disinfectants
NT3 Antiseptics

NT3 Cetylpyridinium chloride
NT3 Chloramines
NT4 Monochloramine
NT3 Chlorates
NT3 Chlorites
NT3 Electrolysed water
NT3 Germicides
NT3 Hexachlorophene
NT3 Hypochlorites
NT3 Iodophors
NT3 Methyl iodide
NT3 Ozone
NT3 Perchlorates
NT3 Quaternary ammonium compounds
NT3 Sanitizers
NT2 Disinfection by-products
NT3 Dichloroacetic acid
NT3 Haloacetic acids
NT3 Trihalomethanes
NT2 Ozonation
NT2 Sanitation
NT1 Hygienic quality
RT Contamination
RT Food safety
RT Fumigation
RT Health
RT Poisoning
RT Pollution
RT Residues
RT Surfactants

Hygienic quality
BT1 Hygiene

Hygrometers
BT1 Humidity

Hygromycins
BT1 Aminoglycoside antibiotics
BT2 Antibiotics
BT3 Drugs
BT4 Residues

Hygroscopic properties
BT1 Physical properties

Hyperactivity
BT1 Diseases

Hypercholesterolaemia
USE **Hyperlipaemia**

Hyperlipaemia
SN includes hypercholesterolaemia
BT1 Diseases
UF Hypercholesterolaemia

Hypermarkets
BT1 Marketing
BT2 Economics

Hypertension
BT1 Diseases

Hyphaene
BT1 Palms
BT2 Plants

Hypoallergenic foods
HN introduced from vol. 41, issue 1 (2009)
BT1 Processed foods
BT2 Foods
RT Allergies

Hypochlorites
BT1 Disinfectants
BT2 Disinfection
BT3 Hygiene

Hypocholesterolaemic activity
USE **Hypolipaemic activity**

Hypoglycaemic activity
HN introduced from vol. 39, issue 1 (2007)
BT1 Health
RT Glucose
RT Glucose tolerance

Hypoglycine A
BT1 Toxins
BT2 Residues

Hypolipaemic activity
SN includes hypocholesterolaemic activity
BT1 Health
RT Lipaemic activity
UF Hypocholesterolaemic activity

Hypoxanthine
BT1 Heterocyclic compounds
BT1 Organic nitrogen compounds

Hyssop
HN under Spices up to vol. 42 (2010)
BT1 Herbs
BT2 Spices
BT3 Flavourings
BT4 Additives

I

I
SN index heading is Iodine
BT1 Iodine
BT2 Halogens
BT3 Elements
BT4 Minerals
BT5 Nutrients

IAA
USE **Indole acetic acid**

Iberian ham
BT1 Ham
BT2 Meat products
BT3 Animal foods
BT4 Foods

Ice
BT1 Physical phases
BT2 Chemistry
BT3 Science
RT Water

Ice cream
BT1 Dairy products
BT2 Animal foods
BT3 Foods
BT1 Frozen foods
BT2 Processed foods
BT3 Foods
NT1 Ice cream bars
NT1 Ice cream factories
NT1 Ice cream mixes
NT1 Ice milk
NT1 Ices
NT1 Mellorine
NT1 Milk ice
RT Frozen yoghurt

Ice cream bars
BT1 Food bars
BT2 Snack foods
BT3 Processed foods
BT4 Foods
BT1 Ice cream
BT2 Dairy products
BT3 Animal foods
BT4 Foods
BT2 Frozen foods
BT3 Processed foods
BT4 Foods

Ice cream cones
BT1 Bakery products
BT2 Cereal products
BT3 Plant foods
BT4 Foods

Ice cream factories
BT1 Ice cream
BT2 Dairy products
BT3 Animal foods
BT4 Foods
BT2 Frozen foods
BT3 Processed foods
BT4 Foods

Ice cream mixes
BT1 Ice cream
BT2 Dairy products
BT3 Animal foods
BT4 Foods
BT2 Frozen foods
BT3 Processed foods
BT4 Foods
BT1 Mixes
BT2 Dried foods
BT3 Processed foods
BT4 Foods
BT2 Instant foods
BT3 Processed foods
BT4 Foods

Ice cream wafers
BT1 Wafers
BT2 Bakery products
BT3 Cereal products
BT4 Plant foods
BT5 Foods

Iced coffee
BT1 Coffee beverages
BT2 Coffee products
BT3 Coffee
BT4 Beverages
BT4 Crops
BT5 Plants
BT4 Plant foods
BT5 Foods

Iced tea
BT1 Tea beverages
BT2 Teas
BT3 Beverages
BT3 Crops
BT4 Plants
BT3 Plant foods
BT4 Foods

Iceland
BT1 Europe
RT Organization for Economic Cooperation and Development

Ice lollies
HN under Ice cream up to vol. 24 (1992)
BT1 Frozen foods
BT2 Processed foods
BT3 Foods
BT1 Sugar confectionery
BT2 Plant foods
BT3 Foods
RT Water ices

Ice milk
BT1 Ice cream
BT2 Dairy products
BT3 Animal foods
BT4 Foods
BT2 Frozen foods
BT3 Processed foods
BT4 Foods

Ice nucleation activity
BT1 Freezing
BT2 Thermal processing
BT3 Processing thermal
BT4 Processing
BT5 Technology

Ices
BT1 Ice cream
BT2 Dairy products
BT3 Animal foods
BT4 Foods
BT2 Frozen foods
BT3 Processed foods
BT4 Foods

Ice wines
HN introduced from vol. 41, issue 1 (2009)
BT1 Wines
BT2 Alcoholic beverages
BT3 Beverages alcoholic
BT4 Beverages
NT1 Eiswein

Icings
BT1 Toppings

Icing sugar
BT1 Sugar
BT2 Plant foods
BT3 Foods

ICP-AES
BT1 Atomic emission spectroscopy
BT2 Spectroscopy
BT3 Analytical techniques
UF Inductively coupled plasma atomic emission spectroscopy

ICP-MS
HN inductively coupled plasma mass spectroscopy used in the index up to vol. 35, issue 6 (2003)
BT1 Mass spectroscopy
BT2 Spectroscopy
BT3 Analytical techniques
UF Inductively coupled plasma mass spectroscopy

ICP-OES
HN introduced from vol. 39, issue 1 (2007)
BT1 Spectroscopy
BT2 Analytical techniques
UF Inductively coupled plasma optical emission spectroscopy

Ictalurus punctatus
BT1 Channel catfish
BT2 Catfish
BT3 Freshwater fish
BT4 Fish
BT5 Animals
BT5 Sea foods
BT6 Aquatic foods
BT7 Animal foods
BT8 Foods

IDF
USE **International Dairy Federation**

Idiazabal cheese
BT1 Cheese varieties
BT2 Cheese
BT3 Dairy products
BT4 Animal foods
BT5 Foods

L-Iditol 2-dehydrogenases
SN EC 1.1.1.14
BT1 Dehydrogenases
BT2 Oxidoreductases
BT3 Enzymes
UF Sorbitol dehydrogenases

Idli
BT1 Fermented foods
BT2 Processed foods
BT3 Foods
BT1 Legumes
BT2 Vegetables specific
BT3 Vegetables
BT4 Crops
BT5 Plants
BT4 Plant foods
BT5 Foods
BT1 Rice
BT2 Cereals
BT3 Crops
BT4 Plants
BT3 Seeds
BT4 Plant foods
BT5 Foods

IEF
HN isoelectric focusing used in the index up to vol. 35, issue 6 (2003)
BT1 Electrophoresis
BT2 Analytical techniques
UF Isoelectric focusing

Ika shiokara
HN under Sea foods up to vol. 42 (2010)
BT1 Shiokara
BT2 Fermented foods
BT3 Processed foods
BT4 Foods
BT2 Sea foods
BT3 Aquatic foods
BT4 Animal foods
BT5 Foods
BT1 Squid
BT2 Cephalopods
BT3 Molluscs
BT4 Shellfish
BT5 Animals
BT5 Sea foods
BT6 Aquatic foods
BT7 Animal foods
BT8 Foods
UF Squid ika shiokara

Ilex paraguariensis
HN under Beverages up to vol. 42 (2010)
BT1 Yerba mate
BT2 Mate
BT3 Herb tea
BT4 Teas
BT5 Beverages
BT5 Crops
BT6 Plants
BT5 Plant foods
BT6 Foods

Illex argentinus
BT1 Squid
BT2 Cephalopods
BT3 Molluscs
BT4 Shellfish
BT5 Animals
BT5 Sea foods
BT6 Aquatic foods
BT7 Animal foods
BT8 Foods

Illipe butter
BT1 Vegetable fats
BT2 Fats vegetable
BT3 Fats
BT4 Lipids
BT5 Nutrients
BT3 Vegetable products

BT4 Plant foods
BT5 Foods

Illipe nuts
BT1 Oilseeds
BT2 Seeds
BT3 Plant foods
BT4 Foods

Image analysis
BT1 Analytical techniques

Image processing
BT1 Quality control
BT2 Technology

Imaging
BT1 Analytical techniques
RT Cameras

Imazalil
BT1 Fungicides
BT2 Pesticides
BT3 Biocides
BT3 Residues

Imbibition
BT1 Soaking
BT2 Processing
BT3 Technology

Imidacloprid
BT1 Insecticides
BT2 Pesticides
BT3 Biocides
BT3 Residues

Imidan
USE **Phosmet**

Imidazoles
BT1 Heterocyclic compounds
BT1 Organic nitrogen compounds
NT1 Allantoin

Imitation cheese
BT1 Imitation dairy products
BT2 Imitation foods
BT3 Simulated foods
BT4 Processed foods
BT5 Foods
RT Cheese substitutes

Imitation crab meat
BT1 Imitation foods
BT2 Simulated foods
BT3 Processed foods
BT4 Foods

Imitation cream
BT1 Imitation dairy products
BT2 Imitation foods
BT3 Simulated foods
BT4 Processed foods
BT5 Foods

Imitation dairy products
BT1 Imitation foods
BT2 Simulated foods
BT3 Processed foods
BT4 Foods
NT1 Imitation cheese
NT1 Imitation cream

Imitation foods
BT1 Simulated foods
BT2 Processed foods
BT3 Foods
NT1 Imitation crab meat
NT1 Imitation dairy products
NT2 Imitation cheese
NT2 Imitation cream

Immersion freezing
HN introduced from vol. 39, issue 1 (2007)
BT1 Freezing
BT2 Thermal processing
BT3 Processing thermal
BT4 Processing
BT5 Technology

Immobilization
BT1 Biotechnology
BT2 Technology
RT Immobilized cells
RT Immobilized enzymes

Immobilized cells
HN heading from vol. 24 (1992)
BT1 Biotechnology
BT2 Technology
BT1 Cells
RT Bioreactors
RT Immobilization

Immobilized enzymes
BT1 Biotechnology
BT2 Technology
BT1 Enzymes
RT Immobilization

Immune response
BT1 Immunology
RT Immunological response

Immunoaffinity chromatography
BT1 Chromatography
BT2 Analytical techniques

Immunoassay
BT1 Immunological techniques
BT2 Analytical techniques

Immunochemical analysis
BT1 Immunological techniques
BT2 Analytical techniques

Immunodiffusion
BT1 Immunological techniques
BT2 Analytical techniques

Immunoelectrophoresis
BT1 Electrophoresis
BT2 Analytical techniques
BT1 Immunological techniques
BT2 Analytical techniques

Immunofluorescence
BT1 Immunological techniques
BT2 Analytical techniques

Immunogenicity
BT1 Immunology
RT Antigenicity

Immunoglobulin A
HN introduced from vol. 37, issue 5 (2005)
BT1 Immunoglobulins
BT2 Animal proteins
BT3 Proteins animal
BT4 Proteins
BT5 Nutrients
BT2 Globulins
BT3 Proteins
BT4 Nutrients

Immunoglobulin E
BT1 Immunoglobulins
BT2 Animal proteins
BT3 Proteins animal
BT4 Proteins
BT5 Nutrients
BT2 Globulins
BT3 Proteins
BT4 Nutrients

Immunoglobulin G
BT1 Immunoglobulins
BT2 Animal proteins
BT3 Proteins animal
BT4 Proteins
BT5 Nutrients
BT2 Globulins
BT3 Proteins
BT4 Nutrients

Immunoglobulins
BT1 Animal proteins
BT2 Proteins animal
BT3 Proteins
BT4 Nutrients
BT1 Globulins
BT2 Proteins
BT3 Nutrients
NT1 Immunoglobulin A
NT1 Immunoglobulin E
NT1 Immunoglobulin G
NT1 Immunoglobulin Y
RT Antibodies
RT γ-Globulins

Immunoglobulin Y
HN introduced from vol. 37, issue 5 (2005)
BT1 Immunoglobulins
BT2 Animal proteins
BT3 Proteins animal
BT4 Proteins
BT5 Nutrients
BT2 Globulins
BT3 Proteins
BT4 Nutrients

Immunological effects
BT1 Immunology

Immunological response
BT1 Immunology
RT Immune response

Immunological techniques
BT1 Analytical techniques
NT1 Agglutination tests
NT1 ELISA
NT1 Enzyme immunoassay
NT1 Immunoassay
NT1 Immunochemical analysis
NT1 Immunodiffusion
NT1 Immunoelectrophoresis
NT1 Immunofluorescence
NT1 Immunomagnetic separation
NT1 Radioimmunoassay
NT1 Serological tests
NT1 Serology
NT1 Serotyping
RT Antisera
RT Cross-reactivity
RT Immunology

Immunology
HN heading up to vol. 22 (1990) and from vol. 25 (1993)
NT1 Allergenicity
NT1 Allergens
NT1 Antibodies
NT1 Antigenicity
NT1 Antigens
NT1 Antisera
NT1 Cross-reactivity
NT1 Cytokines
NT1 Haemolysins
NT1 Immune response
NT1 Immunogenicity
NT1 Immunological effects
NT1 Immunological response
NT1 Immunomodulation
NT1 Immunotherapy
NT1 Monoclonal antibodies
NT1 Serology
NT1 Serotype
NT1 Vaccination
RT Immunological techniques

Immunomagnetic separation
BT1 Immunological techniques
BT2 Analytical techniques
BT1 Separation
BT2 Processing
BT3 Technology

Immunomodulation
BT1 Immunology

Immunotherapy
HN introduced from vol. 39, issue 1 (2007)
BT1 Immunology
BT1 Therapy
RT Allergies

IMP
BT1 Nucleotides
UF Inosine monophosphate

Impala
BT1 Animals

Impedance
HN under Microbiological techniques up to vol. 42 (2010)
BT1 Analytical techniques
BT1 Electrical properties
BT2 Physical properties

Impellers
BT1 Equipment
BT2 Technology
BT1 Mixing
BT2 Processing
BT3 Technology

Impingement drying
BT1 Drying
BT2 Thermal processing
BT3 Processing thermal
BT4 Processing
BT5 Technology

Imports
BT1 Trade
BT2 Economics

Improvements
RT Modification

Improvers
BT1 Additives
RT Flour improvers

Impurities
BT1 Contaminants
BT2 Contamination
RT Purity

Incaparina
BT1 Protein products

Incubation
RT Cell culture
RT Media

India
HN heading up to vol. 24 (1992)
BT1 Asia

Indian mackerel
BT1 Mackerel
BT2 Marine fish
BT3 Fish
BT4 Animals
BT4 Sea foods
BT5 Aquatic foods
BT6 Animal foods
BT7 Foods
BT2 Oily fish
BT3 Fish
BT4 Animals
BT4 Sea foods
BT5 Aquatic foods
BT6 Animal foods
BT7 Foods

Indian mulberries
USE **Noni**

Indian mustard
BT1 Mustard greens
BT2 Vegetables specific
BT3 Vegetables
BT4 Crops
BT5 Plants
BT4 Plant foods
BT5 Foods
BT1 Mustard seeds
BT2 Oilseeds
BT3 Seeds
BT4 Plant foods
BT5 Foods
BT2 Spices
BT3 Flavourings
BT4 Additives

Indian shad
BT1 Shad
BT2 Marine fish
BT3 Fish
BT4 Animals
BT4 Sea foods
BT5 Aquatic foods
BT6 Animal foods
BT7 Foods

Indian spinach
BT1 Vegetables specific
BT2 Vegetables
BT3 Crops
BT4 Plants
BT3 Plant foods
BT4 Foods
NT1 *Basella*

Indigo carmine
BT1 Colorants
BT2 Additives

Indigotine
BT1 Colorants
BT2 Additives

Indole acetic acid
HN introduced from vol. 43, issue 1 (2011); non-descriptor up to 2010 (USE indol-3-ylacetic acid)
BT1 Auxins
BT2 Plant growth regulators
BT3 Cultivation
BT4 Agriculture
NT1 Indol-3-ylacetic acid
UF IAA

Indole-3-carbinol
HN introduced from vol. 41, issue 1 (2009)
BT1 Indoles
BT2 Heterocyclic compounds
BT2 Organic nitrogen compounds
RT Glucobrassicin

Indoles
BT1 Heterocyclic compounds
BT1 Organic nitrogen compounds
NT1 Indole-3-carbinol
RT Alkaloids

Indol-3-ylacetic acid
BT1 Indole acetic acid
BT2 Auxins
BT3 Plant growth regulators
BT4 Cultivation
BT5 Agriculture

Indonesia
BT1 Asia

Induction heating
BT1 Heating
BT2 Thermal processing
BT3 Processing thermal
BT4 Processing
BT5 Technology

Inductively coupled plasma atomic emission spectroscopy
USE **ICP-AES**

Inductively coupled plasma mass spectroscopy
HN ICPMS used in the index from vol. 35, issue 6 (2003))
USE **ICP-MS**

Inductively coupled plasma optical emission spectroscopy
USE **ICP-OES**

Industries
HN heading up to vol. 24 (1992)
NT1 Food industry
NT2 Baking industry
NT2 Beet sugar industry
NT2 Beverages industry
NT2 Brewing industry
NT2 Cane sugar industry
NT2 Canning industry
NT2 Catering industry
NT2 Chocolate industry
NT2 Cocoa industry
NT2 Coffee industry
NT2 Confectionery industry
NT2 Dairy industry
NT2 Distilling industry
NT2 Fish industry
NT2 Flavourings industry
NT2 Fresh produce industry
NT2 Industry attitudes
NT2 Meat industry
NT2 Poultry meat industry
NT2 Sea foods industry
NT2 Sugar confectionery industry
NT2 Sugar industry
NT2 Wine industry
NT1 Pet foods industry

Industry attitudes
HN introduced from vol. 39, issue 1 (2007)
BT1 Food industry
BT2 Industries
RT Consumer attitudes

Infant foods
BT1 Processed foods
BT2 Foods
NT1 Humanized milk
NT1 Infant formulas
NT2 Milk infant formulas
NT1 Soy infant formulas
NT1 Weaning foods
RT Nutrition
UF Baby foods

Infant formulae
USE **Infant formulas**

Infant formulas
BT1 Infant foods
BT2 Processed foods
BT3 Foods
NT1 Milk infant formulas
UF Human milk substitutes
UF Infant formulae

Infant milk formulas
USE **Milk infant formulas**

Infants
SN children <1 year of age
BT1 Population groups
UF Babies

Infection
BT1 Diseases
RT Infectivity

Infectivity
BT1 Virulence factors
RT Infection

Infestation
BT1 Pests

Inflammation
HN introduced from vol. 39, issue 1 (2007)
BT1 Diseases
RT Anti-inflammatory activity

Inflammatory bowel disease
HN introduced from vol. 38, issue 8 (2006)
BT1 Diseases
NT1 Crohns disease
NT1 Ulcerative colitis

Information
NT1 Consumer information
NT2 Health promotion
NT1 Risk communication
RT Advertising
RT Education

Information processing
HN heading up to vol. 24 (1992)
USE **Information technology**

Information technology
HN heading from vol. 25 (1993); under Information processing up to vol. 24 (1992)
BT1 Technology
NT1 Artificial neural networks
NT1 Computerized data processing
NT1 Computer software
NT1 Databanks
NT1 Databases
NT1 Data processing
NT1 E-commerce
NT1 Electronic data processing
NT1 Expert systems
NT1 Food information
NT1 Internet
NT2 World Wide Web
RT Computers
UF Information processing

Infrared
HN heading up to vol. 24 (1992); heading is Infrared radiation from vol. 25 (1993)
USE **IR**

Infrared irradiation
USE **IR irradiation**

Infrared radiation
HN heading from vol. 25 (1993)
BT1 Radiation
NT1 IR radiation
NT2 IR
NT1 NIR

Infrared spectrophotometry
USE **IR spectroscopy**

Infusions
BT1 Extracts
BT2 Flavourings
BT3 Additives

Ingredients

Inheritance
BT1 Genetics

Inhibition
SN includes inhibition of microorganisms and prions
NT1 Antimicrobial activity
NT2 Antibacterial activity
NT2 Antifungal activity
NT2 Antiviral activity
RT Antibiotics
RT Antiseptics
RT Bactericides
RT Bacteriostats

Injection
HN introduced from vol. 39, issue 1 (2007)
BT1 Processing
BT2 Technology

Injectors
BT1 Equipment
BT2 Technology

Injera
BT1 Bread
BT2 Bakery products
BT3 Cereal products
BT4 Plant foods
BT5 Foods

Injury
BT1 Damage

Ink jet printers
BT1 Printers
BT2 Printing
BT3 Labelling
BT4 Packaging
BT5 Technology
UF Printers ink jet

Ink jet technology
BT1 Labelling
BT2 Packaging
BT3 Technology

Inks
BT1 Labelling
BT2 Packaging
BT3 Technology
RT Edible inks

Inn breweries
BT1 Breweries
BT2 Brewing
BT3 Processing
BT4 Technology
RT Pubs

Inorganic acids
BT1 Acids
BT1 Inorganic compounds

Inorganic compounds
NT1 Ammonia
NT2 NH_3
NT1 Carbon dioxide
NT2 CO_2
NT2 Dry Ice
NT2 Supercritical CO_2 extraction
NT1 Carbon monoxide
NT1 Chlorine dioxide
NT1 Inorganic acids
NT1 Nitrous oxide
NT1 Peroxides
NT2 H_2O_2
NT2 Hydroperoxides

Inosine
BT1 Nucleosides

Inosine monophosphate
USE **IMP**

Inositol
BT1 Antinutritional factors
BT2 Nutritional values
BT1 Polyols
BT2 Alcohols
BT2 Carbohydrates
BT3 Nutrients
BT3 Organic compounds
NT1 Inositol phosphates
NT1 Phytates
NT1 Phytic acid

Inositol phosphates
BT1 Inositol
BT2 Antinutritional factors
BT3 Nutritional values
BT2 Polyols
BT3 Alcohols
BT3 Carbohydrates
BT4 Nutrients
BT4 Organic compounds
BT1 Phosphates
BT2 Salts
RT Phytic acid

Insect foods
SN insects eaten as foods
BT1 Animal foods
BT2 Foods
NT1 Phane

Insecticides
BT1 Pesticides
BT2 Biocides
BT2 Residues
NT1 Amitraz
NT1 Avermectins
NT2 Emamectin
NT1 Chlordimeform
NT1 Diflubenzuron
NT1 Dimetilan
NT1 Dinocap
NT1 Fenazaflor
NT1 Imidacloprid
NT1 Methoprene
NT1 *N*-Methylcarbamate insecticides
NT2 Aldicarb
NT2 Carbaryl
NT2 Carbofuran
NT2 Ethiofencarb
NT2 Methomyl
NT2 Oxamyl
NT2 Pirimicarb
NT2 Propoxur
NT1 Organochlorine insecticides
NT2 Aldrin
NT2 Bromocyclen
NT2 Camphechlor
NT2 Chlordane
NT3 Nonachlor
NT2 Chlordecone
NT2 DDT
NT3 DDE
NT3 TDE
NT2 Dichlorobenzene
NT2 Dieldrin
NT2 Dilor
NT2 Endosulfan
NT2 Endrin
NT2 HCH
NT2 Heptachlor
NT3 Heptachlor epoxide
NT2 Kelevan
NT2 Methoxychlor
NT2 Mirex
NT2 Perthane
NT1 Organophosphorus insecticides
NT2 Acephate
NT2 Azinphos-methyl
NT2 Bromophos
NT2 Butonate
NT2 Carbophenothion
NT2 Chlorfenvinphos
NT2 Chlorphoxim
NT2 Chlorpyrifos
NT2 Chlorpyrifos-methyl
NT2 Coumaphos
NT2 Crotoxyphos
NT2 Demeton
NT2 Demeton-*S*-methyl
NT2 Dialifos
NT2 Diazinon
NT2 Dichlorvos
NT2 Dimethoate
NT2 Dioxathion
NT2 Disulfoton
NT2 Ethion
NT2 Ethoprophos
NT2 Etrimfos
NT2 Famphur
NT2 Fenchlorphos
NT2 Fenitrothion
NT2 Fensulfothion
NT2 Fenthion
NT2 Fonofos
NT2 Formothion
NT2 Iodofenphos
NT2 Leptophos
NT2 Malathion
NT3 Malaoxon
NT2 Methamidophos
NT2 Methidathion
NT2 Mevinphos
NT2 Monocrotophos
NT2 Naled
NT2 Omethoate
NT2 Oxydemeton-methyl
NT2 Parathion
NT3 Paraoxon
NT2 Parathion-methyl
NT2 Phenthoate
NT2 Phorate
NT2 Phosalone
NT2 Phosmet
NT2 Phosphamidon
NT2 Phoxim
NT2 Pirimiphos-methyl
NT2 Quinalphos
NT2 Temephos
NT2 Terbufos
NT2 Tetrachlorvinphos
NT2 Triazophos
NT2 Trichlorfon
NT1 Piperonyl butoxide
NT1 Pyrethroid insecticides
NT2 Allethrin
NT2 Cypermethrin
NT2 Deltamethrin
NT2 Fenvalerate
NT2 Fluvalinate
NT2 Permethrin
NT2 Pyrethrins
NT2 Resmethrin
NT1 Rotenone
NT1 Spinosad

Insects
HN heading from vol. 30 (1998); under Pests up to vol. 29 (1997)
BT1 Pests
NT1 Ants
NT1 Aphids
NT1 Bees
NT1 Beetles
NT2 *Ahasverus advena*
NT1 Cockroaches
NT1 *Eurygaster*
NT1 Flies
NT1 Fruit flies
NT1 Grain borers
NT1 *Liposcelis*
NT2 *Liposcelis bostrychophila*
NT1 Moths
NT1 *Oryzaephilus*
NT1 *Phylloxera*

NT1 Psocids
NT1 *Sitophilus*
NT2 Rice weevils
NT3 *Sitophilus oryzae*
NT2 *Sitophilus granarius*
NT2 *Sitophilus zeamais*
NT1 Stink bugs
NT1 Termites
NT1 Thrips
NT1 *Tribolium*
NT1 *Tyrophagus*
NT1 Weevils

Insertion sequences
BT1 Genetics
RT Transposition

Insoluble fibre
HN introduced from vol. 39, issue 1 (2007)
BT1 Dietary fibre
BT2 Fibre

Inspection
BT1 Quality control
BT2 Technology
RT Carcass condemnation

Instant beverages
BT1 Beverages
BT1 Instant foods
BT2 Processed foods
BT3 Foods
NT1 Instant cocoa
NT1 Instant coffee
NT2 Coffee granules
NT1 Instant tea

Instant cocoa
BT1 Cocoa products
BT2 Plant foods
BT3 Foods
BT1 Instant beverages
BT2 Beverages
BT2 Instant foods
BT3 Processed foods
BT4 Foods

Instant coffee
BT1 Coffee products
BT2 Coffee
BT3 Beverages
BT3 Crops
BT4 Plants
BT3 Plant foods
BT4 Foods
BT1 Instant beverages
BT2 Beverages
BT2 Instant foods
BT3 Processed foods
BT4 Foods
NT1 Coffee granules
RT Coffee powders

Instant foods
BT1 Processed foods
BT2 Foods
NT1 Gravy powders
NT1 Instant beverages
NT2 Instant cocoa
NT2 Instant coffee
NT3 Coffee granules
NT2 Instant tea
NT1 Instant noodles
NT1 Instant soups
NT1 Mixes
NT2 Bakery product mixes
NT2 Beverage mixes
NT2 Cake mixes
NT2 Dessert mixes
NT2 Ice cream mixes
NT2 Soup mixes
NT1 Powders
NT2 Beverage powders
NT2 Chocolate powders
NT2 Cocoa powders
NT2 Coffee powders
NT2 Dried dairy products
NT3 Dried milk
NT3 Dried skim milk
NT3 Dried whey
NT2 Dried egg products
NT2 Dried eggs
NT2 Milk powders
NT2 Rice powders
NT2 Skim milk powders
NT2 Tea powders
NT2 Tomato powders
NT1 Tea granules
RT Dried foods
RT Granules
RT Instantization
RT Reconstituted foods
RT Soups
RT Whiteners

Instantization
BT1 Processing
BT2 Technology
RT Instant foods

Instant noodles
BT1 Instant foods
BT2 Processed foods
BT3 Foods
BT1 Noodles
BT2 Pasta
BT3 Cereal products
BT4 Plant foods
BT5 Foods

Instant soups
BT1 Instant foods
BT2 Processed foods
BT3 Foods
BT1 Soups
BT2 Processed foods
BT3 Foods

Instant tea
BT1 Instant beverages
BT2 Beverages
BT2 Instant foods
BT3 Processed foods
BT4 Foods
BT1 Teas
BT2 Beverages
BT2 Crops
BT3 Plants
BT2 Plant foods
BT3 Foods

Institutions
HN heading up to vol. 24 (1992)
NT1 Hospitals
NT1 Schools

Instruments
BT1 Apparatus
BT2 Technology

Insulation
HN heading up to vol. 24

Insulin
BT1 Hormones
BT2 Residues
NT1 Insulin resistance
RT Diabetes

Insulin-like growth factors
HN introduced from vol. 39, issue 1 (2007)
BT1 Hormones
BT2 Residues

Insulin resistance
HN introduced from vol. 38, issue 8 (2006)
BT1 Diseases
BT1 Insulin
BT2 Hormones
BT3 Residues
RT Diabetes

Intake
HN introduced from vol. 43, issue 1 (2011)

Integrated pest management
BT1 Pests

Integrins
HN introduced from vol. 41, issue 1 (2009)
BT1 Proteins
BT2 Nutrients
RT Binding

Intelligent packaging
HN introduced from vol. 39, issue 1 (2007)
BT1 Packaging
BT2 Technology

Interesterification
BT1 Esterification

Interfacial properties
HN introduced from vol. 39, issue 1 (2007)
BT1 Physical properties
RT Physical phases

Interfacial tension
BT1 Physical properties
RT Physical phases

Interferometry
BT1 Analytical techniques

Intermediate moisture foods
BT1 Processed foods
BT2 Foods

BT1 Water activity
NT1 Intermediate moisture pet foods

Intermediate moisture pet foods
HN introduced from vol. 39, issue 1 (2007)
BT1 Intermediate moisture foods
BT2 Processed foods
BT3 Foods
BT2 Water activity
BT1 Pet foods

Intermittent warming
BT1 Storage

International
RT Countries
RT World

International Dairy Federation
RT Dairy industry
UF IDF

International Organization for Standardization
HN heading up to vol. 24 (1992)
UF ISO

Internet
BT1 Information technology
BT2 Technology
NT1 World Wide Web

Intestines
BT1 Offal
BT2 Animal foods
BT3 Foods
RT Chitterlings

Intimins
HN introduced from vol. 39, issue 1 (2007)
BT1 Microbial proteins
BT2 Microorganisms
BT2 Proteins
BT3 Nutrients
BT1 Virulence factors
RT Adherence
RT Adhesins

Intolerance
BT1 Diseases
NT1 Food intolerance
NT2 Lactose intolerance
RT Allergies

Intramuscular fat
HN introduced from vol. 41, issue 1 (2009)
BT1 Animal fats
BT2 Fats animal
BT3 Animal foods
BT4 Foods
BT3 Fats
BT4 Lipids
BT5 Nutrients
RT Marbling

Introns
BT1 Genes
BT2 Chromosomes
BT3 Genetics
BT2 Genomes
BT3 Genetics

Inulases
USE **Inulinases**

Inulases II
USE **Inulin fructotransferases (DFA-III-forming)**

Inulin
BT1 Fructans
BT2 Polysaccharides
BT3 Carbohydrates
BT4 Nutrients
BT4 Organic compounds
RT Prebiotics
RT Raftiline

Inulinases
SN EC 3.2.1.7
BT1 Glycosidases
BT2 Hydrolases
BT3 Enzymes
UF Inulases

Inulin fructotransferases (depolymerizing)
USE **Inulin fructotransferases (DFA-III-forming)**

Inulin fructotransferases (DFA-III-forming)
HN introduced from vol. 39, issue 1 (2007)
SN EC 4.2.2.18
BT1 Lyases
BT2 Enzymes
UF Inulases II
UF Inulin fructotransferases (depolymerizing)

Invasins
HN introduced from vol. 39, issue 1 (2007)
BT1 Microbial proteins
BT2 Microorganisms
BT2 Proteins
BT3 Nutrients
BT1 Virulence factors
RT Invasion

Invasion
BT1 Virulence factors
RT Invasins

Invertases
HN heading up to vol. 24 (1992)
USE **β-Fructofuranosidases**

Invert sugar
BT1 Sugar syrups
BT2 Plant foods
BT3 Foods

Iodates
BT1 Oxidizing agents
BT2 Additives
RT Iodine
RT Iodized salt

Iodides
BT1 Salts
RT Iodine
RT Iodized salt

Iodine
SN symbol I is also used in the index
BT1 Halogens
BT2 Elements
BT3 Minerals
BT4 Nutrients
NT1 I
NT1 Iodized salt
RT Goitre
RT Iodates
RT Iodides
RT Iodophors

Iodine values
RT Fats
RT Oxidation

Iodized salt
BT1 Iodine
BT2 Halogens
BT3 Elements
BT4 Minerals
BT5 Nutrients
BT1 Salt
BT2 Condiments
BT3 Flavourings
BT4 Additives
RT Iodates
RT Iodides

Iodoacetic acid
HN under Plant growth regulators up to vol. 42 (2010)
BT1 Organic halogen compounds

Iodofenphos
BT1 Organophosphorus insecticides
BT2 Insecticides
BT3 Pesticides
BT4 Biocides
BT4 Residues
BT2 Organophosphorus pesticides
BT3 Pesticides
BT4 Biocides
BT4 Residues

Iodometry
BT1 Analytical techniques

Iodophors
BT1 Disinfectants
BT2 Disinfection
BT3 Hygiene
RT Iodine

Ion chromatography
BT1 Chromatography
BT2 Analytical techniques

Ion exchange
NT1 Anion exchange
RT Ion exchange chromatography
RT Ions
RT Sorption

Ion exchange chromatography
BT1 Chromatography
BT2 Analytical techniques
RT Ion exchange

Ionic strength
BT1 Physical properties

Ionization
BT1 Ions

Ionol
USE **BHT**

Ionones
BT1 Ketones
BT2 Carbonyl compounds
BT3 Organic compounds
BT1 Norisoprenoids
BT2 Aroma compounds
BT3 Flavour compounds
BT3 Volatile compounds
BT2 Carotenoids
BT3 Pigments
BT3 Terpenoids
BT4 Lipids
BT5 Nutrients

Ions
NT1 Anions
NT1 Cations
NT1 Ionization
RT Electrolytes
RT Ion exchange

Ion selective electrodes
BT1 Electrodes
BT2 Apparatus
BT3 Technology

Ipomeamarone
BT1 Bitter compounds
BT2 Flavour compounds
BT1 Sesquiterpenoids
BT2 Terpenoids
BT3 Lipids
BT4 Nutrients

Ipomoea batatas
HN used up to vol. 39 (2007)
USE **Sweet potatoes**

Iprodione
BT1 Dicarboximide fungicides
BT2 Fungicides
BT3 Pesticides
BT4 Biocides
BT4 Residues
UF Rovral

Ipronidazole
BT1 Drugs
BT2 Residues

IR
SN heading is Infrared radiation
BT1 IR radiation
BT2 Infrared radiation
BT3 Radiation
RT NIR
UF Infrared

Iran
SN full name is Islamic Republic of Iran
BT1 Asia
BT1 Middle East

IR analysis
BT1 IR spectroscopy
BT2 Spectroscopy
BT3 Analytical techniques

Iraq
BT1 Asia
BT1 Middle East

IR drying
HN introduced from vol. 39, issue 1 (2007)
BT1 Drying
BT2 Thermal processing
BT3 Processing thermal
BT4 Processing
BT5 Technology

Ireland, Republic of
HN heading up to vol. 24 (1992)
USE **Republic of Ireland**

IR heating
HN introduced from vol. 42, issue 1 (2010)
BT1 Heating
BT2 Thermal processing
BT3 Processing thermal
BT4 Processing
BT5 Technology

Iridaea
BT1 Seaweeds
BT2 Algae
BT3 Microorganisms
BT2 Sea foods
BT3 Aquatic foods
BT4 Animal foods
BT5 Foods

IR irradiation
BT1 Irradiation
BT2 Processing
BT3 Technology
RT IR radiation
UF Infrared irradiation

Irish Republic
HN used in the index from vol. 25 (1993) to vol. 35, issue 6 (2003)
USE **Republic of Ireland**

Iron
SN symbol Fe is also used in the index
BT1 Metals
BT2 Elements
BT3 Minerals
BT4 Nutrients
NT1 Fe
NT1 Ferritin

Irpex
BT1 Fungi
BT2 Microorganisms

Irradiated foods
BT1 Processed foods
BT2 Foods

IR radiation
SN heading is Infrared radiation
BT1 Infrared radiation
BT2 Radiation
NT1 IR
RT IR irradiation

Irradiation
BT1 Processing
BT2 Technology
NT1 Electron beam irradiation
NT1 Gamma irradiation
NT1 Gamma rays
NT1 IR irradiation
NT1 Radurization
NT1 UV irradiation
RT Radiation

Irrigation
BT1 Cultivation
BT2 Agriculture
NT1 Water stress

Irritable bowel syndrome
HN introduced from vol. 40, issue 1 (2008)
BT1 Diseases

IR spectra
BT1 IR spectroscopy
BT2 Spectroscopy
BT3 Analytical techniques

IR spectroscopy
BT1 Spectroscopy
BT2 Analytical techniques
NT1 IR analysis
NT1 IR spectra
UF Infrared spectrophotometry

Iru
BT1 African locust beans
BT2 Oilseeds
BT3 Seeds
BT4 Plant foods
BT5 Foods
BT1 Fermented foods
BT2 Processed foods
BT3 Foods
RT Dawadawa

Ishiru
BT1 Fermented foods
BT2 Processed foods
BT3 Foods
BT1 Fish sauces
BT2 Fish products
BT3 Sea foods
BT4 Aquatic foods
BT5 Animal foods

BT6 Foods
BT2 Sauces
BT3 Condiments
BT4 Flavourings
BT5 Additives

Isinglass
BT1 Gelatin
BT2 Animal proteins
BT3 Proteins animal
BT4 Proteins
BT5 Nutrients

Isle of Man
USE **United Kingdom**

ISO
USE **International Organization for Standardization**

Iso-α-acids
BT1 Bitter acids
BT2 Bitter compounds
BT3 Flavour compounds
BT2 Organic acids
BT3 Acids
NT1 Isohumulones

Isoamyl acetate
BT1 Acetates
BT1 Aroma compounds
BT2 Flavour compounds
BT2 Volatile compounds
BT1 Esters
BT2 Organic compounds

Isoamyl alcohol
SN syn. methyl butanol; syn. isopentyl alcohol
BT1 Alcohols
BT1 Aroma compounds
BT2 Flavour compounds
BT2 Volatile compounds
NT1 Isopentyl alcohol
NT1 Methyl butanol

Isoamylamine
BT1 Amines
BT2 Organic nitrogen compounds

Isoamylases
SN EC 3.2.1.68
BT1 Amylases
BT2 Glycosidases
BT3 Hydrolases
BT4 Enzymes

Isoascorbic acid
SN syn. erythorbic acid
BT1 Antioxidants
BT2 Additives

Isobutanol
SN syn. isobutyl alcohol; syn. methyl propanol
BT1 Alcohols
BT1 Aroma compounds
BT2 Flavour compounds
BT2 Volatile compounds
NT1 Isobutyl alcohol
NT1 Methyl propanol

Isobutyl alcohol
SN syn. isobutanol; syn. methyl propanol
BT1 Isobutanol
BT2 Alcohols
BT2 Aroma compounds
BT3 Flavour compounds
BT3 Volatile compounds

Isobutyraldehyde
HN also under Volatile compounds up to vol. 42 (2010)
SN syn. 2-methylpropanal
BT1 Aldehydes
BT2 Carbonyl compounds
BT3 Organic compounds
BT1 Aroma compounds
BT2 Flavour compounds
BT2 Volatile compounds
NT1 2-Methylpropanal

Isobutyric acid
BT1 Aroma compounds
BT2 Flavour compounds
BT2 Volatile compounds
BT1 Branched chain fatty acids
BT2 Fatty acids
BT3 Lipids
BT4 Nutrients
BT3 Organic acids
BT4 Acids
BT1 Short chain fatty acids
BT2 Volatile fatty acids
BT3 Fatty acids
BT4 Lipids
BT5 Nutrients
BT4 Organic acids
BT5 Acids
BT3 Volatile compounds

Isocaproic acid
BT1 Aroma compounds
BT2 Flavour compounds
BT2 Volatile compounds
BT1 Branched chain fatty acids
BT2 Fatty acids
BT3 Lipids
BT4 Nutrients
BT3 Organic acids
BT4 Acids
BT1 Short chain fatty acids
BT2 Volatile fatty acids
BT3 Fatty acids
BT4 Lipids
BT5 Nutrients
BT4 Organic acids
BT5 Acids
BT3 Volatile compounds

Isochlorogenic acid
BT1 Organic acids
BT2 Acids
BT1 Phenols
BT2 Alcohols
BT2 Aromatic compounds
BT3 Organic compounds

Isocitrases
USE **Isocitrate lyases**

Isocitrate dehydrogenases
SN EC 1.1.1.41 or 1.1.1.42
BT1 Dehydrogenases
BT2 Oxidoreductases
BT3 Enzymes

Isocitrate lyases
SN EC 4.1.3.1
BT1 Lyases
BT2 Enzymes
UF Isocitrases

Isocitric acid
BT1 Organic acids
BT2 Acids
RT Citric acid

Isoelectric focusing
HN IEF used in the index from vol. 35, issue 6 (2003)
USE **IEF**

Isoelectric points
BT1 pH
BT2 Physical properties

Isoenzymes
BT1 Enzymes
UF Isozymes

Isoeugenol
HN introduced from vol. 39, issue 1 (2007)
BT1 Phenols
BT2 Alcohols
BT2 Aromatic compounds
BT3 Organic compounds
BT1 Volatile compounds

Isoflavones
BT1 Isoflavonoids
BT2 Flavonoids
BT3 Aromatic compounds
BT4 Organic compounds
BT3 Pigments
NT1 Daidzein
NT1 Equol
NT1 Genistein
NT1 Glycitein
NT1 Puerarin

Isoflavonoids
BT1 Flavonoids
BT2 Aromatic compounds
BT3 Organic compounds
BT2 Pigments
NT1 Coumestrol
NT1 Isoflavones
NT2 Daidzein
NT2 Equol
NT2 Genistein
NT2 Glycitein
NT2 Puerarin

Isoglucose
BT1 Corn syrups
BT2 Sugar syrups

BT3 Plant foods
BT4 Foods

Isohumulones
BT1 Iso-α-acids
BT2 Bitter acids
BT3 Bitter compounds
BT4 Flavour compounds
BT3 Organic acids
BT4 Acids

Isoleucine
BT1 Amino acids
BT2 Nutrients
BT2 Organic acids
BT3 Acids
BT2 Organic nitrogen compounds

Isomalt
BT1 Sweeteners
BT2 Additives
UF Palatinit

Isomaltooligosaccharides
HN under Sugars and Polysaccharides up to vol. 42 (2010)
BT1 Glucooligosaccharides
BT2 Oligosaccharides
BT3 Polysaccharides
BT4 Carbohydrates
BT5 Nutrients
BT5 Organic compounds
BT3 Sugars
BT4 Carbohydrates
BT5 Nutrients
BT5 Organic compounds
BT4 Plant foods
BT5 Foods
RT Maltooligosaccharides

Isomaltose
HN under Sugars up to vol. 42 (2010)
BT1 Disaccharides
BT2 Sugars
BT3 Carbohydrates
BT4 Nutrients
BT4 Organic compounds
BT3 Plant foods
BT4 Foods

Isomaltulose
HN reinstated from vol. 43, issue 1 (2011); Palatinose used previously
BT1 Disaccharides
BT2 Sugars
BT3 Carbohydrates
BT4 Nutrients
BT4 Organic compounds
BT3 Plant foods
BT4 Foods
NT1 Palatinose

Isomerases
SN EC 5
BT1 Enzymes
NT1 Arabinose isomerases
NT1 Epimerases
NT2 Aldose 1-epimerases
NT1 Glucose isomerases
NT1 Phosphoglucomutases
NT1 Racemases
NT1 Xylose isomerases
RT Isomerization

Isomerization
RT Isomerases
RT Isomers

Isomers
HN heading from vol. 25 (1993)
NT1 Enantiomers
NT1 Enantioselectivity
NT1 Stereoisomers
RT Isomerization

Isoniazid
HN introduced from vol. 37, issue 5 (2005)
BT1 Antibiotics
BT2 Drugs
BT3 Residues

Isopentyl alcohol
SN syn. methyl butanol; syn. isoamyl alcohol
BT1 Isoamyl alcohol
BT2 Alcohols
BT2 Aroma compounds
BT3 Flavour compounds
BT3 Volatile compounds

Isoprene
BT1 Hydrocarbons
BT2 Organic compounds
BT1 Terpenoids
BT2 Lipids
BT3 Nutrients

Isoprenoids
BT1 Hydrocarbons
BT2 Organic compounds
BT1 Terpenoids
BT2 Lipids
BT3 Nutrients

Isopropanol
SN syn. isopropyl alcohol; syn. 2-propanol
BT1 Alcohols
BT1 Solvents

Isopropyl alcohol
SN syn. 2-propanol; syn. isopropanol
BT1 Alcohols
BT1 Solvents

Isorhamnetin
HN introduced from vol. 41, issue 1 (2009)
BT1 Flavonols
BT2 Alcohols
BT2 Flavonoids
BT3 Aromatic compounds
BT4 Organic compounds
BT3 Pigments

Isospora
BT1 Parasites
BT2 Pests

Isosyrups
BT1 Corn syrups
BT2 Sugar syrups
BT3 Plant foods
BT4 Foods

Isotachophoresis
BT1 Electrophoresis
BT2 Analytical techniques

Isothiocyanates
BT1 Organic nitrogen compounds
BT1 Organic sulfur compounds
BT1 Volatile sulfur compounds
BT2 Volatile compounds
NT1 Allyl isothiocyanate
NT1 Benzyl isothiocyanate
NT1 Phenethyl isothiocyanate
NT1 Sulforaphane
UF Thiocyanates

Isotonic drinks
BT1 Health beverages
BT2 Beverages
BT2 Health foods
BT3 Processed foods
BT4 Foods
BT1 Soft drinks
BT2 Beverages
RT Energy drinks

Isotopes
HN under Minerals up to vol. 42 (2010)
BT1 Elements
BT2 Minerals
BT3 Nutrients
NT1 Radioelements
NT2 Cs
NT2 Po
NT2 Pu
NT2 Ra
NT2 Radionuclides
NT3 Radioisotopes
NT2 Rn
NT2 Sr
NT2 Tc
NT2 Tritium
NT2 U
RT Stable isotope techniques

Isovaleraldehyde
HN also under Volatile compounds up to vol. 42 (2010)
SN syn. 3-methylbutanal
BT1 3-Methylbutanal
BT2 Aldehydes
BT3 Carbonyl compounds
BT4 Organic compounds
BT2 Aroma compounds
BT3 Flavour compounds
BT3 Volatile compounds

Isovaleric acid
BT1 Aroma compounds
BT2 Flavour compounds
BT2 Volatile compounds
BT1 Branched chain fatty acids
BT2 Fatty acids
BT3 Lipids
BT4 Nutrients
BT3 Organic acids
BT4 Acids
BT1 Short chain fatty acids

BT2 Volatile fatty acids
BT3 Fatty acids
BT4 Lipids
BT5 Nutrients
BT4 Organic acids
BT5 Acids
BT3 Volatile compounds

Isozymes
USE **Isoenzymes**

Israel
BT1 Asia
BT1 Middle East

Issatchenkia
HN introduced from vol. 43, issue 1 (2011)
BT1 Yeasts
BT2 Fungi
BT3 Microorganisms
NT1 *Issatchenkia orientalis*

Issatchenkia orientalis
HN introduced from vol. 41, issue 1 (2009)
SN teleomorph of Candida krusei and synonymous with Pichia kudriavzevii
BT1 *Issatchenkia*
BT2 Yeasts
BT3 Fungi
BT4 Microorganisms

Itaconic acid
BT1 Organic acids
BT2 Acids

Italy
HN heading up to vol. 24
BT1 Europe
BT1 European Union
RT Organization for Economic Cooperation and Development

Ivermectin
BT1 Anthelmintics
BT2 Drugs
BT3 Residues

Ivory Coast
USE **Cote d'Ivoire**

Izvara
BT1 Curd
BT2 Dairy products
BT3 Animal foods
BT4 Foods

J

Jaboticaba
BT1 Fruits specific
BT2 Fruits
BT3 Crops
BT4 Plants
BT3 Plant foods
BT4 Foods

Jack beans
BT1 Legumes
BT2 Vegetables specific
BT3 Vegetables
BT4 Crops
BT5 Plants
BT4 Plant foods
BT5 Foods
NT1 *Canavalia ensiformis*

Jack fruits
USE **Jak fruits**

Jack mackerel
SN syn. horse mackerel
BT1 Mackerel
BT2 Marine fish
BT3 Fish
BT4 Animals
BT4 Sea foods
BT5 Aquatic foods
BT6 Animal foods
BT7 Foods
BT2 Oily fish
BT3 Fish
BT4 Animals
BT4 Sea foods
BT5 Aquatic foods
BT6 Animal foods
BT7 Foods
NT1 *Trachurus japonicus*
NT1 *Trachurus murphyi*

Jaggery
HN under Sugars up to vol. 42 (2010)
SN syn. gur
BT1 Sugar
BT2 Plant foods
BT3 Foods
NT1 Gur

Jak fruits
BT1 Fruits specific
BT2 Fruits
BT3 Crops
BT4 Plants
BT3 Plant foods
BT4 Foods
UF Jack fruits

Jalapeno peppers
HN introduced from vol. 37, issue 5 (2005)
BT1 Chillies
BT2 Capsicums
BT3 Vegetables specific
BT4 Vegetables
BT5 Crops
BT6 Plants
BT5 Plant foods
BT6 Foods

Jamaica
BT1 West Indies
BT2 America

Jams
BT1 Fruit preserves
BT2 Fruit products
BT3 Plant foods
BT4 Foods
BT2 Preserves
BT3 Processed foods
BT4 Foods
NT1 Apricot jams
NT1 Grape jams
NT1 Jelly
NT1 Mango jams
NT1 Marmalades
NT1 Quince jams
NT1 Strawberry jams

Japan
HN heading up to vol. 24 (1992)
BT1 Asia
RT Organization for Economic Cooperation and Development

Japanese apricots
BT1 Fruits specific
BT2 Fruits
BT3 Crops
BT4 Plants
BT3 Plant foods
BT4 Foods
NT1 *Prunus mume*
UF Ume

Japanese chestnuts
BT1 Chestnuts
BT2 Nuts
BT3 Fruits
BT4 Crops
BT5 Plants
BT4 Plant foods
BT5 Foods
BT3 Oilseeds
BT4 Seeds
BT5 Plant foods
BT6 Foods

Japanese flounders
BT1 Flounders
BT2 Flatfish
BT3 Marine fish
BT4 Fish
BT5 Animals
BT5 Sea foods
BT6 Aquatic foods
BT7 Animal foods
BT8 Foods
NT1 *Paralichthys olivaceus*
RT Bastard halibut

Japanese pears
SN syn. Asian pears
BT1 Pears
BT2 Fruits specific
BT3 Fruits
BT4 Crops
BT5 Plants
BT4 Plant foods
BT5 Foods

Japanese pepper
BT1 Spices

BT2 Flavourings
BT3 Additives

Japanese plums
BT1 Plums
BT2 Fruits specific
BT3 Fruits
BT4 Crops
BT5 Plants
BT4 Plant foods
BT5 Foods

Japanese radishes
BT1 Radishes
BT2 Vegetables specific
BT3 Vegetables
BT4 Crops
BT5 Plants
BT4 Plant foods
BT5 Foods

Jarlsberg cheese
BT1 Cheese varieties
BT2 Cheese
BT3 Dairy products
BT4 Animal foods
BT5 Foods

Jars
BT1 Containers

Jasmine
BT1 Flavourings
BT2 Additives

Jasmonic acid
BT1 Methyl jasmonate
BT2 Plant growth regulators
BT3 Cultivation
BT4 Agriculture

Jellied milk
BT1 Milk
BT2 Dairy products
BT3 Animal foods
BT4 Foods

Jellies
BT1 Jelly confectionery
BT2 Sugar confectionery
BT3 Plant foods
BT4 Foods

Jelly
HN under Sugar confectionery up to vol. 29 (1997)
BT1 Desserts
BT2 Processed foods
BT3 Foods
BT1 Jams
BT2 Fruit preserves
BT3 Fruit products
BT4 Plant foods
BT5 Foods
BT3 Preserves
BT4 Processed foods
BT5 Foods

Jelly babies
BT1 Jelly confectionery
BT2 Sugar confectionery
BT3 Plant foods
BT4 Foods

Jelly confectionery
BT1 Sugar confectionery
BT2 Plant foods
BT3 Foods
NT1 Fruit gums
NT1 Jellies
NT1 Jelly babies
NT1 Wine gums

Jelly figs
BT1 Fruits specific
BT2 Fruits
BT3 Crops
BT4 Plants
BT3 Plant foods
BT4 Foods
NT1 *Ficus awkeotsang*

Jellyfish
BT1 Sea foods
BT2 Aquatic foods
BT3 Animal foods
BT4 Foods

Jelly rolls
USE **Swiss rolls**

Jeotgal
BT1 Fermented foods
BT2 Processed foods
BT3 Foods
BT1 Sea foods
BT2 Aquatic foods
BT3 Animal foods
BT4 Foods
RT Shiokara

Jerky
BT1 Meat products
BT2 Animal foods
BT3 Foods

Jerusalem artichokes
HN heading from vol. 30 (1998); under Vegetables specific up to vol. 29 (1997)
BT1 Vegetables specific
BT2 Vegetables
BT3 Crops
BT4 Plants
BT3 Plant foods
BT4 Foods
RT Artichokes
UF Topinambour

Jicama
BT1 Vegetables specific
BT2 Vegetables
BT3 Crops
BT4 Plants
BT3 Plant foods
BT4 Foods

Jobs tears
BT1 Cereals
BT2 Crops
BT3 Plants
BT2 Seeds
BT3 Plant foods
BT4 Foods
UF Adlay

Jointing
BT1 Cutting
BT2 Processing
BT3 Technology

Jojoba oils
BT1 Vegetable oils
BT2 Oils vegetable
BT3 Oils
BT4 Lipids
BT5 Nutrients
BT3 Vegetable products
BT4 Plant foods
BT5 Foods
RT Jojoba seeds
RT Simmondsin

Jojoba seeds
HN introduced from vol. 37, issue 5 (2005)
BT1 Oilseeds
BT2 Seeds
BT3 Plant foods
BT4 Foods
RT Jojoba oils

Jordan
BT1 Asia
BT1 Middle East

Jowar
BT1 Sorghum
BT2 Cereals
BT3 Crops
BT4 Plants
BT3 Seeds
BT4 Plant foods
BT5 Foods

Juices
BT1 Liquids
BT2 Physical phases
BT3 Chemistry
BT4 Science
NT1 Stocks
RT Juiciness

Juiciness
BT1 Sensory properties
NT1 Succulence
RT Juices

Jujubes
HN heading from vol. 30 (1998); under Fruits specificup to vol. 29 (1997)
BT1 Fruits specific
BT2 Fruits
BT3 Crops
BT4 Plants
BT3 Plant foods
BT4 Foods
UF Ber fruits
UF Chinese dates

Juniper
BT1 Spices

BT2 Flavourings
BT3 Additives

Junket
BT1 Dairy products
BT2 Animal foods
BT3 Foods
BT1 Desserts
BT2 Processed foods
BT3 Foods

Jute
BT1 Packaging materials

Jute seeds
BT1 Oilseeds
BT2 Seeds
BT3 Plant foods
BT4 Foods

K

K
SN index heading is Potassium
BT1 Potassium
BT2 Metals
BT3 Elements
BT4 Minerals
BT5 Nutrients

Kachkaval cheese
BT1 Cheese varieties
BT2 Cheese
BT3 Dairy products
BT4 Animal foods
BT5 Foods

Kaempferol
BT1 Flavonols
BT2 Alcohols
BT2 Flavonoids
BT3 Aromatic compounds
BT4 Organic compounds
BT3 Pigments

Kafirins
BT1 Cereal proteins
BT2 Proteins cereal
BT3 Vegetable proteins
BT4 Proteins vegetable
BT5 Proteins
BT6 Nutrients
BT5 Vegetable products
BT6 Plant foods
BT7 Foods

Kahweol
BT1 Alcohols
BT1 Diterpenoids
BT2 Terpenoids
BT3 Lipids
BT4 Nutrients

Kajmak cheese
BT1 Cheese varieties
BT2 Cheese
BT3 Dairy products
BT4 Animal foods
BT5 Foods

Kakdugi
BT1 Kimchies
BT2 Fermented foods
BT3 Processed foods
BT4 Foods
BT2 Vegetable products
BT3 Plant foods
BT4 Foods
BT1 Radishes
BT2 Vegetables specific
BT3 Vegetables
BT4 Crops
BT5 Plants
BT4 Plant foods
BT5 Foods

Kaki figs
USE **Persimmons**

Kaki fruits
USE **Persimmons**

Kalakand
BT1 Dairy products
BT2 Animal foods
BT3 Foods

Kale
BT1 Vegetables specific
BT2 Vegetables
BT3 Crops
BT4 Plants
BT3 Plant foods
BT4 Foods
UF Collards

Kamaboko
BT1 Fish products
BT2 Sea foods
BT3 Aquatic foods
BT4 Animal foods
BT5 Foods

Kampuchea
USE **Cambodia**

Kanamycin
BT1 Aminoglycoside antibiotics
BT2 Antibiotics
BT3 Drugs
BT4 Residues

Kangaroo meat
BT1 Kangaroos
BT2 Animals
BT1 Meat specific
BT2 Meat
BT3 Animal foods
BT4 Foods

Kangaroos
BT1 Animals
NT1 Kangaroo meat

Kanjan
USE **Kanjang**

Kanjang
BT1 Soy sauces
BT2 Fermented foods
BT3 Processed foods
BT4 Foods
BT2 Sauces
BT3 Condiments
BT4 Flavourings
BT5 Additives
BT2 Soy products
BT3 Vegetable products
BT4 Plant foods
BT5 Foods
UF Kanjan

Kapok oils
BT1 Vegetable oils
BT2 Oils vegetable
BT3 Oils
BT4 Lipids
BT5 Nutrients
BT3 Vegetable products
BT4 Plant foods
BT5 Foods

Karaya gums
BT1 Gums
BT2 Polysaccharides
BT3 Carbohydrates
BT4 Nutrients
BT4 Organic compounds
BT2 Stabilizers
BT3 Additives
BT2 Thickeners
BT3 Additives

Kareish cheese
BT1 Cheese varieties
BT2 Cheese
BT3 Dairy products
BT4 Animal foods
BT5 Foods

Kashar cheese
BT1 Cheese varieties
BT2 Cheese
BT3 Dairy products
BT4 Animal foods
BT5 Foods

Kasseler
BT1 Meat products
BT2 Animal foods
BT3 Foods
RT Ham
RT Pork
RT Swine

Kasseri cheese
BT1 Cheese varieties
BT2 Cheese
BT3 Dairy products
BT4 Animal foods
BT5 Foods

Katemfe
BT1 Plants
RT Thaumatin

Katsuobushi
BT1 Fermented foods
BT2 Processed foods
BT3 Foods
BT1 Fish products
BT2 Sea foods
BT3 Aquatic foods
BT4 Animal foods
BT5 Foods
BT1 Skipjack tuna
BT2 Tuna
BT3 Marine fish
BT4 Fish
BT5 Animals
BT5 Sea foods
BT6 Aquatic foods
BT7 Animal foods
BT8 Foods
BT3 Oily fish
BT4 Fish
BT5 Animals
BT5 Sea foods
BT6 Aquatic foods
BT7 Animal foods
BT8 Foods

Katyk
BT1 Fermented cream
BT2 Cream
BT3 Dairy products
BT4 Animal foods
BT5 Foods
BT2 Fermented dairy products
BT3 Dairy products
BT4 Animal foods
BT5 Foods
BT3 Fermented foods
BT4 Processed foods
BT5 Foods

Kava
BT1 Beverages
BT1 Plants

Kawal
BT1 Fermented foods
BT2 Processed foods
BT3 Foods
BT1 Legumes
BT2 Vegetables specific
BT3 Vegetables
BT4 Crops
BT5 Plants
BT4 Plant foods
BT5 Foods

Kazakhstan
BT1 Asia

KCl
BT1 Chlorides
BT2 Salts

Kebabs
BT1 Meat products
BT2 Animal foods
BT3 Foods

Kecap
BT1 Soy sauces
BT2 Fermented foods
BT3 Processed foods
BT4 Foods
BT2 Sauces
BT3 Condiments
BT4 Flavourings
BT5 Additives
BT2 Soy products
BT3 Vegetable products
BT4 Plant foods
BT5 Foods
UF Ketjap
UF Kicap

Keeping quality
HN heading up to vol. 18 (1986)
USE **Shelf life**

Kefalograviera cheese
BT1 Cheese varieties
BT2 Cheese
BT3 Dairy products
BT4 Animal foods
BT5 Foods

Kefalotyri cheese
BT1 Cheese varieties
BT2 Cheese
BT3 Dairy products
BT4 Animal foods
BT5 Foods

Kefir
BT1 Fermented milk
BT2 Fermented dairy products
BT3 Dairy products
BT4 Animal foods
BT5 Foods
BT3 Fermented foods
BT4 Processed foods
BT5 Foods
BT2 Milk
BT3 Dairy products
BT4 Animal foods
BT5 Foods
NT1 Kefir grains
RT Kefiran

Kefiran
BT1 Polysaccharides
BT2 Carbohydrates
BT3 Nutrients
BT3 Organic compounds
RT Exopolysaccharides
RT Kefir
RT Kefir grains
RT *Lactobacillus kefiranofaciens*

Kefir grains
BT1 Kefir
BT2 Fermented milk
BT3 Fermented dairy products
BT4 Dairy products
BT5 Animal foods
BT6 Foods
BT4 Fermented foods
BT5 Processed foods
BT6 Foods
BT3 Milk
BT4 Dairy products
BT5 Animal foods
BT6 Foods
RT Kefiran

Kegs
BT1 Barrels
BT2 Containers

Kelevan
BT1 Organochlorine insecticides
BT2 Insecticides
BT3 Pesticides
BT4 Biocides
BT4 Residues
BT2 Organochlorine pesticides
BT3 Pesticides
BT4 Biocides
BT4 Residues

Kelp
USE ***Laminaria***

Kelthane
USE **Dicofol**

Kenaf seeds
BT1 Oilseeds
BT2 Seeds
BT3 Plant foods
BT4 Foods

Kenkey
BT1 Corn
BT2 Cereals
BT3 Crops
BT4 Plants
BT3 Seeds
BT4 Plant foods
BT5 Foods
BT1 Fermented foods
BT2 Processed foods
BT3 Foods

Kenya
BT1 East Africa
BT2 Africa

Kepone
USE **Chlordecone**

Keratin
BT1 Animal proteins
BT2 Proteins animal
BT3 Proteins
BT4 Nutrients

Keratinases
HN introduced from vol. 41, issue 1 (2009)
BT1 Proteinases
BT2 Hydrolases
BT3 Enzymes

Kesari dhal
USE **Grass peas**

Kestose
HN under Sugars up to vol. 42 (2010)
BT1 Fructooligosaccharides
BT2 Oligosaccharides
BT3 Polysaccharides
BT4 Carbohydrates

BT5 Nutrients
BT5 Organic compounds
BT3 Sugars
BT4 Carbohydrates
BT5 Nutrients
BT5 Organic compounds
BT4 Plant foods
BT5 Foods

Keta salmon
SN syn. chum salmon
BT1 Chum salmon
BT2 Pacific salmon
BT3 Salmon
BT4 Oily fish
BT5 Fish
BT6 Animals
BT6 Sea foods
BT7 Aquatic foods
BT8 Animal foods
BT9 Foods

Ketchups
SN syn. catsups
BT1 Sauces
BT2 Condiments
BT3 Flavourings
BT4 Additives
NT1 Catsups
NT2 Tomato catsups
NT1 Tomato ketchups
NT2 Tomato catsups

Ketjap
USE **Kecap**

Keto acids
BT1 Ketones
BT2 Carbonyl compounds
BT3 Organic compounds
BT1 Organic acids
BT2 Acids

Ketogenic diet
HN introduced from vol. 42, issue 1 (2010)
BT1 Diet therapy
BT2 Diet
BT3 Nutrition
BT2 Therapy

α-Ketoglutaric acid
BT1 Organic acids
BT2 Acids

Ketones
BT1 Carbonyl compounds
BT2 Organic compounds
NT1 Acetoin
NT2 Acetylmethylcarbinol
NT2 3-Hydroxy-2-butanone
NT1 α-Acetolactate
NT1 Acetone
NT1 Acetophenone
NT1 Alkylcyclobutanones
NT1 Aloin
NT1 Benzophenone
NT1 Butanone
NT1 Camphor
NT1 Carvone
NT1 β-Damascenone
NT1 Dihydroxyacetone
NT1 Diketones
NT2 Diacetyl
NT3 2,3-Butanedione
NT1 Filbertone
NT1 Furanones
NT2 Furaneol
NT3 2,5-Dimethyl-4-hydroxy-3(2*H*)-furanone
NT2 Sotolon
NT1 2-Heptanone
NT1 Ionones
NT1 Keto acids
NT1 Nonanone
NT1 Nootkatone
NT1 Octanone
NT1 Pentanedione
NT2 Acetylacetone
NT1 Propanone
NT1 Thujone
NT1 Undecanone
NT1 Zingerone
RT Aroma compounds

Ketoses
HN under Sugars up to vol. 42 (2010)
BT1 Monosaccharides
BT2 Sugars
BT3 Carbohydrates
BT4 Nutrients
BT4 Organic compounds
BT3 Plant foods
BT4 Foods

Kettles
BT1 Equipment
BT2 Technology

Khoa
BT1 Dairy products
BT2 Animal foods
BT3 Foods

Kicap
USE **Kecap**

Kidney beans
HN heading up to vol. 24 (1992)
BT1 Common beans
BT2 Legumes
BT3 Vegetables specific
BT4 Vegetables
BT5 Crops
BT6 Plants
BT5 Plant foods
BT6 Foods

Kidneys
BT1 Offal
BT2 Animal foods
BT3 Foods
NT1 Cattle kidneys
NT1 Lamb kidneys
NT1 Swine kidneys

Kidney stones
HN introduced from vol. 42, issue 1 (2010)
BT1 Diseases

Kids
HN type of goat not specified in the index from vol. 25 (1993)
USE **Goats**

Kieselguhr
HN heading up to vol. 24 (1992)
BT1 Filter aids
BT2 Filtration
BT3 Processing
BT4 Technology

Kilka
BT1 Marine fish
BT2 Fish
BT3 Animals
BT3 Sea foods
BT4 Aquatic foods
BT5 Animal foods
BT6 Foods
UF Black sea sprat

Killer toxins
HN introduced from vol. 39, issue 1 (2007)
BT1 Toxins
BT2 Residues
RT Killer yeasts

Killer yeasts
BT1 Yeasts
BT2 Fungi
BT3 Microorganisms
RT Killer toxins
RT Winemaking
RT Wines

Kilning
BT1 Malting

Kilns
HN heading up to vol. 24 (1992)
BT1 Ovens
BT2 Equipment
BT3 Technology
RT Malting

Kimchies
HN heading from vol. 30 (1998); under Fermented foods and Vegetable products up to vol. 29 (1997)
BT1 Fermented foods
BT2 Processed foods
BT3 Foods
BT1 Vegetable products
BT2 Plant foods
BT3 Foods
NT1 Kakdugi

Ki-mikan
HN introduced from vol. 37, issue 5 (2005)
BT1 Citrus fruits
BT2 Fruits specific
BT3 Fruits
BT4 Crops
BT5 Plants
BT4 Plant foods
BT5 Foods

Kinases
SN includes members of EC 2.7

BT1 Phosphotransferases
BT2 Transferases
BT3 Enzymes
NT1 Aspartate kinases
NT1 Fructokinases
NT1 Glucokinases
NT1 Hexokinases
UF Protein kinases

Kinema
BT1 Fermented foods
BT2 Processed foods
BT3 Foods
BT1 Soy products
BT2 Vegetable products
BT3 Plant foods
BT4 Foods

Kinetics
HN heading up to vol. 24

Kinetin
HN kinetins used in the index up to vol. 35, issue 6 (2003)
BT1 Cytokinins
BT2 Plant growth regulators
BT3 Cultivation
BT4 Agriculture
UF Kinetins

Kinetins
HN kinetin used in the index from vol. 35, issue 6 (2003)
USE **Kinetin**

Kingklip
BT1 Marine fish
BT2 Fish
BT3 Animals
BT3 Sea foods
BT4 Aquatic foods
BT5 Animal foods
BT6 Foods

King salmon
SN syn. chinook salmon
BT1 Chinook salmon
BT2 Pacific salmon
BT3 Salmon
BT4 Oily fish
BT5 Fish
BT6 Animals
BT6 Sea foods
BT7 Aquatic foods
BT8 Animal foods
BT9 Foods

Kinnow mandarins
BT1 Mandarins
BT2 Oranges
BT3 Citrus fruits
BT4 Fruits specific
BT5 Fruits
BT6 Crops
BT7 Plants
BT6 Plant foods
BT7 Foods

Kippers
BT1 Herring
BT2 Marine fish
BT3 Fish
BT4 Animals
BT4 Sea foods
BT5 Aquatic foods
BT6 Animal foods
BT7 Foods
BT2 Oily fish
BT3 Fish
BT4 Animals
BT4 Sea foods
BT5 Aquatic foods
BT6 Animal foods
BT7 Foods
BT1 Smoked fish
BT2 Fish products
BT3 Sea foods
BT4 Aquatic foods
BT5 Animal foods
BT6 Foods
BT2 Smoked foods
BT3 Processed foods
BT4 Foods

Kiribati
BT1 Oceania

Kirsch
BT1 Fruit brandies
BT2 Brandies
BT3 Spirits
BT4 Alcoholic beverages
BT5 Beverages alcoholic
BT6 Beverages
RT Cherry brandy

Kishk
BT1 Cereal products
BT2 Plant foods
BT3 Foods
BT1 Dairy products
BT2 Animal foods
BT3 Foods
BT1 Fermented foods
BT2 Processed foods
BT3 Foods
RT Tarhana
RT Trahanas

Kisra
BT1 Bread
BT2 Bakery products
BT3 Cereal products
BT4 Plant foods
BT5 Foods

Kissel
BT1 Desserts
BT2 Processed foods
BT3 Foods

Kitchens
BT1 Catering

Kitten foods
HN introduced from vol. 39, issue 1 (2007)
BT1 Cat foods
BT2 Pet foods
RT Cats

Kitten milks
HN introduced from vol. 39, issue 1 (2007)
BT1 Cat milks
BT2 Cat foods
BT3 Pet foods
RT Cats

Kiwano
BT1 Fruits specific
BT2 Fruits
BT3 Crops
BT4 Plants
BT3 Plant foods
BT4 Foods

Kiwifruit
HN heading from vol. 25 (1993); under Fruits specific up to vol. 24 (1992)
BT1 Fruits specific
BT2 Fruits
BT3 Crops
BT4 Plants
BT3 Plant foods
BT4 Foods
NT1 *Actinidia chinensis*
NT1 *Actinidia deliciosa*
NT1 *Actinidia polygama*
RT *Actinidia arguta*
RT Kiwifruit juices
UF Chinese gooseberries

Kiwifruit juices
BT1 Fruit juices
BT2 Fruit products
BT3 Plant foods
BT4 Foods
BT2 Soft drinks
BT3 Beverages
RT Kiwifruit

Kjeldahl
BT1 Analytical techniques
RT Kjeldahl nitrogen

Kjeldahl nitrogen
BT1 Proteins
BT2 Nutrients
RT Kjeldahl

Klebsiella
HN heading from vol. 25 (1993); under Enterobacteriaceae up to vol. 24 (1992); Aerobacter also used in the index up to vol. 42 (2010)
BT1 Bacteria
BT2 Microorganisms
NT1 *Klebsiella aerogenes*
NT1 *Klebsiella oxytoca*
NT1 *Klebsiella pneumoniae*
NT1 *Klebsiella terrigena*
UF *Aerobacter*

Klebsiella aerogenes
SN unapproved name; some strains now Klebsiella pneumoniae
BT1 *Klebsiella*
BT2 Bacteria
BT3 Microorganisms

Klebsiella oxytoca
BT1 *Klebsiella*
BT2 Bacteria
BT3 Microorganisms

Klebsiella pneumoniae
BT1 *Klebsiella*
BT2 Bacteria
BT3 Microorganisms

Klebsiella terrigena
SN synonymous with Raoultella terrigena
BT1 *Klebsiella*
BT2 Bacteria
BT3 Microorganisms

Kloeckera
SN mitosporic Hanseniaspora
BT1 Yeasts
BT2 Fungi
BT3 Microorganisms
NT1 *Kloeckera apiculata*

Kloeckera apiculata
SN anamorph of Hanseniaspora uvarum
BT1 *Kloeckera*
BT2 Yeasts
BT3 Fungi
BT4 Microorganisms

Kluyveromyces
HN heading from vol. 25 (1993); under Yeasts up to vol. 24 (1992)
BT1 Yeasts
BT2 Fungi
BT3 Microorganisms
NT1 *Kluyveromyces bulgaricus*
NT1 *Kluyveromyces fragilis*
NT1 *Kluyveromyces lactis*
NT1 *Kluyveromyces marxianus*
NT1 *Kluyveromyces phaffii*
NT1 *Kluyveromyces thermotolerans*

Kluyveromyces bulgaricus
BT1 *Kluyveromyces*
BT2 Yeasts
BT3 Fungi
BT4 Microorganisms

Kluyveromyces fragilis
SN obsolete species, synonymous with Kluyveromyces marxianus
BT1 *Kluyveromyces*
BT2 Yeasts
BT3 Fungi
BT4 Microorganisms

Kluyveromyces lactis
BT1 *Kluyveromyces*
BT2 Yeasts
BT3 Fungi
BT4 Microorganisms

Kluyveromyces marxianus
HN introduced from vol. 39, issue 1 (2007)
SN teleomorph of Candida kefyr; synonymous with the obsolete species Kluyveromyces fragilis and with Candida pseudotropicalis
BT1 *Kluyveromyces*
BT2 Yeasts
BT3 Fungi
BT4 Microorganisms

Kluyveromyces phaffii
SN synonymous with Tetrapisispora phaffii
BT1 *Kluyveromyces*
BT2 Yeasts
BT3 Fungi
BT4 Microorganisms

Kluyveromyces thermotolerans
SN synonymous with Lachancea thermotolerans
BT1 *Kluyveromyces*
BT2 Yeasts
BT3 Fungi
BT4 Microorganisms

Knackwurst
BT1 Sausages
BT2 Meat products
BT3 Animal foods
BT4 Foods

Kneading
BT1 Mixing
BT2 Processing
BT3 Technology
RT Breadmaking

Knives
BT1 Cutting
BT2 Processing
BT3 Technology
BT1 Equipment
BT2 Technology

Kobuvirus
HN introduced from vol. 43, issue 1 (2011)
BT1 Viruses
BT2 Microorganisms
NT1 Aichi virus

Kocho
BT1 Bakery products
BT2 Cereal products
BT3 Plant foods
BT4 Foods

Kochujang
HN under Soybeans up to vol. 42 (2010)
BT1 Capsicums
BT2 Vegetables specific
BT3 Vegetables
BT4 Crops
BT5 Plants
BT4 Plant foods
BT5 Foods
BT1 Fermented foods
BT2 Processed foods
BT3 Foods
BT1 Soy products
BT2 Vegetable products
BT3 Plant foods
BT4 Foods

Kochwurst
BT1 Sausages
BT2 Meat products
BT3 Animal foods
BT4 Foods

Kocuria
HN introduced from vol. 43, issue 1 (2011)
BT1 Bacteria
BT2 Microorganisms
NT1 *Kocuria varians*

Kocuria varians
HN introduced from vol. 39, issue 1 (2007)
SN formerly Micrococcus varians
BT1 *Kocuria*
BT2 Bacteria
BT3 Microorganisms

KOH
HN introduced from vol. 39, issue 1 (2007)
BT1 Alkalies
BT1 Hydroxides
BT2 Salts
UF Potassium hydroxide

Kohlrabi
BT1 Vegetables specific
BT2 Vegetables
BT3 Crops
BT4 Plants
BT3 Plant foods
BT4 Foods

Koji
HN heading up to vol. 24 (1992)
BT1 Cereal products
BT2 Plant foods
BT3 Foods
BT1 Fermented foods
BT2 Processed foods
BT3 Foods
BT1 Legumes
BT2 Vegetables specific
BT3 Vegetables
BT4 Crops
BT5 Plants
BT4 Plant foods
BT5 Foods
NT1 Rice koji

Kojic acid
BT1 Browning inhibitors
BT2 Browning
BT1 Mycotoxins
BT2 Toxins
BT3 Residues
BT1 Pyrones
BT2 Heterocyclic compounds

Koko
BT1 Cassava
BT2 Vegetables specific
BT3 Vegetables
BT4 Crops

BT5 Plants
BT4 Plant foods
BT5 Foods
BT1 Fermented foods
BT2 Processed foods
BT3 Foods
BT1 Porridges
BT2 Cereal products
BT3 Plant foods
BT4 Foods
RT Uji

Kokum
HN introduced from vol. 37, issue 5 (2005)
BT1 Spices
BT2 Flavourings
BT3 Additives
BT1 Vegetable fats
BT2 Fats vegetable
BT3 Fats
BT4 Lipids
BT5 Nutrients
BT3 Vegetable products
BT4 Plant foods
BT5 Foods

Komatsuna
BT1 Vegetables specific
BT2 Vegetables
BT3 Crops
BT4 Plants
BT3 Plant foods
BT4 Foods

Kombu
BT1 *Laminaria*
BT2 Seaweeds
BT3 Algae
BT4 Microorganisms
BT3 Sea foods
BT4 Aquatic foods
BT5 Animal foods
BT6 Foods

Kombucha
BT1 Tea beverages
BT2 Teas
BT3 Beverages
BT3 Crops
BT4 Plants
BT3 Plant foods
BT4 Foods

Konjac
USE **Elephant yams**

Konjac glucomannans
BT1 Elephant yams
BT2 Vegetables specific
BT3 Vegetables
BT4 Crops
BT5 Plants
BT4 Plant foods
BT5 Foods
BT1 Glucomannans
BT2 Mannans
BT3 Polysaccharides
BT4 Carbohydrates
BT5 Nutrients
BT5 Organic compounds

Konnyaku
USE **Elephant yams**

Korea
BT1 Asia
RT North Korea
RT Organization for Economic Cooperation and Development
RT South Korea

Kosher foods
BT1 Processed foods
BT2 Foods

Kostroma cheese
BT1 Cheese varieties
BT2 Cheese
BT3 Dairy products
BT4 Animal foods
BT5 Foods

Koumiss
BT1 Fermented milk
BT2 Fermented dairy products
BT3 Dairy products
BT4 Animal foods
BT5 Foods
BT3 Fermented foods
BT4 Processed foods
BT5 Foods
BT2 Milk
BT3 Dairy products
BT4 Animal foods
BT5 Foods
BT1 Mare milk
BT2 Horses
BT3 Animals
BT2 Milk
BT3 Dairy products
BT4 Animal foods
BT5 Foods
RT Shubat

Krill
BT1 Crustacea
BT2 Shellfish
BT3 Animals
BT3 Sea foods
BT4 Aquatic foods
BT5 Animal foods
BT6 Foods

Krokant
USE **Croquant**

Kudzu
BT1 Vegetables specific
BT2 Vegetables
BT3 Crops
BT4 Plants
BT3 Plant foods
BT4 Foods
RT Puerarin

Kulfi
BT1 Dairy products
BT2 Animal foods
BT3 Foods

Kumquats
BT1 Citrus fruits
BT2 Fruits specific
BT3 Fruits
BT4 Crops
BT5 Plants
BT4 Plant foods
BT5 Foods

Kunun zaki
BT1 Beverages

Kurakkan
USE **Finger millet**

Kurthia
BT1 Bacteria
BT2 Microorganisms

Kuruma prawns
BT1 Prawns
BT2 Crustacea
BT3 Shellfish
BT4 Animals
BT4 Sea foods
BT5 Aquatic foods
BT6 Animal foods
BT7 Foods

Kusaya
BT1 Fish products
BT2 Sea foods
BT3 Aquatic foods
BT4 Animal foods
BT5 Foods

Kusum
BT1 Oilseeds
BT2 Seeds
BT3 Plant foods
BT4 Foods

Kuth
BT1 Plants
UF Costus

Kuwait
HN heading up to vol. 21 (1989)
BT1 Asia
BT1 Middle East

Kvass
BT1 Alcoholic beverages
BT2 Beverages alcoholic
BT3 Beverages

Kwoka
BT1 Corn
BT2 Cereals
BT3 Crops
BT4 Plants
BT3 Seeds
BT4 Plant foods
BT5 Foods

Kylar
USE **Daminozide**

Kyrgyzstan
BT1 Asia

L

La
HN under Minerals up to vol. 42 (2010)
BT1 Lanthanides
BT2 Metals
BT3 Elements
BT4 Minerals
BT5 Nutrients
UF Lanthanum

Laban
USE **Leben**

Labban
USE **Leben**

Labelling
BT1 Packaging
BT2 Technology
NT1 Bar codes
NT1 Branding
NT1 Brands
NT1 Date marking
NT1 Dating
NT1 Health claims
NT1 Ink jet technology
NT1 Inks
NT1 Labels
NT1 Marking
NT1 Nutritional labelling
NT1 Printing
NT2 Printers
NT3 Ink jet printers
NT1 Private labels
NT1 Trademarks

Labels
BT1 Labelling
BT2 Packaging
BT3 Technology

Labeo rohita
BT1 Rohu
BT2 Carp
BT3 Freshwater fish
BT4 Fish
BT5 Animals
BT5 Sea foods
BT6 Aquatic foods
BT7 Animal foods
BT8 Foods
BT3 Oily fish
BT4 Fish
BT5 Animals
BT5 Sea foods
BT6 Aquatic foods
BT7 Animal foods
BT8 Foods

Lablab beans
BT1 Legumes
BT2 Vegetables specific
BT3 Vegetables
BT4 Crops
BT5 Plants
BT4 Plant foods
BT5 Foods
UF Hyacinth beans

Labneh
BT1 Fermented milk
BT2 Fermented dairy products
BT3 Dairy products
BT4 Animal foods
BT5 Foods
BT3 Fermented foods
BT4 Processed foods
BT5 Foods
BT2 Milk
BT3 Dairy products
BT4 Animal foods
BT5 Foods

Laboratories
HN introduced from vol. 39, issue 1 (2007)
BT1 Science

Laccases
SN EC 1.10.3.2
BT1 Phenolases
BT2 Oxidoreductases
BT3 Enzymes

Lacon
BT1 Pork
BT2 Meat specific
BT3 Meat
BT4 Animal foods
BT5 Foods

Lacquers
BT1 Surfaces
NT1 Varnishes

Lactacins
BT1 Bacteriocins
BT2 Antibiotics
BT3 Drugs
BT4 Residues
RT *Lactobacillus*

α-Lactalbumin
BT1 Lactalbumins
BT2 Albumins
BT3 Proteins
BT4 Nutrients
BT2 Milk proteins
BT3 Proteins milk
BT4 Animal proteins
BT5 Proteins animal
BT6 Proteins
BT7 Nutrients

Lactalbumins
BT1 Albumins
BT2 Proteins
BT3 Nutrients
BT1 Milk proteins
BT2 Proteins milk
BT3 Animal proteins
BT4 Proteins animal
BT5 Proteins
BT6 Nutrients
NT1 α-Lactalbumin

β-Lactam antibiotics
HN reinstated vol. 43, issue 1 (2011); antibiotics used 2000-2010 inclusive
BT1 Antibiotics
BT2 Drugs
BT3 Residues
NT1 Cephalosporins
NT2 Ceftazidime
NT2 Ceftiofur
NT2 Cephapirin
NT1 Penicillins
NT2 Amoxicillin
NT2 Ampicillin
NT2 Benzylpenicillin
NT2 Cloxacillin
NT2 Dicloxacillin
NT2 Oxacillin
NT2 Penicillin G

β-Lactamases
SN EC 3.5.2.6
BT1 Hydrolases
BT2 Enzymes
UF Penicillinases

Lactarius
BT1 Edible fungi
BT2 Fungi edible
BT3 Vegetables specific
BT4 Vegetables
BT5 Crops
BT6 Plants
BT5 Plant foods
BT6 Foods

Lactases
USE **β-Galactosidases**

Lactate dehydrogenases
SN EC 1.1.1.27 and 1.1.1.28
BT1 Dehydrogenases
BT2 Oxidoreductases
BT3 Enzymes

D-Lactate dehydrogenases
SN EC 1.1.1.28
BT1 Dehydrogenases
BT2 Oxidoreductases
BT3 Enzymes

L-Lactate dehydrogenases
SN EC 1.1.1.27
BT1 Dehydrogenases
BT2 Oxidoreductases
BT3 Enzymes

Lactate 2-monooxygenases
SN EC 1.13.12.4; formerly EC 1.1.3.2
BT1 Oxidases
BT2 Oxidoreductases
BT3 Enzymes
UF Lactate oxidases

Lactate oxidases
USE **Lactate 2-monooxygenases**

Lactates
BT1 Preservatives
BT2 Additives
BT1 Salts
NT1 Calcium lactate
NT1 Potassium lactate
NT1 Sodium lactate
RT Lactic acid

Lactation
SN used for lactation in animals; for lactation in humans use human lactation
BT1 Physiology
BT2 Science
RT Milking
UF Lactation number
UF Lactation stage

Lactation number
USE **Lactation**

Lactation stage
USE **Lactation**

Lactic acid
BT1 Organic acids
BT2 Acids
BT1 Preservatives
BT2 Additives
RT Lactates
RT Lactic fermentation
RT Sodium lactate

Lactic acid bacteria
BT1 Bacteria
BT2 Microorganisms
RT *Bifidobacterium*
RT *Lactobacillus*
RT *Lactococcus*
RT *Leuconostoc*
RT *Pediococcus*

Lactic beverages
BT1 Dairy beverages
BT2 Beverages
BT2 Dairy products
BT3 Animal foods
BT4 Foods
BT1 Fermented milk
BT2 Fermented dairy products
BT3 Dairy products
BT4 Animal foods
BT5 Foods
BT3 Fermented foods
BT4 Processed foods
BT5 Foods
BT2 Milk
BT3 Dairy products
BT4 Animal foods
BT5 Foods

Lactic fermentation
BT1 Fermentation
RT Lactic acid

Lacticins
BT1 Bacteriocins
BT2 Antibiotics
BT3 Drugs
BT4 Residues
RT *Lactococcus lactis*
RT Lantibiotics

Lactic starters
HN starters lactic also used in the index up to vol. 29 (1997)
BT1 Starters
BT2 Bacteria
BT3 Microorganisms

Lactic streptococci
BT1 *Streptococcus*
BT2 Bacteria
BT3 Microorganisms

Lactitol
BT1 Polyols
BT2 Alcohols
BT2 Carbohydrates
BT3 Nutrients
BT3 Organic compounds

Lactobacillaceae
HN heading up to vol. 24 (1992)
BT1 Bacteria
BT2 Microorganisms
RT *Lactobacillus*
RT *Pediococcus*

Lactobacillus
BT1 Bacteria
BT2 Microorganisms
NT1 *Lactobacillus acidophilus*
NT1 *Lactobacillus alimentarius*
NT1 *Lactobacillus amylophilus*
NT1 *Lactobacillus amylovorus*
NT1 *Lactobacillus brevis*
NT1 *Lactobacillus buchneri*
NT1 *Lactobacillus casei*
NT1 *Lactobacillus collinoides*
NT1 *Lactobacillus crispatus*
NT1 *Lactobacillus curvatus*
NT1 *Lactobacillus delbrueckii*
NT2 *Lactobacillus bulgaricus*
NT2 *Lactobacillus lactis*
NT1 *Lactobacillus fermentum*
NT1 *Lactobacillus fructivorans*
NT1 *Lactobacillus gasseri*
NT1 *Lactobacillus helveticus*
NT1 *Lactobacillus hilgardii*
NT1 *Lactobacillus johnsonii*
NT1 *Lactobacillus kefiranofaciens*
NT1 *Lactobacillus kefiri*
NT1 *Lactobacillus leichmannii*
NT1 *Lactobacillus lindneri*
NT1 *Lactobacillus paracasei*
NT1 *Lactobacillus paraplantarum*
NT1 *Lactobacillus pentosus*
NT1 *Lactobacillus plantarum*
NT1 *Lactobacillus pontis*
NT1 *Lactobacillus reuteri*
NT1 *Lactobacillus rhamnosus*
NT1 *Lactobacillus sakei*
NT1 *Lactobacillus salivarius*
NT1 *Lactobacillus sanfranciscensis*
NT1 *Lactobacillus viridescens*
RT Bavaricins
RT Hiochi bacteria
RT Lactacins
RT Lactic acid bacteria
RT Lactobacillaceae
RT Lactocins
RT Probiotic bacteria

Lactobacillus acidophilus
BT1 *Lactobacillus*
BT2 Bacteria
BT3 Microorganisms
RT Acidocins

Lactobacillus alimentarius
BT1 *Lactobacillus*
BT2 Bacteria
BT3 Microorganisms

Lactobacillus amylophilus
HN introduced from vol. 39, issue 1 (2007)
BT1 *Lactobacillus*
BT2 Bacteria
BT3 Microorganisms

Lactobacillus amylovorus
BT1 *Lactobacillus*
BT2 Bacteria
BT3 Microorganisms
RT Amylovorins

Lactobacillus brevis
BT1 *Lactobacillus*
BT2 Bacteria
BT3 Microorganisms

Lactobacillus buchneri
BT1 *Lactobacillus*
BT2 Bacteria
BT3 Microorganisms

Lactobacillus bulgaricus
SN current name is Lactobacillus delbrueckii subsp. bulgaricus
BT1 *Lactobacillus delbrueckii*
BT2 *Lactobacillus*
BT3 Bacteria
BT4 Microorganisms

Lactobacillus casei
BT1 *Lactobacillus*
BT2 Bacteria
BT3 Microorganisms

Lactobacillus collinoides
HN introduced from vol. 39, issue 1 (2007)
BT1 *Lactobacillus*
BT2 Bacteria
BT3 Microorganisms

Lactobacillus crispatus
BT1 *Lactobacillus*
BT2 Bacteria
BT3 Microorganisms

Lactobacillus curvatus
BT1 *Lactobacillus*

BT2 Bacteria
BT3 Microorganisms

Lactobacillus delbrueckii
BT1 *Lactobacillus*
BT2 Bacteria
BT3 Microorganisms
NT1 *Lactobacillus bulgaricus*
NT1 *Lactobacillus lactis*

Lactobacillus fermentum
BT1 *Lactobacillus*
BT2 Bacteria
BT3 Microorganisms

Lactobacillus fructivorans
BT1 *Lactobacillus*
BT2 Bacteria
BT3 Microorganisms

Lactobacillus gasseri
BT1 *Lactobacillus*
BT2 Bacteria
BT3 Microorganisms
RT Gassericins

Lactobacillus helveticus
BT1 *Lactobacillus*
BT2 Bacteria
BT3 Microorganisms

Lactobacillus hilgardii
BT1 *Lactobacillus*
BT2 Bacteria
BT3 Microorganisms

Lactobacillus johnsonii
BT1 *Lactobacillus*
BT2 Bacteria
BT3 Microorganisms

Lactobacillus kefiranofaciens
BT1 *Lactobacillus*
BT2 Bacteria
BT3 Microorganisms
RT Kefiran

Lactobacillus kefiri
HN introduced from vol. 39, issue 1 (2007)
SN synonymous with Lactobacillus kefir
BT1 *Lactobacillus*
BT2 Bacteria
BT3 Microorganisms

Lactobacillus lactis
SN current name is Lactobacillus delbrueckii subsp. lactis
BT1 *Lactobacillus delbrueckii*
BT2 *Lactobacillus*
BT3 Bacteria
BT4 Microorganisms

Lactobacillus leichmannii
BT1 *Lactobacillus*
BT2 Bacteria
BT3 Microorganisms

Lactobacillus lindneri
HN introduced from vol. 41, issue 1 (2009)
BT1 *Lactobacillus*
BT2 Bacteria
BT3 Microorganisms

Lactobacillus paracasei
BT1 *Lactobacillus*
BT2 Bacteria
BT3 Microorganisms

Lactobacillus paraplantarum
BT1 *Lactobacillus*
BT2 Bacteria
BT3 Microorganisms

Lactobacillus pentosus
BT1 *Lactobacillus*
BT2 Bacteria
BT3 Microorganisms

Lactobacillus plantarum
BT1 *Lactobacillus*
BT2 Bacteria
BT3 Microorganisms
RT Plantaricins

Lactobacillus pontis
BT1 *Lactobacillus*
BT2 Bacteria
BT3 Microorganisms

Lactobacillus reuteri
BT1 *Lactobacillus*
BT2 Bacteria
BT3 Microorganisms

Lactobacillus rhamnosus
BT1 *Lactobacillus*
BT2 Bacteria
BT3 Microorganisms

Lactobacillus sake
USE ***Lactobacillus sakei***

Lactobacillus sakei
SN formerly Lactobacillus sake
BT1 *Lactobacillus*
BT2 Bacteria
BT3 Microorganisms
RT Sakacins
UF *Lactobacillus sake*

Lactobacillus salivarius
BT1 *Lactobacillus*
BT2 Bacteria
BT3 Microorganisms

Lactobacillus sanfranciscensis
BT1 *Lactobacillus*
BT2 Bacteria
BT3 Microorganisms

Lactobacillus viridescens
SN synonymous with Weissella viridescens
BT1 *Lactobacillus*
BT2 Bacteria
BT3 Microorganisms

Lactobionic acid
HN introduced from vol. 39, issue 1 (2007)
BT1 Organic acids
BT2 Acids
RT Lactose

Lactocins
BT1 Bacteriocins
BT2 Antibiotics
BT3 Drugs
BT4 Residues
RT *Lactobacillus*

Lactococcins
BT1 Bacteriocins
BT2 Antibiotics
BT3 Drugs
BT4 Residues
RT *Lactococcus*

Lactococcus
HN heading from vol. 25 (1993); under Streptococcus up to vol. 24 (1992)
BT1 Bacteria
BT2 Microorganisms
NT1 *Lactococcus lactis*
NT1 *Lactococcus raffinolactis*
RT Lactic acid bacteria
RT Lactococcins
RT *Streptococcus*

Lactococcus lactis
BT1 *Lactococcus*
BT2 Bacteria
BT3 Microorganisms
RT Lacticins
RT Lantibiotics
RT Nisin

Lactococcus raffinolactis
HN introduced from vol. 39, issue 1 (2007)
BT1 *Lactococcus*
BT2 Bacteria
BT3 Microorganisms

Lactoferricin
HN introduced from vol. 41, issue 1 (2009)
BT1 Peptides
BT2 Proteins
BT3 Nutrients
RT Lactoferrin

Lactoferrin
BT1 Animal proteins
BT2 Proteins animal
BT3 Proteins
BT4 Nutrients
BT1 Globulins
BT2 Proteins
BT3 Nutrients
RT Lactoferricin
RT Milk proteins

β-Lactoglobulin
BT1 Lactoglobulins
BT2 Globulins
BT3 Proteins
BT4 Nutrients
BT2 Milk proteins
BT3 Proteins milk
BT4 Animal proteins
BT5 Proteins animal

BT6 Proteins
BT7 Nutrients

Lactoglobulins
BT1 Globulins
BT2 Proteins
BT3 Nutrients
BT1 Milk proteins
BT2 Proteins milk
BT3 Animal proteins
BT4 Proteins animal
BT5 Proteins
BT6 Nutrients
NT1 β-Lactoglobulin

Lactones
BT1 Esters
BT2 Organic compounds
BT1 Heterocyclic compounds
NT1 Coumarins
NT2 Coumarin
NT2 Coumestrol
NT2 Esculetin
NT2 Furocoumarins
NT3 Bergapten
NT3 Psoralens
NT3 Xanthotoxin
NT2 Scopoletin
NT1 γ-Decalactone
NT1 Glucono-δ-lactone
RT Aroma compounds

Lactoperoxidase systems
BT1 Peroxidases
BT2 Oxidoreductases
BT3 Enzymes

Lactose
BT1 Disaccharides
BT2 Sugars
BT3 Carbohydrates
BT4 Nutrients
BT4 Organic compounds
BT3 Plant foods
BT4 Foods
NT1 Lactose low foods
RT Dairy products
RT Lactobionic acid

Lactose intolerance
BT1 Food intolerance
BT2 Intolerance
BT3 Diseases

Lactose low foods
HN introduced from vol. 41, issue 1 (2009)
BT1 Lactose
BT2 Disaccharides
BT3 Sugars
BT4 Carbohydrates
BT5 Nutrients
BT5 Organic compounds
BT4 Plant foods
BT5 Foods
UF Low lactose foods

Lactose synthases
SN EC 2.4.1.22
BT1 Glycosyltransferases
BT2 Transferases
BT3 Enzymes
UF *N*-Acetyllactosamine synthases

Lactose syrups
BT1 Sugar syrups
BT2 Plant foods
BT3 Foods

Lactosucrose
HN under Sugars up to vol. 42 (2010)
BT1 Oligosaccharides
BT2 Polysaccharides
BT3 Carbohydrates
BT4 Nutrients
BT4 Organic compounds
BT2 Sugars
BT3 Carbohydrates
BT4 Nutrients
BT4 Organic compounds
BT3 Plant foods
BT4 Foods

Lactulose
HN under Sugars up to vol. 42 (2010)
BT1 Disaccharides
BT2 Sugars
BT3 Carbohydrates
BT4 Nutrients
BT4 Organic compounds
BT3 Plant foods
BT4 Foods

Lactylates
BT1 Emulsifiers
BT2 Additives
NT1 Stearoyl lactylates

Laevulose
USE **Fructose**

Lager
BT1 Beer
BT2 Alcoholic beverages
BT3 Beverages alcoholic
BT4 Beverages

Lagerstroemia speciosa
BT1 Banaba
BT2 Plants

Lairage
HN introduced from vol. 39, issue 1 (2007)
BT1 Housing
BT2 Agriculture
BT1 Slaughter
RT Slaughterhouses

Lake water
BT1 Water

Lamb
BT1 Meat specific
BT2 Meat
BT3 Animal foods
BT4 Foods
NT1 Lamb carcasses
NT1 Lamb chops
NT1 Lamb mince
RT Lambs
RT Mutton

Lambanog
BT1 Spirits
BT2 Alcoholic beverages
BT3 Beverages alcoholic
BT4 Beverages

Lamb carcasses
BT1 Carcasses
BT2 Meat
BT3 Animal foods
BT4 Foods
BT1 Lamb
BT2 Meat specific
BT3 Meat
BT4 Animal foods
BT5 Foods

Lamb chops
BT1 Lamb
BT2 Meat specific
BT3 Meat
BT4 Animal foods
BT5 Foods

Lambic
BT1 Beer
BT2 Alcoholic beverages
BT3 Beverages alcoholic
BT4 Beverages

Lamb kidneys
BT1 Kidneys
BT2 Offal
BT3 Animal foods
BT4 Foods
BT1 Lambs
BT2 Animals

Lamb livers
HN introduced from vol. 39, issue 1 (2007)
BT1 Lambs
BT2 Animals
BT1 Livers
BT2 Offal
BT3 Animal foods
BT4 Foods

Lamb mince
BT1 Lamb
BT2 Meat specific
BT3 Meat
BT4 Animal foods
BT5 Foods

Lambs
HN introduced from vol. 39, issue 1 (2007); heading
BT1 Animals
NT1 Lamb kidneys
NT1 Lamb livers
RT Lamb
RT Sheep

Lamb sausages
BT1 Sausages
BT2 Meat products

BT3 Animal foods
BT4 Foods

Laminaria
BT1 Seaweeds
BT2 Algae
BT3 Microorganisms
BT2 Sea foods
BT3 Aquatic foods
BT4 Animal foods
BT5 Foods
NT1 Kombu
RT Laminarin
UF Kelp
UF Tangle

Laminarin
BT1 Glucans
BT2 Polysaccharides
BT3 Carbohydrates
BT4 Nutrients
BT4 Organic compounds
RT *Laminaria*

Laminarinases
USE **Endo-1,3(4)-β-glucanases**
USE **Glucan endo-1,3-β-D-glucosidases**

Laminates
BT1 Packaging materials

LAMP
HN introduced from vol. 43, issue 1 (2011)
BT1 Genetic techniques
BT2 Genetics
UF Loop-mediated isothermal amplification

Lamprey
BT1 Fish
BT2 Animals
BT2 Sea foods
BT3 Aquatic foods
BT4 Animal foods
BT5 Foods

Land snails
BT1 Snails
BT2 Gastropods
BT3 Molluscs
BT4 Shellfish
BT5 Animals
BT5 Sea foods
BT6 Aquatic foods
BT7 Animal foods
BT8 Foods

Langoustines
BT1 Norway lobsters
BT2 Crustacea
BT3 Shellfish
BT4 Animals
BT4 Sea foods
BT5 Aquatic foods
BT6 Animal foods
BT7 Foods

Langsat
BT1 Fruits specific
BT2 Fruits
BT3 Crops
BT4 Plants
BT3 Plant foods
BT4 Foods
UF Lanzones

Lannate
USE **Methomyl**

Lanternfish
BT1 Marine fish
BT2 Fish
BT3 Animals
BT3 Sea foods
BT4 Aquatic foods
BT5 Animal foods
BT6 Foods

Lanthanides
HN under Minerals up to vol. 42 (2010)
BT1 Metals
BT2 Elements
BT3 Minerals
BT4 Nutrients
NT1 La
NT1 Yb

Lanthanum
USE **La**

Lanthionine
BT1 Amino acids
BT2 Nutrients
BT2 Organic acids
BT3 Acids
BT2 Organic nitrogen compounds
BT1 Organic sulfur compounds

Lantibiotics
BT1 Bacteriocins
BT2 Antibiotics
BT3 Drugs
BT4 Residues
RT Lacticins
RT *Lactococcus lactis*
RT Nisin

Lanzones
USE **Langsat**

Lao-chao
BT1 Fermented foods
BT2 Processed foods
BT3 Foods
BT1 Rice
BT2 Cereals
BT3 Crops
BT4 Plants
BT3 Seeds
BT4 Plant foods
BT5 Foods

Laos
SN conventional long form of the name is Lao People's Democratic Republic
BT1 Asia

Lard
BT1 Animal fats
BT2 Fats animal
BT3 Animal foods
BT4 Foods
BT3 Fats
BT4 Lipids
BT5 Nutrients

Lasagne
BT1 Pasta
BT2 Cereal products
BT3 Plant foods
BT4 Foods

Lasalocids
BT1 Antibiotics
BT2 Drugs
BT3 Residues
BT1 Coccidiostats
BT2 Drugs
BT3 Residues

La Serena cheese
BT1 Cheese varieties
BT2 Cheese
BT3 Dairy products
BT4 Animal foods
BT5 Foods

Laser light scattering
HN introduced from vol. 39, issue 1 (2007)
SN includes dynamic light scattering and multiple angle laser light scattering (MALLS)
BT1 Analytical techniques

Lasers
HN introduced from vol. 39, issue 1 (2007)
BT1 Apparatus
BT2 Technology
BT1 Equipment
BT2 Technology

Lassi
BT1 Fermented milk
BT2 Fermented dairy products
BT3 Dairy products
BT4 Animal foods
BT5 Foods
BT3 Fermented foods
BT4 Processed foods
BT5 Foods
BT2 Milk
BT3 Dairy products
BT4 Animal foods
BT5 Foods

Latex
HN introduced from vol. 39, issue 1 (2007)
BT1 Biopolymers
RT Rubber

Lathyrogens
BT1 Toxins
BT2 Residues

Lathyrus maritimus
BT1 Beach peas
BT2 Legumes
BT3 Vegetables specific
BT4 Vegetables
BT5 Crops
BT6 Plants
BT5 Plant foods
BT6 Foods

Latin America
HN heading up to vol. 24 (1992)
BT1 America

Latvia
BT1 Europe
BT1 European Union

Laurel
HN under Spices up to vol. 42 (2010)
SN syn. bay
BT1 Bay
BT2 Herbs
BT3 Spices
BT4 Flavourings
BT5 Additives

Lauric acid
HN under Fatty acids up to vol. 42 (2010)
SN syn. dodecanoic acid
BT1 Dodecanoic acid
BT2 Aroma compounds
BT3 Flavour compounds
BT3 Volatile compounds
BT2 Saturated fatty acids
BT3 Fatty acids
BT4 Lipids
BT5 Nutrients
BT4 Organic acids
BT5 Acids

Lautering
BT1 Mashing
BT2 Processing
BT3 Technology
NT1 Lauter tuns

Lauter tuns
BT1 Equipment
BT2 Technology
BT1 Lautering
BT2 Mashing
BT3 Processing
BT4 Technology

Lavender
BT1 Plants

Laver
BT1 Seaweeds
BT2 Algae
BT3 Microorganisms
BT2 Sea foods
BT3 Aquatic foods
BT4 Animal foods
BT5 Foods
UF Laverbread

Laverbread
USE **Laver**

Laws
USE **Legislation**

Lben
USE **Leben**

LC
HN liquid chromatography used in the index up to vol. 35, issue 6 (2003)
BT1 High performance liquid chromatography
BT2 Chromatography
BT3 Analytical techniques
UF Liquid chromatography

LC-MS
HN introduced from vol. 39, issue 1 (2007)
BT1 High performance liquid chromatography
BT2 Chromatography
BT3 Analytical techniques
BT1 Mass spectroscopy
BT2 Spectroscopy
BT3 Analytical techniques

LDPE
BT1 Polyethylene
BT2 Plastics
BT3 Packaging materials
UF Low density polyethylene

Lead
SN symbol Pb is also used in the index
BT1 Metals
BT2 Elements
BT3 Minerals
BT4 Nutrients
NT1 Pb

Leaf beet
SN syn. swiss chard
BT1 Swiss chard
BT2 Vegetables specific
BT3 Vegetables
BT4 Crops
BT5 Plants
BT4 Plant foods
BT5 Foods

Leaf proteins
BT1 Vegetable proteins
BT2 Proteins vegetable
BT3 Proteins
BT4 Nutrients
BT3 Vegetable products
BT4 Plant foods
BT5 Foods

Leaf vegetables
HN used up to vol. 39 (2007)
USE **Leafy vegetables**

Leafy vegetables
BT1 Vegetables specific
BT2 Vegetables
BT3 Crops
BT4 Plants
BT3 Plant foods
BT4 Foods
UF Leaf vegetables

Lean
RT Meat

Leavening
BT1 Fermentation

Leaves
HN introduced from vol. 39, issue 1 (2007)
BT1 Plants

Leban
USE **Leben**

Lebanon
BT1 Asia
BT1 Middle East

Lebaycid
USE **Fenthion**

Leben
BT1 Fermented milk
BT2 Fermented dairy products
BT3 Dairy products
BT4 Animal foods
BT5 Foods
BT3 Fermented foods
BT4 Processed foods
BT5 Foods
BT2 Milk
BT3 Dairy products
BT4 Animal foods
BT5 Foods
UF Laban
UF Labban
UF Lben
UF Leban

Leccinum
HN introduced from vol. 39, issue 1 (2007)
BT1 Edible fungi
BT2 Fungi edible
BT3 Vegetables specific
BT4 Vegetables
BT5 Crops
BT6 Plants
BT5 Plant foods
BT6 Foods

Lecithinases
SN term used in non-preferred names for 3 phospholipases and lysophospholipase
BT1 Lipases
BT2 Esterases
BT3 Hydrolases
BT4 Enzymes

Lecithins
BT1 Emulsifiers
BT2 Additives
BT1 Phospholipids
BT2 Lipids
BT3 Nutrients
NT1 Lysolecithin
NT1 Soy lecithins
UF Phosphatidylcholine

Lectins
HN heading from vol. 25 (1993); under Agglutinins up to vol. 24 (1992)
- BT1 Glycoproteins
  - BT2 Proteins
    - BT3 Nutrients
- BT1 Vegetable proteins
  - BT2 Proteins vegetable
    - BT3 Proteins
      - BT4 Nutrients
    - BT3 Vegetable products
      - BT4 Plant foods
        - BT5 Foods
- NT1 Concanavalin A
- NT1 Haemagglutinins
- NT1 Phytohaemagglutinins
- NT1 Ricin
- UF Agglutinins

Leeks
- BT1 Vegetables specific
  - BT2 Vegetables
    - BT3 Crops
      - BT4 Plants
    - BT3 Plant foods
      - BT4 Foods

Lees
- BT1 By-products

Legionella
- BT1 Bacteria
  - BT2 Microorganisms
- NT1 *Legionella pneumophila*
- RT Legionellosis

Legionella pneumophila
HN introduced from vol. 39, issue 1 (2007)
- BT1 *Legionella*
  - BT2 Bacteria
    - BT3 Microorganisms

Legionellosis
- BT1 Diseases
- BT1 Poisoning
- RT *Legionella*
- UF Legionnaires disease

Legionnaires disease
- USE **Legionellosis**

Legislation
- RT Regulations
- RT Standards
- RT Tolerance
- UF Laws

Legume meal
- BT1 Flours
  - BT2 Plant foods
    - BT3 Foods
- BT1 Legumes
  - BT2 Vegetables specific
    - BT3 Vegetables
      - BT4 Crops
        - BT5 Plants
      - BT4 Plant foods
        - BT5 Foods

Legume proteins
- BT1 Legumes
  - BT2 Vegetables specific
    - BT3 Vegetables
      - BT4 Crops
        - BT5 Plants
      - BT4 Plant foods
        - BT5 Foods
- BT1 Vegetable proteins
  - BT2 Proteins vegetable
    - BT3 Proteins
      - BT4 Nutrients
    - BT3 Vegetable products
      - BT4 Plant foods
        - BT5 Foods

Legumes
- BT1 Vegetables specific
  - BT2 Vegetables
    - BT3 Crops
      - BT4 Plants
    - BT3 Plant foods
      - BT4 Foods
- NT1 Adzuki beans
- NT1 African oil beans
  - NT2 Ugba
- NT1 African yam beans
- NT1 Alfalfa
  - NT2 Alfalfa seeds
  - NT2 Lucerne
  - NT2 *Medicago sativa*
- NT1 American groundnuts
- NT1 Asparagus beans
- NT1 Asparagus peas
- NT1 Bambara groundnuts
- NT1 Beach peas
  - NT2 *Lathyrus maritimus*
- NT1 Beans
  - NT2 Bean curd
  - NT2 Bean pastes
- NT1 Black gram
  - NT2 Dosai
- NT1 Carob beans
- NT1 Carob pods
- NT1 *Cassia* seeds
- NT1 Chick peas
  - NT2 Bengal gram
    - NT3 Boondi
  - NT2 Humous
- NT1 Common beans
  - NT2 Anasazi
  - NT2 Black beans
  - NT2 Dry beans
  - NT2 French beans
  - NT2 Green beans
  - NT2 Haricot beans
    - NT3 Baked beans
  - NT2 Kidney beans
  - NT2 Navy beans
  - NT2 Pea beans
  - NT2 Pinto beans
  - NT2 Pole beans
  - NT2 Snap beans
  - NT2 String beans
  - NT2 Wax beans
  - NT2 White beans
- NT1 Cowpeas
  - NT2 Akara
  - NT2 Blackeyed peas
  - NT2 Cowpea meal
  - NT2 Moinmoin
  - NT2 Southern peas
- NT1 *Detarium microcarpum*
- NT1 Dhal
- NT1 Dhokla
- NT1 Djenkol beans
- NT1 Faba beans
  - NT2 Broad beans
  - NT2 Field beans
  - NT2 Horse beans
- NT1 Grass peas
- NT1 Groundbeans
- NT1 Guar beans
  - NT2 Cluster beans
- NT1 Horse gram
- NT1 Idli
- NT1 Jack beans
  - NT2 *Canavalia ensiformis*
- NT1 Kawal
- NT1 Koji
  - NT2 Rice koji
- NT1 Lablab beans
- NT1 Legume meal
- NT1 Legume proteins
- NT1 Legume sprouts
  - NT2 Alfalfa sprouts
  - NT2 Bean sprouts
  - NT2 Soybean sprouts
- NT1 Legume starch
- NT1 Lentils
- NT1 *Leucaena*
- NT1 Lima beans
- NT1 Lupins
  - NT2 Lupin proteins
  - NT2 White lupins
- NT1 Mesquite pods
- NT1 Moth beans
- NT1 Mung beans
  - NT2 Mung bean starch
- NT1 Peas
  - NT2 Dried peas
  - NT2 Field peas
  - NT2 Green peas
  - NT2 Pea meal
  - NT2 Pea protein concentrates
  - NT2 Pea proteins
  - NT2 Pea starch
  - NT2 Snow peas
- NT1 Pigeon peas
- NT1 Pulses
- NT1 Red beans
- NT1 Rice beans
- NT1 Runner beans
- NT1 Siljo
- NT1 Soybeans
  - NT2 Black soybeans
  - NT2 Soybean sprouts
- NT1 Sword beans
  - NT2 *Canavalia gladiata*
- NT1 Tepary beans
- NT1 Velvet beans
- NT1 Vetch seeds
- NT1 Winged beans
- NT1 Yam beans
  - NT2 *Pachyrhizus ahipa*
- UF Grams

Legume sprouts
BT1 Legumes
BT2 Vegetables specific
BT3 Vegetables
BT4 Crops
BT5 Plants
BT4 Plant foods
BT5 Foods
BT1 Sprouts
BT2 Vegetables specific
BT3 Vegetables
BT4 Crops
BT5 Plants
BT4 Plant foods
BT5 Foods
NT1 Alfalfa sprouts
NT1 Bean sprouts
NT1 Soybean sprouts

Legume starch
HN introduced from vol. 41, issue 1 (2009)
BT1 Legumes
BT2 Vegetables specific
BT3 Vegetables
BT4 Crops
BT5 Plants
BT4 Plant foods
BT5 Foods
BT1 Starch
BT2 Glucans
BT3 Polysaccharides
BT4 Carbohydrates
BT5 Nutrients
BT5 Organic compounds
BT2 Thickeners
BT3 Additives

Legumin
BT1 Globulins
BT2 Proteins
BT3 Nutrients
BT1 Vegetable proteins
BT2 Proteins vegetable
BT3 Proteins
BT4 Nutrients
BT3 Vegetable products
BT4 Plant foods
BT5 Foods

Legurame
USE **Carbetamide**

Lemonade
BT1 Soft drinks
BT2 Beverages

Lemon balm
HN under Spices up to vol. 42 (2010)
BT1 Herbs
BT2 Spices
BT3 Flavourings
BT4 Additives

Lemon essential oils
BT1 Citrus essential oils
BT2 Essential oils
BT3 Flavourings
BT4 Additives
BT3 Vegetable oils
BT4 Oils vegetable
BT5 Oils
BT6 Lipids
BT7 Nutrients
BT5 Vegetable products
BT6 Plant foods
BT7 Foods
RT Lemons

Lemon grass
HN used up to vol. 39 (2007)
USE **Lemongrass**

Lemongrass
HN under Spices up to vol. 42 (2010)
BT1 Herbs
BT2 Spices
BT3 Flavourings
BT4 Additives
RT Lemongrass oils
UF Lemon grass

Lemon grass oils
HN used up to vol. 39 (2007)
USE **Lemongrass oils**

Lemongrass oils
BT1 Essential oils
BT2 Flavourings
BT3 Additives
BT2 Vegetable oils
BT3 Oils vegetable
BT4 Oils
BT5 Lipids
BT6 Nutrients
BT4 Vegetable products
BT5 Plant foods
BT6 Foods
RT Lemongrass
UF Lemon grass oils

Lemon juices
BT1 Citrus juices
BT2 Fruit juices
BT3 Fruit products
BT4 Plant foods
BT5 Foods
BT3 Soft drinks
BT4 Beverages

Lemon peel
BT1 Lemons
BT2 Citrus fruits
BT3 Fruits specific
BT4 Fruits
BT5 Crops
BT6 Plants
BT5 Plant foods
BT6 Foods
BT1 Peel
RT Fruit peel

Lemons
BT1 Citrus fruits
BT2 Fruits specific
BT3 Fruits
BT4 Crops
BT5 Plants
BT4 Plant foods
BT5 Foods
NT1 Lemon peel
RT Galgals
RT Lemon essential oils

Lemon tea
BT1 Tea beverages
BT2 Teas
BT3 Beverages
BT3 Crops
BT4 Plants
BT3 Plant foods
BT4 Foods

Lenacil
BT1 Herbicides
BT2 Pesticides
BT3 Biocides
BT3 Residues

Lenthionine
BT1 Aroma compounds
BT2 Flavour compounds
BT2 Volatile compounds
BT1 Heterocyclic compounds
BT1 Organic sulfur compounds

Lentils
HN heading from vol. 30 (1998); under Legumes up to vol. 29 (1997)
BT1 Legumes
BT2 Vegetables specific
BT3 Vegetables
BT4 Crops
BT5 Plants
BT4 Plant foods
BT5 Foods

Lentinula edodes
SN formerly called Lentinus edodes
BT1 Edible fungi
BT2 Fungi edible
BT3 Vegetables specific
BT4 Vegetables
BT5 Crops
BT6 Plants
BT5 Plant foods
BT6 Foods
UF *Lentinus edodes*
UF Shiitake

Lentinus
HN heading from vol. 30 (1998); under Fungi edible up to vol. 29 (1997)
BT1 Edible fungi
BT2 Fungi edible
BT3 Vegetables specific
BT4 Vegetables
BT5 Crops
BT6 Plants
BT5 Plant foods
BT6 Foods

Lentinus edodes
SN former name given to Lentinula edodes
USE ***Lentinula edodes***

Lentivirus
HN introduced from vol. 43, issue 1 (2011)
BT1 Viruses
BT2 Microorganisms

NT1 Bovine immunodeficiency virus
NT1 Human immunodeficiency virus

Lepidorhombus boscii
BT1 Megrim
BT2 Flatfish
BT3 Marine fish
BT4 Fish
BT5 Animals
BT5 Sea foods
BT6 Aquatic foods
BT7 Animal foods
BT8 Foods

Lepista
HN introduced from vol. 39, issue 1 (2007)
BT1 Edible fungi
BT2 Fungi edible
BT3 Vegetables specific
BT4 Vegetables
BT5 Crops
BT6 Plants
BT5 Plant foods
BT6 Foods
NT1 *Lepista nuda*

Lepista nuda
HN introduced from vol. 39, issue 1 (2007)
BT1 *Lepista*
BT2 Edible fungi
BT3 Fungi edible
BT4 Vegetables specific
BT5 Vegetables
BT6 Crops
BT7 Plants
BT6 Plant foods
BT7 Foods

Leptin
HN introduced from vol. 39, issue 1 (2007)
BT1 Hormones
BT2 Residues

Leptophos
BT1 Organophosphorus insecticides
BT2 Insecticides
BT3 Pesticides
BT4 Biocides
BT4 Residues
BT2 Organophosphorus pesticides
BT3 Pesticides
BT4 Biocides
BT4 Residues
UF Phosvel

Leptospira
BT1 Bacteria
BT2 Microorganisms
RT Leptospirosis
RT Parasites

Leptospirosis
BT1 Diseases
BT1 Poisoning
RT *Leptospira*

Lesotho
BT1 Southern Africa
BT2 Africa

Lethrinus lentjan
BT1 Redspot emperor
BT2 Marine fish
BT3 Fish
BT4 Animals
BT4 Sea foods
BT5 Aquatic foods
BT6 Animal foods
BT7 Foods

Lettuces
HN heading from vol. 25 (1993); under Vegetables specific up to vol. 24 (1992)
BT1 Vegetables specific
BT2 Vegetables
BT3 Crops
BT4 Plants
BT3 Plant foods
BT4 Foods

Leucaena
BT1 Legumes
BT2 Vegetables specific
BT3 Vegetables
BT4 Crops
BT5 Plants
BT4 Plant foods
BT5 Foods
BT1 Plants

Leucine
BT1 Amino acids
BT2 Nutrients
BT2 Organic acids
BT3 Acids
BT2 Organic nitrogen compounds

Leuciscus cephalus
BT1 Chub
BT2 Freshwater fish
BT3 Fish
BT4 Animals
BT4 Sea foods
BT5 Aquatic foods
BT6 Animal foods
BT7 Foods

Leucoanthocyanidins
BT1 Anthocyanidins
BT2 Flavonoids
BT3 Aromatic compounds
BT4 Organic compounds
BT3 Pigments
NT1 Leucocyanidin

Leucoanthocyanins
BT1 Anthocyanins
BT2 Flavonoids
BT3 Aromatic compounds
BT4 Organic compounds
BT3 Pigments
NT1 Anthocyanogens

Leucocins
HN introduced from vol. 39, issue 1 (2007)
BT1 Bacteriocins
BT2 Antibiotics
BT3 Drugs
BT4 Residues
RT *Leuconostoc*

Leucocyanidin
BT1 Leucoanthocyanidins
BT2 Anthocyanidins
BT3 Flavonoids
BT4 Aromatic compounds
BT5 Organic compounds
BT4 Pigments

Leucocytes
USE **Leukocytes**

Leuconostoc
HN heading from vol. 25 (1993); under Lactobacillaceae up to vol. 24 (1992)
BT1 Bacteria
BT2 Microorganisms
NT1 *Leuconostoc carnosum*
NT1 *Leuconostoc citreum*
NT1 *Leuconostoc mesenteroides*
NT1 *Leuconostoc oenos*
RT Lactic acid bacteria
RT Leucocins
UF *Betacoccus*

Leuconostoc carnosum
BT1 *Leuconostoc*
BT2 Bacteria
BT3 Microorganisms

Leuconostoc citreum
BT1 *Leuconostoc*
BT2 Bacteria
BT3 Microorganisms

Leuconostoc mesenteroides
BT1 *Leuconostoc*
BT2 Bacteria
BT3 Microorganisms
RT Mesentericins

Leuconostoc oenos
SN synonymous with Oenococcus oeni
BT1 *Leuconostoc*
BT2 Bacteria
BT3 Microorganisms

Leukocytes
BT1 Cells
UF Leucocytes

Levamisoles
BT1 Anthelmintics
BT2 Drugs
BT3 Residues

Levanases
SN EC 3.2.1.65
BT1 Glycosidases
BT2 Hydrolases
BT3 Enzymes

Levans
BT1 Fructans
BT2 Polysaccharides
BT3 Carbohydrates
BT4 Nutrients
BT4 Organic compounds

Levansucrases
SN EC 2.4.1.10
BT1 Glycosyltransferases
BT2 Transferases
BT3 Enzymes

Li
HN under Minerals up to vol. 42 (2010)
BT1 Metals
BT2 Elements
BT3 Minerals
BT4 Nutrients
UF Lithium

Liberia
BT1 West Africa
BT2 Africa

Libya
SN full name is Great Socialist People's Libyan Arab Jamahiriya
BT1 North Africa
BT2 Africa

Lichenases
USE **Licheninases**

Licheninases
SN EC 3.2.1.73
BT1 Glycosidases
BT2 Hydrolases
BT3 Enzymes
UF Lichenases

Lichens
BT1 Plants

Lids
BT1 Closures
BT2 Packaging
BT3 Technology

Liechtenstein
BT1 Europe

Life cycle assessment
BT1 Ecology
BT2 Science

Ligases
HN heading from vol. 25 (1993); under Enzymes up to vol. 24 (1992)
SN EC 6
BT1 Enzymes
NT1 Acetyl-CoA carboxylases
NT1 Pyruvate carboxylases

Light
BT1 Radiation
NT1 Fluorescent light
NT1 Sunlight

Lignans
BT1 Phenols
BT2 Alcohols
BT2 Aromatic compounds
BT3 Organic compounds
NT1 Sesamin
NT1 Sesamolin
RT Polyphenols

Lignin
BT1 Biopolymers
NT1 Lignocelluloses
RT Celluloses
RT Fibre

Ligninases
BT1 Peroxidases
BT2 Oxidoreductases
BT3 Enzymes

Lignin peroxidases
BT1 Peroxidases
BT2 Oxidoreductases
BT3 Enzymes

Lignocelluloses
BT1 Celluloses
BT2 Glucans
BT3 Polysaccharides
BT4 Carbohydrates
BT5 Nutrients
BT5 Organic compounds
BT1 Lignin
BT2 Biopolymers

Lignoceric acid
HN introduced from vol. 39, issue 1 (2007)
BT1 Saturated fatty acids
BT2 Fatty acids
BT3 Lipids
BT4 Nutrients
BT3 Organic acids
BT4 Acids

Lily bulbs
HN introduced from vol. 39, issue 1 (2007)
SN belonging to the genus Lilium
BT1 Vegetables specific
BT2 Vegetables
BT3 Crops
BT4 Plants
BT3 Plant foods
BT4 Foods

Lima beans
BT1 Legumes
BT2 Vegetables specific
BT3 Vegetables
BT4 Crops
BT5 Plants
BT4 Plant foods
BT5 Foods
UF Butter beans
UF Sieva beans

Limburg cheese
BT1 Cheese varieties
BT2 Cheese
BT3 Dairy products
BT4 Animal foods
BT5 Foods

Lime essential oils
BT1 Citrus essential oils
BT2 Essential oils
BT3 Flavourings
BT4 Additives
BT3 Vegetable oils
BT4 Oils vegetable
BT5 Oils
BT6 Lipids
BT7 Nutrients
BT5 Vegetable products
BT6 Plant foods
BT7 Foods
RT Limes

Lime juices
BT1 Citrus juices
BT2 Fruit juices
BT3 Fruit products
BT4 Plant foods
BT5 Foods
BT3 Soft drinks
BT4 Beverages

Limes
BT1 Citrus fruits
BT2 Fruits specific
BT3 Fruits
BT4 Crops
BT5 Plants
BT4 Plant foods
BT5 Foods
RT Lime essential oils

Liming
BT1 Sugar processes
BT2 Processing
BT3 Technology

Limit dextrinases
SN EC 3.2.1.142
BT1 Glycosidases
BT2 Hydrolases
BT3 Enzymes

Limoncello
BT1 Fruit liqueurs
BT2 Liqueurs
BT3 Alcoholic beverages
BT4 Beverages alcoholic
BT5 Beverages

Limonene
BT1 Aroma compounds
BT2 Flavour compounds
BT2 Volatile compounds
BT1 Monoterpenes
BT2 Hydrocarbons
BT3 Organic compounds
BT2 Monoterpenoids
BT3 Terpenoids
BT4 Lipids
BT5 Nutrients

Limonin
HN under Lactones up to vol. 42 (2010)
BT1 Limonoids
BT2 Bitter compounds
BT3 Flavour compounds
BT2 Triterpenoids

BT3 Terpenoids
BT4 Lipids
BT5 Nutrients

Limonoid glucosides
BT1 Glucosides
BT2 Glycosides
BT3 Carbohydrates
BT4 Nutrients
BT4 Organic compounds
BT1 Limonoids
BT2 Bitter compounds
BT3 Flavour compounds
BT2 Triterpenoids
BT3 Terpenoids
BT4 Lipids
BT5 Nutrients

Limonoids
BT1 Bitter compounds
BT2 Flavour compounds
BT1 Triterpenoids
BT2 Terpenoids
BT3 Lipids
BT4 Nutrients
NT1 Limonin
NT1 Limonoid glucosides
NT1 Nomilin

Limpets
BT1 Gastropods
BT2 Molluscs
BT3 Shellfish
BT4 Animals
BT4 Sea foods
BT5 Aquatic foods
BT6 Animal foods
BT7 Foods

Linalool
BT1 Alcohols
BT1 Aroma compounds
BT2 Flavour compounds
BT2 Volatile compounds
BT1 Monoterpenoids
BT2 Terpenoids
BT3 Lipids
BT4 Nutrients

Linalyl acetate
HN also under Flavour compounds up to vol. 42 (2010)
BT1 Acetates
BT1 Aroma compounds
BT2 Flavour compounds
BT2 Volatile compounds
BT1 Esters
BT2 Organic compounds

Linamarases
USE **β-Glucosidases**

Linamarin
BT1 Glycosides
BT2 Carbohydrates
BT3 Nutrients
BT3 Organic compounds
RT Toxins

Lincomycin
BT1 Antibiotics
BT2 Drugs
BT3 Residues

Lindane
USE **HCH**

Ling
BT1 Marine fish
BT2 Fish
BT3 Animals
BT3 Sea foods
BT4 Aquatic foods
BT5 Animal foods
BT6 Foods
NT1 *Molva molva*

Ling cod
BT1 Marine fish
BT2 Fish
BT3 Animals
BT3 Sea foods
BT4 Aquatic foods
BT5 Animal foods
BT6 Foods
NT1 *Ophiodon elongatus*

Lingonberries
SN syn. cowberries
BT1 Berries
BT2 Fruits specific
BT3 Fruits
BT4 Crops
BT5 Plants
BT4 Plant foods
BT5 Foods
NT1 Cowberries

Linoleates
BT1 Fatty acid esters
BT2 Esters
BT3 Organic compounds
NT1 Methyl linoleate

Linoleic acid
BT1 ω-6 Fatty acids
BT2 PUFA
BT3 Unsaturated fatty acids
BT4 Fatty acids
BT5 Lipids
BT6 Nutrients
BT5 Organic acids
BT6 Acids
NT1 CLA
RT Essential fatty acids

Linolenic acid
BT1 PUFA
BT2 Unsaturated fatty acids
BT3 Fatty acids
BT4 Lipids
BT5 Nutrients
BT4 Organic acids
BT5 Acids
NT1 Eleostearic acid
NT1 α-Linolenic acid
NT1 γ-Linolenic acid

α-Linolenic acid
HN introduced from vol. 43, issue 1 (2011)
BT1 ω-3 Fatty acids
BT2 PUFA
BT3 Unsaturated fatty acids
BT4 Fatty acids
BT5 Lipids
BT6 Nutrients
BT5 Organic acids
BT6 Acids
BT1 Linolenic acid
BT2 PUFA
BT3 Unsaturated fatty acids
BT4 Fatty acids
BT5 Lipids
BT6 Nutrients
BT5 Organic acids
BT6 Acids
RT Essential fatty acids

γ-Linolenic acid
HN introduced from vol. 43, issue 1 (2011)
BT1 ω-6 Fatty acids
BT2 PUFA
BT3 Unsaturated fatty acids
BT4 Fatty acids
BT5 Lipids
BT6 Nutrients
BT5 Organic acids
BT6 Acids
BT1 Linolenic acid
BT2 PUFA
BT3 Unsaturated fatty acids
BT4 Fatty acids
BT5 Lipids
BT6 Nutrients
BT5 Organic acids
BT6 Acids

Linseed oils
BT1 Flax seed oils
BT2 Vegetable oils
BT3 Oils vegetable
BT4 Oils
BT5 Lipids
BT6 Nutrients
BT4 Vegetable products
BT5 Plant foods
BT6 Foods

Linseeds
BT1 Flax seeds
BT2 Oilseeds
BT3 Seeds
BT4 Plant foods
BT5 Foods

Linuron
BT1 Herbicides
BT2 Pesticides
BT3 Biocides
BT3 Residues
UF Afalon

Lipaemic activity
BT1 Human physiology
BT2 Physiology
BT3 Science
RT Hypolipaemic activity

Lipases
BT1 Esterases

BT2 Hydrolases
BT3 Enzymes
NT1 Lecithinases
NT1 Lipoprotein lipases
NT1 Lysophospholipases
NT1 Phospholipases
NT1 Triacylglycerol lipases
RT Lipolysis
UF Lipolytic enzymes

Lipids
BT1 Nutrients
NT1 Fats
NT2 Cooking fats
NT2 Fats animal
NT3 Animal fats
NT4 Adipose tissues
NT4 Backfat
NT4 Belly fat
NT4 Blubber
NT5 Seal blubber
NT4 Dripping
NT4 Fatness
NT4 Intramuscular fat
NT4 Lard
NT4 Marbling
NT4 Subcutaneous fat
NT4 Suet
NT4 Tallow
NT3 Fats milk
NT4 Milk fats
NT5 Anhydrous milk fats
NT5 Butterfat
NT5 Butter oils
NT5 Milk fat globule membranes
NT5 Milk fat globules
NT2 Fats high diet
NT2 Fats low diet
NT2 Fats low foods
NT3 Fats low spreads
NT2 Fat substitutes
NT3 Dairy-lo
NT3 Litesse
NT3 Microcrystalline celluloses
NT3 Oatrim
NT3 Raftiline
NT3 Salatrim
NT3 Simplesse
NT3 Sucrose polyesters
NT4 Olestra
NT3 Z-Trim
NT2 Fats vegetable
NT3 Vegetable fats
NT4 Borneo tallow
NT4 Cocoa butter
NT5 Cocoa butter equivalents
NT5 Cocoa butter extenders
NT5 Cocoa butter substitutes
NT4 Coconut butter
NT4 Illipe butter
NT4 Kokum
NT4 Sal fats
NT4 Shea nut butter
NT4 Vanaspati
NT2 Frying fats
NT2 Hydrogenated fats
NT2 Margarines
NT3 Halvarine
NT2 Polyunsaturated fats
NT2 Saturated fats
NT2 Shortenings
NT2 Unsaturated fats
NT1 Fatty acids
NT2 Branched chain fatty acids
NT3 Isobutyric acid
NT3 Isocaproic acid
NT3 Isovaleric acid
NT2 Cyclic fatty acids
NT2 Eicosanoids
NT3 Prostaglandins
NT2 Malvalic acid
NT2 Saturated fatty acids
NT3 Arachidic acid
NT3 Behenic acid
NT3 Butanoic acid
NT4 Butyric acid
NT3 Decanoic acid
NT4 Capric acid
NT3 Dodecanoic acid
NT4 Lauric acid
NT3 Heptadecanoic acid
NT4 Margaric acid
NT3 Heptanoic acid
NT3 Hexadecanoic acid
NT4 Palmitic acid
NT3 Hexanoic acid
NT4 Caproic acid
NT3 Lignoceric acid
NT3 Myristic acid
NT3 Octadecanoic acid
NT4 Stearic acid
NT5 Hydroxystearic acid
NT3 Octanoic acid
NT4 Caprylic acid
NT3 Pentanoic acid
NT4 Valeric acid
NT2 Sterculic acid
NT2 Unsaturated fatty acids
NT3 Essential fatty acids
NT3 Monounsaturated fatty acids
NT4 Decenoic acid
NT4 Docosenoic acid
NT5 Erucic acid
NT4 Eicosenoic acid
NT4 Hexadecenoic acid
NT5 Palmitoleic acid
NT4 Octadecenoic acid
NT5 Elaidic acid
NT5 Oleic acid
NT5 Petroselinic acid
NT5 Vaccenic acid
NT4 Ricinoleic acid
NT3 PUFA
NT4 Conjugated fatty acids
NT5 CLA
NT5 Eleostearic acid
NT4 Eicosatetraenoic acid
NT5 Arachidonic acid
NT4 ω-3 Fatty acids
NT5 Docosahexaenoic acid
NT5 Docosapentaenoic acid
NT5 Eicosapentaenoic acid
NT5 α-Linolenic acid
NT5 Stearidonic acid
NT4 ω-6 Fatty acids
NT5 Arachidonic acid
NT5 Linoleic acid
NT6 CLA
NT5 γ-Linolenic acid
NT4 Linolenic acid
NT5 Eleostearic acid
NT5 α-Linolenic acid
NT5 γ-Linolenic acid
NT3 *trans* Fatty acids
NT4 Elaidic acid
NT4 Vaccenic acid
NT2 Volatile fatty acids
NT3 Short chain fatty acids
NT4 Butanoic acid
NT5 Butyric acid
NT4 Hexanoic acid
NT5 Caproic acid
NT4 Hydroxybutyric acid
NT4 Isobutyric acid
NT4 Isocaproic acid
NT4 Isovaleric acid
NT4 Pentanoic acid
NT5 Valeric acid
NT1 Glycerides
NT2 Acylglycerols
NT2 Diglycerides
NT3 Diacylglycerols
NT2 Glycerol monostearate
NT2 Glyceryl monostearate
NT2 Monoglycerides
NT3 Monoacylglycerols
NT3 Monolaurin
NT2 Phosphoglycerides
NT2 Triglycerides
NT3 Olein
NT4 Palm olein
NT3 Stearin
NT4 Palm stearin
NT3 Triacetin
NT3 Triacylglycerols
NT3 Tricaprylin
NT3 Trilinolein
NT3 Triolein
NT3 Tripalmitin
NT3 Tristearin
NT1 Glycolipids
NT2 Cerebrosides
NT2 Galactolipids
NT2 Gangliosides
NT1 Lipopolysaccharides
NT1 Oils
NT2 Algal oils
NT2 Cooking oils
NT2 Frying oils
NT2 Marine oils
NT3 Oils fish
NT4 Fish oils
NT5 Anchovy oils
NT5 Cod liver oils
NT5 Fish liver oils
NT5 Menhaden oils
NT5 Salmon oils
NT5 Sardine oils
NT5 Tuna oils
NT3 Seal blubber oils
NT3 Seal oils
NT3 Squid oils
NT3 Whale oils
NT2 Mineral oils

NT2 Oils vegetable
NT3 Vegetable oils
NT4 Argemone oils
NT4 Avocado oils
NT4 Baobab oils
NT4 Borage oils
NT4 Camelina oils
NT4 Castor oils
NT4 Coffee oils
NT4 Corn oils
NT5 Corn fibre oils
NT4 Cottonseed oils
NT4 Essential oils
NT5 Bitter almond oils
NT5 Buchu oils
NT5 Cinnamon oils
NT5 Citronella essential oils
NT5 Citrus essential oils
NT6 Bergamot essential oils
NT7 Bergamot oils
NT6 Bitter orange essential oils
NT6 Citrus oils
NT6 Lemon essential oils
NT6 Lime essential oils
NT6 Neroli oils
NT6 Orange essential oils
NT5 Clary sage essential oils
NT5 Clove oils
NT5 Garlic oils
NT5 Hop essential oils
NT5 Lemongrass oils
NT5 Mint oils
NT5 Nutmeg oils
NT5 Oleoresins
NT5 Oregano oils
NT5 Peppermint essential oils
NT5 Petitgrain oils
NT5 Rosemary essential oils
NT5 Sage essential oils
NT5 Tea tree oils
NT5 Thyme oils
NT4 Evening primrose oils
NT4 Flax seed oils
NT5 Linseed oils
NT4 Grape seed oils
NT4 Jojoba oils
NT4 Kapok oils
NT4 Lupin seed oils
NT4 Meadowfoam oils
NT4 Millet oils
NT4 Mustard seed oils
NT4 Nut oils
NT5 Almond oils
NT5 Beech nut oils
NT5 Brazil nut oils
NT5 Coconut oils
NT5 Groundnut oils
NT5 Hazelnut oils
NT5 Pecan oils
NT5 Walnut oils
NT4 Oat oils
NT4 Olive oils
NT5 Olive oil mills effluents
NT5 Olive pomace oils
NT6 Sansa oils
NT4 Palm oils
NT5 Babassu oils
NT5 Palm kernel oils
NT5 Palm oil mills effluents
NT5 Palm olein
NT5 Palm stearin
NT4 Perilla oils
NT4 Pumpkin seed oils
NT4 Rapeseed oils
NT4 Rice bran oils
NT4 Rice germ oils
NT4 Safflower oils
NT4 Sea buckthorn oils
NT4 Sesame oils
NT4 Soybean oils
NT4 Sunflower oils
NT4 Tea seed oils
NT4 Tomato seed oils
NT4 Wheat germ oils
NT2 Salad oils
NT1 Phospholipids
NT2 Cephalins
NT2 Ceramides
NT2 Lecithins
NT3 Lysolecithin
NT3 Soy lecithins
NT2 Lysophospholipids
NT2 Phosphatides
NT2 Phosphatidic acid
NT2 Phosphatidylethanolamine
NT2 Phosphatidylinositol
NT2 Phosphatidylserine
NT1 Proteolipids
NT1 Rhamnolipids
NT1 Sphingolipids
NT2 Sphingomyelin
NT1 Steroids
NT2 Brassinosteroids
NT2 Cortisol
NT2 Sapogenins
NT2 Sterols
NT3 Avenasterol
NT3 Brassicasterol
NT3 Campesterol
NT3 Cholesterol
NT4 Cholesterol low foods
NT4 Cholesterol oxidation products
NT5 Cholesterol oxides
NT3 Cucurbitacins
NT3 Desmosterol
NT3 Ergosterol
NT3 Phytosterols
NT3 Sitosterol
NT3 Stanols
NT4 Phytostanols
NT5 Sitostanol
NT4 Stanol esters
NT3 Sterol esters
NT3 Stigmastadienes
NT3 Stigmasterol
NT1 Structured lipids
NT1 Terpenoids
NT2 Carotenoids
NT3 Apocarotenal
NT3 Astacene
NT3 Bixin
NT3 Capsanthin
NT3 Carotenes
NT4 α-Carotene
NT4 β-Carotene
NT4 Provitamin A
NT3 Crocin
NT4 Crocetin
NT3 Lycopene
NT3 Norisoprenoids
NT4 β-Damascenone
NT4 Ionones
NT3 Phytoene
NT3 Phytofluene
NT3 Xanthophylls
NT4 Astaxanthin
NT4 Canthaxanthin
NT4 Cryptoxanthin
NT4 Diatoxanthin
NT4 Fucoxanthin
NT4 Lutein
NT4 Neoxanthin
NT4 Tunaxanthin
NT4 Violaxanthin
NT4 Zeaxanthin
NT2 Diterpenoids
NT3 Cafestol
NT3 Carnosic acid
NT3 Carnosol
NT3 Diterpenes
NT3 Kahweol
NT3 Rebaudiosides
NT3 Steviol
NT3 Stevioside
NT2 Isoprene
NT2 Isoprenoids
NT2 Monoterpenoids
NT3 Borneol
NT3 Camphor
NT3 Carvacrol
NT3 Carveol
NT3 Carvone
NT3 Cineole
NT4 Eucalyptol
NT3 Citral
NT4 Geranial
NT4 Neral
NT3 Citronellal
NT3 Citronellol
NT3 Dill ether
NT3 Geraniol
NT3 Hotrienol
NT3 Linalool
NT3 Menthol
NT3 Menthone
NT3 2-Methylisoborneol
NT3 Monoterpenes
NT4 Camphene
NT4 Limonene
NT4 Myrcene
NT4 Pinenes
NT4 Terpinene
NT3 Nerol
NT3 Safranal
NT3 Terpineol
NT3 Terpinyl acetate
NT3 Thujone
NT3 Thymol
NT2 Rishitin
NT2 Sesquiterpenoids
NT3 Farnesol
NT3 Ipomeamarone
NT3 Nootkatone

NT3 Sesquiterpenes
NT4 Caryophyllene
NT4 Farnesene
NT4 Humulene
NT2 Terpenes
NT2 Triterpenoids
NT3 Amyrin
NT3 Cucurbitacins
NT3 Glycyrrhizic acid
NT3 Glycyrrhizin
NT3 Limonoids
NT4 Limonin
NT4 Limonoid glucosides
NT4 Nomilin
NT3 Oleanolic acid
NT3 Quassin
NT3 Sapogenins
NT3 Triterpenes
NT4 Squalene
NT3 Ursolic acid
NT2 Vitamin E
NT3 Tocols
NT4 Tocopherols
NT5 α-Tocopherol
NT5 Tocotrienol
NT5 Vitamin E acetate
NT1 Unsaponifiable matter
RT Liposomes
RT Macronutrients
RT Waxes

α-Lipoic acid
HN introduced from vol. 41, issue 1 (2009)
BT1 Organic acids
BT2 Acids

Lipolysis
BT1 Hydrolysis
RT Fatty acids
RT Lipases
RT Rancidity

Lipolytic enzymes
USE **Lipases**

Lipopolysaccharides
BT1 Lipids
BT2 Nutrients
BT1 Polysaccharides
BT2 Carbohydrates
BT3 Nutrients
BT3 Organic compounds

Lipoprotein lipases
SN EC 3.1.1.34
BT1 Lipases
BT2 Esterases
BT3 Hydrolases
BT4 Enzymes

Lipoproteins
SN for use in both food and physiology contexts
BT1 Proteins
BT2 Nutrients
NT1 High density lipoproteins
NT1 Lipovitellins
NT1 Low density lipoproteins
NT1 Purothionin

Liposcelis
BT1 Insects
BT2 Pests
NT1 *Liposcelis bostrychophila*
RT Psocids

Liposcelis bostrychophila
BT1 *Liposcelis*
BT2 Insects
BT3 Pests

Liposomes
HN introduced from vol. 39, issue 1 (2007)
RT Lipids

Lipovitellins
BT1 Lipoproteins
BT2 Proteins
BT3 Nutrients

Lipoxidases
USE **Lipoxygenases**

Lipoxygenases
SN EC 1.13.11.12 and also other members of EC 1.13.11
BT1 Oxygenases
BT2 Oxidoreductases
BT3 Enzymes
UF Lipoxidases

Lippia alba
BT1 Plants

Liquefaction
HN introduced from vol. 41, issue 1 (2009)
BT1 Processing
BT2 Technology

Liqueurs
BT1 Alcoholic beverages
BT2 Beverages alcoholic
BT3 Beverages
NT1 Anisette
NT1 Cordials
NT1 Cream liqueurs
NT1 Fruit liqueurs
NT2 Cassis
NT2 Cherry brandy
NT2 Limoncello
NT1 Pernod
RT Spirits

Liquid chromatography
HN LC used in the index from vol. 35, issue 6 (2003)
USE **LC**

Liquid egg
BT1 Egg products
BT2 Animal foods
BT3 Foods
RT Liquid whole egg

Liquid egg whites
BT1 Egg products
BT2 Animal foods
BT3 Foods
RT Egg whites

Liquid egg yolks
BT1 Egg products
BT2 Animal foods
BT3 Foods
RT Egg yolks

Liquid foods
BT1 Liquids
BT2 Physical phases
BT3 Chemistry
BT4 Science

Liquid membranes
BT1 Membranes

Liquid nitrogen
BT1 Freezing
BT2 Thermal processing
BT3 Processing thermal
BT4 Processing
BT5 Technology
BT1 Nitrogen
BT2 Elements
BT3 Minerals
BT4 Nutrients

Liquid phase microextraction
HN introduced from vol. 41, issue 1 (2009)
BT1 Analytical techniques

Liquids
BT1 Physical phases
BT2 Chemistry
BT3 Science
NT1 Fluids
NT2 Supercritical fluids
NT1 Juices
NT2 Stocks
NT1 Liquid foods

Liquid smoke
HN smoke liquid also used in the index up to vol. 29 (1997)
BT1 Flavourings
BT2 Additives
RT Smoking

Liquid whole egg
BT1 Egg products
BT2 Animal foods
BT3 Foods
RT Liquid egg

Liquorice
BT1 Flavourings
BT2 Additives
BT1 Sugar confectionery
BT2 Plant foods
BT3 Foods
RT Glycyrrhizic acid
RT Glycyrrhizin

Listeria
HN heading from vol. 25 (1993); under Corynebacteriaceae up to vol. 24 (1992)
BT1 Bacteria
BT2 Microorganisms
NT1 *Listeria innocua*
NT1 *Listeria ivanovii*

NT1 *Listeria monocytogenes*
NT1 *Listeria seeligeri*
NT1 *Listeria welshimeri*
RT Listeriolysins
RT Listeriosis

Listeria innocua
BT1 *Listeria*
BT2 Bacteria
BT3 Microorganisms

Listeria ivanovii
BT1 *Listeria*
BT2 Bacteria
BT3 Microorganisms

Listeria monocytogenes
BT1 *Listeria*
BT2 Bacteria
BT3 Microorganisms

Listeria seeligeri
HN introduced from vol. 39, issue 1 (2007)
BT1 *Listeria*
BT2 Bacteria
BT3 Microorganisms

Listeria welshimeri
BT1 *Listeria*
BT2 Bacteria
BT3 Microorganisms

Listeriolysins
BT1 Toxins
BT2 Residues
RT *Listeria*

Listeriosis
BT1 Diseases
BT1 Poisoning
RT *Listeria*

Litchis
HN heading from vol. 30 (1998); under Fruits specific up to vol. 29 (1997)
BT1 Fruits specific
BT2 Fruits
BT3 Crops
BT4 Plants
BT3 Plant foods
BT4 Foods
UF Lychees

Lite beverages
BT1 Beverages
RT Alcohol low beverages
RT Beverages alcohol low
RT Calories low beverages

Lite foods
BT1 Processed foods
BT2 Foods
RT Calories low foods
RT Fats low foods
RT Sugar low foods

Litesse
BT1 Fat substitutes
BT2 Fats
BT3 Lipids
BT4 Nutrients
RT Polydextrose

Lithium
USE **Li**

Lithospermum erythrorhizon
BT1 Plants

Lithuania
BT1 Europe
BT1 European Union

Liver flukes
BT1 Flukes
BT2 Parasites
BT3 Pests
BT1 Parasites
BT2 Pests

Liver pates
BT1 Pates
BT2 Fish products
BT3 Sea foods
BT4 Aquatic foods
BT5 Animal foods
BT6 Foods
BT2 Meat products
BT3 Animal foods
BT4 Foods

Livers
BT1 Offal
BT2 Animal foods
BT3 Foods
NT1 Cattle livers
NT1 Chicken livers
NT1 Duck livers
NT1 Fish livers
NT2 Cod livers
NT1 Foie gras
NT1 Goose livers
NT1 Lamb livers
NT1 Swine livers
NT1 Turkey livers

Liver sausages
BT1 Sausages
BT2 Meat products
BT3 Animal foods
BT4 Foods
UF Liverwurst

Liverwurst
USE **Liver sausages**

Livestock
USE **Animals**

Lizardfish
BT1 Marine fish
BT2 Fish
BT3 Animals
BT3 Sea foods
BT4 Aquatic foods
BT5 Animal foods
BT6 Foods

Loaf vol.
BT1 Breadmaking properties
BT2 Breadmaking
BT3 Bread
BT4 Bakery products
BT5 Cereal products
BT6 Plant foods
BT7 Foods
BT3 Processing
BT4 Technology

Lobsters
HN heading from vol. 25 (1993); under Crustacea up tovol. 24 (1992)
BT1 Crustacea
BT2 Shellfish
BT3 Animals
BT3 Sea foods
BT4 Aquatic foods
BT5 Animal foods
BT6 Foods
NT1 American lobsters

Locust bean gums
HN under Legumes up to vol. 42 (2010)
BT1 Gums
BT2 Polysaccharides
BT3 Carbohydrates
BT4 Nutrients
BT4 Organic compounds
BT2 Stabilizers
BT3 Additives
BT2 Thickeners
BT3 Additives
NT1 Carob gums
RT Carob beans

Locust beans
USE **Carob beans**

Loganberries
BT1 Berries
BT2 Fruits specific
BT3 Fruits
BT4 Crops
BT5 Plants
BT4 Plant foods
BT5 Foods

Logistics
RT Distribution
RT Management

Lokum
USE **Turkish delight**

Lollipops
BT1 Sugar confectionery
BT2 Plant foods
BT3 Foods

Longaniza
BT1 Sausages
BT2 Meat products
BT3 Animal foods
BT4 Foods

Longans
BT1 Fruits specific
BT2 Fruits
BT3 Crops
BT4 Plants
BT3 Plant foods
BT4 Foods

Long life foods
BT1 Shelf life

Loop-mediated isothermal amplification
USE **LAMP**

Loquats
BT1 Fruits specific
BT2 Fruits
BT3 Crops
BT4 Plants
BT3 Plant foods
BT4 Foods

Lorries
BT1 Transport
RT Trucks

Los Pedroches cheese
HN introduced from vol. 37, issue 5 (2005)
BT1 Cheese varieties
BT2 Cheese
BT3 Dairy products
BT4 Animal foods
BT5 Foods

Lotus roots
BT1 Vegetables specific
BT2 Vegetables
BT3 Crops
BT4 Plants
BT3 Plant foods
BT4 Foods

Loukanka
BT1 Sausages
BT2 Meat products
BT3 Animal foods
BT4 Foods

Lovage
BT1 Spices
BT2 Flavourings
BT3 Additives

Low alcohol beer
USE **Alcohol low beer**

Low alcohol beverages
USE **Alcohol low beverages**

Low alcohol wines
USE **Alcohol low wines**

Low calorie beverages
USE **Calories low beverages**

Low calorie diet
USE **Calories low diet**

Low calorie foods
USE **Calories low foods**

Low calorie spreads
USE **Calories low spreads**

Low cholesterol foods
USE **Cholesterol low foods**

Low density lipoproteins
HN introduced from vol. 39, issue 1 (2007)
BT1 Lipoproteins
BT2 Proteins
BT3 Nutrients

Low density polyethylene
USE **LDPE**

Low fat diet
USE **Fats low diet**

Low fat foods
USE **Fats low foods**

Low fat spreads
USE **Fats low spreads**

Low lactose foods
USE **Lactose low foods**

Low sodium diet
USE **Sodium low diet**

Low sodium foods
USE **Sodium low foods**

Low sugar confectionery
USE **Sugar low confectionery**

Low sugar foods
USE **Sugar low foods**

Lozenges
BT1 Sugar confectionery
BT2 Plant foods
BT3 Foods

LTLT pasteurization
SN low temperature long time pasteurization
BT1 Pasteurization
BT2 Thermal processing
BT3 Processing thermal
BT4 Processing
BT5 Technology
RT HTST pasteurization

Lubricants
RT Equipment

Lucerne
HN heading up to vol. 24 (1992)
SN syn. alfalfa
BT1 Alfalfa
BT2 Legumes
BT3 Vegetables specific
BT4 Vegetables
BT5 Crops
BT6 Plants
BT5 Plant foods
BT6 Foods

Lukum
USE **Turkish delight**

Lulo
SN syn. naranjilla
BT1 Naranjilla
BT2 Fruits specific
BT3 Fruits
BT4 Crops
BT5 Plants
BT4 Plant foods
BT5 Foods

Luminescence
SN syn. phosphorescence
BT1 Fluorescence
BT2 Analytical techniques
BT2 Optical properties
BT3 Physical properties
NT1 Phosphorescence

Lumpfish
BT1 Marine fish
BT2 Fish
BT3 Animals
BT3 Sea foods
BT4 Aquatic foods
BT5 Animal foods
BT6 Foods
NT1 *Cyclopterus lumpus*

Lumpiness
BT1 Consistency
BT2 Texture
BT3 Sensory properties

Luncheon meat
BT1 Meat products
BT2 Animal foods
BT3 Foods

Lunches
BT1 Meals
BT2 Processed foods
BT3 Foods

Lung cancer
HN introduced from vol. 39, issue 1 (2007)
BT1 Cancer
BT2 Diseases

Lungs
BT1 Offal
BT2 Animal foods
BT3 Foods

Lupanine
BT1 Alkaloids
BT2 Organic nitrogen compounds

Lupin meal
HN introduced from vol. 41, issue 1 (2009)
BT1 Flours
BT2 Plant foods
BT3 Foods
BT1 Lupin seeds
BT2 Oilseeds
BT3 Seeds
BT4 Plant foods
BT5 Foods

Lupin proteins
BT1 Lupins
BT2 Legumes
BT3 Vegetables specific
BT4 Vegetables

BT5 Crops
BT6 Plants
BT5 Plant foods
BT6 Foods
BT1 Vegetable proteins
BT2 Proteins vegetable
BT3 Proteins
BT4 Nutrients
BT3 Vegetable products
BT4 Plant foods
BT5 Foods

Lupins
HN heading from vol. 30 (1998); under Legumes up to vol. 29 (1997)
BT1 Legumes
BT2 Vegetables specific
BT3 Vegetables
BT4 Crops
BT5 Plants
BT4 Plant foods
BT5 Foods
NT1 Lupin proteins
NT1 White lupins

Lupin seed oils
BT1 Vegetable oils
BT2 Oils vegetable
BT3 Oils
BT4 Lipids
BT5 Nutrients
BT3 Vegetable products
BT4 Plant foods
BT5 Foods

Lupin seeds
BT1 Oilseeds
BT2 Seeds
BT3 Plant foods
BT4 Foods
NT1 Lupin meal

Lupulin
BT1 Bitter acids
BT2 Bitter compounds
BT3 Flavour compounds
BT2 Organic acids
BT3 Acids

Lupulones
BT1 β-Acids
BT2 Bitter acids
BT3 Bitter compounds
BT4 Flavour compounds
BT3 Organic acids
BT4 Acids
NT1 Colupulone

Lutein
BT1 Xanthophylls
BT2 Carotenoids
BT3 Pigments
BT3 Terpenoids
BT4 Lipids
BT5 Nutrients

Luteolin
BT1 Flavones
BT2 Flavonoids
BT3 Aromatic compounds
BT4 Organic compounds
BT3 Pigments

Luteoskyrin
BT1 Mycotoxins
BT2 Toxins
BT3 Residues

Luxembourg
HN heading up to vol. 24 (1992)
BT1 Europe
BT1 European Union
RT Organization for Economic Cooperation and Development

Lyases
HN heading from vol. 25 (1993); under Enzymes up to vol. 24 (1992)
SN EC 4
BT1 Enzymes
NT1 Alliin lyases
NT1 1-Aminocyclopropane-1-carboxylate synthases
NT1 Decarboxylases
NT2 Acetolactate decarboxylases
NT2 Glutamate decarboxylases
NT2 Histidine decarboxylases
NT1 Fructose-bisphosphate aldolases
NT1 Fumarate hydratases
NT1 Hydroperoxide lyases
NT1 Inulin fructotransferases (DFA-III-forming)
NT1 Isocitrate lyases
NT1 Pectate lyases
NT1 Pectin lyases
NT1 Phenylalanine ammonia-lyases
NT1 Phosphoenolpyruvate carboxylases
NT1 Poly(β-D-mannuronate) lyases
NT1 Pyruvate decarboxylases

Lycasin
BT1 Hydrolysed starch syrups
BT2 Sugar syrups
BT3 Plant foods
BT4 Foods
BT1 Sweeteners
BT2 Additives

Lychees
USE **Litchis**

Lycopene
BT1 Carotenoids
BT2 Pigments
BT2 Terpenoids
BT3 Lipids
BT4 Nutrients

Lycoperdon
BT1 Edible fungi
BT2 Fungi edible
BT3 Vegetables specific
BT4 Vegetables
BT5 Crops
BT6 Plants
BT5 Plant foods
BT6 Foods
UF Puff balls

Lyes
BT1 Alkalies

Lymeswold cheese
BT1 Cheese varieties
BT2 Cheese
BT3 Dairy products
BT4 Animal foods
BT5 Foods

Lyophilization
USE **Freeze drying**

Lysine
BT1 Amino acids
BT2 Nutrients
BT2 Organic acids
BT3 Acids
BT2 Organic nitrogen compounds
NT1 Polylysine

Lysinoalanine
BT1 Peptides
BT2 Proteins
BT3 Nutrients

Lysins
SN includes members of EC 3.4.24
BT1 Proteinases
BT2 Hydrolases
BT3 Enzymes
NT1 Autolysins
NT1 Thermolysins

Lysis
HN heading from vol. 41 (2009); under Decomposition up to vol. 40 (2008)
BT1 Decomposition
NT1 Autolysis
NT1 Haemolysis
NT1 Photolysis
NT1 Pyrolysis

Lysolecithin
BT1 Lecithins
BT2 Emulsifiers
BT3 Additives
BT2 Phospholipids
BT3 Lipids
BT4 Nutrients

Lysophospholipases
SN EC 3.1.1.5; syn. lecithinase B; syn. phospholipase B
BT1 Lipases
BT2 Esterases
BT3 Hydrolases
BT4 Enzymes

Lysophospholipids
BT1 Phospholipids
BT2 Lipids
BT3 Nutrients

Lysozymes
HN heading from vol. 28 (1996)
SN EC 3.2.1.17

BT1 Glycosidases
BT2 Hydrolases
BT3 Enzymes
NT1 Eggs lysozymes
NT1 Egg whites lysozymes
RT Mutanolysins
UF Muramidases

M

Maca
BT1 Vegetables specific
BT2 Vegetables
BT3 Crops
BT4 Plants
BT3 Plant foods
BT4 Foods

Macadamia nuts
HN heading from vol. 30 (1998); under Nuts up to vol. 29 (1997)
BT1 Nuts
BT2 Fruits
BT3 Crops
BT4 Plants
BT3 Plant foods
BT4 Foods
BT2 Oilseeds
BT3 Seeds
BT4 Plant foods
BT5 Foods

Macaroni
BT1 Pasta
BT2 Cereal products
BT3 Plant foods
BT4 Foods

Macaroons
BT1 Bakery products
BT2 Cereal products
BT3 Plant foods
BT4 Foods

Mace
BT1 Spices
BT2 Flavourings
BT3 Additives

Macedonia
SN full name is the Former Yugoslav Republic of Macedonia
BT1 Europe

Maceration
BT1 Processing
BT2 Technology
NT1 Carbonic maceration
RT Comminution
RT Winemaking

Machinery
USE **Equipment**

Machines
USE **Equipment**

Machine vision
BT1 Analytical techniques

Mackerel
HN heading from vol. 30 (1998); under Fishes up to vol. 29 (1997)
BT1 Marine fish
BT2 Fish
BT3 Animals
BT3 Sea foods
BT4 Aquatic foods
BT5 Animal foods
BT6 Foods
BT1 Oily fish
BT2 Fish
BT3 Animals
BT3 Sea foods
BT4 Aquatic foods
BT5 Animal foods
BT6 Foods
NT1 Atlantic mackerel
NT2 *Scomber scombrus*
NT1 Chub mackerel
NT2 *Scomber japonicus*
NT1 Frigate mackerel
NT1 Horse mackerel
NT1 Indian mackerel
NT1 Jack mackerel
NT2 *Trachurus japonicus*
NT2 *Trachurus murphyi*
NT1 Pacific mackerel
NT1 Scad
NT1 Seer fish
NT1 Smoked mackerel
NT1 Spanish mackerel
UF Mackerels

Mackerels
HN heading up to vol. 24 (1992)
USE **Mackerel**

Macrococcus
HN introduced from vol. 43, issue 1 (2011)
BT1 Bacteria
BT2 Microorganisms
NT1 *Macrococcus caseolyticus*

Macrococcus caseolyticus
HN introduced from vol. 39, issue 1 (2007)
BT1 *Macrococcus*
BT2 Bacteria
BT3 Microorganisms

Macrocystis
BT1 Seaweeds
BT2 Algae
BT3 Microorganisms
BT2 Sea foods
BT3 Aquatic foods
BT4 Animal foods
BT5 Foods

Macrolide antibiotics
HN introduced from vol. 43, issue 1 (2011)
BT1 Antibiotics
BT2 Drugs
BT3 Residues
NT1 Erythromycin
NT1 Nystatin
NT1 Oleandomycin
NT1 Spiramycin
NT1 Tilmicosin
NT1 Tylosin

Macronutrients
HN introduced from vol. 43, issue 1 (2011)
SN general use only; see also other specific macronutrients
BT1 Nutrients
RT Carbohydrates
RT Lipids
RT Proteins

Madagascar
HN Malagasy Republic used in the index up to vol. 35, issue 6 (2003)
SN formerly Malagasy Republic
BT1 Southern Africa
BT2 Africa
UF Malagasy Republic

Madeira
BT1 Fortified wines
BT2 Wines
BT3 Alcoholic beverages
BT4 Beverages alcoholic
BT5 Beverages

Madeirization
BT1 Winemaking
BT2 Processing
BT3 Technology

Madhuca seeds
BT1 Oilseeds
BT2 Seeds
BT3 Plant foods
BT4 Foods

Magnesium
HN heading up to vol. 24 (1992) and from vol. 30 (1998)
SN symbol Mg also used in the index
BT1 Metals
BT2 Elements
BT3 Minerals
BT4 Nutrients
NT1 Mg

Magnetic fields
BT1 Energy
RT Electromagnetic fields

Magnetic resonance imaging
BT1 Nuclear magnetic resonance
BT2 Spectroscopy
BT3 Analytical techniques

Mahewu
BT1 Beverages

Mahimahi
SN syn. dolphinfish
BT1 Dolphinfish
BT2 Marine fish
BT3 Fish

BT4 Animals
BT4 Sea foods
BT5 Aquatic foods
BT6 Animal foods
BT7 Foods

Mahon cheese
BT1 Cheese varieties
BT2 Cheese
BT3 Dairy products
BT4 Animal foods
BT5 Foods

Maida
BT1 Cereal flours
BT2 Flours cereal
BT3 Cereal products
BT4 Plant foods
BT5 Foods
BT1 Wheat
BT2 Cereals
BT3 Crops
BT4 Plants
BT3 Seeds
BT4 Plant foods
BT5 Foods

Maillard reaction
NT1 Amadori compounds
NT1 Maillard reaction products
NT2 Melanoidins
RT Caramelization
RT Nonenzymic browning

Maillard reaction products
BT1 Maillard reaction
NT1 Melanoidins
RT Glyoxal
RT Pyrazines
RT Pyrroles

Maitake
USE ***Grifola frondosa***

Maize
USE **Corn**

Maize meal
USE **Corn flour**

Maize oils
USE **Corn oils**

Makhana
USE **Gorgon nuts**

Malabar nightshade
USE **Ceylon spinach**

Malabsorption
HN introduced from vol. 39, issue 1 (2007)
BT1 Diseases
BT1 Gastrointestinal tract
BT2 Human physiology
BT3 Physiology
BT4 Science

Malachite green
BT1 Fungicides
BT2 Pesticides
BT3 Biocides
BT3 Residues

Malagasy Republic
HN used in the index up to vol. 35, issue 6 (2003)
SN former name for Madagascar
USE **Madagascar**

Malaoxon
BT1 Malathion
BT2 Acaricides
BT3 Pesticides
BT4 Biocides
BT4 Residues
BT2 Organophosphorus insecticides
BT3 Insecticides
BT4 Pesticides
BT5 Biocides
BT5 Residues
BT3 Organophosphorus pesticides
BT4 Pesticides
BT5 Biocides
BT5 Residues

Malate dehydrogenases
SN includes EC 1.1.1.37 to EC 1.1.1.40
BT1 Oxidoreductases
BT2 Enzymes
UF Malic enzymes

Malathion
HN heading up to vol. 24 (1992)
BT1 Acaricides
BT2 Pesticides
BT3 Biocides
BT3 Residues
BT1 Organophosphorus insecticides
BT2 Insecticides
BT3 Pesticides
BT4 Biocides
BT4 Residues
BT2 Organophosphorus pesticides
BT3 Pesticides
BT4 Biocides
BT4 Residues
NT1 Malaoxon
UF Carbofos

Malawi
BT1 Southern Africa
BT2 Africa

Malay apples
BT1 Fruits specific
BT2 Fruits
BT3 Crops
BT4 Plants
BT3 Plant foods
BT4 Foods
UF Mountain apples

Malaysia
HN heading up to vol. 24 (1992)
BT1 Asia

MALDI-TOF-MS
SN abbreviation for matrix-assisted desorption/ionization time-of-flight mass spectroscopy
BT1 Mass spectroscopy
BT2 Spectroscopy
BT3 Analytical techniques

Maleic acid
BT1 Organic acids
BT2 Acids

Maleic hydrazide
BT1 Antisprouting agents
BT2 Plant growth regulators
BT3 Cultivation
BT4 Agriculture

Mali
BT1 West Africa
BT2 Africa

Malic acid
BT1 Organic acids
BT2 Acids

Malic enzymes
USE **Malate dehydrogenases**

Malignant hyperthermia
BT1 Animal diseases
BT2 Diseases animal
BT3 Diseases
BT1 Genetic disorders

Mallards
USE **Ducks**

Malnutrition
SN includes both overnutrition and undernutrition
BT1 Diseases
RT Antinutritional factors

Malolactic fermentation
BT1 Fermentation
RT Winemaking

Malonaldehyde
SN syn. malondialdehyde
BT1 Aldehydes
BT2 Carbonyl compounds
BT3 Organic compounds
BT1 TBA values
BT2 Thiobarbituric acid values

Malondialdehyde
BT1 Aldehydes
BT2 Carbonyl compounds
BT3 Organic compounds
BT1 TBA values
BT2 Thiobarbituric acid values

Malonic acid
BT1 Organic acids
BT2 Acids

Malt
BT1 Cereal products
BT2 Plant foods
BT3 Foods
NT1 Barley malt

NT1 Rye malt
NT1 Sorghum malt
NT1 Wheat malt
RT Barley
RT Beer
RT Diastatic activity
RT Malting

Malta
BT1 Europe
BT1 European Union

Maltases
USE **α-Glucosidases**

Malt beverages
BT1 Beer
BT2 Alcoholic beverages
BT3 Beverages alcoholic
BT4 Beverages

Malthouses
BT1 Malting

Malting
NT1 Kilning
NT1 Malthouses
NT1 Malting properties
RT Brewing
RT Germination
RT Kilns
RT Malt

Malting barley
HN heading from vol. 30 (1998); under Barley up to vol. 29 (1997)
BT1 Barley
BT2 Cereals
BT3 Crops
BT4 Plants
BT3 Seeds
BT4 Plant foods
BT5 Foods

Malting properties
BT1 Malting

Maltitol
BT1 Polyols
BT2 Alcohols
BT2 Carbohydrates
BT3 Nutrients
BT3 Organic compounds

Maltodextrins
SN syn. maltooligosaccharides
BT1 Dextrins
BT2 Starch
BT3 Glucans
BT4 Polysaccharides
BT5 Carbohydrates
BT6 Nutrients
BT6 Organic compounds
BT3 Thickeners
BT4 Additives
RT Maltooligosaccharides

Maltohexaose
HN under Sugars up to vol. 42 (2010)
BT1 Maltooligosaccharides
BT2 Glucooligosaccharides
BT3 Oligosaccharides
BT4 Polysaccharides
BT5 Carbohydrates
BT6 Nutrients
BT6 Organic compounds
BT4 Sugars
BT5 Carbohydrates
BT6 Nutrients
BT6 Organic compounds
BT5 Plant foods
BT6 Foods

Maltol
HN also under Flavourings up to vol. 42 (2010)
BT1 Aroma compounds
BT2 Flavour compounds
BT2 Volatile compounds
BT1 Pyrones
BT2 Heterocyclic compounds

Maltooligosaccharides
HN under Sugars and Polysaccharides up to vol. 42 (2010)
SN syn. maltodextrins
BT1 Glucooligosaccharides
BT2 Oligosaccharides
BT3 Polysaccharides
BT4 Carbohydrates
BT5 Nutrients
BT5 Organic compounds
BT3 Sugars
BT4 Carbohydrates
BT5 Nutrients
BT5 Organic compounds
BT4 Plant foods
BT5 Foods
NT1 Maltohexaose
NT1 Maltotetraose
NT1 Maltotriose
RT Isomaltooligosaccharides
RT Maltodextrins

Maltose
BT1 Disaccharides
BT2 Sugars
BT3 Carbohydrates
BT4 Nutrients
BT4 Organic compounds
BT3 Plant foods
BT4 Foods

Maltose syrups
BT1 Sugar syrups
BT2 Plant foods
BT3 Foods

Maltotetraose
HN under Sugars up to vol. 42 (2010)
BT1 Maltooligosaccharides
BT2 Glucooligosaccharides
BT3 Oligosaccharides
BT4 Polysaccharides
BT5 Carbohydrates
BT6 Nutrients
BT6 Organic compounds
BT4 Sugars
BT5 Carbohydrates
BT6 Nutrients
BT6 Organic compounds
BT5 Plant foods
BT6 Foods

Maltotriose
HN under Sugars up to vol. 42 (2010)
BT1 Maltooligosaccharides
BT2 Glucooligosaccharides
BT3 Oligosaccharides
BT4 Polysaccharides
BT5 Carbohydrates
BT6 Nutrients
BT6 Organic compounds
BT4 Sugars
BT5 Carbohydrates
BT6 Nutrients
BT6 Organic compounds
BT5 Plant foods
BT6 Foods

Malt vinegar
BT1 Vinegar
BT2 Condiments
BT3 Flavourings
BT4 Additives
BT2 Fermented foods
BT3 Processed foods
BT4 Foods

Malvalic acid
BT1 Fatty acids
BT2 Lipids
BT3 Nutrients
BT2 Organic acids
BT3 Acids

Malvidin
BT1 Anthocyanidins
BT2 Flavonoids
BT3 Aromatic compounds
BT4 Organic compounds
BT3 Pigments

Mamastrovirus
HN introduced from vol. 43, issue 1 (2011)
BT1 Astroviruses
BT2 Viruses
BT3 Microorganisms
NT1 Human astrovirus

Mamey
BT1 Fruits specific
BT2 Fruits
BT3 Crops
BT4 Plants
BT3 Plant foods
BT4 Foods

Management
HN heading up to vol. 27 (1995)
RT Economics
RT Logistics

Manchego cheese
BT1 Cheese varieties
BT2 Cheese
BT3 Dairy products
BT4 Animal foods
BT5 Foods

Mancozeb
BT1 Dithiocarbamate fungicides
BT2 Fungicides
BT3 Pesticides
BT4 Biocides
BT4 Residues

Mandarin juices
BT1 Orange juices
BT2 Citrus juices
BT3 Fruit juices
BT4 Fruit products
BT5 Plant foods
BT6 Foods
BT4 Soft drinks
BT5 Beverages
NT1 Tangerine juices

Mandarins
HN heading from vol. 25 (1993); under Oranges up to vol. 24 (1992)
BT1 Oranges
BT2 Citrus fruits
BT3 Fruits specific
BT4 Fruits
BT5 Crops
BT6 Plants
BT5 Plant foods
BT6 Foods
NT1 Clementines
NT1 Kinnow mandarins
NT1 Ponkans
NT1 Satsuma mandarins
NT1 Satsumas
NT1 Tangerines

Maneb
BT1 Dithiocarbamate fungicides
BT2 Fungicides
BT3 Pesticides
BT4 Biocides
BT4 Residues

Manganese
HN non-descriptor from 1993 to 2010 (USE Mn); reinstated (as heading) from vol. 43, issue 1 (2011)
BT1 Metals
BT2 Elements
BT3 Minerals
BT4 Nutrients
NT1 Mn

Manganese peroxidases
SN EC 1.11.1.13
BT1 Peroxidases
BT2 Oxidoreductases
BT3 Enzymes

Mangiferin
HN introduced from vol. 42, issue 1 (2010)
BT1 Xanthones
BT2 Heterocyclic compounds

Mangoes
BT1 Fruits specific
BT2 Fruits
BT3 Crops
BT4 Plants
BT3 Plant foods
BT4 Foods
NT1 African mangoes
NT1 Mango jams
NT1 Mango kernels
NT1 Mango pickles
NT1 Mango pulps
NT1 Mango purees
RT Mango juices
RT Mango nectars

Mango jams
BT1 Jams
BT2 Fruit preserves
BT3 Fruit products
BT4 Plant foods
BT5 Foods
BT3 Preserves
BT4 Processed foods
BT5 Foods
BT1 Mangoes
BT2 Fruits specific
BT3 Fruits
BT4 Crops
BT5 Plants
BT4 Plant foods
BT5 Foods

Mango juices
BT1 Fruit juices
BT2 Fruit products
BT3 Plant foods
BT4 Foods
BT2 Soft drinks
BT3 Beverages
RT Mangoes
RT Mango nectars

Mango kernels
BT1 Mangoes
BT2 Fruits specific
BT3 Fruits
BT4 Crops
BT5 Plants
BT4 Plant foods
BT5 Foods

Mango nectars
BT1 Fruit nectars
BT2 Fruit juices
BT3 Fruit products
BT4 Plant foods
BT5 Foods
BT3 Soft drinks
BT4 Beverages
RT Mangoes
RT Mango juices

Mango pickles
BT1 Mangoes
BT2 Fruits specific
BT3 Fruits
BT4 Crops
BT5 Plants
BT4 Plant foods
BT5 Foods
BT1 Pickles
BT2 Fermented foods
BT3 Processed foods
BT4 Foods

Mango pulps
BT1 Fruit pulps
BT2 Fruit products
BT3 Plant foods
BT4 Foods
BT2 Pulps
BT3 Processed foods
BT4 Foods
BT1 Mangoes
BT2 Fruits specific
BT3 Fruits
BT4 Crops
BT5 Plants
BT4 Plant foods
BT5 Foods

Mango purees
BT1 Fruit purees
BT2 Fruit products
BT3 Plant foods
BT4 Foods
BT2 Purees
BT3 Pulps
BT4 Processed foods
BT5 Foods
BT1 Mangoes
BT2 Fruits specific
BT3 Fruits
BT4 Crops
BT5 Plants
BT4 Plant foods
BT5 Foods

Mangosteens
BT1 Fruits specific
BT2 Fruits
BT3 Crops
BT4 Plants
BT3 Plant foods
BT4 Foods

Manioc
BT1 Cassava
BT2 Vegetables specific
BT3 Vegetables
BT4 Crops
BT5 Plants
BT4 Plant foods
BT5 Foods

Mannanases
USE **Mannosidases**
USE **β-Mannosidases**

Mannan endo-1,4-β-mannosidases
SN EC 3.2.1.78
BT1 Glycosidases
BT2 Hydrolases
BT3 Enzymes

Mannans
BT1 Polysaccharides
BT2 Carbohydrates
BT3 Nutrients
BT3 Organic compounds
NT1 Galactomannans
NT1 Glucomannans
NT2 Konjac glucomannans

Mannases
USE **Mannosidases**
USE **β-Mannosidases**

Mannitol
HN heading from vol. 30 (1998); under Sugar alcohols up to vol. 29 (1997)
BT1 Polyols
BT2 Alcohols
BT2 Carbohydrates
BT3 Nutrients
BT3 Organic compounds

Mannoproteins
BT1 Glycoproteins
BT2 Proteins
BT3 Nutrients

Mannose
HN under Sugars up to vol. 42 (2010)
BT1 Monosaccharides
BT2 Sugars
BT3 Carbohydrates
BT4 Nutrients
BT4 Organic compounds
BT3 Plant foods
BT4 Foods

Mannosidases
SN used for mannosidases generally if specific enzyme name not given
BT1 Glycosidases
BT2 Hydrolases
BT3 Enzymes
UF Mannanases
UF Mannases

α-Mannosidases
SN EC 3.2.1.24
BT1 Glycosidases
BT2 Hydrolases
BT3 Enzymes

β-Mannosidases
SN EC 3.2.1.25
BT1 Glycosidases
BT2 Hydrolases
BT3 Enzymes
UF Mannanases
UF Mannases

Manometers
BT1 Pressure

Manometry
BT1 Analytical techniques

Maple saps
BT1 Maple syrups
BT2 Sugar syrups
BT3 Plant foods
BT4 Foods

Maple syrups
BT1 Sugar syrups
BT2 Plant foods
BT3 Foods
NT1 Maple saps

Mapping
BT1 Analytical techniques

Marbling
BT1 Animal fats
BT2 Fats animal
BT3 Animal foods
BT4 Foods
BT3 Fats
BT4 Lipids
BT5 Nutrients
RT Intramuscular fat

Marc
BT1 By-products
NT1 Grape marc

Mare milk
BT1 Horses
BT2 Animals
BT1 Milk
BT2 Dairy products
BT3 Animal foods
BT4 Foods
NT1 Koumiss
UF Horse milk

Margaric acid
SN syn. heptadecanoic acid
BT1 Heptadecanoic acid
BT2 Saturated fatty acids
BT3 Fatty acids
BT4 Lipids
BT5 Nutrients
BT4 Organic acids
BT5 Acids

Margarine
HN heading up to vol. 24 (1992)
USE **Margarines**

Margarines
HN heading from vol. 25 (1993); Margarine up to vol. 24 (1992)
BT1 Fats
BT2 Lipids
BT3 Nutrients
NT1 Halvarine
RT Spreads
UF Margarine

Maribo cheese
BT1 Cheese varieties
BT2 Cheese
BT3 Dairy products
BT4 Animal foods
BT5 Foods

Marigolds
BT1 Edible flowers
BT2 Plants
BT2 Vegetables specific
BT3 Vegetables
BT4 Crops
BT5 Plants
BT4 Plant foods
BT5 Foods

Marinades
BT1 Marination
BT2 Soaking
BT3 Processing
BT4 Technology

Marination
BT1 Soaking
BT2 Processing
BT3 Technology
NT1 Marinades

Marine fish
BT1 Fish
BT2 Animals
BT2 Sea foods
BT3 Aquatic foods
BT4 Animal foods
BT5 Foods
NT1 Alaska pollock
NT2 Alaska pollack
NT2 *Theragra chalcogramma*
NT2 Walleye pollack
NT1 Alewife
NT1 Anchovy
NT2 Anchovy pastes
NT2 Budu
NT2 *Engraulis encrasicholus*
NT1 Barracuda
NT1 Barramundi
NT1 Bigeye snapper
NT2 *Priacanthus macracanthus*
NT1 Bluefish
NT1 Blue whiting
NT2 *Micromesistius poutassou*
NT1 Bombay duck
NT1 Capelin
NT1 Coalfish
NT1 Cod
NT2 Cod livers
NT2 *Gadus morhua*
NT2 Rock cod
NT1 Conger eels
NT1 Croakers
NT1 Cutlassfish
NT1 Dogfish
NT1 Dolphinfish
NT2 Mahimahi
NT1 Drum
NT1 Filefish
NT1 Flatfish
NT2 Arrowtooth flounder
NT2 Bastard halibut
NT3 *Paralichthys olivaceus*
NT2 Dab
NT2 Flounders
NT3 Japanese flounders
NT4 *Paralichthys olivaceus*
NT3 *Platichthys flesus*
NT2 Halibut
NT3 Atlantic halibut
NT3 Greenland halibut
NT3 *Reinhardtius hippoglossoides*
NT2 Megrim
NT3 *Lepidorhombus boscii*
NT2 Plaice
NT3 *Pleuronectes platessa*
NT2 Sole
NT2 Turbot
NT1 Flying fish
NT1 Grenadier
NT1 Groundfish
NT1 Grouper
NT2 *Epinephelus guaza*

NT1 Gurnard
NT1 Haddock
NT1 Hagfish
NT1 Hairtail
NT1 Hake
NT2 *Merluccius australis*
NT2 *Merluccius hubbsi*
NT2 *Merluccius merluccius*
NT2 Pacific hake
NT3 *Merluccius productus*
NT3 Pacific whiting
NT2 Red hake
NT1 Herring
NT2 *Clupea harengus*
NT2 Kippers
NT2 Matjes
NT2 Rollmops
NT1 Hilsa
NT1 Hoki
NT1 Kilka
NT1 Kingklip
NT1 Lanternfish
NT1 Ling
NT2 *Molva molva*
NT1 Ling cod
NT2 *Ophiodon elongatus*
NT1 Lizardfish
NT1 Lumpfish
NT2 *Cyclopterus lumpus*
NT1 Mackerel
NT2 Atlantic mackerel
NT3 *Scomber scombrus*
NT2 Chub mackerel
NT3 *Scomber japonicus*
NT2 Frigate mackerel
NT2 Horse mackerel
NT2 Indian mackerel
NT2 Jack mackerel
NT3 *Trachurus japonicus*
NT3 *Trachurus murphyi*
NT2 Pacific mackerel
NT2 Scad
NT2 Seer fish
NT2 Smoked mackerel
NT2 Spanish mackerel
NT1 Marlins
NT1 Menhaden
NT2 *Brevoortia tyrannus*
NT1 Milkfish
NT2 *Chanos chanos*
NT1 Monkfish
NT1 Morwong
NT1 Mullet
NT2 *Mugil cephalus*
NT1 Orange roughy
NT1 Paddlefish
NT2 *Polyodon spathula*
NT1 Pilchards
NT1 Pollack
NT1 Pollock
NT1 Pomfret
NT2 Butterfish
NT1 *Priacanthus tayenus*
NT1 Pufferfish
NT1 Rabbitfish
NT1 Ray
NT1 Redfish
NT1 Redspot emperor
NT2 *Lethrinus lentjan*
NT1 Rockfish
NT1 Sablefish
NT1 Sailfish
NT1 Saithe
NT1 Sand lance
NT1 Sardine
NT2 Monterey sardine
NT2 *Sardina pilchardus*
NT1 *Sardinella*
NT1 Saury
NT1 Sculpin
NT1 Sea bass
NT2 Striped bass
NT3 *Morone saxatilis*
NT1 Sea bream
NT2 Bogue
NT3 *Boops boops*
NT2 Red sea bream
NT3 *Pagrus major*
NT2 *Sparus aurata*
NT1 Sea fish
NT1 Sea perch
NT1 Shad
NT2 Indian shad
NT1 Sharks
NT2 Shark fins
NT1 Sheatfish
NT1 Skate
NT1 Snapper
NT1 Sprat
NT1 Swordfish
NT1 Threadfin bream
NT1 Tuna
NT2 Bigeye tuna
NT2 Bonito
NT2 Skipjack tuna
NT3 Katsuobushi
NT2 White tuna
NT3 Albacore
NT2 Yellowfin tuna
NT1 Whitebait
NT1 White fish
NT1 Whiting
NT1 Wreckfish
NT2 *Polyprion americanus*
NT1 Yellowfin
NT1 Yellowtail

Marine oils
HN oils marine also used in the index up to vol. 29 (1997)
BT1 Oils
BT2 Lipids
BT3 Nutrients
NT1 Oils fish
NT2 Fish oils
NT3 Anchovy oils
NT3 Cod liver oils
NT3 Fish liver oils
NT3 Menhaden oils
NT3 Salmon oils
NT3 Sardine oils
NT3 Tuna oils
NT1 Seal blubber oils
NT1 Seal oils
NT1 Squid oils
NT1 Whale oils

Marjoram
HN under Spices up to vol. 42 (2010)
BT1 Herbs
BT2 Spices
BT3 Flavourings
BT4 Additives

Marker genes
BT1 Cloning technology
BT2 Gene cloning
BT3 Genetic techniques
BT4 Genetics
BT2 Technology
BT1 Genes
BT2 Chromosomes
BT3 Genetics
BT2 Genomes
BT3 Genetics
RT Gene expression
RT Marker proteins
RT Reporter genes

Marker proteins
HN introduced from vol. 39, issue 1 (2007)
BT1 Cloning technology
BT2 Gene cloning
BT3 Genetic techniques
BT4 Genetics
BT2 Technology
BT1 Proteins
BT2 Nutrients
NT1 Green fluorescent protein
RT Marker genes
RT Reporter genes

Marketing
BT1 Economics
NT1 Advertising
NT1 Consumer research
NT1 Consumer spending
NT1 Consumer surveys
NT1 Cooperatives
NT1 Display cabinets
NT1 E-commerce
NT1 Grocery stores
NT1 Hypermarkets
NT1 Market research
NT1 Presentation
NT1 Retail
NT2 Product recalls
NT1 Shops
NT1 Supermarkets
NT1 Vending machines
NT1 Wholesale
RT Consumption
RT Distribution
RT Fair trade
RT Markets
RT Pricing
RT Trade

Market research
BT1 Marketing
BT2 Economics
RT Consumer research

Markets
BT1 Economics
NT1 Purchase
NT1 Single market
RT Fair trade

RT Marketing
RT Pricing
RT Sales
RT Trade

Marking
BT1 Labelling
BT2 Packaging
BT3 Technology

Marlins
BT1 Marine fish
BT2 Fish
BT3 Animals
BT3 Sea foods
BT4 Aquatic foods
BT5 Animal foods
BT6 Foods

Marmalades
BT1 Jams
BT2 Fruit preserves
BT3 Fruit products
BT4 Plant foods
BT5 Foods
BT3 Preserves
BT4 Processed foods
BT5 Foods

Marrons glaces
BT1 Sugar confectionery
BT2 Plant foods
BT3 Foods

Marrows
BT1 Vegetables specific
BT2 Vegetables
BT3 Crops
BT4 Plants
BT3 Plant foods
BT4 Foods

Marsala
HN introduced from vol. 39, issue 1 (2007)
BT1 Fortified wines
BT2 Wines
BT3 Alcoholic beverages
BT4 Beverages alcoholic
BT5 Beverages

Marshmallows
BT1 Sugar confectionery
BT2 Plant foods
BT3 Foods

Martinique
BT1 West Indies
BT2 America

Marula
BT1 Fruits specific
BT2 Fruits
BT3 Crops
BT4 Plants
BT3 Plant foods
BT4 Foods
NT1 *Sclerocarya birrea*

Marzipan
BT1 Sugar confectionery
BT2 Plant foods
BT3 Foods

Mascarpone cheese
BT1 Cheese varieties
BT2 Cheese
BT3 Dairy products
BT4 Animal foods
BT5 Foods

Mashed potatoes
HN introduced from vol. 41, issue 1 (2009)
BT1 Potato products
BT2 Potatoes
BT3 Vegetables specific
BT4 Vegetables
BT5 Crops
BT6 Plants
BT5 Plant foods
BT6 Foods

Mashes
BT1 Mashing
BT2 Processing
BT3 Technology

Mashing
BT1 Processing
BT2 Technology
NT1 Decoction
NT1 Lautering
NT2 Lauter tuns
NT1 Mashes
NT1 Moromi
RT Brewing
RT Extraction
RT Worts

Mashua
USE **Anu**

Massecuites
BT1 Sugar juices
BT2 Plant foods
BT3 Foods
RT Sugar processes

Mass spectrometry
HN heading up to vol. 24 (1992)
USE **MS**

Mass spectroscopy
HN heading from vol. 25 (1993); Mass spectrometry up to vol. 24 (1992)
SN abbrev. MS is also used in the index
BT1 Spectroscopy
BT2 Analytical techniques
NT1 Electrospray ionization MS
NT1 GC-MS
NT1 ICP-MS
NT1 LC-MS
NT1 MALDI-TOF-MS
NT1 MS

Mass transfer
BT1 Physical properties

Mastadenovirus
HN introduced from vol. 43, issue 1 (2011)
BT1 Adenoviruses
BT2 Viruses
BT3 Microorganisms
NT1 Human adenovirus

Mastication
BT1 Human physiology
BT2 Physiology
BT3 Science

Mastitis
BT1 Animal diseases
BT2 Diseases animal
BT3 Diseases

Masu salmon
SN syn. cherry salmon
BT1 Cherry salmon
BT2 Pacific salmon
BT3 Salmon
BT4 Oily fish
BT5 Fish
BT6 Animals
BT6 Sea foods
BT7 Aquatic foods
BT8 Animal foods
BT9 Foods

Mate
HN under Beverages up to vol. 42 (2010)
BT1 Herb tea
BT2 Teas
BT3 Beverages
BT3 Crops
BT4 Plants
BT3 Plant foods
BT4 Foods
NT1 Yerba mate
NT2 *Ilex paraguariensis*

Mathematics
BT1 Science
NT1 Equations
NT1 Formulae
NT1 Nomograms
NT1 Principal component analysis
NT1 Statistical analysis
NT2 Chemometrics
RT Modelling

Matjes
BT1 Fish products
BT2 Sea foods
BT3 Aquatic foods
BT4 Animal foods
BT5 Foods
BT1 Herring
BT2 Marine fish
BT3 Fish
BT4 Animals
BT4 Sea foods
BT5 Aquatic foods
BT6 Animal foods
BT7 Foods
BT2 Oily fish
BT3 Fish
BT4 Animals
BT4 Sea foods
BT5 Aquatic foods
BT6 Animal foods
BT7 Foods

Matrix solid-phase dispersion
HN introduced from vol. 39, issue 1 (2007)
BT1 Analytical techniques

Matsutake
USE ***Tricholoma***

Maturation
USE **Ageing**
USE **Ripening**

Maturity
USE **Age**
USE **Ripeness**

Mauritania
BT1 West Africa
BT2 Africa

Mauritia
BT1 Palms
BT2 Plants

Mauritius
BT1 Southern Africa
BT2 Africa

Mawa
BT1 Condensed milk
BT2 Milk
BT3 Dairy products
BT4 Animal foods
BT5 Foods

Mawe
BT1 Porridges
BT2 Cereal products
BT3 Plant foods
BT4 Foods

Maximum residue limits
USE **MRL**

Mayonnaise
BT1 Condiments
BT2 Flavourings
BT3 Additives

MCPA
BT1 Phenoxy herbicides
BT2 Herbicides
BT3 Pesticides
BT4 Biocides
BT4 Residues

Mead
BT1 Alcoholic beverages
BT2 Beverages alcoholic
BT3 Beverages
RT Honey beverages
RT Melomel

Meadowfoam
BT1 Oilseeds
BT2 Seeds
BT3 Plant foods
BT4 Foods

Meadowfoam oils
BT1 Vegetable oils
BT2 Oils vegetable
BT3 Oils
BT4 Lipids
BT5 Nutrients
BT3 Vegetable products
BT4 Plant foods
BT5 Foods

Meal
HN heading up to vol. 24 (1992) for non-cereal flours
SN used for non-cereal flours
BT1 Flours
BT2 Plant foods
BT3 Foods

Mealiness
BT1 Sensory properties

Meal replacers
BT1 Meals
BT2 Processed foods
BT3 Foods

Meals
BT1 Processed foods
BT2 Foods
NT1 Airline meals
NT1 Army rations
NT1 Breakfast
NT2 Breakfast foods
NT1 Canteen meals
NT1 Casseroles
NT1 Curries
NT1 Dinners
NT1 Dishes
NT2 Meat dishes
NT2 Side dishes
NT1 Entrees
NT1 Frozen meals
NT1 Goulash
NT1 Gouter
NT1 Hospital meals
NT1 Lunches
NT1 Meal replacers
NT1 Military rations
NT1 Prepared dishes
NT1 Prepared meals
NT1 Pub meals
NT1 Ready meals
NT1 Ready to eat meals
NT1 School meals
NT1 Sous vide meals
NT1 Space flight foods
RT Catering
RT Menus

Meat
SN use for meat in general; meat from defined species is under Meat specific
BT1 Animal foods
BT2 Foods
NT1 Carcasses
NT2 Animal carcasses
NT2 Antelope carcasses
NT2 Bison carcasses
NT2 Buffalo carcasses
NT2 Calf carcasses
NT2 Camel carcasses
NT2 Carcass condemnation
NT2 Cattle carcasses
NT2 Chicken carcasses
NT2 Deer carcasses
NT2 Duck carcasses
NT2 Emu carcasses
NT2 Game carcasses
NT2 Gazelle carcasses
NT2 Goat carcasses
NT2 Goose carcasses
NT2 Hare carcasses
NT2 Horse carcasses
NT2 Lamb carcasses
NT2 Ostrich carcasses
NT2 Partridge carcasses
NT2 Pheasant carcasses
NT2 Pigeon carcasses
NT2 Poultry carcasses
NT2 Quail carcasses
NT2 Rabbit carcasses
NT2 Ram carcasses
NT2 Reindeer carcasses
NT2 Rhea carcasses
NT2 Seal carcasses
NT2 Sheep carcasses
NT2 Swine carcasses
NT2 Turkey carcasses
NT2 Veal calf carcasses
NT2 Whale carcasses
NT2 Wild boar carcasses
NT2 Yak carcasses
NT1 Dried meat
NT1 Meat extenders
NT1 Meat factories
NT1 Meat industry
NT1 Meat mince
NT1 Meat specific
NT2 Alligator meat
NT2 Antelope meat
NT3 Antelope carcasses
NT2 Bear meat
NT2 Beef
NT3 Beefburgers
NT3 Beef extracts
NT3 Beef loaf
NT3 Beef mince
NT3 Beef products
NT4 Beef patties
NT3 Beef roasts
NT3 Beef steaks
NT3 Calf carcasses
NT3 Cattle carcasses
NT3 Corned beef
NT3 Oxtail
NT2 Bison meat
NT3 Bison carcasses
NT2 Buffalo meat
NT3 Buffalo carcasses
NT2 Camel meat
NT3 Camel carcasses
NT2 Crocodile meat
NT2 Elk meat
NT2 Game meat
NT3 Game carcasses
NT2 Gazelle meat
NT3 Gazelle carcasses
NT2 Goat meat
NT3 Capretto
NT3 Chevon
NT3 Goat carcasses
NT2 Hare meat

NT3 Hare carcasses
NT2 Horse meat
NT3 Horse carcasses
NT2 Kangaroo meat
NT2 Lamb
NT3 Lamb carcasses
NT3 Lamb chops
NT3 Lamb mince
NT2 Moose meat
NT2 Mutton
NT3 Ram carcasses
NT3 Sheep carcasses
NT2 Partridge meat
NT3 Partridge carcasses
NT2 Pheasant meat
NT3 Pheasant carcasses
NT2 Pigeon meat
NT3 Pigeon carcasses
NT2 Pork
NT3 Boar meat
NT3 Lacon
NT3 Pork bellies
NT3 Pork chops
NT3 Pork mince
NT3 Pork products
NT4 Charcuterie products
NT4 Pork patties
NT3 Swine carcasses
NT3 Wild boar meat
NT4 Wild boar carcasses
NT2 Poultry meat
NT3 Chicken meat
NT4 Chicken carcasses
NT4 Chicken drumsticks
NT4 Chicken mince
NT4 Chicken nuggets
NT4 Chicken products
NT5 Chicken patties
NT3 Duck meat
NT4 Duck carcasses
NT3 Emu meat
NT4 Emu carcasses
NT3 Goose meat
NT4 Goose carcasses
NT3 Ostrich meat
NT4 Ostrich carcasses
NT3 Poultry breast
NT3 Poultry carcasses
NT3 Poultry meat industry
NT3 Poultry products
NT3 Quail meat
NT4 Quail carcasses
NT3 Rhea meat
NT4 Rhea carcasses
NT3 Turkey meat
NT4 Turkey carcasses
NT4 Turkey mince
NT4 Turkey products
NT5 Turkey ham
NT5 Turkey patties
NT2 Rabbit meat
NT3 Rabbit carcasses
NT2 Reindeer meat
NT3 Reindeer carcasses
NT2 Seal meat
NT3 Seal carcasses
NT2 Snail meat
NT2 Veal
NT3 Veal calf carcasses
NT2 Venison
NT3 Deer carcasses
NT2 Whale meat
NT3 Whale carcasses
NT2 Yak meat
NT3 Yak carcasses
NT1 Mechanically recovered meat
NT1 Red meat
NT1 Steaks
RT Connective tissues
RT Lean
RT Meat products
RT Offal
RT Tenderization
RT Tumbling
RT Tylose
UF Animal tissues
UF Muscles
UF Myofibrils

Meat alternatives
USE **Meat substitutes**

Meat analogues
BT1 Simulated foods
BT2 Processed foods
BT3 Foods
RT Meat substitutes

Meat balls
BT1 Meat products
BT2 Animal foods
BT3 Foods

Meat dishes
BT1 Dishes
BT2 Meals
BT3 Processed foods
BT4 Foods
BT1 Meat products
BT2 Animal foods
BT3 Foods

Meat emulsions
BT1 Meat products
BT2 Animal foods
BT3 Foods

Meat extenders
BT1 Meat
BT2 Animal foods
BT3 Foods

Meat extracts
BT1 Extracts
BT2 Flavourings
BT3 Additives
BT1 Meat products
BT2 Animal foods
BT3 Foods

Meat factories
BT1 Food factories
BT1 Meat
BT2 Animal foods
BT3 Foods

Meat industry
BT1 Food industry
BT2 Industries
BT1 Meat
BT2 Animal foods
BT3 Foods

Meat loaf
BT1 Meat products
BT2 Animal foods
BT3 Foods

Meat mince
BT1 Meat
BT2 Animal foods
BT3 Foods
UF Ground meat
UF Minced meat

Meat pastes
BT1 Meat products
BT2 Animal foods
BT3 Foods
BT1 Pastes
BT2 Processed foods
BT3 Foods

Meat patties
BT1 Patties
BT2 Meat products
BT3 Animal foods
BT4 Foods
NT1 Beef patties
NT1 Chicken patties
NT1 Pork patties
NT1 Turkey patties

Meat pies
HN heading up to vol. 24 (1992)
BT1 Meat products
BT2 Animal foods
BT3 Foods
BT1 Pies
BT2 Bakery products
BT3 Cereal products
BT4 Plant foods
BT5 Foods
NT1 Cornish pasties

Meat products
BT1 Animal foods
BT2 Foods
NT1 Bacon
NT2 Baconburgers
NT1 Beef loaf
NT1 Biltong
NT1 Brawn
NT1 Bresaola
NT1 Brined meat
NT1 Burgers
NT2 Baconburgers
NT2 Beefburgers
NT2 Cheeseburgers
NT2 Hamburgers
NT1 Cevapcici
NT1 Charqui
NT1 Chicken nuggets
NT1 Corned beef
NT1 Cornish pasties
NT1 Cured meat
NT1 Doner kebabs
NT1 Dried meat products
NT1 Fricadelles
NT1 Frogs legs

NT1 Gravy
NT2 Gravy powders
NT1 Gyros
NT1 Haggis
NT1 Ham
NT2 Boiled ham
NT2 Dry cured ham
NT2 Dry ham
NT2 Gammon
NT2 Iberian ham
NT2 Parma ham
NT2 Serrano ham
NT1 Jerky
NT1 Kasseler
NT1 Kebabs
NT1 Luncheon meat
NT1 Meat balls
NT1 Meat dishes
NT1 Meat emulsions
NT1 Meat extracts
NT1 Meat loaf
NT1 Meat pastes
NT1 Meat pies
NT2 Cornish pasties
NT1 Pastirma
NT2 Pasterma
NT1 Pastrami
NT1 Pates
NT2 Fish pates
NT2 Liver pates
NT2 Terrines
NT1 Patties
NT2 Meat patties
NT3 Beef patties
NT3 Chicken patties
NT3 Pork patties
NT3 Turkey patties
NT1 Pemmican
NT1 Ragout
NT1 Restructured meat products
NT1 Rissoles
NT1 Sausages
NT2 Ambaritsa
NT2 Androlla
NT2 Beef sausages
NT2 Bierschinken
NT2 Bierwurst
NT2 Blood sausages
NT3 Black puddings
NT2 Bockwurst
NT2 Boiled sausages
NT2 Bologna
NT2 Bratwurst
NT2 Bruehwurst
NT2 Capocollo
NT2 Cervelat
NT2 Chicken sausages
NT2 Chinese sausages
NT2 Chistorra
NT2 Chorizo
NT2 Coppas
NT2 Corn dogs
NT2 Dry sausages
NT2 Fermented sausages
NT2 Fleischwurst
NT2 Frankfurters
NT3 Hot dogs
NT3 Turkey frankfurters
NT3 Wieners
NT2 Knackwurst
NT2 Kochwurst
NT2 Lamb sausages
NT2 Liver sausages
NT2 Longaniza
NT2 Loukanka
NT2 Merguez
NT2 Mettwurst
NT2 Mortadella
NT2 Mutton sausages
NT2 Pepperoni
NT2 Pork sausages
NT2 Poultry sausages
NT2 Rohwurst
NT2 Salami
NT2 Salchichon
NT2 Saucisson
NT2 Sausage emulsions
NT2 Sausagemeat
NT2 Soudjouk
NT2 Sucuk
NT2 Summer sausages
NT2 Turkey sausages
NT2 Vienna sausages
NT2 Weisswurst
NT2 Wuerstel
NT1 Schmalzfleisch
NT1 Shashlik
NT1 Speck
NT1 Surimi
RT Meat

Meat sauces
BT1 Sauces
BT2 Condiments
BT3 Flavourings
BT4 Additives

Meat specific
BT1 Meat
BT2 Animal foods
BT3 Foods
NT1 Alligator meat
NT1 Antelope meat
NT2 Antelope carcasses
NT1 Bear meat
NT1 Beef
NT2 Beefburgers
NT2 Beef extracts
NT2 Beef loaf
NT2 Beef mince
NT2 Beef products
NT3 Beef patties
NT2 Beef roasts
NT2 Beef steaks
NT2 Calf carcasses
NT2 Cattle carcasses
NT2 Corned beef
NT2 Oxtail
NT1 Bison meat
NT2 Bison carcasses
NT1 Buffalo meat
NT2 Buffalo carcasses
NT1 Camel meat
NT2 Camel carcasses
NT1 Crocodile meat
NT1 Elk meat
NT1 Game meat
NT2 Game carcasses
NT1 Gazelle meat
NT2 Gazelle carcasses
NT1 Goat meat
NT2 Capretto
NT2 Chevon
NT2 Goat carcasses
NT1 Hare meat
NT2 Hare carcasses
NT1 Horse meat
NT2 Horse carcasses
NT1 Kangaroo meat
NT1 Lamb
NT2 Lamb carcasses
NT2 Lamb chops
NT2 Lamb mince
NT1 Moose meat
NT1 Mutton
NT2 Ram carcasses
NT2 Sheep carcasses
NT1 Partridge meat
NT2 Partridge carcasses
NT1 Pheasant meat
NT2 Pheasant carcasses
NT1 Pigeon meat
NT2 Pigeon carcasses
NT1 Pork
NT2 Boar meat
NT2 Lacon
NT2 Pork bellies
NT2 Pork chops
NT2 Pork mince
NT2 Pork products
NT3 Charcuterie products
NT3 Pork patties
NT2 Swine carcasses
NT2 Wild boar meat
NT3 Wild boar carcasses
NT1 Poultry meat
NT2 Chicken meat
NT3 Chicken carcasses
NT3 Chicken drumsticks
NT3 Chicken mince
NT3 Chicken nuggets
NT3 Chicken products
NT4 Chicken patties
NT2 Duck meat
NT3 Duck carcasses
NT2 Emu meat
NT3 Emu carcasses
NT2 Goose meat
NT3 Goose carcasses
NT2 Ostrich meat
NT3 Ostrich carcasses
NT2 Poultry breast
NT2 Poultry carcasses
NT2 Poultry meat industry
NT2 Poultry products
NT2 Quail meat
NT3 Quail carcasses
NT2 Rhea meat
NT3 Rhea carcasses
NT2 Turkey meat
NT3 Turkey carcasses
NT3 Turkey mince
NT3 Turkey products
NT4 Turkey ham
NT4 Turkey patties
NT1 Rabbit meat
NT2 Rabbit carcasses
NT1 Reindeer meat

NT2 Reindeer carcasses
NT1 Seal meat
NT2 Seal carcasses
NT1 Snail meat
NT1 Veal
NT2 Veal calf carcasses
NT1 Venison
NT2 Deer carcasses
NT1 Whale meat
NT2 Whale carcasses
NT1 Yak meat
NT2 Yak carcasses

Meat substitutes
BT1 Simulated foods
BT2 Processed foods
BT3 Foods
RT Meat analogues
UF Meat alternatives

Mechanical boning
HN boning mechanical also used in the index up to vol. 29 (1997)
BT1 Boning
BT2 Processing
BT3 Technology

Mechanical harvesting
HN harvesting mechanical also used in the index up tovol. 29 (1997)
BT1 Harvesting
BT2 Agriculture

Mechanically recovered meat
BT1 Meat
BT2 Animal foods
BT3 Foods

Mechanical properties
BT1 Physical properties
NT1 Airflow properties
NT1 Fracture properties
NT1 Hardness
NT1 Residence time distribution
NT1 Rheological properties
NT2 Compressibility
NT2 Creep
NT2 Deformation
NT2 Elasticity
NT2 Extensibility
NT2 Flow
NT3 Flow meters
NT3 Gushing
NT2 Friction
NT2 Rheology
NT2 Rheometers
NT2 Rigidity
NT2 Shear
NT2 Shear values
NT2 Stickiness
NT2 Stiffness
NT2 Stress relaxation
NT2 Stretch
NT2 Surface tension
NT2 Thixotropy
NT2 Viscoelasticity
NT2 Viscosity
NT3 Viscometers
NT2 Yield stress
NT1 Shear strength
NT1 Strength
NT1 Tensile strength
RT Sensory properties

Mechanization
BT1 Technology
RT Automation

Media
HN heading up to vol. 24
BT1 Microbiological techniques
RT Agar
RT Cell culture
RT Incubation
RT Plate counts
UF Culture media

Medicago sativa
BT1 Alfalfa
BT2 Legumes
BT3 Vegetables specific
BT4 Vegetables
BT5 Crops
BT6 Plants
BT5 Plant foods
BT6 Foods

Medical foods
SN foods formulated for specific dietary management of diseases
BT1 Novel foods
BT2 Foods
RT Functional foods
RT Nutraceutical foods
RT Nutrition

Medicinal plants
HN introduced from vol. 39, issue 1 (2007)
BT1 Plants
RT Health

Mediterranean diet
BT1 Diet
BT2 Nutrition

Medlars
BT1 Fruits specific
BT2 Fruits
BT3 Crops
BT4 Plants
BT3 Plant foods
BT4 Foods

Megasphaera
BT1 Bacteria
BT2 Microorganisms

Megrim
HN under Fish up to vol. 42 (2010)
BT1 Flatfish
BT2 Marine fish
BT3 Fish
BT4 Animals
BT4 Sea foods
BT5 Aquatic foods
BT6 Animal foods
BT7 Foods
NT1 *Lepidorhombus boscii*

Meitauza
BT1 Fermented foods
BT2 Processed foods
BT3 Foods
BT1 Okara
BT2 Soy products
BT3 Vegetable products
BT4 Plant foods
BT5 Foods

Meju
BT1 Dried foods
BT2 Processed foods
BT3 Foods
BT1 Soy products
BT2 Vegetable products
BT3 Plant foods
BT4 Foods

Melamine
BT1 Heterocyclic compounds
BT1 Organic nitrogen compounds
BT1 Plastics
BT2 Packaging materials

Melanins
BT1 Pigments

Melanoidins
BT1 Maillard reaction products
BT2 Maillard reaction
BT1 Organic compounds
BT1 Pigments

Melanosis
BT1 Discoloration
RT Blackspot

Melatonin
BT1 Heterocyclic compounds
BT1 Organic nitrogen compounds

Melengestrol
BT1 Hormones
BT2 Residues

Melezitose
HN under Sugars up to vol. 42 (2010)
BT1 Oligosaccharides
BT2 Polysaccharides
BT3 Carbohydrates
BT4 Nutrients
BT4 Organic compounds
BT2 Sugars
BT3 Carbohydrates
BT4 Nutrients
BT4 Organic compounds
BT3 Plant foods
BT4 Foods

Melibiases
USE **α-Galactosidases**

Melibiose
HN under Sugars up to vol. 42 (2010)
BT1 Disaccharides
BT2 Sugars
BT3 Carbohydrates
BT4 Nutrients
BT4 Organic compounds

BT3 Plant foods
BT4 Foods

Mellorine
BT1 Ice cream
BT2 Dairy products
BT3 Animal foods
BT4 Foods
BT2 Frozen foods
BT3 Processed foods
BT4 Foods

Melomel
BT1 Alcoholic beverages
BT2 Beverages alcoholic
BT3 Beverages
RT Honey beverages
RT Mead

Melon juices
HN introduced from vol. 39, issue 1 (2007)
BT1 Fruit juices
BT2 Fruit products
BT3 Plant foods
BT4 Foods
BT2 Soft drinks
BT3 Beverages
RT Melons

Melons
BT1 Fruits specific
BT2 Fruits
BT3 Crops
BT4 Plants
BT3 Plant foods
BT4 Foods
NT1 Cantaloupes
NT1 Honeydew melons
NT1 Muskmelons
RT Melon juices

Melon seeds
BT1 Oilseeds
BT2 Seeds
BT3 Plant foods
BT4 Foods

Melting
BT1 Thermophysical properties
BT2 Physical properties

Melting point
USE **m.p.**

Membrane bioreactors
BT1 Bioreactors
BT2 Fermentation technology
BT3 Biotechnology
BT4 Technology
BT3 Process control
BT4 Technology

Membrane distillation
HN introduced from vol. 39, issue 1 (2007)
BT1 Processing
BT2 Technology

Membranes
NT1 Ceramic membranes
NT1 Liquid membranes
RT Biological membranes
RT Dialysis
RT Filtration
RT Fouling
RT Ultrafiltration

Memory
HN introduced from vol. 39, issue 1 (2007)
BT1 Cognitive performance
BT2 Behavioural effects
BT3 Human physiology
BT4 Physiology
BT5 Science

Men
BT1 Population groups

Menadione
BT1 Vitamins
BT2 Nutrients
UF Vitamin K_3

Menaquinones
BT1 Vitamins
BT2 Nutrients
UF Vitamin K_2 series

Menhaden
BT1 Marine fish
BT2 Fish
BT3 Animals
BT3 Sea foods
BT4 Aquatic foods
BT5 Animal foods
BT6 Foods
NT1 *Brevoortia tyrannus*

Menhaden oils
BT1 Fish oils
BT2 Oils fish
BT3 Fish products
BT4 Sea foods
BT5 Aquatic foods
BT6 Animal foods
BT7 Foods
BT3 Marine oils
BT4 Oils
BT5 Lipids
BT6 Nutrients

Menopause
BT1 Reproduction
BT2 Human physiology
BT3 Physiology
BT4 Science

Menstrual cycle
SN includes premenstrual syndrome
BT1 Reproduction
BT2 Human physiology
BT3 Physiology
BT4 Science

Mental health
HN introduced from vol. 39, issue 1 (2007)
BT1 Health
RT Psychiatric disorders

Menthol
HN also under Flavourings up to vol. 42 (2010)
BT1 Alcohols
BT1 Aroma compounds
BT2 Flavour compounds
BT2 Volatile compounds
BT1 Monoterpenoids
BT2 Terpenoids
BT3 Lipids
BT4 Nutrients

Menthone
BT1 Aroma compounds
BT2 Flavour compounds
BT2 Volatile compounds
BT1 Monoterpenoids
BT2 Terpenoids
BT3 Lipids
BT4 Nutrients

Menus
HN introduced from vol. 41, issue 1 (2009)
RT Catering
RT Meals

Mercaptans
SN syn. thiols
BT1 Thiols
BT2 Organic sulfur compounds
NT1 Methyl mercaptan

Mercaptoethanol
BT1 Thiols
BT2 Organic sulfur compounds

Mercaptophos
USE **Fenthion**

Mercosur
BT1 Trade
BT2 Economics

Mercury
SN symbol Hg is also used in the index
BT1 Metals
BT2 Elements
BT3 Minerals
BT4 Nutrients
NT1 Hg
NT1 Methylmercury

Mergers
BT1 Food business
BT2 Economics

Merguez
BT1 Sausages
BT2 Meat products
BT3 Animal foods
BT4 Foods

Meringues
BT1 Egg products
BT2 Animal foods
BT3 Foods
RT Egg whites

Merissa
BT1 Beer
BT2 Alcoholic beverages

BT3 Beverages alcoholic
BT4 Beverages

Merluccius australis
BT1 Hake
BT2 Marine fish
BT3 Fish
BT4 Animals
BT4 Sea foods
BT5 Aquatic foods
BT6 Animal foods
BT7 Foods

Merluccius hubbsi
BT1 Hake
BT2 Marine fish
BT3 Fish
BT4 Animals
BT4 Sea foods
BT5 Aquatic foods
BT6 Animal foods
BT7 Foods

Merluccius merluccius
BT1 Hake
BT2 Marine fish
BT3 Fish
BT4 Animals
BT4 Sea foods
BT5 Aquatic foods
BT6 Animal foods
BT7 Foods

Merluccius productus
BT1 Pacific hake
BT2 Hake
BT3 Marine fish
BT4 Fish
BT5 Animals
BT5 Sea foods
BT6 Aquatic foods
BT7 Animal foods
BT8 Foods

Mesentericins
BT1 Bacteriocins
BT2 Antibiotics
BT3 Drugs
BT4 Residues
RT *Leuconostoc mesenteroides*

Mesona procumbens
BT1 Hsian-tsao
BT2 Plants

Mesophiles
SN organisms with optimum growth between 20 and 45 C
BT1 Microorganisms
RT Psychrophiles
RT Psychrotrophs
RT Thermophiles

Mesquite pods
BT1 Legumes
BT2 Vegetables specific
BT3 Vegetables
BT4 Crops
BT5 Plants
BT4 Plant foods
BT5 Foods

Mesquite seed gums
HN under Legumes up to vol. 42 (2010)
BT1 Gums
BT2 Polysaccharides
BT3 Carbohydrates
BT4 Nutrients
BT4 Organic compounds
BT2 Stabilizers
BT3 Additives
BT2 Thickeners
BT3 Additives

Metabisulfites
BT1 Preservatives
BT2 Additives
BT1 Sulfites
BT2 Salts
NT1 Potassium metabisulfite
NT1 Sodium metabisulfite
NT1 Sodium pyrosulfite
UF Metabisulphites

Metabisulphites
HN used for metabisulfites up to vol. 35, issue 6 (2003)
USE **Metabisulfites**

Metabolic disorders
SN includes disorders of amino acid, carbohydrate and mineral metabolism
BT1 Diseases
RT Allergies
RT Diet
RT Nutrition

Metabolic engineering
HN introduced from vol. 39, issue 1 (2007)
BT1 Genetic techniques
BT2 Genetics

Metabolic rate
HN introduced from vol. 39, issue 1 (2007)
BT1 Metabolism
BT2 Physiology
BT3 Science
RT Thermogenesis

Metabolic syndrome
HN introduced from vol. 39, issue 1 (2007)
BT1 Diseases

Metabolism
HN introduced from vol. 38, issue 8 (2006)
BT1 Physiology
BT2 Science
NT1 Bioaccumulation
NT1 Biohydrogenation
NT1 Biomagnification
NT1 Metabolic rate
NT1 Metabolomics
RT Human metabolism

Metabolomics
HN introduced from vol. 39, issue 1 (2007)
BT1 Analytical techniques
BT1 Metabolism
BT2 Physiology
BT3 Science
RT Genomics
RT Proteomics

Metacercariae
BT1 Parasites
BT2 Pests

Metalaxyl
HN introduced from vol. 37, issue 5 (2005)
BT1 Fungicides
BT2 Pesticides
BT3 Biocides
BT3 Residues

Metaldehyde
BT1 Molluscicides
BT2 Pesticides
BT3 Biocides
BT3 Residues

Metal detectors
BT1 Equipment
BT2 Technology

Metalloenzymes
BT1 Enzymes

Metallothioneins
BT1 Proteins
BT2 Nutrients

Metals
HN heading up to vol. 24 (1992); non-descriptor from 1993 (USE Minerals); reinstated (as heading) from vol. 43, issue 1 (2011)
BT1 Elements
BT2 Minerals
BT3 Nutrients
NT1 Ag
NT1 Aluminium
NT2 Al
NT2 Al compounds
NT1 Au
NT1 Ba
NT1 Be
NT1 Bi
NT1 Cadmium
NT2 Cd
NT1 Calcium
NT2 Ca
NT1 Ce
NT1 Cobalt
NT2 Co
NT1 Copper
NT2 Cu
NT1 Cr
NT1 Ga
NT1 Heavy metals
NT1 Iron
NT2 Fe
NT2 Ferritin
NT1 Lanthanides
NT2 La
NT2 Yb
NT1 Lead
NT2 Pb
NT1 Li

NT1 Magnesium
NT2 Mg
NT1 Manganese
NT2 Mn
NT1 Mercury
NT2 Hg
NT2 Methylmercury
NT1 Mo
NT1 Nb
NT1 Ni
NT1 Os
NT1 Pd
NT1 Potassium
NT2 K
NT1 Pt
NT1 Rb
NT1 Re
NT1 Rhodium
NT1 Ru
NT1 Sc
NT1 Sodium
NT2 Na
NT2 Sodium low diet
NT2 Sodium low foods
NT1 Sr
NT1 Th
NT1 Ti
NT1 Tin
NT2 Sn
NT1 Tl
NT1 V
NT1 W
NT1 Y
NT1 Zinc
NT2 Zn
NT1 Zr
UF Trace metals

Metanil yellow
BT1 Colorants
BT2 Additives

Metaphos
USE **Parathion-methyl**

Metasystox
USE **Demeton-*S*-methyl**

Meters
BT1 Apparatus
BT2 Technology

Methabenzthiazuron
BT1 Herbicides
BT2 Pesticides
BT3 Biocides
BT3 Residues
UF Tribunil

Methamidophos
BT1 Acaricides
BT2 Pesticides
BT3 Biocides
BT3 Residues
BT1 Organophosphorus insecticides
BT2 Insecticides
BT3 Pesticides
BT4 Biocides
BT4 Residues
BT2 Organophosphorus pesticides
BT3 Pesticides
BT4 Biocides
BT4 Residues
UF Monitor

Methanal
SN syn. formaldehyde
BT1 Formaldehyde
BT2 Aldehydes
BT3 Carbonyl compounds
BT4 Organic compounds
BT2 Preservatives
BT3 Additives
RT Disinfection

Methane
BT1 Gases
BT2 Physical phases
BT3 Chemistry
BT4 Science
BT1 Hydrocarbons
BT2 Organic compounds
RT Biogas

Methanearsonic acid
USE **Methylarsonic acid**

Methanethiol
SN syn. methyl mercaptan
BT1 Aroma compounds
BT2 Flavour compounds
BT2 Volatile compounds
BT1 Thiols
BT2 Organic sulfur compounds
BT1 Volatile sulfur compounds
BT2 Volatile compounds
NT1 Methyl mercaptan
RT Off odour

Methanol
BT1 Alcohols
BT1 Solvents
UF Methyl alcohol

Methanolysis
HN introduced from vol. 39, issue 1 (2007)
BT1 Alcoholysis
BT2 Esterification

Methazole
BT1 Herbicides
BT2 Pesticides
BT3 Biocides
BT3 Residues

Methidathion
BT1 Organophosphorus insecticides
BT2 Insecticides
BT3 Pesticides
BT4 Biocides
BT4 Residues
BT2 Organophosphorus pesticides
BT3 Pesticides
BT4 Biocides
BT4 Residues
UF Supracide

Methimazole
BT1 Antithyroid agents
BT2 Drugs
BT3 Residues
UF Tapazole

Methional
BT1 Aldehydes
BT2 Carbonyl compounds
BT3 Organic compounds
BT1 Aroma compounds
BT2 Flavour compounds
BT2 Volatile compounds
BT1 Thiols
BT2 Organic sulfur compounds

Methionine
BT1 Amino acids
BT2 Nutrients
BT2 Organic acids
BT3 Acids
BT2 Organic nitrogen compounds
BT1 Organic sulfur compounds
NT1 *S*-Adenosyl-L-methionine
NT1 *S*-Methylmethionine
NT1 Selenomethionine

Methionol
HN also under Flavour compounds up to vol. 42 (2010)
BT1 Alcohols
BT1 Aroma compounds
BT2 Flavour compounds
BT2 Volatile compounds
BT1 Thiols
BT2 Organic sulfur compounds

Methomyl
BT1 Acaricides
BT2 Pesticides
BT3 Biocides
BT3 Residues
BT1 *N*-Methylcarbamate insecticides
BT2 Insecticides
BT3 Pesticides
BT4 Biocides
BT4 Residues
BT2 *N*-Methylcarbamate pesticides
BT3 Carbamate pesticides
BT4 Pesticides
BT5 Biocides
BT5 Residues
UF Lannate

Methoprene
BT1 Insecticides
BT2 Pesticides
BT3 Biocides
BT3 Residues

Methoxychlor
BT1 Organochlorine insecticides
BT2 Insecticides
BT3 Pesticides
BT4 Biocides
BT4 Residues
BT2 Organochlorine pesticides

BT3 Pesticides
BT4 Biocides
BT4 Residues
UF DMDT

Methyl alcohol
USE **Methanol**

Methylamine
HN heading up to vol. 24 (1992)
BT1 Amines
BT2 Organic nitrogen compounds

Methylarsonic acid
BT1 Arsenicals
BT2 Arsenic
BT3 Contaminants
BT4 Contamination
BT3 Elements
BT4 Minerals
BT5 Nutrients
BT1 Herbicides
BT2 Pesticides
BT3 Biocides
BT3 Residues
UF Methanearsonic acid

Methylation
BT1 Modification

Methyl benzoate
HN introduced from vol. 39, issue 1 (2007)
BT1 Aroma compounds
BT2 Flavour compounds
BT2 Volatile compounds
BT1 Esters
BT2 Organic compounds

Methyl bromide
BT1 Fumigants
BT2 Biocides
UF Bromomethane

3-Methylbutanal
HN also under Volatile compounds up to vol. 42 (2010)
SN syn. isovaleraldehyde
BT1 Aldehydes
BT2 Carbonyl compounds
BT3 Organic compounds
BT1 Aroma compounds
BT2 Flavour compounds
BT2 Volatile compounds
NT1 Isovaleraldehyde
RT Off odour

Methyl butanol
SN syn. isopentyl alcohol; syn. isoamyl alcohol
BT1 Isoamyl alcohol
BT2 Alcohols
BT2 Aroma compounds
BT3 Flavour compounds
BT3 Volatile compounds

Methyl carbamate
BT1 Carcinogens
BT2 Mutagens
BT1 Esters
BT2 Organic compounds
BT1 Organic nitrogen compounds

***N*-Methylcarbamate insecticides**
HN insecticides N-methylcarbamate also used in the index up to vol. 29 (1997)
BT1 Insecticides
BT2 Pesticides
BT3 Biocides
BT3 Residues
BT1 *N*-Methylcarbamate pesticides
BT2 Carbamate pesticides
BT3 Pesticides
BT4 Biocides
BT4 Residues
NT1 Aldicarb
NT1 Carbaryl
NT1 Carbofuran
NT1 Ethiofencarb
NT1 Methomyl
NT1 Oxamyl
NT1 Pirimicarb
NT1 Propoxur

***N*-Methylcarbamate pesticides**
HN pesticides N-methylcarbamate also used in the index up to vol. 29 (1997)
BT1 Carbamate pesticides
BT2 Pesticides
BT3 Biocides
BT3 Residues
NT1 *N*-Methylcarbamate insecticides
NT2 Aldicarb
NT2 Carbaryl
NT2 Carbofuran
NT2 Ethiofencarb
NT2 Methomyl
NT2 Oxamyl
NT2 Pirimicarb
NT2 Propoxur

Methylcellulose
BT1 Bulking agents
BT2 Thickeners
BT3 Additives
BT1 Celluloses
BT2 Glucans
BT3 Polysaccharides
BT4 Carbohydrates
BT5 Nutrients
BT5 Organic compounds

1-Methylcyclopropene
BT1 Plant growth regulators
BT2 Cultivation
BT3 Agriculture

Methylene chloride
SN syn. dichloromethane
BT1 Chlorinated hydrocarbons
BT2 Organic halogen compounds
BT1 Solvents

Methylglyoxal
SN syn. pyruvaldehyde
BT1 Aldehydes
BT2 Carbonyl compounds
BT3 Organic compounds

Methylhistidine
BT1 Amino acids
BT2 Nutrients
BT2 Organic acids
BT3 Acids
BT2 Organic nitrogen compounds

Methyl iodide
BT1 Disinfectants
BT2 Disinfection
BT3 Hygiene
BT1 Organic halogen compounds

2-Methylisoborneol
BT1 Monoterpenoids
BT2 Terpenoids
BT3 Lipids
BT4 Nutrients
RT Taints

Methyl jasmonate
BT1 Plant growth regulators
BT2 Cultivation
BT3 Agriculture
NT1 Jasmonic acid

Methyl linoleate
HN introduced from vol. 37, issue 5 (2005)
BT1 Linoleates
BT2 Fatty acid esters
BT3 Esters
BT4 Organic compounds

Methyl mercaptan
SN syn. methanethiol
BT1 Mercaptans
BT2 Thiols
BT3 Organic sulfur compounds
BT1 Methanethiol
BT2 Aroma compounds
BT3 Flavour compounds
BT3 Volatile compounds
BT2 Thiols
BT3 Organic sulfur compounds
BT2 Volatile sulfur compounds
BT3 Volatile compounds

Methylmercaptofos
USE **Demeton-*S*-methyl**

Methylmercury
BT1 Mercury
BT2 Metals
BT3 Elements
BT4 Minerals
BT5 Nutrients

***S*-Methylmethionine**
HN under Nutrients, Organic nitrogen compounds and Organic sulfur compounds up to vol. 42 (2010)
BT1 Methionine
BT2 Amino acids
BT3 Nutrients
BT3 Organic acids

BT4 Acids
BT3 Organic nitrogen compounds
BT2 Organic sulfur compounds
UF Vitamin U

Methylnitrophos
USE **Fenitrothion**

Methylobacillus
BT1 Bacteria
BT2 Microorganisms

Methylococcus
BT1 Bacteria
BT2 Microorganisms

Methylomonas
BT1 Bacteria
BT2 Microorganisms

Methylparaben
BT1 Parabens
BT2 Hydroxybenzoic acid esters
BT3 Esters
BT4 Organic compounds
BT3 Preservatives
BT4 Additives

Methylparathion
USE **Parathion-methyl**

2-Methylpropanal
HN also under Volatile compounds up to vol. 42 (2010)
SN syn. isobutyraldehyde
BT1 Isobutyraldehyde
BT2 Aldehydes
BT3 Carbonyl compounds
BT4 Organic compounds
BT2 Aroma compounds
BT3 Flavour compounds
BT3 Volatile compounds

Methyl propanol
SN syn. isobutyl alcohol; syn. isobutanol
BT1 Isobutanol
BT2 Alcohols
BT2 Aroma compounds
BT3 Flavour compounds
BT3 Volatile compounds

Methyl sulfide
SN syn. dimethyl sulfide
BT1 Dimethyl sulfide
BT2 Organic sulfur compounds
BT2 Solvents
BT2 Sulfides
BT3 Salts
UF Methyl sulphide

Methyl sulphide
HN used for methyl sulfide up to vol. 35, issue 6 (2003)
USE **Methyl sulfide**

Methylthiophanate
USE **Thiophanate-methyl**

Methylthiouracil
BT1 Antithyroid agents
BT2 Drugs
BT3 Residues

Methyltransferases
HN introduced from vol. 39, issue 1 (2007)
BT1 Transferases
BT2 Enzymes

Methylxanthines
BT1 Alkaloids
BT2 Organic nitrogen compounds

Metmyoglobin
BT1 Myoglobin
BT2 Animal proteins
BT3 Proteins animal
BT4 Proteins
BT5 Nutrients
BT2 Pigments

Metolachlor
BT1 Herbicides
BT2 Pesticides
BT3 Biocides
BT3 Residues

Metribuzin
BT1 Herbicides
BT2 Pesticides
BT3 Biocides
BT3 Residues
UF Sencor

Metronidazole
HN introduced from vol. 39, issue 1 (2007)
BT1 Antibiotics
BT2 Drugs
BT3 Residues

Metroxylon
BT1 Palms
BT2 Plants
RT Sago

Metschnikowia
HN introduced from vol. 39, issue 1 (2007)
BT1 Yeasts
BT2 Fungi
BT3 Microorganisms
NT1 *Metschnikowia pulcherrima*

Metschnikowia pulcherrima
BT1 *Metschnikowia*
BT2 Yeasts
BT3 Fungi
BT4 Microorganisms

Mettwurst
BT1 Sausages
BT2 Meat products
BT3 Animal foods
BT4 Foods

Mevalonic acid
BT1 Organic acids
BT2 Acids

Mevinphos
BT1 Acaricides
BT2 Pesticides
BT3 Biocides
BT3 Residues
BT1 Organophosphorus insecticides
BT2 Insecticides
BT3 Pesticides
BT4 Biocides
BT4 Residues
BT2 Organophosphorus pesticides
BT3 Pesticides
BT4 Biocides
BT4 Residues
UF Phosdrin

Mexico
BT1 Central America
BT2 America
RT Organization for Economic Cooperation and Development

Mezcal
BT1 Spirits
BT2 Alcoholic beverages
BT3 Beverages alcoholic
BT4 Beverages

Mg
SN index heading is Magnesium
BT1 Magnesium
BT2 Metals
BT3 Elements
BT4 Minerals
BT5 Nutrients

$MgCl_2$
HN introduced from vol. 39, issue 1 (2007); also under Magnesium up to vol. 42 (2010)
BT1 Additives
BT1 Chlorides
BT2 Salts

Micellar electrokinetic chromatography
BT1 Chromatography
BT2 Analytical techniques

Microalgae
BT1 Algae
BT2 Microorganisms
NT1 *Chlamydomonas*
NT1 *Chlorella*
NT2 *Chlorella vulgaris*
NT1 *Chlorococcum*
NT1 *Crypthecodinium*
NT2 *Crypthecodinium cohnii*
NT1 Dinoflagellates
NT2 *Alexandrium*
NT3 *Alexandrium catenella*
NT3 *Alexandrium minutum*
NT3 *Alexandrium tamarense*
NT1 *Dunaliella*
NT2 *Dunaliella salina*
NT1 *Euglena*
NT2 *Euglena gracilis*

NT1 *Haematococcus*
NT2 *Haematococcus pluvialis*
NT1 *Nitzschia*
NT2 *Nitzschia laevis*
NT1 *Phaeodactylum*
NT2 *Phaeodactylum tricornutum*
NT1 *Porphyridium*
NT1 *Scenedesmus*

Microarrays
HN introduced from vol. 39, issue 1 (2007)
BT1 Analytical techniques
RT DNA microarrays
RT Proteomics

Microbacterium
BT1 Bacteria
BT2 Microorganisms

Microbial biomass
BT1 Biomass
BT2 Fermentation products
BT3 Biotechnology
BT4 Technology
BT1 Microorganisms
NT1 Bacterial biomass
NT1 Yeast biomass

Microbial contamination
BT1 Contamination
BT1 Microorganisms
NT1 Bacterial contamination
RT Microbial spoilage
RT Poisoning
RT Wild yeasts

Microbial counts
BT1 Microbiological techniques
RT Plate counts

Microbial proteins
HN heading from vol. 43 (2011); under Proteins up to vol. 42 (2010)
BT1 Microorganisms
BT1 Proteins
BT2 Nutrients
NT1 Adhesins
NT1 Aerolysins
NT1 Flagellins
NT1 Fungal proteins
NT1 Intimins
NT1 Invasins
NT1 Pilins
NT1 Porins
NT1 Siderophores
NT1 Yeast proteins

Microbial rennets
BT1 Rennets
BT2 Milk clotting enzymes
BT3 Enzymes milk clotting
BT4 Proteinases
BT5 Hydrolases
BT6 Enzymes

Microbial spoilage
HN spoilage microbial also used in the index up to vol. 29 (1997)
BT1 Spoilage
NT1 Decay
RT Bacterial contamination
RT Microbial contamination
RT Wild yeasts

Microbial spores
HN heading from vol. 28 (1996)
BT1 Spores
NT1 Bacterial spores
NT1 Fungal spores
RT Sporulation

Microbicidal compounds
BT1 Biocides
RT Antibiotics

Microbiological quality
HN heading from vol. 25 (1993)
NT1 Bacteriological quality
RT Food safety

Microbiological techniques
HN heading from vol. 25 (1993)
NT1 Ames test
NT1 Bacterial counts
NT1 Cell counts
NT1 Colony counting
NT1 Colony counts
NT1 Enrichment techniques
NT1 Flow cytometry
NT1 Fungal counts
NT1 Media
NT1 Microbial counts
NT1 MPN
NT1 Plate counts
NT1 Predictive modelling
NT2 Survival curves
NT1 Somatic cells counts
RT Cell culture
RT Gram negative bacteria
RT Gram positive bacteria
RT Microbiology

Microbiology
NT1 Bacteriology
NT2 Bacteriostats
NT1 Predictive microbiology
RT Microbiological techniques
RT Microorganisms

Microbreweries
HN introduced from vol. 37, issue 5 (2005)
BT1 Breweries
BT2 Brewing
BT3 Processing
BT4 Technology

Microchip technology
HN introduced from vol. 39, issue 1 (2007)
BT1 Apparatus
BT2 Technology
BT1 Equipment
BT2 Technology

Micrococcaceae
BT1 Bacteria
BT2 Microorganisms

Micrococcus
HN heading up to vol. 24 (1992)
BT1 Bacteria
BT2 Microorganisms
NT1 *Micrococcus luteus*

Micrococcus luteus
BT1 *Micrococcus*
BT2 Bacteria
BT3 Microorganisms

Microcrystalline celluloses
BT1 Celluloses
BT2 Glucans
BT3 Polysaccharides
BT4 Carbohydrates
BT5 Nutrients
BT5 Organic compounds
BT1 Fat substitutes
BT2 Fats
BT3 Lipids
BT4 Nutrients

Microcystins
BT1 Toxins
BT2 Residues
RT *Microcystis*

Microcystis
BT1 Cyanobacteria
BT2 Bacteria
BT3 Microorganisms
RT Microcystins

Microemulsions
BT1 Emulsions
BT2 Physical phases
BT3 Chemistry
BT4 Science

Microencapsulation
BT1 Encapsulation
BT2 Technology

Microfiltration
BT1 Filtration
BT2 Processing
BT3 Technology

Microflora
BT1 Microorganisms

Microfluidic technology
HN introduced from vol. 42, issue 1 (2010)
BT1 Technology
RT Fluids
RT Microfluidization

Microfluidization
BT1 Fluidization
BT2 Processing
BT3 Technology
RT Microfluidic technology

Micromesistius poutassou
BT1 Blue whiting
BT2 Marine fish
BT3 Fish
BT4 Animals
BT4 Sea foods
BT5 Aquatic foods
BT6 Animal foods
BT7 Foods

Micrometers
BT1 Apparatus
BT2 Technology

Micromonospora
BT1 Bacteria
BT2 Microorganisms

Micronization
BT1 Processing
BT2 Technology
RT Cereals

Micronutrients
HN introduced from vol. 43, issue 1 (2011)
SN general use only; see also other specific micronutrients
BT1 Nutrients
RT Minerals
RT Vitamins

Microorganisms
NT1 Aerobes
NT1 Algae
NT2 Microalgae
NT3 *Chlamydomonas*
NT3 *Chlorella*
NT4 *Chlorella vulgaris*
NT3 *Chlorococcum*
NT3 *Crypthecodinium*
NT4 *Crypthecodinium cohnii*
NT3 Dinoflagellates
NT4 *Alexandrium*
NT5 *Alexandrium catenella*
NT5 *Alexandrium minutum*
NT5 *Alexandrium tamarense*
NT3 *Dunaliella*
NT4 *Dunaliella salina*
NT3 *Euglena*
NT4 *Euglena gracilis*
NT3 *Haematococcus*
NT4 *Haematococcus pluvialis*
NT3 *Nitzschia*
NT4 *Nitzschia laevis*
NT3 *Phaeodactylum*
NT4 *Phaeodactylum tricornutum*
NT3 *Porphyridium*
NT3 *Scenedesmus*
NT2 Seaweeds
NT3 *Caulerpa*
NT3 *Chondrus*
NT4 *Chondrus crispus*
NT3 *Cystoseira*
NT3 Dulse
NT4 *Palmaria palmata*
NT3 *Ecklonia*
NT3 *Eucheuma*
NT3 *Fucus*
NT3 *Furcellaria*
NT3 *Gigartina*
NT3 *Gracilaria*
NT3 *Hizikia*
NT3 *Iridaea*
NT3 *Laminaria*
NT4 Kombu
NT3 Laver
NT3 *Macrocystis*
NT3 Onigusa
NT3 *Phyllophora*
NT3 *Porphyra*
NT4 Nori
NT4 *Porphyra yezoensis*
NT3 *Sargassum*
NT3 *Ulva*
NT4 Sea lettuces
NT4 *Ulva lactuca*
NT3 *Undaria*
NT4 *Undaria pinnatifida*
NT4 Wakame
NT1 Anaerobes
NT1 Antimicrobial activity
NT2 Antibacterial activity
NT2 Antifungal activity
NT2 Antiviral activity
NT1 Archaea
NT2 *Pyrococcus*
NT3 *Pyrococcus furiosus*
NT2 *Sulfolobus*
NT3 *Sulfolobus solfataricus*
NT2 *Thermococcus*
NT3 *Thermococcus kodakaraensis*
NT1 Bacteria
NT2 Acetic acid bacteria
NT2 *Acetobacter*
NT3 *Acetobacter aceti*
NT3 *Acetobacter diazotrophicus*
NT3 *Acetobacter pasteurianus*
NT3 *Acetobacter suboxydans*
NT3 *Acetobacter xylinum*
NT2 *Achromobacter*
NT2 *Acinetobacter*
NT3 *Acinetobacter calcoaceticus*
NT3 *Acinetobacter haemolyticus*
NT3 *Acinetobacter radioresistens*
NT2 *Actinobacillus*
NT2 *Actinobacteria*
NT3 Actinomycetes
NT2 *Actinomyces*
NT2 Actinomycetales
NT2 *Actinoplanes*
NT2 *Aerococcus*
NT2 *Aeromonas*
NT3 *Aeromonas caviae*
NT3 *Aeromonas hydrophila*
NT2 *Agrobacterium*
NT3 *Agrobacterium tumefaciens*
NT4 *Agrobacterium radiobacter*
NT2 *Alcaligenes*
NT3 *Alcaligenes eutrophus*
NT3 *Alcaligenes faecalis*
NT3 *Alcaligenes xylosoxydans*
NT2 *Alicyclobacillus*
NT3 *Alicyclobacillus acidocaldarius*
NT3 *Alicyclobacillus acidoterrestris*
NT2 *Alteromonas*
NT2 *Amycolatopsis*
NT2 Antibacterial activity
NT2 *Arcobacter*
NT3 *Arcobacter butzleri*
NT2 *Arthrobacter*
NT3 *Arthrobacter globiformis*
NT3 *Arthrobacter protophormiae*
NT2 *Azotobacter*
NT3 *Azotobacter chroococcum*
NT3 *Azotobacter vinelandii*
NT2 Bacilli
NT2 *Bacillus*
NT3 *Bacillus acidopullulyticus*
NT3 *Bacillus agaradhaerens*
NT3 *Bacillus alcalophilus*
NT3 *Bacillus amyloliquefaciens*
NT3 *Bacillus anthracis*
NT3 *Bacillus brevis*
NT3 *Bacillus cereus*
NT3 *Bacillus circulans*
NT3 *Bacillus coagulans*
NT3 *Bacillus firmus*
NT3 *Bacillus halodurans*
NT3 *Bacillus lentus*
NT3 *Bacillus licheniformis*
NT3 *Bacillus macerans*
NT3 *Bacillus megaterium*
NT3 *Bacillus mojavensis*
NT3 *Bacillus polymyxa*
NT3 *Bacillus pumilus*
NT3 *Bacillus sphaericus*
NT3 *Bacillus sporothermodurans*
NT3 *Bacillus stearothermophilus*
NT3 *Bacillus subtilis*
NT4 *Bacillus natto*
NT3 *Bacillus thermoleovorans*
NT3 *Bacillus thermoproteolyticus*
NT3 *Bacillus thuringiensis*
NT2 Bacterial biomass
NT2 Bacterial contamination
NT2 *Bacteroides*
NT2 *Bdellovibrio*
NT2 *Beijerinckia*
NT2 *Bifidobacterium*
NT3 *Bifidobacterium adolescentis*
NT3 *Bifidobacterium animalis*
NT3 *Bifidobacterium bifidum*
NT3 *Bifidobacterium breve*
NT3 *Bifidobacterium infantis*
NT3 *Bifidobacterium lactis*
NT3 *Bifidobacterium longum*
NT3 *Bifidobacterium pseudolongum*
NT3 *Bifidobacterium thermophilum*
NT2 *Brevibacillus*
NT2 *Brevibacterium*
NT3 *Brevibacterium flavum*
NT3 *Brevibacterium helvolum*
NT3 *Brevibacterium lactofermentum*
NT3 *Brevibacterium linens*
NT2 *Brochothrix*
NT3 *Brochothrix thermosphacta*
NT2 *Brucella*
NT2 *Burkholderia*

NT3 *Burkholderia cepacia*
NT3 *Burkholderia gladioli*
NT2 *Butyrivibrio*
NT3 *Butyrivibrio fibrisolvens*
NT2 *Campylobacter*
NT3 *Campylobacter coli*
NT3 *Campylobacter fetus*
NT3 *Campylobacter jejuni*
NT3 *Campylobacter lari*
NT2 *Carnobacterium*
NT3 *Carnobacterium divergens*
NT3 *Carnobacterium maltaromaticum*
NT4 *Carnobacterium piscicola*
NT2 *Cellulomonas*
NT3 *Cellulomonas fimi*
NT3 *Cellulomonas flavigena*
NT2 *Cellvibrio*
NT2 *Chromobacterium*
NT3 *Chromobacterium violaceum*
NT3 *Chromobacterium viscosum*
NT2 *Chryseobacterium*
NT2 *Citrobacter*
NT3 *Citrobacter freundii*
NT2 *Clostridium*
NT3 *Clostridium absonum*
NT3 *Clostridium acetobutylicum*
NT3 *Clostridium beijerinckii*
NT3 *Clostridium botulinum*
NT3 *Clostridium butyricum*
NT3 *Clostridium cellulolyticum*
NT3 *Clostridium difficile*
NT3 *Clostridium josui*
NT3 *Clostridium lentocellum*
NT3 *Clostridium perfringens*
NT3 *Clostridium sporogenes*
NT3 *Clostridium stercorarium*
NT4 *Clostridium thermolacticum*
NT3 *Clostridium thermoaceticum*
NT3 *Clostridium thermocellum*
NT3 *Clostridium thermosuccinogenes*
NT3 *Clostridium thermosulfurogenes*
NT3 *Clostridium tyrobutyricum*
NT2 Cocci
NT2 Coliforms
NT2 *Comamonas*
NT2 Corynebacteriaceae
NT2 *Corynebacterium*
NT3 *Corynebacterium casei*
NT3 *Corynebacterium glutamicum*
NT2 *Coxiella*
NT2 Cyanobacteria
NT3 *Anabaena*
NT3 Blue green algae
NT3 *Microcystis*
NT3 *Nostoc*
NT3 *Spirulina*
NT4 *Spirulina maxima*
NT4 *Spirulina platensis*
NT3 *Synechococcus*
NT3 *Synechocystis*
NT2 *Cytophaga*
NT2 *Desulfovibrio*
NT2 *Edwardsiella*
NT2 *Enterobacter*
NT3 *Enterobacter aerogenes*
NT3 *Enterobacter cloacae*
NT3 *Enterobacter sakazakii*
NT2 Enterobacteria
NT2 Enterobacteriaceae
NT2 *Enterococcus*
NT3 *Enterococcus casseliflavus*
NT3 *Enterococcus faecalis*
NT3 *Enterococcus faecium*
NT3 *Enterococcus gallinarum*
NT2 *Erwinia*
NT3 *Erwinia carotovora*
NT3 *Erwinia chrysanthemi*
NT3 *Erwinia herbicola*
NT2 *Erysipelothrix*
NT2 *Escherichia*
NT3 *Escherichia coli*
NT2 *Fibrobacter*
NT2 *Flavimonas oryzihabitans*
NT2 *Flavobacterium*
NT3 *Flavobacterium aurantiacum*
NT3 *Flavobacterium meningosepticum*
NT2 *Francisella*
NT3 *Francisella tularensis*
NT2 *Geobacillus*
NT3 *Geobacillus stearothermophilus*
NT3 *Geobacillus thermoleovorans*
NT2 *Gluconacetobacter*
NT2 *Gluconobacter*
NT3 *Acetomonas*
NT3 *Gluconobacter frateurii*
NT3 *Gluconobacter oxydans*
NT2 Gram negative bacteria
NT2 Gram positive bacteria
NT2 *Hafnia*
NT3 *Hafnia alvei*
NT2 *Halomonas*
NT2 *Helicobacter*
NT3 *Helicobacter canadensis*
NT3 *Helicobacter pylori*
NT2 Hiochi bacteria
NT2 *Klebsiella*
NT3 *Klebsiella aerogenes*
NT3 *Klebsiella oxytoca*
NT3 *Klebsiella pneumoniae*
NT3 *Klebsiella terrigena*
NT2 *Kocuria*
NT3 *Kocuria varians*
NT2 *Kurthia*
NT2 Lactic acid bacteria
NT2 Lactobacillaceae
NT2 *Lactobacillus*
NT3 *Lactobacillus acidophilus*
NT3 *Lactobacillus alimentarius*
NT3 *Lactobacillus amylophilus*
NT3 *Lactobacillus amylovorus*
NT3 *Lactobacillus brevis*
NT3 *Lactobacillus buchneri*
NT3 *Lactobacillus casei*
NT3 *Lactobacillus collinoides*
NT3 *Lactobacillus crispatus*
NT3 *Lactobacillus curvatus*
NT3 *Lactobacillus delbrueckii*
NT4 *Lactobacillus bulgaricus*
NT4 *Lactobacillus lactis*
NT3 *Lactobacillus fermentum*
NT3 *Lactobacillus fructivorans*
NT3 *Lactobacillus gasseri*
NT3 *Lactobacillus helveticus*
NT3 *Lactobacillus hilgardii*
NT3 *Lactobacillus johnsonii*
NT3 *Lactobacillus kefiranofaciens*
NT3 *Lactobacillus kefiri*
NT3 *Lactobacillus leichmannii*
NT3 *Lactobacillus lindneri*
NT3 *Lactobacillus paracasei*
NT3 *Lactobacillus paraplantarum*
NT3 *Lactobacillus pentosus*
NT3 *Lactobacillus plantarum*
NT3 *Lactobacillus pontis*
NT3 *Lactobacillus reuteri*
NT3 *Lactobacillus rhamnosus*
NT3 *Lactobacillus sakei*
NT3 *Lactobacillus salivarius*
NT3 *Lactobacillus sanfranciscensis*
NT3 *Lactobacillus viridescens*
NT2 *Lactococcus*
NT3 *Lactococcus lactis*
NT3 *Lactococcus raffinolactis*
NT2 *Legionella*
NT3 *Legionella pneumophila*
NT2 *Leptospira*
NT2 *Leuconostoc*
NT3 *Leuconostoc carnosum*
NT3 *Leuconostoc citreum*
NT3 *Leuconostoc mesenteroides*
NT3 *Leuconostoc oenos*
NT2 *Listeria*
NT3 *Listeria innocua*
NT3 *Listeria ivanovii*
NT3 *Listeria monocytogenes*
NT3 *Listeria seeligeri*
NT3 *Listeria welshimeri*
NT2 *Macrococcus*
NT3 *Macrococcus caseolyticus*
NT2 *Megasphaera*
NT2 *Methylobacillus*
NT2 *Methylococcus*
NT2 *Methylomonas*
NT2 *Microbacterium*
NT2 Micrococcaceae
NT2 *Micrococcus*
NT3 *Micrococcus luteus*
NT2 *Micromonospora*
NT2 *Moraxella*
NT2 *Morganella*
NT3 *Morganella morganii*
NT2 *Mycobacterium*
NT3 *Mycobacterium avium*
NT4 *Mycobacterium paratuberculosis*
NT3 *Mycobacterium bovis*
NT3 *Mycobacterium tuberculosis*
NT2 *Mycoplasma*

NT2 *Nitrosomonas*
NT2 *Nocardia*
NT2 *Nocardiopsis*
NT2 *Obesumbacterium*
NT2 *Oenococcus*
NT3 *Oenococcus oeni*
NT2 *Paenibacillus*
NT3 *Paenibacillus amylolyticus*
NT3 *Paenibacillus polymyxa*
NT2 *Pantoea*
NT3 *Pantoea agglomerans*
NT2 *Paracoccus*
NT2 *Pasteurella*
NT2 *Pectinatus*
NT3 *Pectinatus frisingensis*
NT2 *Pediococcus*
NT3 *Pediococcus acidilactici*
NT3 *Pediococcus damnosus*
NT3 *Pediococcus pentosaceus*
NT2 *Peptococcus*
NT2 *Photobacterium*
NT3 *Photobacterium phosphoreum*
NT2 *Plesiomonas*
NT3 *Plesiomonas shigelloides*
NT2 Probiotic bacteria
NT2 Propionibacteriaceae
NT2 *Propionibacterium*
NT3 *Propionibacterium acidipropionici*
NT4 *Propionibacterium acidi-propionici*
NT3 *Propionibacterium freudenreichii*
NT4 *Propionibacterium shermanii*
NT3 *Propionibacterium jensenii*
NT3 *Propionibacterium thoenii*
NT2 Propionic acid bacteria
NT2 Proteobacteria
NT2 *Proteus*
NT3 *Proteus mirabilis*
NT3 *Proteus vulgaris*
NT2 *Providencia*
NT2 *Pseudoalteromonas*
NT2 Pseudomonadaceae
NT2 *Pseudomonas*
NT3 *Pseudomonas aeruginosa*
NT3 *Pseudomonas cellulosa*
NT3 *Pseudomonas cepacia*
NT3 *Pseudomonas fluorescens*
NT3 *Pseudomonas fragi*
NT3 *Pseudomonas marginalis*
NT3 *Pseudomonas pseudoalcaligenes*
NT3 *Pseudomonas putida*
NT3 *Pseudomonas stutzeri*
NT3 *Pseudomonas syringae*
NT2 *Psychrobacter*
NT3 *Psychrobacter immobilis*
NT2 *Rahnella*
NT3 *Rahnella aquatilis*
NT2 *Rhizobium*
NT2 *Rhodobacter*
NT2 *Rhodococcus*
NT3 *Rhodococcus equi*
NT3 *Rhodococcus erythropolis*
NT3 *Rhodococcus opacus*
NT2 *Rhodothermus*
NT3 *Rhodothermus marinus*
NT2 *Rickettsia*
NT2 Ropy bacteria
NT2 *Ruminococcus*
NT2 *Salmonella*
NT3 *Salmonella* Agona
NT3 *Salmonella* Blockley
NT3 *Salmonella* Bredeney
NT3 *Salmonella* Choleraesuis
NT3 *Salmonella* Cubana
NT3 *Salmonella* Derby
NT3 *Salmonella* Diarizonae
NT3 *Salmonella* Dublin
NT3 Salmonellae
NT3 *Salmonella enterica*
NT3 *Salmonella* Enteritidis
NT3 *Salmonella* Gallinarum
NT3 *Salmonella* Heidelberg
NT3 *Salmonella* Indiana
NT3 *Salmonella* Infantis
NT3 *Salmonella* Java
NT3 *Salmonella* Kottbus
NT3 *Salmonella* Mbandaka
NT3 *Salmonella* Montevideo
NT3 *Salmonella* Muenchen
NT3 *Salmonella* Muenster
NT3 *Salmonella* Newport
NT3 *Salmonella* Ohio
NT3 *Salmonella* Oranienburg
NT3 *Salmonella* Panama
NT3 *Salmonella* Paratyphi
NT3 *Salmonella* Poona
NT3 *Salmonella* Pullorum
NT3 *Salmonella* Senftenberg
NT3 *Salmonella* Stanley
NT3 *Salmonella* Thompson
NT3 *Salmonella* Typhi
NT3 *Salmonella* Typhimurium
NT3 *Salmonella* Virchow
NT2 *Sarcina*
NT2 *Serratia*
NT3 *Serratia liquefaciens*
NT3 *Serratia marcescens*
NT2 *Shewanella*
NT3 *Shewanella putrefaciens*
NT2 *Shigella*
NT3 *Shigella boydii*
NT3 *Shigella dysenteriae*
NT3 *Shigella flexneri*
NT3 *Shigella sonnei*
NT2 Slime bacteria
NT2 *Sphingomonas*
NT3 *Sphingomonas paucimobilis*
NT2 Spoilage bacteria
NT2 *Staphylococcus*
NT3 *Staphylococcus aureus*
NT3 *Staphylococcus carnosus*
NT3 *Staphylococcus epidermidis*
NT3 *Staphylococcus equorum*
NT3 *Staphylococcus intermedius*
NT3 *Staphylococcus saprophyticus*
NT3 *Staphylococcus sciuri*
NT3 *Staphylococcus simulans*
NT3 *Staphylococcus xylosus*
NT2 Starters
NT3 Adjunct cultures
NT3 Butter starters
NT3 Cheese starters
NT3 Dairy starters
NT3 Lactic starters
NT3 Nuruk
NT3 Yoghurt starters
NT2 *Stenotrophomonas*
NT3 *Stenotrophomonas maltophilia*
NT2 *Streptococcus*
NT3 Lactic streptococci
NT3 *Streptococcus bovis*
NT3 *Streptococcus faecalis*
NT3 *Streptococcus faecium*
NT3 *Streptococcus macedonicus*
NT3 *Streptococcus mutans*
NT3 *Streptococcus pyogenes*
NT3 *Streptococcus salivarius*
NT3 *Streptococcus suis*
NT3 *Streptococcus thermophilus*
NT3 *Streptococcus uberis*
NT2 *Streptomyces*
NT3 *Streptomyces albulus*
NT3 *Streptomyces coelicolor*
NT3 *Streptomyces diastaticus*
NT3 *Streptomyces globisporus*
NT3 *Streptomyces griseus*
NT3 *Streptomyces lividans*
NT3 *Streptomyces murinus*
NT3 *Streptomyces olivaceoviridis*
NT3 *Streptomyces thermoviolaceus*
NT2 *Streptoverticillium*
NT3 *Streptoverticillium mobaraense*
NT2 *Tetragenococcus*
NT3 *Tetragenococcus halophilus*
NT2 *Thermoactinomyces*
NT3 *Thermoactinomyces vulgaris*
NT2 *Thermoanaerobacter*
NT3 *Thermoanaerobacter brockii*
NT3 *Thermoanaerobacter ethanolicus*
NT2 *Thermoanaerobacterium*
NT3 *Thermoanaerobacterium thermosulfurigenes*
NT2 *Thermobifida*
NT3 *Thermobifida fusca*
NT2 *Thermomonospora*
NT3 *Thermomonospora fusca*
NT2 *Thermotoga*
NT3 *Thermotoga maritima*
NT2 *Thermus*
NT3 *Thermus aquaticus*
NT3 *Thermus nonproteolyticus*
NT3 *Thermus thermophilus*
NT2 *Thiobacillus thiooxidans*
NT2 *Veillonella*
NT2 *Vibrio*
NT3 *Vibrio alginolyticus*
NT3 *Vibrio cholerae*
NT3 *Vibrio fischeri*

NT3 *Vibrio lentus*
NT3 *Vibrio metschnikovii*
NT3 *Vibrio mimicus*
NT3 *Vibrio parahaemolyticus*
NT3 *Vibrio vulnificus*
NT2 *Weissella*
NT3 *Weissella confusa*
NT3 *Weissella kimchii*
NT3 *Weissella paramesenteroides*
NT3 *Weissella viridescens*
NT2 *Xanthomonas*
NT3 *Xanthomonas campestris*
NT2 *Yersinia*
NT3 *Yersinia enterocolitica*
NT3 *Yersinia pseudotuberculosis*
NT3 *Yersinia ruckeri*
NT2 *Zymomonas*
NT3 *Zymomonas mobilis*
NT1 Biofilms
NT1 Chromista
NT2 *Phytophthora*
NT2 *Schizochytrium*
NT2 *Thraustochytrium*
NT1 Fungi
NT2 *Absidia*
NT3 *Absidia corymbifera*
NT2 *Acremonium*
NT3 *Acremonium cellulolyticus*
NT3 *Cephalosporium*
NT2 *Actinomucor*
NT3 *Actinomucor elegans*
NT2 *Alternaria*
NT3 *Alternaria alternata*
NT3 *Alternaria citri*
NT2 *Amylomyces*
NT3 *Amylomyces rouxii*
NT2 Antifungal activity
NT2 Ascomycetes
NT2 *Aspergillus*
NT3 *Aspergillus aculeatus*
NT3 *Aspergillus awamori*
NT3 *Aspergillus candidus*
NT3 *Aspergillus carbonarius*
NT3 *Aspergillus clavatus*
NT3 *Aspergillus ficuum*
NT3 *Aspergillus flavus*
NT3 *Aspergillus foetidus*
NT3 *Aspergillus fumigatus*
NT3 *Aspergillus japonicus*
NT3 *Aspergillus kawachii*
NT3 *Aspergillus melleus*
NT3 *Aspergillus nidulans*
NT3 *Aspergillus niger*
NT3 *Aspergillus ochraceus*
NT3 *Aspergillus oryzae*
NT3 *Aspergillus parasiticus*
NT3 *Aspergillus phoenicis*
NT4 *Aspergillus saitoi*
NT3 *Aspergillus repens*
NT3 *Aspergillus sojae*
NT3 *Aspergillus terreus*
NT3 *Aspergillus tubingensis*
NT3 *Aspergillus ustus*
NT3 *Aspergillus versicolor*
NT2 *Aureobasidium*
NT3 *Aureobasidium pullulans*
NT2 Basidiomycetes
NT2 *Beauveria*
NT3 *Beauveria bassiana*
NT2 *Blakeslea*
NT3 *Blakeslea trispora*
NT2 *Botrytis*
NT3 *Botrytis cinerea*
NT2 *Byssochlamys*
NT3 *Byssochlamys fulva*
NT2 *Ceratocystis*
NT3 *Ceratocystis fimbriata*
NT2 *Chaetomium*
NT2 *Chrysosporium*
NT2 *Cladosporium*
NT2 *Claviceps*
NT3 *Claviceps purpurea*
NT2 *Colletotrichum*
NT3 *Colletotrichum acutatum*
NT3 *Colletotrichum gloeosporioides*
NT2 *Cryphonectria*
NT3 *Cryphonectria parasitica*
NT2 *Cunninghamella*
NT2 *Curvularia*
NT2 *Diplodia*
NT2 *Endomyces*
NT2 *Endothia*
NT2 *Eurotium*
NT2 *Fomes*
NT2 Fungal proteins
NT2 *Fusarium*
NT3 *Fusarium avenaceum*
NT3 *Fusarium culmorum*
NT3 *Fusarium equiseti*
NT3 *Fusarium graminearum*
NT3 *Fusarium moniliforme*
NT3 *Fusarium oxysporum*
NT3 *Fusarium proliferatum*
NT3 *Fusarium sambucinum*
NT3 *Fusarium solani*
NT4 *Fusarium solani pisi*
NT3 *Fusarium sporotrichioides*
NT3 *Fusarium verticillioides*
NT2 *Fusidium*
NT2 *Geotrichum*
NT3 *Geotrichum candidum*
NT3 *Geotrichum klebahnii*
NT2 *Gibberella*
NT3 *Gibberella fujikuroi* complex
NT4 *Gibberella fujikuroi*
NT2 *Gliocladium*
NT2 *Helminthosporium*
NT2 *Humicola*
NT3 *Humicola grisea*
NT3 *Humicola insolens*
NT3 *Humicola lanuginosa*
NT2 *Irpex*
NT2 *Monascus*
NT3 *Monascus purpureus*
NT3 *Monascus ruber*
NT2 *Monilia*
NT2 *Monilinia*
NT3 *Monilinia fructicola*
NT3 *Monilinia fructigena*
NT3 *Monilinia laxa*
NT2 *Mortierella*
NT3 *Mortierella alliacea*
NT3 *Mortierella alpina*
NT3 *Mortierella isabellina*
NT2 *Mucor*
NT3 *Mucor circinelloides*
NT3 *Mucor miehei*
NT3 *Mucor rouxii*
NT2 *Myrothecium*
NT2 *Neocallimastix*
NT3 *Neocallimastix patriciarum*
NT2 *Neosartorya*
NT2 *Neurospora*
NT2 *Paecilomyces*
NT3 *Paecilomyces japonica*
NT3 *Paecilomyces sinclairii*
NT2 *Penicillium*
NT3 *Penicillium aurantiogriseum*
NT3 *Penicillium brasilianum*
NT3 *Penicillium camemberti*
NT3 *Penicillium canescens*
NT3 *Penicillium chrysogenum*
NT3 *Penicillium citrinum*
NT3 *Penicillium corylophilum*
NT3 *Penicillium crustosum*
NT3 *Penicillium decumbens*
NT3 *Penicillium digitatum*
NT3 *Penicillium expansum*
NT3 *Penicillium funiculosum*
NT3 *Penicillium glabrum*
NT3 *Penicillium griseoroseum*
NT3 *Penicillium italicum*
NT3 *Penicillium janthinellum*
NT3 *Penicillium nalgiovense*
NT3 *Penicillium olsonii*
NT3 *Penicillium oxalicum*
NT3 *Penicillium palitans*
NT3 *Penicillium purpurogenum*
NT3 *Penicillium restrictum*
NT3 *Penicillium roqueforti*
NT3 *Penicillium simplicissimum*
NT3 *Penicillium spinulosum*
NT3 *Penicillium verrucosum*
NT3 *Penicillium viridicatum*
NT2 *Phanerochaete*
NT3 *Phanerochaete chrysosporium*
NT2 *Phlebia*
NT3 *Phlebia radiata*
NT2 *Phoma*
NT2 *Pithomyces*
NT2 *Polyporus*
NT2 *Pycnoporus*
NT3 *Pycnoporus cinnabarinus*
NT2 *Rhizoctonia*
NT2 *Rhizomucor*
NT3 *Rhizomucor miehei*
NT2 *Rhizopus*
NT3 *Rhizopus arrhizus*
NT3 *Rhizopus chinensis*
NT3 *Rhizopus cohnii*
NT3 *Rhizopus delemar*
NT3 *Rhizopus japonicus*
NT3 *Rhizopus microsporus*
NT3 *Rhizopus niveus*
NT3 *Rhizopus oligosporus*
NT3 *Rhizopus oryzae*
NT3 *Rhizopus stolonifer*
NT4 *Rhizopus nigricans*
NT2 *Sclerotinia*
NT2 *Sclerotium*
NT2 *Scopulariopsis*

NT2 *Septoria*
NT2 Spoilage fungi
NT2 *Sporotrichum*
NT2 *Stachybotrys*
NT2 *Talaromyces*
NT3 *Talaromyces avellaneus*
NT3 *Talaromyces macrosporus*
NT2 *Thermoascus*
NT3 *Thermoascus aurantiacus*
NT2 *Thermomyces*
NT3 *Thermomyces lanuginosus*
NT2 *Thielaviopsis*
NT2 *Trametes*
NT3 *Trametes hirsuta*
NT3 *Trametes versicolor*
NT2 *Trichoderma*
NT3 *Trichoderma harzianum*
NT3 *Trichoderma koningii*
NT3 *Trichoderma longibrachiatum*
NT3 *Trichoderma reesei*
NT3 *Trichoderma viride*
NT2 *Trichophyton*
NT2 *Trichothecium*
NT2 *Verticillium*
NT2 *Wallemia*
NT3 *Wallemia sebi*
NT2 Yeasts
NT3 *Arxula*
NT4 *Arxula adeninivorans*
NT3 *Ashbya*
NT4 *Ashbya gossypii*
NT3 *Brettanomyces*
NT4 *Brettanomyces anomalus*
NT4 *Brettanomyces bruxellensis*
NT4 *Brettanomyces intermedius*
NT3 *Candida*
NT4 *Candida albicans*
NT4 *Candida antarctica*
NT4 *Candida boidinii*
NT4 *Candida bombicola*
NT4 *Candida cylindracea*
NT4 *Candida famata*
NT4 *Candida glycerinogenes*
NT4 *Candida guilliermondii*
NT4 *Candida humilis*
NT5 *Candida milleri*
NT4 *Candida intermedia*
NT4 *Candida kefyr*
NT5 *Candida pseudotropicalis*
NT4 *Candida krusei*
NT4 *Candida lipolytica*
NT4 *Candida magnoliae*
NT4 *Candida maltosa*
NT4 *Candida mogii*
NT4 *Candida molischiana*
NT4 *Candida oleophila*
NT4 *Candida parapsilosis*
NT4 *Candida rugosa*
NT4 *Candida saitoana*
NT4 *Candida sake*
NT4 *Candida shehatae*
NT4 *Candida stellata*
NT4 *Candida tropicalis*
NT4 *Candida utilis*
NT4 *Candida valida*
NT4 *Candida versatilis*
NT4 *Candida wickerhamii*
NT4 *Candida zeylanoides*
NT4 Torula yeast
NT3 Cider yeasts
NT3 *Cryptococcus*
NT4 *Cryptococcus albidus*
NT4 *Cryptococcus curvatus*
NT4 *Cryptococcus laurentii*
NT4 *Cryptococcus nodaensis*
NT3 *Debaryomyces*
NT4 *Debaryomyces hansenii*
NT3 *Dekkera*
NT4 *Dekkera anomala*
NT4 *Dekkera bruxellensis*
NT3 Distillers yeasts
NT3 Dried yeasts
NT3 *Endomycopsis*
NT3 *Eremothecium*
NT3 *Hanseniaspora*
NT4 *Hanseniaspora guilliermondii*
NT4 *Hanseniaspora osmophila*
NT4 *Hanseniaspora uvarum*
NT3 *Hansenula*
NT4 *Hansenula polymorpha*
NT3 *Issatchenkia*
NT4 *Issatchenkia orientalis*
NT3 Killer yeasts
NT3 *Kloeckera*
NT4 *Kloeckera apiculata*
NT3 *Kluyveromyces*
NT4 *Kluyveromyces bulgaricus*
NT4 *Kluyveromyces fragilis*
NT4 *Kluyveromyces lactis*
NT4 *Kluyveromyces marxianus*
NT4 *Kluyveromyces phaffii*
NT4 *Kluyveromyces thermotolerans*
NT3 *Metschnikowia*
NT4 *Metschnikowia pulcherrima*
NT3 *Pachysolen*
NT3 *Phaffia*
NT4 *Phaffia rhodozyma*
NT3 *Pichia*
NT4 *Pichia anomala*
NT4 *Pichia fermentans*
NT4 *Pichia guilliermondii*
NT4 *Pichia heedii*
NT4 *Pichia membranifaciens*
NT5 *Pichia membranefaciens*
NT4 *Pichia methanolica*
NT4 *Pichia pastoris*
NT4 *Pichia stipitis*
NT4 *Pichia subpelliculosa*
NT3 *Rhodosporidium*
NT4 *Rhodosporidium toruloides*
NT3 *Rhodotorula*
NT4 *Rhodotorula glutinis*
NT4 *Rhodotorula gracilis*
NT4 *Rhodotorula mucilaginosa*
NT5 *Rhodotorula rubra*
NT3 *Saccharomyces*
NT4 *Saccharomyces bayanus*
NT4 *Saccharomyces boulardii*
NT4 *Saccharomyces carlsbergensis*
NT4 *Saccharomyces cerevisiae*
NT4 *Saccharomyces diastaticus*
NT4 *Saccharomyces exiguus*
NT4 *Saccharomyces pastorianus*
NT4 *Saccharomyces uvarum*
NT4 Yeasts bakers
NT5 Bakers yeasts
NT4 Yeasts brewers
NT5 Brewers yeasts
NT6 Bottom fermenting yeasts
NT6 Top fermenting yeasts
NT4 Yeasts wine
NT5 Wine yeasts
NT6 Sake yeasts
NT3 *Saccharomycodes*
NT3 *Saccharomycopsis*
NT4 *Saccharomycopsis fibuligera*
NT3 *Schizosaccharomyces*
NT4 *Schizosaccharomyces pombe*
NT3 *Schwanniomyces*
NT3 Spoilage yeasts
NT3 *Sporobolomyces*
NT3 *Torulaspora*
NT4 *Torulaspora delbrueckii*
NT3 *Torulopsis*
NT4 *Torulopsis glabrata*
NT3 *Trichosporon*
NT4 *Trichosporon cutaneum*
NT4 *Trichosporon pullulans*
NT3 Wild yeasts
NT3 *Xanthophyllomyces*
NT4 *Xanthophyllomyces dendrorhous*
NT3 *Yarrowia*
NT4 *Yarrowia lipolytica*
NT3 Yeast biomass
NT3 Yeast extracts
NT3 Yeast proteins
NT3 *Zygosaccharomyces*
NT4 *Zygosaccharomyces bailii*
NT4 *Zygosaccharomyces rouxii*
NT1 GM microorganisms
NT1 Growth promoters (microbial)
NT1 Halophiles
NT1 Mesophiles
NT1 Microbial biomass
NT2 Bacterial biomass
NT2 Yeast biomass
NT1 Microbial contamination
NT2 Bacterial contamination
NT1 Microbial proteins
NT2 Adhesins
NT2 Aerolysins
NT2 Flagellins
NT2 Fungal proteins

NT2 Intimins
NT2 Invasins
NT2 Pilins
NT2 Porins
NT2 Siderophores
NT2 Yeast proteins
NT1 Microflora
NT1 Pathogens
NT1 Probiotic microorganisms
NT2 Probiotic bacteria
NT1 Prokaryotes
NT1 Protozoa
NT1 Psychrophiles
NT1 Psychrotrophs
NT1 Recombinant microorganisms
NT1 Thermophiles
NT1 Viruses
NT2 Adenoviruses
NT3 Mastadenovirus
NT4 Human adenovirus
NT2 Antiviral activity
NT2 Apthovirus
NT3 Foot and mouth disease virus
NT2 Astroviruses
NT3 Mamastrovirus
NT4 Human astrovirus
NT2 Bacteriophages
NT3 Bacteriophages resistance
NT3 Coliphages
NT2 Caliciviruses
NT3 Noroviruses
NT4 Norovirus
NT5 Norwalk virus
NT6 Norwalk-like virus
NT6 Small round structured virus
NT3 Sapoviruses
NT4 Sapovirus
NT5 Sapporo virus
NT2 Coronavirus
NT2 Coxsackieviruses
NT2 Enteric viruses
NT2 Enterovirus
NT3 Echovirus
NT3 Human enterovirus
NT4 Human coxsackievirus
NT3 Poliovirus
NT2 Hepatitis viruses
NT3 Hepatovirus
NT4 Hepatitis A virus
NT3 Hepevirus
NT4 Hepatitis E virus
NT2 Herpesviruses
NT2 Kobuvirus
NT3 Aichi virus
NT2 Lentivirus
NT3 Bovine immunodeficiency virus
NT3 Human immunodeficiency virus
NT2 Orthopoxvirus
NT3 Vaccinia virus
NT2 Parvoviruses
NT3 Parvovirus
NT2 Rotaviruses
NT3 Rotavirus
RT Microbiology

Microprocessors
BT1 Computers
BT2 Equipment
BT3 Technology

Microsatellite markers
BT1 Genetic techniques
BT2 Genetics

Microsatellites
BT1 Genetic techniques
BT2 Genetics

Microscopes
BT1 Microscopy
BT2 Analytical techniques

Microscopy
BT1 Analytical techniques
NT1 Atomic force microscopy
NT1 Electron microscopy
NT2 EM
NT2 SEM
NT2 TEM
NT1 Fluorescence microscopy
NT1 Microscopes

Microstructure
RT Physical properties

Microwaveable containers
HN containers microwaveable used up to vol. 29 (1997)
BT1 Containers

Microwaveable foods
BT1 Foods
RT Microwaves

Microwaveable packaging
BT1 Packaging
BT2 Technology

Microwave cooking
HN introduced from vol. 39, issue 1 (2007)
BT1 Cooking
BT2 Thermal processing
BT3 Processing thermal
BT4 Processing
BT5 Technology
BT1 Microwaves
BT2 Radiation

Microwave ovens
BT1 Ovens
BT2 Equipment
BT3 Technology

Microwave popcorn
BT1 Popcorn
BT2 Corn
BT3 Cereals
BT4 Crops
BT5 Plants
BT4 Seeds
BT5 Plant foods
BT6 Foods
BT2 Snack foods
BT3 Processed foods
BT4 Foods

Microwaves
BT1 Radiation
NT1 Microwave cooking
NT1 Microwave susceptors
RT Microwaveable foods

Microwave susceptors
BT1 Microwaves
BT2 Radiation
UF Browning susceptors
UF Susceptors

Middle East
HN heading from vol. 22 (1991) to vol. 24 (1992)
NT1 Bahrain
NT1 Cyprus
NT1 Egypt
NT1 Gaza Strip
NT1 Iran
NT1 Iraq
NT1 Israel
NT1 Jordan
NT1 Kuwait
NT1 Lebanon
NT1 Oman
NT1 Qatar
NT1 Saudi Arabia
NT1 Syria
NT1 Turkey
NT1 United Arab Emirates
NT1 West Bank
NT1 Yemen
RT Africa
RT Asia
RT Europe

Migraine
BT1 Diseases

Migration
HN heading from vol. 25 (1993); under Contamination up to vol. 24 (1992)
SN used for migration of undesirable compounds, e.g. plasticizers, into foods
RT Contamination
RT Food safety additives
RT Packaging materials
RT Plasticizers

Military rations
BT1 Meals
BT2 Processed foods
BT3 Foods
RT Army rations
RT Space flight foods

Milk
SN cow milk unless other species specified
BT1 Dairy products
BT2 Animal foods
BT3 Foods
NT1 Ass milk
NT1 Buffalo milk
NT2 Shrikhand
NT1 Camel milk
NT2 Shubat
NT1 Cheesemaking milk
NT1 Cheese milk

NT1 Chocolate milk
NT1 Colostrum
NT1 Concentrated milk
NT1 Condensed milk
NT2 Mawa
NT1 Cream milk
NT1 Dried milk
NT1 Evaporated milk
NT1 Ewe milk
NT1 Farm milk
NT1 Fermented milk
NT2 Acidophilin
NT2 Acidophilus milk
NT2 Amasi
NT2 Bifidus milk
NT2 Biogarde
NT2 Bioghurt
NT2 Dahi
NT2 Kefir
NT3 Kefir grains
NT2 Koumiss
NT2 Labneh
NT2 Lactic beverages
NT2 Lassi
NT2 Leben
NT2 Nono
NT2 Prostokvasha
NT2 Ryazhenka
NT2 Shrikhand
NT2 Shubat
NT2 Skyr
NT2 Snezhok
NT2 Sour milk
NT2 Tarag
NT2 Tykmaelk
NT2 Yakult
NT2 Ymer
NT2 Yoghurt
NT3 Buffalo yoghurt
NT3 Ewe yoghurt
NT3 Flavoured yoghurt
NT3 Frozen yoghurt
NT3 Fruit yoghurt
NT3 Goat yoghurt
NT3 Yoghurt beverages
NT4 Drinking yoghurt
NT2 Zabady
NT3 Zabadi
NT1 Flavoured milk
NT1 Goat milk
NT1 Half and half milk
NT1 Homogenized milk
NT1 Human milk
NT1 Jellied milk
NT1 Mare milk
NT2 Koumiss
NT1 Milk beverages
NT1 Milk powders
NT1 Milkshakes
NT1 Miltone
NT1 Pasteurized milk
NT1 Raw milk
NT1 Recombined milk
NT1 Semi skimmed milk
NT1 Skim milk
NT2 Dried skim milk
NT2 Skim milk powders
NT1 Sterilized milk
NT1 UHT milk
NT1 Whole milk
NT1 Yak milk
UF Cow milk

Milk beverages
BT1 Dairy beverages
BT2 Beverages
BT2 Dairy products
BT3 Animal foods
BT4 Foods
BT1 Milk
BT2 Dairy products
BT3 Animal foods
BT4 Foods
UF Milk drinks

Milk chocolate
BT1 Chocolate products
BT2 Chocolate
BT3 Sugar confectionery
BT4 Plant foods
BT5 Foods

Milk clotting
BT1 Clotting
BT2 Coagulation
BT3 Processing
BT4 Technology

Milk clotting enzymes
SN index heading is Enzymes milk clotting
BT1 Enzymes milk clotting
BT2 Proteinases
BT3 Hydrolases
BT4 Enzymes
NT1 Chymosin
NT1 Rennets
NT2 Animal rennets
NT2 Calf rennets
NT2 Microbial rennets
NT2 Vegetable rennets
NT1 Rennet substitutes

Milk drinks
USE **Milk beverages**

Milk fat globule membranes
BT1 Milk fats
BT2 Fats milk
BT3 Fats animal
BT4 Animal foods
BT5 Foods
BT4 Fats
BT5 Lipids
BT6 Nutrients

Milk fat globules
BT1 Milk fats
BT2 Fats milk
BT3 Fats animal
BT4 Animal foods
BT5 Foods
BT4 Fats
BT5 Lipids
BT6 Nutrients

Milk fats
SN index heading is Fats milk
BT1 Fats milk
BT2 Fats animal
BT3 Animal foods
BT4 Foods
BT3 Fats
BT4 Lipids
BT5 Nutrients
NT1 Anhydrous milk fats
NT1 Butterfat
NT1 Butter oils
NT1 Milk fat globule membranes
NT1 Milk fat globules
RT Butter
RT Cream
RT Ghee

Milkfish
BT1 Marine fish
BT2 Fish
BT3 Animals
BT3 Sea foods
BT4 Aquatic foods
BT5 Animal foods
BT6 Foods
NT1 *Chanos chanos*

Milk ice
BT1 Ice cream
BT2 Dairy products
BT3 Animal foods
BT4 Foods
BT2 Frozen foods
BT3 Processed foods
BT4 Foods

Milk infant formulas
BT1 Infant formulas
BT2 Infant foods
BT3 Processed foods
BT4 Foods
UF Human milk substitutes
UF Infant milk formulas

Milking
BT1 Husbandry
BT2 Agriculture
RT Lactation
UF Milking frequency
UF Milking interval

Milking frequency
USE **Milking**

Milking interval
USE **Milking**

Milking machines
BT1 Equipment
BT2 Technology

Milk powders
BT1 Milk
BT2 Dairy products
BT3 Animal foods
BT4 Foods
BT1 Powders
BT2 Dried foods
BT3 Processed foods
BT4 Foods
BT2 Instant foods
BT3 Processed foods
BT4 Foods
RT Dried milk

RT Dried skim milk
RT Skim milk powders

Milk products
USE **Dairy products**

Milk protein concentrates
BT1 Milk proteins
BT2 Proteins milk
BT3 Animal proteins
BT4 Proteins animal
BT5 Proteins
BT6 Nutrients
BT1 Protein concentrates
BT2 Concentrates
BT3 Processed foods
BT4 Foods
BT2 Protein products

Milk proteins
SN index heading is Proteins milk
BT1 Proteins milk
BT2 Animal proteins
BT3 Proteins animal
BT4 Proteins
BT5 Nutrients
NT1 Butyrophilin
NT1 Casein
NT2 Acid casein
NT2 α_s-Casein
NT2 α_{s1}-Casein
NT2 α_{s2}-Casein
NT2 β-Casein
NT2 γ-Casein
NT2 κ-Casein
NT2 Casein micelles
NT1 β-Casomorphins
NT1 Lactalbumins
NT2 α-Lactalbumin
NT1 Lactoglobulins
NT2 β-Lactoglobulin
NT1 Milk protein concentrates
NT1 Proteose peptones
NT1 Whey proteins
NT2 Whey protein concentrates
RT Lactoferrin

Milk puddings
BT1 Desserts
BT2 Processed foods
BT3 Foods

Milkshakes
BT1 Dairy beverages
BT2 Beverages
BT2 Dairy products
BT3 Animal foods
BT4 Foods
BT1 Milk
BT2 Dairy products
BT3 Animal foods
BT4 Foods

Milk substitutes
BT1 Simulated foods
BT2 Processed foods
BT3 Foods

Millet
HN heading from vol. 25 (1993); heading was Millets up to vol. 24 (1992)
BT1 Cereals
BT2 Crops
BT3 Plants
BT2 Seeds
BT3 Plant foods
BT4 Foods
NT1 Bajra
NT1 Common millet
NT1 Finger millet
NT1 Fonio
NT1 Foxtail millet
NT1 Millet flour
NT1 Millet starch
NT1 Pearl millet
NT1 Ragi
NT1 Teff
UF Millets

Millet flour
HN introduced from vol. 41, issue 1 (2009)
BT1 Cereal flours
BT2 Flours cereal
BT3 Cereal products
BT4 Plant foods
BT5 Foods
BT1 Millet
BT2 Cereals
BT3 Crops
BT4 Plants
BT3 Seeds
BT4 Plant foods
BT5 Foods

Millet oils
BT1 Vegetable oils
BT2 Oils vegetable
BT3 Oils
BT4 Lipids
BT5 Nutrients
BT3 Vegetable products
BT4 Plant foods
BT5 Foods

Millets
HN heading up to vol. 24 (1992)
USE **Millet**

Millet starch
HN introduced from vol. 39, issue 1 (2007)
BT1 Millet
BT2 Cereals
BT3 Crops
BT4 Plants
BT3 Seeds
BT4 Plant foods
BT5 Foods
BT1 Starch
BT2 Glucans
BT3 Polysaccharides
BT4 Carbohydrates
BT5 Nutrients
BT5 Organic compounds
BT2 Thickeners
BT3 Additives

Milling
BT1 Processing
BT2 Technology
NT1 Milling properties
NT1 Mills
NT2 Flour mills
NT2 Roller mills
NT1 Wet milling
RT Comminution
RT Polishing

Milling properties
BT1 Milling
BT2 Processing
BT3 Technology

Mills
BT1 Equipment
BT2 Technology
BT1 Milling
BT2 Processing
BT3 Technology
NT1 Flour mills
NT1 Roller mills

Milo
BT1 Sorghum
BT2 Cereals
BT3 Crops
BT4 Plants
BT3 Seeds
BT4 Plant foods
BT5 Foods

Milt
BT1 Roes
BT2 Fish products
BT3 Sea foods
BT4 Aquatic foods
BT5 Animal foods
BT6 Foods

Miltone
BT1 Milk
BT2 Dairy products
BT3 Animal foods
BT4 Foods

Minas cheese
BT1 Cheese varieties
BT2 Cheese
BT3 Dairy products
BT4 Animal foods
BT5 Foods

Minas Frescal cheese
BT1 Cheese varieties
BT2 Cheese
BT3 Dairy products
BT4 Animal foods
BT5 Foods

Minced beef
USE **Beef mince**

Minced meat
USE **Meat mince**

Mincers
BT1 Equipment
BT2 Technology

BT1 Mincing
 BT2 Comminution
  BT3 Processing
   BT4 Technology

Mincing
BT1 Comminution
 BT2 Processing
  BT3 Technology
NT1 Mincers

Mineral oils
BT1 Oils
 BT2 Lipids
  BT3 Nutrients

Minerals
BT1 Nutrients
NT1 Asbestos
NT1 Ash
NT1 Demineralization
NT1 Elements
 NT2 Ar
 NT2 Arsenic
  NT3 Arsenicals
   NT4 Arsenobetaine
   NT4 Dimethylarsinic acid
   NT4 Methylarsonic acid
  NT3 As
 NT2 B
 NT2 Carbon
  NT3 Activated C
   NT4 Activated carbon
  NT3 C
  NT3 Charcoal
 NT2 Ge
 NT2 Halogens
  NT3 Br
  NT3 Chlorine
   NT4 Cl
  NT3 F
  NT3 Iodine
   NT4 I
   NT4 Iodized salt
 NT2 He
 NT2 Hydrogen
  NT3 Deuterium
  NT3 H_2
  NT3 Tritium
 NT2 Isotopes
  NT3 Radioelements
   NT4 Cs
   NT4 Po
   NT4 Pu
   NT4 Ra
   NT4 Radionuclides
    NT5 Radioisotopes
   NT4 Rn
   NT4 Sr
   NT4 Tc
   NT4 Tritium
   NT4 U
 NT2 Metals
  NT3 Ag
  NT3 Aluminium
   NT4 Al
   NT4 Al compounds
  NT3 Au
  NT3 Ba
  NT3 Be
  NT3 Bi
  NT3 Cadmium
   NT4 Cd
  NT3 Calcium
   NT4 Ca
  NT3 Ce
  NT3 Cobalt
   NT4 Co
  NT3 Copper
   NT4 Cu
  NT3 Cr
  NT3 Ga
  NT3 Heavy metals
  NT3 Iron
   NT4 Fe
   NT4 Ferritin
  NT3 Lanthanides
   NT4 La
   NT4 Yb
  NT3 Lead
   NT4 Pb
  NT3 Li
  NT3 Magnesium
   NT4 Mg
  NT3 Manganese
   NT4 Mn
  NT3 Mercury
   NT4 Hg
   NT4 Methylmercury
  NT3 Mo
  NT3 Nb
  NT3 Ni
  NT3 Os
  NT3 Pd
  NT3 Potassium
   NT4 K
  NT3 Pt
  NT3 Rb
  NT3 Re
  NT3 Rhodium
  NT3 Ru
  NT3 Sc
  NT3 Sodium
   NT4 Na
   NT4 Sodium low diet
   NT4 Sodium low foods
  NT3 Sr
  NT3 Th
  NT3 Ti
  NT3 Tin
   NT4 Sn
  NT3 Tl
  NT3 V
  NT3 W
  NT3 Y
  NT3 Zinc
   NT4 Zn
  NT3 Zr
 NT2 Nitrogen
  NT3 Amino N
   NT4 α-Amino N
  NT3 Liquid nitrogen
  NT3 N
  NT3 N_2
  NT3 Nitrogen compounds
   NT4 N compounds
 NT2 Oxygen
  NT3 O_2
  NT3 Oxygen absorbers
   NT4 Oxygen scavengers
  NT3 Ozone
 NT2 Phosphorus
  NT3 P
 NT2 Sb
 NT2 Selenium
  NT3 Se
  NT3 Selenites
  NT3 Selenomethionine
  NT3 Selenoproteins
 NT2 Si
 NT2 Sulfur
  NT3 S
 NT2 Te
 NT2 Trace elements
 NT2 Xe
NT1 Silica
RT Micronutrients

Mineral waters
HN heading from vol. 25 (1993); under Beverages up to vol. 24 (1992)
BT1 Soft drinks
 BT2 Beverages
BT1 Water
NT1 Bottled mineral waters
NT1 Soda water
NT1 Spring waters
RT Drinking water

Minimally processed foods
BT1 Processed foods
 BT2 Foods
RT Minimal processing

Minimal processing
BT1 Processing
 BT2 Technology
RT Minimally processed foods

Mint
HN under Spices up to vol. 42 (2010)
BT1 Herbs
 BT2 Spices
  BT3 Flavourings
   BT4 Additives
NT1 Peppermint
NT1 Spearmint
RT Mint oils

Mint oils
BT1 Essential oils
 BT2 Flavourings
  BT3 Additives
 BT2 Vegetable oils
  BT3 Oils vegetable
   BT4 Oils
    BT5 Lipids
     BT6 Nutrients
   BT4 Vegetable products
    BT5 Plant foods
     BT6 Foods
RT Mint

Mints
BT1 Sugar confectionery
 BT2 Plant foods
  BT3 Foods

Miraculin
BT1 Glycoproteins

BT2 Proteins
BT3 Nutrients
RT Sweet proteins

Mirex
BT1 Organochlorine insecticides
BT2 Insecticides
BT3 Pesticides
BT4 Biocides
BT4 Residues
BT2 Organochlorine pesticides
BT3 Pesticides
BT4 Biocides
BT4 Residues

Mirin
BT1 Condiments
BT2 Flavourings
BT3 Additives

Mirliton
USE **Chayote**

Miso
BT1 Fermented foods
BT2 Processed foods
BT3 Foods
BT1 Soy products
BT2 Vegetable products
BT3 Plant foods
BT4 Foods
RT Soy sauces

Mistletoe
BT1 Plants

Mites
BT1 Pests

Mitochondria
HN introduced from vol. 39, issue 1 (2007)
BT1 Cells
RT Mitochondrial DNA

Mitochondrial DNA
HN introduced from vol. 39, issue 1 (2007)
BT1 DNA
BT2 Nucleic acids
BT3 Organic acids
BT4 Acids
RT Mitochondria

Mitosis
HN introduced from vol. 39, issue 1 (2007)
BT1 Cell cycle
BT2 Physiology
BT3 Science

Mixer pet foods
HN introduced from vol. 39, issue 1 (2007)
BT1 Pet foods

Mixers
BT1 Equipment
BT2 Technology
BT1 Mixing
BT2 Processing
BT3 Technology

Mixes
BT1 Dried foods
BT2 Processed foods
BT3 Foods
BT1 Instant foods
BT2 Processed foods
BT3 Foods
NT1 Bakery product mixes
NT1 Beverage mixes
NT1 Cake mixes
NT1 Dessert mixes
NT1 Ice cream mixes
NT1 Soup mixes

Mixing
BT1 Processing
BT2 Technology
NT1 Agitation
NT1 Blending
NT1 Conching
NT1 Impellers
NT1 Kneading
NT1 Mixers
NT1 Stirring
RT Emulsification
RT Homogenization

Mixographs
BT1 Apparatus
BT2 Technology

Mn
HN under Minerals up to vol. 42 (2010)
BT1 Manganese
BT2 Metals
BT3 Elements
BT4 Minerals
BT5 Nutrients

Mo
HN under Minerals up to vol. 42 (2010)
BT1 Metals
BT2 Elements
BT3 Minerals
BT4 Nutrients
UF Molybdenum

Model foods
HN introduced from vol. 39, issue 1 (2007)
NT1 Tylose

Modelling
HN heading up to vol. 24 (1992); heading from vol. 43 (2011)
NT1 Artificial neural networks
RT Computers
RT Mathematics

Modification
HN heading from vol. 42 (2010)
NT1 Acetylation
NT1 Acylation
NT1 Amidation
NT1 Carboxymethylation
NT1 Cross-linking
NT1 Deacetylation
NT1 Deamidation
NT1 Decarboxylation
NT1 Depolymerization
NT1 Desaturation
NT1 Etherification
NT1 Fucosylation
NT1 Glycation
NT1 Glycosylation
NT2 Transglycosylation
NT1 Hydroxylation
NT1 Hydroxypropylation
NT1 Methylation
NT1 Mutagenesis
NT2 Site directed mutagenesis
NT1 Phosphorylation
NT1 Polymerization
NT1 Protein engineering
NT2 Site directed mutagenesis
NT1 Succinylation
RT Esterification
RT Improvements

Modified atmosphere packaging
HN packaging modified atm used in the index up to vol. 24 (1992) and packaging modified atmosphere up to vol. 31 (1999)
BT1 Packaging
BT2 Technology
RT Controlled atmosphere packaging
UF Packaging modified atm
UF Packaging modified atmosphere

Modified starches
BT1 Starch
BT2 Glucans
BT3 Polysaccharides
BT4 Carbohydrates
BT5 Nutrients
BT5 Organic compounds
BT2 Thickeners
BT3 Additives

Modori
BT1 Degradation
BT2 Decomposition

Moinmoin
BT1 Cowpeas
BT2 Legumes
BT3 Vegetables specific
BT4 Vegetables
BT5 Crops
BT6 Plants
BT5 Plant foods
BT6 Foods

Moistness
BT1 Humidity

Moisture
BT1 Moisture content

Moisture content
NT1 Hydration
NT1 Moisture
RT a_w
RT Humidity
RT Moisture retention
RT Moisture transfer
RT Sorption

RT Water
RT Water activity

Moisture retention
HN introduced from vol. 39, issue 1 (2007)
BT1 Functional properties
BT2 Physical properties
RT Moisture content

Moisture sorption
BT1 Sorption
RT Water sorption

Moisture transfer
RT Diffusivity
RT Moisture content

Molasses
BT1 Sugar
BT2 Plant foods
BT3 Foods
NT1 Beet molasses
NT1 Cane molasses
RT Sugar processes

Moldavia
USE **Moldova**

Moldova
SN full name is Republic of Moldova
BT1 Europe
UF Moldavia

Molecular distillation
USE **Vacuum distillation**

Molecular weight
USE **Mol. wt.**

Molinate
BT1 Herbicides
BT2 Pesticides
BT3 Biocides
BT3 Residues

Molluscicides
BT1 Pesticides
BT2 Biocides
BT2 Residues
NT1 Metaldehyde

Molluscs
BT1 Shellfish
BT2 Animals
BT2 Sea foods
BT3 Aquatic foods
BT4 Animal foods
BT5 Foods
NT1 Bivalves
NT2 Arkshells
NT2 Carpet shells
NT2 Clams
NT3 Freshwater clams
NT3 *Pseudocardium sachalinensis*
NT3 *Tapes philippinarum*
NT2 Cockles
NT2 Mussels
NT3 Blue mussels
NT3 Green mussels
NT3 *Mytilus edulis*
NT3 *Mytilus galloprovincialis*
NT3 *Mytilus trossulus*
NT2 Oysters
NT3 *Crassostrea gigas*
NT3 *Crassostrea virginica*
NT3 Oyster sauces
NT2 Razor shells
NT2 Scallops
NT3 *Patinopecten yessoensis*
NT1 Cephalopods
NT2 Cuttlefish
NT2 Octopus
NT2 Squid
NT3 Ika shiokara
NT3 *Illex argentinus*
NT3 *Ommastrephes bartrami*
NT1 Gastropods
NT2 Abalones
NT2 Limpets
NT2 Periwinkles
NT2 Snails
NT3 Land snails
NT3 Snail meat
NT2 Top shells
NT2 Trumpet shells
NT2 Turban shells
NT2 Whelks

Molva molva
BT1 Ling
BT2 Marine fish
BT3 Fish
BT4 Animals
BT4 Sea foods
BT5 Aquatic foods
BT6 Animal foods
BT7 Foods

Mol. wt.
BT1 Physical properties
UF Molecular weight

Molybdenum
USE **Mo**

Momoni
HN introduced from vol. 37, issue 5 (2005)
BT1 Fermented foods
BT2 Processed foods
BT3 Foods
BT1 Fish products
BT2 Sea foods
BT3 Aquatic foods
BT4 Animal foods
BT5 Foods

Monaco
BT1 Europe

Monascus
BT1 Fungi
BT2 Microorganisms
NT1 *Monascus purpureus*
NT1 *Monascus ruber*
RT Colorants

Monascus purpureus
BT1 *Monascus*
BT2 Fungi
BT3 Microorganisms

Monascus ruber
BT1 *Monascus*
BT2 Fungi
BT3 Microorganisms

Monatin
HN introduced from vol. 39, issue 1 (2007)
BT1 Sweeteners
BT2 Additives

Monellin
BT1 Sweet proteins
BT2 Proteins
BT3 Nutrients
BT2 Sweeteners
BT3 Additives

Monensin
BT1 Antibiotics
BT2 Drugs
BT3 Residues
BT1 Coccidiostats
BT2 Drugs
BT3 Residues

Mongolia
BT1 Asia

Monilia
SN obsolete genus name for Candida spp.
BT1 Fungi
BT2 Microorganisms

Moniliformin
BT1 Mycotoxins
BT2 Toxins
BT3 Residues

Monilinia
BT1 Fungi
BT2 Microorganisms
NT1 *Monilinia fructicola*
NT1 *Monilinia fructigena*
NT1 *Monilinia laxa*

Monilinia fructicola
BT1 *Monilinia*
BT2 Fungi
BT3 Microorganisms

Monilinia fructigena
BT1 *Monilinia*
BT2 Fungi
BT3 Microorganisms

Monilinia laxa
BT1 *Monilinia*
BT2 Fungi
BT3 Microorganisms

Monitor
USE **Methamidophos**

Monkfish
BT1 Marine fish
BT2 Fish
BT3 Animals

BT3 Sea foods
BT4 Aquatic foods
BT5 Animal foods
BT6 Foods

Monoacylglycerols
SN syn. monoglycerides
BT1 Monoglycerides
BT2 Glycerides
BT3 Emulsifiers
BT4 Additives
BT3 Fatty acid esters
BT4 Esters
BT5 Organic compounds
BT3 Lipids
BT4 Nutrients

Monoamine oxidases
USE **Amine oxidases**

Monochloramine
HN introduced from vol. 39, issue 1 (2007)
BT1 Chloramines
BT2 Amines
BT3 Organic nitrogen compounds
BT2 Chlorides
BT3 Salts
BT2 Disinfectants
BT3 Disinfection
BT4 Hygiene

Monoclonal antibodies
HN antibodies monoclonal also used in the index up to vol. 29 (1997)
BT1 Immunology

Monocrotophos
BT1 Acaricides
BT2 Pesticides
BT3 Biocides
BT3 Residues
BT1 Organophosphorus insecticides
BT2 Insecticides
BT3 Pesticides
BT4 Biocides
BT4 Residues
BT2 Organophosphorus pesticides
BT3 Pesticides
BT4 Biocides
BT4 Residues
UF Azodrin

Monoglycerides
HN heading from vol. 25 (1993); under Glycerides up to vol. 24 (1992)
SN syn. monoacylglycerols
BT1 Glycerides
BT2 Emulsifiers
BT3 Additives
BT2 Fatty acid esters
BT3 Esters
BT4 Organic compounds
BT2 Lipids
BT3 Nutrients
NT1 Monoacylglycerols
NT1 Monolaurin

Monolaurin
BT1 Monoglycerides
BT2 Glycerides
BT3 Emulsifiers
BT4 Additives
BT3 Fatty acid esters
BT4 Esters
BT5 Organic compounds
BT3 Lipids
BT4 Nutrients
BT1 Preservatives
BT2 Additives
UF Glycerol monolaurate

Monooxygenases
BT1 Oxidoreductases
BT2 Enzymes

Monophenol monooxygenases
SN EC 1.14.18.1; also catalyses the reaction of catechol oxidase (EC 1.10.3.1) under certain conditions
BT1 Phenolases
BT2 Oxidoreductases
BT3 Enzymes

Monosaccharides
HN heading from vol. 43 (2011); under Sugars up to vol. 42 (2010)
BT1 Sugars
BT2 Carbohydrates
BT3 Nutrients
BT3 Organic compounds
BT2 Plant foods
BT3 Foods
NT1 Aldoses
NT1 Arabinose
NT1 Fructose
NT1 Fucose
NT1 Galactose
NT1 Glucose
NT2 Glucose-6-phosphate
NT1 Hexoses
NT1 Ketoses
NT1 Mannose
NT1 Pentoses
NT1 Psicose
NT1 Rhamnose
NT1 Ribose
NT1 Sorbose
NT1 Tagatose
NT1 Xylose
NT1 Xylulose

Monosodium glutamate
BT1 Glutamates
BT2 Flavourings
BT3 Additives
BT2 Salts
RT Flavour enhancers

Monoterpenes
BT1 Hydrocarbons
BT2 Organic compounds
BT1 Monoterpenoids
BT2 Terpenoids
BT3 Lipids
BT4 Nutrients
NT1 Camphene
NT1 Limonene
NT1 Myrcene
NT1 Pinenes
NT1 Terpinene

Monoterpenoids
BT1 Terpenoids
BT2 Lipids
BT3 Nutrients
NT1 Borneol
NT1 Camphor
NT1 Carvacrol
NT1 Carveol
NT1 Carvone
NT1 Cineole
NT2 Eucalyptol
NT1 Citral
NT2 Geranial
NT2 Neral
NT1 Citronellal
NT1 Citronellol
NT1 Dill ether
NT1 Geraniol
NT1 Hotrienol
NT1 Linalool
NT1 Menthol
NT1 Menthone
NT1 2-Methylisoborneol
NT1 Monoterpenes
NT2 Camphene
NT2 Limonene
NT2 Myrcene
NT2 Pinenes
NT2 Terpinene
NT1 Nerol
NT1 Safranal
NT1 Terpineol
NT1 Terpinyl acetate
NT1 Thujone
NT1 Thymol

Monounsaturated fatty acids
HN heading from vol. 43 (2011); under Fatty acids up to vol. 42 (2010)
BT1 Unsaturated fatty acids
BT2 Fatty acids
BT3 Lipids
BT4 Nutrients
BT3 Organic acids
BT4 Acids
NT1 Decenoic acid
NT1 Docosenoic acid
NT2 Erucic acid
NT1 Eicosenoic acid
NT1 Hexadecenoic acid
NT2 Palmitoleic acid
NT1 Octadecenoic acid
NT2 Elaidic acid
NT2 Oleic acid
NT2 Petroselinic acid
NT2 Vaccenic acid
NT1 Ricinoleic acid
RT Unsaturation

Montasio cheese
BT1 Cheese varieties
BT2 Cheese
BT3 Dairy products
BT4 Animal foods
BT5 Foods

Montenegro
HN introduced from vol. 39, issue 1 (2007)
BT1 Europe

Monterey Jack cheese
HN introduced from vol. 39, issue 1 (2007)
BT1 Cheese varieties
BT2 Cheese
BT3 Dairy products
BT4 Animal foods
BT5 Foods

Monterey sardine
HN introduced from vol. 37, issue 5 (2005)
BT1 Sardine
BT2 Marine fish
BT3 Fish
BT4 Animals
BT4 Sea foods
BT5 Aquatic foods
BT6 Animal foods
BT7 Foods
BT2 Oily fish
BT3 Fish
BT4 Animals
BT4 Sea foods
BT5 Aquatic foods
BT6 Animal foods
BT7 Foods

Monuron
BT1 Herbicides
BT2 Pesticides
BT3 Biocides
BT3 Residues

Mood
BT1 Behavioural effects
BT2 Human physiology
BT3 Physiology
BT4 Science
RT Psychiatric disorders

Moose
BT1 Animals
NT1 Moose meat

Moose meat
BT1 Meat specific
BT2 Meat
BT3 Animal foods
BT4 Foods
BT1 Moose
BT2 Animals

Moraxella
BT1 Bacteria
BT2 Microorganisms

Morchella
BT1 Edible fungi
BT2 Fungi edible
BT3 Vegetables specific
BT4 Vegetables
BT5 Crops
BT6 Plants
BT5 Plant foods
BT6 Foods
NT1 *Morchella esculenta*
UF Morels

Morchella esculenta
HN introduced from vol. 39, issue 1 (2007)
BT1 *Morchella*
BT2 Edible fungi
BT3 Fungi edible
BT4 Vegetables specific
BT5 Vegetables
BT6 Crops
BT7 Plants
BT6 Plant foods
BT7 Foods

Morello cherries
BT1 Cherries
BT2 Fruits specific
BT3 Fruits
BT4 Crops
BT5 Plants
BT4 Plant foods
BT5 Foods

Morels
USE ***Morchella***

Morestan
USE **Quinomethionate**

Morganella
BT1 Bacteria
BT2 Microorganisms
NT1 *Morganella morganii*

Morganella morganii
BT1 *Morganella*
BT2 Bacteria
BT3 Microorganisms

Morin
BT1 Flavonols
BT2 Alcohols
BT2 Flavonoids
BT3 Aromatic compounds
BT4 Organic compounds
BT3 Pigments

Moringa
BT1 Oilseeds
BT2 Seeds
BT3 Plant foods
BT4 Foods
BT1 Vegetables specific
BT2 Vegetables
BT3 Crops
BT4 Plants
BT3 Plant foods
BT4 Foods

Morning goods
BT1 Bakery products
BT2 Cereal products
BT3 Plant foods
BT4 Foods
RT Breakfast

Moroccan smen
USE **Smen**

Morocco
BT1 North Africa
BT2 Africa

Moromi
BT1 Mashing
BT2 Processing
BT3 Technology
RT Sake
RT Soy sauces

Morone saxatilis
BT1 Striped bass
BT2 Sea bass
BT3 Marine fish
BT4 Fish
BT5 Animals
BT5 Sea foods
BT6 Aquatic foods
BT7 Animal foods
BT8 Foods

Morpholine
BT1 Amines
BT2 Organic nitrogen compounds
BT1 Heterocyclic compounds

Morphology
BT1 Histology
BT2 Science

Mortadella
BT1 Sausages
BT2 Meat products
BT3 Animal foods
BT4 Foods

Mortierella
BT1 Fungi
BT2 Microorganisms
NT1 *Mortierella alliacea*
NT1 *Mortierella alpina*
NT1 *Mortierella isabellina*

Mortierella alliacea
BT1 *Mortierella*
BT2 Fungi
BT3 Microorganisms

Mortierella alpina
BT1 *Mortierella*
BT2 Fungi
BT3 Microorganisms

Mortierella isabellina
BT1 *Mortierella*
BT2 Fungi
BT3 Microorganisms

Morwong
BT1 Marine fish
BT2 Fish
BT3 Animals
BT3 Sea foods
BT4 Aquatic foods
BT5 Animal foods
BT6 Foods

Moth beans
BT1 Legumes

BT2 Vegetables specific
BT3 Vegetables
BT4 Crops
BT5 Plants
BT4 Plant foods
BT5 Foods

Moths
BT1 Insects
BT2 Pests

Motility
HN introduced from vol. 39, issue 1 (2007)
BT1 Physiology
BT2 Science
BT1 Virulence factors
RT Chemotaxis
RT Flagella

Mottling
BT1 Discoloration

Moufflon
BT1 Animals

Mould counts
USE **Fungal counts**

Moulding
BT1 Processing
BT2 Technology
NT1 Shaping

Moulds
USE **Fungi**

Mountain apples
USE **Malay apples**

Mousses
BT1 Desserts
BT2 Processed foods
BT3 Foods

Mouthfeel
BT1 Sensory properties
NT1 Grittiness

Moxidectin
HN introduced from vol. 37, issue 5 (2005)
BT1 Anthelmintics
BT2 Drugs
BT3 Residues

Mozambique
BT1 Southern Africa
BT2 Africa

Mozzarella cheese
BT1 Cheese varieties
BT2 Cheese
BT3 Dairy products
BT4 Animal foods
BT5 Foods
NT1 Buffalo mozzarella cheese

m.p.
BT1 Thermophysical properties
BT2 Physical properties
UF Melting point

MPN
BT1 Microbiological techniques

MRL
RT Nutrition
UF Maximum residue limits

mRNA
BT1 RNA
BT2 Nucleic acids
BT3 Organic acids
BT4 Acids

MS
SN index heading is Mass spectroscopy
BT1 Mass spectroscopy
BT2 Spectroscopy
BT3 Analytical techniques
UF Mass spectrometry

Mucic acid
BT1 Organic acids
BT2 Acids

Mucilage
BT1 Gums
BT2 Polysaccharides
BT3 Carbohydrates
BT4 Nutrients
BT4 Organic compounds
BT2 Stabilizers
BT3 Additives
BT2 Thickeners
BT3 Additives

Mucins
BT1 Animal proteins
BT2 Proteins animal
BT3 Proteins
BT4 Nutrients
BT1 Glycoproteins
BT2 Proteins
BT3 Nutrients

Mucoids
BT1 Glycoproteins
BT2 Proteins
BT3 Nutrients

Mucopolysaccharides
SN syn. glycosaminoglycans
BT1 Glycosaminoglycans
BT2 Polysaccharides
BT3 Carbohydrates
BT4 Nutrients
BT4 Organic compounds

Mucor
BT1 Fungi
BT2 Microorganisms
NT1 *Mucor circinelloides*
NT1 *Mucor miehei*
NT1 *Mucor rouxii*

Mucor circinelloides
HN introduced from vol. 41, issue 1 (2009)
BT1 *Mucor*
BT2 Fungi
BT3 Microorganisms

Mucor miehei
SN Genbank common name for Rhizomucor miehei
BT1 *Mucor*
BT2 Fungi
BT3 Microorganisms

Mucor rouxii
SN synonymous with Amylomyces rouxii
BT1 *Mucor*
BT2 Fungi
BT3 Microorganisms

Mud crabs
BT1 Crabs
BT2 Crustacea
BT3 Shellfish
BT4 Animals
BT4 Sea foods
BT5 Aquatic foods
BT6 Animal foods
BT7 Foods

Muenster cheese
SN syn. Munster cheese
BT1 Cheese varieties
BT2 Cheese
BT3 Dairy products
BT4 Animal foods
BT5 Foods

Muesli
BT1 Cereal products
BT2 Plant foods
BT3 Foods
RT Muesli bars

Muesli bars
BT1 Cereal bars
BT2 Food bars
BT3 Snack foods
BT4 Processed foods
BT5 Foods
RT Muesli

Muffins
SN UK usage - bakery products; US usage - cakes
BT1 Bakery products
BT2 Cereal products
BT3 Plant foods
BT4 Foods
BT1 Cakes
BT2 Bakery products
BT3 Cereal products
BT4 Plant foods
BT5 Foods
RT English muffins

Mugil cephalus
BT1 Mullet
BT2 Marine fish
BT3 Fish
BT4 Animals
BT4 Sea foods
BT5 Aquatic foods
BT6 Animal foods
BT7 Foods

Mugwort
HN under Spices up to vol. 42 (2010)
BT1 Herbs
BT2 Spices
BT3 Flavourings
BT4 Additives
NT1 *Artemisia vulgaris*

Mulberries
BT1 Berries
BT2 Fruits specific
BT3 Fruits
BT4 Crops
BT5 Plants
BT4 Plant foods
BT5 Foods

Mulberry leaves
BT1 Plants

Mulching
BT1 Cultivation
BT2 Agriculture

Mullet
BT1 Marine fish
BT2 Fish
BT3 Animals
BT3 Sea foods
BT4 Aquatic foods
BT5 Animal foods
BT6 Foods
NT1 *Mugil cephalus*

Multipacks
BT1 Packs
BT2 Containers

Mung beans
HN heading from vol. 30 (1998); under Legumes up to vol. 29 (1997)
BT1 Legumes
BT2 Vegetables specific
BT3 Vegetables
BT4 Crops
BT5 Plants
BT4 Plant foods
BT5 Foods
NT1 Mung bean starch
UF Green gram

Mung bean starch
HN introduced from vol. 39, issue 1 (2007)
BT1 Mung beans
BT2 Legumes
BT3 Vegetables specific
BT4 Vegetables
BT5 Crops
BT6 Plants
BT5 Plant foods
BT6 Foods
BT1 Starch
BT2 Glucans
BT3 Polysaccharides
BT4 Carbohydrates
BT5 Nutrients
BT5 Organic compounds
BT2 Thickeners
BT3 Additives

Munggo
USE **Black gram**

Munster cheese
SN syn. Muenster cheese
BT1 Cheese varieties
BT2 Cheese
BT3 Dairy products
BT4 Animal foods
BT5 Foods

Muramidases
USE **Lysozymes**

Murraya koenigii
HN under Spices up to vol. 42 (2010)
BT1 Curry leaves
BT2 Herbs
BT3 Spices
BT4 Flavourings
BT5 Additives

Musa cavendishii
BT1 Bananas
BT2 Fruits specific
BT3 Fruits
BT4 Crops
BT5 Plants
BT4 Plant foods
BT5 Foods

Muscadine grapes
BT1 Grapes
BT2 Berries
BT3 Fruits specific
BT4 Fruits
BT5 Crops
BT6 Plants
BT5 Plant foods
BT6 Foods

Muscles
USE **Meat**

Mushrooms
BT1 Edible fungi
BT2 Fungi edible
BT3 Vegetables specific
BT4 Vegetables
BT5 Crops
BT6 Plants
BT5 Plant foods
BT6 Foods
NT1 Wild mushrooms

Muskmelons
BT1 Melons
BT2 Fruits specific
BT3 Fruits
BT4 Crops
BT5 Plants
BT4 Plant foods
BT5 Foods

Mussel poisoning
BT1 Diseases
BT1 Poisoning
RT Mussels
RT Paralytic shellfish poisoning

Mussels
HN heading from vol. 25 (1993); under Molluscs up to vol. 24 (1992)
BT1 Bivalves
BT2 Molluscs
BT3 Shellfish
BT4 Animals
BT4 Sea foods
BT5 Aquatic foods
BT6 Animal foods
BT7 Foods
NT1 Blue mussels
NT1 Green mussels
NT1 *Mytilus edulis*
NT1 *Mytilus galloprovincialis*
NT1 *Mytilus trossulus*
RT Mussel poisoning
UF Himegai

Mustard
BT1 Condiments
BT2 Flavourings
BT3 Additives

Mustard greens
BT1 Vegetables specific
BT2 Vegetables
BT3 Crops
BT4 Plants
BT3 Plant foods
BT4 Foods
NT1 Ethiopian mustard
NT2 *Brassica carinata*
NT1 Indian mustard

Mustard seed oils
BT1 Vegetable oils
BT2 Oils vegetable
BT3 Oils
BT4 Lipids
BT5 Nutrients
BT3 Vegetable products
BT4 Plant foods
BT5 Foods

Mustard seeds
HN heading from vol. 30 (1998); under Oilseeds or Spices up to vol. 29 (1997)
BT1 Oilseeds
BT2 Seeds
BT3 Plant foods
BT4 Foods
BT1 Spices
BT2 Flavourings
BT3 Additives
NT1 Ethiopian mustard
NT2 *Brassica carinata*
NT1 Indian mustard

Musts
BT1 Fruit juices
BT2 Fruit products
BT3 Plant foods
BT4 Foods
BT2 Soft drinks
BT3 Beverages
NT1 Apple musts
NT1 Grape musts

NT2 Concentrated rectified musts
RT Grape juices
RT Winemaking
RT Wines

Mutagenesis
BT1 Genetic techniques
BT2 Genetics
BT1 Modification
NT1 Site directed mutagenesis
RT Mutations

Mutagenicity
HN heading from vol. 25 (1993); under Carcinogens up to vol. 24 (1992)
NT1 Clastogenicity
NT1 Genotoxicity
RT Ames test
RT Antimutagenicity
RT Carcinogenicity
RT Carcinogens
RT Genetics
RT Mutagens
RT Mutants
RT Mutations
RT Teratogenicity

Mutagens
HN heading from vol. 25 (1993); under Carcinogens up to vol. 24 (1992)
NT1 Carcinogens
NT2 Agaritine
NT2 Benzopyrene
NT2 Cycasin
NT2 Dioxane
NT2 Ethyl carbamate
NT2 Methyl carbamate
NT2 Urethane
RT Antimutagens
RT Cancer
RT Carcinogenicity
RT Mutagenicity
RT Mutants
RT Mutations
RT Teratogenesis

Mutanolysins
BT1 Glycosidases
BT2 Hydrolases
BT3 Enzymes
RT Lysozymes

Mutants
BT1 Mutations
BT2 Genetics
RT Carcinogenicity
RT Carcinogens
RT Mutagenicity
RT Mutagens
RT Teratogenicity

Mutarotases
USE **Aldose 1-epimerases**

Mutation
HN heading up to vol. 23 (1991)
USE **Mutations**

Mutations
HN heading from vol. 24 (1992)
BT1 Genetics
NT1 Mutants
RT Carcinogenicity
RT Carcinogens
RT Mutagenesis
RT Mutagenicity
RT Mutagens
RT Teratogenicity
UF Mutation

Mutton
BT1 Meat specific
BT2 Meat
BT3 Animal foods
BT4 Foods
NT1 Ram carcasses
NT1 Sheep carcasses
RT Lamb
RT Sheep
UF Ram meat
UF Ram muscles
UF Sheep meat
UF Sheep muscles

Mutton sausages
BT1 Sausages
BT2 Meat products
BT3 Animal foods
BT4 Foods

Myanmar
HN used from vol. 30 (1998)
BT1 Asia
UF Burma

Mycobacterium
BT1 Bacteria
BT2 Microorganisms
NT1 *Mycobacterium avium*
NT2 *Mycobacterium paratuberculosis*
NT1 *Mycobacterium bovis*
NT1 *Mycobacterium tuberculosis*
RT Tuberculosis

Mycobacterium avium
BT1 *Mycobacterium*
BT2 Bacteria
BT3 Microorganisms
NT1 *Mycobacterium paratuberculosis*

Mycobacterium bovis
HN introduced from vol. 39, issue 1 (2007)
BT1 *Mycobacterium*
BT2 Bacteria
BT3 Microorganisms

Mycobacterium paratuberculosis
SN current name is Mycobacterium avium subsp. paratuberculosis
BT1 *Mycobacterium avium*
BT2 *Mycobacterium*
BT3 Bacteria
BT4 Microorganisms

Mycobacterium tuberculosis
BT1 *Mycobacterium*
BT2 Bacteria
BT3 Microorganisms

Mycoplasma
BT1 Bacteria
BT2 Microorganisms

Mycoprotein
BT1 Biomass
BT2 Fermentation products
BT3 Biotechnology
BT4 Technology
BT1 Proteins
BT2 Nutrients
NT1 Quorn
RT Fungal proteins

Mycostatin
USE **Nystatin**

Mycotoxicosis
BT1 Diseases
BT1 Poisoning
NT1 Aflatoxicosis
RT Fungi
RT Mycotoxins
RT Toxins

Mycotoxins
BT1 Toxins
BT2 Residues
NT1 Aflatoxins
NT2 Aflatoxin B_1
NT2 Aflatoxin B_2
NT2 Aflatoxin B_3
NT2 Aflatoxin D_1
NT2 Aflatoxin G_1
NT2 Aflatoxin G_2
NT2 Aflatoxin M_1
NT2 Aflatoxin M_2
NT2 Aflatoxin P_1
NT2 Aflatoxin Q_1
NT1 Agaritine
NT1 Alternariol
NT1 Amatoxins
NT2 Amanitins
NT1 Beauvericin
NT1 Byssochlamic acid
NT1 Citreoviridin
NT1 Citrinin
NT1 Cyclochlorotine
NT1 Cyclopiazonic acid
NT1 Cytochalasins
NT1 Enniatins
NT1 Eremofortin
NT1 F2 toxin
NT1 Fumagillin
NT1 Fumonisins
NT2 Fumonisin B_1
NT2 Fumonisin B_2
NT2 Fumonisin B_3
NT1 Fusaproliferin
NT1 Fusarin C
NT1 Gliotoxin
NT1 Griseofulvin
NT1 Gyromitrin
NT1 Kojic acid
NT1 Luteoskyrin
NT1 Moniliformin
NT1 β-Nitropropionic acid

NT1 Ochratoxins
 NT2 Ochratoxin A
NT1 Patulin
NT1 Penicillic acid
NT1 Penitrems
NT1 Polyketides
NT1 Roquefortine
NT1 Rubratoxins
NT1 Rugulosin
NT1 Sterigmatocystins
NT1 Tenuazonic acid
NT1 Terreic acid
NT1 Tremorgens
NT1 Tremortins
NT1 Trichothecenes
 NT2 Deoxynivalenol
 NT2 Diacetoxyscirpenol
 NT2 Fusarenon X
 NT2 Nivalenol
 NT2 Trichothecin
 NT2 T2 toxin
 NT2 Vomitoxin
NT1 Verrucosidin
NT1 Verruculogen
NT1 Versicolorin
NT1 Viriditoxin
NT1 Volvatoxins
NT1 Xanthomegnin
NT1 Zearalenol
NT1 Zearalenone
RT Alkaloids
RT Fungi
RT *Fusarium*
RT *Gliocladium*
RT Mycotoxicosis
RT *Myrothecium*
RT *Penicillium*
RT *Pithomyces*
RT *Stachybotrys*
RT *Trichothecium*

Mylar
BT1 Plastics
 BT2 Packaging materials

Myocardial infarction
HN introduced from vol. 41, issue 1 (2009)
BT1 Coronary heart diseases
 BT2 Cardiovascular diseases
  BT3 Diseases

Myofibrillar proteins
BT1 Animal proteins
 BT2 Proteins animal
  BT3 Proteins
   BT4 Nutrients

Myofibrils
USE **Meat**

Myoglobin
BT1 Animal proteins
 BT2 Proteins animal
  BT3 Proteins
   BT4 Nutrients
BT1 Pigments
NT1 Deoxymyoglobin
NT1 Metmyoglobin
NT1 Nitrosylmyoglobin
NT1 Oxymyoglobin

Myosin
HN heading from vol. 25 (1993); under Globulins up to vol. 24 (1992)
BT1 Animal proteins
 BT2 Proteins animal
  BT3 Proteins
   BT4 Nutrients
BT1 Globulins
 BT2 Proteins
  BT3 Nutrients
NT1 Myosin heavy chains
NT1 Myosin light chains

Myosin heavy chains
BT1 Myosin
 BT2 Animal proteins
  BT3 Proteins animal
   BT4 Proteins
    BT5 Nutrients
 BT2 Globulins
  BT3 Proteins
   BT4 Nutrients

Myosin light chains
BT1 Myosin
 BT2 Animal proteins
  BT3 Proteins animal
   BT4 Proteins
    BT5 Nutrients
 BT2 Globulins
  BT3 Proteins
   BT4 Nutrients

Myostatin
HN introduced from vol. 42, issue 1 (2010)
BT1 Growth factors
 BT2 Hormones
  BT3 Residues

Myrcene
BT1 Aroma compounds
 BT2 Flavour compounds
 BT2 Volatile compounds
BT1 Monoterpenes
 BT2 Hydrocarbons
  BT3 Organic compounds
 BT2 Monoterpenoids
  BT3 Terpenoids
   BT4 Lipids
    BT5 Nutrients

Myricetin
BT1 Flavonols
 BT2 Alcohols
 BT2 Flavonoids
  BT3 Aromatic compounds
   BT4 Organic compounds
  BT3 Pigments

Myristic acid
BT1 Saturated fatty acids
 BT2 Fatty acids
  BT3 Lipids
   BT4 Nutrients
  BT3 Organic acids
   BT4 Acids

Myristicin
BT1 Aroma compounds
 BT2 Flavour compounds
 BT2 Volatile compounds
BT1 Aromatic compounds
 BT2 Organic compounds

Myrobalans
HN introduced from vol. 39, issue 1 (2007)
BT1 Fruits specific
 BT2 Fruits
  BT3 Crops
   BT4 Plants
  BT3 Plant foods
   BT4 Foods

Myrosinases
USE **Thioglucosidases**

Myrothecium
BT1 Fungi
 BT2 Microorganisms
RT Mycotoxins

Myrrh
BT1 Flavourings
 BT2 Additives

Myrtle
BT1 Fruits specific
 BT2 Fruits
  BT3 Crops
   BT4 Plants
  BT3 Plant foods
   BT4 Foods

Mytilus edulis
BT1 Mussels
 BT2 Bivalves
  BT3 Molluscs
   BT4 Shellfish
    BT5 Animals
    BT5 Sea foods
     BT6 Aquatic foods
      BT7 Animal foods
       BT8 Foods

Mytilus galloprovincialis
BT1 Mussels
 BT2 Bivalves
  BT3 Molluscs
   BT4 Shellfish
    BT5 Animals
    BT5 Sea foods
     BT6 Aquatic foods
      BT7 Animal foods
       BT8 Foods

Mytilus trossulus
BT1 Mussels
 BT2 Bivalves
  BT3 Molluscs
   BT4 Shellfish
    BT5 Animals
    BT5 Sea foods
     BT6 Aquatic foods
      BT7 Animal foods
       BT8 Foods

N

N
SN index heading is Nitrogen
BT1 Nitrogen
BT2 Elements
BT3 Minerals
BT4 Nutrients

N_2
SN use for gaseous form
BT1 Gases
BT2 Physical phases
BT3 Chemistry
BT4 Science
BT1 Nitrogen
BT2 Elements
BT3 Minerals
BT4 Nutrients

Na
SN index heading is Sodium
BT1 Sodium
BT2 Metals
BT3 Elements
BT4 Minerals
BT5 Nutrients

NAA
SN index heading is Neutron activation analysis
BT1 Neutron activation analysis
BT2 Analytical techniques

NaCl
SN index heading is Salt
BT1 Chlorides
BT2 Salts
BT1 Salt
BT2 Condiments
BT3 Flavourings
BT4 Additives
UF Sodium chloride

NAD(P)
BT1 Nucleotides
UF Nicotinamide adenine dinucleotide (phosphate)

Naegleria
BT1 Parasites
BT2 Pests

NAFTA
BT1 Trade agreements
BT2 Trade
BT3 Economics
UF North American Free Trade Agreement

Naled
BT1 Acaricides
BT2 Pesticides
BT3 Biocides
BT3 Residues
BT1 Organophosphorus insecticides
BT2 Insecticides
BT3 Pesticides
BT4 Biocides
BT4 Residues
BT2 Organophosphorus pesticides
BT3 Pesticides
BT4 Biocides
BT4 Residues

Nalidixic acid
BT1 Quinolones
BT2 Antibiotics
BT3 Drugs
BT4 Residues

Namibia
BT1 Southern Africa
BT2 Africa
UF South West Africa

Nan
BT1 Bread
BT2 Bakery products
BT3 Cereal products
BT4 Plant foods
BT5 Foods

Nanofiltration
BT1 Filtration
BT2 Processing
BT3 Technology

Nanoparticles
HN introduced from vol. 42, issue 1 (2010)
BT1 Nanotechnology
BT2 Technology
BT1 Particles

Nanotechnology
HN introduced from vol. 39, issue 1 (2007)
BT1 Technology
NT1 Nanoparticles

NaOH
BT1 Alkalies
BT1 Hydroxides
BT2 Salts
UF Sodium hydroxide

Naphthalene
BT1 Aromatic compounds
BT2 Organic compounds

Naphthaleneacetic acid
HN introduced from vol. 43, issue 1 (2011); non-descriptor up to 2010 (USE 2-(1-Naphthyl)acetic acid)
BT1 Auxins
BT2 Plant growth regulators
BT3 Cultivation
BT4 Agriculture
NT1 2-(1-Naphthyl)acetic acid
NT1 (2-Naphthyloxy)acetic acid

Naphthol
BT1 Phenols
BT2 Alcohols
BT2 Aromatic compounds
BT3 Organic compounds
RT Carbaryl

β-Naphthoxyacetic acid
USE **(2-Naphthyloxy)acetic acid**

2-(1-Naphthyl)acetic acid
BT1 Naphthaleneacetic acid
BT2 Auxins
BT3 Plant growth regulators
BT4 Cultivation
BT5 Agriculture

Naphthylmethylcarbamate
USE **Carbaryl**

(2-Naphthyloxy)acetic acid
BT1 Naphthaleneacetic acid
BT2 Auxins
BT3 Plant growth regulators
BT4 Cultivation
BT5 Agriculture
UF β-Naphthoxyacetic acid

Napins
BT1 Vegetable proteins
BT2 Proteins vegetable
BT3 Proteins
BT4 Nutrients
BT3 Vegetable products
BT4 Plant foods
BT5 Foods

Naranjilla
SN syn. lulo
BT1 Fruits specific
BT2 Fruits
BT3 Crops
BT4 Plants
BT3 Plant foods
BT4 Foods
NT1 Lulo
UF Quito orange

Narazuke
BT1 Sake
BT2 Rice wines
BT3 Cereal wines
BT4 Alcoholic beverages
BT5 Beverages alcoholic
BT6 Beverages
BT1 Vegetable pickles
BT2 Pickles
BT3 Fermented foods
BT4 Processed foods
BT5 Foods
BT2 Vegetable products
BT3 Plant foods
BT4 Foods

Naringenin
BT1 Flavanones
BT2 Flavonoids
BT3 Aromatic compounds
BT4 Organic compounds
BT3 Pigments
BT1 Glycosides
BT2 Carbohydrates
BT3 Nutrients
BT3 Organic compounds

Naringin
BT1 Bitter compounds

BT2 Flavour compounds
BT1 Flavanones
BT2 Flavonoids
BT3 Aromatic compounds
BT4 Organic compounds
BT3 Pigments
BT1 Glycosides
BT2 Carbohydrates
BT3 Nutrients
BT3 Organic compounds
RT Bitterness
RT Citrus fruits

Naringinases
BT1 Enzymes

Narirutin
HN introduced from vol. 39, issue 1 (2007)
BT1 Flavanones
BT2 Flavonoids
BT3 Aromatic compounds
BT4 Organic compounds
BT3 Pigments

Nata
BT1 Coconuts
BT2 Nuts
BT3 Fruits
BT4 Crops
BT5 Plants
BT4 Plant foods
BT5 Foods
BT3 Oilseeds
BT4 Seeds
BT5 Plant foods
BT6 Foods
BT1 Desserts
BT2 Processed foods
BT3 Foods
BT1 Fermented foods
BT2 Processed foods
BT3 Foods

Natamycin
SN syn. pimaricin
BT1 Fungicides
BT2 Pesticides
BT3 Biocides
BT3 Residues
BT1 Preservatives
BT2 Additives
NT1 Pimaricin

Natto
BT1 Fermented foods
BT2 Processed foods
BT3 Foods
BT1 Soy products
BT2 Vegetable products
BT3 Plant foods
BT4 Foods

Natural colorants
HN colorants natural also used in the index up to vol. 29 (1997)
BT1 Colorants
BT2 Additives

Natural flavourings
HN flavourings natural also used in the index up to vol. 29 (1997)
BT1 Flavourings
BT2 Additives

Natural foods
BT1 Foods
RT Organic foods

Natural sweeteners
HN sweeteners natural also used in the index up to vol. 29 (1997)
BT1 Sweeteners
BT2 Additives

Navy beans
BT1 Common beans
BT2 Legumes
BT3 Vegetables specific
BT4 Vegetables
BT5 Crops
BT6 Plants
BT5 Plant foods
BT6 Foods

Nb
HN under Minerals up to vol. 42 (2010)
BT1 Metals
BT2 Elements
BT3 Minerals
BT4 Nutrients
UF Niobium

N compounds
HN also under Organic nitrogen compounds up to vol. 42 (2010)
BT1 Nitrogen compounds
BT2 Nitrogen
BT3 Elements
BT4 Minerals
BT5 Nutrients

NDGA
SN abbreviation for nordihydroguaiaretic acid
BT1 Nordihydroguaiaretic acid
BT2 Antioxidants
BT3 Additives
BT2 Phenols
BT3 Alcohols
BT3 Aromatic compounds
BT4 Organic compounds

Near infrared
USE **NIR**

Nectarines
BT1 Peaches
BT2 Fruits specific
BT3 Fruits
BT4 Crops
BT5 Plants
BT4 Plant foods
BT5 Foods

Neem
HN introduced from vol. 41, issue 1 (2009)
BT1 Plants

Nematocides
BT1 Pesticides
BT2 Biocides
BT2 Residues
NT1 Aldicarb
NT1 Carbaryl
NT1 Carbofuran
NT1 Chlorpyrifos
NT1 Dimethoate
NT1 Ethoprophos
NT1 Fensulfothion
NT1 Oxamyl
NT1 Phorate
NT1 Phosphamidon
NT1 Terbufos
NT1 Triazophos

Nematodes
BT1 Parasites
BT2 Pests

Neocallimastix
BT1 Fungi
BT2 Microorganisms
NT1 *Neocallimastix patriciarum*

Neocallimastix patriciarum
BT1 *Neocallimastix*
BT2 Fungi
BT3 Microorganisms

Neohesperidin
HN under Sweeteners up to vol. 42 (2010)
BT1 Flavanones
BT2 Flavonoids
BT3 Aromatic compounds
BT4 Organic compounds
BT3 Pigments
BT1 Glycosides
BT2 Carbohydrates
BT3 Nutrients
BT3 Organic compounds
RT Neohesperidin dihydrochalcone

Neohesperidin dihydrochalcone
BT1 Dihydrochalcones
BT2 Chalcones
BT3 Antioxidants
BT4 Additives
BT3 Flavonoids
BT4 Aromatic compounds
BT5 Organic compounds
BT4 Pigments
BT2 Glycosides
BT3 Carbohydrates
BT4 Nutrients
BT4 Organic compounds
BT1 Sweeteners
BT2 Additives
RT Neohesperidin

Neomycin
BT1 Aminoglycoside antibiotics
BT2 Antibiotics
BT3 Drugs
BT4 Residues

Neopullulanases
SN EC 3.2.1.135
BT1 Glycosidases
BT2 Hydrolases
BT3 Enzymes

Neosartorya
BT1 Fungi
BT2 Microorganisms

Neotame
BT1 Sweeteners
BT2 Additives
RT Aspartame

Neoxanthin
HN introduced from vol. 39, issue 1 (2007)
BT1 Xanthophylls
BT2 Carotenoids
BT3 Pigments
BT3 Terpenoids
BT4 Lipids
BT5 Nutrients

Nepal
BT1 Asia

Nephelometry
BT1 Analytical techniques

Neral
HN also under Flavour compounds up to vol. 42 (2010)
BT1 Citral
BT2 Aldehydes
BT3 Carbonyl compounds
BT4 Organic compounds
BT2 Aroma compounds
BT3 Flavour compounds
BT3 Volatile compounds
BT2 Monoterpenoids
BT3 Terpenoids
BT4 Lipids
BT5 Nutrients
RT Geranial

Nerol
BT1 Alcohols
BT1 Aroma compounds
BT2 Flavour compounds
BT2 Volatile compounds
BT1 Monoterpenoids
BT2 Terpenoids
BT3 Lipids
BT4 Nutrients
RT Geraniol

Neroli oils
BT1 Citrus essential oils
BT2 Essential oils
BT3 Flavourings
BT4 Additives
BT3 Vegetable oils
BT4 Oils vegetable
BT5 Oils
BT6 Lipids
BT7 Nutrients
BT5 Vegetable products
BT6 Plant foods
BT7 Foods
RT Citrus fruits

Netherlands
HN heading up to vol. 24 (1992)
BT1 Europe
BT1 European Union
RT Organization for Economic Cooperation and Development
UF Holland

Net protein ratio
USE **NPR**

Net protein utilization
USE **NPU**

Nettings
HN introduced from vol. 39, issue 1 (2007)
BT1 Packs
BT2 Containers

Nettles
BT1 Vegetables specific
BT2 Vegetables
BT3 Crops
BT4 Plants
BT3 Plant foods
BT4 Foods

Neural networks
HN used up to vol. 39 (2007)
USE **Artificial neural networks**

Neural tube defects
BT1 Diseases
NT1 Spina bifida
UF Anencephaly

Neurodegenerative diseases
HN introduced from vol. 39, issue 1 (2007)
SN includes Alzheimer's disease, Parkinson's disease, dementia, etc.
BT1 Diseases
RT Psychiatric disorders
UF Alzheimer's disease
UF Dementia
UF Parkinson's disease

Neurological shellfish poisoning
BT1 Diseases
BT1 Poisoning
RT Sea foods

Neurospora
BT1 Fungi
BT2 Microorganisms

Neurotoxicity
BT1 Toxicity
RT Neurotoxins

Neurotoxins
BT1 Toxins
BT2 Residues
NT1 Anatoxins
RT Neurotoxicity

Neutralization
NT1 Deacidification
RT Acidity
RT Alkalinity
RT pH
RT Titration

Neutron activation analysis
SN abbrev. NAA is also used in the index
BT1 Analytical techniques
NT1 NAA

New Caledonia
BT1 Australasia
BT2 Oceania

New Guinea
HN used in the index up to vol. 35, issue 6 (2003)
USE **Papua New Guinea**

New Zealand
HN heading up to vol. 24 (1992)
BT1 Oceania
RT Organization for Economic Cooperation and Development

NH_3
SN index heading is Ammonia
BT1 Ammonia
BT2 Gases
BT3 Physical phases
BT4 Chemistry
BT5 Science
BT2 Inorganic compounds

Ni
HN under Minerals up to vol. 42 (2010)
BT1 Metals
BT2 Elements
BT3 Minerals
BT4 Nutrients
UF Nickel

Niacin
SN syn. nicotinic acid; syn. nicotinamide
BT1 Nicotinic acid
BT2 Vitamin B group
BT3 Vitamins
BT4 Nutrients
UF Vitamin PP

Niacinamide
SN syn. nicotinamide; syn. nicotinic acid amide
BT1 Nicotinic acid
BT2 Vitamin B group
BT3 Vitamins
BT4 Nutrients

Nicaragua
BT1 Central America
BT2 America

Nicarbazin
BT1 Coccidiostats
BT2 Drugs
BT3 Residues

Nickel
USE **Ni**

Nicotinamide
SN syn. niacinamide; syn. nicotinic acid amide
BT1 Nicotinic acid
BT2 Vitamin B group
BT3 Vitamins
BT4 Nutrients

Nicotinamide adenine dinucleotide (phosphate)
USE **NAD(P)**

Nicotine
HN introduced from vol. 39, issue 1 (2007)
BT1 Alkaloids
BT2 Organic nitrogen compounds
RT Cigarette smoking

Nicotinic acid
SN syn. niacin
BT1 Vitamin B group
BT2 Vitamins
BT3 Nutrients
NT1 Niacin
NT1 Niacinamide
NT1 Nicotinamide
NT1 Nicotinic acid amide

Nicotinic acid amide
SN syn. nicotinamide; syn. niacinamide
BT1 Nicotinic acid
BT2 Vitamin B group
BT3 Vitamins
BT4 Nutrients

Niger
BT1 West Africa
BT2 Africa

Nigeria
BT1 West Africa
BT2 Africa

Nigerose
HN under Sugars up to vol. 42 (2010)
BT1 Disaccharides
BT2 Sugars
BT3 Carbohydrates
BT4 Nutrients
BT4 Organic compounds
BT3 Plant foods
BT4 Foods

Niger seeds
BT1 Oilseeds
BT2 Seeds
BT3 Plant foods
BT4 Foods

Nile perch
BT1 Freshwater fish
BT2 Fish
BT3 Animals
BT3 Sea foods
BT4 Aquatic foods
BT5 Animal foods
BT6 Foods

Nile tilapia
BT1 Tilapia
BT2 Freshwater fish
BT3 Fish
BT4 Animals
BT4 Sea foods
BT5 Aquatic foods
BT6 Animal foods
BT7 Foods
NT1 Bolti
NT1 *Oreochromis niloticus*
NT1 *Tilapia nilotica*

Niobium
USE **Nb**

NIR
BT1 Infrared radiation
BT2 Radiation
RT IR
UF Near infrared

NIR spectroscopy
BT1 Spectroscopy
BT2 Analytical techniques

Nisin
BT1 Bacteriocins
BT2 Antibiotics
BT3 Drugs
BT4 Residues
BT1 Preservatives
BT2 Additives
RT *Lactococcus lactis*
RT Lantibiotics

Nitrate reductases
BT1 Reductases
BT2 Oxidoreductases
BT3 Enzymes

Nitrates
BT1 Salts
RT Curing
RT Denitrification
RT Preservatives

Nitric acid
BT1 Acids

Nitric oxide
BT1 Gases
BT2 Physical phases
BT3 Chemistry
BT4 Science
BT1 Oxides
BT1 Reactive nitrogen species
BT2 Free radicals
BT3 Radicals
BT2 Nitroso compounds
BT3 Organic nitrogen compounds
UF Nitrogen monoxide

Nitrification
BT1 Processing
BT2 Technology
RT Denitrification

Nitrites
BT1 Salts
NT1 Peroxynitrite
RT Curing
RT Preservatives

Nitrobenzene
BT1 Organic nitrogen compounds

Nitrofen
BT1 Herbicides
BT2 Pesticides
BT3 Biocides
BT3 Residues

Nitrofurans
HN introduced from vol. 39, issue 1 (2007)
BT1 Antibiotics
BT2 Drugs
BT3 Residues
NT1 Furazolidone
NT1 Nitrofurazone
NT1 Nitrovin

Nitrofurazone
BT1 Nitrofurans
BT2 Antibiotics
BT3 Drugs
BT4 Residues

5-Nitrofurylacrylic acid
BT1 Organic acids
BT2 Acids
BT1 Preservatives
BT2 Additives

Nitrogen
HN also under Gases up to vol. 42 (2010)
SN use generally for this element; use N2 for gaseous form
BT1 Elements
BT2 Minerals
BT3 Nutrients
NT1 Amino N
NT2 α-Amino N
NT1 Liquid nitrogen
NT1 N
NT1 N_2
NT1 Nitrogen compounds
NT2 N compounds
RT Flushing

Nitrogen compounds
HN heading up to vol. 24 (1992)
BT1 Nitrogen
BT2 Elements
BT3 Minerals
BT4 Nutrients
NT1 N compounds
RT Organic nitrogen compounds

Nitrogen dioxide
USE **NO_2**

Nitrogen monoxide
USE **Nitric oxide**

Nonenal
BT1 Aldehydes
BT2 Carbonyl compounds
BT3 Organic compounds
BT1 Aroma compounds
BT2 Flavour compounds
BT2 Volatile compounds
RT Off odour

Nonenzymic browning
HN browning nonenymic also used in the index up to vol. 29 (1997)
BT1 Browning
RT Caramelization
RT Maillard reaction

Noni
HN introduced from vol. 39, issue 1 (2007)
BT1 Fruits specific
BT2 Fruits
BT3 Crops
BT4 Plants
BT3 Plant foods
BT4 Foods
RT Noni juices
UF Indian mulberries

Noni juices
HN introduced from vol. 41, issue 1 (2009)
BT1 Fruit juices
BT2 Fruit products
BT3 Plant foods
BT4 Foods
BT2 Soft drinks
BT3 Beverages
RT Noni

Nono
BT1 Fermented milk
BT2 Fermented dairy products
BT3 Dairy products
BT4 Animal foods
BT5 Foods
BT3 Fermented foods
BT4 Processed foods
BT5 Foods
BT2 Milk
BT3 Dairy products
BT4 Animal foods
BT5 Foods

Nonreducing sugars
HN sugars nonreducing also used in the index up to vol. 29 (1997)
BT1 Sugars
BT2 Carbohydrates
BT3 Nutrients
BT3 Organic compounds
BT2 Plant foods
BT3 Foods
UF Sugars nonreducing

Nonstarch polysaccharides
HN introduced from vol. 39, issue 1 (2007)
BT1 Dietary fibre
BT2 Fibre
BT1 Polysaccharides
BT2 Carbohydrates
BT3 Nutrients
BT3 Organic compounds

Nonthermal processes
BT1 Processing
BT2 Technology

Noodles
HN heading from vol. 30 (1998); under Pasta up to vol. 29 (1997)
BT1 Pasta
BT2 Cereal products
BT3 Plant foods
BT4 Foods
NT1 Instant noodles
RT Rice noodles

Nootkatone
BT1 Aroma compounds
BT2 Flavour compounds
BT2 Volatile compounds
BT1 Ketones
BT2 Carbonyl compounds
BT3 Organic compounds
BT1 Sesquiterpenoids
BT2 Terpenoids
BT3 Lipids
BT4 Nutrients

Noradrenaline
HN introduced from vol. 39, issue 1 (2007)
BT1 Catecholamines
BT2 Biogenic amines
BT3 Amines
BT4 Organic nitrogen compounds
BT2 Hormones
BT3 Residues
UF Norepinephrine

Norbixin
BT1 Colorants
BT2 Additives

Nordihydroguaiaretic acid
SN abbrev. NDGA is also used in the index
BT1 Antioxidants
BT2 Additives
BT1 Phenols
BT2 Alcohols
BT2 Aromatic compounds
BT3 Organic compounds
NT1 NDGA

Norepinephrine
USE **Noradrenaline**

Norflurazon
BT1 Herbicides
BT2 Pesticides
BT3 Biocides
BT3 Residues

Norharman
BT1 Alkaloids
BT2 Organic nitrogen compounds
RT Carbolines
RT Carcinogens
RT Harman

Nori
BT1 *Porphyra*
BT2 Seaweeds
BT3 Algae
BT4 Microorganisms
BT3 Sea foods
BT4 Aquatic foods
BT5 Animal foods
BT6 Foods

Norisoprenoids
HN introduced from vol. 39, issue 1 (2007)
BT1 Aroma compounds
BT2 Flavour compounds
BT2 Volatile compounds
BT1 Carotenoids
BT2 Pigments
BT2 Terpenoids
BT3 Lipids
BT4 Nutrients
NT1 β-Damascenone
NT1 Ionones

Norovirus
HN introduced from vol. 43, issue 1 (2011)
BT1 Noroviruses
BT2 Caliciviruses
BT3 Viruses
BT4 Microorganisms
NT1 Norwalk virus
NT2 Norwalk-like virus
NT2 Small round structured virus

Noroviruses
HN introduced from vol. 39, issue 1 (2007); under Enteric viruses up to vol. 42 (2010)
SN for descriptive use only
BT1 Caliciviruses
BT2 Viruses
BT3 Microorganisms
NT1 Norovirus
NT2 Norwalk virus
NT3 Norwalk-like virus
NT3 Small round structured virus

North Africa
BT1 Africa
NT1 Algeria
NT1 Egypt
NT1 Libya
NT1 Morocco
NT1 Tunisia

North America
HN heading up to vol. 24 (1992)
BT1 America
NT1 Bermuda
NT1 Canada
NT1 Greenland
NT1 United States of America

North American Free Trade Agreement
USE **NAFTA**

Northern blotting
BT1 Blotting
BT2 Hybridization
BT3 Genetic techniques
BT4 Genetics

Northern Ireland
BT1 United Kingdom
BT2 Europe
BT2 European Union

North Korea
SN full name is Democratic People's Republic of Korea
BT1 Asia
RT Korea

Norvegia cheese
BT1 Cheese varieties
BT2 Cheese
BT3 Dairy products
BT4 Animal foods
BT5 Foods

Norwalk-like virus
HN introduced from vol. 43, issue 1 (2011); Norwalk-like viruses also used in the index up to vol. 42 (2010)
BT1 Norwalk virus
BT2 Norovirus
BT3 Noroviruses
BT4 Caliciviruses
BT5 Viruses
BT6 Microorganisms
UF Norwalk-like viruses

Norwalk-like viruses
HN introduced from vol. 39, issue 1 (2007); Norwalk-like virus used in the index from vol. 43 (2011)
USE **Norwalk-like virus**

Norwalk virus
HN introduced from vol. 43, issue 1 (2011); Norwalk viruses also used in the index up to vol. 42 (2010)
BT1 Norovirus
BT2 Noroviruses
BT3 Caliciviruses
BT4 Viruses
BT5 Microorganisms
NT1 Norwalk-like virus
NT1 Small round structured virus
UF Norwalk viruses

Norwalk viruses
HN Norwalk virus used in the index from vol. 43 (2011)
USE **Norwalk virus**

Norway
HN heading up to vol. 24 (1992)
BT1 Europe
RT Organization for Economic Cooperation and Development

Norway lobsters
BT1 Crustacea
BT2 Shellfish
BT3 Animals
BT3 Sea foods
BT4 Aquatic foods
BT5 Animal foods
BT6 Foods
NT1 Langoustines
NT1 Scampi

Nostoc
BT1 Cyanobacteria
BT2 Bacteria
BT3 Microorganisms

Nougat
BT1 Sugar confectionery
BT2 Plant foods
BT3 Foods

Novel foods
HN heading from vol. 28 (1996)
SN foods prepared by unconventional processes, derived from unconventional sources or offering non-nutritional benefits
BT1 Foods
NT1 Beauty foods
NT1 Biotechnologically derived foods
NT1 Cloned animal foods
NT1 Designer foods
NT1 Functional foods
NT2 Functional beverages
NT2 Nutraceutical foods
NT1 Genetically engineered foods
NT1 GM foods
NT1 Medical foods
NT1 Prebiotic foods
NT1 Probiotic foods
NT1 Synbiotic foods
RT Transgenic animals
RT Transgenic plants

Novobiocin
BT1 Antibiotics
BT2 Drugs
BT3 Residues

NPR
BT1 Nutritional values
UF Net protein ratio

NPU
BT1 Nutritional values
UF Net protein utilization

Nuclear magnetic resonance
SN abbrev. NMR is also used in the index
BT1 Spectroscopy
BT2 Analytical techniques
NT1 Magnetic resonance imaging
NT1 NMR
NT1 Proton magnetic resonance
NT1 Proton resonance

Nuclear power
BT1 Energy

Nuclear reactor accidents
BT1 Radioactivity

Nucleases
SN EC 3.1.11-3.1.16 and 3.1.21-3.1.31
BT1 Esterases
BT2 Hydrolases
BT3 Enzymes
NT1 Deoxyribonucleases
NT1 Endonucleases
NT1 Restriction endonucleases
NT1 Restriction enzymes
NT1 Ribonucleases
NT2 Angiogenin

Nucleic acids
BT1 Organic acids
BT2 Acids
NT1 DNA
NT2 cDNA
NT2 Mitochondrial DNA
NT2 RAPD
NT1 RNA
NT2 mRNA
NT2 rRNA
RT Nucleotides

Nucleosides
NT1 Adenosine
NT2 *S*-Adenosyl-L-methionine
NT1 Cytidine
NT1 Guanosine
NT1 Inosine
NT1 Ribonucleosides
NT1 Uridine
RT Nucleotides

Nucleotidases
SN EC 3.1.3.31
BT1 Phosphatases
BT2 Esterases
BT3 Hydrolases
BT4 Enzymes

Nucleotides
NT1 ADP
NT1 AMP
NT1 ATP
NT1 cAMP
NT1 GMP
NT1 IMP
NT1 NAD(P)
NT1 Oligonucleotides
NT1 Ribonucleotides
NT1 UMP
RT Nucleic acids
RT Nucleosides

Nucleotide sequences
HN introduced from vol. 39, issue 1 (2007)
SN includes DNA, RNA sequence data, etc.
BT1 Genetics

Nukazuke
HN under Sea foods up to vol. 42 (2010)
BT1 Fermented foods
BT2 Processed foods
BT3 Foods
BT1 Fish products
BT2 Sea foods
BT3 Aquatic foods
BT4 Animal foods
BT5 Foods

Nuoc-mam
BT1 Fermented foods
BT2 Processed foods
BT3 Foods
BT1 Fish sauces
BT2 Fish products
BT3 Sea foods
BT4 Aquatic foods
BT5 Animal foods
BT6 Foods
BT2 Sauces
BT3 Condiments
BT4 Flavourings
BT5 Additives

Nuruk
BT1 Starters
BT2 Bacteria
BT3 Microorganisms

Nutmeg
BT1 Spices
BT2 Flavourings
BT3 Additives
RT Nutmeg oils

Nutmeg oils
HN introduced from vol. 39, issue 1 (2007)
BT1 Essential oils
BT2 Flavourings
BT3 Additives
BT2 Vegetable oils
BT3 Oils vegetable
BT4 Oils
BT5 Lipids
BT6 Nutrients
BT4 Vegetable products
BT5 Plant foods
BT6 Foods
RT Nutmeg

Nut oils
BT1 Vegetable oils
BT2 Oils vegetable
BT3 Oils
BT4 Lipids
BT5 Nutrients
BT3 Vegetable products
BT4 Plant foods
BT5 Foods
NT1 Almond oils
NT1 Beech nut oils
NT1 Brazil nut oils
NT1 Coconut oils
NT1 Groundnut oils
NT1 Hazelnut oils
NT1 Pecan oils
NT1 Walnut oils

Nut pastes
HN under Sugar confectionery up to vol. 42 (2010)
BT1 Nuts
BT2 Fruits
BT3 Crops
BT4 Plants
BT3 Plant foods
BT4 Foods
BT2 Oilseeds
BT3 Seeds
BT4 Plant foods
BT5 Foods
BT1 Pastes
BT2 Processed foods
BT3 Foods
NT1 Peanut pastes
RT Confectionery pastes
RT Tahini

Nut products
HN introduced from vol. 41, issue 1 (2009)
BT1 Nuts
BT2 Fruits
BT3 Crops
BT4 Plants
BT3 Plant foods
BT4 Foods
BT2 Oilseeds
BT3 Seeds
BT4 Plant foods
BT5 Foods

Nutraceutical foods
HN under Novel foods up to vol. 42 (2010)
SN syn. functional foods
BT1 Functional foods
BT2 Novel foods
BT3 Foods
RT Designer foods
RT Health
RT Medical foods
RT Nutrition
RT Phytochemicals

NutraSweet
BT1 Aspartame
BT2 Sweeteners
BT3 Additives

Nutria
SN syn. coypu
BT1 Coypu
BT2 Animals

Nutrient density
HN introduced from vol. 43, issue 1 (2011)
BT1 Nutritional values

Nutrient requirements
HN introduced from vol. 38, issue 8 (2006)
BT1 Nutrients
BT1 Nutrition
NT1 DRI
NT2 RDA
NT1 DRV
NT1 RDI

Nutrients
HN heading from vol. 25 (1993); under Nutrition up to vol. 24 (1992)
NT1 Amino acids
NT1 Carbohydrates
NT1 Gene-nutrient interactions
NT1 Lipids
NT1 Macronutrients
NT1 Micronutrients
NT1 Minerals
NT1 Nutrient requirements
NT1 Proteins
NT1 Vitamins
RT Antinutritional factors
RT Nutrition
RT Nutritional values

Nutrigenetics
HN introduced from vol. 39, issue 1 (2007)
BT1 Genetics
BT1 Nutrition
RT Gene-nutrient interactions
RT Nutrigenomics

Nutrigenomics
HN introduced from vol. 39, issue 1 (2007)
BT1 Genomics
BT2 Genetics
BT1 Nutrition
RT Nutrigenetics

Nutrition
NT1 Calories
NT2 Calories high foods
NT2 Calories low beverages
NT2 Calories low diet
NT2 Calories low foods
NT3 Calories low spreads
NT1 Diet
NT2 Dietary study techniques
NT3 Food frequency questionnaires
NT2 Diet therapy
NT3 Calories low diet
NT3 Carbohydrates low diet
NT3 Diabetic diet
NT3 Fats low diet
NT3 Ketogenic diet
NT3 Sodium low diet
NT3 Wt. loss diet
NT2 Fats high diet
NT2 Mediterranean diet
NT2 Proteins high diet
NT2 Vegan diet
NT2 Vegetarian diet
NT1 Digestibility
NT1 Food composition tables
NT1 Food guide pyramids
NT1 Nutrient requirements
NT2 DRI
NT3 RDA
NT2 DRV
NT2 RDI
NT1 Nutrigenetics
NT1 Nutrigenomics
NT1 Nutritional assessment
NT1 Nutritional status
NT2 Antioxidant status
NT2 Hydration status
NT1 Prenatal nutrition
NT1 Sports nutrition
RT ADI
RT Anticarcinogenicity
RT Anticarcinogens
RT Antimutagenicity
RT Antimutagens
RT Antinutritional factors
RT Cholesterol

RT Dietetic foods
RT Food supplements
RT Functional foods
RT Health
RT Health foods
RT Infant foods
RT Medical foods
RT Metabolic disorders
RT MRL
RT Nutraceutical foods
RT Nutrients
RT Nutritional values
RT Probiotic foods
RT RDA
RT RDI
RT Teratogenicity

Nutritional assessment
HN introduced from vol. 39, issue 1 (2007)
BT1 Nutrition
RT Dietary study techniques

Nutritional labelling
HN labelling nutritional used up to vol. 29 (1997)
BT1 Labelling
BT2 Packaging
BT3 Technology
RT Consumer information

Nutritional status
HN introduced from vol. 38, issue 8 (2006)
BT1 Nutrition
NT1 Antioxidant status
NT1 Hydration status
RT Deficiency diseases
RT Human physiology

Nutritional values
NT1 Antinutritional factors
NT2 Amylases inhibitors
NT3 α-Amylases inhibitors
NT2 Inositol
NT3 Inositol phosphates
NT3 Phytates
NT3 Phytic acid
NT2 Proteinases inhibitors
NT3 Calpastatins
NT3 Chymotrypsin inhibitors
NT3 Cystatins
NT3 Trypsin inhibitors
NT2 Vitamin antagonists
NT1 Bioavailability
NT2 Availability
NT1 Biological values
NT1 Calorific values
NT2 Energy density
NT1 Glycaemic index values
NT1 Glycaemic load
NT1 NPR
NT1 NPU
NT1 Nutrient density
NT1 PER
NT1 Protein values
RT Calories
RT Diet
RT Food enrichment
RT Nutrients
RT Nutrition

Nuts
BT1 Fruits
BT2 Crops
BT3 Plants
BT2 Plant foods
BT3 Foods
BT1 Oilseeds
BT2 Seeds
BT3 Plant foods
BT4 Foods
NT1 Acorns
NT1 Almonds
NT2 Sweet almonds
NT1 Australian chestnuts
NT1 Brazil nuts
NT1 Butternuts
NT1 Cashew nuts
NT1 Cedar nuts
NT1 Chestnuts
NT2 Japanese chestnuts
NT2 Sweet chestnuts
NT1 Chilean hazelnuts
NT1 Coconuts
NT2 Bongkrek
NT2 Coconut cream
NT2 Coconut milk
NT2 Coconut water
NT2 Copra
NT2 Desiccated coconut
NT2 Nata
NT1 Cola nuts
NT2 *Cola nitida*
NT1 Conophor nuts
NT1 Ginkgo nuts
NT1 Gorgon nuts
NT1 Hazelnuts
NT1 Hickory nuts
NT1 Macadamia nuts
NT1 Nut pastes
NT2 Peanut pastes
NT1 Nut products
NT1 Peanuts
NT2 Ontjom
NT2 Peanut butter
NT2 Peanut meal
NT2 Peanut milk
NT2 Peanut pastes
NT2 Peanut products
NT2 Peanut proteins
NT2 Roasted peanuts
NT1 Pecan nuts
NT1 Pine nuts
NT1 Pistachio nuts
NT1 Walnuts

Nylon
BT1 Plastics
BT2 Packaging materials

Nystatin
BT1 Macrolide antibiotics
BT2 Antibiotics
BT3 Drugs
BT4 Residues
UF Mycostatin

Nystose
HN under Sugars up to vol. 42 (2010)
BT1 Fructooligosaccharides
BT2 Oligosaccharides
BT3 Polysaccharides
BT4 Carbohydrates
BT5 Nutrients
BT5 Organic compounds
BT3 Sugars
BT4 Carbohydrates
BT5 Nutrients
BT5 Organic compounds
BT4 Plant foods
BT5 Foods

O

O_2
SN use for gaseous molecular form
BT1 Gases
BT2 Physical phases
BT3 Chemistry
BT4 Science
BT1 Oxygen
BT2 Elements
BT3 Minerals
BT4 Nutrients

O_2 absorbers
USE **Oxygen absorbers**

Oak
BT1 Wood
BT2 Packaging materials

Oat bran
BT1 Bran
BT2 Cereal products
BT3 Plant foods
BT4 Foods
BT1 Oats
BT2 Cereals
BT3 Crops
BT4 Plants
BT3 Seeds
BT4 Plant foods
BT5 Foods

Oat fibre
BT1 Fibre
BT1 Oats
BT2 Cereals
BT3 Crops
BT4 Plants
BT3 Seeds
BT4 Plant foods
BT5 Foods

Oat flakes
HN introduced from vol. 39, issue 1 (2007)
BT1 Oats
BT2 Cereals
BT3 Crops
BT4 Plants
BT3 Seeds
BT4 Plant foods
BT5 Foods

Oat flour
BT1 Cereal flours
BT2 Flours cereal
BT3 Cereal products
BT4 Plant foods
BT5 Foods
BT1 Oats
BT2 Cereals
BT3 Crops
BT4 Plants
BT3 Seeds
BT4 Plant foods
BT5 Foods

Oatmeal
SN use only for milling product; use porridge for the food prepared from oatmeal
BT1 Cereal flours
BT2 Flours cereal
BT3 Cereal products
BT4 Plant foods
BT5 Foods
BT1 Oats
BT2 Cereals
BT3 Crops
BT4 Plants
BT3 Seeds
BT4 Plant foods
BT5 Foods

Oat oils
BT1 Vegetable oils
BT2 Oils vegetable
BT3 Oils
BT4 Lipids
BT5 Nutrients
BT3 Vegetable products
BT4 Plant foods
BT5 Foods

Oatrim
BT1 Fat substitutes
BT2 Fats
BT3 Lipids
BT4 Nutrients

Oats
BT1 Cereals
BT2 Crops
BT3 Plants
BT2 Seeds
BT3 Plant foods
BT4 Foods
NT1 *Avena fatua*
NT1 Oat bran
NT1 Oat fibre
NT1 Oat flakes
NT1 Oat flour
NT1 Oatmeal
NT1 Oat starch
NT1 Porridge
RT Avenanthramides

Oat starch
BT1 Oats
BT2 Cereals
BT3 Crops
BT4 Plants
BT3 Seeds
BT4 Plant foods
BT5 Foods
BT1 Starch
BT2 Glucans
BT3 Polysaccharides
BT4 Carbohydrates
BT5 Nutrients
BT5 Organic compounds
BT2 Thickeners
BT3 Additives

Obesity
BT1 Diseases
RT Anthropometric parameters
RT Body composition
RT Body wt.
RT Food portions
RT Overweight
RT Portion sizes
RT Wt. loss diet

Obesumbacterium
BT1 Bacteria
BT2 Microorganisms

Oca
BT1 Vegetables specific
BT2 Vegetables
BT3 Crops
BT4 Plants
BT3 Plant foods
BT4 Foods
NT1 *Oxalis tuberosa*

Oceania
HN heading up to vol. 24 (1992)
NT1 American Samoa
NT1 Australasia
NT2 New Caledonia
NT1 Australia
NT1 Fiji
NT1 Guam
NT1 Kiribati
NT1 New Zealand
NT1 Papua New Guinea
NT1 Samoa
NT1 Solomon Islands
NT1 Tonga

Ochratoxin A
HN included as ochratoxins up to vol. 29 (1997)
BT1 Ochratoxins
BT2 Mycotoxins
BT3 Toxins
BT4 Residues

Ochratoxins
HN heading from vol. 30 (1998); under Mycotoxins up to vol. 29 (1997)
BT1 Mycotoxins
BT2 Toxins
BT3 Residues
NT1 Ochratoxin A

Octadecanoic acid
SN syn. stearic acid
BT1 Saturated fatty acids
BT2 Fatty acids
BT3 Lipids
BT4 Nutrients
BT3 Organic acids
BT4 Acids
NT1 Stearic acid
NT2 Hydroxystearic acid

Octadecenoic acid
BT1 Monounsaturated fatty acids
BT2 Unsaturated fatty acids
BT3 Fatty acids
BT4 Lipids
BT5 Nutrients
BT4 Organic acids
BT5 Acids
NT1 Elaidic acid
NT1 Oleic acid
NT1 Petroselinic acid
NT1 Vaccenic acid

Octanal
HN also under Flavour compounds up to vol. 42 (2010)
BT1 Aldehydes
BT2 Carbonyl compounds
BT3 Organic compounds
BT1 Aroma compounds
BT2 Flavour compounds
BT2 Volatile compounds

Octanoic acid
HN under Flavour compounds and Fatty acids up to vol. 42 (2010)
SN syn. caprylic acid
BT1 Aroma compounds
BT2 Flavour compounds
BT2 Volatile compounds
BT1 Saturated fatty acids
BT2 Fatty acids
BT3 Lipids
BT4 Nutrients
BT3 Organic acids
BT4 Acids
NT1 Caprylic acid

Octanol
BT1 Alcohols

Octanone
HN also under Flavour compounds up to vol. 42 (2010)
BT1 Aroma compounds
BT2 Flavour compounds
BT2 Volatile compounds
BT1 Ketones
BT2 Carbonyl compounds
BT3 Organic compounds

1-Octen-3-ol
HN introduced from vol. 39, issue 1 (2007); also under Flavour compounds up to vol. 42 (2010)
BT1 Alcohols
BT1 Aroma compounds
BT2 Flavour compounds
BT2 Volatile compounds

Octopine
BT1 Amino acids
BT2 Nutrients
BT2 Organic acids

BT3 Acids
BT2 Organic nitrogen compounds

Octopus
BT1 Cephalopods
BT2 Molluscs
BT3 Shellfish
BT4 Animals
BT4 Sea foods
BT5 Aquatic foods
BT6 Animal foods
BT7 Foods

Octyl gallate
HN introduced from vol. 39, issue 1 (2007)
BT1 Antioxidants
BT2 Additives
BT1 Esters
BT2 Organic compounds

Odorant
USE **Aroma compounds**

Odour
USE **Aroma**

Odour activity values
BT1 Aroma
BT2 Sensory properties
RT Odour threshold values

Odour threshold values
BT1 Aroma
BT2 Sensory properties
RT Odour activity values

OECD
USE **Organization for Economic Cooperation and Development**

Oedema
BT1 Diseases
UF Dropsy

Oenococcus
BT1 Bacteria
BT2 Microorganisms
NT1 *Oenococcus oeni*

Oenococcus oeni
SN synonymous with Leuconostoc oenos
BT1 *Oenococcus*
BT2 Bacteria
BT3 Microorganisms

Oenocyanins
BT1 Anthocyanins
BT2 Flavonoids
BT3 Aromatic compounds
BT4 Organic compounds
BT3 Pigments

Oenological properties
BT1 Winemaking
BT2 Processing
BT3 Technology

Oestradiol
BT1 Oestrogens
BT2 Hormones
BT3 Residues

Oestrogenic activity
HN introduced from vol. 39, issue 1 (2007)
BT1 Health
BT1 Oestrogens
BT2 Hormones
BT3 Residues

Oestrogens
BT1 Hormones
BT2 Residues
NT1 Oestradiol
NT1 Oestrogenic activity
NT1 Oestrone
RT Diethylstilboestrol
RT Phytoestrogens

Oestrone
BT1 Oestrogens
BT2 Hormones
BT3 Residues

Offal
BT1 Animal foods
BT2 Foods
NT1 Bladders
NT1 Bowels
NT1 Brains
NT1 Chicken gizzard pickles
NT1 Chitterlings
NT1 Giblets
NT1 Gizzards
NT1 Hearts
NT1 Intestines
NT1 Kidneys
NT2 Cattle kidneys
NT2 Lamb kidneys
NT2 Swine kidneys
NT1 Livers
NT2 Cattle livers
NT2 Chicken livers
NT2 Duck livers
NT2 Fish livers
NT3 Cod livers
NT2 Foie gras
NT2 Goose livers
NT2 Lamb livers
NT2 Swine livers
NT2 Turkey livers
NT1 Lungs
NT1 Pancreas
NT1 Spleens
NT1 Stomachs
NT1 Sweetbreads
NT1 Tongues
NT1 Tripe
RT By-products
RT Carcasses
RT Meat
UF Carcass by-products
UF Slaughter by-products

Off flavour
BT1 Taints
BT2 Flavour
BT3 Sensory properties
RT Flavour
RT Flavour compounds

Off odour
BT1 Taints
BT2 Flavour
BT3 Sensory properties
RT Aldehydes
RT Aroma
RT Aroma compounds
RT Dimethyl sulfide
RT Methanethiol
RT 3-Methylbutanal
RT Nonenal
RT Pentanal
RT Trimethylamine

Ogi
BT1 Cereal products
BT2 Plant foods
BT3 Foods
BT1 Fermented foods
BT2 Processed foods
BT3 Foods

Ogiri
BT1 Fermented foods
BT2 Processed foods
BT3 Foods
BT1 Seeds
BT2 Plant foods
BT3 Foods

Ohmic heating
BT1 Sterilization
BT2 Thermal processing
BT3 Processing thermal
BT4 Processing
BT5 Technology

Oil absorption capacity
HN introduced from vol. 42, issue 1 (2010)
BT1 Functional properties
BT2 Physical properties
RT Absorption
RT Oils

Oil expellers
BT1 Equipment
BT2 Technology
BT1 Pressing
BT2 Processing
BT3 Technology

Oil palms
RT Palm oils
RT Palms

Oils
BT1 Lipids
BT2 Nutrients
NT1 Algal oils
NT1 Cooking oils
NT1 Frying oils
NT1 Marine oils
NT2 Oils fish
NT3 Fish oils
NT4 Anchovy oils
NT4 Cod liver oils

NT4 Fish liver oils
NT4 Menhaden oils
NT4 Salmon oils
NT4 Sardine oils
NT4 Tuna oils
NT2 Seal blubber oils
NT2 Seal oils
NT2 Squid oils
NT2 Whale oils
NT1 Mineral oils
NT1 Oils vegetable
NT2 Vegetable oils
NT3 Argemone oils
NT3 Avocado oils
NT3 Baobab oils
NT3 Borage oils
NT3 Camelina oils
NT3 Castor oils
NT3 Coffee oils
NT3 Corn oils
NT4 Corn fibre oils
NT3 Cottonseed oils
NT3 Essential oils
NT4 Bitter almond oils
NT4 Buchu oils
NT4 Cinnamon oils
NT4 Citronella essential oils
NT4 Citrus essential oils
NT5 Bergamot essential oils
NT6 Bergamot oils
NT5 Bitter orange essential oils
NT5 Citrus oils
NT5 Lemon essential oils
NT5 Lime essential oils
NT5 Neroli oils
NT5 Orange essential oils
NT4 Clary sage essential oils
NT4 Clove oils
NT4 Garlic oils
NT4 Hop essential oils
NT4 Lemongrass oils
NT4 Mint oils
NT4 Nutmeg oils
NT4 Oleoresins
NT4 Oregano oils
NT4 Peppermint essential oils
NT4 Petitgrain oils
NT4 Rosemary essential oils
NT4 Sage essential oils
NT4 Tea tree oils
NT4 Thyme oils
NT3 Evening primrose oils
NT3 Flax seed oils
NT4 Linseed oils
NT3 Grape seed oils
NT3 Jojoba oils
NT3 Kapok oils
NT3 Lupin seed oils
NT3 Meadowfoam oils
NT3 Millet oils
NT3 Mustard seed oils
NT3 Nut oils
NT4 Almond oils
NT4 Beech nut oils
NT4 Brazil nut oils
NT4 Coconut oils
NT4 Groundnut oils
NT4 Hazelnut oils
NT4 Pecan oils
NT4 Walnut oils
NT3 Oat oils
NT3 Olive oils
NT4 Olive oil mills effluents
NT4 Olive pomace oils
NT5 Sansa oils
NT3 Palm oils
NT4 Babassu oils
NT4 Palm kernel oils
NT4 Palm oil mills effluents
NT4 Palm olein
NT4 Palm stearin
NT3 Perilla oils
NT3 Pumpkin seed oils
NT3 Rapeseed oils
NT3 Rice bran oils
NT3 Rice germ oils
NT3 Safflower oils
NT3 Sea buckthorn oils
NT3 Sesame oils
NT3 Soybean oils
NT3 Sunflower oils
NT3 Tea seed oils
NT3 Tomato seed oils
NT3 Wheat germ oils
NT1 Salad oils
RT Fats
RT Hydrogenation
RT Oil absorption capacity
UF Edible oils

Oilseed proteins
BT1 Vegetable proteins
BT2 Proteins vegetable
BT3 Proteins
BT4 Nutrients
BT3 Vegetable products
BT4 Plant foods
BT5 Foods

Oilseeds
BT1 Seeds
BT2 Plant foods
BT3 Foods
NT1 African locust beans
NT2 Dawadawa
NT2 Iru
NT1 African mango seeds
NT2 Dika nuts
NT1 African oil beans
NT2 Ugba
NT1 Aiele fruits
NT1 Babassu palm kernels
NT1 *Brassica* seeds
NT1 *Camelina sativa*
NT1 Castor beans
NT1 Cottonseeds
NT2 Cottonseed meal
NT2 Cottonseed proteins
NT2 Gossypol
NT1 Crambe seeds
NT2 *Crambe abyssinica*
NT1 Cucumber seeds
NT1 *Cuphea*
NT1 Egusi
NT1 *Euphorbia*
NT1 Evening primrose seeds
NT1 Flax seeds
NT2 Linseeds
NT1 Gourd seeds
NT1 *Guizotia*
NT1 Hemp seeds
NT1 Illipe nuts
NT1 Jojoba seeds
NT1 Jute seeds
NT1 Kenaf seeds
NT1 Kusum
NT1 Lupin seeds
NT2 Lupin meal
NT1 Madhuca seeds
NT1 Meadowfoam
NT1 Melon seeds
NT1 *Moringa*
NT1 Mustard seeds
NT2 Ethiopian mustard
NT3 *Brassica carinata*
NT2 Indian mustard
NT1 Niger seeds
NT1 Nuts
NT2 Acorns
NT2 Almonds
NT3 Sweet almonds
NT2 Australian chestnuts
NT2 Brazil nuts
NT2 Butternuts
NT2 Cashew nuts
NT2 Cedar nuts
NT2 Chestnuts
NT3 Japanese chestnuts
NT3 Sweet chestnuts
NT2 Chilean hazelnuts
NT2 Coconuts
NT3 Bongkrek
NT3 Coconut cream
NT3 Coconut milk
NT3 Coconut water
NT3 Copra
NT3 Desiccated coconut
NT3 Nata
NT2 Cola nuts
NT3 *Cola nitida*
NT2 Conophor nuts
NT2 Ginkgo nuts
NT2 Gorgon nuts
NT2 Hazelnuts
NT2 Hickory nuts
NT2 Macadamia nuts
NT2 Nut pastes
NT3 Peanut pastes
NT2 Nut products
NT2 Peanuts
NT3 Ontjom
NT3 Peanut butter
NT3 Peanut meal
NT3 Peanut milk
NT3 Peanut pastes
NT3 Peanut products
NT3 Peanut proteins
NT3 Roasted peanuts
NT2 Pecan nuts
NT2 Pine nuts
NT2 Pistachio nuts
NT2 Walnuts
NT1 Olives
NT2 Black olives
NT2 Table olives
NT1 Perilla seeds
NT1 Pumpkin seeds

NT1 Rapeseeds
NT2 Bird rape
NT2 *Brassica napus*
NT2 Rapeseed meal
NT1 Raya seeds
NT1 Rubber seeds
NT1 Safflower seeds
NT1 Sal seeds
NT1 Sesame seeds
NT2 Halva
NT2 Sesame
NT2 Sesame seed meal
NT2 Tahini
NT3 Tehineh
NT1 Shea nuts
NT1 Soybeans
NT2 Black soybeans
NT2 Soybean sprouts
NT1 Squash seeds
NT1 Sunflower seeds
NT2 Sunflower meal
NT2 Sunflowers
NT1 Tomato seeds
NT1 *Vernonia*
NT1 Watermelon seeds
NT1 White mustard
NT1 Yellow mustard
RT Fats vegetable
RT Oils vegetable
RT Vegetable fats
RT Vegetable oils

Oils fish
SN fish oils is also used in the index
BT1 Fish products
BT2 Sea foods
BT3 Aquatic foods
BT4 Animal foods
BT5 Foods
BT1 Marine oils
BT2 Oils
BT3 Lipids
BT4 Nutrients
NT1 Fish oils
NT2 Anchovy oils
NT2 Cod liver oils
NT2 Fish liver oils
NT2 Menhaden oils
NT2 Salmon oils
NT2 Sardine oils
NT2 Tuna oils
RT Animal fats

Oils vegetable
SN vegetable oils is also used in the index
BT1 Oils
BT2 Lipids
BT3 Nutrients
BT1 Vegetable products
BT2 Plant foods
BT3 Foods
NT1 Vegetable oils
NT2 Argemone oils
NT2 Avocado oils
NT2 Baobab oils
NT2 Borage oils
NT2 Camelina oils
NT2 Castor oils
NT2 Coffee oils
NT2 Corn oils
NT3 Corn fibre oils
NT2 Cottonseed oils
NT2 Essential oils
NT3 Bitter almond oils
NT3 Buchu oils
NT3 Cinnamon oils
NT3 Citronella essential oils
NT3 Citrus essential oils
NT4 Bergamot essential oils
NT5 Bergamot oils
NT4 Bitter orange essential oils
NT4 Citrus oils
NT4 Lemon essential oils
NT4 Lime essential oils
NT4 Neroli oils
NT4 Orange essential oils
NT3 Clary sage essential oils
NT3 Clove oils
NT3 Garlic oils
NT3 Hop essential oils
NT3 Lemongrass oils
NT3 Mint oils
NT3 Nutmeg oils
NT3 Oleoresins
NT3 Oregano oils
NT3 Peppermint essential oils
NT3 Petitgrain oils
NT3 Rosemary essential oils
NT3 Sage essential oils
NT3 Tea tree oils
NT3 Thyme oils
NT2 Evening primrose oils
NT2 Flax seed oils
NT3 Linseed oils
NT2 Grape seed oils
NT2 Jojoba oils
NT2 Kapok oils
NT2 Lupin seed oils
NT2 Meadowfoam oils
NT2 Millet oils
NT2 Mustard seed oils
NT2 Nut oils
NT3 Almond oils
NT3 Beech nut oils
NT3 Brazil nut oils
NT3 Coconut oils
NT3 Groundnut oils
NT3 Hazelnut oils
NT3 Pecan oils
NT3 Walnut oils
NT2 Oat oils
NT2 Olive oils
NT3 Olive oil mills effluents
NT3 Olive pomace oils
NT4 Sansa oils
NT2 Palm oils
NT3 Babassu oils
NT3 Palm kernel oils
NT3 Palm oil mills effluents
NT3 Palm olein
NT3 Palm stearin
NT2 Perilla oils
NT2 Pumpkin seed oils
NT2 Rapeseed oils
NT2 Rice bran oils
NT2 Rice germ oils
NT2 Safflower oils
NT2 Sea buckthorn oils
NT2 Sesame oils
NT2 Soybean oils
NT2 Sunflower oils
NT2 Tea seed oils
NT2 Tomato seed oils
NT2 Wheat germ oils
RT Fats vegetable
RT Oilseeds

Oily fish
HN introduced from vol. 40, issue 1 (2008)
BT1 Fish
BT2 Animals
BT2 Sea foods
BT3 Aquatic foods
BT4 Animal foods
BT5 Foods
NT1 Anchovy
NT2 Anchovy pastes
NT2 Budu
NT2 *Engraulis encrasicholus*
NT1 Carp
NT2 Bighead carp
NT3 *Aristichthys nobilis*
NT2 Crucian carp
NT2 *Cyprinus carpio*
NT2 Grass carp
NT3 White amur
NT2 Rohu
NT3 *Labeo rohita*
NT2 Silver carp
NT1 Eels
NT1 Herring
NT2 *Clupea harengus*
NT2 Kippers
NT2 Matjes
NT2 Rollmops
NT1 Hilsa
NT1 Mackerel
NT2 Atlantic mackerel
NT3 *Scomber scombrus*
NT2 Chub mackerel
NT3 *Scomber japonicus*
NT2 Frigate mackerel
NT2 Horse mackerel
NT2 Indian mackerel
NT2 Jack mackerel
NT3 *Trachurus japonicus*
NT3 *Trachurus murphyi*
NT2 Pacific mackerel
NT2 Scad
NT2 Seer fish
NT2 Smoked mackerel
NT2 Spanish mackerel
NT1 Orange roughy
NT1 Pilchards
NT1 Salmon
NT2 Atlantic salmon
NT3 *Salmo salar*
NT2 Pacific salmon
NT3 Cherry salmon
NT4 Masu salmon
NT3 Chinook salmon
NT4 King salmon
NT3 Chum salmon
NT4 Keta salmon
NT4 *Oncorhynchus keta*
NT3 Coho salmon

NT3 Pink salmon
NT3 Sockeye salmon
NT4 Red salmon
NT2 Smoked salmon
NT1 Sardine
NT2 Monterey sardine
NT2 *Sardina pilchardus*
NT1 Sprat
NT1 Swordfish
NT1 Trout
NT2 Brook trout
NT2 Brown trout
NT2 Rainbow trout
NT3 *Oncorhynchus mykiss*
NT2 Sea trout
NT2 Smoked trout
NT1 Tuna
NT2 Bigeye tuna
NT2 Bonito
NT2 Skipjack tuna
NT3 Katsuobushi
NT2 White tuna
NT3 Albacore
NT2 Yellowfin tuna
NT1 Whitebait

Okadaic acid
BT1 Toxins
BT2 Residues
RT Diarrhoetic shellfish toxins

Okara
BT1 Soy products
BT2 Vegetable products
BT3 Plant foods
BT4 Foods
NT1 Meitauza

Okenia hypogaea
BT1 Plants

Okra
BT1 Vegetables specific
BT2 Vegetables
BT3 Crops
BT4 Plants
BT3 Plant foods
BT4 Foods

Oleandomycin
BT1 Macrolide antibiotics
BT2 Antibiotics
BT3 Drugs
BT4 Residues

Oleanolic acid
HN introduced from vol. 41, issue 1 (2009)
BT1 Organic acids
BT2 Acids
BT1 Triterpenoids
BT2 Terpenoids
BT3 Lipids
BT4 Nutrients

Olefins
BT1 Hydrocarbons
BT2 Organic compounds
BT3 Organic compounds
RT Olives

Oleic acid
HN heading up to vol. 42 (2010); under Monounsaturated fatty acids from vol. 43 (2011)
BT1 Octadecenoic acid
BT2 Monounsaturated fatty acids
BT3 Unsaturated fatty acids
BT4 Fatty acids
BT5 Lipids
BT6 Nutrients
BT5 Organic acids
BT6 Acids

Olein
SN syn. triolein
BT1 Triglycerides
BT2 Glycerides
BT3 Emulsifiers
BT4 Additives
BT3 Fatty acid esters
BT4 Esters
BT5 Organic compounds
BT3 Lipids
BT4 Nutrients
NT1 Palm olein

Oleoresins
BT1 Essential oils
BT2 Flavourings
BT3 Additives
BT2 Vegetable oils
BT3 Oils vegetable
BT4 Oils
BT5 Lipids
BT6 Nutrients
BT4 Vegetable products
BT5 Plant foods
BT6 Foods

Oleosins
BT1 Vegetable proteins
BT2 Proteins vegetable
BT3 Proteins
BT4 Nutrients
BT3 Vegetable products
BT4 Plant foods
BT5 Foods

Olestra
BT1 Sucrose polyesters
BT2 Additives
BT2 Esters
BT3 Organic compounds
BT2 Fat substitutes
BT3 Fats
BT4 Lipids
BT5 Nutrients

Oleuropein
BT1 Bitter compounds
BT2 Flavour compounds
BT1 Glycosides
BT2 Carbohydrates
BT3 Nutrients
BT3 Organic compounds
BT1 Phenols
BT2 Alcohols
BT2 Aromatic compounds

Olfactometry
BT1 Sensory analysis
BT2 Analytical techniques

Oligofructose
USE **Fructooligosaccharides**

Oligo-1,6-glucosidases
SN EC 3.2.1.10
BT1 Glycosidases
BT2 Hydrolases
BT3 Enzymes

Oligonucleotide probes
USE **Gene probes**

Oligonucleotides
BT1 Nucleotides
RT DNA probes
RT Gene probes

Oligopeptides
HN introduced from vol. 41, issue 1 (2009)
BT1 Peptides
BT2 Proteins
BT3 Nutrients

Oligosaccharides
HN heading from vol. 43 (2011); under Polysaccharides and Sugars up to vol. 42 (2010)
BT1 Polysaccharides
BT2 Carbohydrates
BT3 Nutrients
BT3 Organic compounds
BT1 Sugars
BT2 Carbohydrates
BT3 Nutrients
BT3 Organic compounds
BT2 Plant foods
BT3 Foods
NT1 Chitooligosaccharides
NT1 Fructooligosaccharides
NT2 Kestose
NT2 Nystose
NT1 Galactooligosaccharides
NT1 Glucooligosaccharides
NT2 Isomaltooligosaccharides
NT2 Maltooligosaccharides
NT3 Maltohexaose
NT3 Maltotetraose
NT3 Maltotriose
NT2 Panose
NT1 Lactosucrose
NT1 Melezitose
NT1 Raffinose
NT1 Stachyose
NT1 Verbascose
NT1 Xylooligosaccharides
RT Cyclodextrins
RT Prebiotics

Olive oil mills effluents
BT1 Effluents
BT2 Waste water
BT3 Wastes
BT3 Water

BT1 Olive oils
BT2 Vegetable oils
BT3 Oils vegetable
BT4 Oils
BT5 Lipids
BT6 Nutrients
BT4 Vegetable products
BT5 Plant foods
BT6 Foods

Olive oils
BT1 Vegetable oils
BT2 Oils vegetable
BT3 Oils
BT4 Lipids
BT5 Nutrients
BT3 Vegetable products
BT4 Plant foods
BT5 Foods
NT1 Olive oil mills effluents
NT1 Olive pomace oils
NT2 Sansa oils
RT Olives

Olive pomace oils
HN introduced from vol. 39, issue 1 (2007)
BT1 Olive oils
BT2 Vegetable oils
BT3 Oils vegetable
BT4 Oils
BT5 Lipids
BT6 Nutrients
BT4 Vegetable products
BT5 Plant foods
BT6 Foods
NT1 Sansa oils
RT Pomaces

Olives
BT1 Fruits specific
BT2 Fruits
BT3 Crops
BT4 Plants
BT3 Plant foods
BT4 Foods
BT1 Oilseeds
BT2 Seeds
BT3 Plant foods
BT4 Foods
NT1 Black olives
NT1 Table olives
RT Oleuropein
RT Olive oils

Oman
BT1 Asia
BT1 Middle East

Omelettes
BT1 Egg products
BT2 Animal foods
BT3 Foods

Omethoate
BT1 Acaricides
BT2 Pesticides
BT3 Biocides
BT3 Residues
BT1 Organophosphorus insecticides
BT2 Insecticides
BT3 Pesticides
BT4 Biocides
BT4 Residues
BT2 Organophosphorus pesticides
BT3 Pesticides
BT4 Biocides
BT4 Residues
UF Folimat

Omija
BT1 Fruits specific
BT2 Fruits
BT3 Crops
BT4 Plants
BT3 Plant foods
BT4 Foods

Omite
USE **Propargite**

Ommastrephes bartrami
BT1 Squid
BT2 Cephalopods
BT3 Molluscs
BT4 Shellfish
BT5 Animals
BT5 Sea foods
BT6 Aquatic foods
BT7 Animal foods
BT8 Foods

Oncom
USE **Ontjom**

Oncorhynchus keta
BT1 Chum salmon
BT2 Pacific salmon
BT3 Salmon
BT4 Oily fish
BT5 Fish
BT6 Animals
BT6 Sea foods
BT7 Aquatic foods
BT8 Animal foods
BT9 Foods

Oncorhynchus mykiss
BT1 Rainbow trout
BT2 Trout
BT3 Oily fish
BT4 Fish
BT5 Animals
BT5 Sea foods
BT6 Aquatic foods
BT7 Animal foods
BT8 Foods

Onigusa
BT1 Seaweeds
BT2 Algae
BT3 Microorganisms
BT2 Sea foods
BT3 Aquatic foods
BT4 Animal foods
BT5 Foods
UF *Gelidium*

Onions
BT1 Vegetables specific
BT2 Vegetables
BT3 Crops
BT4 Plants
BT3 Plant foods
BT4 Foods
NT1 Pickled onions
NT1 Red onions

Ontjom
BT1 Fermented foods
BT2 Processed foods
BT3 Foods
BT1 Peanuts
BT2 Nuts
BT3 Fruits
BT4 Crops
BT5 Plants
BT4 Plant foods
BT5 Foods
BT3 Oilseeds
BT4 Seeds
BT5 Plant foods
BT6 Foods
UF Oncom

Oocysts
BT1 Parasites
BT2 Pests
RT Eukaryotes
RT Protozoa

Oolong tea
HN under Teas up to vol. 42 (2010)
BT1 Tea
BT2 Teas
BT3 Beverages
BT3 Crops
BT4 Plants
BT3 Plant foods
BT4 Foods

Opacity
BT1 Optical properties
BT2 Physical properties

Opalescence
BT1 Optical properties
BT2 Physical properties

Opaque 2
BT1 Cereal proteins
BT2 Proteins cereal
BT3 Vegetable proteins
BT4 Proteins vegetable
BT5 Proteins
BT6 Nutrients
BT5 Vegetable products
BT6 Plant foods
BT7 Foods

Openings
BT1 Packaging
BT2 Technology
RT Closures

Operators
BT1 Operons
BT2 Genetics

RT Gene expression
RT Genes

Operons
BT1 Genetics
NT1 Operators
NT1 Promoters
NT1 Structural genes
RT Gene expression
RT Genes

Ophiodon elongatus
BT1 Ling cod
BT2 Marine fish
BT3 Fish
BT4 Animals
BT4 Sea foods
BT5 Aquatic foods
BT6 Animal foods
BT7 Foods

Optical density
BT1 Optical properties
BT2 Physical properties

Optical properties
BT1 Physical properties
NT1 Birefringence
NT1 Brightness
NT1 Brilliance
NT1 Chalkiness
NT1 Clarity
NT1 Colour
NT1 Diffraction
NT1 Fluorescence
NT2 Autofluorescence
NT2 Bioluminescence
NT2 Chemiluminescence
NT2 Green fluorescent protein
NT2 Luminescence
NT3 Phosphorescence
NT2 Thermoluminescence
NT1 Glassiness
NT1 Gloss
NT1 Opacity
NT1 Opalescence
NT1 Optical density
NT1 Optical rotation
NT1 Pigmentation
NT1 Polarization
NT1 Reflectance
NT1 Reflectivity
NT1 Refractive index
NT1 Specific rotation
NT1 Translucency
NT1 Transmittance
NT1 Transparency
NT1 Turbidity
NT2 Cloud
NT3 Clouding agents
NT2 Cloudiness
NT2 Haze
NT1 Vitreosity
NT1 Whiteness

Optical rotation
BT1 Optical properties
BT2 Physical properties

Opuntia ficus-indica
BT1 Prickly pears
BT2 Fruits specific
BT3 Fruits
BT4 Crops
BT5 Plants
BT4 Plant foods
BT5 Foods

Oral food challenges
HN introduced from vol. 39, issue 1 (2007)
BT1 Clinical techniques

Orange beverages
BT1 Soft drinks
BT2 Beverages

Orange essential oils
BT1 Citrus essential oils
BT2 Essential oils
BT3 Flavourings
BT4 Additives
BT3 Vegetable oils
BT4 Oils vegetable
BT5 Oils
BT6 Lipids
BT7 Nutrients
BT5 Vegetable products
BT6 Plant foods
BT7 Foods
RT Oranges

Orange juice beverages
BT1 Fruit juice beverages
BT2 Soft drinks
BT3 Beverages

Orange juice concentrates
BT1 Citrus juice concentrates
BT2 Citrus juices
BT3 Fruit juices
BT4 Fruit products
BT5 Plant foods
BT6 Foods
BT4 Soft drinks
BT5 Beverages
BT2 Fruit juice concentrates
BT3 Concentrates
BT4 Processed foods
BT5 Foods
BT3 Fruit juices
BT4 Fruit products
BT5 Plant foods
BT6 Foods
BT4 Soft drinks
BT5 Beverages
BT1 Orange juices
BT2 Citrus juices
BT3 Fruit juices
BT4 Fruit products
BT5 Plant foods
BT6 Foods
BT4 Soft drinks
BT5 Beverages

Orange juices
BT1 Citrus juices
BT2 Fruit juices
BT3 Fruit products
BT4 Plant foods
BT5 Foods
BT3 Soft drinks
BT4 Beverages
NT1 Mandarin juices
NT2 Tangerine juices
NT1 Orange juice concentrates
RT Oranges

Orange peel
BT1 Oranges
BT2 Citrus fruits
BT3 Fruits specific
BT4 Fruits
BT5 Crops
BT6 Plants
BT5 Plant foods
BT6 Foods
BT1 Peel
RT Fruit peel

Orange roughy
BT1 Marine fish
BT2 Fish
BT3 Animals
BT3 Sea foods
BT4 Aquatic foods
BT5 Animal foods
BT6 Foods
BT1 Oily fish
BT2 Fish
BT3 Animals
BT3 Sea foods
BT4 Aquatic foods
BT5 Animal foods
BT6 Foods

Oranges
BT1 Citrus fruits
BT2 Fruits specific
BT3 Fruits
BT4 Crops
BT5 Plants
BT4 Plant foods
BT5 Foods
NT1 Mandarins
NT2 Clementines
NT2 Kinnow mandarins
NT2 Ponkans
NT2 Satsuma mandarins
NT2 Satsumas
NT2 Tangerines
NT1 Orange peel
RT Orange essential oils
RT Orange juices

Orange wines
BT1 Fruit wines
BT2 Alcoholic beverages
BT3 Beverages alcoholic
BT4 Beverages

Oregano
HN under Spices up to vol. 42 (2010)
BT1 Herbs
BT2 Spices
BT3 Flavourings
BT4 Additives
RT Oregano oils

Oregano oils
BT1 Essential oils
BT2 Flavourings
BT3 Additives
BT2 Vegetable oils
BT3 Oils vegetable
BT4 Oils
BT5 Lipids
BT6 Nutrients
BT4 Vegetable products
BT5 Plant foods
BT6 Foods
RT Oregano

Oreochromis
BT1 Tilapia
BT2 Freshwater fish
BT3 Fish
BT4 Animals
BT4 Sea foods
BT5 Aquatic foods
BT6 Animal foods
BT7 Foods
NT1 *Oreochromis niloticus*

Oreochromis niloticus
BT1 Nile tilapia
BT2 Tilapia
BT3 Freshwater fish
BT4 Fish
BT5 Animals
BT5 Sea foods
BT6 Aquatic foods
BT7 Animal foods
BT8 Foods
BT1 *Oreochromis*
BT2 Tilapia
BT3 Freshwater fish
BT4 Fish
BT5 Animals
BT5 Sea foods
BT6 Aquatic foods
BT7 Animal foods
BT8 Foods

Organic acids
HN heading from vol. 25; under Acids up to vol. 24
BT1 Acids
NT1 Acetic acid
NT1 *N*-Acetylneuraminic acid
NT1 Aconitic acid
NT1 Adipic acid
NT1 Amino acids
NT2 Alanine
NT2 D-Amino acids
NT2 Arginine
NT2 Asparagine
NT2 Aspartic acid
NT2 Canavanine
NT2 Citrulline
NT2 Cysteine
NT3 *N*-Acetyl-L-cysteine
NT2 Cystine
NT2 DOPA
NT2 Glutamic acid
NT3 Poly(γ-glutamic acid)
NT2 Glutamine
NT2 Glycine
NT2 Histidine
NT2 Homocysteine
NT2 Homoserine
NT2 Hydroxyproline
NT2 Isoleucine
NT2 Lanthionine
NT2 Leucine
NT2 Lysine
NT3 Polylysine
NT2 Methionine
NT3 *S*-Adenosyl-L-methionine
NT3 *S*-Methylmethionine
NT3 Selenomethionine
NT2 Methylhistidine
NT2 Octopine
NT2 Ornithine
NT2 Phenylalanine
NT2 Pipecolic acid
NT2 Proline
NT2 Pyroglutamic acid
NT2 Serine
NT2 Taurine
NT2 Theanine
NT2 Threonine
NT2 Tryptophan
NT2 Tyrosine
NT2 Valine
NT1 Aminobenzoic acid
NT1 Aminobutyric acid
NT1 Anthranilic acid
NT1 Barbituric acid
NT1 Benzoic acid
NT1 Bitter acids
NT2 α-Acids
NT3 Humulones
NT4 Adhumulone
NT4 Cohumulone
NT4 Humulinic acid
NT2 β-Acids
NT3 Hulupones
NT3 Lupulones
NT4 Colupulone
NT2 Iso-α-acids
NT3 Isohumulones
NT2 Lupulin
NT1 Caffeic acid
NT1 Carboxylic acids
NT1 Chlorogenic acid
NT2 Caffeoylquinic acid
NT1 Cinnamic acid
NT1 Citramalic acid
NT1 Citric acid
NT1 Cyclamic acid
NT1 Dehydroacetic acid
NT1 Diethylpyrocarbonate
NT1 Dipicolinic acid
NT1 EDTA
NT1 Ellagic acid
NT1 Erythorbic acid
NT1 Fatty acids
NT2 Branched chain fatty acids
NT3 Isobutyric acid
NT3 Isocaproic acid
NT3 Isovaleric acid
NT2 Cyclic fatty acids
NT2 Eicosanoids
NT3 Prostaglandins
NT2 Malvalic acid
NT2 Saturated fatty acids
NT3 Arachidic acid
NT3 Behenic acid
NT3 Butanoic acid
NT4 Butyric acid
NT3 Decanoic acid
NT4 Capric acid
NT3 Dodecanoic acid
NT4 Lauric acid
NT3 Heptadecanoic acid
NT4 Margaric acid
NT3 Heptanoic acid
NT3 Hexadecanoic acid
NT4 Palmitic acid
NT3 Hexanoic acid
NT4 Caproic acid
NT3 Lignoceric acid
NT3 Myristic acid
NT3 Octadecanoic acid
NT4 Stearic acid
NT5 Hydroxystearic acid
NT3 Octanoic acid
NT4 Caprylic acid
NT3 Pentanoic acid
NT4 Valeric acid
NT2 Sterculic acid
NT2 Unsaturated fatty acids
NT3 Essential fatty acids
NT3 Monounsaturated fatty acids
NT4 Decenoic acid
NT4 Docosenoic acid
NT5 Erucic acid
NT4 Eicosenoic acid
NT4 Hexadecenoic acid
NT5 Palmitoleic acid
NT4 Octadecenoic acid
NT5 Elaidic acid
NT5 Oleic acid
NT5 Petroselinic acid
NT5 Vaccenic acid
NT4 Ricinoleic acid
NT3 PUFA
NT4 Conjugated fatty acids
NT5 CLA
NT5 Eleostearic acid
NT4 Eicosatetraenoic acid
NT5 Arachidonic acid
NT4 ω-3 Fatty acids
NT5 Docosahexaenoic acid
NT5 Docosapentaenoic acid
NT5 Eicosapentaenoic acid
NT5 α-Linolenic acid
NT5 Stearidonic acid
NT4 ω-6 Fatty acids
NT5 Arachidonic acid
NT5 Linoleic acid
NT6 CLA
NT5 γ-Linolenic acid
NT4 Linolenic acid
NT5 Eleostearic acid
NT5 α-Linolenic acid
NT5 γ-Linolenic acid
NT3 *trans* Fatty acids
NT4 Elaidic acid
NT4 Vaccenic acid
NT2 Volatile fatty acids
NT3 Short chain fatty acids
NT4 Butanoic acid
NT5 Butyric acid
NT4 Hexanoic acid

NT5 Caproic acid
NT4 Hydroxybutyric acid
NT4 Isobutyric acid
NT4 Isocaproic acid
NT4 Isovaleric acid
NT4 Pentanoic acid
NT5 Valeric acid
NT1 Ferulic acid
NT1 Feruloylquinic acid
NT1 Formic acid
NT1 Fumaric acid
NT1 Gallic acid
NT1 Gluconic acid
NT1 Glutaric acid
NT1 Glycolic acid
NT1 Hippuric acid
NT1 Humic acids
NT1 Hydroxybenzoic acid
NT1 Hydroxycinnamic acid
NT2 Coumaric acid
NT1 Hydroxycitric acid
NT1 Isochlorogenic acid
NT1 Isocitric acid
NT1 Itaconic acid
NT1 Keto acids
NT1 α-Ketoglutaric acid
NT1 Lactic acid
NT1 Lactobionic acid
NT1 α-Lipoic acid
NT1 Maleic acid
NT1 Malic acid
NT1 Malonic acid
NT1 Mevalonic acid
NT1 Mucic acid
NT1 5-Nitrofurylacrylic acid
NT1 Nucleic acids
NT2 DNA
NT3 cDNA
NT3 Mitochondrial DNA
NT3 RAPD
NT2 RNA
NT3 mRNA
NT3 rRNA
NT1 Oleanolic acid
NT1 Orotic acid
NT1 Oxalic acid
NT1 Oxaloacetic acid
NT1 Peracetic acid
NT1 Phenylacetic acid
NT1 Phosphatidic acid
NT1 Phthalic acid
NT1 Propionic acid
NT1 Protocatechuic acid
NT1 Pyruvic acid
NT1 Quinic acid
NT1 Salicylic acid
NT1 Shikimic acid
NT1 Sialic acid
NT1 Sinapic acid
NT1 Sorbic acid
NT1 Succinic acid
NT1 Syringic acid
NT1 Tannins
NT2 Ellagitannins
NT2 Proanthocyanidins
NT3 Procyanidins
NT2 Tannic acid
NT1 Tartaric acid
NT1 Thioglycolic acid
NT1 Uronic acids
NT2 Galacturonic acid
NT2 Glucuronic acid
NT2 Polyuronides
NT1 Ursolic acid
NT1 Vanillic acid

Organic beverages
HN introduced from vol. 42, issue 1 (2010)
BT1 Beverages
RT Organic foods

Organic compounds
HN heading up to vol. 24 (1992)
NT1 Aliphatic compounds
NT1 Aromatic compounds
NT1 Carbohydrates
NT1 Carbonyl compounds
NT1 Esters
NT1 Ethers
NT1 Geosmin
NT1 Hydrocarbons
NT1 Melanoidins
NT1 Organotin compounds
NT1 Volatile organic compounds
RT Heterocyclic compounds
RT Organic halogen compounds
RT Organic nitrogen compounds
RT Organic sulfur compounds

Organic foods
HN heading from vol. 25 (1993); under Health foods up to vol. 24 (1992)
BT1 Foods
NT1 Organic pet foods
RT Natural foods
RT Organic beverages

Organic halogen compounds
HN heading from vol. 25 (1993); under Halogenated compounds up to vol. 24 (1992)
NT1 Chlorinated hydrocarbons
NT2 Carbon tetrachloride
NT2 Chloroform
NT2 Dichloroacetic acid
NT2 Dichloromethane
NT2 Epichlorohydrin
NT2 Hexachlorobutadiene
NT2 Methylene chloride
NT2 Polychlorinated biphenyls
NT3 Arochlor
NT3 Hexachlorobiphenyl
NT3 PCB
NT2 Tetrachloromethane
NT2 Trichloromethane
NT1 Chlorophenol
NT1 Haloacetic acids
NT1 Haloanisoles
NT2 Trichloroanisole
NT1 Halogenated compounds
NT1 Iodoacetic acid
NT1 Methyl iodide
NT1 Organobromine compounds
NT2 Bromophenols
NT2 Polybrominated biphenyls
NT2 Polybrominated diphenyl ethers
NT1 Organochlorine compounds
NT2 Chloropropanols
NT1 Polychlorinated dibenzodioxins
NT1 Polychlorinated dibenzofurans
NT1 Polychlorinated dibenzo-*p*-dioxins
NT2 Tetrachlorodibenzo-*p*-dioxins
NT1 Trihalomethanes
RT Heterocyclic compounds
RT Hydrocarbons
RT Organic compounds
RT Organic nitrogen compounds
RT Organic sulfur compounds

Organic nitrogen compounds
HN heading from vol. 25 (1993); under Nitrogen compounds up to vol. 24 (1992)
NT1 Acetonitrile
NT1 Agaritine
NT1 Alkaloids
NT2 Caffeine
NT2 Carbolines
NT2 Ergotamine
NT2 Glycoalkaloids
NT3 Chaconine
NT3 Solanine
NT2 Harman
NT2 Lupanine
NT2 Methylxanthines
NT2 Nicotine
NT2 Norharman
NT2 Piperine
NT2 Pyrrolizidine alkaloids
NT2 Quinine
NT2 Sanguinarine
NT2 Solanidine
NT2 Theanine
NT2 Theobromine
NT2 Theophylline
NT2 Tomatine
NT2 Trigonelline
NT1 Amides
NT2 Acrylamide
NT2 Avenanthramides
NT2 Azodicarbonamide
NT2 Capsaicinoids
NT3 Capsaicin
NT2 Carbamide
NT2 Dimethylformamide
NT2 Formamide
NT2 Urea
NT1 Amines
NT2 Agmatine
NT2 Aminoethanol
NT2 Aniline
NT2 Anisidine
NT2 Benzidine
NT2 Biogenic amines
NT3 Cadaverine
NT3 Catecholamines
NT4 Adrenaline
NT4 Noradrenaline
NT3 Choline
NT3 Dopamine
NT3 Histamine
NT3 Hordenine
NT3 5-Hydroxytryptamine
NT3 Putrescine

NT3 Serotonin
NT3 Skatole
NT3 Spermine
NT3 Tryptamine
NT3 Tyramine
NT2 Chloramines
NT3 Monochloramine
NT2 Cyclohexylamine
NT2 Diethylamine
NT2 Dimethylamine
NT2 Ethanolamine
NT2 Ethylamine
NT2 Ethylenediamine
NT2 Heterocyclic amines
NT2 Heterocyclic aromatic amines
NT2 Hexylamine
NT2 Hydroxylamine
NT2 Isoamylamine
NT2 Methylamine
NT2 Morpholine
NT2 Nitrosamines
NT3 Diethylnitrosamine
NT3 Dimethylnitrosamine
NT3 *N*-Nitrosodiethylamine
NT3 *N*-Nitrosodimethylamine
NT2 Polyamines
NT3 Putrescine
NT3 Spermidine
NT3 Spermine
NT2 Propylamine
NT2 Trimethylamine
NT1 Amino acids
NT2 Alanine
NT2 D-Amino acids
NT2 Arginine
NT2 Asparagine
NT2 Aspartic acid
NT2 Canavanine
NT2 Citrulline
NT2 Cysteine
NT3 *N*-Acetyl-L-cysteine
NT2 Cystine
NT2 DOPA
NT2 Glutamic acid
NT3 Poly(γ-glutamic acid)
NT2 Glutamine
NT2 Glycine
NT2 Histidine
NT2 Homocysteine
NT2 Homoserine
NT2 Hydroxyproline
NT2 Isoleucine
NT2 Lanthionine
NT2 Leucine
NT2 Lysine
NT3 Polylysine
NT2 Methionine
NT3 *S*-Adenosyl-L-methionine
NT3 *S*-Methylmethionine
NT3 Selenomethionine
NT2 Methylhistidine
NT2 Octopine
NT2 Ornithine
NT2 Phenylalanine
NT2 Pipecolic acid
NT2 Proline
NT2 Pyroglutamic acid
NT2 Serine
NT2 Taurine
NT2 Theanine
NT2 Threonine
NT2 Tryptophan
NT2 Tyrosine
NT2 Valine
NT1 Aminobenzoic acid
NT1 Aminobutyric acid
NT1 Anthranilic acid
NT1 Benzothiazole
NT1 Betaine
NT1 Betalains
NT2 Betacyanins
NT3 Betanin
NT3 Betanine
NT2 Betalaines
NT2 Betaxanthin
NT1 Carnitine
NT1 Cetylpyridinium chloride
NT1 Creatine
NT1 Creatinine
NT1 Ethyl carbamate
NT1 Glycine betaine
NT1 Guanidine
NT1 Hydrazine
NT1 Hypoxanthine
NT1 Imidazoles
NT2 Allantoin
NT1 Indoles
NT2 Indole-3-carbinol
NT1 Isothiocyanates
NT2 Allyl isothiocyanate
NT2 Benzyl isothiocyanate
NT2 Phenethyl isothiocyanate
NT2 Sulforaphane
NT1 Melamine
NT1 Melatonin
NT1 Methyl carbamate
NT1 Nitrobenzene
NT1 Nitroso compounds
NT2 Nitrosamines
NT3 Diethylnitrosamine
NT3 Dimethylnitrosamine
NT3 *N*-Nitrosodiethylamine
NT3 *N*-Nitrosodimethylamine
NT2 Nitroso pigments
NT2 *N*-Nitrosopyrrolidine
NT2 Reactive nitrogen species
NT3 Nitric oxide
NT3 Peroxynitrite
NT1 Phytoalexins
NT1 Piperidine
NT1 Porphyrins
NT2 Chlorophylls
NT2 Haem
NT2 Haematin
NT2 Haemin
NT1 Purines
NT2 Adenine
NT2 Caffeine
NT2 Theobromine
NT2 Theophylline
NT2 Uric acid
NT1 Pyrazines
NT1 Pyridine
NT1 Pyrimidines
NT2 Barbituric acid
NT2 Cytosine
NT2 Propylthiouracil
NT2 Thymine
NT2 Uracil
NT1 Pyrroles
NT1 Resazurin
NT1 Sarcosine
NT1 Semicarbazide
NT1 Tetrazoles
NT1 Thiourea
NT1 Urethane
RT Heterocyclic compounds
RT Hydrocarbons
RT Nitrogen compounds
RT Organic compounds
RT Organic halogen compounds
RT Organic sulfur compounds

Organic pet foods
HN introduced from vol. 39, issue 1 (2007)
BT1 Organic foods
BT2 Foods
BT1 Pet foods

Organic solvents
BT1 Solvents

Organic sulfur compounds
HN heading from vol. 35, issue 7 (2003)
NT1 Allicin
NT1 Alliin
NT1 *S*-Allylcysteine
NT1 Allyl sulfides
NT2 Diallyl disulfide
NT1 Benzothiazole
NT1 Cysteine sulfoxides
NT1 Dimethyl disulfide
NT1 Dimethyl sulfide
NT2 Methyl sulfide
NT1 Dimethyl sulfoxide
NT1 Dimethyl trisulfide
NT1 Glutathione
NT1 Homocysteine
NT1 Isothiocyanates
NT2 Allyl isothiocyanate
NT2 Benzyl isothiocyanate
NT2 Phenethyl isothiocyanate
NT2 Sulforaphane
NT1 Lanthionine
NT1 Lenthionine
NT1 Methionine
NT2 *S*-Adenosyl-L-methionine
NT2 *S*-Methylmethionine
NT2 Selenomethionine
NT1 SDS
NT1 Thiazoles
NT1 Thiols
NT2 Dithiothreitol
NT2 Mercaptans
NT3 Methyl mercaptan
NT2 Mercaptoethanol
NT2 Methanethiol
NT3 Methyl mercaptan
NT2 Methional
NT2 Methionol
NT2 Sulfhydryl groups
NT2 Thioesters
NT2 Thioglycolic acid
NT2 Thioglycosides
NT1 Thiophenes
NT1 Thiourea

RT Aroma compounds
RT Heterocyclic compounds
RT Hydrocarbons
RT Organic compounds
RT Organic halogen compounds
RT Organic nitrogen compounds
UF Organic sulphur compounds

Organic sulphur compounds
HN used for organic sulfur compounds up to vol. 35, issue 6 (2003)
USE **Organic sulfur compounds**

Organization for Economic Cooperation and Development
HN heading up to vol. 24 (1992)
RT Australia
RT Austria
RT Belgium
RT Canada
RT Czech Republic
RT Denmark
RT Finland
RT France
RT Germany
RT Greece
RT Hungary
RT Iceland
RT Italy
RT Japan
RT Korea
RT Luxembourg
RT Mexico
RT Netherlands
RT New Zealand
RT Norway
RT Poland
RT Portugal
RT Republic of Ireland
RT Slovakia
RT Spain
RT Sweden
RT Switzerland
RT Turkey
RT United Kingdom
RT United States of America
UF OECD

Organobromine compounds
BT1 Organic halogen compounds
NT1 Bromophenols
NT1 Polybrominated biphenyls
NT1 Polybrominated diphenyl ethers
RT Br

Organochlorine compounds
BT1 Organic halogen compounds
NT1 Chloropropanols
RT Chlorinated hydrocarbons
RT Chlorine

Organochlorine insecticides
HN insecticides organochlorine also used in the index up to vol. 29 (1997)
BT1 Insecticides
BT2 Pesticides
BT3 Biocides
BT3 Residues
BT1 Organochlorine pesticides
BT2 Pesticides
BT3 Biocides
BT3 Residues
NT1 Aldrin
NT1 Bromocyclen
NT1 Camphechlor
NT1 Chlordane
NT2 Nonachlor
NT1 Chlordecone
NT1 DDT
NT2 DDE
NT2 TDE
NT1 Dichlorobenzene
NT1 Dieldrin
NT1 Dilor
NT1 Endosulfan
NT1 Endrin
NT1 HCH
NT1 Heptachlor
NT2 Heptachlor epoxide
NT1 Kelevan
NT1 Methoxychlor
NT1 Mirex
NT1 Perthane

Organochlorine pesticides
HN pesticides organochlorine also used in the index up to vol. 29 (1997)
BT1 Pesticides
BT2 Biocides
BT2 Residues
NT1 Chlorobenzilate
NT1 Dicofol
NT1 Organochlorine insecticides
NT2 Aldrin
NT2 Bromocyclen
NT2 Camphechlor
NT2 Chlordane
NT3 Nonachlor
NT2 Chlordecone
NT2 DDT
NT3 DDE
NT3 TDE
NT2 Dichlorobenzene
NT2 Dieldrin
NT2 Dilor
NT2 Endosulfan
NT2 Endrin
NT2 HCH
NT2 Heptachlor
NT3 Heptachlor epoxide
NT2 Kelevan
NT2 Methoxychlor
NT2 Mirex
NT2 Perthane

Organoleptic evaluation
HN heading up to vol. 18 (1986)
USE **Sensory analysis**

Organoleptic properties
HN heading up to vol. 18 (1986)
USE **Sensory properties**

Organophosphorus insecticides
HN insecticides organophosphorus also used in the index up to vol. 29 (1997)
BT1 Insecticides
BT2 Pesticides
BT3 Biocides
BT3 Residues
BT1 Organophosphorus pesticides
BT2 Pesticides
BT3 Biocides
BT3 Residues
NT1 Acephate
NT1 Azinphos-methyl
NT1 Bromophos
NT1 Butonate
NT1 Carbophenothion
NT1 Chlorfenvinphos
NT1 Chlorphoxim
NT1 Chlorpyrifos
NT1 Chlorpyrifos-methyl
NT1 Coumaphos
NT1 Crotoxyphos
NT1 Demeton
NT1 Demeton-*S*-methyl
NT1 Dialifos
NT1 Diazinon
NT1 Dichlorvos
NT1 Dimethoate
NT1 Dioxathion
NT1 Disulfoton
NT1 Ethion
NT1 Ethoprophos
NT1 Etrimfos
NT1 Famphur
NT1 Fenchlorphos
NT1 Fenitrothion
NT1 Fensulfothion
NT1 Fenthion
NT1 Fonofos
NT1 Formothion
NT1 Iodofenphos
NT1 Leptophos
NT1 Malathion
NT2 Malaoxon
NT1 Methamidophos
NT1 Methidathion
NT1 Mevinphos
NT1 Monocrotophos
NT1 Naled
NT1 Omethoate
NT1 Oxydemeton-methyl
NT1 Parathion
NT2 Paraoxon
NT1 Parathion-methyl
NT1 Phenthoate
NT1 Phorate
NT1 Phosalone
NT1 Phosmet
NT1 Phosphamidon
NT1 Phoxim
NT1 Pirimiphos-methyl
NT1 Quinalphos
NT1 Temephos
NT1 Terbufos
NT1 Tetrachlorvinphos

NT1 Triazophos
NT1 Trichlorfon

Organophosphorus pesticides
HN pesticides organophosphorus also used in the index up to vol. 29 (1997)
BT1 Pesticides
BT2 Biocides
BT2 Residues
NT1 Edifenphos
NT1 Glyphosate
NT1 Organophosphorus insecticides
NT2 Acephate
NT2 Azinphos-methyl
NT2 Bromophos
NT2 Butonate
NT2 Carbophenothion
NT2 Chlorfenvinphos
NT2 Chlorphoxim
NT2 Chlorpyrifos
NT2 Chlorpyrifos-methyl
NT2 Coumaphos
NT2 Crotoxyphos
NT2 Demeton
NT2 Demeton-*S*-methyl
NT2 Dialifos
NT2 Diazinon
NT2 Dichlorvos
NT2 Dimethoate
NT2 Dioxathion
NT2 Disulfoton
NT2 Ethion
NT2 Ethoprophos
NT2 Etrimfos
NT2 Famphur
NT2 Fenchlorphos
NT2 Fenitrothion
NT2 Fensulfothion
NT2 Fenthion
NT2 Fonofos
NT2 Formothion
NT2 Iodofenphos
NT2 Leptophos
NT2 Malathion
NT3 Malaoxon
NT2 Methamidophos
NT2 Methidathion
NT2 Mevinphos
NT2 Monocrotophos
NT2 Naled
NT2 Omethoate
NT2 Oxydemeton-methyl
NT2 Parathion
NT3 Paraoxon
NT2 Parathion-methyl
NT2 Phenthoate
NT2 Phorate
NT2 Phosalone
NT2 Phosmet
NT2 Phosphamidon
NT2 Phoxim
NT2 Pirimiphos-methyl
NT2 Quinalphos
NT2 Temephos
NT2 Terbufos
NT2 Tetrachlorvinphos
NT2 Triazophos
NT2 Trichlorfon

Organotin compounds
BT1 Contaminants
BT2 Contamination
BT1 Organic compounds
NT1 Butyltins
NT2 Tributyltin

Origin
NT1 Botanical origin
NT1 Geographical origin
NT1 Species identification
NT1 Strain identification
RT Traceability

Original gravity
BT1 Density
BT2 Physical properties

Ormetoprim
BT1 Drugs
BT2 Residues

Ornithine
BT1 Amino acids
BT2 Nutrients
BT2 Organic acids
BT3 Acids
BT2 Organic nitrogen compounds

Orotic acid
HN under Nutrients up to vol. 42 (2010)
BT1 Organic acids
BT2 Acids
UF Vitamin B_{13}

Ortanique
BT1 Citrus fruits
BT2 Fruits specific
BT3 Fruits
BT4 Crops
BT5 Plants
BT4 Plant foods
BT5 Foods

Orthocide
USE **Captan**

Orthophenylphenol
USE **2-Phenylphenol**

Orthopoxvirus
HN introduced from vol. 43, issue 1 (2011)
BT1 Viruses
BT2 Microorganisms
NT1 Vaccinia virus

Oryzaephilus
BT1 Insects
BT2 Pests

Oryzalin
BT1 Herbicides
BT2 Pesticides
BT3 Biocides
BT3 Residues
UF Ryzelan

Oryzanols
BT1 Antioxidants
BT2 Additives
BT1 Aromatic compounds
BT2 Organic compounds

Oryzenin
BT1 Cereal proteins
BT2 Proteins cereal
BT3 Vegetable proteins
BT4 Proteins vegetable
BT5 Proteins
BT6 Nutrients
BT5 Vegetable products
BT6 Plant foods
BT7 Foods

Os
HN under Minerals up to vol. 42 (2010)
BT1 Metals
BT2 Elements
BT3 Minerals
BT4 Nutrients
UF Osmium

O_2 scavengers
USE **Oxygen scavengers**

Osmium
USE **Os**

Osmolality
RT Osmotic pressure

Osmolarity
RT Osmotic pressure

Osmoregulation
RT Osmotic pressure
RT Osmotic stress

Osmosis
HN heading from vol. 25 (1993)
RT Diffusion
RT Osmotic pressure
RT Osmotic stress
RT Reverse osmosis

Osmotic dehydration
USE **Osmotic drying**

Osmotic drying
HN drying osmotic also used in the index up to vol. 29 (1997)
BT1 Drying
BT2 Thermal processing
BT3 Processing thermal
BT4 Processing
BT5 Technology
UF Osmotic dehydration

Osmotic pressure
HN introduced from vol. 39, issue 1 (2007)
BT1 Pressure
RT Osmolality
RT Osmolarity
RT Osmoregulation
RT Osmosis
RT Osmotic stress
RT Permeability
UF Turgor

Osmotic stress
BT1 Stress
RT Osmoregulation
RT Osmosis
RT Osmotic pressure

Osteoporosis
BT1 Diseases

Ostiepok cheese
BT1 Cheese varieties
BT2 Cheese
BT3 Dairy products
BT4 Animal foods
BT5 Foods

Ostrich carcasses
BT1 Carcasses
BT2 Meat
BT3 Animal foods
BT4 Foods
BT1 Ostrich meat
BT2 Ostriches
BT3 Poultry
BT4 Birds
BT2 Poultry meat
BT3 Meat specific
BT4 Meat
BT5 Animal foods
BT6 Foods

Ostriches
BT1 Poultry
BT2 Birds
NT1 Ostrich meat
NT2 Ostrich carcasses

Ostrich fern
BT1 Ferns

Ostrich meat
BT1 Ostriches
BT2 Poultry
BT3 Birds
BT1 Poultry meat
BT2 Meat specific
BT3 Meat
BT4 Animal foods
BT5 Foods
NT1 Ostrich carcasses

Ouzo
HN under Liqueurs up to vol. 42 (2010)
BT1 Spirits
BT2 Alcoholic beverages
BT3 Beverages alcoholic
BT4 Beverages

Ovalbumins
BT1 Albumins
BT2 Proteins
BT3 Nutrients
BT1 Egg proteins
BT2 Animal proteins
BT3 Proteins animal
BT4 Proteins
BT5 Nutrients

Ovarian cancer
HN introduced from vol. 42, issue 1 (2010)
BT1 Cancer
BT2 Diseases

Ovens
BT1 Equipment
BT2 Technology
NT1 Baking ovens
NT1 Kilns
NT1 Microwave ovens
UF Stoves

Overrun
HN introduced from vol. 39, issue 1 (2007)
BT1 Physical properties

Overweight
HN introduced from vol. 41, issue 1 (2009)
BT1 Body wt.
BT2 Anthropometric parameters
BT3 Health
RT Obesity

Overwrapping
BT1 Packaging
BT2 Technology

Ovine
USE **Sheep**

Ovomucins
BT1 Egg proteins
BT2 Animal proteins
BT3 Proteins animal
BT4 Proteins
BT5 Nutrients
BT1 Glycoproteins
BT2 Proteins
BT3 Nutrients
RT Egg whites

Ovomucoid
BT1 Egg proteins
BT2 Animal proteins
BT3 Proteins animal
BT4 Proteins
BT5 Nutrients
BT1 Glycoproteins
BT2 Proteins
BT3 Nutrients
RT Egg whites

Ovotransferrin
BT1 Egg proteins
BT2 Animal proteins
BT3 Proteins animal
BT4 Proteins
BT5 Nutrients
BT1 Glycoproteins
BT2 Proteins
BT3 Nutrients
RT Egg whites

Oxacillin
BT1 Penicillins
BT2 β-Lactam antibiotics
BT3 Antibiotics
BT4 Drugs
BT5 Residues

Oxadiazon
BT1 Herbicides
BT2 Pesticides
BT3 Biocides
BT3 Residues

Oxalates
BT1 Salts
RT Oxalic acid

Oxalic acid
HN heading up to vol. 24 (1992)
BT1 Organic acids
BT2 Acids
RT Oxalates

Oxalis tuberosa
BT1 Oca
BT2 Vegetables specific
BT3 Vegetables
BT4 Crops
BT5 Plants
BT4 Plant foods
BT5 Foods

Oxaloacetic acid
BT1 Organic acids
BT2 Acids

Oxamyl
BT1 Acaricides
BT2 Pesticides
BT3 Biocides
BT3 Residues
BT1 *N*-Methylcarbamate insecticides
BT2 Insecticides
BT3 Pesticides
BT4 Biocides
BT4 Residues
BT2 *N*-Methylcarbamate pesticides
BT3 Carbamate pesticides
BT4 Pesticides
BT5 Biocides
BT5 Residues
BT1 Nematocides
BT2 Pesticides
BT3 Biocides
BT3 Residues

Oxen
USE **Cattle**

Oxidants
BT1 Oxidizing agents
BT2 Additives
RT Oxygen
RT Ozone

Oxidases
SN EC 1.-.3
BT1 Oxidoreductases
BT2 Enzymes
NT1 Alcohol oxidases
NT2 Aryl-alcohol oxidases
NT1 Amine oxidases
NT1 Amino acid oxidases
NT1 1-Aminocyclopropane-1-carboxylate oxidases
NT1 L-Ascorbate oxidases

NT1 Cholesterol oxidases
NT1 Glucose oxidases
NT1 L-Glutamate oxidases
NT1 Lactate 2-monooxygenases
NT1 Xanthine oxidases

Oxidation
NT1 Antioxidative activity
NT1 Autoxidation
NT1 Oxidative stability
NT1 Oxidative stress
NT1 Peroxidation
NT2 Peroxide values
NT1 Photooxidation
NT1 Prooxidative activity
RT Free radicals
RT Iodine values
RT Oxidizing agents
RT Oxygen
RT Peroxides
RT Radicals
RT Rancidity
RT Reactive oxygen species
RT Redox potential
RT Reduction
RT Spoilage
RT TBA values
RT Thiobarbituric acid values

Oxidation reduction potential
USE **Redox potential**

Oxidative stability
BT1 Oxidation
BT1 Stability
BT2 Physical properties

Oxidative stress
HN introduced from vol. 39, issue 1 (2007)
BT1 Oxidation
BT1 Stress
RT Free radicals

Oxides
HN introduced from vol. 39, issue 1 (2007)
NT1 Carbon dioxide
NT2 CO_2
NT2 Dry Ice
NT2 Supercritical CO_2 extraction
NT1 Carbon monoxide
NT1 Chlorine dioxide
NT1 Cysteine sulfoxides
NT1 Dimethyl sulfoxide
NT1 Ethylene oxide
NT1 Nitric oxide
NT1 Nitrous oxide
NT1 NO_2
NT1 Peroxides
NT2 H_2O_2
NT2 Hydroperoxides
NT1 Propylene oxide
NT1 Sulfur dioxide
NT2 SO_2
NT1 Superoxides

Oxidizing agents
BT1 Additives
NT1 Chlorine dioxide
NT1 Iodates
NT1 Oxidants
NT1 Peracetic acid
NT1 Peroxynitrite
RT Oxidation
RT Ozone
RT Reactive oxygen species

Oxidoreductases
HN heading from vol. 25 (1993); under Oxidases up to vol. 24 (1992)
SN EC 1
BT1 Enzymes
NT1 Cyclooxygenases
NT1 Dehydrogenases
NT2 Alcohol dehydrogenases
NT2 Aldehyde dehydrogenases
NT2 Aldehyde reductases
NT2 Glutamate dehydrogenases
NT2 L-Iditol 2-dehydrogenases
NT2 Isocitrate dehydrogenases
NT2 Lactate dehydrogenases
NT2 D-Lactate dehydrogenases
NT2 L-Lactate dehydrogenases
NT2 Xanthine dehydrogenases
NT2 D-Xylulose reductases
NT1 Desaturases
NT1 Dioxygenases
NT1 Malate dehydrogenases
NT1 Monooxygenases
NT1 Oxidases
NT2 Alcohol oxidases
NT3 Aryl-alcohol oxidases
NT2 Amine oxidases
NT2 Amino acid oxidases
NT2 1-Aminocyclopropane-1-carboxylate oxidases
NT2 L-Ascorbate oxidases
NT2 Cholesterol oxidases
NT2 Glucose oxidases
NT2 L-Glutamate oxidases
NT2 Lactate 2-monooxygenases
NT2 Xanthine oxidases
NT1 Oxygenases
NT2 Lipoxygenases
NT1 Peroxidases
NT2 Catalases
NT2 Glutathione peroxidases
NT2 Lactoperoxidase systems
NT2 Ligninases
NT2 Lignin peroxidases
NT2 Manganese peroxidases
NT1 Phenolases
NT2 Catechol oxidases
NT2 Laccases
NT2 Monophenol monooxygenases
NT2 Tyrosinases
NT1 Prostaglandin-endoperoxide synthases
NT1 Reductases
NT2 Nitrate reductases
NT1 Superoxide dismutases

Oxolinic acid
BT1 Quinolones
BT2 Antibiotics
BT3 Drugs
BT4 Residues

Oxtail
BT1 Beef
BT2 Meat specific
BT3 Meat
BT4 Animal foods
BT5 Foods

Oxydemeton-methyl
BT1 Organophosphorus insecticides
BT2 Insecticides
BT3 Pesticides
BT4 Biocides
BT4 Residues
BT2 Organophosphorus pesticides
BT3 Pesticides
BT4 Biocides
BT4 Residues

Oxygen
HN also under Gases up to vol. 42 (2010)
SN use generally for this element; use O2 for gaseous, molecular form
BT1 Elements
BT2 Minerals
BT3 Nutrients
NT1 O_2
NT1 Oxygen absorbers
NT2 Oxygen scavengers
NT1 Ozone
RT Oxidants
RT Oxidation
RT Reactive oxygen species
RT Respiration

Oxygen absorbers
SN syn. oxygen scavengers
BT1 Oxygen
BT2 Elements
BT3 Minerals
BT4 Nutrients
BT1 Packaging
BT2 Technology
NT1 Oxygen scavengers
UF O_2 absorbers

Oxygenases
BT1 Oxidoreductases
BT2 Enzymes
NT1 Lipoxygenases

Oxygen scavengers
SN syn. oxygen absorbers
BT1 Oxygen absorbers
BT2 Oxygen
BT3 Elements
BT4 Minerals
BT5 Nutrients
BT2 Packaging
BT3 Technology
UF O_2 scavengers

Oxymyoglobin
BT1 Myoglobin
BT2 Animal proteins
BT3 Proteins animal
BT4 Proteins
BT5 Nutrients
BT2 Pigments

Oxysterols
USE **Cholesterol oxidation products**

Oxytetracycline
BT1 Tetracyclines
BT2 Antibiotics
BT3 Drugs
BT4 Residues
UF Terramycin

Oxytocin
BT1 Hormones
BT2 Residues

Oyster mushrooms
USE ***Pleurotus***

Oyster plant
USE **Salsify**

Oysters
HN heading from vol. 25 (1993); under Molluscs up to vol. 24 (1992)
BT1 Bivalves
BT2 Molluscs
BT3 Shellfish
BT4 Animals
BT4 Sea foods
BT5 Aquatic foods
BT6 Animal foods
BT7 Foods
NT1 *Crassostrea gigas*
NT1 *Crassostrea virginica*
NT1 Oyster sauces

Oyster sauces
BT1 Oysters
BT2 Bivalves
BT3 Molluscs
BT4 Shellfish
BT5 Animals
BT5 Sea foods
BT6 Aquatic foods
BT7 Animal foods
BT8 Foods
BT1 Sauces
BT2 Condiments
BT3 Flavourings
BT4 Additives

Ozonation
BT1 Disinfection
BT2 Hygiene
RT Ozone

Ozone
BT1 Disinfectants
BT2 Disinfection
BT3 Hygiene
BT1 Gases
BT2 Physical phases
BT3 Chemistry
BT4 Science
BT1 Oxygen
BT2 Elements
BT3 Minerals
BT4 Nutrients
RT Oxidants
RT Oxidizing agents
RT Ozonation

P

P
SN index heading is Phosphorus
BT1 Phosphorus
BT2 Elements
BT3 Minerals
BT4 Nutrients

Pachyrhizus ahipa
BT1 Yam beans
BT2 Legumes
BT3 Vegetables specific
BT4 Vegetables
BT5 Crops
BT6 Plants
BT5 Plant foods
BT6 Foods

Pachysolen
BT1 Yeasts
BT2 Fungi
BT3 Microorganisms

Pacific hake
BT1 Hake
BT2 Marine fish
BT3 Fish
BT4 Animals
BT4 Sea foods
BT5 Aquatic foods
BT6 Animal foods
BT7 Foods
NT1 *Merluccius productus*
NT1 Pacific whiting

Pacific mackerel
SN syn. chub mackerel; syn. Spanish mackerel
BT1 Mackerel
BT2 Marine fish
BT3 Fish
BT4 Animals
BT4 Sea foods
BT5 Aquatic foods
BT6 Animal foods
BT7 Foods
BT2 Oily fish
BT3 Fish
BT4 Animals
BT4 Sea foods
BT5 Aquatic foods
BT6 Animal foods
BT7 Foods

Pacific salmon
BT1 Salmon
BT2 Oily fish
BT3 Fish
BT4 Animals
BT4 Sea foods
BT5 Aquatic foods
BT6 Animal foods
BT7 Foods
NT1 Cherry salmon
NT2 Masu salmon
NT1 Chinook salmon
NT2 King salmon
NT1 Chum salmon
NT2 Keta salmon
NT2 *Oncorhynchus keta*
NT1 Coho salmon
NT1 Pink salmon
NT1 Sockeye salmon
NT2 Red salmon

Pacific whiting
BT1 Pacific hake
BT2 Hake
BT3 Marine fish
BT4 Fish
BT5 Animals
BT5 Sea foods
BT6 Aquatic foods
BT7 Animal foods
BT8 Foods

Packages
USE **Packs**

Packaging
BT1 Technology
NT1 Active packaging
NT1 Bag in box packaging
NT1 Bottling
NT1 Canning
NT2 Canneries
NT2 Canning equipment
NT2 Canning industry
NT2 Canning quality
NT1 Cartoning
NT1 Closures
NT2 Caps
NT3 Screw caps
NT2 Corks
NT2 Crown corks
NT2 Lids
NT2 Stoppers
NT2 Tamper evident closures
NT1 Controlled atmosphere packaging
NT1 Filling
NT2 Fillers
NT2 Filling equipment
NT1 Intelligent packaging
NT1 Labelling
NT2 Bar codes
NT2 Branding
NT2 Brands
NT2 Date marking
NT2 Dating
NT2 Health claims
NT2 Ink jet technology
NT2 Inks
NT2 Labels
NT2 Marking
NT2 Nutritional labelling
NT2 Printing
NT3 Printers
NT4 Ink jet printers
NT2 Private labels
NT2 Trademarks
NT1 Microwaveable packaging
NT1 Modified atmosphere packaging
NT1 Openings
NT1 Overwrapping
NT1 Oxygen absorbers

NT2 Oxygen scavengers
NT1 Packaging aseptic
NT2 Aseptic packaging
NT1 Packinghouses
NT1 Sealing
NT2 Seaming
NT1 Shrink packaging
NT1 Tamper evident packaging
NT1 Vacuum packaging
NT1 Wrapping
RT Adhesives
RT Containers
RT Packaging materials
RT Packs
UF Packing

Packaging aseptic
HN aseptic packaging also used in the index from vol.30 (1998)
BT1 Packaging
BT2 Technology
NT1 Aseptic packaging

Packaging bag in box
HN used in addition to bag in box packaging up to vol. 29 (1997)
USE **Bag in box packaging**

Packaging controlled atm
HN used for controlled atmosphere packaging up to vol. 24 (1992)
USE **Controlled atmosphere packaging**

Packaging controlled atmosphere
HN used for controlled atmosphere packaging up to vol. 31 (1999)
USE **Controlled atmosphere packaging**

Packaging films
BT1 Packaging materials
NT1 Antimicrobial packaging films

Packaging materials
NT1 Aluminium
NT2 Al
NT2 Al compounds
NT1 Board
NT2 Cardboard
NT2 Cartonboard
NT2 Fibreboard
NT2 Paperboard
NT2 Pulpboard
NT1 Environment friendly packaging materials
NT1 Foils
NT2 Al foils
NT1 Glass
NT2 Glass bottles
NT2 Glass containers
NT1 Jute
NT1 Laminates
NT1 Packaging films
NT2 Antimicrobial packaging films
NT1 Paper
NT2 Glassine
NT2 Parchment paper
NT1 Plasticizers
NT1 Plastics
NT2 Acrylonitrile
NT2 Cryovac
NT2 Epoxides
NT2 Foamed plastics
NT2 Melamine
NT2 Mylar
NT2 Nylon
NT2 PET
NT2 Plastics bags
NT2 Plastics bottles
NT2 Plastics films
NT3 Cellulose films
NT4 Cellophane
NT2 Polyacrylamides
NT2 Polyamides
NT2 Polycarbonates
NT2 Polyesters
NT2 Polyethylene
NT3 HDPE
NT3 LDPE
NT3 Polyethylene bags
NT3 Polyethylene films
NT2 Polyethylene naphthalate
NT2 Polyolefins
NT2 Polypropylene
NT2 Polystyrene
NT3 Styrene
NT2 Polyurethane
NT2 Polyvinyl alcohol
NT2 Polyvinyl chloride
NT3 PVC
NT3 Vinyl chloride
NT2 Polyvinylpyrrolidinone
NT2 Polyvinylpyrrolidone
NT2 PTFE
NT2 PVDC
NT2 Saran
NT2 Vinylidene chloride
NT1 Rubber
NT1 Steel
NT2 Stainless steel
NT1 Tin
NT2 Sn
NT1 Tin plate
NT1 Wood
NT2 Oak
NT2 Timber
RT Contact Materials
RT Containers
RT Migration
RT Packaging

Packaging modified atm
HN used for packaging modified atmosphere up to vol. 24 (1992)
USE **Modified atmosphere packaging**

Packaging modified atmosphere
HN used for modified atmosphere packaging up to vol. 31 (1999)
USE **Modified atmosphere packaging**

Packed bed bioreactors
HN introduced from vol. 39, issue 1 (2007)
BT1 Bioreactors
BT2 Fermentation technology
BT3 Biotechnology
BT4 Technology
BT3 Process control
BT4 Technology

Packing
USE **Packaging**

Packinghouses
BT1 Packaging
BT2 Technology

Packs
BT1 Containers
NT1 Aerosol packs
NT1 Edible packs
NT1 Flexible packs
NT1 Multipacks
NT1 Nettings
NT1 Portion packs
NT1 Punnets
RT Packaging
UF Packages

Packs flexible
HN used up to vol. 31 (1999)
USE **Flexible packs**

Paclobutrazol
BT1 Plant growth regulators
BT2 Cultivation
BT3 Agriculture

Pacu
HN introduced from vol. 37, issue 5 (2005)
BT1 Freshwater fish
BT2 Fish
BT3 Animals
BT3 Sea foods
BT4 Aquatic foods
BT5 Animal foods
BT6 Foods

Paddlefish
BT1 Marine fish
BT2 Fish
BT3 Animals
BT3 Sea foods
BT4 Aquatic foods
BT5 Animal foods
BT6 Foods
NT1 *Polyodon spathula*

Paddy
BT1 Rice
BT2 Cereals
BT3 Crops
BT4 Plants
BT3 Seeds
BT4 Plant foods
BT5 Foods

Padi straw mushrooms
USE ***Volvariella***

Paecilomyces
SN teleomorph is Talaromyces
BT1 Fungi
BT2 Microorganisms

NT1 *Paecilomyces japonica*
NT1 *Paecilomyces sinclairii*

Paecilomyces japonica
BT1 *Paecilomyces*
BT2 Fungi
BT3 Microorganisms

Paecilomyces sinclairii
BT1 *Paecilomyces*
BT2 Fungi
BT3 Microorganisms

Paenibacillus
HN introduced from vol. 37, issue 5 (2005)
BT1 Bacteria
BT2 Microorganisms
NT1 *Paenibacillus amylolyticus*
NT1 *Paenibacillus polymyxa*

Paenibacillus amylolyticus
BT1 *Paenibacillus*
BT2 Bacteria
BT3 Microorganisms

Paenibacillus polymyxa
SN synonymous with Bacillus polymyxa
BT1 *Paenibacillus*
BT2 Bacteria
BT3 Microorganisms

PAGE
BT1 Electrophoresis
BT2 Analytical techniques
RT Gel electrophoresis
UF Polyacrylamide gel electrophoresis

Pagrus major
BT1 Red sea bream
BT2 Sea bream
BT3 Marine fish
BT4 Fish
BT5 Animals
BT5 Sea foods
BT6 Aquatic foods
BT7 Animal foods
BT8 Foods

PAH
BT1 Hydrocarbons
BT2 Organic compounds
UF Polycyclic aromatic hydrocarbons
UF Polynuclear aromatic hydrocarbons

Paints
HN heading up to vol. 24 (1992)
BT1 Surfaces

Pak choi
BT1 Chinese cabbages
BT2 Vegetables specific
BT3 Vegetables
BT4 Crops
BT5 Plants
BT4 Plant foods
BT5 Foods

Pakistan
BT1 Asia

Pakoras
BT1 Snack foods
BT2 Processed foods
BT3 Foods

Palatability
HN heading up to vol. 24 (1992)
BT1 Sensory properties

Palatinit
USE **Isomalt**

Palatinose
HN under Sugars up to vol. 42 (2010)
BT1 Isomaltulose
BT2 Disaccharides
BT3 Sugars
BT4 Carbohydrates
BT5 Nutrients
BT5 Organic compounds
BT4 Plant foods
BT5 Foods

Pale soft exudative defect
USE **PSE defect**

Palladium
USE **Pd**

Palletization
BT1 Pallets

Pallets
NT1 Palletization
RT Handling
RT Transport

Palmaria palmata
BT1 Dulse
BT2 Seaweeds
BT3 Algae
BT4 Microorganisms
BT3 Sea foods
BT4 Aquatic foods
BT5 Animal foods
BT6 Foods

Palmarosa
HN under Spices up to vol. 42 (2010)
BT1 Herbs
BT2 Spices
BT3 Flavourings
BT4 Additives

Palm hearts
BT1 Palms
BT2 Plants
BT1 Vegetables specific
BT2 Vegetables
BT3 Crops
BT4 Plants
BT3 Plant foods
BT4 Foods

Palmitic acid
HN heading from vol. 25 (1993) up to vol. 42 (2010); under Fatty acids up to vol. 24 (1992) and under Saturated fatty acids from vol. 43 (2011)
SN syn. hexadecanoic acid
BT1 Hexadecanoic acid
BT2 Saturated fatty acids
BT3 Fatty acids
BT4 Lipids
BT5 Nutrients
BT4 Organic acids
BT5 Acids

Palmitoleic acid
BT1 Hexadecenoic acid
BT2 Monounsaturated fatty acids
BT3 Unsaturated fatty acids
BT4 Fatty acids
BT5 Lipids
BT6 Nutrients
BT5 Organic acids
BT6 Acids

Palm kernel oils
BT1 Palm oils
BT2 Palms
BT3 Plants
BT2 Vegetable oils
BT3 Oils vegetable
BT4 Oils
BT5 Lipids
BT6 Nutrients
BT4 Vegetable products
BT5 Plant foods
BT6 Foods

Palm oil mills effluents
BT1 Effluents
BT2 Waste water
BT3 Wastes
BT3 Water
BT1 Palm oils
BT2 Palms
BT3 Plants
BT2 Vegetable oils
BT3 Oils vegetable
BT4 Oils
BT5 Lipids
BT6 Nutrients
BT4 Vegetable products
BT5 Plant foods
BT6 Foods

Palm oils
BT1 Palms
BT2 Plants
BT1 Vegetable oils
BT2 Oils vegetable
BT3 Oils
BT4 Lipids
BT5 Nutrients
BT3 Vegetable products
BT4 Plant foods
BT5 Foods
NT1 Babassu oils
NT1 Palm kernel oils
NT1 Palm oil mills effluents

NT1 Palm olein
NT1 Palm stearin
RT *Elaeis*
RT Oil palms
UF *Elaeis* oils

Palm olein
BT1 Olein
BT2 Triglycerides
BT3 Glycerides
BT4 Emulsifiers
BT5 Additives
BT4 Fatty acid esters
BT5 Esters
BT6 Organic compounds
BT4 Lipids
BT5 Nutrients
BT1 Palm oils
BT2 Palms
BT3 Plants
BT2 Vegetable oils
BT3 Oils vegetable
BT4 Oils
BT5 Lipids
BT6 Nutrients
BT4 Vegetable products
BT5 Plant foods
BT6 Foods

Palms
HN heading up to vol. 24 (1992) and from vol. 39, issue 1 (2007)
BT1 Plants
NT1 Acai
NT1 *Acrocomia*
NT1 *Areca*
NT2 *Areca catechu*
NT1 *Arenga*
NT1 *Astrocaryum*
NT1 Babassu palm kernels
NT1 *Bactris*
NT1 *Borassus*
NT1 *Elaeis*
NT1 *Hyphaene*
NT1 *Mauritia*
NT1 *Metroxylon*
NT1 Palm hearts
NT1 Palm oils
NT2 Babassu oils
NT2 Palm kernel oils
NT2 Palm oil mills effluents
NT2 Palm olein
NT2 Palm stearin
NT1 Palmyra
NT2 Palmyrah
NT1 *Phoenix*
NT1 *Raphia*
NT1 *Syagrus*
NT1 Wines palm
NT2 Palm wines
NT3 Coconut toddy
NT3 Toddy
NT3 Tuba
RT Oil palms
RT Sago

Palm stearin
BT1 Palm oils
BT2 Palms
BT3 Plants
BT2 Vegetable oils
BT3 Oils vegetable
BT4 Oils
BT5 Lipids
BT6 Nutrients
BT4 Vegetable products
BT5 Plant foods
BT6 Foods
BT1 Stearin
BT2 Triglycerides
BT3 Glycerides
BT4 Emulsifiers
BT5 Additives
BT4 Fatty acid esters
BT5 Esters
BT6 Organic compounds
BT4 Lipids
BT5 Nutrients

Palm wines
SN index heading is Wines palm
BT1 Wines palm
BT2 Alcoholic beverages
BT3 Beverages alcoholic
BT4 Beverages
BT2 Palms
BT3 Plants
NT1 Coconut toddy
NT1 Toddy
NT1 Tuba

Palmyra
SN syn. palmyrah
BT1 Palms
BT2 Plants
NT1 Palmyrah

Palmyrah
SN syn. palmyra
BT1 Palmyra
BT2 Palms
BT3 Plants

Palytoxin
BT1 Toxins
BT2 Residues

Panama
BT1 Central America
BT2 America

Panax notoginseng
BT1 Ginseng
BT2 Plants

Pancakes
BT1 Bakery products
BT2 Cereal products
BT3 Plant foods
BT4 Foods

Pancreas
BT1 Offal
BT2 Animal foods
BT3 Foods

Pancreatins
BT1 Hydrolases
BT2 Enzymes

Pandalus borealis
BT1 Shrimps
BT2 Crustacea
BT3 Shellfish
BT4 Animals
BT4 Sea foods
BT5 Aquatic foods
BT6 Animal foods
BT7 Foods

Paneer
BT1 Curd
BT2 Dairy products
BT3 Animal foods
BT4 Foods

Panellists
BT1 Sensory analysis
BT2 Analytical techniques
RT Taste panels

Panettone
BT1 Bakery products
BT2 Cereal products
BT3 Plant foods
BT4 Foods

Panning
BT1 Coating
BT2 Processing
BT3 Technology
RT Chocolate

Panose
HN under Sugars up to vol. 42 (2010)
BT1 Glucooligosaccharides
BT2 Oligosaccharides
BT3 Polysaccharides
BT4 Carbohydrates
BT5 Nutrients
BT5 Organic compounds
BT3 Sugars
BT4 Carbohydrates
BT5 Nutrients
BT5 Organic compounds
BT4 Plant foods
BT5 Foods

Pans
BT1 Equipment
BT2 Technology

Pantoea
HN introduced from vol. 39, issue 1 (2007)
BT1 Bacteria
BT2 Microorganisms
NT1 *Pantoea agglomerans*

Pantoea agglomerans
SN synonymous with Erwinia herbicola
BT1 *Pantoea*
BT2 Bacteria
BT3 Microorganisms

Pantothenic acid
BT1 Vitamin B group
BT2 Vitamins
BT3 Nutrients

Papads
BT1 Bakery products
BT2 Cereal products
BT3 Plant foods
BT4 Foods

Papain
HN heading up to vol. 24 (1992)
SN EC 3.4.22.2
BT1 Proteinases
BT2 Hydrolases
BT3 Enzymes

Papaya nectars
BT1 Fruit nectars
BT2 Fruit juices
BT3 Fruit products
BT4 Plant foods
BT5 Foods
BT3 Soft drinks
BT4 Beverages
RT Papayas

Papayas
HN heading from vol. 25 (1993); under Pawpaws up to vol. 24 (1992)
BT1 Fruits specific
BT2 Fruits
BT3 Crops
BT4 Plants
BT3 Plant foods
BT4 Foods
NT1 Pawpaws
RT Papaya nectars

Paper
BT1 Packaging materials
NT1 Glassine
NT1 Parchment paper

Paperboard
BT1 Board
BT2 Packaging materials

Paper chromatography
HN heading up to vol. 18 (1986)
BT1 Chromatography
BT2 Analytical techniques

Paprika
BT1 Spices
BT2 Flavourings
BT3 Additives

Paps
BT1 Cereal products
BT2 Plant foods
BT3 Foods

Papua New Guinea
BT1 Oceania
UF New Guinea

Parabens
SN syn. hydroxybenzoic acid esters
BT1 Hydroxybenzoic acid esters
BT2 Esters
BT3 Organic compounds
BT2 Preservatives
BT3 Additives
NT1 Methylparaben
NT1 Propylparaben

Paracoccus
BT1 Bacteria
BT2 Microorganisms

Paraffins
BT1 Hydrocarbons
BT2 Organic compounds

Paraformaldehyde
HN under Insecticides up to vol. 42 (2010)
BT1 Aldehydes
BT2 Carbonyl compounds
BT3 Organic compounds
BT1 Fumigants
BT2 Biocides

Paraguay
BT1 South America
BT2 America

Paralichthys olivaceus
BT1 Bastard halibut
BT2 Flatfish
BT3 Marine fish
BT4 Fish
BT5 Animals
BT5 Sea foods
BT6 Aquatic foods
BT7 Animal foods
BT8 Foods
BT1 Japanese flounders
BT2 Flounders
BT3 Flatfish
BT4 Marine fish
BT5 Fish
BT6 Animals
BT6 Sea foods
BT7 Aquatic foods
BT8 Animal foods
BT9 Foods

Paralytic shellfish poisoning
BT1 Diseases
BT1 Poisoning
NT1 PSP
RT Brevetoxins
RT Diarrhoetic shellfish poisoning
RT Dinoflagellate toxins
RT Mussel poisoning
RT Paralytic shellfish toxins
RT Saxitoxin
RT Sea foods

Paralytic shellfish toxins
BT1 Toxins
BT2 Residues
RT Brevetoxins
RT Diarrhoetic shellfish toxins
RT Dinoflagellates
RT Paralytic shellfish poisoning

Paraoxon
BT1 Parathion
BT2 Acaricides
BT3 Pesticides
BT4 Biocides
BT4 Residues
BT2 Organophosphorus insecticides
BT3 Insecticides
BT4 Pesticides
BT5 Biocides
BT5 Residues
BT3 Organophosphorus pesticides
BT4 Pesticides
BT5 Biocides
BT5 Residues

Paraquat
BT1 Herbicides
BT2 Pesticides
BT3 Biocides
BT3 Residues

Parasites
BT1 Pests
NT1 Amoebae
NT2 *Acanthamoeba*
NT1 *Anisakis*
NT2 *Anisakis simplex*
NT1 Cestodes
NT1 *Clonorchis sinensis*
NT1 *Cryptosporidium*
NT2 *Cryptosporidium hominis*
NT2 *Cryptosporidium parvum*
NT1 *Cyclospora*
NT2 *Cyclospora cayetanensis*
NT1 *Cysticercus*
NT1 *Diphyllobothrium*
NT1 *Echinococcus*
NT1 *Entamoeba*
NT2 *Entamoeba histolytica*
NT1 *Fasciola*
NT1 Flukes
NT2 Liver flukes
NT1 *Giardia*
NT2 *Giardia intestinalis*
NT2 *Giardia lamblia*
NT2 *Giardia muris*
NT1 Helminths
NT1 *Isospora*
NT1 Liver flukes
NT1 Metacercariae
NT1 *Naegleria*
NT1 Nematodes
NT1 Oocysts
NT1 *Pseudoterranova*
NT1 *Sarcocystis*
NT1 *Sarcosporidia*
NT1 *Taenia*
NT1 Tapeworms
NT1 *Toxoplasma*
NT2 *Toxoplasma gondii*
NT1 Trematodes
NT1 Trichinae
NT1 *Trichinella*
NT2 *Trichinella spiralis*
RT Food safety
RT *Leptospira*
RT *Rickettsia*

Parasiticol
USE **Aflatoxin B_3**

Parathas
HN introduced from vol. 39, issue 1 (2007)
BT1 Bakery products
BT2 Cereal products
BT3 Plant foods
BT4 Foods

Parathion
HN heading up to vol. 18 (1986)
BT1 Acaricides
BT2 Pesticides
BT3 Biocides
BT3 Residues
BT1 Organophosphorus insecticides
BT2 Insecticides
BT3 Pesticides
BT4 Biocides
BT4 Residues
BT2 Organophosphorus pesticides
BT3 Pesticides
BT4 Biocides
BT4 Residues
NT1 Paraoxon

Parathion-methyl
BT1 Acaricides
BT2 Pesticides
BT3 Biocides
BT3 Residues
BT1 Organophosphorus insecticides
BT2 Insecticides
BT3 Pesticides
BT4 Biocides
BT4 Residues
BT2 Organophosphorus pesticides
BT3 Pesticides
BT4 Biocides
BT4 Residues
UF Metaphos
UF Methylparathion

Paratyphoid
BT1 Diseases
RT *Salmonella* Paratyphi

Parboiling
BT1 Boiling
BT2 Cooking
BT3 Thermal processing
BT4 Processing thermal
BT5 Processing
BT6 Technology

Parching
BT1 Drying
BT2 Thermal processing
BT3 Processing thermal
BT4 Processing
BT5 Technology

Parchment paper
BT1 Paper
BT2 Packaging materials

Parental response
HN introduced from vol. 43, issue 1 (2011)
BT1 Consumer response

Parkinson's disease
USE **Neurodegenerative diseases**

Parma ham
BT1 Ham
BT2 Meat products
BT3 Animal foods
BT4 Foods

Parmesan cheese
BT1 Cheese varieties
BT2 Cheese
BT3 Dairy products
BT4 Animal foods
BT5 Foods

Parmigiano Reggiano cheese
BT1 Cheese varieties
BT2 Cheese
BT3 Dairy products
BT4 Animal foods
BT5 Foods

Parottas
HN introduced from vol. 39, issue 1 (2007)
BT1 Bread
BT2 Bakery products
BT3 Cereal products
BT4 Plant foods
BT5 Foods

Parsley
HN under Spices up to vol. 42 (2010)
BT1 Herbs
BT2 Spices
BT3 Flavourings
BT4 Additives

Parsnips
BT1 Vegetables specific
BT2 Vegetables
BT3 Crops
BT4 Plants
BT3 Plant foods
BT4 Foods

Parthenocarpy
BT1 Seeds
BT2 Plant foods
BT3 Foods

Particles
HN heading from vol. 25 (1993)
NT1 Nanoparticles
NT1 Particulate foods
RT Granules

Particulate foods
BT1 Particles

Partitioning
BT1 Separation
BT2 Processing
BT3 Technology

Partridge carcasses
BT1 Carcasses
BT2 Meat
BT3 Animal foods
BT4 Foods
BT1 Partridge meat
BT2 Meat specific
BT3 Meat
BT4 Animal foods
BT5 Foods
BT2 Partridges
BT3 Birds

Partridge meat
BT1 Meat specific
BT2 Meat
BT3 Animal foods
BT4 Foods
BT1 Partridges
BT2 Birds
NT1 Partridge carcasses

Partridges
BT1 Birds
NT1 Partridge meat
NT2 Partridge carcasses

Parvovirus
HN introduced from vol. 43, issue 1 (2011)
BT1 Parvoviruses
BT2 Viruses
BT3 Microorganisms

Parvoviruses
HN introduced from vol. 39, issue 1 (2007); under Enteric viruses up to vol. 42 (2010)
SN for descriptive use only
BT1 Viruses
BT2 Microorganisms
NT1 Parvovirus

Passiflora edulis
BT1 Passion fruits
BT2 Fruits specific
BT3 Fruits
BT4 Crops
BT5 Plants
BT4 Plant foods
BT5 Foods

Passion fruit juices
BT1 Fruit juices
BT2 Fruit products
BT3 Plant foods
BT4 Foods
BT2 Soft drinks
BT3 Beverages
RT Passion fruits

Passion fruits
HN heading from vol. 30 (1998); under Fruits specific up to vol. 29 (1997)
BT1 Fruits specific
BT2 Fruits
BT3 Crops
BT4 Plants
BT3 Plant foods
BT4 Foods
NT1 *Passiflora edulis*

RT Passion fruit juices
UF Granadillas

Pasta
BT1 Cereal products
BT2 Plant foods
BT3 Foods
NT1 Alimentary pastes
NT1 Canneloni
NT1 Egg pasta
NT1 Lasagne
NT1 Macaroni
NT1 Noodles
NT2 Instant noodles
NT1 Ravioli
NT1 Somen
NT1 Spaghetti
NT1 Tagliatelli
NT1 Tortellini
NT1 Udon
NT1 Vermicelli
RT Pasta sauces
RT Semolina

Pasta filata cheese
BT1 Cheese varieties
BT2 Cheese
BT3 Dairy products
BT4 Animal foods
BT5 Foods

Pasta sauces
HN introduced from vol. 39, issue 1 (2007)
BT1 Sauces
BT2 Condiments
BT3 Flavourings
BT4 Additives
NT1 Pesto
RT Pasta

Pasterma
SN syn. pastirma
BT1 Pastirma
BT2 Meat products
BT3 Animal foods
BT4 Foods

Pastes
BT1 Processed foods
BT2 Foods
NT1 Bean pastes
NT1 Confectionery pastes
NT1 Fish pastes
NT2 Anchovy pastes
NT1 Fruit pastes
NT1 Meat pastes
NT1 Nut pastes
NT2 Peanut pastes
NT1 Soy pastes
NT1 Tahini
NT2 Tehineh
NT1 Tomato pastes
RT Pates
RT Spreads

Pasteurella
BT1 Bacteria
BT2 Microorganisms
RT Pasteurellosis

Pasteurellosis
BT1 Diseases
RT *Pasteurella*

Pasteurization
BT1 Thermal processing
BT2 Processing thermal
BT3 Processing
BT4 Technology
NT1 HTST pasteurization
NT1 LTLT pasteurization
NT1 Pasteurizers
NT1 Surface pasteurization
NT1 Ultrapasteurization
RT Heating
RT Pasteurized milk
RT Sterilization

Pasteurization HTST
HN used up to vol. 31 (1999)
USE **HTST pasteurization**

Pasteurized milk
BT1 Milk
BT2 Dairy products
BT3 Animal foods
BT4 Foods
RT Pasteurization
UF Pasteurized milks

Pasteurized milks
HN heading up to vol. 24 (1992)
USE **Pasteurized milk**

Pasteurizers
BT1 Equipment
BT2 Technology
BT1 Pasteurization
BT2 Thermal processing
BT3 Processing thermal
BT4 Processing
BT5 Technology

Pastila
USE **Pastilles**

Pastilles
BT1 Sugar confectionery
BT2 Plant foods
BT3 Foods
UF Pastila

Pastiness
BT1 Consistency
BT2 Texture
BT3 Sensory properties

Pasting properties
BT1 Functional properties
BT2 Physical properties

Pastirma
SN syn. pasterma
BT1 Meat products
BT2 Animal foods
BT3 Foods
NT1 Pasterma

Pastrami
BT1 Meat products
BT2 Animal foods
BT3 Foods
RT Beef

Pastries
BT1 Bakery products
BT2 Cereal products
BT3 Plant foods
BT4 Foods
NT1 Cream puffs
NT1 Danish pastries
NT1 Eclairs
NT1 Strudels
RT Pies

Pastry
BT1 Bakery products
BT2 Cereal products
BT3 Plant foods
BT4 Foods
NT1 Puff pastry

Pastures
BT1 Feeds

Patagras cheese
BT1 Cheese varieties
BT2 Cheese
BT3 Dairy products
BT4 Animal foods
BT5 Foods

Patatin
BT1 Vegetable proteins
BT2 Proteins vegetable
BT3 Proteins
BT4 Nutrients
BT3 Vegetable products
BT4 Plant foods
BT5 Foods
RT Potatoes

Pate
HN heading up to vol. 24 (1992)
USE **Pates**

Patents
HN heading from vol. 24 (1992)

Pates
HN heading from vol. 25 (1993); Pate up to vol. 24 (1992)
BT1 Fish products
BT2 Sea foods
BT3 Aquatic foods
BT4 Animal foods
BT5 Foods
BT1 Meat products
BT2 Animal foods
BT3 Foods
NT1 Fish pates
NT1 Liver pates
NT1 Terrines
RT Pastes
RT Spreads
UF Pate

Pathogenesis
BT1 Pathogenicity
RT Pathogens
RT Virulence
RT Virulence factors

Pathogenic bacteria
USE **Pathogens**

Pathogenicity
HN heading from vol. 28 (1996)
NT1 Pathogenesis
NT1 Pathogenicity islands
RT Pathogens
RT Virulence
RT Virulence factors

Pathogenicity islands
BT1 Pathogenicity

Pathogenic microorganisms
USE **Pathogens**

Pathogens
HN heading from vol. 25 (1993)
BT1 Microorganisms
RT Diseases
RT Food safety
RT Pathogenesis
RT Pathogenicity
RT Virulence
RT Virulence factors
UF Pathogenic bacteria
UF Pathogenic microorganisms

Patinopecten yessoensis
BT1 Scallops
BT2 Bivalves
BT3 Molluscs
BT4 Shellfish
BT5 Animals
BT5 Sea foods
BT6 Aquatic foods
BT7 Animal foods
BT8 Foods

Patis
BT1 Fermented foods
BT2 Processed foods
BT3 Foods
BT1 Fish sauces
BT2 Fish products
BT3 Sea foods
BT4 Aquatic foods
BT5 Animal foods
BT6 Foods
BT2 Sauces
BT3 Condiments
BT4 Flavourings
BT5 Additives

Patisserie products
BT1 Bakery products
BT2 Cereal products
BT3 Plant foods
BT4 Foods

Patties
BT1 Meat products
BT2 Animal foods
BT3 Foods
NT1 Meat patties
NT2 Beef patties
NT2 Chicken patties
NT2 Pork patties
NT2 Turkey patties

Patulin
BT1 Mycotoxins
BT2 Toxins
BT3 Residues
RT *Byssochlamys*

Pauas
USE **Abalones**

Paullinia cupana
BT1 Guarana
BT2 Soft drinks
BT3 Beverages

Pawpaws
HN heading up to vol. 24 (1992)
BT1 Papayas
BT2 Fruits specific
BT3 Fruits
BT4 Crops
BT5 Plants
BT4 Plant foods
BT5 Foods

Payment
BT1 Pricing
BT2 Food policy
BT3 Economics

Payzone
USE **Nitrovin**

Pb
SN index heading is Lead
BT1 Lead
BT2 Metals
BT3 Elements
BT4 Minerals
BT5 Nutrients

PCB
SN index heading is Polychlorinated biphenyls
BT1 Polychlorinated biphenyls
BT2 Chlorinated hydrocarbons
BT3 Organic halogen compounds

PCR
HN heading from vol. 43 (2011); under Genetic techniques up to vol. 42 (2010)
BT1 Genetic techniques
BT2 Genetics
RT RAPD
RT RFLP
UF Polymerase chain reaction

Pd
HN under Minerals up to vol. 42 (2010)
BT1 Metals
BT2 Elements
BT3 Minerals
BT4 Nutrients
UF Palladium

Pea beans
BT1 Common beans
BT2 Legumes
BT3 Vegetables specific
BT4 Vegetables
BT5 Crops
BT6 Plants
BT5 Plant foods
BT6 Foods

Peaches
BT1 Fruits specific
BT2 Fruits
BT3 Crops
BT4 Plants
BT3 Plant foods
BT4 Foods
NT1 Nectarines
NT1 Peach pulps
NT1 Peach purees
RT Peach juices
RT Peach nectars

Peach juices
BT1 Fruit juices
BT2 Fruit products
BT3 Plant foods
BT4 Foods
BT2 Soft drinks
BT3 Beverages
RT Peaches
RT Peach nectars

Peach nectars
BT1 Fruit nectars
BT2 Fruit juices
BT3 Fruit products
BT4 Plant foods
BT5 Foods
BT3 Soft drinks
BT4 Beverages
RT Peaches
RT Peach juices

Peach pulps
BT1 Fruit pulps
BT2 Fruit products
BT3 Plant foods
BT4 Foods
BT2 Pulps
BT3 Processed foods
BT4 Foods
BT1 Peaches
BT2 Fruits specific
BT3 Fruits
BT4 Crops
BT5 Plants
BT4 Plant foods
BT5 Foods

Peach purees
HN introduced from vol. 39, issue 1 (2007)
BT1 Fruit purees
BT2 Fruit products
BT3 Plant foods
BT4 Foods
BT2 Purees
BT3 Pulps
BT4 Processed foods
BT5 Foods
BT1 Peaches
BT2 Fruits specific
BT3 Fruits
BT4 Crops
BT5 Plants

BT4 Plant foods
BT5 Foods

Pea flour
USE **Pea meal**

Pea meal
BT1 Flours
BT2 Plant foods
BT3 Foods
BT1 Peas
BT2 Legumes
BT3 Vegetables specific
BT4 Vegetables
BT5 Crops
BT6 Plants
BT5 Plant foods
BT6 Foods
UF Pea flour

Peanut butter
BT1 Peanuts
BT2 Nuts
BT3 Fruits
BT4 Crops
BT5 Plants
BT4 Plant foods
BT5 Foods
BT3 Oilseeds
BT4 Seeds
BT5 Plant foods
BT6 Foods
BT1 Spreads
BT2 Processed foods
BT3 Foods
RT Peanut pastes

Peanut meal
BT1 Flours
BT2 Plant foods
BT3 Foods
BT1 Peanuts
BT2 Nuts
BT3 Fruits
BT4 Crops
BT5 Plants
BT4 Plant foods
BT5 Foods
BT3 Oilseeds
BT4 Seeds
BT5 Plant foods
BT6 Foods

Peanut milk
BT1 Peanuts
BT2 Nuts
BT3 Fruits
BT4 Crops
BT5 Plants
BT4 Plant foods
BT5 Foods
BT3 Oilseeds
BT4 Seeds
BT5 Plant foods
BT6 Foods

Peanut oils
USE **Groundnut oils**

Peanut pastes
BT1 Nut pastes
BT2 Nuts
BT3 Fruits
BT4 Crops
BT5 Plants
BT4 Plant foods
BT5 Foods
BT3 Oilseeds
BT4 Seeds
BT5 Plant foods
BT6 Foods
BT2 Pastes
BT3 Processed foods
BT4 Foods
BT1 Peanuts
BT2 Nuts
BT3 Fruits
BT4 Crops
BT5 Plants
BT4 Plant foods
BT5 Foods
BT3 Oilseeds
BT4 Seeds
BT5 Plant foods
BT6 Foods
RT Peanut butter

Peanut products
BT1 Peanuts
BT2 Nuts
BT3 Fruits
BT4 Crops
BT5 Plants
BT4 Plant foods
BT5 Foods
BT3 Oilseeds
BT4 Seeds
BT5 Plant foods
BT6 Foods

Peanut proteins
BT1 Peanuts
BT2 Nuts
BT3 Fruits
BT4 Crops
BT5 Plants
BT4 Plant foods
BT5 Foods
BT3 Oilseeds
BT4 Seeds
BT5 Plant foods
BT6 Foods
BT1 Vegetable proteins
BT2 Proteins vegetable
BT3 Proteins
BT4 Nutrients
BT3 Vegetable products
BT4 Plant foods
BT5 Foods
RT Arachin
RT Conarachin

Peanuts
HN heading from vol. 25 (1993); use Groundnuts up to vol. 24 (1992)
BT1 Nuts
BT2 Fruits
BT3 Crops
BT4 Plants
BT3 Plant foods
BT4 Foods
BT2 Oilseeds
BT3 Seeds
BT4 Plant foods
BT5 Foods
NT1 Ontjom
NT1 Peanut butter
NT1 Peanut meal
NT1 Peanut milk
NT1 Peanut pastes
NT1 Peanut products
NT1 Peanut proteins
NT1 Roasted peanuts
RT Arachin
UF Groundnuts

Pea protein concentrates
BT1 Peas
BT2 Legumes
BT3 Vegetables specific
BT4 Vegetables
BT5 Crops
BT6 Plants
BT5 Plant foods
BT6 Foods
BT1 Protein concentrates
BT2 Concentrates
BT3 Processed foods
BT4 Foods
BT2 Protein products

Pea proteins
BT1 Peas
BT2 Legumes
BT3 Vegetables specific
BT4 Vegetables
BT5 Crops
BT6 Plants
BT5 Plant foods
BT6 Foods
BT1 Vegetable proteins
BT2 Proteins vegetable
BT3 Proteins
BT4 Nutrients
BT3 Vegetable products
BT4 Plant foods
BT5 Foods

Pear juices
BT1 Fruit juices
BT2 Fruit products
BT3 Plant foods
BT4 Foods
BT2 Soft drinks
BT3 Beverages
RT Pears

Pearl barley
BT1 Barley
BT2 Cereals
BT3 Crops
BT4 Plants
BT3 Seeds
BT4 Plant foods
BT5 Foods

Pearling
BT1 Processing
BT2 Technology

Pearl millet
BT1 Millet
BT2 Cereals
BT3 Crops
BT4 Plants
BT3 Seeds
BT4 Plant foods
BT5 Foods

Pears
BT1 Fruits specific
BT2 Fruits
BT3 Crops
BT4 Plants
BT3 Plant foods
BT4 Foods
NT1 Asian pears
NT1 Chinese pears
NT1 Japanese pears
RT Pear juices

Peas
BT1 Legumes
BT2 Vegetables specific
BT3 Vegetables
BT4 Crops
BT5 Plants
BT4 Plant foods
BT5 Foods
NT1 Dried peas
NT1 Field peas
NT1 Green peas
NT1 Pea meal
NT1 Pea protein concentrates
NT1 Pea proteins
NT1 Pea starch
NT1 Snow peas

Pea starch
BT1 Peas
BT2 Legumes
BT3 Vegetables specific
BT4 Vegetables
BT5 Crops
BT6 Plants
BT5 Plant foods
BT6 Foods
BT1 Starch
BT2 Glucans
BT3 Polysaccharides
BT4 Carbohydrates
BT5 Nutrients
BT5 Organic compounds
BT2 Thickeners
BT3 Additives

Pecan nuts
HN heading from vol. 30 (1998); under Nuts up to vol.29 (1997)
BT1 Nuts
BT2 Fruits
BT3 Crops
BT4 Plants
BT3 Plant foods
BT4 Foods
BT2 Oilseeds
BT3 Seeds
BT4 Plant foods
BT5 Foods

Pecan oils
BT1 Nut oils
BT2 Vegetable oils
BT3 Oils vegetable
BT4 Oils
BT5 Lipids
BT6 Nutrients
BT4 Vegetable products
BT5 Plant foods
BT6 Foods

Pecorino cheese
BT1 Cheese varieties
BT2 Cheese
BT3 Dairy products
BT4 Animal foods
BT5 Foods

Pecorino Sardo cheese
BT1 Cheese varieties
BT2 Cheese
BT3 Dairy products
BT4 Animal foods
BT5 Foods

Pectate lyases
SN EC 4.2.2.2
BT1 Lyases
BT2 Enzymes
BT1 Pectic enzymes
BT2 Enzymes
UF Pectate transeliminases

Pectate transeliminases
USE **Pectate lyases**

Pectic enzymes
BT1 Enzymes
NT1 Pectate lyases
NT1 Pectinesterases
NT1 Pectin lyases
NT1 Pectolytic enzymes
NT1 Polygalacturonases

Pectic substances
BT1 Polysaccharides
BT2 Carbohydrates
BT3 Nutrients
BT3 Organic compounds
NT1 Galacturonic acid
NT1 Pectins
NT2 Apple pectins
NT2 Citrus pectins
NT2 Sugar beet pectins
NT1 Polyuronides
NT1 Rhamnogalacturonans

Pectinases
USE **Polygalacturonases**

Pectinatus
BT1 Bacteria
BT2 Microorganisms
NT1 *Pectinatus frisingensis*

Pectinatus frisingensis
BT1 *Pectinatus*
BT2 Bacteria
BT3 Microorganisms

Pectinesterases
SN EC 3.1.1.11
BT1 Esterases
BT2 Hydrolases
BT3 Enzymes
BT1 Pectic enzymes
BT2 Enzymes
UF Pectin methylesterases

Pectin lyases
SN EC 4.2.2.10
BT1 Lyases
BT2 Enzymes
BT1 Pectic enzymes
BT2 Enzymes

Pectin methylesterases
USE **Pectinesterases**

Pectins
BT1 Pectic substances
BT2 Polysaccharides
BT3 Carbohydrates
BT4 Nutrients
BT4 Organic compounds
NT1 Apple pectins
NT1 Citrus pectins
NT1 Sugar beet pectins

Pectolytic enzymes
BT1 Pectic enzymes
BT2 Enzymes

Peda
BT1 Dairy products
BT2 Animal foods
BT3 Foods

Pediocins
BT1 Bacteriocins
BT2 Antibiotics
BT3 Drugs
BT4 Residues
RT *Pediococcus*

Pediococcus
HN heading from vol. 25 (1993); under Lactobacillaceae up to vol. 24 (1992)
BT1 Bacteria
BT2 Microorganisms
NT1 *Pediococcus acidilactici*
NT1 *Pediococcus damnosus*
NT1 *Pediococcus pentosaceus*
RT Lactic acid bacteria
RT Lactobacillaceae
RT Pediocins

Pediococcus acidilactici
BT1 *Pediococcus*
BT2 Bacteria
BT3 Microorganisms

Pediococcus damnosus
BT1 *Pediococcus*
BT2 Bacteria
BT3 Microorganisms

Pediococcus pentosaceus
BT1 *Pediococcus*

BT2 Bacteria
BT3 Microorganisms

Peel
NT1 Apple peel
NT1 Banana peel
NT1 Citrus peel
NT1 Fruit peel
NT1 Grapefruit peel
NT1 Grape skins
NT1 Lemon peel
NT1 Orange peel
NT1 Potato peel
NT1 Tomato skins
RT Peeling
UF Rind

Peeling
BT1 Processing
BT2 Technology
RT Peel

Pekmez
BT1 Fruit products
BT2 Plant foods
BT3 Foods
RT Grape juices

Pelargonidin
BT1 Anthocyanidins
BT2 Flavonoids
BT3 Aromatic compounds
BT4 Organic compounds
BT3 Pigments

Pelargonium
BT1 Plants

Pelmeni
BT1 Bakery products
BT2 Cereal products
BT3 Plant foods
BT4 Foods

Pelshenke values
RT Cereals

Pelt 44
USE **Thiophanate-methyl**

Pemmican
BT1 Meat products
BT2 Animal foods
BT3 Foods

Penamellera cheese
BT1 Cheese varieties
BT2 Cheese
BT3 Dairy products
BT4 Animal foods
BT5 Foods

Penetration
HN heading up to vol. 24 (1992)
RT Permeability
RT Rheological properties

Penetrometers
BT1 Apparatus
BT2 Technology
BT1 Firmness
BT2 Texture
BT3 Sensory properties

Penetrometry
BT1 Analytical techniques

Penicillic acid
BT1 Antibiotics
BT2 Drugs
BT3 Residues
BT1 Mycotoxins
BT2 Toxins
BT3 Residues

Penicillinases
USE **β-Lactamases**

Penicillin G
SN syn. benzylpenicillin
BT1 Penicillins
BT2 β-Lactam antibiotics
BT3 Antibiotics
BT4 Drugs
BT5 Residues

Penicillins
BT1 β-Lactam antibiotics
BT2 Antibiotics
BT3 Drugs
BT4 Residues
NT1 Amoxicillin
NT1 Ampicillin
NT1 Benzylpenicillin
NT1 Cloxacillin
NT1 Dicloxacillin
NT1 Oxacillin
NT1 Penicillin G

Penicillium
BT1 Fungi
BT2 Microorganisms
NT1 *Penicillium aurantiogriseum*
NT1 *Penicillium brasilianum*
NT1 *Penicillium camemberti*
NT1 *Penicillium canescens*
NT1 *Penicillium chrysogenum*
NT1 *Penicillium citrinum*
NT1 *Penicillium corylophilum*
NT1 *Penicillium crustosum*
NT1 *Penicillium decumbens*
NT1 *Penicillium digitatum*
NT1 *Penicillium expansum*
NT1 *Penicillium funiculosum*
NT1 *Penicillium glabrum*
NT1 *Penicillium griseoroseum*
NT1 *Penicillium italicum*
NT1 *Penicillium janthinellum*
NT1 *Penicillium nalgiovense*
NT1 *Penicillium olsonii*
NT1 *Penicillium oxalicum*
NT1 *Penicillium palitans*
NT1 *Penicillium purpurogenum*
NT1 *Penicillium restrictum*
NT1 *Penicillium roqueforti*
NT1 *Penicillium simplicissimum*
NT1 *Penicillium spinulosum*
NT1 *Penicillium verrucosum*
NT1 *Penicillium viridicatum*
RT Mycotoxins

Penicillium aurantiogriseum
BT1 *Penicillium*
BT2 Fungi
BT3 Microorganisms

Penicillium brasilianum
BT1 *Penicillium*
BT2 Fungi
BT3 Microorganisms

Penicillium camemberti
BT1 *Penicillium*
BT2 Fungi
BT3 Microorganisms

Penicillium canescens
BT1 *Penicillium*
BT2 Fungi
BT3 Microorganisms

Penicillium chrysogenum
BT1 *Penicillium*
BT2 Fungi
BT3 Microorganisms

Penicillium citrinum
HN introduced from vol. 39, issue 1 (2007)
BT1 *Penicillium*
BT2 Fungi
BT3 Microorganisms

Penicillium corylophilum
BT1 *Penicillium*
BT2 Fungi
BT3 Microorganisms

Penicillium crustosum
HN introduced from vol. 39, issue 1 (2007)
BT1 *Penicillium*
BT2 Fungi
BT3 Microorganisms

Penicillium decumbens
BT1 *Penicillium*
BT2 Fungi
BT3 Microorganisms

Penicillium digitatum
BT1 *Penicillium*
BT2 Fungi
BT3 Microorganisms

Penicillium expansum
BT1 *Penicillium*
BT2 Fungi
BT3 Microorganisms

Penicillium funiculosum
BT1 *Penicillium*
BT2 Fungi
BT3 Microorganisms

Penicillium glabrum
BT1 *Penicillium*
BT2 Fungi
BT3 Microorganisms

Penicillium griseoroseum
BT1 *Penicillium*

BT2 Fungi
BT3 Microorganisms

Penicillium italicum
BT1 *Penicillium*
BT2 Fungi
BT3 Microorganisms

Penicillium janthinellum
BT1 *Penicillium*
BT2 Fungi
BT3 Microorganisms

Penicillium nalgiovense
BT1 *Penicillium*
BT2 Fungi
BT3 Microorganisms

Penicillium olsonii
BT1 *Penicillium*
BT2 Fungi
BT3 Microorganisms

Penicillium oxalicum
HN introduced from vol. 39, issue 1 (2007)
BT1 *Penicillium*
BT2 Fungi
BT3 Microorganisms

Penicillium palitans
HN introduced from vol. 39, issue 1 (2007)
BT1 *Penicillium*
BT2 Fungi
BT3 Microorganisms

Penicillium purpurogenum
HN introduced from vol. 39, issue 1 (2007)
BT1 *Penicillium*
BT2 Fungi
BT3 Microorganisms

Penicillium restrictum
BT1 *Penicillium*
BT2 Fungi
BT3 Microorganisms

Penicillium roqueforti
BT1 *Penicillium*
BT2 Fungi
BT3 Microorganisms

Penicillium simplicissimum
BT1 *Penicillium*
BT2 Fungi
BT3 Microorganisms

Penicillium spinulosum
BT1 *Penicillium*
BT2 Fungi
BT3 Microorganisms

Penicillium verrucosum
BT1 *Penicillium*
BT2 Fungi
BT3 Microorganisms

Penicillium viridicatum
HN introduced from vol. 39, issue 1 (2007)
BT1 *Penicillium*
BT2 Fungi
BT3 Microorganisms

Penitrems
HN introduced from vol. 39, issue 1 (2007)
BT1 Mycotoxins
BT2 Toxins
BT3 Residues

Pentachlorobenzene
BT1 Fungicides
BT2 Pesticides
BT3 Biocides
BT3 Residues

Pentachloronitrobenzene
USE **Quintozene**

Pentanal
HN also under Volatile compounds up to vol. 42 (2010)
SN syn. valeraldehyde
BT1 Aldehydes
BT2 Carbonyl compounds
BT3 Organic compounds
BT1 Aroma compounds
BT2 Flavour compounds
BT2 Volatile compounds
NT1 Valeraldehyde
RT Off odour

Pentane
BT1 Hydrocarbons
BT2 Organic compounds
BT1 Solvents

Pentanedione
HN also under Flavour compounds up to vol. 42 (2010)
SN syn. acetylacetone
BT1 Aroma compounds
BT2 Flavour compounds
BT2 Volatile compounds
BT1 Ketones
BT2 Carbonyl compounds
BT3 Organic compounds
NT1 Acetylacetone

Pentanoic acid
SN syn. valeric acid
BT1 Aroma compounds
BT2 Flavour compounds
BT2 Volatile compounds
BT1 Saturated fatty acids
BT2 Fatty acids
BT3 Lipids
BT4 Nutrients
BT3 Organic acids
BT4 Acids
BT1 Short chain fatty acids
BT2 Volatile fatty acids
BT3 Fatty acids
BT4 Lipids
BT5 Nutrients
BT4 Organic acids
BT5 Acids
BT3 Volatile compounds
NT1 Valeric acid

Pentanol
SN syn. amyl alcohol
BT1 Amyl alcohol
BT2 Alcohols
BT2 Aroma compounds
BT3 Flavour compounds
BT3 Volatile compounds

Pentosanases
BT1 Glycosidases
BT2 Hydrolases
BT3 Enzymes

Pentosans
BT1 Polysaccharides
BT2 Carbohydrates
BT3 Nutrients
BT3 Organic compounds
NT1 Arabinans
NT1 Arabinoxylans

Pentoses
HN under Sugars up to vol. 42 (2010)
BT1 Monosaccharides
BT2 Sugars
BT3 Carbohydrates
BT4 Nutrients
BT4 Organic compounds
BT3 Plant foods
BT4 Foods

Peonidin
BT1 Anthocyanidins
BT2 Flavonoids
BT3 Aromatic compounds
BT4 Organic compounds
BT3 Pigments

Pepino
BT1 Fruits specific
BT2 Fruits
BT3 Crops
BT4 Plants
BT3 Plant foods
BT4 Foods

Pepper
BT1 Spices
BT2 Flavourings
BT3 Additives
NT1 Black pepper
NT1 Peppercorns
NT1 *Piper longum*
NT1 White pepper
RT Piperidine
RT Piperine

Peppercorns
BT1 Pepper
BT2 Spices
BT3 Flavourings
BT4 Additives

Peppermint
HN under Spices up to vol. 42 (2010)
BT1 Mint
BT2 Herbs
BT3 Spices
BT4 Flavourings
BT5 Additives
RT Peppermint essential oils

Peppermint essential oils
BT1 Essential oils
 BT2 Flavourings
  BT3 Additives
 BT2 Vegetable oils
  BT3 Oils vegetable
   BT4 Oils
    BT5 Lipids
     BT6 Nutrients
   BT4 Vegetable products
    BT5 Plant foods
     BT6 Foods
RT Peppermint

Pepperoni
BT1 Sausages
 BT2 Meat products
  BT3 Animal foods
   BT4 Foods

Peppers
HN heading up to vol. 24 (1992)
BT1 Capsicums
 BT2 Vegetables specific
  BT3 Vegetables
   BT4 Crops
    BT5 Plants
   BT4 Plant foods
    BT5 Foods

Pepsin
HN heading up to vol. 24 (1992)
USE **Pepsins**

Pepsins
SN includes EC 3.4.23.1 and EC 3.4.23.2
BT1 Proteinases
 BT2 Hydrolases
  BT3 Enzymes
UF Pepsin

Peptidases
BT1 Proteinases
 BT2 Hydrolases
  BT3 Enzymes

Peptides
BT1 Proteins
 BT2 Nutrients
NT1 Anserine
NT1 Balenine
NT1 Bioactive peptides
NT1 Bitter peptides
NT1 Carnosine
NT1 Caseinomacropeptides
NT1 Dipeptides
 NT2 Dipeptide sweeteners
NT1 Glutathione
NT1 Glycomacropeptides
NT1 Glycopeptides
NT1 Lactoferricin
NT1 Lysinoalanine
NT1 Oligopeptides
NT1 Phosphopeptides
NT1 Polylysine
NT1 Polypeptides
RT Protein hydrolysates

Peptidyl-dipeptidase A
SN EC 3.4.15.1
BT1 Proteinases
 BT2 Hydrolases
  BT3 Enzymes
RT ACE inhibitors
UF Angiotensin I-converting enzymes

Peptococcus
BT1 Bacteria
 BT2 Microorganisms

Peptones
BT1 Protein hydrolysates
 BT2 Proteins
  BT3 Nutrients

PER
BT1 Nutritional values
UF Protein efficiency ratios

Pera
BT1 Dairy products
 BT2 Animal foods
  BT3 Foods
BT1 Desserts
 BT2 Processed foods
  BT3 Foods

Peracetic acid
BT1 Organic acids
 BT2 Acids
BT1 Oxidizing agents
 BT2 Additives

Perca fluviatilis
BT1 Perch
 BT2 Freshwater fish
  BT3 Fish
   BT4 Animals
   BT4 Sea foods
    BT5 Aquatic foods
     BT6 Animal foods
      BT7 Foods

Perch
BT1 Freshwater fish
 BT2 Fish
  BT3 Animals
  BT3 Sea foods
   BT4 Aquatic foods
    BT5 Animal foods
     BT6 Foods
NT1 *Perca fluviatilis*
NT1 Yellow perch

Perchlorates
HN introduced from vol. 39, issue 1 (2007)
BT1 Contaminants
 BT2 Contamination
BT1 Disinfectants
 BT2 Disinfection
  BT3 Hygiene
RT Chlorates

Perfluidone
BT1 Herbicides
 BT2 Pesticides
  BT3 Biocides
  BT3 Residues
UF Destun

Performance drinks
BT1 Soft drinks
 BT2 Beverages
RT Cognitive performance
RT Exercise performance
RT Sports drinks

Perilla
BT1 Vegetables specific
 BT2 Vegetables
  BT3 Crops
   BT4 Plants
  BT3 Plant foods
   BT4 Foods

Perilla oils
BT1 Vegetable oils
 BT2 Oils vegetable
  BT3 Oils
   BT4 Lipids
    BT5 Nutrients
  BT3 Vegetable products
   BT4 Plant foods
    BT5 Foods

Perilla seeds
BT1 Oilseeds
 BT2 Seeds
  BT3 Plant foods
   BT4 Foods

Perishability
BT1 Shelf life

Perishable foods
BT1 Foods

Periwinkles
BT1 Gastropods
 BT2 Molluscs
  BT3 Shellfish
   BT4 Animals
   BT4 Sea foods
    BT5 Aquatic foods
     BT6 Animal foods
      BT7 Foods

Permeability
NT1 Barrier properties
NT1 Permeation
NT1 Porosity
RT Diffusion
RT Osmotic pressure
RT Penetration

Permeation
BT1 Permeability

Permethrin
BT1 Acaricides
 BT2 Pesticides
  BT3 Biocides
  BT3 Residues
BT1 Pyrethroid insecticides
 BT2 Insecticides
  BT3 Pesticides
   BT4 Biocides
   BT4 Residues

Permissible levels
BT1 Tolerance

Pernod
BT1 Liqueurs
BT2 Alcoholic beverages
BT3 Beverages alcoholic
BT4 Beverages

Peroxidases
SN includes EC 1.11.1.7 and other members of subclass EC 1.11.1
BT1 Oxidoreductases
BT2 Enzymes
NT1 Catalases
NT1 Glutathione peroxidases
NT1 Lactoperoxidase systems
NT1 Ligninases
NT1 Lignin peroxidases
NT1 Manganese peroxidases

Peroxidation
BT1 Oxidation
NT1 Peroxide values
RT Peroxides
RT Rancidity

Peroxides
BT1 Inorganic compounds
BT1 Oxides
BT1 Reactive oxygen species
BT2 Free radicals
BT3 Radicals
NT1 H_2O_2
NT1 Hydroperoxides
RT Oxidation
RT Peroxidation
RT Peroxide values
RT Rancidity

Peroxide values
BT1 Peroxidation
BT2 Oxidation
RT Peroxides
RT Rancidity

Peroxynitrite
HN introduced from vol. 39, issue 1 (2007)
BT1 Nitrites
BT2 Salts
BT1 Oxidizing agents
BT2 Additives
BT1 Reactive nitrogen species
BT2 Free radicals
BT3 Radicals
BT2 Nitroso compounds
BT3 Organic nitrogen compounds

Perry
BT1 Alcoholic beverages
BT2 Beverages alcoholic
BT3 Beverages
RT Cider

Persimmon juices
BT1 Fruit juices
BT2 Fruit products
BT3 Plant foods
BT4 Foods
BT2 Soft drinks
BT3 Beverages
RT Persimmons

Persimmons
HN heading from vol. 25 (1993); under Fruits specificup to vol. 24 (1992)
BT1 Fruits specific
BT2 Fruits
BT3 Crops
BT4 Plants
BT3 Plant foods
BT4 Foods
RT Persimmon juices
UF Kaki figs
UF Kaki fruits
UF Sharon fruit

Persipan
BT1 Sugar confectionery
BT2 Plant foods
BT3 Foods

Persulfates
BT1 Bakery additives
BT2 Additives
BT1 Salts
UF Persulphates

Persulphates
HN used for persulfates up to vol. 35, issue 6 (2003)
USE **Persulfates**

Perthane
BT1 Organochlorine insecticides
BT2 Insecticides
BT3 Pesticides
BT4 Biocides
BT4 Residues
BT2 Organochlorine pesticides
BT3 Pesticides
BT4 Biocides
BT4 Residues

Peru
BT1 South America
BT2 America

Peruvian carrots
USE **Arracacha**

Peruvian parsnips
USE **Arracacha**

Pervaporation
BT1 Separation
BT2 Processing
BT3 Technology

Perylene
BT1 Aromatic compounds
BT2 Organic compounds

Pesticides
BT1 Biocides
BT1 Residues
NT1 Acaricides
NT1 Algicides
NT1 Carbamate pesticides
NT1 Fungicides
NT1 Herbicides
NT1 Insecticides
NT1 Molluscicides
NT1 Nematocides
NT1 Organochlorine pesticides
NT1 Organophosphorus pesticides
NT1 Rodenticides
RT Agriculture
RT Fumigants
RT Pests

Pesto
BT1 Pasta sauces
BT2 Sauces
BT3 Condiments
BT4 Flavourings
BT5 Additives

Pests
NT1 Disinfestation
NT2 Biocontrol
NT2 Entoleters
NT1 Infestation
NT1 Insects
NT2 Ants
NT2 Aphids
NT2 Bees
NT2 Beetles
NT3 *Ahasverus advena*
NT2 Cockroaches
NT2 *Eurygaster*
NT2 Flies
NT2 Fruit flies
NT2 Grain borers
NT2 *Liposcelis*
NT3 *Liposcelis bostrychophila*
NT2 Moths
NT2 *Oryzaephilus*
NT2 *Phylloxera*
NT2 Psocids
NT2 *Sitophilus*
NT3 Rice weevils
NT4 *Sitophilus oryzae*
NT3 *Sitophilus granarius*
NT3 *Sitophilus zeamais*
NT2 Stink bugs
NT2 Termites
NT2 Thrips
NT2 *Tribolium*
NT2 *Tyrophagus*
NT2 Weevils
NT1 Integrated pest management
NT1 Mites
NT1 Parasites
NT2 Amoebae
NT3 *Acanthamoeba*
NT2 *Anisakis*
NT3 *Anisakis simplex*
NT2 Cestodes
NT2 *Clonorchis sinensis*
NT2 *Cryptosporidium*
NT3 *Cryptosporidium hominis*
NT3 *Cryptosporidium parvum*
NT2 *Cyclospora*
NT3 *Cyclospora cayetanensis*
NT2 *Cysticercus*
NT2 *Diphyllobothrium*
NT2 *Echinococcus*
NT2 *Entamoeba*
NT3 *Entamoeba histolytica*
NT2 *Fasciola*
NT2 Flukes
NT3 Liver flukes

NT2 *Giardia*
NT3 *Giardia intestinalis*
NT3 *Giardia lamblia*
NT3 *Giardia muris*
NT2 Helminths
NT2 *Isospora*
NT2 Liver flukes
NT2 Metacercariae
NT2 *Naegleria*
NT2 Nematodes
NT2 Oocysts
NT2 *Pseudoterranova*
NT2 *Sarcocystis*
NT2 *Sarcosporidia*
NT2 *Taenia*
NT2 Tapeworms
NT2 *Toxoplasma*
NT3 *Toxoplasma gondii*
NT2 Trematodes
NT2 Trichinae
NT2 *Trichinella*
NT3 *Trichinella spiralis*
NT1 Rodents
NT1 Slugs
RT Food safety
RT Pesticides

PET
BT1 Plastics
BT2 Packaging materials
UF Polyethyleneterephthalate

Pet birds
HN introduced from vol. 39, issue 1 (2007)
BT1 Pets
RT Bird foods

Pet chews
HN introduced from vol. 40, issue 1 (2008)
BT1 Pet foods

Pet fish
HN introduced from vol. 39, issue 1 (2007)
BT1 Pets
RT Fish foods

Pet food additives
HN introduced from vol. 39, issue 1 (2007)
BT1 Additives
BT1 Pet foods

Pet foods
HN introduced from vol. 39, issue 1 (2007); heading
NT1 Bird foods
NT1 Canned pet foods
NT1 Cat foods
NT2 Cat milks
NT3 Kitten milks
NT2 Kitten foods
NT1 Dog foods
NT2 Dog biscuits
NT2 Puppy foods
NT1 Dried pet foods
NT1 Extruded pet foods
NT1 Fish foods
NT1 Frozen pet foods
NT1 Intermediate moisture pet foods
NT1 Mixer pet foods
NT1 Organic pet foods
NT1 Pet chews
NT1 Pet food additives
NT1 Pet foods industry
NT1 Pet treats
NT1 Soft pet foods
NT1 Wet pet foods

Pet foods industry
HN introduced from vol. 39, issue 1 (2007)
BT1 Industries
BT1 Pet foods

Petitgrain oils
BT1 Essential oils
BT2 Flavourings
BT3 Additives
BT2 Vegetable oils
BT3 Oils vegetable
BT4 Oils
BT5 Lipids
BT6 Nutrients
BT4 Vegetable products
BT5 Plant foods
BT6 Foods

Pet nutrition
HN introduced from vol. 39, issue 1 (2007)
BT1 Pets

Petroleum
BT1 Hydrocarbons
BT2 Organic compounds
BT1 Solvents

Petroselinic acid
BT1 Octadecenoic acid
BT2 Monounsaturated fatty acids
BT3 Unsaturated fatty acids
BT4 Fatty acids
BT5 Lipids
BT6 Nutrients
BT5 Organic acids
BT6 Acids

Pets
HN introduced from vol. 39, issue 1 (2007); heading
NT1 Cats
NT1 Dogs
NT1 Pet birds
NT1 Pet fish
NT1 Pet nutrition
RT Animals
RT Birds

Pet treats
HN introduced from vol. 39, issue 1 (2007)
BT1 Pet foods

Petunidin
BT1 Anthocyanidins
BT2 Flavonoids
BT3 Aromatic compounds
BT4 Organic compounds
BT3 Pigments

PFGE
HN pulsed field gel electrophoresis used in the index up to vol. 35, issue 6 (2003)
BT1 Gel electrophoresis
BT2 Electrophoresis
BT3 Analytical techniques
UF Pulsed field gel electrophoresis

pH
BT1 Physical properties
NT1 Isoelectric points
NT1 pH meters
RT Acidification
RT Alkalization
RT Neutralization
UF Hydrogen ion concentration

Phaeodactylum
HN introduced from vol. 43, issue 1 (2011)
BT1 Microalgae
BT2 Algae
BT3 Microorganisms
NT1 *Phaeodactylum tricornutum*

Phaeodactylum tricornutum
HN introduced from vol. 39, issue 1 (2007)
BT1 *Phaeodactylum*
BT2 Microalgae
BT3 Algae
BT4 Microorganisms

Phaeophytins
BT1 Pigments

Phaffia
BT1 Yeasts
BT2 Fungi
BT3 Microorganisms
NT1 *Phaffia rhodozyma*

Phaffia rhodozyma
BT1 *Phaffia*
BT2 Yeasts
BT3 Fungi
BT4 Microorganisms

Phages
USE **Bacteriophages**

Phalsa
BT1 Fruits specific
BT2 Fruits
BT3 Crops
BT4 Plants
BT3 Plant foods
BT4 Foods

Phaltan
USE **Folpet**

Phane
BT1 Insect foods
BT2 Animal foods
BT3 Foods

Phanerochaete
BT1 Fungi
BT2 Microorganisms
NT1 *Phanerochaete chrysosporium*

Phanerochaete chrysosporium
BT1 *Phanerochaete*
BT2 Fungi
BT3 Microorganisms

Pharmacological properties
RT Drugs

Phase behaviour
BT1 Physical properties
RT Physical phases

Phaseolins
BT1 Vegetable proteins
BT2 Proteins vegetable
BT3 Proteins
BT4 Nutrients
BT3 Vegetable products
BT4 Plant foods
BT5 Foods
RT Common beans

Pheasant carcasses
BT1 Carcasses
BT2 Meat
BT3 Animal foods
BT4 Foods
BT1 Pheasant meat
BT2 Meat specific
BT3 Meat
BT4 Animal foods
BT5 Foods
BT2 Pheasants
BT3 Birds

Pheasant meat
BT1 Meat specific
BT2 Meat
BT3 Animal foods
BT4 Foods
BT1 Pheasants
BT2 Birds
NT1 Pheasant carcasses

Pheasants
BT1 Birds
NT1 Pheasant meat
NT2 Pheasant carcasses

Phellinus linteus
BT1 Edible fungi
BT2 Fungi edible
BT3 Vegetables specific
BT4 Vegetables
BT5 Crops
BT6 Plants
BT5 Plant foods
BT6 Foods

Phenanthrene
BT1 Aromatic compounds
BT2 Organic compounds

Phenethyl alcohol
SN syn. phenylethanol
BT1 Phenylethanol
BT2 Alcohols
BT2 Aroma compounds
BT3 Flavour compounds
BT3 Volatile compounds

Phenethyl isothiocyanate
HN introduced from vol. 39, issue 1 (2007)
SN syn. phenylethyl isothiocyanate
BT1 Isothiocyanates
BT2 Organic nitrogen compounds
BT2 Organic sulfur compounds
BT2 Volatile sulfur compounds
BT3 Volatile compounds

Phenmedipham
BT1 Carbamate pesticides
BT2 Pesticides
BT3 Biocides
BT3 Residues
BT1 Herbicides
BT2 Pesticides
BT3 Biocides
BT3 Residues
UF Betanal

Phenobarbital
BT1 Barbiturates
BT2 Drugs
BT3 Residues

Phenolases
SN term also used in narrow sense as syn. for catechol oxidases and tyrosinases
BT1 Oxidoreductases
BT2 Enzymes
NT1 Catechol oxidases
NT1 Laccases
NT1 Monophenol monooxygenases
NT1 Tyrosinases

Phenolic compounds
USE **Phenols**

Phenols
BT1 Alcohols
BT1 Aromatic compounds
BT2 Organic compounds
NT1 Alkylphenols
NT1 Alkylresorcinols
NT1 Anisole
NT1 Arbutin
NT1 Avenanthramides
NT1 Bisphenol A
NT1 Bisphenol A diglycidyl ether
NT1 Bisphenol F diglycidyl ether
NT1 Bromophenols
NT1 Caffeic acid
NT1 Carvacrol
NT1 Catechols
NT2 Catechin
NT2 Epicatechin
NT2 Epicatechin gallate
NT2 Epicatechol
NT2 Epigallocatechin
NT2 Epigallocatechin gallate
NT2 Gallocatechin gallate
NT2 Pyrocatechol
NT1 Chlorogenic acid
NT2 Caffeoylquinic acid
NT1 Chlorophenol
NT1 Cinnamic acid
NT1 Coumarins
NT2 Coumarin
NT2 Coumestrol
NT2 Esculetin
NT2 Furocoumarins
NT3 Bergapten
NT3 Psoralens
NT3 Xanthotoxin
NT2 Scopoletin
NT1 Cresols
NT1 Curcuminoids
NT2 Curcumin
NT1 Ellagic acid
NT1 Ellagitannins
NT1 Estragole
NT1 Eugenol
NT1 Ferulic acid
NT1 Feruloylquinic acid
NT1 Gingerols
NT1 Guaiacol
NT1 4-Hexylresorcinol
NT1 Hydroquinone
NT1 Hydroxycinnamic acid
NT2 Coumaric acid
NT1 Hydroxytyrosol
NT1 Isochlorogenic acid
NT1 Isoeugenol
NT1 Lignans
NT2 Sesamin
NT2 Sesamolin
NT1 Naphthol
NT1 Nordihydroguaiaretic acid
NT2 NDGA
NT1 Oleuropein
NT1 Phenylpropanoids
NT1 Phloroglucinol
NT1 Polyphenols
NT1 Protocatechuic acid
NT1 Pyrogallol
NT1 Resorcinol
NT1 Rosmarinic acid
NT1 Sesamol
NT1 Stilbenes
NT2 Piceatannol
NT2 Piceid
NT2 Resveratrol
NT1 Syringic acid
NT1 Thymol
NT1 Tyrosol
NT1 Vanillic acid
NT1 Vanillin
NT1 Zingerone
UF Phenolic compounds

Phenothiazine
HN under Pesticides up to vol. 42 (2010)
BT1 Drugs
BT2 Residues

Phenotype
BT1 Genetics

Phenoxy herbicides
HN introduced from vol. 43, issue 1 (2011)
BT1 Herbicides
BT2 Pesticides
BT3 Biocides
BT3 Residues
NT1 Chlorophenoxyacetic acid
NT1 2,4-D
NT1 Dichlorprop
NT1 Fenoprop
NT1 MCPA
NT1 2,4,5-T

Phenthoate
BT1 Organophosphorus insecticides
BT2 Insecticides
BT3 Pesticides
BT4 Biocides
BT4 Residues
BT2 Organophosphorus pesticides
BT3 Pesticides
BT4 Biocides
BT4 Residues

Phenylacetaldehyde
BT1 Aldehydes
BT2 Carbonyl compounds
BT3 Organic compounds
BT1 Aroma compounds
BT2 Flavour compounds
BT2 Volatile compounds

Phenylacetic acid
BT1 Aromatic compounds
BT2 Organic compounds
BT1 Organic acids
BT2 Acids
BT1 Volatile compounds
RT Aroma compounds

Phenylalanine
BT1 Amino acids
BT2 Nutrients
BT2 Organic acids
BT3 Acids
BT2 Organic nitrogen compounds

Phenylalanine ammonia-lyases
SN EC 4.3.1.24, formerly 4.3.1.5
BT1 Lyases
BT2 Enzymes

Phenylethanol
SN syn. phenethyl alcohol
BT1 Alcohols
BT1 Aroma compounds
BT2 Flavour compounds
BT2 Volatile compounds
NT1 Phenethyl alcohol

Phenylketonuria
USE **PKU**

2-Phenylphenol
BT1 Fungicides
BT2 Pesticides
BT3 Biocides
BT3 Residues
UF Dowicide A
UF Orthophenylphenol
UF Sodium *o*-phenylphenate
UF SOPP

Phenylpropanoids
HN introduced from vol. 39, issue 1 (2007)
BT1 Phenols
BT2 Alcohols
BT2 Aromatic compounds
BT3 Organic compounds

Pheromones
RT Hormones

Philippines
BT1 Asia

Phlebia
HN introduced from vol. 43, issue 1 (2011)
BT1 Fungi
BT2 Microorganisms
NT1 *Phlebia radiata*

Phlebia radiata
BT1 *Phlebia*
BT2 Fungi
BT3 Microorganisms

Phloretin
HN introduced from vol. 39, issue 1 (2007)
BT1 Dihydrochalcones
BT2 Chalcones
BT3 Antioxidants
BT4 Additives
BT3 Flavonoids
BT4 Aromatic compounds
BT5 Organic compounds
BT4 Pigments
BT2 Glycosides
BT3 Carbohydrates
BT4 Nutrients
BT4 Organic compounds

Phloroglucinol
BT1 Phenols
BT2 Alcohols
BT2 Aromatic compounds
BT3 Organic compounds

Phloxine
BT1 Colorants
BT2 Additives

pH meters
BT1 pH
BT2 Physical properties

Phoenix
BT1 Palms
BT2 Plants
RT Dates

Pholiota
HN introduced from vol. 39, issue 1 (2007)
BT1 Edible fungi
BT2 Fungi edible
BT3 Vegetables specific
BT4 Vegetables
BT5 Crops
BT6 Plants
BT5 Plant foods
BT6 Foods

Phoma
BT1 Fungi
BT2 Microorganisms

Phorate
BT1 Acaricides
BT2 Pesticides
BT3 Biocides
BT3 Residues
BT1 Nematocides
BT2 Pesticides
BT3 Biocides
BT3 Residues
BT1 Organophosphorus insecticides
BT2 Insecticides
BT3 Pesticides
BT4 Biocides
BT4 Residues
BT2 Organophosphorus pesticides
BT3 Pesticides
BT4 Biocides
BT4 Residues

Phosalone
BT1 Acaricides
BT2 Pesticides
BT3 Biocides
BT3 Residues
BT1 Organophosphorus insecticides
BT2 Insecticides
BT3 Pesticides
BT4 Biocides
BT4 Residues
BT2 Organophosphorus pesticides
BT3 Pesticides
BT4 Biocides
BT4 Residues
UF Zolone

Phosdrin
USE **Mevinphos**

Phosmet
BT1 Acaricides
BT2 Pesticides
BT3 Biocides
BT3 Residues
BT1 Organophosphorus insecticides
BT2 Insecticides
BT3 Pesticides
BT4 Biocides
BT4 Residues
BT2 Organophosphorus pesticides
BT3 Pesticides
BT4 Biocides

BT4 Residues
UF Imidan

Phosphamide
USE **Dimethoate**

Phosphamidon
BT1 Nematocides
BT2 Pesticides
BT3 Biocides
BT3 Residues
BT1 Organophosphorus insecticides
BT2 Insecticides
BT3 Pesticides
BT4 Biocides
BT4 Residues
BT2 Organophosphorus pesticides
BT3 Pesticides
BT4 Biocides
BT4 Residues

Phosphatases
HN heading up to vol. 24 (1992)
SN includes members of EC 3.1.3
BT1 Esterases
BT2 Hydrolases
BT3 Enzymes
NT1 Acid phosphatases
NT1 Alkaline phosphatases
NT1 Nucleotidases
NT1 Phytases
NT2 3-Phytases
NT2 4-Phytases

Phosphates
BT1 Salts
NT1 Inositol phosphates
NT1 Phytates
NT1 Phytic acid
NT1 Polyphosphates
NT1 Pyrophosphates
NT1 Sodium tripolyphosphate
NT1 Tripolyphosphates
NT1 Trisodium phosphate
RT Phosphoric acid

Phosphatides
BT1 Phospholipids
BT2 Lipids
BT3 Nutrients

Phosphatidic acid
BT1 Organic acids
BT2 Acids
BT1 Phospholipids
BT2 Lipids
BT3 Nutrients

Phosphatidylcholine
USE **Lecithins**

Phosphatidylethanolamine
BT1 Phospholipids
BT2 Lipids
BT3 Nutrients

Phosphatidylinositol
BT1 Phospholipids
BT2 Lipids
BT3 Nutrients

Phosphatidylserine
BT1 Phospholipids
BT2 Lipids
BT3 Nutrients

Phosphine
BT1 Fumigants
BT2 Biocides

Phosphodiesterases
HN introduced from vol. 39, issue 1 (2007)
BT1 Esterases
BT2 Hydrolases
BT3 Enzymes

Phosphoenolpyruvate carboxylases
SN EC 4.1.1.31
BT1 Lyases
BT2 Enzymes

Phosphoglucomutases
SN EC 5.4.2.2 and 5.4.2.6
BT1 Isomerases
BT2 Enzymes

Phosphoglycerides
BT1 Glycerides
BT2 Emulsifiers
BT3 Additives
BT2 Fatty acid esters
BT3 Esters
BT4 Organic compounds
BT2 Lipids
BT3 Nutrients

Phospholipases
SN includes phospholipase A1 (EC 3.1.1.32), A2 (3.1.1.4), C (3.1.4.3) and D (3.1.4.4); for A2, C, D, syn. lecithinases A, C, D; for phospholipase B see lysophospholipases
BT1 Lipases
BT2 Esterases
BT3 Hydrolases
BT4 Enzymes

Phospholipids
BT1 Lipids
BT2 Nutrients
NT1 Cephalins
NT1 Ceramides
NT1 Lecithins
NT2 Lysolecithin
NT2 Soy lecithins
NT1 Lysophospholipids
NT1 Phosphatides
NT1 Phosphatidic acid
NT1 Phosphatidylethanolamine
NT1 Phosphatidylinositol
NT1 Phosphatidylserine
RT Sphingolipids

Phosphopeptides
BT1 Peptides
BT2 Proteins
BT3 Nutrients

Phosphorescence
SN syn. luminescence
BT1 Luminescence
BT2 Fluorescence
BT3 Analytical techniques
BT3 Optical properties
BT4 Physical properties

Phosphoric acid
BT1 Acids
RT Phosphates

Phosphorus
SN symbol P is also used in the index
BT1 Elements
BT2 Minerals
BT3 Nutrients
NT1 P

Phosphorylases
SN members of EC 2.4
BT1 Transferases
BT2 Enzymes

Phosphorylation
BT1 Modification

Phosphotransferases
SN EC 2.7
BT1 Transferases
BT2 Enzymes
NT1 Kinases
NT2 Aspartate kinases
NT2 Fructokinases
NT2 Glucokinases
NT2 Hexokinases

Phostoxin
SN syn. aluminium phosphide
BT1 Fumigants
BT2 Biocides

Phosvel
USE **Leptophos**

Phosvitin
BT1 Egg proteins
BT2 Animal proteins
BT3 Proteins animal
BT4 Proteins
BT5 Nutrients
RT Egg yolks

Photobacterium
BT1 Bacteria
BT2 Microorganisms
NT1 *Photobacterium phosphoreum*

Photobacterium phosphoreum
BT1 *Photobacterium*
BT2 Bacteria
BT3 Microorganisms

Photocolorimetry
BT1 Colorimetry
BT2 Analytical techniques

Photodensitometry
BT1 Analytical techniques

Photography
BT1 Analytical techniques
RT Cameras

Photolysis
BT1 Lysis
BT2 Decomposition

Photometry
BT1 Analytical techniques
NT1 Flame photometry

Photooxidation
BT1 Oxidation

Phoxim
BT1 Acaricides
BT2 Pesticides
BT3 Biocides
BT3 Residues
BT1 Organophosphorus insecticides
BT2 Insecticides
BT3 Pesticides
BT4 Biocides
BT4 Residues
BT2 Organophosphorus pesticides
BT3 Pesticides
BT4 Biocides
BT4 Residues

Phthalic acid
BT1 Aromatic compounds
BT2 Organic compounds
BT1 Organic acids
BT2 Acids

Phthalic acid esters
BT1 Contaminants
BT2 Contamination
BT1 Esters
BT2 Organic compounds

Phycocyanin
BT1 Pigments

Phycoerythrin
BT1 Pigments
BT1 Proteins
BT2 Nutrients

R-phycoerythrin
BT1 Pigments
BT1 Proteins
BT2 Nutrients

Phyllophora
BT1 Seaweeds
BT2 Algae
BT3 Microorganisms
BT2 Sea foods
BT3 Aquatic foods
BT4 Animal foods
BT5 Foods

Phylloquinone
BT1 Vitamins
BT2 Nutrients
UF Vitamin K_1

Phylloxera
BT1 Insects
BT2 Pests

Physalis
USE **Cape gooseberries**

Physical activity
HN introduced from vol. 38, issue 8 (2006); heading
BT1 Health
NT1 Exercise performance
RT Sports nutrition

Physical phases
HN introduced from vol. 42, issue 1 (2010)
BT1 Chemistry
BT2 Science
NT1 Colloids
NT2 Colloidal stability
NT2 Hydrocolloids
NT1 Crystals
NT1 Dispersions
NT2 Dispersion
NT1 Emulsions
NT2 Food emulsions
NT2 Microemulsions
NT1 Gases
NT2 Acetylene
NT2 Air
NT3 Airborne
NT3 Air conditioning
NT3 Air speed
NT3 Atmosphere
NT2 Ammonia
NT3 NH_3
NT2 Ar
NT2 Biogas
NT2 Butane
NT2 Carbon dioxide
NT3 CO_2
NT3 Dry Ice
NT3 Supercritical CO_2 extraction
NT2 Carbon monoxide
NT2 Chlorine dioxide
NT2 Ethane
NT2 Ethylene
NT3 ACC
NT3 Ethephon
NT2 H_2
NT2 He
NT2 H_2S
NT2 Methane
NT2 N_2
NT2 Nitric oxide
NT2 Nitrous oxide
NT2 NO_2
NT2 O_2
NT2 Ozone
NT2 Propane
NT2 Sulfur dioxide
NT3 SO_2
NT2 Vapours
NT3 Water vapour
NT2 Xe
NT1 Gels
NT2 Agar gels
NT2 Alginate gels
NT2 Aspic
NT2 Carrageenan gels
NT2 Silica gels
NT1 Ice
NT1 Liquids
NT2 Fluids
NT3 Supercritical fluids
NT2 Juices
NT3 Stocks
NT2 Liquid foods
NT1 Solids
NT2 SNF
NT2 Soluble solids
NT2 TS
NT2 TSS
NT1 Vapours
NT2 Water vapour
RT Interfacial properties
RT Interfacial tension
RT Phase behaviour

Physical properties
NT1 Acidity
NT2 Acid values
NT2 Titratable acidity
NT1 Activation energy
NT1 Adhesion
NT2 Sticking
NT1 Alkalinity
NT1 Crystallinity
NT1 Density
NT2 Apparent density
NT2 Brix values
NT2 Bulk density
NT2 Gravity
NT2 Original gravity
NT2 sp. gr.
NT3 Relative density
NT1 Electrical properties
NT2 Capacitance
NT2 Dielectric constant
NT2 Dielectric properties
NT2 Electrical conductivity
NT2 Electrical resistance
NT2 Electrostatic interactions
NT2 Impedance
NT2 Specific conductivity
NT1 Expansion
NT1 Functional properties
NT2 Binding capacity
NT2 Buffering capacity
NT2 Chipping properties
NT2 Dispersibility
NT2 Emulsification properties
NT2 Emulsifying capacity
NT2 Foaming
NT3 Foaming agents
NT2 Foaming capacity
NT2 Foaming properties
NT2 Gelling capacity
NT2 Moisture retention
NT2 Oil absorption capacity
NT2 Pasting properties
NT2 Surface active properties
NT2 Swelling
NT2 Water binding capacity
NT2 Water holding capacity
NT2 Whipping properties
NT3 Whipping capacity

NT1 Hydrophobicity
NT1 Hygroscopic properties
NT1 Interfacial properties
NT1 Interfacial tension
NT1 Ionic strength
NT1 Mass transfer
NT1 Mechanical properties
NT2 Airflow properties
NT2 Fracture properties
NT2 Hardness
NT2 Residence time distribution
NT2 Rheological properties
NT3 Compressibility
NT3 Creep
NT3 Deformation
NT3 Elasticity
NT3 Extensibility
NT3 Flow
NT4 Flow meters
NT4 Gushing
NT3 Friction
NT3 Rheology
NT3 Rheometers
NT3 Rigidity
NT3 Shear
NT3 Shear values
NT3 Stickiness
NT3 Stiffness
NT3 Stress relaxation
NT3 Stretch
NT3 Surface tension
NT3 Thixotropy
NT3 Viscoelasticity
NT3 Viscosity
NT4 Viscometers
NT3 Yield stress
NT2 Shear strength
NT2 Strength
NT2 Tensile strength
NT1 Mol. wt.
NT1 Optical properties
NT2 Birefringence
NT2 Brightness
NT2 Brilliance
NT2 Chalkiness
NT2 Clarity
NT2 Colour
NT2 Diffraction
NT2 Fluorescence
NT3 Autofluorescence
NT3 Bioluminescence
NT3 Chemiluminescence
NT3 Green fluorescent protein
NT3 Luminescence
NT4 Phosphorescence
NT3 Thermoluminescence
NT2 Glassiness
NT2 Gloss
NT2 Opacity
NT2 Opalescence
NT2 Optical density
NT2 Optical rotation
NT2 Pigmentation
NT2 Polarization
NT2 Reflectance
NT2 Reflectivity
NT2 Refractive index
NT2 Specific rotation
NT2 Translucency
NT2 Transmittance
NT2 Transparency
NT2 Turbidity
NT3 Cloud
NT4 Clouding agents
NT3 Cloudiness
NT3 Haze
NT2 Vitreosity
NT2 Whiteness
NT1 Overrun
NT1 pH
NT2 Isoelectric points
NT2 pH meters
NT1 Phase behaviour
NT1 Physicochemical properties
NT2 Nitrogen solubility index
NT1 Redox potential
NT1 Roughness
NT1 Shape
NT1 Size
NT1 Solubility
NT2 Solubilization
NT1 Stability
NT2 Colloidal stability
NT2 Freeze-thaw stability
NT2 Heat stability
NT2 Oxidative stability
NT2 Stabilization
NT2 Thermal stability
NT1 Thermophysical properties
NT2 b.p.
NT2 Cryoscopes
NT2 Enthalpy
NT2 Entropy
NT2 f.p.
NT2 Glass transition
NT2 Glass transition temp.
NT2 Heat resistance
NT2 Heat stability
NT2 Melting
NT2 m.p.
NT2 Specific heat
NT2 Thermal capacity
NT2 Thermal conductivity
NT2 Thermal diffusivity
NT2 Thermal expansion
NT2 Thermal properties
NT2 Thermal stability
NT2 Thermodynamic properties
NT1 Thickness
NT1 Weight
NT2 Weighing
NT2 Weighing machines
NT2 Wt.
NT1 Wettability
RT Microstructure
RT Structure
RT Ultrastructure

Physicochemical properties
BT1 Physical properties
NT1 Nitrogen solubility index

Physics
BT1 Science

Physiological effects
BT1 Human physiology
BT2 Physiology
BT3 Science

Physiology
HN heading from vol. 42 (2010); under Science up to vol. 41 (2009)
BT1 Science
NT1 Adipogenesis
NT1 Cell cycle
NT2 Apoptosis
NT2 Mitosis
NT1 Chemotaxis
NT1 Endocrine system
NT1 Human physiology
NT2 Angiogenesis
NT2 Appetite
NT2 Behavioural effects
NT3 Cognitive performance
NT4 Cognitive development
NT4 Memory
NT3 Cravings
NT3 Mood
NT2 Body fats
NT2 Breast feeding
NT2 Cardiovascular physiology
NT3 Blood pressure
NT2 Digestion
NT2 Exercise performance
NT2 Flatulence
NT3 Flatulence factors
NT2 Gastrointestinal tract
NT3 Malabsorption
NT2 Glucose tolerance
NT2 Human lactation
NT2 Human metabolism
NT2 Hunger
NT2 Lipaemic activity
NT2 Mastication
NT2 Physiological effects
NT2 Postprandial response
NT2 Psychophysiological effects
NT2 Reproduction
NT3 Menopause
NT3 Menstrual cycle
NT3 Pregnancy
NT2 Saliva
NT2 Satiety
NT2 Sensory perception
NT2 Sleep
NT2 Swallowing
NT2 Thermogenesis
NT2 Thirst
NT2 Vision
NT2 Weaning
NT1 Lactation
NT1 Metabolism
NT2 Bioaccumulation
NT2 Biohydrogenation
NT2 Biomagnification
NT2 Metabolic rate
NT2 Metabolomics
NT1 Motility
NT1 Puberty
NT1 Quorum sensing
NT1 Secretion
NT1 Starvation
NT1 Stress resistance
NT1 Viability

Phytases
SN EC 3.1.3.8 and 3.1.3.26
BT1 Phosphatases
BT2 Esterases

BT3 Hydrolases
BT4 Enzymes
NT1 3-Phytases
NT1 4-Phytases

3-Phytases
SN EC 3.1.3.8
BT1 Phytases
BT2 Phosphatases
BT3 Esterases
BT4 Hydrolases
BT5 Enzymes
RT 4-Phytases

4-Phytases
HN 6-Phytases used up to vol. 39 (2007)
SN EC 3.1.3.26
BT1 Phytases
BT2 Phosphatases
BT3 Esterases
BT4 Hydrolases
BT5 Enzymes
RT 3-Phytases

Phytates
BT1 Inositol
BT2 Antinutritional factors
BT3 Nutritional values
BT2 Polyols
BT3 Alcohols
BT3 Carbohydrates
BT4 Nutrients
BT4 Organic compounds
BT1 Phosphates
BT2 Salts
RT Phytic acid

Phytic acid
BT1 Inositol
BT2 Antinutritional factors
BT3 Nutritional values
BT2 Polyols
BT3 Alcohols
BT3 Carbohydrates
BT4 Nutrients
BT4 Organic compounds
BT1 Phosphates
BT2 Salts
RT Inositol phosphates
RT Phytates

Phytoalexins
BT1 Organic nitrogen compounds

Phytochemicals
RT Elicitation
RT Functional foods
RT Health
RT Health foods
RT Nutraceutical foods
RT Phytoestrogens

Phytochrome
BT1 Pigments

Phytoene
HN introduced from vol. 39, issue 1 (2007)
BT1 Carotenoids
BT2 Pigments
BT2 Terpenoids
BT3 Lipids
BT4 Nutrients

Phytoestrogens
RT Oestrogens
RT Phytochemicals

Phytofluene
BT1 Carotenoids
BT2 Pigments
BT2 Terpenoids
BT3 Lipids
BT4 Nutrients

Phytohaemagglutinins
BT1 Lectins
BT2 Glycoproteins
BT3 Proteins
BT4 Nutrients
BT2 Vegetable proteins
BT3 Proteins vegetable
BT4 Proteins
BT5 Nutrients
BT4 Vegetable products
BT5 Plant foods
BT6 Foods
RT Toxins

Phytohormones
BT1 Plant growth regulators
BT2 Cultivation
BT3 Agriculture

Phytophthora
BT1 Chromista
BT2 Microorganisms

Phytostanols
BT1 Stanols
BT2 Sterols
BT3 Alcohols
BT3 Steroids
BT4 Lipids
BT5 Nutrients
NT1 Sitostanol
RT Phytosterols

Phytosterols
BT1 Sterols
BT2 Alcohols
BT2 Steroids
BT3 Lipids
BT4 Nutrients
RT Phytostanols

Picante cheese
BT1 Cheese varieties
BT2 Cheese
BT3 Dairy products
BT4 Animal foods
BT5 Foods

Piceatannol
HN introduced from vol. 39, issue 1 (2007)
BT1 Stilbenes
BT2 Phenols
BT3 Alcohols
BT3 Aromatic compounds
BT4 Organic compounds

Piceid
HN introduced from vol. 42, issue 1 (2010)
BT1 Glucosides
BT2 Glycosides
BT3 Carbohydrates
BT4 Nutrients
BT4 Organic compounds
BT1 Stilbenes
BT2 Phenols
BT3 Alcohols
BT3 Aromatic compounds
BT4 Organic compounds
RT Resveratrol

Pichia
HN heading from vol. 25 (1993); under Yeasts up to vol. 24 (1992)
SN synonymous with Hansenula
BT1 Yeasts
BT2 Fungi
BT3 Microorganisms
NT1 *Pichia anomala*
NT1 *Pichia fermentans*
NT1 *Pichia guilliermondii*
NT1 *Pichia heedii*
NT1 *Pichia membranifaciens*
NT2 *Pichia membranefaciens*
NT1 *Pichia methanolica*
NT1 *Pichia pastoris*
NT1 *Pichia stipitis*
NT1 *Pichia subpelliculosa*

Pichia anomala
BT1 *Pichia*
BT2 Yeasts
BT3 Fungi
BT4 Microorganisms

Pichia fermentans
HN introduced from vol. 39, issue 1 (2007)
BT1 *Pichia*
BT2 Yeasts
BT3 Fungi
BT4 Microorganisms

Pichia guilliermondii
SN anamorph is Candida guilliermondii
BT1 *Pichia*
BT2 Yeasts
BT3 Fungi
BT4 Microorganisms

Pichia heedii
BT1 *Pichia*
BT2 Yeasts
BT3 Fungi
BT4 Microorganisms

Pichia membranefaciens
SN preferred spelling is Pichia membranifaciens; alternative spellings are Pichia membranaefaciens and Pichia membranefaciens
BT1 *Pichia membranifaciens*
BT2 *Pichia*
BT3 Yeasts
BT4 Fungi
BT5 Microorganisms

Pichia membranifaciens
HN introduced from vol. 43, issue 1 (2011)
SN preferred spelling is Pichia membranifaciens; alternative spellings are Pichia membranaefaciens and Pichia membranefaciens; Genbank anamorph is Candida valida
BT1 *Pichia*
BT2 Yeasts
BT3 Fungi
BT4 Microorganisms
NT1 *Pichia membranefaciens*

Pichia methanolica
BT1 *Pichia*
BT2 Yeasts
BT3 Fungi
BT4 Microorganisms

Pichia pastoris
BT1 *Pichia*
BT2 Yeasts
BT3 Fungi
BT4 Microorganisms

Pichia stipitis
BT1 *Pichia*
BT2 Yeasts
BT3 Fungi
BT4 Microorganisms

Pichia subpelliculosa
BT1 *Pichia*
BT2 Yeasts
BT3 Fungi
BT4 Microorganisms

Picking
BT1 Harvesting
BT2 Agriculture

Pickled cheese
BT1 Cheese varieties
BT2 Cheese
BT3 Dairy products
BT4 Animal foods
BT5 Foods

Pickled cucumbers
USE **Cucumber pickles**

Pickled eggs
BT1 Egg products
BT2 Animal foods
BT3 Foods

Pickled onions
BT1 Onions
BT2 Vegetables specific
BT3 Vegetables
BT4 Crops
BT5 Plants
BT4 Plant foods
BT5 Foods
BT1 Vegetable pickles
BT2 Pickles
BT3 Fermented foods
BT4 Processed foods
BT5 Foods
BT2 Vegetable products
BT3 Plant foods
BT4 Foods

Pickles
BT1 Fermented foods
BT2 Processed foods
BT3 Foods
NT1 Chicken gizzard pickles
NT1 Chutneys
NT1 Mango pickles
NT1 Vegetable pickles
NT2 Cucumber pickles
NT2 Narazuke
NT2 Pickled onions
RT Pickling
RT Vegetable products

Pickling
BT1 Processing
BT2 Technology
RT Brining
RT Curing
RT Pickles

Picloram
BT1 Herbicides
BT2 Pesticides
BT3 Biocides
BT3 Residues
UF Tordon

Pidan
BT1 Duck eggs
BT2 Ducks
BT3 Poultry
BT4 Birds
BT2 Eggs
BT3 Animal foods
BT4 Foods
BT1 Fermented foods
BT2 Processed foods
BT3 Foods

Pie fillings
BT1 Fillings
BT1 Pies
BT2 Bakery products
BT3 Cereal products
BT4 Plant foods
BT5 Foods

Pies
BT1 Bakery products
BT2 Cereal products
BT3 Plant foods
BT4 Foods
NT1 Fruit pies
NT1 Meat pies
NT2 Cornish pasties
NT1 Pie fillings
NT1 Quiches
NT1 Tarts
RT Pastries

Pigeon carcasses
BT1 Carcasses
BT2 Meat
BT3 Animal foods
BT4 Foods
BT1 Pigeon meat
BT2 Meat specific
BT3 Meat
BT4 Animal foods
BT5 Foods
BT2 Pigeons
BT3 Birds

Pigeon meat
BT1 Meat specific
BT2 Meat
BT3 Animal foods
BT4 Foods
BT1 Pigeons
BT2 Birds
NT1 Pigeon carcasses

Pigeon peas
HN heading from vol. 30 (1998); under Legumes up to vol. 29 (1997)
BT1 Legumes
BT2 Vegetables specific
BT3 Vegetables
BT4 Crops
BT5 Plants
BT4 Plant foods
BT5 Foods
UF Red gram

Pigeons
BT1 Birds
NT1 Pigeon meat
NT2 Pigeon carcasses

Pigging
RT Cleaning
RT Pipes

Pigmentation
BT1 Optical properties
BT2 Physical properties
RT Colour

Pigments
NT1 Anthraquinones
NT2 Emodin
NT1 Betalains
NT2 Betacyanins
NT3 Betanin
NT3 Betanine
NT2 Betalaines
NT2 Betaxanthin
NT1 Carotenoids
NT2 Apocarotenal
NT2 Astacene
NT2 Bixin
NT2 Capsanthin
NT2 Carotenes
NT3 α-Carotene
NT3 β-Carotene
NT3 Provitamin A
NT2 Crocin
NT3 Crocetin
NT2 Lycopene
NT2 Norisoprenoids
NT3 β-Damascenone
NT3 Ionones
NT2 Phytoene
NT2 Phytofluene
NT2 Xanthophylls

NT3 Astaxanthin
NT3 Canthaxanthin
NT3 Cryptoxanthin
NT3 Diatoxanthin
NT3 Fucoxanthin
NT3 Lutein
NT3 Neoxanthin
NT3 Tunaxanthin
NT3 Violaxanthin
NT3 Zeaxanthin
NT1 Curcuminoids
NT2 Curcumin
NT1 Flavins
NT1 Flavonoids
NT2 Anthocyanidins
NT3 Cyanidin
NT3 Delphinidin
NT3 Leucoanthocyanidins
NT4 Leucocyanidin
NT3 Malvidin
NT3 Pelargonidin
NT3 Peonidin
NT3 Petunidin
NT3 Proanthocyanidins
NT4 Procyanidins
NT2 Anthocyanins
NT3 Leucoanthocyanins
NT4 Anthocyanogens
NT3 Oenocyanins
NT3 Pyranoanthocyanins
NT2 Bioflavonoids
NT2 Chalcones
NT3 Dihydrochalcones
NT4 Neohesperidin dihydrochalcone
NT4 Phloretin
NT3 Xanthohumol
NT2 Flavanols
NT3 Catechols
NT4 Catechin
NT4 Epicatechin
NT4 Epicatechin gallate
NT4 Epicatechol
NT4 Epigallocatechin
NT4 Epigallocatechin gallate
NT4 Gallocatechin gallate
NT4 Pyrocatechol
NT2 Flavanones
NT3 Hesperetin
NT3 Hesperidin
NT3 Naringenin
NT3 Naringin
NT3 Narirutin
NT3 Neohesperidin
NT2 Flavones
NT3 Apigenin
NT3 Chrysin
NT3 Luteolin
NT2 Flavonols
NT3 Dihydroquercetin
NT3 Fisetin
NT3 Isorhamnetin
NT3 Kaempferol
NT3 Morin
NT3 Myricetin
NT3 Quercetin
NT3 Quercitrin
NT3 Rutin
NT2 Isoflavonoids
NT3 Coumestrol
NT3 Isoflavones
NT4 Daidzein
NT4 Equol
NT4 Genistein
NT4 Glycitein
NT4 Puerarin
NT2 Theaflavins
NT2 Thearubigins
NT1 Gossypol
NT1 Haemoglobin
NT1 Haemoproteins
NT1 Hordeumin
NT1 Melanins
NT1 Melanoidins
NT1 Myoglobin
NT2 Deoxymyoglobin
NT2 Metmyoglobin
NT2 Nitrosylmyoglobin
NT2 Oxymyoglobin
NT1 Nitroso pigments
NT1 Phaeophytins
NT1 Phycocyanin
NT1 Phycoerythrin
NT1 R-phycoerythrin
NT1 Phytochrome
NT1 Porphyrins
NT2 Chlorophylls
NT2 Haem
NT2 Haematin
NT2 Haemin
RT Colorants
RT Colour
RT Glycosides
RT Pyrroles

Pigs
USE **Swine**

Pike
BT1 Freshwater fish
BT2 Fish
BT3 Animals
BT3 Sea foods
BT4 Aquatic foods
BT5 Animal foods
BT6 Foods

Pilchards
BT1 Marine fish
BT2 Fish
BT3 Animals
BT3 Sea foods
BT4 Aquatic foods
BT5 Animal foods
BT6 Foods
BT1 Oily fish
BT2 Fish
BT3 Animals
BT3 Sea foods
BT4 Aquatic foods
BT5 Animal foods
BT6 Foods

Pili
HN introduced from vol. 39, issue 1 (2007)
BT1 Cells
BT1 Virulence factors
RT Adherence
RT Pilins

Pilins
HN introduced from vol. 39, issue 1 (2007)
BT1 Microbial proteins
BT2 Microorganisms
BT2 Proteins
BT3 Nutrients
BT1 Virulence factors
RT Pili

Pimaricin
SN syn. natamycin
BT1 Natamycin
BT2 Fungicides
BT3 Pesticides
BT4 Biocides
BT4 Residues
BT2 Preservatives
BT3 Additives

Pimento
USE **Allspice**

Pimento peppers
SN syn. pimiento peppers
BT1 Capsicums
BT2 Vegetables specific
BT3 Vegetables
BT4 Crops
BT5 Plants
BT4 Plant foods
BT5 Foods
NT1 Pimiento peppers

Pimiento peppers
SN syn. pimento peppers
BT1 Pimento peppers
BT2 Capsicums
BT3 Vegetables specific
BT4 Vegetables
BT5 Crops
BT6 Plants
BT5 Plant foods
BT6 Foods

Pineapple juices
BT1 Fruit juices
BT2 Fruit products
BT3 Plant foods
BT4 Foods
BT2 Soft drinks
BT3 Beverages
RT Pineapple nectars
RT Pineapples

Pineapple nectars
BT1 Fruit nectars
BT2 Fruit juices
BT3 Fruit products
BT4 Plant foods
BT5 Foods
BT3 Soft drinks
BT4 Beverages
RT Pineapple juices
RT Pineapples

Pineapples
BT1 Fruits specific

BT2 Fruits
BT3 Crops
BT4 Plants
BT3 Plant foods
BT4 Foods
RT Pineapple juices
RT Pineapple nectars

Pine needles
BT1 Plants

Pinenes
HN also under Volatile compounds up to vol. 42 (2010)
BT1 Aroma compounds
BT2 Flavour compounds
BT2 Volatile compounds
BT1 Monoterpenes
BT2 Hydrocarbons
BT3 Organic compounds
BT2 Monoterpenoids
BT3 Terpenoids
BT4 Lipids
BT5 Nutrients

Pine nuts
BT1 Nuts
BT2 Fruits
BT3 Crops
BT4 Plants
BT3 Plant foods
BT4 Foods
BT2 Oilseeds
BT3 Seeds
BT4 Plant foods
BT5 Foods

Pink salmon
BT1 Pacific salmon
BT2 Salmon
BT3 Oily fish
BT4 Fish
BT5 Animals
BT5 Sea foods
BT6 Aquatic foods
BT7 Animal foods
BT8 Foods

Pinto beans
BT1 Common beans
BT2 Legumes
BT3 Vegetables specific
BT4 Vegetables
BT5 Crops
BT6 Plants
BT5 Plant foods
BT6 Foods

Pinus
HN introduced from vol. 39, issue 1 (2007)
BT1 Plants
NT1 *Pinus densiflora*

Pinus densiflora
BT1 *Pinus*
BT2 Plants

Pipecolic acid
BT1 Amino acids
BT2 Nutrients
BT2 Organic acids
BT3 Acids
BT2 Organic nitrogen compounds
BT1 Heterocyclic compounds

Piperidine
BT1 Aroma compounds
BT2 Flavour compounds
BT2 Volatile compounds
BT1 Heterocyclic compounds
BT1 Organic nitrogen compounds
RT Pepper
RT Piperine

Piperine
BT1 Alkaloids
BT2 Organic nitrogen compounds
BT1 Aroma compounds
BT2 Flavour compounds
BT2 Volatile compounds
BT1 Pungent principles
BT2 Flavour compounds
RT Pepper
RT Piperidine

Piper longum
BT1 Pepper
BT2 Spices
BT3 Flavourings
BT4 Additives

Piperonyl butoxide
BT1 Insecticides
BT2 Pesticides
BT3 Biocides
BT3 Residues

Pipes
BT1 Equipment
BT2 Technology
RT Pigging

Pips
USE **Seeds**

Pirimicarb
BT1 *N*-Methylcarbamate insecticides
BT2 Insecticides
BT3 Pesticides
BT4 Biocides
BT4 Residues
BT2 *N*-Methylcarbamate pesticides
BT3 Carbamate pesticides
BT4 Pesticides
BT5 Biocides
BT5 Residues

Pirimiphos-methyl
BT1 Acaricides
BT2 Pesticides
BT3 Biocides
BT3 Residues
BT1 Organophosphorus insecticides
BT2 Insecticides
BT3 Pesticides
BT4 Biocides
BT4 Residues
BT2 Organophosphorus pesticides
BT3 Pesticides
BT4 Biocides
BT4 Residues

Piscicolins
BT1 Bacteriocins
BT2 Antibiotics
BT3 Drugs
BT4 Residues
RT *Carnobacterium piscicola*

Pisco
HN under Spirits up to vol. 42 (2010)
BT1 Brandies
BT2 Spirits
BT3 Alcoholic beverages
BT4 Beverages alcoholic
BT5 Beverages

Pistachio nuts
HN heading from vol. 30 (1998); under Nuts up to vol. 29 (1997)
BT1 Nuts
BT2 Fruits
BT3 Crops
BT4 Plants
BT3 Plant foods
BT4 Foods
BT2 Oilseeds
BT3 Seeds
BT4 Plant foods
BT5 Foods

Pita bread
BT1 Bread
BT2 Bakery products
BT3 Cereal products
BT4 Plant foods
BT5 Foods
UF Pitta bread

Pitayos
BT1 Fruits specific
BT2 Fruits
BT3 Crops
BT4 Plants
BT3 Plant foods
BT4 Foods

Pithomyces
BT1 Fungi
BT2 Microorganisms
RT Mycotoxins

Pito
HN under Beverages alcoholic up to vol. 42 (2010)
BT1 Beer
BT2 Alcoholic beverages
BT3 Beverages alcoholic
BT4 Beverages

Pitta bread
USE **Pita bread**

Pitting disorders
HN introduced from vol. 42, issue 1 (2010)

BT1 Plant disorders
BT2 Diseases plant
BT3 Diseases

Pizza dough
BT1 Dough
BT2 Bakery products
BT3 Cereal products
BT4 Plant foods
BT5 Foods
BT1 Pizzas
BT2 Bakery products
BT3 Cereal products
BT4 Plant foods
BT5 Foods

Pizza fillings
BT1 Fillings
BT1 Pizzas
BT2 Bakery products
BT3 Cereal products
BT4 Plant foods
BT5 Foods

Pizzas
BT1 Bakery products
BT2 Cereal products
BT3 Plant foods
BT4 Foods
NT1 Pizza dough
NT1 Pizza fillings

PKU
BT1 Diseases
UF Phenylketonuria

Plaice
BT1 Flatfish
BT2 Marine fish
BT3 Fish
BT4 Animals
BT4 Sea foods
BT5 Aquatic foods
BT6 Animal foods
BT7 Foods
NT1 *Pleuronectes platessa*

Plain chocolate
USE **Dark chocolate**

Plankton
BT1 Sea foods
BT2 Aquatic foods
BT3 Animal foods
BT4 Foods

Planning
RT Food business

Plantains
BT1 Bananas
BT2 Fruits specific
BT3 Fruits
BT4 Crops
BT5 Plants
BT4 Plant foods
BT5 Foods

Plantaricins
BT1 Bacteriocins
BT2 Antibiotics
BT3 Drugs
BT4 Residues
RT *Lactobacillus plantarum*

Plant density
BT1 Cultivation
BT2 Agriculture

Plant diseases
SN index heading is Diseases plant
BT1 Diseases plant
BT2 Diseases
NT1 Anthracnose
NT1 Blights
NT1 Disease resistance
NT1 Ergot
NT1 Fungal decay
NT1 Rots
NT2 Brown rot
NT1 Rusts
NT1 Scab
RT Elicitation
RT Plant disorders

Plant disorders
BT1 Diseases plant
BT2 Diseases
NT1 Bitter pit
NT1 Blossom end rot
NT1 Brown heart
NT1 Cork spots
NT1 Pitting disorders
NT1 Russeting
NT1 Scald
NT1 Skin spot
NT1 Sunburn
NT1 Tipburn
NT1 Watercore
NT1 Woolliness
RT Elicitation
RT Plant diseases

Plant extracts
HN introduced from vol. 39, issue 1 (2007)
BT1 Plants

Plant foods
HN heading from vol. 25 (1993); under Plants up to vol. 24 (1992)
SN general use only
BT1 Foods
NT1 Cereal products
NT1 Cocoa
NT1 Cocoa products
NT1 Coffee
NT1 Flours
NT1 Fruit products
NT1 Fruits
NT1 Seeds
NT1 Sugar
NT1 Sugar confectionery
NT1 Sugar juices
NT1 Sugars
NT1 Sugar syrups
NT1 Teas
NT1 Vegetable products
NT1 Vegetables
RT Plants
UF Plant products

Plant growth regulators
BT1 Cultivation
BT2 Agriculture
NT1 Abscisic acid
NT1 Acetylene
NT1 Aminoethoxyvinylglycine
NT1 Antisprouting agents
NT2 Maleic hydrazide
NT1 Antitranspirants
NT1 Auxins
NT2 Indole acetic acid
NT3 Indol-3-ylacetic acid
NT2 Naphthaleneacetic acid
NT3 2-(1-Naphthyl)acetic acid
NT3 (2-Naphthyloxy)acetic acid
NT1 Chlormequat
NT1 CPTA
NT1 Cytokinins
NT2 Benzyladenine
NT3 6-Benzylaminopurine
NT2 Kinetin
NT2 Thidiazuron
NT2 Zeatin
NT1 Daminozide
NT1 Ethylene
NT2 ACC
NT2 Ethephon
NT1 Gibberellins
NT2 Gibberellic acid
NT1 Growth promoters (plant)
NT1 1-Methylcyclopropene
NT1 Methyl jasmonate
NT2 Jasmonic acid
NT1 Paclobutrazol
NT1 Phytohormones
NT1 Propylene
NT1 Triiodobenzoic acid
RT Herbicides

Planting
BT1 Cultivation
BT2 Agriculture

Plant (machinery)
USE **Equipment**

Plant products
USE **Plant foods**

Plant proteins
BT1 Vegetable proteins
BT2 Proteins vegetable
BT3 Proteins
BT4 Nutrients
BT3 Vegetable products
BT4 Plant foods
BT5 Foods

Plants
NT1 *Acacia*
NT1 Agave
NT1 Aloe
NT1 *Angelica keiskei*
NT1 *Arabidopsis*
NT1 *Atractylodes lancea*
NT1 Banaba
NT1 Betel leaves
NT1 Borage
NT1 *Boronia*
NT1 *Cadaba farinosa*

NT1 Calamus
NT1 *Calendula officinalis*
NT1 *Camelina sativa*
NT1 *Catharanthus roseus*
NT1 *Chrysanthemum*
NT1 Citronella
NT1 Crops
NT1 Cycad seeds
NT1 *Decalepis hamiltonii*
NT1 *Echinacea*
NT1 Edible flowers
NT1 Eucalyptus
NT1 *Eucommia ulmoides*
NT1 Flowers
NT1 *Gardenia*
NT1 Gentians
NT1 *Gevuina avellana*
NT1 *Ginkgo biloba*
NT1 Ginseng
NT1 Hemp
NT1 *Hovenia dulcis*
NT1 Hsian-tsao
NT1 Katemfe
NT1 Kava
NT1 Kuth
NT1 Lavender
NT1 Leaves
NT1 *Leucaena*
NT1 Lichens
NT1 *Lippia alba*
NT1 *Lithospermum erythrorhizon*
NT1 Medicinal plants
NT1 Mistletoe
NT1 Mulberry leaves
NT1 Neem
NT1 *Okenia hypogaea*
NT1 Palms
NT1 *Pelargonium*
NT1 Pine needles
NT1 *Pinus*
NT1 Plant extracts
NT1 *Pulsatilla cernua*
NT1 *Quercus mongolica*
NT1 *Quillaja saponaria*
NT1 Red clover
NT1 Roots
NT1 Roselle
NT1 Roses
NT1 *Scutellaria baicalensis*
NT1 Seed coats
NT1 *Sideritis*
NT1 Stems
NT1 *Stevia rebaudiana*
NT1 *Tagetes maxima*
NT1 *Tagetes minuta*
NT1 Tanshen
NT1 Thistles
NT1 Tobacco
NT1 Transgenic plants
NT1 *Treculia africana*
NT1 Trees
NT1 Yarrow
NT1 Yucca
RT Eukaryotes
RT Plant foods

Plasma
USE **Blood**

Plasmids
HN heading from vol. 24 (1992)
BT1 Genetics
RT Cloning vectors
RT Food safety
RT Shuttle vectors

Plasmin
SN EC 3.4.21.7
BT1 Proteinases
BT2 Hydrolases
BT3 Enzymes
RT Plasminogen
UF Fibrinolysin

Plasminogen
BT1 Proteinases
BT2 Hydrolases
BT3 Enzymes
RT Plasmin
RT Plasminogen activators

Plasminogen activators
SN includes both EC 3.4.21.68 and 3.4.21.73
BT1 Proteinases
BT2 Hydrolases
BT3 Enzymes
RT Plasminogen

Plasteins
BT1 Proteins
BT2 Nutrients

Plasticity
BT1 Consistency
BT2 Texture
BT3 Sensory properties

Plasticizers
BT1 Packaging materials
RT Food safety additives
RT Migration

Plastics
BT1 Packaging materials
NT1 Acrylonitrile
NT1 Cryovac
NT1 Epoxides
NT1 Foamed plastics
NT1 Melamine
NT1 Mylar
NT1 Nylon
NT1 PET
NT1 Plastics bags
NT1 Plastics bottles
NT1 Plastics films
NT2 Cellulose films
NT3 Cellophane
NT1 Polyacrylamides
NT1 Polyamides
NT1 Polycarbonates
NT1 Polyesters
NT1 Polyethylene
NT2 HDPE
NT2 LDPE
NT2 Polyethylene bags
NT2 Polyethylene films
NT1 Polyethylene naphthalate
NT1 Polyolefins
NT1 Polypropylene
NT1 Polystyrene
NT2 Styrene
NT1 Polyurethane
NT1 Polyvinyl alcohol
NT1 Polyvinyl chloride
NT2 PVC
NT2 Vinyl chloride
NT1 Polyvinylpyrrolidinone
NT1 Polyvinylpyrrolidone
NT1 PTFE
NT1 PVDC
NT1 Saran
NT1 Vinylidene chloride

Plastics bags
BT1 Bags
BT2 Containers
BT1 Plastics
BT2 Packaging materials
RT Polyethylene bags

Plastics bottles
BT1 Bottles
BT2 Containers
BT1 Plastics
BT2 Packaging materials

Plastics films
BT1 Plastics
BT2 Packaging materials
NT1 Cellulose films
NT2 Cellophane
RT Polyethylene films

Plate counts
BT1 Microbiological techniques
RT Agar
RT Bacterial counts
RT Cell counts
RT Fungal counts
RT Media
RT Microbial counts

Platelets
HN introduced from vol. 39, issue 1 (2007)
BT1 Cells

Platichthys flesus
BT1 Flounders
BT2 Flatfish
BT3 Marine fish
BT4 Fish
BT5 Animals
BT5 Sea foods
BT6 Aquatic foods
BT7 Animal foods
BT8 Foods

Platinum
USE **Pt**

Plesiomonas
BT1 Bacteria
BT2 Microorganisms
NT1 *Plesiomonas shigelloides*

Plesiomonas shigelloides
BT1 *Plesiomonas*
BT2 Bacteria
BT3 Microorganisms

Pleuronectes platessa
BT1 Plaice
BT2 Flatfish
BT3 Marine fish
BT4 Fish
BT5 Animals
BT5 Sea foods
BT6 Aquatic foods
BT7 Animal foods
BT8 Foods

Pleurotus
HN heading from vol. 30 (1998); under Fungi edible up to vol. 29 (1997)
BT1 Edible fungi
BT2 Fungi edible
BT3 Vegetables specific
BT4 Vegetables
BT5 Crops
BT6 Plants
BT5 Plant foods
BT6 Foods
NT1 *Pleurotus citrinopileatus*
NT1 *Pleurotus eryngii*
NT1 *Pleurotus florida*
NT1 *Pleurotus ostreatus*
NT1 *Pleurotus sajor-caju*
NT1 *Pleurotus tuberregium*
UF Oyster mushrooms

Pleurotus citrinopileatus
BT1 *Pleurotus*
BT2 Edible fungi
BT3 Fungi edible
BT4 Vegetables specific
BT5 Vegetables
BT6 Crops
BT7 Plants
BT6 Plant foods
BT7 Foods

Pleurotus eryngii
BT1 *Pleurotus*
BT2 Edible fungi
BT3 Fungi edible
BT4 Vegetables specific
BT5 Vegetables
BT6 Crops
BT7 Plants
BT6 Plant foods
BT7 Foods

Pleurotus florida
HN introduced from vol. 39, issue 1 (2007)
BT1 *Pleurotus*
BT2 Edible fungi
BT3 Fungi edible
BT4 Vegetables specific
BT5 Vegetables
BT6 Crops
BT7 Plants
BT6 Plant foods
BT7 Foods

Pleurotus ostreatus
BT1 *Pleurotus*
BT2 Edible fungi
BT3 Fungi edible
BT4 Vegetables specific
BT5 Vegetables
BT6 Crops
BT7 Plants
BT6 Plant foods
BT7 Foods

Pleurotus sajor-caju
HN introduced from vol. 39, issue 1 (2007)
BT1 *Pleurotus*
BT2 Edible fungi
BT3 Fungi edible
BT4 Vegetables specific
BT5 Vegetables
BT6 Crops
BT7 Plants
BT6 Plant foods
BT7 Foods

Pleurotus tuberregium
BT1 *Pleurotus*
BT2 Edible fungi
BT3 Fungi edible
BT4 Vegetables specific
BT5 Vegetables
BT6 Crops
BT7 Plants
BT6 Plant foods
BT7 Foods

Plictran
USE **Cyhexatin**

Plucking
USE **Defeathering**

Plum juices
BT1 Fruit juices
BT2 Fruit products
BT3 Plant foods
BT4 Foods
BT2 Soft drinks
BT3 Beverages
RT Plums

Plums
BT1 Fruits specific
BT2 Fruits
BT3 Crops
BT4 Plants
BT3 Plant foods
BT4 Foods
NT1 Damsons
NT1 Greengages
NT1 Japanese plums
RT Plum juices
RT Prunes

Plutonium
USE **Pu**

Pneumatic conveyors
HN conveyors pneumatic used in the index up to vol. 31 (1999)
BT1 Conveyors
BT2 Equipment
BT3 Technology
UF Conveyors pneumatic

Po
BT1 Radioelements
BT2 Isotopes
BT3 Elements
BT4 Minerals
BT5 Nutrients
BT2 Residues
UF Polonium

Pogonias
USE **Drum**

Poi
HN also under Vegetables specific up to vol. 42 (2010)
BT1 Fermented foods
BT2 Processed foods
BT3 Foods
BT1 Taro
BT2 Vegetables specific
BT3 Vegetables
BT4 Crops
BT5 Plants
BT4 Plant foods
BT5 Foods

Poisoning
NT1 Amnesic shellfish poisoning
NT1 Amoebiasis
NT1 Anisakiasis
NT2 Anisakidosis
NT1 Botulism
NT1 Campylobacteriosis
NT1 Ciguatera
NT1 Cryptosporidiosis
NT1 Cyclosporiasis
NT1 Diarrhoetic shellfish poisoning
NT1 Food poisoning
NT1 Giardiasis
NT1 Legionellosis
NT1 Leptospirosis
NT1 Listeriosis
NT1 Mussel poisoning
NT1 Mycotoxicosis
NT2 Aflatoxicosis
NT1 Neurological shellfish poisoning
NT1 Paralytic shellfish poisoning
NT2 PSP
NT1 Poisons
NT1 Salmonellosis
NT1 Scombroid poisoning
NT1 Shigellosis
NT1 Toxoplasmosis
NT1 Trichinosis
NT1 Yersiniosis
NT1 Yusho
RT Bacterial contamination
RT Contamination
RT Diseases
RT Food safety
RT Glucosinolates
RT Gossypol
RT Hexachlorobiphenyl
RT Hygiene
RT Microbial contamination
RT Toxicity
RT Toxins

Poisons
BT1 Poisoning
RT Toxins

Poland
HN heading up to vol. 24
BT1 Europe
BT1 European Union
RT Organization for Economic Cooperation and Development

Polar compounds

Polarimetry
BT1 Analytical techniques

Polarization
BT1 Optical properties
BT2 Physical properties

Polarography
BT1 Analytical techniques

Pole beans
BT1 Common beans
BT2 Legumes
BT3 Vegetables specific
BT4 Vegetables
BT5 Crops
BT6 Plants
BT5 Plant foods
BT6 Foods

Polenta
BT1 Porridges
BT2 Cereal products
BT3 Plant foods
BT4 Foods

Policies
BT1 Food policy
BT2 Economics

Policosanols
HN introduced from vol. 39, issue 1 (2007)
BT1 Alcohols

Policy
BT1 Food policy
BT2 Economics
RT Health promotion

Poliomyelitis
BT1 Diseases
RT Polioviruses

Poliovirus
HN introduced from vol. 43, issue 1 (2011); polioviruses also used in the index up to vol. 42 (2010)
BT1 Enterovirus
BT2 Viruses
BT3 Microorganisms
UF Polioviruses

Polioviruses
HN Poliovirus used in the index from vol. 43 (2011)
USE **Poliovirus**

Polishing
BT1 Processing
BT2 Technology
RT Milling
RT Rice

Pollack
BT1 Marine fish
BT2 Fish
BT3 Animals
BT3 Sea foods
BT4 Aquatic foods
BT5 Animal foods
BT6 Foods

Pollen
BT1 Honeys
BT2 Sugar
BT3 Plant foods
BT4 Foods
RT Pollination

Pollination
RT Cultivation
RT Pollen

Pollock
BT1 Marine fish
BT2 Fish
BT3 Animals
BT3 Sea foods
BT4 Aquatic foods
BT5 Animal foods
BT6 Foods
RT Alaska pollock

Pollutants
BT1 Pollution
BT2 Contamination
NT1 Air pollutants
NT2 Exhaust gases
NT2 Factory fumes

Pollution
HN heading up to vol. 24 (1992)
BT1 Contamination
NT1 Environmental pollution
NT2 Air pollution
NT3 Air pollutants
NT4 Exhaust gases
NT4 Factory fumes
NT2 Water pollution
NT1 Pollutants
NT2 Air pollutants
NT3 Exhaust gases
NT3 Factory fumes
RT Chemical contamination
RT Hygiene
RT Radioelements
RT Wastes

Polonium
USE **Po**

Polyacetylenes
HN introduced from vol. 39, issue 1 (2007)
BT1 Hydrocarbons
BT2 Organic compounds

Polyacrylamide gel electrophoresis
USE **PAGE**

Polyacrylamides
BT1 Plastics
BT2 Packaging materials

Polyamides
BT1 Plastics
BT2 Packaging materials

Polyamines
BT1 Amines
BT2 Organic nitrogen compounds
NT1 Putrescine
NT1 Spermidine
NT1 Spermine

Polybrominated biphenyls
BT1 Organobromine compounds
BT2 Organic halogen compounds
RT Carcinogens
RT Toxins

Polybrominated diphenyl ethers
BT1 Organobromine compounds
BT2 Organic halogen compounds

Polycarbonates
BT1 Plastics
BT2 Packaging materials
RT Bisphenol A

Polychlorinated biphenyls
SN abbrev. PCB is also used in the index
BT1 Chlorinated hydrocarbons
BT2 Organic halogen compounds
NT1 Arochlor
NT1 Hexachlorobiphenyl
NT1 PCB
RT Carcinogens
RT Toxins
RT Yusho

Polychlorinated dibenzodioxins
BT1 Contaminants
BT2 Contamination
BT1 Organic halogen compounds
RT Polychlorinated dibenzo-*p*-dioxins

Polychlorinated dibenzofurans
BT1 Contaminants
BT2 Contamination
BT1 Organic halogen compounds

Polychlorinated dibenzo-*p*-dioxins
BT1 Contaminants
BT2 Contamination
BT1 Organic halogen compounds

NT1 Tetrachlorodibenzo-*p*-dioxins
RT Polychlorinated dibenzodioxins

Polycyclic aromatic hydrocarbons
USE **PAH**

Polydextrose
HN under Polysaccharides up to vol. 42 (2010)
BT1 Glucans
BT2 Polysaccharides
BT3 Carbohydrates
BT4 Nutrients
BT4 Organic compounds
RT Litesse

Polydimethylsiloxane
BT1 Additives

Polyesters
BT1 Plastics
BT2 Packaging materials

Polyethylene
BT1 Plastics
BT2 Packaging materials
NT1 HDPE
NT1 LDPE
NT1 Polyethylene bags
NT1 Polyethylene films
UF Polythene

Polyethylene bags
BT1 Bags
BT2 Containers
BT1 Polyethylene
BT2 Plastics
BT3 Packaging materials
RT Plastics bags

Polyethylene films
BT1 Polyethylene
BT2 Plastics
BT3 Packaging materials
RT Plastics films

Polyethylene glycol
BT1 Glycols
BT2 Alcohols

Polyethylene naphthalate
BT1 Plastics
BT2 Packaging materials

Polyethyleneterephthalate
USE **PET**

Polygalacturonases
SN EC 3.2.1.15
BT1 Glycosidases
BT2 Hydrolases
BT3 Enzymes
BT1 Pectic enzymes
BT2 Enzymes
UF Endopolygalacturonases
UF Pectinases

Poly(γ-glutamic acid)
BT1 Glutamic acid
BT2 Amino acids
BT3 Nutrients
BT3 Organic acids
BT4 Acids
BT3 Organic nitrogen compounds
BT2 Flavourings
BT3 Additives

Polyglycerol fatty acid esters
HN introduced from vol. 39, issue 1 (2007)
BT1 Emulsifiers
BT2 Additives
BT1 Fatty acid esters
BT2 Esters
BT3 Organic compounds
RT Glycerol

Polyglycerol polyricinoleate
BT1 Emulsifiers
BT2 Additives

Polyhydroxyalkanoates
BT1 Hydrocarbons
BT2 Organic compounds

Polyketides
BT1 Mycotoxins
BT2 Toxins
BT3 Residues

Polylysine
HN introduced from vol. 39, issue 1 (2007)
BT1 Lysine
BT2 Amino acids
BT3 Nutrients
BT3 Organic acids
BT4 Acids
BT3 Organic nitrogen compounds
BT1 Peptides
BT2 Proteins
BT3 Nutrients
BT1 Preservatives
BT2 Additives

Poly(β-D-mannuronate) lyases
SN EC 4.2.2.3
BT1 Lyases
BT2 Enzymes
UF Alginate lyases

Polymerase chain reaction
USE **PCR**

Polymerization
BT1 Modification
RT Polymers

Polymers
SN use for food polymers only, not plastics
RT Biopolymers
RT Polymerization
RT Resins

Polymorphism
BT1 Genetics
RT Genetic variants

Polymyxins
BT1 Antibiotics
BT2 Drugs
BT3 Residues

Polynuclear aromatic hydrocarbons
USE **PAH**

Polyodon spathula
BT1 Paddlefish
BT2 Marine fish
BT3 Fish
BT4 Animals
BT4 Sea foods
BT5 Aquatic foods
BT6 Animal foods
BT7 Foods

Polyolefins
BT1 Plastics
BT2 Packaging materials

Polyols
BT1 Alcohols
BT1 Carbohydrates
BT2 Nutrients
BT2 Organic compounds
NT1 Alditols
NT1 Arabitol
NT1 Dulcitol
NT1 Erythritol
NT1 Galactitol
NT1 Glycerol
NT2 Glycerin
NT2 Glycerine
NT1 Inositol
NT2 Inositol phosphates
NT2 Phytates
NT2 Phytic acid
NT1 Lactitol
NT1 Maltitol
NT1 Mannitol
NT1 Sorbitol
NT1 Sugar alcohols
NT1 Xylitol
RT Sweeteners

Polypeptides
BT1 Peptides
BT2 Proteins
BT3 Nutrients

Polyphenol oxidases
USE **Catechol oxidases**

Polyphenols
SN general use only; see also other specified polyphenols
BT1 Phenols
BT2 Alcohols
BT2 Aromatic compounds
BT3 Organic compounds
RT Curcuminoids
RT Flavonoids
RT Lignans
RT Stilbenes

Polyphosphates
BT1 Phosphates
BT2 Salts

Polyporus
SN lignicolous fungi
BT1 Fungi
BT2 Microorganisms

Polyprion americanus
BT1 Wreckfish
BT2 Marine fish
BT3 Fish
BT4 Animals
BT4 Sea foods
BT5 Aquatic foods
BT6 Animal foods
BT7 Foods

Polypropylene
BT1 Plastics
BT2 Packaging materials

Polysaccharides
BT1 Carbohydrates
BT2 Nutrients
BT2 Organic compounds
NT1 Agar
NT2 Agar gels
NT2 Agarose
NT1 Alginates
NT2 Alginate gels
NT2 Alginic acid
NT1 Arabinogalactans
NT1 Carrageenans
NT2 Carrageenan gels
NT1 Chitin
NT2 Chitosan
NT1 Exopolysaccharides
NT1 Fructans
NT2 Inulin
NT2 Levans
NT1 Fucoidans
NT1 Galactans
NT1 Gellan
NT2 Gellan gums
NT1 Glucans
NT2 Alternan
NT2 Celluloses
NT3 Carboxymethylcellulose
NT3 Cellulose acetate
NT3 Cellulose ether
NT3 Cellulose sausage casings
NT3 Hydroxypropylcellulose
NT3 Hydroxypropylmethylcellulose
NT3 Lignocelluloses
NT3 Methylcellulose
NT3 Microcrystalline celluloses
NT3 Regenerated cellulose
NT3 Tylose
NT2 Curdlan
NT2 Dextran
NT2 β-Glucans
NT2 Glycogen
NT2 Laminarin
NT2 Polydextrose
NT2 Pullulan
NT2 Starch
NT3 Amaranth starch
NT3 Amylopectins
NT3 Amyloses
NT3 Arrowroot
NT3 Barley starch
NT3 Buckwheat starch
NT3 Canna starch
NT3 Cassava starch
NT4 Tapioca
NT3 Corn starch
NT4 High amylose corn starch
NT3 Dextrins
NT4 Amylodextrins
NT4 Cyclodextrins
NT4 Maltodextrins
NT4 Pyrodextrins
NT3 Farina
NT3 Legume starch
NT3 Millet starch
NT3 Modified starches
NT3 Mung bean starch
NT3 Oat starch
NT3 Pea starch
NT3 Potato starch
NT3 Resistant starch
NT3 Rice starch
NT3 Rye starch
NT3 Sago
NT3 Sorghum starch
NT3 Starch granules
NT3 Sweet potato starch
NT3 Wheat starch
NT3 Yam starch
NT2 Xyloglucans
NT1 Glycosaminoglycans
NT2 Chondroitin
NT2 Hyaluronic acid
NT2 Mucopolysaccharides
NT1 Gums
NT2 Cassia gums
NT2 Furcellaran
NT2 Gellan gums
NT2 Guar gums
NT2 Gum arabic
NT3 Gum acacia
NT2 Gum ghatti
NT2 Gum kondagogu
NT2 Gum tragacanth
NT2 Karaya gums
NT2 Locust bean gums
NT3 Carob gums
NT2 Mesquite seed gums
NT2 Mucilage
NT2 Psyllium gums
NT2 Tara gums
NT2 Xanthan gums
NT1 Hemicelluloses
NT1 Kefiran
NT1 Lipopolysaccharides
NT1 Mannans
NT2 Galactomannans
NT2 Glucomannans
NT3 Konjac glucomannans
NT1 Nonstarch polysaccharides
NT1 Oligosaccharides
NT2 Chitooligosaccharides
NT2 Fructooligosaccharides
NT3 Kestose
NT3 Nystose
NT2 Galactooligosaccharides
NT2 Glucooligosaccharides
NT3 Isomaltooligosaccharides
NT3 Maltooligosaccharides
NT4 Maltohexaose
NT4 Maltotetraose
NT4 Maltotriose
NT3 Panose
NT2 Lactosucrose
NT2 Melezitose
NT2 Raffinose
NT2 Stachyose
NT2 Verbascose
NT2 Xylooligosaccharides
NT1 Pectic substances
NT2 Galacturonic acid
NT2 Pectins
NT3 Apple pectins
NT3 Citrus pectins
NT3 Sugar beet pectins
NT2 Polyuronides
NT2 Rhamnogalacturonans
NT1 Pentosans
NT2 Arabinans
NT2 Arabinoxylans
NT1 Proteoglycans
NT1 Xanthan
NT2 Xanthan gums
NT1 Xylan
RT Hydrocolloids
UF Glycans

Polysorbate 60
BT1 Emulsifiers
BT2 Additives

Polystyrene
BT1 Plastics
BT2 Packaging materials
NT1 Styrene

Polytetrafluoroethylene
USE **PTFE**

Polythene
USE **Polyethylene**

Polyunsaturated fats
HN fats polyunsaturated also used in the index up to vol. 29 (1997)
BT1 Fats
BT2 Lipids
BT3 Nutrients
RT Unsaturated fats
RT Unsaturation

Polyunsaturated fatty acids
HN fatty acids polyunsaturated also used in the index up to vol. 29 (1997); PUFA used in the index from vol. 35, issue 6 (2003)
USE **PUFA**

Polyurethane
BT1 Plastics
BT2 Packaging materials

Polyuronides
BT1 Pectic substances
BT2 Polysaccharides
BT3 Carbohydrates

BT4 Nutrients
BT4 Organic compounds
BT1 Uronic acids
BT2 Organic acids
BT3 Acids
BT2 Sugars
BT3 Carbohydrates
BT4 Nutrients
BT4 Organic compounds
BT3 Plant foods
BT4 Foods

Polyvinyl acetate
BT1 Acetates
BT1 Chewing gums
BT2 Gum confectionery
BT3 Sugar confectionery
BT4 Plant foods
BT5 Foods
BT1 Coatings

Polyvinyl alcohol
BT1 Plastics
BT2 Packaging materials

Polyvinyl chloride
SN abbrev. PVC is also used in the index
BT1 Plastics
BT2 Packaging materials
NT1 PVC
NT1 Vinyl chloride

Polyvinylidene chloride
USE **PVDC**

Polyvinylpyrrolidinone
BT1 Plastics
BT2 Packaging materials

Polyvinylpyrrolidone
BT1 Plastics
BT2 Packaging materials
UF Povidone

Pomaces
BT1 Wastes
NT1 Apple pomaces
NT1 Grape pomaces
RT Olive pomace oils

Pombe
BT1 Beer
BT2 Alcoholic beverages
BT3 Beverages alcoholic
BT4 Beverages

Pome fruits
BT1 Fruits specific
BT2 Fruits
BT3 Crops
BT4 Plants
BT3 Plant foods
BT4 Foods

Pomegranate juices
BT1 Fruit juices
BT2 Fruit products
BT3 Plant foods
BT4 Foods
BT2 Soft drinks
BT3 Beverages
RT Pomegranates

Pomegranates
BT1 Fruits specific
BT2 Fruits
BT3 Crops
BT4 Plants
BT3 Plant foods
BT4 Foods
RT Pomegranate juices

Pomelos
SN syn. pummelos, shaddocks
BT1 Citrus fruits
BT2 Fruits specific
BT3 Fruits
BT4 Crops
BT5 Plants
BT4 Plant foods
BT5 Foods
NT1 *Citrus grandis*
NT1 Pummelos
NT1 Shaddocks

Pomfret
SN syn. butterfish
BT1 Marine fish
BT2 Fish
BT3 Animals
BT3 Sea foods
BT4 Aquatic foods
BT5 Animal foods
BT6 Foods
NT1 Butterfish
UF Pomfrets

Pomfrets
HN used up to vol. 29 (1997)
USE **Pomfret**

Pommes frites
BT1 Chips
BT2 Processed foods
BT3 Foods
BT1 Potato products
BT2 Potatoes
BT3 Vegetables specific
BT4 Vegetables
BT5 Crops
BT6 Plants
BT5 Plant foods
BT6 Foods

Ponceau
BT1 Colorants
BT2 Additives

Ponkans
BT1 Mandarins
BT2 Oranges
BT3 Citrus fruits
BT4 Fruits specific
BT5 Fruits
BT6 Crops
BT7 Plants
BT6 Plant foods
BT7 Foods

Pont-l'Eveque cheese
BT1 Cheese varieties
BT2 Cheese
BT3 Dairy products
BT4 Animal foods
BT5 Foods

Poori
BT1 Bread
BT2 Bakery products
BT3 Cereal products
BT4 Plant foods
BT5 Foods

Popcorn
SN used for unprocessed kernels and popped kernels
BT1 Corn
BT2 Cereals
BT3 Crops
BT4 Plants
BT3 Seeds
BT4 Plant foods
BT5 Foods
BT1 Snack foods
BT2 Processed foods
BT3 Foods
NT1 Microwave popcorn

Popping
BT1 Processing
BT2 Technology

Poppy seeds
BT1 Spices
BT2 Flavourings
BT3 Additives

Population groups
HN heading from vol. 32 (2000)
NT1 Adolescents
NT1 Adults
NT1 Anthropological groups
NT2 Cultural groups
NT2 Ethnic groups
NT2 Religious groups
NT1 Athletes
NT1 Children
NT1 Elderly
NT1 Fetuses
NT1 Infants
NT1 Men
NT1 Socioeconomic groups
NT1 Women

Porcine
USE **Swine**

Porcine somatotropin
HN introduced from vol. 39, issue 1 (2007)
BT1 Somatotropin
BT2 Hormones
BT3 Residues

Poria cocos
BT1 Edible fungi
BT2 Fungi edible
BT3 Vegetables specific
BT4 Vegetables
BT5 Crops
BT6 Plants

BT5 Plant foods
BT6 Foods

Porins
BT1 Microbial proteins
BT2 Microorganisms
BT2 Proteins
BT3 Nutrients
BT1 Virulence factors

Pork
BT1 Meat specific
BT2 Meat
BT3 Animal foods
BT4 Foods
NT1 Boar meat
NT1 Lacon
NT1 Pork bellies
NT1 Pork chops
NT1 Pork mince
NT1 Pork products
NT2 Charcuterie products
NT2 Pork patties
NT1 Swine carcasses
NT1 Wild boar meat
NT2 Wild boar carcasses
RT Bacon
RT Ham
RT Kasseler
RT Rendement Napole genes
RT Swine
UF Swine muscles

Pork bellies
HN introduced from vol. 37, issue 5 (2005)
BT1 Pork
BT2 Meat specific
BT3 Meat
BT4 Animal foods
BT5 Foods

Pork chops
BT1 Pork
BT2 Meat specific
BT3 Meat
BT4 Animal foods
BT5 Foods

Pork mince
BT1 Pork
BT2 Meat specific
BT3 Meat
BT4 Animal foods
BT5 Foods
UF Ground pork

Pork patties
HN introduced from vol. 39, issue 1 (2007)
BT1 Meat patties
BT2 Patties
BT3 Meat products
BT4 Animal foods
BT5 Foods
BT1 Pork products
BT2 Pork
BT3 Meat specific
BT4 Meat
BT5 Animal foods
BT6 Foods

Pork products
BT1 Pork
BT2 Meat specific
BT3 Meat
BT4 Animal foods
BT5 Foods
NT1 Charcuterie products
NT1 Pork patties

Pork sausages
BT1 Sausages
BT2 Meat products
BT3 Animal foods
BT4 Foods

Porosity
BT1 Permeability

Porphyra
BT1 Seaweeds
BT2 Algae
BT3 Microorganisms
BT2 Sea foods
BT3 Aquatic foods
BT4 Animal foods
BT5 Foods
NT1 Nori
NT1 *Porphyra yezoensis*

Porphyra yezoensis
BT1 *Porphyra*
BT2 Seaweeds
BT3 Algae
BT4 Microorganisms
BT3 Sea foods
BT4 Aquatic foods
BT5 Animal foods
BT6 Foods

Porphyridium
BT1 Microalgae
BT2 Algae
BT3 Microorganisms

Porphyrins
HN heading up to vol. 24 (1992)
BT1 Heterocyclic compounds
BT1 Organic nitrogen compounds
BT1 Pigments
NT1 Chlorophylls
NT1 Haem
NT1 Haematin
NT1 Haemin

Porpoises
BT1 Animals
RT Cetacea

Porridge
SN the food prepared from oatmeal, rolled oats or other oat products
BT1 Oats
BT2 Cereals
BT3 Crops
BT4 Plants
BT3 Seeds
BT4 Plant foods
BT5 Foods
BT1 Porridges
BT2 Cereal products
BT3 Plant foods
BT4 Foods

Porridges
HN introduced from vol. 39, issue 1 (2007)
BT1 Cereal products
BT2 Plant foods
BT3 Foods
NT1 Dalia
NT1 Gruel
NT1 Koko
NT1 Mawe
NT1 Polenta
NT1 Porridge
NT1 Uji

Port
BT1 Fortified wines
BT2 Wines
BT3 Alcoholic beverages
BT4 Beverages alcoholic
BT5 Beverages

Portioning
HN under Cutting up to vol. 42 (2010)
BT1 Processing
BT2 Technology
RT Food portions
RT Portion sizes

Portion packs
BT1 Packs
BT2 Containers

Portion sizes
HN introduced from vol. 43, issue 1 (2011)
BT1 Food portions
BT2 Eating habits
BT3 Consumer behaviour
BT4 Consumer response
RT Obesity
RT Portioning

Port Salut cheese
BT1 Cheese varieties
BT2 Cheese
BT3 Dairy products
BT4 Animal foods
BT5 Foods

Portugal
BT1 Europe
BT1 European Union
RT Organization for Economic Cooperation and Development

Postprandial response
HN introduced from vol. 39, issue 1 (2007)
BT1 Human physiology
BT2 Physiology
BT3 Science

Potable water
BT1 Drinking water
BT2 Water

Potassium
SN symbol K is also used in the index

BT1 Metals
BT2 Elements
BT3 Minerals
BT4 Nutrients
NT1 K

Potassium bromate
BT1 Bromates
BT2 Bakery additives
BT3 Additives
BT2 Salts

Potassium hydroxide
USE **KOH**

Potassium lactate
BT1 Lactates
BT2 Preservatives
BT3 Additives
BT2 Salts

Potassium metabisulfite
HN introduced from vol. 42, issue 1 (2010)
BT1 Metabisulfites
BT2 Preservatives
BT3 Additives
BT2 Sulfites
BT3 Salts
BT1 Preservatives
BT2 Additives

Potato chips
BT1 Chips
BT2 Processed foods
BT3 Foods
BT1 Potato products
BT2 Potatoes
BT3 Vegetables specific
BT4 Vegetables
BT5 Crops
BT6 Plants
BT5 Plant foods
BT6 Foods

Potato crisps
BT1 Chips
BT2 Processed foods
BT3 Foods
BT1 Potato products
BT2 Potatoes
BT3 Vegetables specific
BT4 Vegetables
BT5 Crops
BT6 Plants
BT5 Plant foods
BT6 Foods

Potatoes
BT1 Vegetables specific
BT2 Vegetables
BT3 Crops
BT4 Plants
BT3 Plant foods
BT4 Foods
NT1 Potato peel
NT1 Potato products
NT2 French fries
NT2 Gnocchi
NT2 Mashed potatoes
NT2 Pommes frites
NT2 Potato chips
NT2 Potato crisps
NT2 Potato flakes
NT2 Potato granules
NT2 Potato meal
NT2 Potato purees
NT2 Potato salads
NT2 Potato starch
NT1 *Solanum tuberosum*
RT Chaconine
RT Patatin
RT Solanine

Potato flakes
BT1 Dried foods
BT2 Processed foods
BT3 Foods
BT1 Potato products
BT2 Potatoes
BT3 Vegetables specific
BT4 Vegetables
BT5 Crops
BT6 Plants
BT5 Plant foods
BT6 Foods

Potato granules
HN introduced from vol. 39, issue 1 (2007)
BT1 Potato products
BT2 Potatoes
BT3 Vegetables specific
BT4 Vegetables
BT5 Crops
BT6 Plants
BT5 Plant foods
BT6 Foods

Potato meal
BT1 Flours
BT2 Plant foods
BT3 Foods
BT1 Potato products
BT2 Potatoes
BT3 Vegetables specific
BT4 Vegetables
BT5 Crops
BT6 Plants
BT5 Plant foods
BT6 Foods

Potato peel
BT1 Peel
BT1 Potatoes
BT2 Vegetables specific
BT3 Vegetables
BT4 Crops
BT5 Plants
BT4 Plant foods
BT5 Foods

Potato products
BT1 Potatoes
BT2 Vegetables specific
BT3 Vegetables
BT4 Crops
BT5 Plants
BT4 Plant foods
BT5 Foods
NT1 French fries
NT1 Gnocchi
NT1 Mashed potatoes
NT1 Pommes frites
NT1 Potato chips
NT1 Potato crisps
NT1 Potato flakes
NT1 Potato granules
NT1 Potato meal
NT1 Potato purees
NT1 Potato salads
NT1 Potato starch

Potato purees
BT1 Potato products
BT2 Potatoes
BT3 Vegetables specific
BT4 Vegetables
BT5 Crops
BT6 Plants
BT5 Plant foods
BT6 Foods
BT1 Vegetable purees
BT2 Purees
BT3 Pulps
BT4 Processed foods
BT5 Foods
BT2 Vegetable products
BT3 Plant foods
BT4 Foods

Potato salads
BT1 Potato products
BT2 Potatoes
BT3 Vegetables specific
BT4 Vegetables
BT5 Crops
BT6 Plants
BT5 Plant foods
BT6 Foods
BT1 Vegetable salads
BT2 Salads
BT2 Vegetable products
BT3 Plant foods
BT4 Foods

Potato starch
BT1 Potato products
BT2 Potatoes
BT3 Vegetables specific
BT4 Vegetables
BT5 Crops
BT6 Plants
BT5 Plant foods
BT6 Foods
BT1 Starch
BT2 Glucans
BT3 Polysaccharides
BT4 Carbohydrates
BT5 Nutrients
BT5 Organic compounds
BT2 Thickeners
BT3 Additives

Potentiometry
HN heading from vol. 30 (1998); under Analytical techniques up to vol. 29 (1997)
BT1 Analytical techniques

Pots
BT1 Containers

Pouches
HN heading from vol. 25 (1993); under Packs up to vol. 24 (1992)
BT1 Containers
NT1 Retort pouches
NT1 Sachets

Pouchong tea
BT1 Tea
BT2 Teas
BT3 Beverages
BT3 Crops
BT4 Plants
BT3 Plant foods
BT4 Foods

Poultry
SN domestic or farmed birds
BT1 Birds
NT1 Chickens
NT2 Chicken bones
NT2 Chicken gizzard pickles
NT2 Chicken livers
NT2 Chicken meat
NT3 Chicken carcasses
NT3 Chicken drumsticks
NT3 Chicken mince
NT3 Chicken nuggets
NT3 Chicken products
NT4 Chicken patties
NT2 Chicken skin
NT1 Chukars
NT1 Ducks
NT2 Duck eggs
NT3 Pidan
NT2 Duck livers
NT2 Duck meat
NT3 Duck carcasses
NT1 Emus
NT2 Emu meat
NT3 Emu carcasses
NT1 Fowl
NT1 Geese
NT2 Goose eggs
NT2 Goose livers
NT2 Goose meat
NT3 Goose carcasses
NT1 Guinea fowl
NT1 Ostriches
NT2 Ostrich meat
NT3 Ostrich carcasses
NT1 Quails
NT2 Quail carcasses
NT2 Quail eggs
NT2 Quail meat
NT3 Quail carcasses
NT1 Rheas
NT2 Rhea meat
NT3 Rhea carcasses
NT1 Turkeys
NT2 Turkey meat
NT3 Turkey carcasses
NT3 Turkey mince
NT3 Turkey products
NT4 Turkey ham
NT4 Turkey patties
NT1 Waterfowl
RT Poultry meat

Poultry breast
BT1 Poultry meat
BT2 Meat specific
BT3 Meat
BT4 Animal foods
BT5 Foods

Poultry carcasses
BT1 Carcasses
BT2 Meat
BT3 Animal foods
BT4 Foods
BT1 Poultry meat
BT2 Meat specific
BT3 Meat
BT4 Animal foods
BT5 Foods

Poultry meat
HN heading from vol. 25 (1993); under Meat specific up to vol. 24 (1992)
BT1 Meat specific
BT2 Meat
BT3 Animal foods
BT4 Foods
NT1 Chicken meat
NT2 Chicken carcasses
NT2 Chicken drumsticks
NT2 Chicken mince
NT2 Chicken nuggets
NT2 Chicken products
NT3 Chicken patties
NT1 Duck meat
NT2 Duck carcasses
NT1 Emu meat
NT2 Emu carcasses
NT1 Goose meat
NT2 Goose carcasses
NT1 Ostrich meat
NT2 Ostrich carcasses
NT1 Poultry breast
NT1 Poultry carcasses
NT1 Poultry meat industry
NT1 Poultry products
NT1 Quail meat
NT2 Quail carcasses
NT1 Rhea meat
NT2 Rhea carcasses
NT1 Turkey meat
NT2 Turkey carcasses
NT2 Turkey mince
NT2 Turkey products
NT3 Turkey ham
NT3 Turkey patties
RT Chickens
RT Poultry

Poultry meat industry
HN introduced from vol. 42, issue 1 (2010)
BT1 Food industry
BT2 Industries
BT1 Poultry meat
BT2 Meat specific
BT3 Meat
BT4 Animal foods
BT5 Foods

Poultry products
BT1 Poultry meat
BT2 Meat specific
BT3 Meat
BT4 Animal foods
BT5 Foods

Poultry sausages
BT1 Sausages
BT2 Meat products
BT3 Animal foods
BT4 Foods
RT Chicken sausages
RT Turkey sausages

Poultry science
BT1 Animal science
BT2 Science

Poverty
HN introduced from vol. 39, issue 1 (2007)
BT1 Economics
RT Food security
RT Socioeconomic factors
RT Socioeconomic groups

Povidone
USE **Polyvinylpyrrolidone**

Powders
HN heading up to vol. 24 (1992)
BT1 Dried foods
BT2 Processed foods
BT3 Foods
BT1 Instant foods
BT2 Processed foods
BT3 Foods
NT1 Beverage powders
NT1 Chocolate powders
NT1 Cocoa powders
NT1 Coffee powders
NT1 Dried dairy products
NT2 Dried milk
NT2 Dried skim milk
NT2 Dried whey
NT1 Dried egg products
NT1 Dried eggs
NT1 Milk powders
NT1 Rice powders
NT1 Skim milk powders
NT1 Tea powders
NT1 Tomato powders
RT Granules
UF Food powders

Power
BT1 Energy

Pozol
BT1 Corn
BT2 Cereals
BT3 Crops
BT4 Plants
BT3 Seeds
BT4 Plant foods
BT5 Foods
BT1 Fermented foods
BT2 Processed foods
BT3 Foods

Pralines
BT1 Sugar confectionery
BT2 Plant foods
BT3 Foods

Prato cheese
BT1 Cheese varieties
BT2 Cheese
BT3 Dairy products
BT4 Animal foods
BT5 Foods

Prawn crackers
BT1 Prawns
BT2 Crustacea
BT3 Shellfish
BT4 Animals
BT4 Sea foods
BT5 Aquatic foods
BT6 Animal foods
BT7 Foods
BT1 Snack foods
BT2 Processed foods
BT3 Foods

Prawns
BT1 Crustacea
BT2 Shellfish
BT3 Animals
BT3 Sea foods
BT4 Aquatic foods
BT5 Animal foods
BT6 Foods
NT1 Kuruma prawns
NT1 Prawn crackers
RT Shrimps

Prebiotic foods
BT1 Novel foods
BT2 Foods
RT Prebiotics
RT Probiotic foods

Prebiotics
HN introduced from vol. 39, issue 1 (2007)
BT1 Carbohydrates
BT2 Nutrients
BT2 Organic compounds
RT Difructose anhydride
RT Inulin
RT Oligosaccharides
RT Prebiotic foods
RT Probiotic foods
RT Synbiotic foods

Precipitation
NT1 Sedimentation
RT Crystallization

Predictive microbiology
BT1 Microbiology

Predictive modelling
BT1 Microbiological techniques
NT1 Survival curves

Preference
BT1 Consumer response
NT1 Consumer preference

Pregnancy
BT1 Reproduction
BT2 Human physiology
BT3 Physiology
BT4 Science
RT Prenatal nutrition

Prenatal nutrition
HN introduced from vol. 42, issue 1 (2010)
BT1 Nutrition
RT Fetuses
RT Pregnancy
UF Fetal programming

Prepared dishes
BT1 Meals
BT2 Processed foods
BT3 Foods

Prepared foods
HN heading up to vol. 24 (1992)
USE **Processed foods**

Prepared meals
BT1 Meals
BT2 Processed foods
BT3 Foods

Presentation
BT1 Marketing
BT2 Economics

Preservation
BT1 Technology
NT1 Bottling
NT1 Canning
NT2 Canneries
NT2 Canning equipment
NT2 Canning industry
NT2 Canning quality
NT1 Curing
NT2 Curing agents
NT1 Hurdle technology
NT1 Smoking
NT2 Smoke
NT2 Smokehouses
RT Refrigeration
RT Storage
UF Preserving

Preservatives
BT1 Additives
NT1 Benzoates
NT2 Sodium benzoate
NT1 Benzoic acid
NT1 Dehydroacetic acid
NT1 Diethylpyrocarbonate
NT1 Food preservatives
NT1 Formaldehyde
NT2 Formalin
NT2 Formol
NT2 Methanal
NT1 Formic acid
NT1 Furylfuramide
NT1 H_2O_2
NT1 Hydroxybenzoic acid esters
NT2 Parabens
NT3 Methylparaben
NT3 Propylparaben
NT1 Lactates
NT2 Calcium lactate
NT2 Potassium lactate
NT2 Sodium lactate
NT1 Lactic acid
NT1 Metabisulfites
NT2 Potassium metabisulfite
NT2 Sodium metabisulfite
NT2 Sodium pyrosulfite
NT1 Monolaurin
NT1 Natamycin
NT2 Pimaricin
NT1 Nisin
NT1 5-Nitrofurylacrylic acid
NT1 Polylysine
NT1 Potassium metabisulfite
NT1 Propionic acid
NT1 Pyrocarbonic acid diethyl ester
NT1 Salicylic acid
NT1 Sodium acetate
NT1 Sodium diacetate
NT1 Sodium metabisulfite
NT1 Sodium pyrosulfite
NT1 Sorbates
NT1 Sorbic acid
NT1 Sulfur dioxide
NT2 SO_2
NT1 Sulfurous acid
RT Antibiotics
RT Nitrates
RT Nitrites
RT Tartaric acid

Preserves
BT1 Processed foods
BT2 Foods
NT1 Fish preserves
NT1 Fruit preserves
NT2 Jams
NT3 Apricot jams
NT3 Grape jams
NT3 Jelly
NT3 Mango jams
NT3 Marmalades
NT3 Quince jams
NT3 Strawberry jams
NT1 Vegetable preserves

Preserving
USE **Preservation**

Presses
BT1 Equipment
BT2 Technology
BT1 Pressing
BT2 Processing
BT3 Technology

Pressing
BT1 Processing
BT2 Technology
NT1 Briquetting
NT1 Compression
NT1 Oil expellers
NT1 Presses
RT Pressure

Pressure
NT1 High pressure processing
NT1 Manometers

NT1 Osmotic pressure
NT1 Pressure shift freezing
RT Pressing

Pressure shift freezing
HN introduced from vol. 39, issue 1 (2007)
BT1 Freezing
BT2 Thermal processing
BT3 Processing thermal
BT4 Processing
BT5 Technology
BT1 Pressure

Pretzels
BT1 Bakery products
BT2 Cereal products
BT3 Plant foods
BT4 Foods

Priacanthus macracanthus
BT1 Bigeye snapper
BT2 Marine fish
BT3 Fish
BT4 Animals
BT4 Sea foods
BT5 Aquatic foods
BT6 Animal foods
BT7 Foods

Priacanthus tayenus
BT1 Marine fish
BT2 Fish
BT3 Animals
BT3 Sea foods
BT4 Aquatic foods
BT5 Animal foods
BT6 Foods

Prices
HN under Costs up to vol. 24
BT1 Pricing
BT2 Food policy
BT3 Economics

Pricing
HN heading from vol. 25 (1993)
BT1 Food policy
BT2 Economics
NT1 Payment
NT1 Prices
RT Marketing
RT Markets

Prickly pears
SN syn. cactus pears
BT1 Fruits specific
BT2 Fruits
BT3 Crops
BT4 Plants
BT3 Plant foods
BT4 Foods
NT1 *Opuntia ficus-indica*
UF Barberry figs

Principal component analysis
BT1 Mathematics
BT2 Science

Printers
BT1 Printing
BT2 Labelling
BT3 Packaging
BT4 Technology
NT1 Ink jet printers

Printers ink jet
USE **Ink jet printers**

Printing
BT1 Labelling
BT2 Packaging
BT3 Technology
NT1 Printers
NT2 Ink jet printers

Prion diseases
BT1 Diseases
NT1 BSE
NT1 CJD
NT1 Scrapie
RT Animal diseases
RT Prions
UF Transmissible spongiform encephalopathies

Prion proteins
USE **Prions**

Prions
BT1 Proteins
BT2 Nutrients
RT Prion diseases
UF Prion proteins

Pristane
BT1 Hydrocarbons
BT2 Organic compounds

Private labels
BT1 Labelling
BT2 Packaging
BT3 Technology
RT Branding

Proanthocyanidins
BT1 Anthocyanidins
BT2 Flavonoids
BT3 Aromatic compounds
BT4 Organic compounds
BT3 Pigments
BT1 Tannins
BT2 Aromatic compounds
BT3 Organic compounds
BT2 Glycosides
BT3 Carbohydrates
BT4 Nutrients
BT4 Organic compounds
BT2 Organic acids
BT3 Acids
NT1 Procyanidins

Probiotic bacteria
BT1 Bacteria
BT2 Microorganisms
BT1 Probiotic microorganisms
BT2 Microorganisms
RT *Bifidobacterium*
RT *Lactobacillus*
RT Probiotic foods

Probiotic foods
BT1 Novel foods
BT2 Foods
RT Nutrition
RT Prebiotic foods
RT Prebiotics
RT Probiotic bacteria
RT Probiotic microorganisms

Probiotic microorganisms
BT1 Microorganisms
NT1 Probiotic bacteria
RT Probiotic foods

Procaryotes
USE **Prokaryotes**

Proceedings
RT Books
RT Conference proceedings

Process control
BT1 Technology
NT1 Control systems
NT1 Fermentation technology
NT2 Bioreactors
NT3 Chemostats
NT3 Membrane bioreactors
NT3 Packed bed bioreactors
NT3 Stirred tank bioreactors
NT3 UASB bioreactors
NT2 Cofermentation
NT2 Downstream processing
NT2 Extractive fermentation
NT2 Fermenters
NT2 Simultaneous saccharification and fermentation
NT2 Solid state fermentation
NT2 Submerged fermentation
NT1 Fuzzy control
NT1 Fuzzy logic process control
NT1 Thyristors

Processed cheese
BT1 Cheese varieties
BT2 Cheese
BT3 Dairy products
BT4 Animal foods
BT5 Foods

Processed foods
HN heading from vol. 25 (1993); under Prepared foods up to vol. 24 (1992)
BT1 Foods
NT1 Barbecued foods
NT1 Canned foods
NT1 Chilled foods
NT1 Chips
NT1 Concentrates
NT1 Convenience foods
NT1 Cook chill foods
NT1 Delicatessen foods
NT1 Desserts
NT1 Dietetic foods
NT1 Dips
NT1 Dried foods
NT1 Ethnic foods
NT1 Extruded foods
NT1 Fast foods

NT1 Fermented foods
NT1 Fondues
NT1 Fortified foods
NT1 Fried foods
NT1 Frozen foods
NT1 Halal foods
NT1 Health foods
NT1 Hypoallergenic foods
NT1 Infant foods
NT1 Instant foods
NT1 Intermediate moisture foods
NT1 Irradiated foods
NT1 Kosher foods
NT1 Lite foods
NT1 Meals
NT1 Minimally processed foods
NT1 Pastes
NT1 Preserves
NT1 Pulps
NT1 Ready to eat foods
NT1 Ready to serve foods
NT1 Recombined foods
NT1 Reconstituted foods
NT1 Roasted foods
NT1 Simulated foods
NT1 Smoked foods
NT1 Snack foods
NT1 Soups
NT1 Sous vide foods
NT1 Spreads
NT1 Vegan foods
NT1 Vegetarian foods
UF Prepared foods

Processing
BT1 Technology
NT1 Acidification
NT1 Aeration
NT1 Alkalization
NT1 Aseptic processing
NT1 Basting
NT1 Bleaching
NT2 Bleaching agents
NT1 Boning
NT2 Cold boning
NT2 Hot boning
NT2 Mechanical boning
NT1 Breadmaking
NT2 Breadmaking properties
NT3 Loaf vol.
NT2 Wheat breadmaking
NT1 Brewing
NT2 Breweries
NT3 Breweries effluents
NT3 Inn breweries
NT3 Microbreweries
NT2 Brewing adjuncts
NT2 Brewing industry
NT2 High gravity brewing
NT2 Hopping
NT1 Brining
NT2 Brines
NT2 Curing brines
NT1 Buttermaking
NT2 Butter factories
NT2 Churning
NT1 Carbonation
NT1 Cheesemaking
NT2 Cheddaring
NT1 Clarification
NT2 Clarifiers
NT2 Fining
NT3 Fining agents
NT2 Winterization
NT1 Cleaning
NT2 Cleaning agents
NT2 Cleaning in place
NT2 Depuration
NT2 Descaling
NT2 Dishwashers
NT2 Rinsing
NT2 Washing
NT1 Clipping
NT1 Coagulation
NT2 Clotting
NT3 Milk clotting
NT2 Coagulants
NT2 Rennetability
NT1 Coating
NT2 Breading
NT2 Enrobing
NT2 Glazing
NT2 Panning
NT1 Comminution
NT2 Crumbling
NT2 Crushing
NT2 Flaking
NT2 Grating
NT2 Grinding
NT2 Mincing
NT3 Mincers
NT2 Pulverization
NT2 Shredding
NT1 Concentration
NT2 Freeze concentration
NT1 Condensation
NT1 Continuous processing
NT1 Cracking
NT1 Crystallization
NT1 Cutting
NT2 Chopping
NT3 Chopping boards
NT2 Coring
NT3 Corers
NT2 Cutability
NT2 Dicing
NT2 Filleting
NT2 Jointing
NT2 Knives
NT2 Slicing
NT2 Splitting
NT2 Trimming
NT1 Deaeration
NT1 Debittering
NT1 Debranning
NT1 Decaffeination
NT1 Decarbonation
NT1 Decoloration
NT1 Decoration
NT1 Decortication
NT1 Defeathering
NT1 Degreening
NT1 Degumming
NT1 Dehairing
NT1 Denitrification
NT1 Desulfitation
NT1 Detoxification
NT1 Dewatering
NT1 Dewaxing
NT1 Dialysis
NT2 Electrodialysis
NT1 Dilution
NT1 Dipping
NT1 Distillation
NT2 Corn steep liquor
NT2 Distilleries
NT3 Distilleries effluents
NT2 Distilling industry
NT2 Rectification
NT2 Vacuum distillation
NT1 Dressing
NT1 Emulsification
NT1 Evisceration
NT1 Extraction
NT2 Sonication
NT2 Supercritical CO_2 extraction
NT2 Supercritical fluid extraction
NT1 Extrusion
NT2 Coextrusion
NT2 Extrudates
NT2 Extruders
NT2 Extrusion cooking
NT1 Filtration
NT2 Filter aids
NT3 Bentonite
NT3 Clays
NT3 Diatomaceous earths
NT3 Kieselguhr
NT2 Filters
NT2 Microfiltration
NT2 Nanofiltration
NT2 Racking
NT2 Ultrafiltration
NT3 Diafiltration
NT1 Fluidization
NT2 Fluidized beds
NT2 Microfluidization
NT1 Flushing
NT1 Food technology
NT1 Frothing
NT1 Gutting
NT1 High pressure processing
NT1 Homogenization
NT2 Homogenizers
NT1 Husking
NT2 Dehulling
NT2 Hulling
NT2 Hulls
NT2 Husks
NT1 Hydrogenation
NT2 Hardening
NT1 Injection
NT1 Instantization
NT1 Irradiation
NT2 Electron beam irradiation
NT2 Gamma irradiation
NT2 Gamma rays
NT2 IR irradiation
NT2 Radurization
NT2 UV irradiation
NT1 Liquefaction
NT1 Maceration
NT2 Carbonic maceration
NT1 Mashing
NT2 Decoction
NT2 Lautering
NT3 Lauter tuns

NT2 Mashes
NT2 Moromi
NT1 Membrane distillation
NT1 Micronization
NT1 Milling
NT2 Milling properties
NT2 Mills
NT3 Flour mills
NT3 Roller mills
NT2 Wet milling
NT1 Minimal processing
NT1 Mixing
NT2 Agitation
NT2 Blending
NT2 Conching
NT2 Impellers
NT2 Kneading
NT2 Mixers
NT2 Stirring
NT1 Moulding
NT2 Shaping
NT1 Nitrification
NT1 Nixtamalization
NT1 Nonthermal processes
NT1 Pearling
NT1 Peeling
NT1 Pickling
NT1 Polishing
NT1 Popping
NT1 Portioning
NT1 Pressing
NT2 Briquetting
NT2 Compression
NT2 Oil expellers
NT2 Presses
NT1 Processing equipment
NT1 Processing lines
NT1 Processing thermal
NT2 Thermal processing
NT3 Cook chill processing
NT3 Cooking
NT4 Baking
NT5 Bakeries
NT5 Baking industry
NT5 Baking properties
NT5 Baking quality
NT5 Proofers
NT5 Proofing
NT4 Blanching
NT4 Boiling
NT5 Boilers
NT5 Parboiling
NT4 Braising
NT4 Broiling
NT4 Cookers
NT4 Cooking properties
NT5 Cooking loss
NT4 Frying
NT5 Deep frying
NT5 Frying properties
NT5 Stir frying
NT4 Grilling
NT4 Hard to cook defect
NT4 Microwave cooking
NT4 Roasting
NT4 Sauteing
NT4 Simmering
NT4 Slow cooking
NT4 Sous vide
NT4 Steaming
NT5 Steam
NT4 Stewing
NT4 Toasting
NT3 Cooling
NT4 Air cooling
NT4 Chilling
NT5 Chillers
NT4 Coolers
NT4 Hydrocooling
NT4 Supercooling
NT4 Vacuum cooling
NT3 Drying
NT4 Air drying
NT4 Driers
NT5 Freeze driers
NT5 Solar driers
NT5 Spray driers
NT4 Drum drying
NT4 Freeze drying
NT5 Freeze driers
NT4 Impingement drying
NT4 IR drying
NT4 Osmotic drying
NT4 Parching
NT4 Roller drying
NT4 Solar drying
NT5 Solar driers
NT4 Spray drying
NT5 Spray driers
NT4 Thin layer drying
NT4 Vacuum drying
NT4 Withering
NT3 Evaporation
NT4 Evaporators
NT4 Vacuum evaporation
NT4 Vaporization
NT3 Freezing
NT4 Cryogenics
NT4 Cryopreservation
NT4 Deep freezing
NT4 Freezers
NT4 Freeze-thaw stability
NT4 Ice nucleation activity
NT4 Immersion freezing
NT4 Liquid nitrogen
NT4 Pressure shift freezing
NT3 Heating
NT4 Annealing
NT4 Dielectric heating
NT4 Flaming
NT4 Heat
NT4 Heat distribution
NT4 Heaters
NT4 Heat transfer
NT4 Induction heating
NT4 IR heating
NT4 Reheating
NT4 Thermization
NT4 Warming
NT3 Hydrothermal processing
NT3 Pasteurization
NT4 HTST pasteurization
NT4 LTLT pasteurization
NT4 Pasteurizers
NT4 Surface pasteurization
NT4 Ultrapasteurization
NT3 Refrigeration
NT4 Refrigerants
NT5 Chlorofluorocarbons
NT5 Freons
NT4 Refrigerated storage
NT4 Refrigerated transport
NT4 Refrigerators
NT3 Rendering
NT3 Scalding
NT3 Sterilization
NT4 Autoclaves
NT4 Ohmic heating
NT4 Retorting
NT4 UHT treatment
NT3 Tempering
NT4 Temper
NT3 Thawing
NT4 Defrosting
NT4 Drip
NT4 Freeze-thaw stability
NT4 Purge loss
NT3 Thermal processes
NT1 Process water
NT1 Puffing
NT1 Pulping
NT1 Pulsed electric fields
NT1 Purification
NT2 Defecation
NT2 Deodorization
NT2 Downstream processing
NT2 Epuration
NT2 Refining
NT3 Affination
NT1 Recombination
NT1 Reconstitution
NT2 Rehydration
NT1 Reverse osmosis
NT1 Rolling
NT1 Saccharification
NT1 Salting
NT1 Scaling
NT1 Separation
NT2 Centrifugation
NT3 Bactofugation
NT3 Centrifuges
NT4 Centrifugal separators
NT3 Ultracentrifugation
NT2 Flocculation
NT3 Floc
NT3 Flocculants
NT2 Flotation
NT2 Fractionation
NT3 Foam fractionation
NT2 Immunomagnetic separation
NT2 Partitioning
NT2 Pervaporation
NT2 Separators
NT3 Centrifugal separators
NT2 Sieving
NT3 Sieves
NT3 Sifting
NT4 Sifters
NT2 Strainers
NT1 Skinning
NT1 Soaking
NT2 Imbibition
NT2 Marination
NT3 Marinades
NT2 Steeping
NT1 Spouted bed processing

NT1 Spraying
NT1 Stretching
NT1 Sugar processes
NT2 Carbonatation
NT2 Liming
NT2 Sugar pans
NT2 Vacuum pans
NT1 Sulfitation
NT1 Tenderization
NT1 Texturization
NT2 Spinning
NT2 Texturizers
NT2 Texturizing agents
NT1 Thickening
NT1 Trussing
NT1 Tumbling
NT1 Vacuum impregnation
NT1 Vitrification
NT1 Whipping
NT2 Beating
NT1 Winemaking
NT2 Chaptalization
NT2 Madeirization
NT2 Oenological properties
NT2 Sparkling winemaking
NT3 Champagnization
NT2 Terroir
NT2 Viniculture
NT2 Vintage
NT2 Wineries
UF Product technology

Processing continuous
HN used for continuous processing up to vol. 31 (1999)
USE **Continuous processing**

Processing equipment
SN general use only; see also other specific processing equipment
BT1 Equipment
BT2 Technology
BT1 Processing
BT2 Technology
RT Processing lines

Processing HTST
USE **HTST pasteurization**

Processing lines
BT1 Equipment
BT2 Technology
BT1 Processing
BT2 Technology
RT Processing equipment

Processing thermal
HN heading from vol. 25 (1993); under Thermal processes up to vol. 24 (1992); thermal processing also used in the index from vol. 32 (2000)
BT1 Processing
BT2 Technology
NT1 Thermal processing
NT2 Cook chill processing
NT2 Cooking
NT3 Baking
NT4 Bakeries
NT4 Baking industry
NT4 Baking properties
NT4 Baking quality
NT4 Proofers
NT4 Proofing
NT3 Blanching
NT3 Boiling
NT4 Boilers
NT4 Parboiling
NT3 Braising
NT3 Broiling
NT3 Cookers
NT3 Cooking properties
NT4 Cooking loss
NT3 Frying
NT4 Deep frying
NT4 Frying properties
NT4 Stir frying
NT3 Grilling
NT3 Hard to cook defect
NT3 Microwave cooking
NT3 Roasting
NT3 Sauteing
NT3 Simmering
NT3 Slow cooking
NT3 Sous vide
NT3 Steaming
NT4 Steam
NT3 Stewing
NT3 Toasting
NT2 Cooling
NT3 Air cooling
NT3 Chilling
NT4 Chillers
NT3 Coolers
NT3 Hydrocooling
NT3 Supercooling
NT3 Vacuum cooling
NT2 Drying
NT3 Air drying
NT3 Driers
NT4 Freeze driers
NT4 Solar driers
NT4 Spray driers
NT3 Drum drying
NT3 Freeze drying
NT4 Freeze driers
NT3 Impingement drying
NT3 IR drying
NT3 Osmotic drying
NT3 Parching
NT3 Roller drying
NT3 Solar drying
NT4 Solar driers
NT3 Spray drying
NT4 Spray driers
NT3 Thin layer drying
NT3 Vacuum drying
NT3 Withering
NT2 Evaporation
NT3 Evaporators
NT3 Vacuum evaporation
NT3 Vaporization
NT2 Freezing
NT3 Cryogenics
NT3 Cryopreservation
NT3 Deep freezing
NT3 Freezers
NT3 Freeze-thaw stability
NT3 Ice nucleation activity
NT3 Immersion freezing
NT3 Liquid nitrogen
NT3 Pressure shift freezing
NT2 Heating
NT3 Annealing
NT3 Dielectric heating
NT3 Flaming
NT3 Heat
NT3 Heat distribution
NT3 Heaters
NT3 Heat transfer
NT3 Induction heating
NT3 IR heating
NT3 Reheating
NT3 Thermization
NT3 Warming
NT2 Hydrothermal processing
NT2 Pasteurization
NT3 HTST pasteurization
NT3 LTLT pasteurization
NT3 Pasteurizers
NT3 Surface pasteurization
NT3 Ultrapasteurization
NT2 Refrigeration
NT3 Refrigerants
NT4 Chlorofluorocarbons
NT4 Freons
NT3 Refrigerated storage
NT3 Refrigerated transport
NT3 Refrigerators
NT2 Rendering
NT2 Scalding
NT2 Sterilization
NT3 Autoclaves
NT3 Ohmic heating
NT3 Retorting
NT3 UHT treatment
NT2 Tempering
NT3 Temper
NT2 Thawing
NT3 Defrosting
NT3 Drip
NT3 Freeze-thaw stability
NT3 Purge loss
NT2 Thermal processes

Process water
HN introduced from vol. 39, issue 1 (2007)
BT1 Processing
BT2 Technology
BT1 Water

Procyanidins
BT1 Proanthocyanidins
BT2 Anthocyanidins
BT3 Flavonoids
BT4 Aromatic compounds
BT5 Organic compounds
BT4 Pigments
BT2 Tannins
BT3 Aromatic compounds
BT4 Organic compounds
BT3 Glycosides
BT4 Carbohydrates
BT5 Nutrients
BT5 Organic compounds
BT3 Organic acids
BT4 Acids

Procymidone
BT1 Dicarboximide fungicides
BT2 Fungicides
BT3 Pesticides
BT4 Biocides
BT4 Residues

Production
SN use for economic aspects only
BT1 Economics
RT Sustainability

Product liability
BT1 Food policy
BT2 Economics

Product recalls
HN introduced from vol. 39, issue 1 (2007)
BT1 Retail
BT2 Marketing
BT3 Economics
RT Consumer protection
RT Food safety
RT Risks management
RT Traceability

Product technology
HN heading up to vol. 24, used up to vol. 39 (2007)
USE **Processing**

Profilins
HN introduced from vol. 39, issue 1 (2007)
BT1 Proteins
BT2 Nutrients

Profitability
BT1 Economics

Profits
BT1 Economics

Progesterone
BT1 Hormones
BT2 Residues

Progoitrin
BT1 Bitter compounds
BT2 Flavour compounds
BT1 Glucosinolates
BT2 Glycosides
BT3 Carbohydrates
BT4 Nutrients
BT4 Organic compounds

Prokaryotes
BT1 Microorganisms
RT Bacteria
RT Viruses
UF Procaryotes

Prolactin
BT1 Hormones
BT2 Residues

Prolamins
BT1 Cereal proteins
BT2 Proteins cereal
BT3 Vegetable proteins
BT4 Proteins vegetable
BT5 Proteins
BT6 Nutrients
BT5 Vegetable products
BT6 Plant foods
BT7 Foods

Proline
HN heading from vol. 25 (1993); under Amino acids up to vol. 24 (1992)
BT1 Amino acids
BT2 Nutrients
BT2 Organic acids
BT3 Acids
BT2 Organic nitrogen compounds

Prometryn
BT1 Triazine herbicides
BT2 Herbicides
BT3 Pesticides
BT4 Biocides
BT4 Residues

Promine
BT1 Soy proteins
BT2 Vegetable proteins
BT3 Proteins vegetable
BT4 Proteins
BT5 Nutrients
BT4 Vegetable products
BT5 Plant foods
BT6 Foods

Promoters
BT1 Operons
BT2 Genetics
RT Gene expression
RT Genes

Pronase
BT1 Proteinases
BT2 Hydrolases
BT3 Enzymes

Proofers
BT1 Baking
BT2 Cooking
BT3 Thermal processing
BT4 Processing thermal
BT5 Processing
BT6 Technology

Proofing
BT1 Baking
BT2 Cooking
BT3 Thermal processing
BT4 Processing thermal
BT5 Processing
BT6 Technology

Prooxidative activity
HN introduced from vol. 39, issue 1 (2007)
BT1 Oxidation

Propachlor
BT1 Herbicides
BT2 Pesticides
BT3 Biocides
BT3 Residues
UF Ramrod

Propanal
SN syn. propionaldehyde
BT1 Aldehydes
BT2 Carbonyl compounds
BT3 Organic compounds
BT1 Aroma compounds
BT2 Flavour compounds
BT2 Volatile compounds
NT1 Propionaldehyde

Propane
BT1 Gases
BT2 Physical phases
BT3 Chemistry
BT4 Science
BT1 Hydrocarbons
BT2 Organic compounds

1,2-Propanediol
SN syn. propylene glycol
BT1 Glycols
BT2 Alcohols

Propanil
BT1 Herbicides
BT2 Pesticides
BT3 Biocides
BT3 Residues

Propanol
SN syn. propyl alcohol
BT1 Alcohols
BT1 Solvents
NT1 Chloropropanols

2-Propanol
SN syn. isopropyl alcohol; syn. isopropanol
BT1 Alcohols
BT1 Solvents

Propanone
SN syn. acetone
BT1 Ketones
BT2 Carbonyl compounds
BT3 Organic compounds
BT1 Solvents

Propargite
HN under Insecticides up to vol. 42 (2010)
BT1 Acaricides
BT2 Pesticides
BT3 Biocides
BT3 Residues
UF Omite

Propazine
BT1 Triazine herbicides
BT2 Herbicides
BT3 Pesticides
BT4 Biocides
BT4 Residues

Propenal
SN syn. acrolein
BT1 Acrolein
BT2 Aldehydes
BT3 Carbonyl compounds
BT4 Organic compounds

Propham
BT1 Carbamate pesticides
BT2 Pesticides
BT3 Biocides
BT3 Residues
BT1 Herbicides
BT2 Pesticides
BT3 Biocides
BT3 Residues

Propineb
BT1 Dithiocarbamate fungicides
BT2 Fungicides
BT3 Pesticides
BT4 Biocides
BT4 Residues

Propionaldehyde
SN syn. propanal
BT1 Propanal
BT2 Aldehydes
BT3 Carbonyl compounds
BT4 Organic compounds
BT2 Aroma compounds
BT3 Flavour compounds
BT3 Volatile compounds

Propionibacteria
USE ***Propionibacterium***

Propionibacteriaceae
HN heading up to vol. 24 (1992)
BT1 Bacteria
BT2 Microorganisms
RT *Propionibacterium*

Propionibacterium
HN heading from vol. 30 (1998); under Bacteria up to vol. 29 (1997)
BT1 Bacteria
BT2 Microorganisms
NT1 *Propionibacterium acidipropionici*
NT2 *Propionibacterium acidi-propionici*
NT1 *Propionibacterium freudenreichii*
NT2 *Propionibacterium shermanii*
NT1 *Propionibacterium jensenii*
NT1 *Propionibacterium thoenii*
RT Propionibacteriaceae
RT Propionic acid bacteria
RT Propionicins
UF Propionibacteria

Propionibacterium acidipropionici
HN introduced from vol. 43, issue 1 (2011)
BT1 *Propionibacterium*
BT2 Bacteria
BT3 Microorganisms
NT1 *Propionibacterium acidi-propionici*

Propionibacterium acidi-propionici
SN current name is Propionibacterium acidipropionici
BT1 *Propionibacterium acidipropionici*
BT2 *Propionibacterium*
BT3 Bacteria
BT4 Microorganisms

Propionibacterium freudenreichii
BT1 *Propionibacterium*
BT2 Bacteria
BT3 Microorganisms
NT1 *Propionibacterium shermanii*

Propionibacterium jensenii
HN introduced from vol. 39, issue 1 (2007)
BT1 *Propionibacterium*
BT2 Bacteria
BT3 Microorganisms

Propionibacterium shermanii
SN synonymous with Propionibacterium freudenreichii subsp. shermanii
BT1 *Propionibacterium freudenreichii*
BT2 *Propionibacterium*
BT3 Bacteria
BT4 Microorganisms

Propionibacterium thoenii
HN introduced from vol. 39, issue 1 (2007)
BT1 *Propionibacterium*
BT2 Bacteria
BT3 Microorganisms

Propionic acid
BT1 Organic acids
BT2 Acids
BT1 Preservatives
BT2 Additives
RT Propionic fermentation

Propionic acid bacteria
BT1 Bacteria
BT2 Microorganisms
RT *Propionibacterium*

Propionic fermentation
BT1 Fermentation
RT Propionic acid

Propionicins
BT1 Bacteriocins
BT2 Antibiotics
BT3 Drugs
BT4 Residues
RT *Propionibacterium*

Propolis
BT1 Honeys
BT2 Sugar
BT3 Plant foods
BT4 Foods
RT Apiculture

Propoxur
BT1 Acaricides
BT2 Pesticides
BT3 Biocides
BT3 Residues
BT1 *N*-Methylcarbamate insecticides
BT2 Insecticides
BT3 Pesticides
BT4 Biocides
BT4 Residues
BT2 *N*-Methylcarbamate pesticides
BT3 Carbamate pesticides
BT4 Pesticides
BT5 Biocides
BT5 Residues

Propranolol
BT1 β-Adrenergic agonists
BT2 Drugs
BT3 Residues

Propyl alcohol
SN syn. propanol
BT1 Alcohols
BT1 Solvents

Propylamine
BT1 Amines
BT2 Organic nitrogen compounds

Propylene
BT1 Plant growth regulators
BT2 Cultivation
BT3 Agriculture

Propylene glycol
SN syn. 1,2-propanediol
BT1 Emulsifiers
BT2 Additives
BT1 Glycols
BT2 Alcohols

Propylene oxide
BT1 Fumigants
BT2 Biocides
BT1 Oxides

Propyl gallate
BT1 Antioxidants
BT2 Additives
BT1 Esters
BT2 Organic compounds

Propylparaben
BT1 Parabens
BT2 Hydroxybenzoic acid esters
BT3 Esters
BT4 Organic compounds
BT3 Preservatives
BT4 Additives

Propylthiouracil
HN introduced from vol. 41, issue 1 (2009)
BT1 Bitter compounds
BT2 Flavour compounds
BT1 Pyrimidines
BT2 Heterocyclic compounds
BT2 Organic nitrogen compounds
RT Sensory perception

Proso millet
USE **Common millet**

***Prosopis africana* seeds**
BT1 Seeds
BT2 Plant foods
BT3 Foods

Prostaglandin-endoperoxide synthases
HN introduced from vol. 39, issue 1 (2007)
SN EC 1.14.99.1; cyclooxygenases (non-current EC term) still widely used for this enzyme
BT1 Oxidoreductases
BT2 Enzymes

Prostaglandins
HN under Hormones up to vol. 41 (2009)
BT1 Eicosanoids
BT2 Fatty acids
BT3 Lipids
BT4 Nutrients
BT3 Organic acids
BT4 Acids

Prostate cancer
HN introduced from vol. 39, issue 1 (2007)
BT1 Cancer
BT2 Diseases

Prostokvasha
BT1 Fermented milk
BT2 Fermented dairy products
BT3 Dairy products
BT4 Animal foods
BT5 Foods
BT3 Fermented foods
BT4 Processed foods
BT5 Foods
BT2 Milk
BT3 Dairy products
BT4 Animal foods
BT5 Foods

Protamine
HN under Drugs up to vol. 42 (2010)
BT1 Animal proteins
BT2 Proteins animal
BT3 Proteins
BT4 Nutrients

Proteases
USE **Proteinases**

Proteasomes
USE **Proteinases**

Proteinases
SN includes all peptide hydrolases EC 3.4
BT1 Hydrolases
BT2 Enzymes
NT1 Actinidains
NT1 Aminopeptidases
NT1 Aqualysins
NT1 Bromelains
NT1 Calpains
NT1 Carboxypeptidases
NT1 Caspases
NT1 Cathepsins
NT1 Chymotrypsin
NT1 Collagenases
NT1 Cucumisins
NT1 Dipeptidases
NT1 Elastase
NT1 Endopeptidases
NT1 Enzymes milk clotting
NT2 Milk clotting enzymes
NT3 Chymosin
NT3 Rennets
NT4 Animal rennets
NT4 Calf rennets
NT4 Microbial rennets
NT4 Vegetable rennets
NT3 Rennet substitutes
NT1 Ficains
NT1 γ-Glutamyl hydrolases
NT1 Keratinases
NT1 Lysins
NT2 Autolysins
NT2 Thermolysins
NT1 Papain
NT1 Pepsins
NT1 Peptidases
NT1 Peptidyl-dipeptidase A
NT1 Plasmin
NT1 Plasminogen
NT1 Plasminogen activators
NT1 Pronase
NT1 Subtilisins
NT1 Trypsin
RT Proteolysis
UF Proteases
UF Proteasomes
UF Proteolytic enzymes

Proteinases inhibitors
BT1 Antinutritional factors
BT2 Nutritional values
BT1 Enzyme inhibitors
BT2 Enzymes
NT1 Calpastatins
NT1 Chymotrypsin inhibitors
NT1 Cystatins
NT1 Trypsin inhibitors

Proteinates
BT1 Protein products

Protein concentrates
HN heading from vol. 25 (1993)
BT1 Concentrates
BT2 Processed foods
BT3 Foods
BT1 Protein products
NT1 FPC
NT1 Milk protein concentrates
NT1 Pea protein concentrates
NT1 Soy protein concentrates
NT1 Whey protein concentrates

Protein efficiency ratios
USE **PER**

Protein engineering
HN heading from vol. 24 (1992)
BT1 Genetic techniques
BT2 Genetics
BT1 Modification
NT1 Site directed mutagenesis
RT Genetic engineering
RT Sequencing

Protein-glutamine γ-glutamyltransferases
SN EC 2.3.2.13
BT1 Acyltransferases
BT2 Transferases
BT3 Enzymes
UF Transglutaminases

Protein hydrolysates
BT1 Proteins
BT2 Nutrients
NT1 Peptones
RT Peptides

Protein isolates
BT1 Proteins
BT2 Nutrients

Protein kinases
USE **Kinases**

Protein products
NT1 Caseinates
NT2 Sodium caseinate
NT1 Incaparina
NT1 Proteinates
NT1 Protein concentrates
NT2 FPC
NT2 Milk protein concentrates
NT2 Pea protein concentrates
NT2 Soy protein concentrates
NT2 Whey protein concentrates
RT Proteins
RT Proteins animal
RT Proteins cereal
RT Proteins milk
RT Proteins vegetable

Proteins
BT1 Nutrients
NT1 Albumins
NT2 Bovine serum albumin
NT2 Conalbumin
NT2 Lactalbumins
NT3 α-Lactalbumin
NT2 Ovalbumins
NT1 Angiogenin
NT1 Antifreeze proteins
NT1 Apoproteins
NT1 Calmodulin
NT1 Chaperones
NT1 σ Factors
NT1 Ferritin
NT1 Fusion proteins
NT1 Globulins
NT2 Actins
NT3 F-actin
NT2 Actomyosin
NT2 Arachin
NT2 Edestin
NT2 γ-Globulins
NT2 Immunoglobulins
NT3 Immunoglobulin A
NT3 Immunoglobulin E
NT3 Immunoglobulin G

NT3 Immunoglobulin Y
NT2 Lactoferrin
NT2 Lactoglobulins
NT3 β-Lactoglobulin
NT2 Legumin
NT2 Myosin
NT3 Myosin heavy chains
NT3 Myosin light chains
NT2 11S Globulins
NT2 7S Globulins
NT2 Vicilin
NT1 Glycoproteins
NT2 Avidin
NT2 Bifidus factors
NT2 Lectins
NT3 Concanavalin A
NT3 Haemagglutinins
NT3 Phytohaemagglutinins
NT3 Ricin
NT2 Mannoproteins
NT2 Miraculin
NT2 Mucins
NT2 Mucoids
NT2 Ovomucins
NT2 Ovomucoid
NT2 Ovotransferrin
NT2 Transferrins
NT1 Haemocyanin
NT1 Histones
NT1 Integrins
NT1 Kjeldahl nitrogen
NT1 Lipoproteins
NT2 High density lipoproteins
NT2 Lipovitellins
NT2 Low density lipoproteins
NT2 Purothionin
NT1 Marker proteins
NT2 Green fluorescent protein
NT1 Metallothioneins
NT1 Microbial proteins
NT2 Adhesins
NT2 Aerolysins
NT2 Flagellins
NT2 Fungal proteins
NT2 Intimins
NT2 Invasins
NT2 Pilins
NT2 Porins
NT2 Siderophores
NT2 Yeast proteins
NT1 Mycoprotein
NT2 Quorn
NT1 Peptides
NT2 Anserine
NT2 Balenine
NT2 Bioactive peptides
NT2 Bitter peptides
NT2 Carnosine
NT2 Caseinomacropeptides
NT2 Dipeptides
NT3 Dipeptide sweeteners
NT2 Glutathione
NT2 Glycomacropeptides
NT2 Glycopeptides
NT2 Lactoferricin
NT2 Lysinoalanine
NT2 Oligopeptides
NT2 Phosphopeptides
NT2 Polylysine
NT2 Polypeptides
NT1 Phycoerythrin
NT1 R-phycoerythrin
NT1 Plasteins
NT1 Prions
NT1 Profilins
NT1 Protein hydrolysates
NT2 Peptones
NT1 Protein isolates
NT1 Proteins animal
NT2 Animal proteins
NT3 Actins
NT4 F-actin
NT3 Actomyosin
NT3 Blood proteins
NT3 Bovine serum albumin
NT3 Collagen
NT4 Collagen sausage casings
NT3 Connectin
NT3 Desmin
NT3 Egg proteins
NT4 Avidin
NT4 Conalbumin
NT4 Ovalbumins
NT4 Ovomucins
NT4 Ovomucoid
NT4 Ovotransferrin
NT4 Phosvitin
NT3 Elastin
NT3 Fibrin
NT3 Fibrinogen
NT3 Fish proteins
NT3 Gelatin
NT4 Isinglass
NT3 Globins
NT3 γ-Globulins
NT3 Haemoglobin
NT3 Haemoproteins
NT3 Immunoglobulins
NT4 Immunoglobulin A
NT4 Immunoglobulin E
NT4 Immunoglobulin G
NT4 Immunoglobulin Y
NT3 Keratin
NT3 Lactoferrin
NT3 Mucins
NT3 Myofibrillar proteins
NT3 Myoglobin
NT4 Deoxymyoglobin
NT4 Metmyoglobin
NT4 Nitrosylmyoglobin
NT4 Oxymyoglobin
NT3 Myosin
NT4 Myosin heavy chains
NT4 Myosin light chains
NT3 Protamine
NT3 Proteins milk
NT4 Milk proteins
NT5 Butyrophilin
NT5 Casein
NT6 Acid casein
NT6 α_s-Casein
NT6 α_{s1}-Casein
NT6 α_{s2}-Casein
NT6 β-Casein
NT6 γ-Casein
NT6 κ-Casein
NT6 Casein micelles
NT5 β-Casomorphins
NT5 Lactalbumins
NT6 α-Lactalbumin
NT5 Lactoglobulins
NT6 β-Lactoglobulin
NT5 Milk protein concentrates
NT5 Proteose peptones
NT5 Whey proteins
NT6 Whey protein concentrates
NT3 Sarcoplasmic proteins
NT3 Titin
NT3 Transferrins
NT3 Tropomyosin
NT3 Troponin
NT1 Proteins high diet
NT1 Proteins high foods
NT1 Proteins vegetable
NT2 Vegetable proteins
NT3 Arachin
NT3 Carmin
NT3 Conarachin
NT3 Cottonseed proteins
NT3 Cruciferins
NT3 Dioscorin
NT3 Edestin
NT3 Expansins
NT3 Helianthinin
NT3 Leaf proteins
NT3 Lectins
NT4 Concanavalin A
NT4 Haemagglutinins
NT4 Phytohaemagglutinins
NT4 Ricin
NT3 Legume proteins
NT3 Legumin
NT3 Lupin proteins
NT3 Napins
NT3 Oilseed proteins
NT3 Oleosins
NT3 Patatin
NT3 Peanut proteins
NT3 Pea proteins
NT3 Phaseolins
NT3 Plant proteins
NT3 Proteins cereal
NT4 Cereal proteins
NT5 Avenins
NT5 Friabilins
NT5 Gliadins
NT5 Glutelins
NT5 Gluten
NT6 Gluten low foods
NT7 Gluten low bread
NT6 Vital gluten
NT6 Wheat gluten
NT5 Glutenin
NT5 Hordein
NT5 Hordothionins
NT5 Kafirins
NT5 Opaque 2
NT5 Oryzenin
NT5 Prolamins
NT5 Puroindolines
NT5 Purothionin
NT5 Secalins
NT5 Thionins
NT5 Zein

NT3 11S Globulins
NT3 7S Globulins
NT3 Soy proteins
NT4 Conglycinin
NT4 β-Conglycinin
NT4 Glycinin
NT4 Promine
NT4 Soy globulins
NT4 Soy glycinin
NT4 Soy protein concentrates
NT4 Soy 11S globulins
NT4 Soy 7S globulins
NT3 Storage proteins
NT3 Textured vegetable proteins
NT3 Vicilin
NT1 Proteoglycans
NT1 Proteomics
NT1 Recombinant proteins
NT1 Selenoproteins
NT1 Single cell proteins
NT1 Stress proteins
NT2 Cold shock proteins
NT2 Heat shock proteins
NT1 Sweet proteins
NT2 Brazzein
NT2 Curculin
NT2 Monellin
NT2 Thaumatin
NT1 Thioredoxin
RT Active sites
RT Denaturation
RT Macronutrients
RT Protein products
RT Sequencing
RT Transcription factors

Proteins animal
SN animal proteins also used in the index
BT1 Proteins
BT2 Nutrients
NT1 Animal proteins
NT2 Actins
NT3 F-actin
NT2 Actomyosin
NT2 Blood proteins
NT2 Bovine serum albumin
NT2 Collagen
NT3 Collagen sausage casings
NT2 Connectin
NT2 Desmin
NT2 Egg proteins
NT3 Avidin
NT3 Conalbumin
NT3 Ovalbumins
NT3 Ovomucins
NT3 Ovomucoid
NT3 Ovotransferrin
NT3 Phosvitin
NT2 Elastin
NT2 Fibrin
NT2 Fibrinogen
NT2 Fish proteins
NT2 Gelatin
NT3 Isinglass
NT2 Globins
NT2 γ-Globulins
NT2 Haemoglobin
NT2 Haemoproteins
NT2 Immunoglobulins
NT3 Immunoglobulin A
NT3 Immunoglobulin E
NT3 Immunoglobulin G
NT3 Immunoglobulin Y
NT2 Keratin
NT2 Lactoferrin
NT2 Mucins
NT2 Myofibrillar proteins
NT2 Myoglobin
NT3 Deoxymyoglobin
NT3 Metmyoglobin
NT3 Nitrosylmyoglobin
NT3 Oxymyoglobin
NT2 Myosin
NT3 Myosin heavy chains
NT3 Myosin light chains
NT2 Protamine
NT2 Proteins milk
NT3 Milk proteins
NT4 Butyrophilin
NT4 Casein
NT5 Acid casein
NT5 α_s-Casein
NT5 α_{s1}-Casein
NT5 α_{s2}-Casein
NT5 β-Casein
NT5 γ-Casein
NT5 κ-Casein
NT5 Casein micelles
NT4 β-Casomorphins
NT4 Lactalbumins
NT5 α-Lactalbumin
NT4 Lactoglobulins
NT5 β-Lactoglobulin
NT4 Milk protein concentrates
NT4 Proteose peptones
NT4 Whey proteins
NT5 Whey protein concentrates
NT2 Sarcoplasmic proteins
NT2 Titin
NT2 Transferrins
NT2 Tropomyosin
NT2 Troponin
RT Protein products

Proteins cereal
SN cereal proteins also used in the index
BT1 Vegetable proteins
BT2 Proteins vegetable
BT3 Proteins
BT4 Nutrients
BT3 Vegetable products
BT4 Plant foods
BT5 Foods
NT1 Cereal proteins
NT2 Avenins
NT2 Friabilins
NT2 Gliadins
NT2 Glutelins
NT2 Gluten
NT3 Gluten low foods
NT4 Gluten low bread
NT3 Vital gluten
NT3 Wheat gluten
NT2 Glutenin
NT2 Hordein
NT2 Hordothionins
NT2 Kafirins
NT2 Opaque 2
NT2 Oryzenin
NT2 Prolamins
NT2 Puroindolines
NT2 Purothionin
NT2 Secalins
NT2 Thionins
NT2 Zein
RT Protein products

Proteins high diet
HN introduced from vol. 41, issue 1 (2009)
BT1 Diet
BT2 Nutrition
BT1 Proteins
BT2 Nutrients
UF High protein diet

Proteins high foods
HN introduced from vol. 39, issue 1 (2007)
BT1 Proteins
BT2 Nutrients
UF High protein foods

Proteins milk
SN milk proteins also used in the index
BT1 Animal proteins
BT2 Proteins animal
BT3 Proteins
BT4 Nutrients
NT1 Milk proteins
NT2 Butyrophilin
NT2 Casein
NT3 Acid casein
NT3 α_s-Casein
NT3 α_{s1}-Casein
NT3 α_{s2}-Casein
NT3 β-Casein
NT3 γ-Casein
NT3 κ-Casein
NT3 Casein micelles
NT2 β-Casomorphins
NT2 Lactalbumins
NT3 α-Lactalbumin
NT2 Lactoglobulins
NT3 β-Lactoglobulin
NT2 Milk protein concentrates
NT2 Proteose peptones
NT2 Whey proteins
NT3 Whey protein concentrates
RT Protein products

Proteins vegetable
SN vegetable proteins also used in the index
BT1 Proteins
BT2 Nutrients
BT1 Vegetable products
BT2 Plant foods
BT3 Foods
NT1 Vegetable proteins
NT2 Arachin
NT2 Carmin
NT2 Conarachin
NT2 Cottonseed proteins
NT2 Cruciferins
NT2 Dioscorin
NT2 Edestin

NT2 Expansins
NT2 Helianthinin
NT2 Leaf proteins
NT2 Lectins
NT3 Concanavalin A
NT3 Haemagglutinins
NT3 Phytohaemagglutinins
NT3 Ricin
NT2 Legume proteins
NT2 Legumin
NT2 Lupin proteins
NT2 Napins
NT2 Oilseed proteins
NT2 Oleosins
NT2 Patatin
NT2 Peanut proteins
NT2 Pea proteins
NT2 Phaseolins
NT2 Plant proteins
NT2 Proteins cereal
NT3 Cereal proteins
NT4 Avenins
NT4 Friabilins
NT4 Gliadins
NT4 Glutelins
NT4 Gluten
NT5 Gluten low foods
NT6 Gluten low bread
NT5 Vital gluten
NT5 Wheat gluten
NT4 Glutenin
NT4 Hordein
NT4 Hordothionins
NT4 Kafirins
NT4 Opaque 2
NT4 Oryzenin
NT4 Prolamins
NT4 Puroindolines
NT4 Purothionin
NT4 Secalins
NT4 Thionins
NT4 Zein
NT2 11S Globulins
NT2 7S Globulins
NT2 Soy proteins
NT3 Conglycinin
NT3 β-Conglycinin
NT3 Glycinin
NT3 Promine
NT3 Soy globulins
NT3 Soy glycinin
NT3 Soy protein concentrates
NT3 Soy 11S globulins
NT3 Soy 7S globulins
NT2 Storage proteins
NT2 Textured vegetable proteins
NT2 Vicilin
RT Protein products

Protein values
BT1 Nutritional values

Proteobacteria
HN introduced from vol. 39, issue 1 (2007)
BT1 Bacteria
BT2 Microorganisms

Proteoglycans
HN under Glucans up to vol. 42 (2010)
BT1 Polysaccharides
BT2 Carbohydrates
BT3 Nutrients
BT3 Organic compounds
BT1 Proteins
BT2 Nutrients

Proteolipids
BT1 Lipids
BT2 Nutrients

Proteolysis
BT1 Hydrolysis
RT Proteinases

Proteolytic enzymes
USE **Proteinases**

Proteomics
HN introduced from vol. 39, issue 1 (2007)
BT1 Analytical techniques
BT1 Proteins
BT2 Nutrients
RT Genomics
RT Metabolomics
RT Microarrays

Proteose peptones
BT1 Milk proteins
BT2 Proteins milk
BT3 Animal proteins
BT4 Proteins animal
BT5 Proteins
BT6 Nutrients

Proteus
HN heading from vol. 25 (1993); under Bacteria up to vol. 24 (1992)
BT1 Bacteria
BT2 Microorganisms
NT1 *Proteus mirabilis*
NT1 *Proteus vulgaris*

Proteus mirabilis
HN introduced from vol. 39, issue 1 (2007)
BT1 *Proteus*
BT2 Bacteria
BT3 Microorganisms

Proteus vulgaris
BT1 *Proteus*
BT2 Bacteria
BT3 Microorganisms

Protocatechuic acid
BT1 Organic acids
BT2 Acids
BT1 Phenols
BT2 Alcohols
BT2 Aromatic compounds
BT3 Organic compounds

Proton magnetic resonance
BT1 Nuclear magnetic resonance
BT2 Spectroscopy
BT3 Analytical techniques

Proton resonance
BT1 Nuclear magnetic resonance
BT2 Spectroscopy
BT3 Analytical techniques

Protoplast fusion
BT1 Gene transfer
BT2 Gene cloning
BT3 Genetic techniques
BT4 Genetics

Protoplasts
BT1 Cells

Protozoa
BT1 Microorganisms
RT Eukaryotes
RT Oocysts

Providencia
HN under Enterobacteriaceae up to vol. 24 (1992)
BT1 Bacteria
BT2 Microorganisms

Provitamin A
BT1 Carotenes
BT2 Carotenoids
BT3 Pigments
BT3 Terpenoids
BT4 Lipids
BT5 Nutrients

Provolone cheese
BT1 Cheese varieties
BT2 Cheese
BT3 Dairy products
BT4 Animal foods
BT5 Foods

Prunasin
BT1 Cyanogens
BT2 Cyanides
BT3 Salts
BT1 Glycosides
BT2 Carbohydrates
BT3 Nutrients
BT3 Organic compounds

Prune juices
BT1 Fruit juices
BT2 Fruit products
BT3 Plant foods
BT4 Foods
BT2 Soft drinks
BT3 Beverages
RT Prunes

Prunes
BT1 Dried fruits
BT2 Fruits dried
BT3 Dried foods
BT4 Processed foods
BT5 Foods
BT3 Fruits
BT4 Crops
BT5 Plants
BT4 Plant foods
BT5 Foods
RT Plums
RT Prune juices

Pruning
BT1 Cultivation
BT2 Agriculture

Prunus mume
BT1 Japanese apricots
BT2 Fruits specific
BT3 Fruits
BT4 Crops
BT5 Plants
BT4 Plant foods
BT5 Foods

PSE defect
BT1 Genetic disorders
RT Animal stress
UF Pale soft exudative defect

Pseudoalteromonas
HN introduced from vol. 41, issue 1 (2009)
BT1 Bacteria
BT2 Microorganisms

Pseudocardium sachalinensis
BT1 Clams
BT2 Bivalves
BT3 Molluscs
BT4 Shellfish
BT5 Animals
BT5 Sea foods
BT6 Aquatic foods
BT7 Animal foods
BT8 Foods

Pseudocereals
HN heading from vol. 25 (1993)
BT1 Seeds
BT2 Plant foods
BT3 Foods
NT1 Amaranth grain
NT2 Amaranth flour
NT2 Amaranth starch
NT2 *Amaranthus*
NT2 Grain amaranth
NT1 Buckwheat
NT2 Buckwheat flour
NT2 Buckwheat starch
NT1 Canary grass
NT1 Quinoa
NT2 Quinoa flour

Pseudomonadaceae
HN heading up to vol. 24 (1992)
BT1 Bacteria
BT2 Microorganisms

Pseudomonas
HN heading from vol. 25 (1993); under Pseudomonadaceae up to vol. 24 (1992)
BT1 Bacteria
BT2 Microorganisms
NT1 *Pseudomonas aeruginosa*
NT1 *Pseudomonas cellulosa*
NT1 *Pseudomonas cepacia*
NT1 *Pseudomonas fluorescens*
NT1 *Pseudomonas fragi*
NT1 *Pseudomonas marginalis*
NT1 *Pseudomonas pseudoalcaligenes*
NT1 *Pseudomonas putida*
NT1 *Pseudomonas stutzeri*
NT1 *Pseudomonas syringae*
RT *Burkholderia*

Pseudomonas aeruginosa
BT1 *Pseudomonas*
BT2 Bacteria
BT3 Microorganisms

Pseudomonas cellulosa
SN synonymous with Cellvibrio japonicus
BT1 *Pseudomonas*
BT2 Bacteria
BT3 Microorganisms

Pseudomonas cepacia
SN synonymous with Burkholderia cepacia
BT1 *Pseudomonas*
BT2 Bacteria
BT3 Microorganisms

Pseudomonas fluorescens
BT1 *Pseudomonas*
BT2 Bacteria
BT3 Microorganisms

Pseudomonas fragi
BT1 *Pseudomonas*
BT2 Bacteria
BT3 Microorganisms

Pseudomonas marginalis
BT1 *Pseudomonas*
BT2 Bacteria
BT3 Microorganisms

Pseudomonas pseudoalcaligenes
BT1 *Pseudomonas*
BT2 Bacteria
BT3 Microorganisms

Pseudomonas putida
BT1 *Pseudomonas*
BT2 Bacteria
BT3 Microorganisms

Pseudomonas stutzeri
HN introduced from vol. 39, issue 1 (2007)
BT1 *Pseudomonas*
BT2 Bacteria
BT3 Microorganisms

Pseudomonas syringae
BT1 *Pseudomonas*
BT2 Bacteria
BT3 Microorganisms

Pseudoterranova
BT1 Parasites
BT2 Pests
RT Anisakiasis

Psicose
HN under Sugars up to vol. 42 (2010)
BT1 Monosaccharides
BT2 Sugars
BT3 Carbohydrates
BT4 Nutrients
BT4 Organic compounds
BT3 Plant foods
BT4 Foods

Psocids
BT1 Insects
BT2 Pests
RT *Liposcelis*

Psoralens
BT1 Furocoumarins
BT2 Coumarins
BT3 Lactones
BT4 Esters
BT5 Organic compounds
BT4 Heterocyclic compounds
BT3 Phenols
BT4 Alcohols
BT4 Aromatic compounds
BT5 Organic compounds

PSP
BT1 Paralytic shellfish poisoning
BT2 Diseases
BT2 Poisoning

Psychiatric disorders
HN introduced from vol. 39, issue 1 (2007)
SN includes clinical depression, neuroses, schizophrenia, etc.
BT1 Diseases
NT1 Eating disorders
RT Mental health
RT Mood
RT Neurodegenerative diseases

Psychophysiological effects
BT1 Human physiology
BT2 Physiology
BT3 Science
RT Behavioural effects

Psychrobacter
BT1 Bacteria
BT2 Microorganisms
NT1 *Psychrobacter immobilis*

Psychrobacter immobilis
BT1 *Psychrobacter*
BT2 Bacteria
BT3 Microorganisms

Psychrophiles
SN organisms which grow at less than 15 C
BT1 Microorganisms
RT Mesophiles
RT Psychrotrophs
RT Thermophiles

Psychrotrophs
SN organisms which grow at 0-5 C but which grow optimally between 15 and 20 C
BT1 Microorganisms
RT Mesophiles
RT Psychrophiles
RT Thermophiles

Psyllium
BT1 Seeds
BT2 Plant foods
BT3 Foods
RT Psyllium gums

Psyllium gums
BT1 Gums
BT2 Polysaccharides
BT3 Carbohydrates
BT4 Nutrients
BT4 Organic compounds
BT2 Stabilizers
BT3 Additives
BT2 Thickeners
BT3 Additives
RT Psyllium

Pt
HN under Minerals up to vol. 42 (2010)
BT1 Metals
BT2 Elements
BT3 Minerals
BT4 Nutrients
UF Platinum

Ptarmigans
BT1 Birds

PTFE
BT1 Plastics
BT2 Packaging materials
UF Polytetrafluoroethylene

Pu
BT1 Radioelements
BT2 Isotopes
BT3 Elements
BT4 Minerals
BT5 Nutrients
BT2 Residues
UF Plutonium

Puberty
HN introduced from vol. 39, issue 1 (2007)
BT1 Physiology
BT2 Science

Public health
HN introduced from vol. 39, issue 1 (2007)
RT Food safety

Pub meals
BT1 Meals
BT2 Processed foods
BT3 Foods

Pubs
RT Inn breweries
RT Restaurants

Pudding mixes
BT1 Desserts
BT2 Processed foods
BT3 Foods

Puddings
BT1 Desserts
BT2 Processed foods
BT3 Foods

Puerarin
HN introduced from vol. 41, issue 1 (2009)
BT1 Glucosides
BT2 Glycosides
BT3 Carbohydrates
BT4 Nutrients
BT4 Organic compounds
BT1 Isoflavones
BT2 Isoflavonoids
BT3 Flavonoids
BT4 Aromatic compounds
BT5 Organic compounds
BT4 Pigments
RT Daidzein
RT Kudzu

Pu-erh tea
HN under Teas up to vol. 42 (2010)
BT1 Tea
BT2 Teas
BT3 Beverages
BT3 Crops
BT4 Plants
BT3 Plant foods
BT4 Foods

Puerto Rico
BT1 West Indies
BT2 America

PUFA
HN heading from vol. 43 (2011); under Fatty acids up to vol. 42 (2010); polyunsaturated fatty acids also used in the index up to vol. 35, issue 6 (2003)
BT1 Unsaturated fatty acids
BT2 Fatty acids
BT3 Lipids
BT4 Nutrients
BT3 Organic acids
BT4 Acids
NT1 Conjugated fatty acids
NT2 CLA
NT2 Eleostearic acid
NT1 Eicosatetraenoic acid
NT2 Arachidonic acid
NT1 ω-3 Fatty acids
NT2 Docosahexaenoic acid
NT2 Docosapentaenoic acid
NT2 Eicosapentaenoic acid
NT2 α-Linolenic acid
NT2 Stearidonic acid
NT1 ω-6 Fatty acids
NT2 Arachidonic acid
NT2 Linoleic acid
NT3 CLA
NT2 γ-Linolenic acid
NT1 Linolenic acid
NT2 Eleostearic acid
NT2 α-Linolenic acid
NT2 γ-Linolenic acid
RT Unsaturation
UF Polyunsaturated fatty acids

Puff balls
USE ***Lycoperdon***

Puffed rice
BT1 Rice
BT2 Cereals
BT3 Crops
BT4 Plants
BT3 Seeds
BT4 Plant foods
BT5 Foods

Pufferfish
BT1 Marine fish
BT2 Fish
BT3 Animals
BT3 Sea foods
BT4 Aquatic foods
BT5 Animal foods
BT6 Foods

Puffing
BT1 Processing
BT2 Technology

Puff pastry
BT1 Pastry
BT2 Bakery products
BT3 Cereal products
BT4 Plant foods
BT5 Foods

Pullet eggs
USE **Eggs**

Pullulan
HN under Polysaccharides up to vol. 42 (2010)
BT1 Glucans
BT2 Polysaccharides
BT3 Carbohydrates
BT4 Nutrients
BT4 Organic compounds
RT *Aureobasidium pullulans*
RT Exopolysaccharides

Pullulanases
HN used up to vol. 31 (1999) and from vol. 39 (2007)
SN EC 3.2.1.41
BT1 Glycosidases
BT2 Hydrolases
BT3 Enzymes
UF Debranching enzymes
UF α-Dextrin endo-1,6-α-glucosidases

Pulpboard
BT1 Board
BT2 Packaging materials

Pulping
BT1 Processing
BT2 Technology
RT Comminution

Pulps
BT1 Processed foods
BT2 Foods
NT1 Fruit pulps
NT2 Apple pulps
NT2 Apricot pulps
NT2 Banana pulps
NT2 Guava pulps

NT2 Mango pulps
NT2 Peach pulps
NT2 Strawberry pulps
NT2 Tomato pulps
NT1 Purees
NT2 Fruit purees
NT3 Apple purees
NT3 Apricot purees
NT3 Banana purees
NT3 Guava purees
NT3 Mango purees
NT3 Peach purees
NT3 Strawberry purees
NT3 Tomato purees
NT2 Vegetable purees
NT3 Potato purees
NT3 Soy purees
NT1 Vegetable pulps
NT2 Carrot pulps

Pulque
BT1 Alcoholic beverages
BT2 Beverages alcoholic
BT3 Beverages

Pulsatilla cernua
BT1 Plants

Pulsed electric fields
BT1 Electric fields
BT2 Electricity
BT3 Energy
BT1 Processing
BT2 Technology

Pulsed field gel electrophoresis
HN used in the index up to vol. 35, issue 6 (2003)
USE **PFGE**

Pulses
BT1 Legumes
BT2 Vegetables specific
BT3 Vegetables
BT4 Crops
BT5 Plants
BT4 Plant foods
BT5 Foods

Pulverization
BT1 Comminution
BT2 Processing
BT3 Technology

Pummelos
SN syn. pomelos, shaddocks
BT1 Pomelos
BT2 Citrus fruits
BT3 Fruits specific
BT4 Fruits
BT5 Crops
BT6 Plants
BT5 Plant foods
BT6 Foods

Pumpernickel
BT1 Bread
BT2 Bakery products
BT3 Cereal products
BT4 Plant foods
BT5 Foods

Pumpkins
HN heading from vol. 30 (1998); under Vegetables specific up to vol. 29 (1997)
BT1 Vegetables specific
BT2 Vegetables
BT3 Crops
BT4 Plants
BT3 Plant foods
BT4 Foods
NT1 Fluted pumpkins

Pumpkin seed oils
BT1 Vegetable oils
BT2 Oils vegetable
BT3 Oils
BT4 Lipids
BT5 Nutrients
BT3 Vegetable products
BT4 Plant foods
BT5 Foods

Pumpkin seeds
BT1 Oilseeds
BT2 Seeds
BT3 Plant foods
BT4 Foods

Pumps
BT1 Equipment
BT2 Technology

Pungency
BT1 Aroma
BT2 Sensory properties

Pungent principles
BT1 Flavour compounds
NT1 Allicin
NT1 Allyl isothiocyanate
NT1 Capsaicinoids
NT2 Capsaicin
NT1 Gingerols
NT1 Piperine
NT1 Zingerone

Punnets
BT1 Packs
BT2 Containers

Puppy foods
HN introduced from vol. 39, issue 1 (2007)
BT1 Dog foods
BT2 Pet foods
RT Dogs

Purchase
BT1 Markets
BT2 Economics
RT Purchasing behaviour

Purchasing behaviour
HN introduced from vol. 39, issue 1 (2007)
BT1 Consumer behaviour
BT2 Consumer response
RT Purchase

Purees
BT1 Pulps
BT2 Processed foods
BT3 Foods
NT1 Fruit purees
NT2 Apple purees
NT2 Apricot purees
NT2 Banana purees
NT2 Guava purees
NT2 Mango purees
NT2 Peach purees
NT2 Strawberry purees
NT2 Tomato purees
NT1 Vegetable purees
NT2 Potato purees
NT2 Soy purees

Purge loss
HN introduced from vol. 39, issue 1 (2007)
BT1 Thawing
BT2 Thermal processing
BT3 Processing thermal
BT4 Processing
BT5 Technology

Purification
BT1 Processing
BT2 Technology
NT1 Defecation
NT1 Deodorization
NT1 Downstream processing
NT1 Epuration
NT1 Refining
NT2 Affination

Purines
BT1 Heterocyclic compounds
BT1 Organic nitrogen compounds
NT1 Adenine
NT1 Caffeine
NT1 Theobromine
NT1 Theophylline
NT1 Uric acid

Purity
NT1 Authenticity
RT Adulteration
RT Contamination
RT Impurities

Puroindolines
HN introduced from vol. 37, issue 5 (2005)
BT1 Cereal proteins
BT2 Proteins cereal
BT3 Vegetable proteins
BT4 Proteins vegetable
BT5 Proteins
BT6 Nutrients
BT5 Vegetable products
BT6 Plant foods
BT7 Foods

Purothionin
BT1 Cereal proteins
BT2 Proteins cereal
BT3 Vegetable proteins
BT4 Proteins vegetable
BT5 Proteins
BT6 Nutrients
BT5 Vegetable products
BT6 Plant foods

BT7 Foods
BT1 Lipoproteins
BT2 Proteins
BT3 Nutrients

Purslane
BT1 Vegetables specific
BT2 Vegetables
BT3 Crops
BT4 Plants
BT3 Plant foods
BT4 Foods

Puto
BT1 Fermented foods
BT2 Processed foods
BT3 Foods
BT1 Rice
BT2 Cereals
BT3 Crops
BT4 Plants
BT3 Seeds
BT4 Plant foods
BT5 Foods

Putrefaction
BT1 Spoilage

Putrescine
BT1 Biogenic amines
BT2 Amines
BT3 Organic nitrogen compounds
BT1 Polyamines
BT2 Amines
BT3 Organic nitrogen compounds

PVC
SN index heading is Polyvinyl chloride
BT1 Polyvinyl chloride
BT2 Plastics
BT3 Packaging materials

PVDC
SN syn. Saran
BT1 Plastics
BT2 Packaging materials
UF Polyvinylidene chloride

Pycnometry
BT1 Analytical techniques

Pycnoporus
HN introduced from vol. 43, issue 1 (2011)
BT1 Fungi
BT2 Microorganisms
NT1 *Pycnoporus cinnabarinus*

Pycnoporus cinnabarinus
BT1 *Pycnoporus*
BT2 Fungi
BT3 Microorganisms

Pyramin
USE **Chloridazon**

Pyranoanthocyanins
HN introduced from vol. 41, issue 1 (2009)
BT1 Anthocyanins
BT2 Flavonoids
BT3 Aromatic compounds
BT4 Organic compounds
BT3 Pigments

Pyrazines
HN also under Flavour compounds up to vol. 42 (2010)
BT1 Aroma compounds
BT2 Flavour compounds
BT2 Volatile compounds
BT1 Heterocyclic compounds
BT1 Organic nitrogen compounds
RT Maillard reaction products

Pyrazon
USE **Chloridazon**

Pyrene
BT1 Aromatic compounds
BT2 Organic compounds

Pyrethrins
BT1 Pyrethroid insecticides
BT2 Insecticides
BT3 Pesticides
BT4 Biocides
BT4 Residues

Pyrethroid insecticides
BT1 Insecticides
BT2 Pesticides
BT3 Biocides
BT3 Residues
NT1 Allethrin
NT1 Cypermethrin
NT1 Deltamethrin
NT1 Fenvalerate
NT1 Fluvalinate
NT1 Permethrin
NT1 Pyrethrins
NT1 Resmethrin

Pyridine
BT1 Heterocyclic compounds
BT1 Organic nitrogen compounds
BT1 Solvents
BT1 Volatile compounds

Pyridoxal
BT1 Vitamin B_6
BT2 Vitamin B group
BT3 Vitamins
BT4 Nutrients

Pyridoxamine
BT1 Vitamin B_6
BT2 Vitamin B group
BT3 Vitamins
BT4 Nutrients

Pyridoxine
BT1 Vitamin B_6
BT2 Vitamin B group
BT3 Vitamins
BT4 Nutrients

Pyrimethamine
BT1 Coccidiostats
BT2 Drugs
BT3 Residues

Pyrimethanil
HN introduced from vol. 41, issue 1 (2009)
BT1 Fungicides
BT2 Pesticides
BT3 Biocides
BT3 Residues

Pyrimidines
BT1 Heterocyclic compounds
BT1 Organic nitrogen compounds
NT1 Barbituric acid
NT1 Cytosine
NT1 Propylthiouracil
NT1 Thymine
NT1 Uracil

Pyrocarbonic acid diethyl ester
BT1 Esters
BT2 Organic compounds
BT1 Preservatives
BT2 Additives

Pyrocatechol
BT1 Catechols
BT2 Flavanols
BT3 Flavonoids
BT4 Aromatic compounds
BT5 Organic compounds
BT4 Pigments
BT2 Phenols
BT3 Alcohols
BT3 Aromatic compounds
BT4 Organic compounds

Pyrococcus
BT1 Archaea
BT2 Microorganisms
NT1 *Pyrococcus furiosus*

Pyrococcus furiosus
BT1 *Pyrococcus*
BT2 Archaea
BT3 Microorganisms

Pyrodextrins
HN introduced from vol. 39, issue 1 (2007)
BT1 Dextrins
BT2 Starch
BT3 Glucans
BT4 Polysaccharides
BT5 Carbohydrates
BT6 Nutrients
BT6 Organic compounds
BT3 Thickeners
BT4 Additives

Pyrogallol
BT1 Phenols
BT2 Alcohols
BT2 Aromatic compounds
BT3 Organic compounds

Pyroglutamic acid
BT1 Amino acids
BT2 Nutrients
BT2 Organic acids

BT3 Acids
BT2 Organic nitrogen compounds

Pyrolysis
BT1 Analytical techniques
BT1 Lysis
BT2 Decomposition

Pyrones
BT1 Heterocyclic compounds
NT1 Kojic acid
NT1 Maltol
RT Aroma compounds

Pyrophosphatases
BT1 Hydrolases
BT2 Enzymes

Pyrophosphates
BT1 Phosphates
BT2 Salts

Pyrroles
HN heading up to vol. 24 (1992); also under Aroma compounds up to vol. 42 (2010)
BT1 Heterocyclic compounds
BT1 Organic nitrogen compounds
RT Aroma compounds
RT Maillard reaction products
RT Pigments

Pyrrolizidine alkaloids
HN introduced from vol. 39, issue 1 (2007)
BT1 Alkaloids
BT2 Organic nitrogen compounds
BT1 Toxins
BT2 Residues

Pyruvaldehyde
SN syn. methylglyoxal
BT1 Aldehydes
BT2 Carbonyl compounds
BT3 Organic compounds

Pyruvate carboxylases
SN EC 6.4.1.1
BT1 Ligases
BT2 Enzymes

Pyruvate decarboxylases
SN EC 4.1.1.1
BT1 Lyases
BT2 Enzymes

Pyruvic acid
HN heading up to vol. 24 (1992)
BT1 Organic acids
BT2 Acids

Q

Qatar
BT1 Asia
BT1 Middle East

QTL
BT1 Genes
BT2 Chromosomes
BT3 Genetics
BT2 Genomes
BT3 Genetics
UF Quantitative trait loci

Quail carcasses
BT1 Carcasses
BT2 Meat
BT3 Animal foods
BT4 Foods
BT1 Quail meat
BT2 Poultry meat
BT3 Meat specific
BT4 Meat
BT5 Animal foods
BT6 Foods
BT2 Quails
BT3 Poultry
BT4 Birds
BT1 Quails
BT2 Poultry
BT3 Birds

Quail eggs
BT1 Eggs
BT2 Animal foods
BT3 Foods
BT1 Quails
BT2 Poultry
BT3 Birds

Quail meat
BT1 Poultry meat
BT2 Meat specific
BT3 Meat
BT4 Animal foods
BT5 Foods
BT1 Quails
BT2 Poultry
BT3 Birds
NT1 Quail carcasses

Quails
BT1 Poultry
BT2 Birds
NT1 Quail carcasses
NT1 Quail eggs
NT1 Quail meat
NT2 Quail carcasses

Quality

Quality assurance
BT1 Quality control
BT2 Technology

Quality control
BT1 Technology
NT1 Critical control points
NT1 Good Manufacturing Practice
NT1 HACCP
NT1 Image processing
NT1 Inspection
NT1 Quality assurance
NT1 Time temp. integrators
NT1 Total quality management
NT1 Veterinary inspection
NT1 Vision systems
RT Analytical techniques
RT TBA values
RT Thiobarbituric acid values

Quality of life
HN introduced from vol. 42, issue 1 (2010)
RT Economics
RT Health
RT Socioeconomic factors

Quantitative descriptive analysis
BT1 Sensory analysis
BT2 Analytical techniques

Quantitative trait loci
USE **QTL**

Quarg
BT1 Cheese varieties
BT2 Cheese
BT3 Dairy products
BT4 Animal foods
BT5 Foods
NT1 Tvaroh
NT1 Tvorog
NT1 Twarog
RT Curd

Quartirolo cheese
BT1 Cheese varieties
BT2 Cheese
BT3 Dairy products
BT4 Animal foods
BT5 Foods

Quassin
BT1 Bitter compounds
BT2 Flavour compounds
BT1 Triterpenoids
BT2 Terpenoids
BT3 Lipids
BT4 Nutrients

Quaternary ammonium compounds
BT1 Ammonium compounds
BT1 Disinfectants
BT2 Disinfection
BT3 Hygiene

Quercetin
BT1 Flavonols
BT2 Alcohols
BT2 Flavonoids
BT3 Aromatic compounds
BT4 Organic compounds
BT3 Pigments

Quercitrin
BT1 Flavonols
BT2 Alcohols
BT2 Flavonoids
BT3 Aromatic compounds
BT4 Organic compounds

BT3 Pigments
BT1 Glycosides
BT2 Carbohydrates
BT3 Nutrients
BT3 Organic compounds

Quercus mongolica
BT1 Plants

Queso Blanco cheese
BT1 Cheese varieties
BT2 Cheese
BT3 Dairy products
BT4 Animal foods
BT5 Foods

Queso fresco cheese
BT1 Cheese varieties
BT2 Cheese
BT3 Dairy products
BT4 Animal foods
BT5 Foods

Quiches
BT1 Pies
BT2 Bakery products
BT3 Cereal products
BT4 Plant foods
BT5 Foods

Quillaja saponaria
BT1 Plants
RT Quillaja saponins

Quillaja saponins
BT1 Saponins
BT2 Glycosides
BT3 Carbohydrates
BT4 Nutrients
BT4 Organic compounds
RT *Quillaja saponaria*

Quinalphos
BT1 Acaricides
BT2 Pesticides
BT3 Biocides
BT3 Residues
BT1 Organophosphorus insecticides
BT2 Insecticides
BT3 Pesticides
BT4 Biocides
BT4 Residues
BT2 Organophosphorus pesticides
BT3 Pesticides
BT4 Biocides
BT4 Residues
UF Bayrusil
UF Ekalux

Quince jams
BT1 Jams
BT2 Fruit preserves
BT3 Fruit products
BT4 Plant foods
BT5 Foods
BT3 Preserves
BT4 Processed foods
BT5 Foods
BT1 Quinces
BT2 Fruits specific
BT3 Fruits
BT4 Crops
BT5 Plants
BT4 Plant foods
BT5 Foods

Quince juices
BT1 Fruit juices
BT2 Fruit products
BT3 Plant foods
BT4 Foods
BT2 Soft drinks
BT3 Beverages
RT Quinces

Quinces
BT1 Fruits specific
BT2 Fruits
BT3 Crops
BT4 Plants
BT3 Plant foods
BT4 Foods
NT1 Quince jams
RT Quince juices

Quinic acid
BT1 Organic acids
BT2 Acids

Quinine
BT1 Alkaloids
BT2 Organic nitrogen compounds
BT1 Bitter compounds
BT2 Flavour compounds

Quinoa
BT1 Pseudocereals
BT2 Seeds
BT3 Plant foods
BT4 Foods
NT1 Quinoa flour

Quinoa flour
HN introduced from vol. 39, issue 1 (2007)
BT1 Cereal flours
BT2 Flours cereal
BT3 Cereal products
BT4 Plant foods
BT5 Foods
BT1 Quinoa
BT2 Pseudocereals
BT3 Seeds
BT4 Plant foods
BT5 Foods

Quinolones
BT1 Antibiotics
BT2 Drugs
BT3 Residues
NT1 Ciprofloxacin
NT1 Enrofloxacin
NT1 Flumequine
NT1 Nalidixic acid
NT1 Oxolinic acid

Quinomethionate
HN under Insecticides up to vol. 42 (2010)
SN also known as chinomethionat
BT1 Acaricides
BT2 Pesticides
BT3 Biocides
BT3 Residues
BT1 Fungicides
BT2 Pesticides
BT3 Biocides
BT3 Residues
UF Morestan

Quinones
BT1 Aromatic compounds
BT2 Organic compounds
NT1 Coenzyme Q

Quintozene
BT1 Fungicides
BT2 Pesticides
BT3 Biocides
BT3 Residues
UF Pentachloronitrobenzene

Quito orange
USE **Naranjilla**

Quorn
BT1 Mycoprotein
BT2 Biomass
BT3 Fermentation products
BT4 Biotechnology
BT5 Technology
BT2 Proteins
BT3 Nutrients
RT Fungal proteins
RT Fungi

Quorum sensing
HN introduced from vol. 41, issue 1 (2009)
BT1 Physiology
BT2 Science
RT Bacteria
RT Virulence

R

Ra
BT1 Radioelements
BT2 Isotopes
BT3 Elements
BT4 Minerals
BT5 Nutrients
BT2 Residues
UF Radium

Rabadi
BT1 Buttermilk
BT2 Dairy products
BT3 Animal foods
BT4 Foods
BT1 Cereal products
BT2 Plant foods
BT3 Foods
BT1 Fermented foods

BT2 Processed foods
BT3 Foods

Rabbit carcasses
BT1 Carcasses
BT2 Meat
BT3 Animal foods
BT4 Foods
BT1 Rabbit meat
BT2 Meat specific
BT3 Meat
BT4 Animal foods
BT5 Foods
BT2 Rabbits
BT3 Animals

Rabbitfish
BT1 Marine fish
BT2 Fish
BT3 Animals
BT3 Sea foods
BT4 Aquatic foods
BT5 Animal foods
BT6 Foods

Rabbit meat
HN heading from vol. 30 (1998); under Rabbits and Meat specific up to vol. 29 (1997)
BT1 Meat specific
BT2 Meat
BT3 Animal foods
BT4 Foods
BT1 Rabbits
BT2 Animals
NT1 Rabbit carcasses

Rabbits
BT1 Animals
NT1 Rabbit meat
NT2 Rabbit carcasses

Rabon
USE **Tetrachlorvinphos**

Rabri
BT1 Dairy products
BT2 Animal foods
BT3 Foods

Racemases
SN includes members of the subclass EC 5.1
BT1 Isomerases
BT2 Enzymes

Racking
BT1 Filtration
BT2 Processing
BT3 Technology

Raclette cheese
HN introduced from vol. 39, issue 1 (2007)
BT1 Cheese varieties
BT2 Cheese
BT3 Dairy products
BT4 Animal foods
BT5 Foods

Ractopamine
BT1 β-Adrenergic agonists
BT2 Drugs
BT3 Residues

Radiation
NT1 Infrared radiation
NT2 IR radiation
NT3 IR
NT2 NIR
NT1 Light
NT2 Fluorescent light
NT2 Sunlight
NT1 Microwaves
NT2 Microwave cooking
NT2 Microwave susceptors
NT1 Radiofrequency
NT1 Solar radiation
NT1 Ultraviolet radiation
NT2 UV radiation
NT3 UV
NT1 X-rays
RT Fluorescence
RT Irradiation
RT Radioactivity

Radicals
NT1 Free radicals
NT2 Reactive nitrogen species
NT3 Nitric oxide
NT3 Peroxynitrite
NT2 Reactive oxygen species
NT3 Peroxides
NT4 H_2O_2
NT4 Hydroperoxides
NT3 Superoxides
RT Health
RT Oxidation

Radical scavenging activity
RT Free radicals

Radioactive contamination
BT1 Contamination
BT1 Radioactivity
NT1 Fallout
RT Radioelements

Radioactivity
NT1 Counters
NT1 Dosimeters
NT1 Nuclear reactor accidents
NT1 Radioactive contamination
NT2 Fallout
RT Radiation
RT Radioelements

Radioelements
BT1 Isotopes
BT2 Elements
BT3 Minerals
BT4 Nutrients
BT1 Residues
NT1 Cs
NT1 Po
NT1 Pu
NT1 Ra
NT1 Radionuclides
NT2 Radioisotopes
NT1 Rn
NT1 Sr
NT1 Tc
NT1 Tritium
NT1 U
RT Pollution
RT Radioactive contamination
RT Radioactivity

Radiofrequency
BT1 Radiation

Radioimmunoassay
BT1 Immunological techniques
BT2 Analytical techniques

Radioisotopes
BT1 Radionuclides
BT2 Radioelements
BT3 Isotopes
BT4 Elements
BT5 Minerals
BT6 Nutrients
BT3 Residues

Radiometry
BT1 Analytical techniques

Radionuclides
BT1 Radioelements
BT2 Isotopes
BT3 Elements
BT4 Minerals
BT5 Nutrients
BT2 Residues
NT1 Radioisotopes

Radishes
HN heading from vol. 30 (1998); under Vegetables specific up to vol. 29 (1997)
BT1 Vegetables specific
BT2 Vegetables
BT3 Crops
BT4 Plants
BT3 Plant foods
BT4 Foods
NT1 Dongchimi
NT1 Japanese radishes
NT1 Kakdugi
NT1 Radish sprouts

Radish sprouts
BT1 Radishes
BT2 Vegetables specific
BT3 Vegetables
BT4 Crops
BT5 Plants
BT4 Plant foods
BT5 Foods
BT1 Sprouts
BT2 Vegetables specific
BT3 Vegetables
BT4 Crops
BT5 Plants
BT4 Plant foods
BT5 Foods

Radium
USE **Ra**

Radon
USE **Rn**

Radurization
BT1 Irradiation
BT2 Processing
BT3 Technology

Raffinose
HN under Sugars up to vol. 42 (2010)
BT1 Oligosaccharides
BT2 Polysaccharides
BT3 Carbohydrates
BT4 Nutrients
BT4 Organic compounds
BT2 Sugars
BT3 Carbohydrates
BT4 Nutrients
BT4 Organic compounds
BT3 Plant foods
BT4 Foods
RT Antinutritional factors

Raftiline
BT1 Fat substitutes
BT2 Fats
BT3 Lipids
BT4 Nutrients
RT Inulin

Raftilose
USE **Sweeteners**

Ragi
SN syn. finger millet
BT1 Millet
BT2 Cereals
BT3 Crops
BT4 Plants
BT3 Seeds
BT4 Plant foods
BT5 Foods

Ragout
BT1 Meat products
BT2 Animal foods
BT3 Foods

Ragusano cheese
BT1 Cheese varieties
BT2 Cheese
BT3 Dairy products
BT4 Animal foods
BT5 Foods

Rahat
USE **Turkish delight**

Rahnella
HN introduced from vol. 43, issue 1 (2011)
BT1 Bacteria
BT2 Microorganisms
NT1 *Rahnella aquatilis*

Rahnella aquatilis
BT1 *Rahnella*
BT2 Bacteria
BT3 Microorganisms

Rainbow trout
HN under trouts up to vol. 24 (1992)
BT1 Trout
BT2 Oily fish
BT3 Fish
BT4 Animals
BT4 Sea foods
BT5 Aquatic foods
BT6 Animal foods
BT7 Foods
NT1 *Oncorhynchus mykiss*

Raising agents
BT1 Bakery additives
BT2 Additives

Raisins
BT1 Dried fruits
BT2 Fruits dried
BT3 Dried foods
BT4 Processed foods
BT5 Foods
BT3 Fruits
BT4 Crops
BT5 Plants
BT4 Plant foods
BT5 Foods

Raki
HN under Liqueurs up to vol. 42 (2010)
BT1 Spirits
BT2 Alcoholic beverages
BT3 Beverages alcoholic
BT4 Beverages

Rakia
HN under Liqueurs up to vol. 42 (2010)
BT1 Fruit brandies
BT2 Brandies
BT3 Spirits
BT4 Alcoholic beverages
BT5 Beverages alcoholic
BT6 Beverages

Rakkyo
BT1 Vegetables specific
BT2 Vegetables
BT3 Crops
BT4 Plants
BT3 Plant foods
BT4 Foods

Raman spectroscopy
BT1 Spectroscopy
BT2 Analytical techniques

Rambutan
BT1 Fruits specific
BT2 Fruits
BT3 Crops
BT4 Plants
BT3 Plant foods
BT4 Foods

Ram carcasses
BT1 Carcasses
BT2 Meat
BT3 Animal foods
BT4 Foods
BT1 Mutton
BT2 Meat specific
BT3 Meat
BT4 Animal foods
BT5 Foods

Ram meat
USE **Mutton**

Ram muscles
USE **Mutton**

Ramrod
USE **Propachlor**

Rams
USE **Sheep**

Rancidity
BT1 Flavour
BT2 Sensory properties
RT Acid values
RT Lipolysis
RT Oxidation
RT Peroxidation
RT Peroxides
RT Peroxide values
RT TBA values
RT Thiobarbituric acid values

Randomly amplified polymorphic DNA
USE **RAPD**

RAPD
BT1 DNA
BT2 Nucleic acids
BT3 Organic acids
BT4 Acids
BT1 Genetic techniques
BT2 Genetics
RT PCR
UF Randomly amplified polymorphic DNA

Rapeseed meal
BT1 Flours
BT2 Plant foods
BT3 Foods
BT1 Rapeseeds
BT2 Oilseeds
BT3 Seeds
BT4 Plant foods
BT5 Foods

Rapeseed oils
BT1 Vegetable oils
BT2 Oils vegetable
BT3 Oils
BT4 Lipids
BT5 Nutrients
BT3 Vegetable products
BT4 Plant foods
BT5 Foods
RT Docosenoic acid
RT Erucic acid
UF Canbra oils
UF Canola oils
UF Colza oils

Rapeseeds
BT1 Oilseeds
BT2 Seeds
BT3 Plant foods
BT4 Foods
NT1 Bird rape

NT1 *Brassica napus*
NT1 Rapeseed meal
UF Canola

Raphia
BT1 Palms
BT2 Plants

Ras cheese
BT1 Cheese varieties
BT2 Cheese
BT3 Dairy products
BT4 Animal foods
BT5 Foods

Rasogolla
BT1 Dairy products
BT2 Animal foods
BT3 Foods
BT1 Desserts
BT2 Processed foods
BT3 Foods

Raspberries
BT1 Berries
BT2 Fruits specific
BT3 Fruits
BT4 Crops
BT5 Plants
BT4 Plant foods
BT5 Foods
RT Raspberry juices

Raspberry juices
BT1 Berry juices
BT2 Fruit juices
BT3 Fruit products
BT4 Plant foods
BT5 Foods
BT3 Soft drinks
BT4 Beverages
RT Raspberries

Ravioli
BT1 Pasta
BT2 Cereal products
BT3 Plant foods
BT4 Foods

Raw milk
BT1 Milk
BT2 Dairy products
BT3 Animal foods
BT4 Foods

Ray
BT1 Marine fish
BT2 Fish
BT3 Animals
BT3 Sea foods
BT4 Aquatic foods
BT5 Animal foods
BT6 Foods
RT Skate
UF Rays

Raya seeds
BT1 Oilseeds
BT2 Seeds
BT3 Plant foods
BT4 Foods

Rays
HN used up to vol. 29 (1997)
USE **Ray**

Razor shells
BT1 Bivalves
BT2 Molluscs
BT3 Shellfish
BT4 Animals
BT4 Sea foods
BT5 Aquatic foods
BT6 Animal foods
BT7 Foods

Rb
HN under Minerals up to vol. 42 (2010)
BT1 Metals
BT2 Elements
BT3 Minerals
BT4 Nutrients
UF Rubidium

RDA
BT1 DRI
BT2 Nutrient requirements
BT3 Nutrients
BT3 Nutrition
RT DRV
RT Nutrition
RT RDI
UF Recommended dietary allowance

RDI
BT1 Nutrient requirements
BT2 Nutrients
BT2 Nutrition
RT DRI
RT DRV
RT Nutrition
RT RDA
UF Recommended daily intake

Re
HN under Minerals up to vol. 42 (2010)
BT1 Metals
BT2 Elements
BT3 Minerals
BT4 Nutrients
UF Rhenium

Reactive nitrogen species
HN introduced from vol. 39, issue 1 (2007)
BT1 Free radicals
BT2 Radicals
BT1 Nitroso compounds
BT2 Organic nitrogen compounds
NT1 Nitric oxide
NT1 Peroxynitrite

Reactive oxygen species
HN introduced from vol. 39, issue 1 (2007)
BT1 Free radicals
BT2 Radicals
NT1 Peroxides
NT2 H_2O_2
NT2 Hydroperoxides
NT1 Superoxides
RT Oxidation
RT Oxidizing agents
RT Oxygen

Ready meals
BT1 Meals
BT2 Processed foods
BT3 Foods
RT Ready to eat foods
RT Ready to eat meals
RT Ready to serve foods

Ready to eat foods
BT1 Processed foods
BT2 Foods
RT Ready meals
RT Ready to eat meals
RT Ready to serve foods

Ready to eat meals
BT1 Meals
BT2 Processed foods
BT3 Foods
RT Ready meals
RT Ready to eat foods
RT Ready to serve foods

Ready to serve foods
BT1 Processed foods
BT2 Foods
RT Ready meals
RT Ready to eat foods
RT Ready to eat meals

Rearing
BT1 Agriculture
RT Husbandry

Rebaudiosides
HN introduced from vol. 39, issue 1 (2007)
BT1 Diterpenoids
BT2 Terpenoids
BT3 Lipids
BT4 Nutrients
BT1 Glycosides
BT2 Carbohydrates
BT3 Nutrients
BT3 Organic compounds
BT1 Sweeteners
BT2 Additives
RT *Stevia rebaudiana*
RT Stevioside

Recipes
HN introduced from vol. 41, issue 1 (2009)

Recombinant enzymes
BT1 Enzymes

Recombinant microorganisms
BT1 Genetics
BT1 Microorganisms

Recombinant proteins
BT1 Proteins
BT2 Nutrients

Recombination
BT1 Processing

BT2 Technology
RT Recombined foods
RT Reconstitution

Recombined foods
BT1 Processed foods
BT2 Foods
NT1 Recombined milk
RT Recombination
RT Reconstituted foods

Recombined milk
BT1 Milk
BT2 Dairy products
BT3 Animal foods
BT4 Foods
BT1 Recombined foods
BT2 Processed foods
BT3 Foods

Recommended daily intake
USE **RDI**

Recommended dietary allowance
USE **RDA**

Reconstituted foods
BT1 Processed foods
BT2 Foods
NT1 Rehydrated foods
RT Instant foods
RT Recombined foods
RT Reconstitution

Reconstituted meat products
USE **Restructured meat products**

Reconstitution
BT1 Processing
BT2 Technology
NT1 Rehydration
RT Recombination
RT Reconstituted foods

Rectification
BT1 Distillation
BT2 Processing
BT3 Technology

Recycling
BT1 Ecology
BT2 Science

Red beans
BT1 Legumes
BT2 Vegetables specific
BT3 Vegetables
BT4 Crops
BT5 Plants
BT4 Plant foods
BT5 Foods

Red beets
BT1 Beets
BT2 Vegetables specific
BT3 Vegetables
BT4 Crops
BT5 Plants
BT4 Plant foods
BT5 Foods

Red cabbages
BT1 Cabbages
BT2 Vegetables specific
BT3 Vegetables
BT4 Crops
BT5 Plants
BT4 Plant foods
BT5 Foods

Red chillies
HN introduced from vol. 41, issue 1 (2009)
BT1 Chillies
BT2 Capsicums
BT3 Vegetables specific
BT4 Vegetables
BT5 Crops
BT6 Plants
BT5 Plant foods
BT6 Foods

Red clover
HN introduced from vol. 41, issue 1 (2009)
BT1 Plants

Red crabs
BT1 Crabs
BT2 Crustacea
BT3 Shellfish
BT4 Animals
BT4 Sea foods
BT5 Aquatic foods
BT6 Animal foods
BT7 Foods

Redcurrant juices
BT1 Berry juices
BT2 Fruit juices
BT3 Fruit products
BT4 Plant foods
BT5 Foods
BT3 Soft drinks
BT4 Beverages
RT Redcurrants

Redcurrants
BT1 Berries
BT2 Fruits specific
BT3 Fruits
BT4 Crops
BT5 Plants
BT4 Plant foods
BT5 Foods
RT Redcurrant juices

Reddish pink soft exudative defect
USE **RSE defect**

Redfish
BT1 Marine fish
BT2 Fish
BT3 Animals
BT3 Sea foods
BT4 Aquatic foods
BT5 Animal foods
BT6 Foods

Red ginseng
HN introduced from vol. 41, issue 1 (2009)
BT1 Ginseng
BT2 Plants

Red gram
USE **Pigeon peas**

Red hake
BT1 Hake
BT2 Marine fish
BT3 Fish
BT4 Animals
BT4 Sea foods
BT5 Aquatic foods
BT6 Animal foods
BT7 Foods

Red meat
HN introduced from vol. 39, issue 1 (2007)
SN use for unspecified red meats
BT1 Meat
BT2 Animal foods
BT3 Foods

Red onions
HN introduced from vol. 41, issue 1 (2009)
BT1 Onions
BT2 Vegetables specific
BT3 Vegetables
BT4 Crops
BT5 Plants
BT4 Plant foods
BT5 Foods

Redox potential
HN heading up to vol. 24 (1992)
BT1 Physical properties
RT Oxidation
RT Reduction
UF Oxidation reduction potential

Red peppers
BT1 Capsicums
BT2 Vegetables specific
BT3 Vegetables
BT4 Crops
BT5 Plants
BT4 Plant foods
BT5 Foods

Red rice
SN excludes non-fermented naturally red rice
USE **Angkak**

Red salmon
SN syn. sockeye salmon
BT1 Sockeye salmon
BT2 Pacific salmon
BT3 Salmon
BT4 Oily fish
BT5 Fish
BT6 Animals
BT6 Sea foods
BT7 Aquatic foods
BT8 Animal foods
BT9 Foods

Red sea bream
BT1 Sea bream
BT2 Marine fish
BT3 Fish
BT4 Animals
BT4 Sea foods
BT5 Aquatic foods
BT6 Animal foods
BT7 Foods
NT1 *Pagrus major*

Redspot emperor
BT1 Marine fish
BT2 Fish
BT3 Animals
BT3 Sea foods
BT4 Aquatic foods
BT5 Animal foods
BT6 Foods
NT1 *Lethrinus lentjan*

Reducing agents
BT1 Additives
NT1 Reductones
RT Reducing substances
RT Reduction

Reducing substances
RT Reducing agents

Reducing sugars
HN sugars reducing also used in the index up to vol. 29 (1997)
BT1 Sugars
BT2 Carbohydrates
BT3 Nutrients
BT3 Organic compounds
BT2 Plant foods
BT3 Foods
UF Sugars reducing

Reductases
BT1 Oxidoreductases
BT2 Enzymes
NT1 Nitrate reductases

Reduction
HN heading from vol. 25 (1993)
SN used for chemical process only
RT Hydrogenation
RT Oxidation
RT Redox potential
RT Reducing agents

Reductones
HN heading up to vol. 24 (1992)
BT1 Reducing agents
BT2 Additives

Red wines
BT1 Wines
BT2 Alcoholic beverages
BT3 Beverages alcoholic
BT4 Beverages

Reference materials
NT1 Food reference materials
RT Analytical techniques

Refining
BT1 Purification
BT2 Processing
BT3 Technology
NT1 Affination

Reflectance
BT1 Optical properties
BT2 Physical properties

Reflectivity
BT1 Optical properties
BT2 Physical properties

Reflectometers
BT1 Apparatus
BT2 Technology

Refractive index
BT1 Optical properties
BT2 Physical properties

Refractometry
BT1 Analytical techniques

Refrigerants
BT1 Refrigeration
BT2 Thermal processing
BT3 Processing thermal
BT4 Processing
BT5 Technology
NT1 Chlorofluorocarbons
NT1 Freons

Refrigerated foods
BT1 Chilled foods
BT2 Processed foods
BT3 Foods

Refrigerated storage
HN storage refrigerated also used in the index up to vol. 29 (1997)
BT1 Refrigeration
BT2 Thermal processing
BT3 Processing thermal
BT4 Processing
BT5 Technology
RT Storage cold

Refrigerated transport
HN transport refrigerated also used in the index up to vol. 29 (1997)
BT1 Refrigeration
BT2 Thermal processing
BT3 Processing thermal
BT4 Processing
BT5 Technology
BT1 Transport

Refrigeration
BT1 Thermal processing
BT2 Processing thermal
BT3 Processing
BT4 Technology
NT1 Refrigerants
NT2 Chlorofluorocarbons
NT2 Freons
NT1 Refrigerated storage
NT1 Refrigerated transport
NT1 Refrigerators
RT Cooling
RT Freezing
RT Preservation
RT Storage cold

Refrigerators
BT1 Equipment
BT2 Technology
BT1 Refrigeration
BT2 Thermal processing
BT3 Processing thermal
BT4 Processing
BT5 Technology
RT Chillers

Regenerated cellulose
HN reinstated vol. 43, issue 1 (2011); cellophane used previously
BT1 Celluloses
BT2 Glucans
BT3 Polysaccharides
BT4 Carbohydrates
BT5 Nutrients
BT5 Organic compounds
RT Cellophane

Regeneration
BT1 Cell culture

Reggianito cheese
BT1 Cheese varieties
BT2 Cheese
BT3 Dairy products
BT4 Animal foods
BT5 Foods

Regional foods
HN introduced from vol. 41, issue 1 (2009)
BT1 Foods
RT Ethnic foods

Regulations
SN used for legislation in general; specific pieces of legislation are under Legislation
RT Guidelines
RT Legislation

Reheating
BT1 Heating
BT2 Thermal processing
BT3 Processing thermal
BT4 Processing
BT5 Technology

Rehydrated foods
BT1 Reconstituted foods
BT2 Processed foods
BT3 Foods

Rehydration
BT1 Reconstitution
BT2 Processing
BT3 Technology
RT Hydration

Reindeer
BT1 Animals
NT1 Reindeer meat
NT2 Reindeer carcasses

Reindeer carcasses
BT1 Carcasses

BT2 Meat
BT3 Animal foods
BT4 Foods
BT1 Reindeer meat
BT2 Meat specific
BT3 Meat
BT4 Animal foods
BT5 Foods
BT2 Reindeer
BT3 Animals

Reindeer meat
BT1 Meat specific
BT2 Meat
BT3 Animal foods
BT4 Foods
BT1 Reindeer
BT2 Animals
NT1 Reindeer carcasses

Reinhardtius hippoglossoides
BT1 Halibut
BT2 Flatfish
BT3 Marine fish
BT4 Fish
BT5 Animals
BT5 Sea foods
BT6 Aquatic foods
BT7 Animal foods
BT8 Foods

Relative density
SN syn. sp. gr.
BT1 sp. gr.
BT2 Density
BT3 Physical properties

Relative humidity
USE **RH**

Religious groups
BT1 Anthropological groups
BT2 Population groups

Relishes
BT1 Condiments
BT2 Flavourings
BT3 Additives

Renaturation
RT Denaturation

Rendement Napole genes
HN introduced from vol. 39, issue 1 (2007)
BT1 Genetic disorders
RT Ham
RT Pork
RT Swine

Rendering
BT1 Thermal processing
BT2 Processing thermal
BT3 Processing
BT4 Technology
RT Heating

Rennetability
BT1 Coagulation
BT2 Processing
BT3 Technology
RT Rennets

Rennets
HN heading up to vol. 24 (1992)
BT1 Milk clotting enzymes
BT2 Enzymes milk clotting
BT3 Proteinases
BT4 Hydrolases
BT5 Enzymes
NT1 Animal rennets
NT1 Calf rennets
NT1 Microbial rennets
NT1 Vegetable rennets
RT Rennetability

Rennet substitutes
HN under Rennets up to vol. 24 (1992)
BT1 Milk clotting enzymes
BT2 Enzymes milk clotting
BT3 Proteinases
BT4 Hydrolases
BT5 Enzymes

Rennin
USE **Chymosin**

Report
RT Reviews

Reporter genes
BT1 Cloning technology
BT2 Gene cloning
BT3 Genetic techniques
BT4 Genetics
BT2 Technology
BT1 Genes
BT2 Chromosomes
BT3 Genetics
BT2 Genomes
BT3 Genetics
RT Gene expression
RT Marker genes
RT Marker proteins

Reproduction
HN introduced from vol. 42, issue 1 (2010)
BT1 Human physiology
BT2 Physiology
BT3 Science
NT1 Menopause
NT1 Menstrual cycle
NT1 Pregnancy
RT Reproductive toxicity

Reproductive toxicity
HN introduced from vol. 42, issue 1 (2010)
BT1 Toxicity
RT Reproduction

Republic of Ireland
HN Ireland, Republic of was a heading up to vol. 24 (1992); Irish Republic used from vol. 25 (1993) to vol. 35, issue 6 (2003)
BT1 Europe
BT1 European Union
RT Organization for Economic Cooperation and Development
UF Ireland, Republic of
UF Irish Republic

Republic of the Congo
HN introduced from vol. 39, issue 1 (2007)
BT1 West Africa
BT2 Africa
UF Congo, Republic of the

Resazurin
HN heading up to vol. 24 (1992)
BT1 Heterocyclic compounds
BT1 Organic nitrogen compounds
RT Bacteriology

Reservoir water
BT1 Water

Residence time distribution
BT1 Mechanical properties
BT2 Physical properties

Residues
NT1 Chemicals
NT1 Drugs
NT1 Hormones
NT1 Pesticides
NT1 Radioelements
NT1 Toxins
RT Bioaccumulation
RT Biomagnification
RT Contamination
RT Food safety
RT Health
RT Hygiene

Resins
HN heading up to vol. 24 (1992)
RT Gums
RT Polymers

Resistant starch
BT1 Starch
BT2 Glucans
BT3 Polysaccharides
BT4 Carbohydrates
BT5 Nutrients
BT5 Organic compounds
BT2 Thickeners
BT3 Additives
RT Dietary fibre

Resmethrin
BT1 Pyrethroid insecticides
BT2 Insecticides
BT3 Pesticides
BT4 Biocides
BT4 Residues

Resorcinol
BT1 Phenols
BT2 Alcohols
BT2 Aromatic compounds
BT3 Organic compounds

Respiration
RT Carbon dioxide
RT Oxygen

Response surface

methodology
BT1 Analytical techniques

Restaurants
NT1 Cafeterias
NT1 Canteens
NT1 Coffee bars
NT1 Sandwich bars
RT Catering
RT Pubs

Restriction endonucleases
SN syn. restriction enzymes. Includes EC 3.1.21.3, 3.1.21.4 and 3.1.21.5
BT1 Nucleases
BT2 Esterases
BT3 Hydrolases
BT4 Enzymes

Restriction enzymes
SN syn. restriction endonucleases
BT1 Nucleases
BT2 Esterases
BT3 Hydrolases
BT4 Enzymes

Restriction fragment length polymorphism
USE **RFLP**

Restriction modification systems
BT1 Enzymes

Restructured fish products
HN introduced from vol. 39, issue 1 (2007)
BT1 Fish products
BT2 Sea foods
BT3 Aquatic foods
BT4 Animal foods
BT5 Foods

Restructured meat products
HN under Reconstituted foods and Meat products up to vol. 24 (1992)
BT1 Meat products
BT2 Animal foods
BT3 Foods
UF Reconstituted meat products

Resveratrol
BT1 Stilbenes
BT2 Phenols
BT3 Alcohols
BT3 Aromatic compounds
BT4 Organic compounds
RT Piceid

Retail
BT1 Marketing
BT2 Economics
NT1 Product recalls

Retail display
HN introduced from vol. 39, issue 1 (2007)
BT1 Storage
RT Display cabinets

Retinal
BT1 Retinoids
BT2 Vitamins
BT3 Nutrients

Retinoic acid
BT1 Retinoids
BT2 Vitamins
BT3 Nutrients

Retinoids
HN heading from vol. 35, issue 6 (2003); under Retinols from vol. 25 (1993) and Retinol up to vol. 24 (1992)
BT1 Vitamins
BT2 Nutrients
NT1 Retinal
NT1 Retinoic acid
NT1 Retinol
NT1 Retinols
NT1 Retinyl palmitate
NT1 Vitamin A
RT Carotenoids

Retinol
HN heading up to vol. 24 (1992)
BT1 Retinoids
BT2 Vitamins
BT3 Nutrients
RT Vitamin A

Retinols
HN heading from vol. 25 (1993) to vol. 35, issue 6 (2003); was Retinol up to vol. 24 (1992)
BT1 Retinoids
BT2 Vitamins
BT3 Nutrients
RT Vitamin A

Retinyl palmitate
BT1 Retinoids
BT2 Vitamins
BT3 Nutrients

Retorting
BT1 Sterilization
BT2 Thermal processing
BT3 Processing thermal
BT4 Processing
BT5 Technology

Retort pouches
BT1 Pouches
BT2 Containers

Retrogradation
RT Crystallization
RT Staling
RT Starch

Retsina
BT1 Aromatized wines
BT2 Wines
BT3 Alcoholic beverages
BT4 Beverages alcoholic
BT5 Beverages

Reunion
BT1 Southern Africa
BT2 Africa

Reuterin
SN syn. 3-hydroxypropionaldehyde
BT1 Aldehydes
BT2 Carbonyl compounds
BT3 Organic compounds
BT1 Antibiotics
BT2 Drugs
BT3 Residues

Reverse micelles

Reverse osmosis
BT1 Processing
BT2 Technology
RT Dialysis
RT Osmosis

Reviews
RT Report

RFLP
BT1 Genetic techniques
BT2 Genetics
RT DNA fingerprinting
RT Genetic fingerprinting
RT PCR
UF Restriction fragment length polymorphism

RH
BT1 Humidity
UF Relative humidity

Rhamnogalacturonans
HN introduced from vol. 39, issue 1 (2007)
BT1 Pectic substances
BT2 Polysaccharides
BT3 Carbohydrates
BT4 Nutrients
BT4 Organic compounds

Rhamnolipids
BT1 Lipids
BT2 Nutrients

Rhamnose
HN under Sugars up to vol. 42 (2010)
BT1 Monosaccharides
BT2 Sugars
BT3 Carbohydrates
BT4 Nutrients
BT4 Organic compounds
BT3 Plant foods
BT4 Foods

α-L-rhamnosidases
SN EC 3.2.1.40
BT1 Glycosidases
BT2 Hydrolases
BT3 Enzymes

Rhea carcasses
BT1 Carcasses
BT2 Meat
BT3 Animal foods
BT4 Foods
BT1 Rhea meat
BT2 Poultry meat
BT3 Meat specific
BT4 Meat

BT5 Animal foods
BT6 Foods
BT2 Rheas
BT3 Poultry
BT4 Birds

Rhea meat
BT1 Poultry meat
BT2 Meat specific
BT3 Meat
BT4 Animal foods
BT5 Foods
BT1 Rheas
BT2 Poultry
BT3 Birds
NT1 Rhea carcasses

Rheas
BT1 Poultry
BT2 Birds
NT1 Rhea meat
NT2 Rhea carcasses

Rhenium
USE **Re**

Rheological properties
BT1 Mechanical properties
BT2 Physical properties
NT1 Compressibility
NT1 Creep
NT1 Deformation
NT1 Elasticity
NT1 Extensibility
NT1 Flow
NT2 Flow meters
NT2 Gushing
NT1 Friction
NT1 Rheology
NT1 Rheometers
NT1 Rigidity
NT1 Shear
NT1 Shear values
NT1 Stickiness
NT1 Stiffness
NT1 Stress relaxation
NT1 Stretch
NT1 Surface tension
NT1 Thixotropy
NT1 Viscoelasticity
NT1 Viscosity
NT2 Viscometers
NT1 Yield stress
RT Consistency
RT Firmness
RT Penetration
RT Sensory properties
RT Texture

Rheology
BT1 Rheological properties
BT2 Mechanical properties
BT3 Physical properties

Rheometers
BT1 Rheological properties
BT2 Mechanical properties
BT3 Physical properties

Rhizobium
BT1 Bacteria
BT2 Microorganisms

Rhizoctonia
BT1 Fungi
BT2 Microorganisms
RT Diseases plant

Rhizomucor
HN heading from vol. 30 (1998); under Fungi up to vol. 29 (1997)
BT1 Fungi
BT2 Microorganisms
NT1 *Rhizomucor miehei*

Rhizomucor miehei
SN Genbank common name is Mucor miehei
BT1 *Rhizomucor*
BT2 Fungi
BT3 Microorganisms

Rhizopus
BT1 Fungi
BT2 Microorganisms
NT1 *Rhizopus arrhizus*
NT1 *Rhizopus chinensis*
NT1 *Rhizopus cohnii*
NT1 *Rhizopus delemar*
NT1 *Rhizopus japonicus*
NT1 *Rhizopus microsporus*
NT1 *Rhizopus niveus*
NT1 *Rhizopus oligosporus*
NT1 *Rhizopus oryzae*
NT1 *Rhizopus stolonifer*
NT2 *Rhizopus nigricans*

Rhizopus arrhizus
HN introduced from vol. 39, issue 1 (2007)
SN synonymous with Rhizopus oryzae
BT1 *Rhizopus*
BT2 Fungi
BT3 Microorganisms

Rhizopus chinensis
SN synonymous with Rhizopus microporus var. chinensis
BT1 *Rhizopus*
BT2 Fungi
BT3 Microorganisms

Rhizopus cohnii
SN obsolete species
BT1 *Rhizopus*
BT2 Fungi
BT3 Microorganisms

Rhizopus delemar
SN obsolete species
BT1 *Rhizopus*
BT2 Fungi
BT3 Microorganisms

Rhizopus japonicus
BT1 *Rhizopus*
BT2 Fungi
BT3 Microorganisms

Rhizopus microsporus
BT1 *Rhizopus*
BT2 Fungi
BT3 Microorganisms

Rhizopus nigricans
HN introduced from vol. 41, issue 1 (2009)
SN synonymous with Rhizopus stolonifer
BT1 *Rhizopus stolonifer*
BT2 *Rhizopus*
BT3 Fungi
BT4 Microorganisms

Rhizopus niveus
BT1 *Rhizopus*
BT2 Fungi
BT3 Microorganisms

Rhizopus oligosporus
SN synonymous with Rhizopus microsporus var. oligosporus
BT1 *Rhizopus*
BT2 Fungi
BT3 Microorganisms

Rhizopus oryzae
SN synonymous with Rhizopus arrhizus
BT1 *Rhizopus*
BT2 Fungi
BT3 Microorganisms

Rhizopus stolonifer
SN synonymous with Rhizopus nigricans
BT1 *Rhizopus*
BT2 Fungi
BT3 Microorganisms
NT1 *Rhizopus nigricans*

Rhodesia
USE **Zimbabwe**

Rhodium
HN under Minerals up to vol. 42 (2010)
BT1 Metals
BT2 Elements
BT3 Minerals
BT4 Nutrients

Rhodobacter
BT1 Bacteria
BT2 Microorganisms

Rhodococcus
BT1 Bacteria
BT2 Microorganisms
NT1 *Rhodococcus equi*
NT1 *Rhodococcus erythropolis*
NT1 *Rhodococcus opacus*

Rhodococcus equi
BT1 *Rhodococcus*
BT2 Bacteria
BT3 Microorganisms

Rhodococcus erythropolis
BT1 *Rhodococcus*
BT2 Bacteria
BT3 Microorganisms

Rhodococcus opacus
BT1 *Rhodococcus*

BT2 Bacteria
BT3 Microorganisms

Rhodosporidium
HN introduced from vol. 43, issue 1 (2011)
BT1 Yeasts
BT2 Fungi
BT3 Microorganisms
NT1 *Rhodosporidium toruloides*

Rhodosporidium toruloides
HN introduced from vol. 43, issue 1 (2011)
SN synonymous with Rhodotorula gracilis
BT1 *Rhodosporidium*
BT2 Yeasts
BT3 Fungi
BT4 Microorganisms

Rhodothermus
BT1 Bacteria
BT2 Microorganisms
NT1 *Rhodothermus marinus*

Rhodothermus marinus
BT1 *Rhodothermus*
BT2 Bacteria
BT3 Microorganisms

Rhodotorula
BT1 Yeasts
BT2 Fungi
BT3 Microorganisms
NT1 *Rhodotorula glutinis*
NT1 *Rhodotorula gracilis*
NT1 *Rhodotorula mucilaginosa*
NT2 *Rhodotorula rubra*

Rhodotorula glutinis
BT1 *Rhodotorula*
BT2 Yeasts
BT3 Fungi
BT4 Microorganisms

Rhodotorula gracilis
SN synonymous with Rhodosporidium toruloides
BT1 *Rhodotorula*
BT2 Yeasts
BT3 Fungi
BT4 Microorganisms

Rhodotorula mucilaginosa
HN introduced from vol. 39, issue 1 (2007)
SN synonymous with Rhodotorula rubra
BT1 *Rhodotorula*
BT2 Yeasts
BT3 Fungi
BT4 Microorganisms
NT1 *Rhodotorula rubra*

Rhodotorula rubra
SN synonymous with Rhodotorula mucilaginosa
BT1 *Rhodotorula mucilaginosa*
BT2 *Rhodotorula*
BT3 Yeasts
BT4 Fungi
BT5 Microorganisms

Rhubarb
HN under Fruits specific up to vol. 24 (1992)
BT1 Vegetables specific
BT2 Vegetables
BT3 Crops
BT4 Plants
BT3 Plant foods
BT4 Foods

Riboflavin
BT1 Vitamin B group
BT2 Vitamins
BT3 Nutrients
RT Carotenoids
UF Vitamin B_2
UF Vitamin G

Ribonucleases
SN includes members of EC 3.1.13-3.1.16 and EC 3.1.26-3.1.31
BT1 Nucleases
BT2 Esterases
BT3 Hydrolases
BT4 Enzymes
NT1 Angiogenin
UF RNases

Ribonucleic acids
USE **RNA**

Ribonucleosides
BT1 Nucleosides

Ribonucleotides
BT1 Nucleotides

Ribose
HN under Sugars up to vol. 42 (2010)
BT1 Monosaccharides
BT2 Sugars
BT3 Carbohydrates
BT4 Nutrients
BT4 Organic compounds
BT3 Plant foods
BT4 Foods

Ribotype
BT1 Genetics

Ribotyping
BT1 Genetic techniques
BT2 Genetics

Rice
BT1 Cereals
BT2 Crops
BT3 Plants
BT2 Seeds
BT3 Plant foods
BT4 Foods
NT1 Arare
NT1 Basmati rice
NT1 Black rice
NT1 Brown rice
NT1 Dosai
NT1 Idli
NT1 Lao-chao
NT1 Paddy
NT1 Puffed rice
NT1 Puto
NT1 Rice bran
NT1 Rice bread
NT1 Rice cakes
NT1 Rice crackers
NT1 Rice flour
NT1 Rice koji
NT1 Rice milk
NT1 Rice noodles
NT1 Rice powders
NT1 Rice starch
NT1 Sikhe
NT1 Tape
NT2 Tape ketan
NT1 Yukwa
RT Polishing

Rice beans
BT1 Legumes
BT2 Vegetables specific
BT3 Vegetables
BT4 Crops
BT5 Plants
BT4 Plant foods
BT5 Foods

Rice bran
BT1 Bran
BT2 Cereal products
BT3 Plant foods
BT4 Foods
BT1 Rice
BT2 Cereals
BT3 Crops
BT4 Plants
BT3 Seeds
BT4 Plant foods
BT5 Foods

Rice bran oils
BT1 Vegetable oils
BT2 Oils vegetable
BT3 Oils
BT4 Lipids
BT5 Nutrients
BT3 Vegetable products
BT4 Plant foods
BT5 Foods

Rice bread
BT1 Bread
BT2 Bakery products
BT3 Cereal products
BT4 Plant foods
BT5 Foods
BT1 Rice
BT2 Cereals
BT3 Crops
BT4 Plants
BT3 Seeds
BT4 Plant foods
BT5 Foods

Rice cakes
BT1 Rice
BT2 Cereals
BT3 Crops
BT4 Plants
BT3 Seeds
BT4 Plant foods
BT5 Foods

Rice crackers
BT1 Rice
BT2 Cereals
BT3 Crops
BT4 Plants
BT3 Seeds
BT4 Plant foods
BT5 Foods
BT1 Snack foods
BT2 Processed foods
BT3 Foods

Rice flour
BT1 Cereal flours
BT2 Flours cereal
BT3 Cereal products
BT4 Plant foods
BT5 Foods
BT1 Rice
BT2 Cereals
BT3 Crops
BT4 Plants
BT3 Seeds
BT4 Plant foods
BT5 Foods

Rice germ oils
HN introduced from vol. 37, issue 5 (2005)
BT1 Vegetable oils
BT2 Oils vegetable
BT3 Oils
BT4 Lipids
BT5 Nutrients
BT3 Vegetable products
BT4 Plant foods
BT5 Foods

Rice koji
BT1 Koji
BT2 Cereal products
BT3 Plant foods
BT4 Foods
BT2 Fermented foods
BT3 Processed foods
BT4 Foods
BT2 Legumes
BT3 Vegetables specific
BT4 Vegetables
BT5 Crops
BT6 Plants
BT5 Plant foods
BT6 Foods
BT1 Rice
BT2 Cereals
BT3 Crops
BT4 Plants
BT3 Seeds
BT4 Plant foods
BT5 Foods

Rice milk
HN introduced from vol. 39, issue 1 (2007)
BT1 Beverages
BT1 Rice
BT2 Cereals
BT3 Crops
BT4 Plants
BT3 Seeds
BT4 Plant foods
BT5 Foods

Rice noodles
HN introduced from vol. 39, issue 1 (2007)
BT1 Cereal products
BT2 Plant foods
BT3 Foods
BT1 Rice
BT2 Cereals
BT3 Crops
BT4 Plants
BT3 Seeds
BT4 Plant foods
BT5 Foods
RT Noodles

Rice powders
BT1 Powders
BT2 Dried foods
BT3 Processed foods
BT4 Foods
BT2 Instant foods
BT3 Processed foods
BT4 Foods
BT1 Rice
BT2 Cereals
BT3 Crops
BT4 Plants
BT3 Seeds
BT4 Plant foods
BT5 Foods

Rice starch
BT1 Rice
BT2 Cereals
BT3 Crops
BT4 Plants
BT3 Seeds
BT4 Plant foods
BT5 Foods
BT1 Starch
BT2 Glucans
BT3 Polysaccharides
BT4 Carbohydrates
BT5 Nutrients
BT5 Organic compounds
BT2 Thickeners
BT3 Additives

Rice vinegar
HN introduced from vol. 37, issue 5 (2005)
BT1 Vinegar
BT2 Condiments
BT3 Flavourings
BT4 Additives
BT2 Fermented foods
BT3 Processed foods
BT4 Foods

Rice weevils
BT1 *Sitophilus*
BT2 Insects
BT3 Pests
NT1 *Sitophilus oryzae*

Rice wines
HN heading from vol. 30 (1998); under Beverages alcoholic up to vol. 29 (1997)
BT1 Cereal wines
BT2 Alcoholic beverages
BT3 Beverages alcoholic
BT4 Beverages
NT1 Sake
NT2 Ginjoshu
NT2 Narazuke
NT1 Takju
NT1 Yakju

Ricin
BT1 Lectins
BT2 Glycoproteins
BT3 Proteins
BT4 Nutrients
BT2 Vegetable proteins
BT3 Proteins vegetable
BT4 Proteins
BT5 Nutrients
BT4 Vegetable products
BT5 Plant foods
BT6 Foods
RT Toxins

Ricinoleic acid
BT1 Monounsaturated fatty acids
BT2 Unsaturated fatty acids
BT3 Fatty acids
BT4 Lipids
BT5 Nutrients
BT4 Organic acids
BT5 Acids

Rickettsia
BT1 Bacteria
BT2 Microorganisms
RT Parasites

Ricotta cheese
BT1 Cheese varieties
BT2 Cheese
BT3 Dairy products
BT4 Animal foods
BT5 Foods

Rigidity
BT1 Rheological properties
BT2 Mechanical properties
BT3 Physical properties

Rigor
USE ***Rigor mortis***

Rigor mortis
HN heading up to vol. 24 (1992)
BT1 Firmness
BT2 Texture
BT3 Sensory properties
UF *Rigor*

Rigorometers
BT1 Firmness
BT2 Texture
BT3 Sensory properties

Rind
USE **Cheese rind**
USE **Peel**

Rinsing
BT1 Cleaning
BT2 Hygiene
BT2 Processing
BT3 Technology

Ripened cream
BT1 Fermented cream
BT2 Cream
BT3 Dairy products
BT4 Animal foods
BT5 Foods
BT2 Fermented dairy products
BT3 Dairy products
BT4 Animal foods
BT5 Foods
BT3 Fermented foods
BT4 Processed foods
BT5 Foods

Ripeness
BT1 Ripening
UF Maturity

Ripening
NT1 Ripeness
NT1 Senescence
RT Ageing
UF Maturation

Rishitin
BT1 Terpenoids
BT2 Lipids
BT3 Nutrients

Risk communication
HN introduced from vol. 39, issue 1 (2007)
BT1 Information
RT Food safety
RT Hazards
RT Risk factors
RT Risks management

Risk factors
SN includes diet and nutrition as risk factors for chronic diseases
RT Diseases
RT Risk communication

Risks assessment
RT Food safety
RT Hazards analysis
RT Risks management

Risks management
RT Food safety
RT Product recalls
RT Risk communication
RT Risks assessment

Rissoles
BT1 Meat products
BT2 Animal foods
BT3 Foods

River fish
BT1 Freshwater fish
BT2 Fish
BT3 Animals
BT3 Sea foods
BT4 Aquatic foods
BT5 Animal foods
BT6 Foods

Rn
BT1 Radioelements
BT2 Isotopes
BT3 Elements
BT4 Minerals
BT5 Nutrients
BT2 Residues
UF Radon

RNA
BT1 Nucleic acids
BT2 Organic acids
BT3 Acids
NT1 mRNA
NT1 rRNA
RT Genomes
UF Ribonucleic acids

RNA interference
HN introduced from vol. 41, issue 1 (2009)
BT1 Gene silencing
BT2 Genetic techniques
BT3 Genetics

RNA polymerases
USE **DNA-directed RNA polymerases**

RNases
USE **Ribonucleases**

Roach
BT1 Freshwater fish
BT2 Fish
BT3 Animals
BT3 Sea foods
BT4 Aquatic foods
BT5 Animal foods
BT6 Foods

Roasted coffee
BT1 Coffee
BT2 Beverages
BT2 Crops
BT3 Plants
BT2 Plant foods
BT3 Foods

Roasted foods
BT1 Processed foods
BT2 Foods
NT1 Roasted peanuts

Roasted peanuts
BT1 Peanuts
BT2 Nuts
BT3 Fruits
BT4 Crops
BT5 Plants
BT4 Plant foods
BT5 Foods
BT3 Oilseeds
BT4 Seeds
BT5 Plant foods
BT6 Foods
BT1 Roasted foods
BT2 Processed foods
BT3 Foods

Roasting
BT1 Cooking
BT2 Thermal processing
BT3 Processing thermal
BT4 Processing
BT5 Technology

Roasting coffee
HN heading up to vol. 24 (1992)
BT1 Coffee
BT2 Beverages
BT2 Crops
BT3 Plants
BT2 Plant foods
BT3 Foods

Robiola cheese
BT1 Cheese varieties
BT2 Cheese
BT3 Dairy products
BT4 Animal foods
BT5 Foods

Robotics
BT1 Automation
BT2 Technology

Rock cod
BT1 Cod
BT2 Marine fish
BT3 Fish
BT4 Animals
BT4 Sea foods
BT5 Aquatic foods
BT6 Animal foods
BT7 Foods

Rocket
HN introduced from vol. 37, issue 5 (2005)
BT1 Vegetables specific
BT2 Vegetables
BT3 Crops
BT4 Plants
BT3 Plant foods
BT4 Foods

Rockfish
BT1 Marine fish
BT2 Fish
BT3 Animals
BT3 Sea foods
BT4 Aquatic foods
BT5 Animal foods
BT6 Foods

Rodenticides
BT1 Pesticides
BT2 Biocides
BT2 Residues
NT1 Endrin
NT1 Fluoroacetate

NT1 HCH
NT1 Zinc phosphide

Rodents
BT1 Pests

Roes
BT1 Fish products
BT2 Sea foods
BT3 Aquatic foods
BT4 Animal foods
BT5 Foods
NT1 Caviar
NT1 Caviar substitutes
NT1 Milt

Rohu
BT1 Carp
BT2 Freshwater fish
BT3 Fish
BT4 Animals
BT4 Sea foods
BT5 Aquatic foods
BT6 Animal foods
BT7 Foods
BT2 Oily fish
BT3 Fish
BT4 Animals
BT4 Sea foods
BT5 Aquatic foods
BT6 Animal foods
BT7 Foods
NT1 *Labeo rohita*

Rohwurst
BT1 Sausages
BT2 Meat products
BT3 Animal foods
BT4 Foods

Rokpol cheese
HN introduced from vol. 39, issue 1 (2007)
BT1 Cheese varieties
BT2 Cheese
BT3 Dairy products
BT4 Animal foods
BT5 Foods

Roller drying
HN drying roller also used in the index up to vol. 29(1997)
BT1 Drying
BT2 Thermal processing
BT3 Processing thermal
BT4 Processing
BT5 Technology

Roller mills
BT1 Mills
BT2 Equipment
BT3 Technology
BT2 Milling
BT3 Processing
BT4 Technology

Rolling
BT1 Processing
BT2 Technology

Rollmops
BT1 Fish products
BT2 Sea foods
BT3 Aquatic foods
BT4 Animal foods
BT5 Foods
BT1 Herring
BT2 Marine fish
BT3 Fish
BT4 Animals
BT4 Sea foods
BT5 Aquatic foods
BT6 Animal foods
BT7 Foods
BT2 Oily fish
BT3 Fish
BT4 Animals
BT4 Sea foods
BT5 Aquatic foods
BT6 Animal foods
BT7 Foods
UF Rolmops

Rolls
HN heading up to vol. 24 (1992)
BT1 Bread
BT2 Bakery products
BT3 Cereal products
BT4 Plant foods
BT5 Foods

Rolmops
USE **Rollmops**

Romania
HN heading up to vol. 24 (1992)
BT1 Europe

Romano cheese
HN introduced from vol. 37, issue 5 (2005)
BT1 Cheese varieties
BT2 Cheese
BT3 Dairy products
BT4 Animal foods
BT5 Foods

Roncal cheese
BT1 Cheese varieties
BT2 Cheese
BT3 Dairy products
BT4 Animal foods
BT5 Foods

Ronidazole
BT1 Drugs
BT2 Residues

Ronilan
USE **Vinclozolin**

Ronit
BT1 Herbicides
BT2 Pesticides
BT3 Biocides
BT3 Residues

Ronnel
USE **Fenchlorphos**

Rooibos tea
BT1 Herb tea
BT2 Teas
BT3 Beverages
BT3 Crops
BT4 Plants
BT3 Plant foods
BT4 Foods

Root crops
BT1 Vegetables specific
BT2 Vegetables
BT3 Crops
BT4 Plants
BT3 Plant foods
BT4 Foods

Roots
HN introduced from vol. 39, issue 1 (2007)
BT1 Plants

Rootstocks
BT1 Cultivation
BT2 Agriculture

Root vegetables
BT1 Vegetables specific
BT2 Vegetables
BT3 Crops
BT4 Plants
BT3 Plant foods
BT4 Foods

Ropiness
RT Ropy bacteria

Ropy bacteria
BT1 Bacteria
BT2 Microorganisms
RT Ropiness

Roquefort cheese
BT1 Cheese varieties
BT2 Cheese
BT3 Dairy products
BT4 Animal foods
BT5 Foods

Roquefortine
BT1 Mycotoxins
BT2 Toxins
BT3 Residues

Rose apples
BT1 Fruits specific
BT2 Fruits
BT3 Crops
BT4 Plants
BT3 Plant foods
BT4 Foods

Rose Bengal
BT1 Colorants
BT2 Additives

Rosehips
BT1 Fruits specific
BT2 Fruits
BT3 Crops
BT4 Plants

BT3 Plant foods
BT4 Foods

Roselle
BT1 Colorants
BT2 Additives
BT1 Plants

Rosemary
HN under Spices up to vol. 42 (2010)
BT1 Herbs
BT2 Spices
BT3 Flavourings
BT4 Additives
RT Rosemary essential oils

Rosemary essential oils
HN introduced from vol. 39, issue 1 (2007)
BT1 Essential oils
BT2 Flavourings
BT3 Additives
BT2 Vegetable oils
BT3 Oils vegetable
BT4 Oils
BT5 Lipids
BT6 Nutrients
BT4 Vegetable products
BT5 Plant foods
BT6 Foods
RT Rosemary

Roses
HN heading up to vol. 24 (1992)
BT1 Plants

Rose wines
BT1 Wines
BT2 Alcoholic beverages
BT3 Beverages alcoholic
BT4 Beverages

Rosmarinic acid
BT1 Phenols
BT2 Alcohols
BT2 Aromatic compounds
BT3 Organic compounds

Rossiiskii cheese
BT1 Cheese varieties
BT2 Cheese
BT3 Dairy products
BT4 Animal foods
BT5 Foods

Rotavirus
HN introduced from vol. 43, issue 1 (2011)
BT1 Rotaviruses
BT2 Viruses
BT3 Microorganisms

Rotaviruses
HN under Enteric viruses up to vol. 42 (2010)
SN for descriptive use only
BT1 Viruses
BT2 Microorganisms
NT1 Rotavirus

Rotenone
HN introduced from vol. 39, issue 1 (2007)
BT1 Insecticides
BT2 Pesticides
BT3 Biocides
BT3 Residues

Roti
BT1 Bread
BT2 Bakery products
BT3 Cereal products
BT4 Plant foods
BT5 Foods

Rots
BT1 Plant diseases
BT2 Diseases plant
BT3 Diseases
NT1 Brown rot

Rotting
BT1 Spoilage

Roughage
BT1 Fibre

Roughness
BT1 Physical properties

Roux
BT1 Sauces
BT2 Condiments
BT3 Flavourings
BT4 Additives

Rovral
USE **Iprodione**

Rowanberries
BT1 Berries
BT2 Fruits specific
BT3 Fruits
BT4 Crops
BT5 Plants
BT4 Plant foods
BT5 Foods

Roxarsone
BT1 Drugs
BT2 Residues

Royal jelly
BT1 Health foods
BT2 Processed foods
BT3 Foods
RT Apiculture

rRNA
BT1 RNA
BT2 Nucleic acids
BT3 Organic acids
BT4 Acids

RSE defect
BT1 Genetic disorders
UF Reddish pink soft exudative defect

Ru
HN under Minerals up to vol. 42 (2010)
BT1 Metals
BT2 Elements
BT3 Minerals
BT4 Nutrients
UF Ruthenium

Rubber
HN heading up to vol. 24 (1992)
BT1 Packaging materials
RT Latex

Rubber seeds
BT1 Oilseeds
BT2 Seeds
BT3 Plant foods
BT4 Foods

Rubidium
USE **Rb**

Rubratoxins
BT1 Mycotoxins
BT2 Toxins
BT3 Residues

Rue
HN under Spices up to vol. 42 (2010)
BT1 Herbs
BT2 Spices
BT3 Flavourings
BT4 Additives

Rugulosin
HN heading up to vol. 23 (1991)
BT1 Mycotoxins
BT2 Toxins
BT3 Residues

Rum
BT1 Spirits
BT2 Alcoholic beverages
BT3 Beverages alcoholic
BT4 Beverages
RT Sugar cane spirits

Ruminants
BT1 Animals

Ruminococcus
BT1 Bacteria
BT2 Microorganisms

Runner beans
BT1 Legumes
BT2 Vegetables specific
BT3 Vegetables
BT4 Crops
BT5 Plants
BT4 Plant foods
BT5 Foods

Rusks
BT1 Bakery products
BT2 Cereal products
BT3 Plant foods
BT4 Foods

Russeting
BT1 Plant disorders
BT2 Diseases plant
BT3 Diseases

Russia
BT1 Asia
BT1 Europe

Russula
BT1 Edible fungi
BT2 Fungi edible
BT3 Vegetables specific
BT4 Vegetables
BT5 Crops
BT6 Plants
BT5 Plant foods
BT6 Foods

Rust
BT1 Corrosion

Rusts
BT1 Plant diseases
BT2 Diseases plant
BT3 Diseases

Rutabagas
USE **Swedes**

Ruthenium
USE **Ru**

Rutin
HN under Vitamins up to vol. 42 (2010)
BT1 Flavonols
BT2 Alcohols
BT2 Flavonoids
BT3 Aromatic compounds
BT4 Organic compounds
BT3 Pigments
BT1 Glycosides
BT2 Carbohydrates
BT3 Nutrients
BT3 Organic compounds

Rwanda
BT1 Central Africa
BT2 Africa

Ryazhenka
BT1 Fermented milk
BT2 Fermented dairy products
BT3 Dairy products
BT4 Animal foods
BT5 Foods
BT3 Fermented foods
BT4 Processed foods
BT5 Foods
BT2 Milk
BT3 Dairy products
BT4 Animal foods
BT5 Foods

Rye
BT1 Cereals
BT2 Crops
BT3 Plants
BT2 Seeds
BT3 Plant foods
BT4 Foods
NT1 Rye bran
NT1 Rye bread
NT1 Rye flour
NT1 Rye starch
RT Secalins

Rye bran
BT1 Bran
BT2 Cereal products
BT3 Plant foods
BT4 Foods
BT1 Rye
BT2 Cereals
BT3 Crops
BT4 Plants
BT3 Seeds
BT4 Plant foods
BT5 Foods

Rye bread
BT1 Bread
BT2 Bakery products
BT3 Cereal products
BT4 Plant foods
BT5 Foods
BT1 Rye
BT2 Cereals
BT3 Crops
BT4 Plants
BT3 Seeds
BT4 Plant foods
BT5 Foods

Rye flour
BT1 Cereal flours
BT2 Flours cereal
BT3 Cereal products
BT4 Plant foods
BT5 Foods
BT1 Rye
BT2 Cereals
BT3 Crops
BT4 Plants
BT3 Seeds
BT4 Plant foods
BT5 Foods

Rye malt
BT1 Malt
BT2 Cereal products
BT3 Plant foods
BT4 Foods

Rye starch
HN introduced from vol. 42, issue 1 (2010)
BT1 Rye
BT2 Cereals
BT3 Crops
BT4 Plants
BT3 Seeds
BT4 Plant foods
BT5 Foods
BT1 Starch
BT2 Glucans
BT3 Polysaccharides
BT4 Carbohydrates
BT5 Nutrients
BT5 Organic compounds
BT2 Thickeners
BT3 Additives

Ryzelan
USE **Oryzalin**

S

S
SN index heading is Sulfur
BT1 Sulfur
BT2 Elements
BT3 Minerals
BT4 Nutrients

Sabah
BT1 Asia

Sablefish
BT1 Marine fish
BT2 Fish
BT3 Animals
BT3 Sea foods
BT4 Aquatic foods
BT5 Animal foods
BT6 Foods

Saccharases
USE **β-Fructofuranosidases**

Saccharides
BT1 Sugars
BT2 Carbohydrates
BT3 Nutrients
BT3 Organic compounds
BT2 Plant foods
BT3 Foods

Saccharification
BT1 Processing
BT2 Technology

Saccharin
BT1 Sweeteners
BT2 Additives

Saccharomyces
BT1 Yeasts
BT2 Fungi
BT3 Microorganisms
NT1 *Saccharomyces bayanus*
NT1 *Saccharomyces boulardii*
NT1 *Saccharomyces carlsbergensis*
NT1 *Saccharomyces cerevisiae*
NT1 *Saccharomyces diastaticus*
NT1 *Saccharomyces exiguus*
NT1 *Saccharomyces pastorianus*
NT1 *Saccharomyces uvarum*
NT1 Yeasts bakers
NT2 Bakers yeasts
NT1 Yeasts brewers
NT2 Brewers yeasts
NT3 Bottom fermenting yeasts
NT3 Top fermenting yeasts
NT1 Yeasts wine
NT2 Wine yeasts
NT3 Sake yeasts

Saccharomyces bayanus
BT1 *Saccharomyces*
BT2 Yeasts
BT3 Fungi
BT4 Microorganisms

Saccharomyces boulardii
HN introduced from vol. 41, issue 1 (2009)
BT1 *Saccharomyces*
BT2 Yeasts
BT3 Fungi
BT4 Microorganisms

Saccharomyces carlsbergensis
BT1 *Saccharomyces*
BT2 Yeasts
BT3 Fungi
BT4 Microorganisms

Saccharomyces cerevisiae
BT1 *Saccharomyces*
BT2 Yeasts
BT3 Fungi
BT4 Microorganisms

Saccharomyces diastaticus
BT1 *Saccharomyces*
BT2 Yeasts
BT3 Fungi
BT4 Microorganisms

Saccharomyces exiguus
SN synonymous with Kazachstania exigua
BT1 *Saccharomyces*
BT2 Yeasts
BT3 Fungi
BT4 Microorganisms

Saccharomyces pastorianus
BT1 *Saccharomyces*
BT2 Yeasts
BT3 Fungi
BT4 Microorganisms

Saccharomyces uvarum
BT1 *Saccharomyces*
BT2 Yeasts
BT3 Fungi
BT4 Microorganisms

Saccharomycodes
BT1 Yeasts
BT2 Fungi
BT3 Microorganisms

Saccharomycopsis
HN under Fungi up to vol. 42 (2010)
BT1 Yeasts
BT2 Fungi
BT3 Microorganisms
NT1 *Saccharomycopsis fibuligera*

Saccharomycopsis fibuligera
HN under Fungi up to vol. 42 (2010)
BT1 *Saccharomycopsis*
BT2 Yeasts
BT3 Fungi
BT4 Microorganisms

Saccharose
USE **Sucrose**

Sachets
BT1 Pouches
BT2 Containers

Sacks
BT1 Bags
BT2 Containers

SADH
USE **Daminozide**

Safety
HN heading up to vol. 23 (1991)
SN mechanical and operational aspects of safety; safety aspects of foods under Food safety
RT Explosions
RT Health
RT Health hazards

Safflower oils
BT1 Vegetable oils
BT2 Oils vegetable
BT3 Oils
BT4 Lipids
BT5 Nutrients
BT3 Vegetable products
BT4 Plant foods
BT5 Foods

Safflowers
BT1 Flowers
BT2 Plants
RT Saffron

Safflower seeds
BT1 Oilseeds
BT2 Seeds
BT3 Plant foods
BT4 Foods

Saffron
BT1 Colorants
BT2 Additives
BT1 Spices
BT2 Flavourings
BT3 Additives
RT Carthamin
RT Safflowers
RT Safranal

Safranal
HN introduced from vol. 39, issue 1 (2007)
BT1 Aldehydes
BT2 Carbonyl compounds
BT3 Organic compounds
BT1 Aroma compounds
BT2 Flavour compounds
BT2 Volatile compounds
BT1 Monoterpenoids
BT2 Terpenoids
BT3 Lipids
BT4 Nutrients
RT Saffron

Safrole
HN under Flavour compounds up to vol. 42 (2010)
BT1 Aroma compounds
BT2 Flavour compounds
BT2 Volatile compounds
BT1 Aromatic compounds
BT2 Organic compounds
BT1 Heterocyclic compounds

Sage
HN under Spices up to vol. 42 (2010)
BT1 Herbs
BT2 Spices
BT3 Flavourings
BT4 Additives
RT Sage essential oils

Sage essential oils
HN introduced from vol. 42, issue 1 (2010)
BT1 Essential oils
BT2 Flavourings
BT3 Additives
BT2 Vegetable oils
BT3 Oils vegetable
BT4 Oils
BT5 Lipids
BT6 Nutrients
BT4 Vegetable products
BT5 Plant foods
BT6 Foods
RT Sage

Sago
HN heading up to vol. 24 (1992); under Starches from vol. 25 (1993)
BT1 Starch
BT2 Glucans
BT3 Polysaccharides
BT4 Carbohydrates
BT5 Nutrients
BT5 Organic compounds
BT2 Thickeners
BT3 Additives
RT *Metroxylon*
RT Palms

Sailfish
BT1 Marine fish
BT2 Fish
BT3 Animals
BT3 Sea foods
BT4 Aquatic foods
BT5 Animal foods
BT6 Foods

Saint-Nectaire cheese
BT1 Cheese varieties
BT2 Cheese
BT3 Dairy products
BT4 Animal foods
BT5 Foods

Saint-Paulin cheese
BT1 Cheese varieties
BT2 Cheese
BT3 Dairy products
BT4 Animal foods
BT5 Foods

Saithe
BT1 Marine fish
BT2 Fish
BT3 Animals
BT3 Sea foods

BT4 Aquatic foods
BT5 Animal foods
BT6 Foods

Sakacins
BT1 Bacteriocins
BT2 Antibiotics
BT3 Drugs
BT4 Residues
RT *Lactobacillus sakei*

Sake
BT1 Rice wines
BT2 Cereal wines
BT3 Alcoholic beverages
BT4 Beverages alcoholic
BT5 Beverages
NT1 Ginjoshu
NT1 Narazuke
RT Hiochi bacteria
RT Moromi

Sake yeasts
BT1 Wine yeasts
BT2 Yeasts wine
BT3 *Saccharomyces*
BT4 Yeasts
BT5 Fungi
BT6 Microorganisms

Sakuradai
USE **Sea bream**

Salad cream
BT1 Salad dressings
BT2 Condiments
BT3 Flavourings
BT4 Additives

Salad dressings
BT1 Condiments
BT2 Flavourings
BT3 Additives
NT1 Dressings
NT1 French dressing
NT1 Salad cream
NT1 Salad oils
RT Sauces

Salad oils
BT1 Oils
BT2 Lipids
BT3 Nutrients
BT1 Salad dressings
BT2 Condiments
BT3 Flavourings
BT4 Additives

Salads
NT1 Delicatessen salads
NT1 Fruit salads
NT1 Vegetable salads
NT2 Potato salads
RT Chilled foods
RT Delicatessen foods
RT Fruit products
RT Vegetable products

Salad vegetables
BT1 Vegetables specific
BT2 Vegetables
BT3 Crops
BT4 Plants
BT3 Plant foods
BT4 Foods

Salami
BT1 Sausages
BT2 Meat products
BT3 Animal foods
BT4 Foods

Salatrim
BT1 Fat substitutes
BT2 Fats
BT3 Lipids
BT4 Nutrients

Salbutamol
BT1 β-Adrenergic agonists
BT2 Drugs
BT3 Residues

Salchichon
BT1 Sausages
BT2 Meat products
BT3 Animal foods
BT4 Foods

Salers cheese
BT1 Cheese varieties
BT2 Cheese
BT3 Dairy products
BT4 Animal foods
BT5 Foods

Sales
BT1 Economics
RT Consumption
RT Markets

Sal fats
BT1 Vegetable fats
BT2 Fats vegetable
BT3 Fats
BT4 Lipids
BT5 Nutrients
BT3 Vegetable products
BT4 Plant foods
BT5 Foods

Salicylic acid
BT1 Organic acids
BT2 Acids
BT1 Preservatives
BT2 Additives

Salinity
SN use for salt content of foods, brines, etc., but not soils
BT1 Salt
BT2 Condiments
BT3 Flavourings
BT4 Additives

Salinomycin
BT1 Antibiotics
BT2 Drugs
BT3 Residues
BT1 Coccidiostats
BT2 Drugs
BT3 Residues

Saliva
HN introduced from vol. 39, issue 1 (2007)
BT1 Human physiology
BT2 Physiology
BT3 Science

Salmon
HN heading up to vol. 24 (1992) and from vol. 30 (1998)
BT1 Oily fish
BT2 Fish
BT3 Animals
BT3 Sea foods
BT4 Aquatic foods
BT5 Animal foods
BT6 Foods
NT1 Atlantic salmon
NT2 *Salmo salar*
NT1 Pacific salmon
NT2 Cherry salmon
NT3 Masu salmon
NT2 Chinook salmon
NT3 King salmon
NT2 Chum salmon
NT3 Keta salmon
NT3 *Oncorhynchus keta*
NT2 Coho salmon
NT2 Pink salmon
NT2 Sockeye salmon
NT3 Red salmon
NT1 Smoked salmon

Salmonella
BT1 Bacteria
BT2 Microorganisms
NT1 *Salmonella* Agona
NT1 *Salmonella* Blockley
NT1 *Salmonella* Bredeney
NT1 *Salmonella* Choleraesuis
NT1 *Salmonella* Cubana
NT1 *Salmonella* Derby
NT1 *Salmonella* Diarizonae
NT1 *Salmonella* Dublin
NT1 Salmonellae
NT1 *Salmonella enterica*
NT1 *Salmonella* Enteritidis
NT1 *Salmonella* Gallinarum
NT1 *Salmonella* Heidelberg
NT1 *Salmonella* Indiana
NT1 *Salmonella* Infantis
NT1 *Salmonella* Java
NT1 *Salmonella* Kottbus
NT1 *Salmonella* Mbandaka
NT1 *Salmonella* Montevideo
NT1 *Salmonella* Muenchen
NT1 *Salmonella* Muenster
NT1 *Salmonella* Newport
NT1 *Salmonella* Ohio
NT1 *Salmonella* Oranienburg
NT1 *Salmonella* Panama
NT1 *Salmonella* Paratyphi
NT1 *Salmonella* Poona
NT1 *Salmonella* Pullorum
NT1 *Salmonella* Senftenberg
NT1 *Salmonella* Stanley
NT1 *Salmonella* Thompson
NT1 *Salmonella* Typhi
NT1 *Salmonella* Typhimurium

NT1 *Salmonella* Virchow
RT Salmonellosis

Salmonella Agona
HN introduced from vol. 41, issue 1 (2009)
BT1 *Salmonella*
BT2 Bacteria
BT3 Microorganisms

Salmonella Blockley
BT1 *Salmonella*
BT2 Bacteria
BT3 Microorganisms

Salmonella Bredeney
BT1 *Salmonella*
BT2 Bacteria
BT3 Microorganisms

Salmonella Choleraesuis
BT1 *Salmonella*
BT2 Bacteria
BT3 Microorganisms

Salmonella Cubana
BT1 *Salmonella*
BT2 Bacteria
BT3 Microorganisms

Salmonella Derby
HN introduced from vol. 39, issue 1 (2007)
BT1 *Salmonella*
BT2 Bacteria
BT3 Microorganisms

Salmonella Diarizonae
BT1 *Salmonella*
BT2 Bacteria
BT3 Microorganisms

Salmonella Dublin
HN introduced from vol. 39, issue 1 (2007)
BT1 *Salmonella*
BT2 Bacteria
BT3 Microorganisms

Salmonellae
BT1 *Salmonella*
BT2 Bacteria
BT3 Microorganisms

Salmonella enterica
BT1 *Salmonella*
BT2 Bacteria
BT3 Microorganisms

Salmonella Enteritidis
BT1 *Salmonella*
BT2 Bacteria
BT3 Microorganisms

Salmonella Gallinarum
HN introduced from vol. 41, issue 1 (2009)
BT1 *Salmonella*
BT2 Bacteria
BT3 Microorganisms

Salmonella Heidelberg
HN introduced from vol. 39, issue 1 (2007)
BT1 *Salmonella*
BT2 Bacteria
BT3 Microorganisms

Salmonella Indiana
BT1 *Salmonella*
BT2 Bacteria
BT3 Microorganisms

Salmonella Infantis
BT1 *Salmonella*
BT2 Bacteria
BT3 Microorganisms

Salmonella Java
HN introduced from vol. 39, issue 1 (2007)
BT1 *Salmonella*
BT2 Bacteria
BT3 Microorganisms

Salmonella Kottbus
BT1 *Salmonella*
BT2 Bacteria
BT3 Microorganisms

Salmonella Mbandaka
BT1 *Salmonella*
BT2 Bacteria
BT3 Microorganisms

Salmonella Montevideo
BT1 *Salmonella*
BT2 Bacteria
BT3 Microorganisms

Salmonella Muenchen
BT1 *Salmonella*
BT2 Bacteria
BT3 Microorganisms

Salmonella Muenster
HN introduced from vol. 39, issue 1 (2007)
BT1 *Salmonella*
BT2 Bacteria
BT3 Microorganisms

Salmonella Newport
BT1 *Salmonella*
BT2 Bacteria
BT3 Microorganisms

Salmonella Ohio
BT1 *Salmonella*
BT2 Bacteria
BT3 Microorganisms

Salmonella Oranienburg
HN introduced from vol. 41, issue 1 (2009)
BT1 *Salmonella*
BT2 Bacteria
BT3 Microorganisms

Salmonella Panama
BT1 *Salmonella*
BT2 Bacteria
BT3 Microorganisms

Salmonella Paratyphi
SN includes Paratyphi A, B and C
BT1 *Salmonella*
BT2 Bacteria
BT3 Microorganisms
RT Paratyphoid

Salmonella Poona
HN introduced from vol. 39, issue 1 (2007)
BT1 *Salmonella*
BT2 Bacteria
BT3 Microorganisms

Salmonella Pullorum
BT1 *Salmonella*
BT2 Bacteria
BT3 Microorganisms

Salmonella Senftenberg
BT1 *Salmonella*
BT2 Bacteria
BT3 Microorganisms

Salmonella Stanley
BT1 *Salmonella*
BT2 Bacteria
BT3 Microorganisms

Salmonella Thompson
HN introduced from vol. 39, issue 1 (2007)
BT1 *Salmonella*
BT2 Bacteria
BT3 Microorganisms

Salmonella Typhi
BT1 *Salmonella*
BT2 Bacteria
BT3 Microorganisms
RT Typhoid

Salmonella Typhimurium
BT1 *Salmonella*
BT2 Bacteria
BT3 Microorganisms

Salmonella Virchow
BT1 *Salmonella*
BT2 Bacteria
BT3 Microorganisms

Salmonellosis
BT1 Diseases
BT1 Poisoning
RT *Salmonella*

Salmon oils
BT1 Fish oils
BT2 Oils fish
BT3 Fish products
BT4 Sea foods
BT5 Aquatic foods
BT6 Animal foods
BT7 Foods
BT3 Marine oils
BT4 Oils
BT5 Lipids
BT6 Nutrients

Salmo salar
BT1 Atlantic salmon
BT2 Salmon
BT3 Oily fish
BT4 Fish
BT5 Animals
BT5 Sea foods
BT6 Aquatic foods
BT7 Animal foods
BT8 Foods

Salsa
BT1 Sauces
BT2 Condiments
BT3 Flavourings
BT4 Additives

Sal seeds
BT1 Oilseeds
BT2 Seeds
BT3 Plant foods
BT4 Foods

Salsify
BT1 Vegetables specific
BT2 Vegetables
BT3 Crops
BT4 Plants
BT3 Plant foods
BT4 Foods
UF Oyster plant

Salt
SN symbol NaCl is also used in the index
BT1 Condiments
BT2 Flavourings
BT3 Additives
NT1 Desalination
NT1 Desalting
NT1 Iodized salt
NT1 NaCl
NT1 Salinity
NT1 Salt substitutes
RT Brining
RT Flavour compounds
RT Salting

Salted fish
BT1 Fish products
BT2 Sea foods
BT3 Aquatic foods
BT4 Animal foods
BT5 Foods

Saltine crackers
BT1 Biscuits
BT2 Bakery products
BT3 Cereal products
BT4 Plant foods
BT5 Foods

Saltiness
BT1 Flavour
BT2 Sensory properties

Salting
HN reinstated vol. 39, issue 1 (2007); brining used 1990-2006 inclusive
BT1 Processing
BT2 Technology
RT Brining
RT Salt

Salt replacers
USE **Salt substitutes**

Salts
NT1 Alginates
NT2 Alginate gels
NT2 Alginic acid
NT1 Alum
NT1 Arsenates
NT1 Ascorbates
NT2 Sodium ascorbate
NT1 Benzoates
NT2 Sodium benzoate
NT1 Bicarbonates
NT2 Sodium bicarbonate
NT1 Bromates
NT2 Potassium bromate
NT1 Bromides
NT1 Carbonates
NT1 Chlorides
NT2 $CaCl_2$
NT2 Chloramines
NT3 Monochloramine
NT2 KCl
NT2 $MgCl_2$
NT2 NaCl
NT1 Citrates
NT1 Cyanides
NT2 Acetonitrile
NT2 Cyanogens
NT3 Cyanogenic glycosides
NT3 Prunasin
NT2 Hydrocyanic acid
NT2 Hydrogen cyanide
NT1 Cyclamates
NT2 Sodium cyclamate
NT1 Electrolytes
NT1 Fluorides
NT2 Fluoridation
NT1 Gluconates
NT1 Glutamates
NT2 Monosodium glutamate
NT1 Halides
NT1 Hydroxides
NT2 $Ca(OH)_2$
NT2 KOH
NT2 NaOH
NT1 Iodides
NT1 Lactates
NT2 Calcium lactate
NT2 Potassium lactate
NT2 Sodium lactate
NT1 Nitrates
NT1 Nitrites
NT2 Peroxynitrite
NT1 Oxalates
NT1 Persulfates
NT1 Phosphates
NT2 Inositol phosphates
NT2 Phytates
NT2 Phytic acid
NT2 Polyphosphates
NT2 Pyrophosphates
NT2 Sodium tripolyphosphate
NT2 Tripolyphosphates
NT2 Trisodium phosphate
NT1 Silicates
NT2 Zeolites
NT1 Sodium acetate
NT1 Sodium diacetate
NT1 Sorbates
NT1 Sulfates
NT2 SDS
NT1 Sulfides
NT2 Allyl sulfides
NT3 Diallyl disulfide
NT2 Dimethyl sulfide
NT3 Methyl sulfide
NT2 Dimethyl trisulfide
NT2 Disulfides
NT3 Carbon disulfide
NT3 Diallyl disulfide
NT3 Dimethyl disulfide
NT2 H_2S
NT1 Sulfites
NT2 Bisulfites
NT2 Metabisulfites
NT3 Potassium metabisulfite
NT3 Sodium metabisulfite
NT3 Sodium pyrosulfite
NT1 Tartrates
NT2 Calcium tartrate
NT1 Water hardness
RT Acetates

Salt substitutes
BT1 Salt
BT2 Condiments
BT3 Flavourings
BT4 Additives
UF Salt replacers

Samna
HN under Fats milk up to vol. 42 (2010)
BT1 Butter
BT2 Dairy products
BT3 Animal foods
BT4 Foods

Samoa
BT1 Oceania
UF Western Samoa

Samphire
BT1 Herbs
BT2 Spices
BT3 Flavourings
BT4 Additives
NT1 Sea fennel
NT2 *Crithmum maritimum*

Sampling
RT Analytical techniques

Samso cheese
HN introduced from vol. 37, issue 5 (2005)
BT1 Cheese varieties
BT2 Cheese
BT3 Dairy products
BT4 Animal foods
BT5 Foods

Sandesh
BT1 Dairy products
BT2 Animal foods
BT3 Foods
BT1 Sugar confectionery

BT2 Plant foods
BT3 Foods

Sand lance
BT1 Marine fish
BT2 Fish
BT3 Animals
BT3 Sea foods
BT4 Aquatic foods
BT5 Animal foods
BT6 Foods

Sandwich bars
HN introduced from vol. 42, issue 1 (2010)
BT1 Restaurants

Sandwiches
BT1 Snack foods
BT2 Processed foods
BT3 Foods

Sangak
BT1 Bread
BT2 Bakery products
BT3 Cereal products
BT4 Plant foods
BT5 Foods

Sangria
BT1 Aromatized wines
BT2 Wines
BT3 Alcoholic beverages
BT4 Beverages alcoholic
BT5 Beverages

Sanguinarine
BT1 Alkaloids
BT2 Organic nitrogen compounds

Sanitation
BT1 Disinfection
BT2 Hygiene
RT Sanitizers

Sanitizers
BT1 Disinfectants
BT2 Disinfection
BT3 Hygiene
RT Sanitation

San Marino
BT1 Europe

Sansa oils
BT1 Olive pomace oils
BT2 Olive oils
BT3 Vegetable oils
BT4 Oils vegetable
BT5 Oils
BT6 Lipids
BT7 Nutrients
BT5 Vegetable products
BT6 Plant foods
BT7 Foods

San Simon cheese
BT1 Cheese varieties
BT2 Cheese
BT3 Dairy products
BT4 Animal foods
BT5 Foods

Santoquin
USE **Ethoxyquin**

Sapodillas
BT1 Fruits specific
BT2 Fruits
BT3 Crops
BT4 Plants
BT3 Plant foods
BT4 Foods
UF Sapota

Sapogenins
BT1 Steroids
BT2 Lipids
BT3 Nutrients
BT1 Triterpenoids
BT2 Terpenoids
BT3 Lipids
BT4 Nutrients
RT Saponins

Saponification
BT1 Hydrolysis

Saponins
BT1 Glycosides
BT2 Carbohydrates
BT3 Nutrients
BT3 Organic compounds
NT1 Digitonin
NT1 Ginsenosides
NT1 Quillaja saponins
RT Sapogenins

Sapota
USE **Sapodillas**

Sapovirus
HN introduced from vol. 43, issue 1 (2011)
BT1 Sapoviruses
BT2 Caliciviruses
BT3 Viruses
BT4 Microorganisms
NT1 Sapporo virus

Sapoviruses
HN introduced from vol. 41, issue 1 (2009); under Enteric viruses up to vol. 42 (2010)
SN for descriptive use only
BT1 Caliciviruses
BT2 Viruses
BT3 Microorganisms
NT1 Sapovirus
NT2 Sapporo virus

Sapporo virus
HN introduced from vol. 43, issue 1 (2011)
BT1 Sapovirus
BT2 Sapoviruses
BT3 Caliciviruses
BT4 Viruses
BT5 Microorganisms

Saran
SN syn. PVDC
BT1 Plastics
BT2 Packaging materials

Sarawak
BT1 Asia

Sarcina
BT1 Bacteria
BT2 Microorganisms

Sarcocystis
BT1 Parasites
BT2 Pests

Sarcodon aspratus
BT1 Edible fungi
BT2 Fungi edible
BT3 Vegetables specific
BT4 Vegetables
BT5 Crops
BT6 Plants
BT5 Plant foods
BT6 Foods

Sarcodon imbricatum
BT1 Edible fungi
BT2 Fungi edible
BT3 Vegetables specific
BT4 Vegetables
BT5 Crops
BT6 Plants
BT5 Plant foods
BT6 Foods

Sarcoplasmic proteins
HN introduced from vol. 39, issue 1 (2007)
BT1 Animal proteins
BT2 Proteins animal
BT3 Proteins
BT4 Nutrients

Sarcosine
BT1 Organic nitrogen compounds

Sarcosporidia
BT1 Parasites
BT2 Pests

Sarda
USE **Bonito**

Sardina pilchardus
BT1 Sardine
BT2 Marine fish
BT3 Fish
BT4 Animals
BT4 Sea foods
BT5 Aquatic foods
BT6 Animal foods
BT7 Foods
BT2 Oily fish
BT3 Fish
BT4 Animals
BT4 Sea foods
BT5 Aquatic foods
BT6 Animal foods
BT7 Foods

Sardine
HN heading from vol. 30 (1998); Sardines used up to vol. 29 (1997)
BT1 Marine fish
BT2 Fish
BT3 Animals
BT3 Sea foods
BT4 Aquatic foods
BT5 Animal foods
BT6 Foods
BT1 Oily fish
BT2 Fish
BT3 Animals
BT3 Sea foods
BT4 Aquatic foods
BT5 Animal foods
BT6 Foods
NT1 Monterey sardine
NT1 *Sardina pilchardus*
UF Sardines

Sardinella
BT1 Marine fish
BT2 Fish
BT3 Animals
BT3 Sea foods
BT4 Aquatic foods
BT5 Animal foods
BT6 Foods
UF Sardinellas

Sardinellas
HN used up to vol. 29 (1997)
USE ***Sardinella***

Sardine oils
BT1 Fish oils
BT2 Oils fish
BT3 Fish products
BT4 Sea foods
BT5 Aquatic foods
BT6 Animal foods
BT7 Foods
BT3 Marine oils
BT4 Oils
BT5 Lipids
BT6 Nutrients

Sardines
HN used up to vol. 29 (1997)
USE **Sardine**

Sargassum
BT1 Seaweeds
BT2 Algae
BT3 Microorganisms
BT2 Sea foods
BT3 Aquatic foods
BT4 Animal foods
BT5 Foods

Sarsaparilla
BT1 Spices
BT2 Flavourings
BT3 Additives

Sashimi
HN under Fish up to vol. 42 (2010)
BT1 Fish products
BT2 Sea foods
BT3 Aquatic foods
BT4 Animal foods
BT5 Foods

Saskatoon fruits
BT1 Fruits specific
BT2 Fruits
BT3 Crops
BT4 Plants
BT3 Plant foods
BT4 Foods

Satiety
BT1 Human physiology
BT2 Physiology
BT3 Science

Satsuma mandarins
BT1 Mandarins
BT2 Oranges
BT3 Citrus fruits
BT4 Fruits specific
BT5 Fruits
BT6 Crops
BT7 Plants
BT6 Plant foods
BT7 Foods

Satsumas
BT1 Mandarins
BT2 Oranges
BT3 Citrus fruits
BT4 Fruits specific
BT5 Fruits
BT6 Crops
BT7 Plants
BT6 Plant foods
BT7 Foods

Saturated fats
HN introduced from vol. 41, issue 1 (2009)
BT1 Fats
BT2 Lipids
BT3 Nutrients

Saturated fatty acids
HN heading from vol. 43 (2011); under Fatty acids up to vol. 42 (2010)
BT1 Fatty acids
BT2 Lipids
BT3 Nutrients
BT2 Organic acids
BT3 Acids
NT1 Arachidic acid
NT1 Behenic acid
NT1 Butanoic acid
NT2 Butyric acid
NT1 Decanoic acid
NT2 Capric acid
NT1 Dodecanoic acid
NT2 Lauric acid
NT1 Heptadecanoic acid
NT2 Margaric acid
NT1 Heptanoic acid
NT1 Hexadecanoic acid
NT2 Palmitic acid
NT1 Hexanoic acid
NT2 Caproic acid
NT1 Lignoceric acid
NT1 Myristic acid
NT1 Octadecanoic acid
NT2 Stearic acid
NT3 Hydroxystearic acid
NT1 Octanoic acid
NT2 Caprylic acid
NT1 Pentanoic acid
NT2 Valeric acid

Satureja
HN under Spices up to vol. 42 (2010)
BT1 Savory
BT2 Herbs
BT3 Spices
BT4 Flavourings
BT5 Additives

Sauce mixes
BT1 Sauces
BT2 Condiments
BT3 Flavourings
BT4 Additives

Sauces
BT1 Condiments
BT2 Flavourings
BT3 Additives
NT1 Apple sauces
NT1 Cheese sauces
NT1 Fish sauces
NT2 Budu
NT2 Ishiru
NT2 Nuoc-mam
NT2 Patis
NT1 Fondues
NT1 Gravy
NT2 Gravy powders
NT1 Hollandaise sauces
NT1 Ketchups
NT2 Catsups
NT3 Tomato catsups
NT2 Tomato ketchups
NT3 Tomato catsups
NT1 Meat sauces
NT1 Oyster sauces
NT1 Pasta sauces
NT2 Pesto
NT1 Roux
NT1 Salsa
NT1 Sauce mixes
NT1 Soy sauces
NT2 Kanjang
NT2 Kecap
NT2 Shoyu
NT1 Tomato sauces
NT1 Worcestershire sauces
RT Salad dressings

Saucisson
BT1 Sausages
BT2 Meat products
BT3 Animal foods
BT4 Foods

Saudi Arabia
BT1 Asia
BT1 Middle East

Sauerkraut
HN heading up to vol. 24 (1992)
BT1 Cabbages
BT2 Vegetables specific

BT3 Vegetables
BT4 Crops
BT5 Plants
BT4 Plant foods
BT5 Foods
BT1 Fermented foods
BT2 Processed foods
BT3 Foods

Saury
BT1 Marine fish
BT2 Fish
BT3 Animals
BT3 Sea foods
BT4 Aquatic foods
BT5 Animal foods
BT6 Foods

Sausage casings
BT1 Casings
NT1 Cellulose sausage casings
NT1 Collagen sausage casings
RT Sausages

Sausage emulsions
BT1 Sausages
BT2 Meat products
BT3 Animal foods
BT4 Foods

Sausagemeat
BT1 Sausages
BT2 Meat products
BT3 Animal foods
BT4 Foods

Sausages
HN use for meat sausages only from vol. 25 (1993)
BT1 Meat products
BT2 Animal foods
BT3 Foods
NT1 Ambaritsa
NT1 Androlla
NT1 Beef sausages
NT1 Bierschinken
NT1 Bierwurst
NT1 Blood sausages
NT2 Black puddings
NT1 Bockwurst
NT1 Boiled sausages
NT1 Bologna
NT1 Bratwurst
NT1 Bruehwurst
NT1 Capocollo
NT1 Cervelat
NT1 Chicken sausages
NT1 Chinese sausages
NT1 Chistorra
NT1 Chorizo
NT1 Coppas
NT1 Corn dogs
NT1 Dry sausages
NT1 Fermented sausages
NT1 Fleischwurst
NT1 Frankfurters
NT2 Hot dogs
NT2 Turkey frankfurters
NT2 Wieners
NT1 Knackwurst
NT1 Kochwurst
NT1 Lamb sausages
NT1 Liver sausages
NT1 Longaniza
NT1 Loukanka
NT1 Merguez
NT1 Mettwurst
NT1 Mortadella
NT1 Mutton sausages
NT1 Pepperoni
NT1 Pork sausages
NT1 Poultry sausages
NT1 Rohwurst
NT1 Salami
NT1 Salchichon
NT1 Saucisson
NT1 Sausage emulsions
NT1 Sausagemeat
NT1 Soudjouk
NT1 Sucuk
NT1 Summer sausages
NT1 Turkey sausages
NT1 Vienna sausages
NT1 Weisswurst
NT1 Wuerstel
RT Sausage casings

Sauteing
BT1 Cooking
BT2 Thermal processing
BT3 Processing thermal
BT4 Processing
BT5 Technology

Savory
HN under Spices up to vol. 42 (2010)
BT1 Herbs
BT2 Spices
BT3 Flavourings
BT4 Additives
NT1 *Satureja*

Savoy cabbages
BT1 Cabbages
BT2 Vegetables specific
BT3 Vegetables
BT4 Crops
BT5 Plants
BT4 Plant foods
BT5 Foods

Saxitoxin
BT1 Toxins
BT2 Residues
RT Dinoflagellate toxins
RT Paralytic shellfish poisoning

Sb
HN under Minerals up to vol. 42 (2010)
BT1 Elements
BT2 Minerals
BT3 Nutrients
UF Antimony

Sc
HN under Minerals up to vol. 42 (2010)
BT1 Metals
BT2 Elements
BT3 Minerals
BT4 Nutrients
UF Scandium

Scab
HN introduced from vol. 39, issue 1 (2007)
BT1 Plant diseases
BT2 Diseases plant
BT3 Diseases

Scad
SN syn. horse mackerel
BT1 Mackerel
BT2 Marine fish
BT3 Fish
BT4 Animals
BT4 Sea foods
BT5 Aquatic foods
BT6 Animal foods
BT7 Foods
BT2 Oily fish
BT3 Fish
BT4 Animals
BT4 Sea foods
BT5 Aquatic foods
BT6 Animal foods
BT7 Foods
UF Scads

Scads
HN used up to vol. 29 (1997)
USE **Scad**

Scald
BT1 Plant disorders
BT2 Diseases plant
BT3 Diseases
RT Diphenylamine
RT Farnesene

Scalding
BT1 Thermal processing
BT2 Processing thermal
BT3 Processing
BT4 Technology
RT Heating

Scales
USE **Weighing machines**

Scaling
SN removal of scales from fish
BT1 Processing
BT2 Technology

Scallion
BT1 Vegetables specific
BT2 Vegetables
BT3 Crops
BT4 Plants
BT3 Plant foods
BT4 Foods

Scallops
BT1 Bivalves
BT2 Molluscs
BT3 Shellfish
BT4 Animals
BT4 Sea foods
BT5 Aquatic foods
BT6 Animal foods
BT7 Foods
NT1 *Patinopecten yessoensis*

Scampi
BT1 Norway lobsters
BT2 Crustacea
BT3 Shellfish
BT4 Animals
BT4 Sea foods
BT5 Aquatic foods
BT6 Animal foods
BT7 Foods

Scandinavia
BT1 Europe

Scandium
USE **Sc**

Scanning electron microscopy
USE **SEM**

Scenedesmus
BT1 Microalgae
BT2 Algae
BT3 Microorganisms

Schizochytrium
HN introduced from vol. 39, issue 1 (2007)
BT1 Chromista
BT2 Microorganisms

Schizophyllum
BT1 Edible fungi
BT2 Fungi edible
BT3 Vegetables specific
BT4 Vegetables
BT5 Crops
BT6 Plants
BT5 Plant foods
BT6 Foods
NT1 *Schizophyllum commune*

Schizophyllum commune
HN introduced from vol. 39, issue 1 (2007)
BT1 *Schizophyllum*
BT2 Edible fungi
BT3 Fungi edible
BT4 Vegetables specific
BT5 Vegetables
BT6 Crops
BT7 Plants
BT6 Plant foods
BT7 Foods

Schizosaccharomyces
HN under Fungi up to vol. 42 (2010)
BT1 Yeasts
BT2 Fungi
BT3 Microorganisms
NT1 *Schizosaccharomyces pombe*

Schizosaccharomyces pombe
HN under Fungi up to vol. 42 (2010)
BT1 *Schizosaccharomyces*
BT2 Yeasts
BT3 Fungi
BT4 Microorganisms

Schmalzfleisch
BT1 Meat products
BT2 Animal foods
BT3 Foods

Schnapps
BT1 Spirits
BT2 Alcoholic beverages
BT3 Beverages alcoholic
BT4 Beverages

School meals
BT1 Meals
BT2 Processed foods
BT3 Foods
RT Schools

Schools
HN introduced from vol. 39, issue 1 (2007)
BT1 Institutions
RT School meals

Schwanniomyces
SN synonymous with Debaryomyces
BT1 Yeasts
BT2 Fungi
BT3 Microorganisms

Science
NT1 Animal science
NT2 Poultry science
NT1 Biochemistry
NT1 Biology
NT1 Chemistry
NT2 Histochemistry
NT2 Physical phases
NT3 Colloids
NT4 Colloidal stability
NT4 Hydrocolloids
NT3 Crystals
NT3 Dispersions
NT4 Dispersion
NT3 Emulsions
NT4 Food emulsions
NT4 Microemulsions
NT3 Gases
NT4 Acetylene
NT4 Air
NT5 Airborne
NT5 Air conditioning
NT5 Air speed
NT5 Atmosphere
NT4 Ammonia
NT5 NH_3
NT4 Ar
NT4 Biogas
NT4 Butane
NT4 Carbon dioxide
NT5 CO_2
NT5 Dry Ice
NT5 Supercritical CO_2 extraction
NT4 Carbon monoxide
NT4 Chlorine dioxide
NT4 Ethane
NT4 Ethylene
NT5 ACC
NT5 Ethephon
NT4 H_2
NT4 He
NT4 H_2S
NT4 Methane
NT4 N_2
NT4 Nitric oxide
NT4 Nitrous oxide
NT4 NO_2
NT4 O_2
NT4 Ozone
NT4 Propane
NT4 Sulfur dioxide
NT5 SO_2
NT4 Vapours
NT5 Water vapour
NT4 Xe
NT3 Gels
NT4 Agar gels
NT4 Alginate gels
NT4 Aspic
NT4 Carrageenan gels
NT4 Silica gels
NT3 Ice
NT3 Liquids
NT4 Fluids
NT5 Supercritical fluids
NT4 Juices
NT5 Stocks
NT4 Liquid foods
NT3 Solids
NT4 SNF
NT4 Soluble solids
NT4 TS
NT4 TSS
NT3 Vapours
NT4 Water vapour
NT1 Ecology
NT2 Environmental protection
NT2 Environment friendly packaging materials
NT2 Environment friendly processes
NT2 Life cycle assessment
NT2 Recycling
NT1 Engineering
NT1 Food science
NT2 Dairy science
NT1 Histology
NT2 Morphology
NT1 Laboratories
NT1 Mathematics
NT2 Equations
NT2 Formulae
NT2 Nomograms
NT2 Principal component analysis
NT2 Statistical analysis
NT3 Chemometrics
NT1 Physics
NT1 Physiology
NT2 Adipogenesis
NT2 Cell cycle
NT3 Apoptosis
NT3 Mitosis
NT2 Chemotaxis
NT2 Endocrine system
NT2 Human physiology
NT3 Angiogenesis
NT3 Appetite
NT3 Behavioural effects
NT4 Cognitive performance
NT5 Cognitive development

NT5 Memory
NT4 Cravings
NT4 Mood
NT3 Body fats
NT3 Breast feeding
NT3 Cardiovascular physiology
NT4 Blood pressure
NT3 Digestion
NT3 Exercise performance
NT3 Flatulence
NT4 Flatulence factors
NT3 Gastrointestinal tract
NT4 Malabsorption
NT3 Glucose tolerance
NT3 Human lactation
NT3 Human metabolism
NT3 Hunger
NT3 Lipaemic activity
NT3 Mastication
NT3 Physiological effects
NT3 Postprandial response
NT3 Psychophysiological effects
NT3 Reproduction
NT4 Menopause
NT4 Menstrual cycle
NT4 Pregnancy
NT3 Saliva
NT3 Satiety
NT3 Sensory perception
NT3 Sleep
NT3 Swallowing
NT3 Thermogenesis
NT3 Thirst
NT3 Vision
NT3 Weaning
NT2 Lactation
NT2 Metabolism
NT3 Bioaccumulation
NT3 Biohydrogenation
NT3 Biomagnification
NT3 Metabolic rate
NT3 Metabolomics
NT2 Motility
NT2 Puberty
NT2 Quorum sensing
NT2 Secretion
NT2 Starvation
NT2 Stress resistance
NT2 Viability
NT1 Taxonomy

Sclerocarya birrea
BT1 Marula
BT2 Fruits specific
BT3 Fruits
BT4 Crops
BT5 Plants
BT4 Plant foods
BT5 Foods

Sclerotinia
BT1 Fungi
BT2 Microorganisms
RT Diseases plant

Sclerotium
BT1 Fungi
BT2 Microorganisms

Sclex
USE **Dichlozoline**

Scomber japonicus
BT1 Chub mackerel
BT2 Mackerel
BT3 Marine fish
BT4 Fish
BT5 Animals
BT5 Sea foods
BT6 Aquatic foods
BT7 Animal foods
BT8 Foods
BT3 Oily fish
BT4 Fish
BT5 Animals
BT5 Sea foods
BT6 Aquatic foods
BT7 Animal foods
BT8 Foods

Scomber scombrus
BT1 Atlantic mackerel
BT2 Mackerel
BT3 Marine fish
BT4 Fish
BT5 Animals
BT5 Sea foods
BT6 Aquatic foods
BT7 Animal foods
BT8 Foods
BT3 Oily fish
BT4 Fish
BT5 Animals
BT5 Sea foods
BT6 Aquatic foods
BT7 Animal foods
BT8 Foods

Scombroid poisoning
BT1 Diseases
BT1 Poisoning
RT Histamine

Scones
BT1 Bakery products
BT2 Cereal products
BT3 Plant foods
BT4 Foods

Scoops
HN introduced from vol. 41, issue 1 (2009)
BT1 Containers
BT1 Utensils
BT2 Equipment
BT3 Technology

Scopoletin
BT1 Coumarins
BT2 Lactones
BT3 Esters
BT4 Organic compounds
BT3 Heterocyclic compounds
BT2 Phenols
BT3 Alcohols
BT3 Aromatic compounds
BT4 Organic compounds

Scopulariopsis
BT1 Fungi
BT2 Microorganisms

Scotch whisky
HN introduced from vol. 43, issue 1 (2011)
BT1 Whisky
BT2 Whiskies
BT3 Spirits
BT4 Alcoholic beverages
BT5 Beverages alcoholic
BT6 Beverages

Scotland
BT1 United Kingdom
BT2 Europe
BT2 European Union

Scrambled egg
BT1 Egg products
BT2 Animal foods
BT3 Foods

Scrapie
BT1 Prion diseases
BT2 Diseases

Screw caps
HN introduced from vol. 41, issue 1 (2009)
BT1 Caps
BT2 Closures
BT3 Packaging
BT4 Technology

Scuffing
BT1 Damage

Sculpin
BT1 Marine fish
BT2 Fish
BT3 Animals
BT3 Sea foods
BT4 Aquatic foods
BT5 Animal foods
BT6 Foods
UF Sculpins

Sculpins
HN used up to vol. 29 (1997)
USE **Sculpin**

Scutellaria baicalensis
BT1 Plants

SDS
BT1 Organic sulfur compounds
BT1 Sulfates
BT2 Salts
BT1 Surfactants
UF Sodium dodecyl sulfate
UF Sodium dodecyl sulphate
UF Sodium lauryl sulfate
UF Sodium lauryl sulphate

SDS-PAGE
BT1 Electrophoresis
BT2 Analytical techniques

Se
SN index heading is Selenium

BT1 Selenium
BT2 Elements
BT3 Minerals
BT4 Nutrients

Sea bass
SN syn. sea perch
BT1 Marine fish
BT2 Fish
BT3 Animals
BT3 Sea foods
BT4 Aquatic foods
BT5 Animal foods
BT6 Foods
NT1 Striped bass
NT2 *Morone saxatilis*

Sea bream
BT1 Marine fish
BT2 Fish
BT3 Animals
BT3 Sea foods
BT4 Aquatic foods
BT5 Animal foods
BT6 Foods
NT1 Bogue
NT2 *Boops boops*
NT1 Red sea bream
NT2 *Pagrus major*
NT1 *Sparus aurata*
UF *Dentex*
UF Sakuradai

Sea buckthorn
BT1 Fruits specific
BT2 Fruits
BT3 Crops
BT4 Plants
BT3 Plant foods
BT4 Foods
RT Sea buckthorn juices

Sea buckthorn juices
HN introduced from vol. 41, issue 1 (2009)
BT1 Fruit juices
BT2 Fruit products
BT3 Plant foods
BT4 Foods
BT2 Soft drinks
BT3 Beverages
RT Sea buckthorn

Sea buckthorn oils
BT1 Vegetable oils
BT2 Oils vegetable
BT3 Oils
BT4 Lipids
BT5 Nutrients
BT3 Vegetable products
BT4 Plant foods
BT5 Foods

Sea cucumbers
BT1 Sea foods
BT2 Aquatic foods
BT3 Animal foods
BT4 Foods
UF Beche de mer
UF Sea slugs

Sea fennel
HN under Spices up to vol. 42 (2010)
BT1 Samphire
BT2 Herbs
BT3 Spices
BT4 Flavourings
BT5 Additives
NT1 *Crithmum maritimum*

Sea fish
BT1 Marine fish
BT2 Fish
BT3 Animals
BT3 Sea foods
BT4 Aquatic foods
BT5 Animal foods
BT6 Foods

Sea food products
HN introduced from vol. 39, issue 1 (2007)
BT1 Sea foods
BT2 Aquatic foods
BT3 Animal foods
BT4 Foods

Sea foods
BT1 Aquatic foods
BT2 Animal foods
BT3 Foods
NT1 Ascidians
NT2 Sea squirts
NT1 Dried sea foods
NT2 Dried fish
NT1 Echinoderms
NT1 Fish
NT2 Bass
NT2 Char
NT3 Arctic char
NT2 Dried fish
NT2 Farmed fish
NT2 Finfish
NT2 Fish bones
NT2 Fish factories
NT2 Fish fillets
NT2 Fish industry
NT2 Fish livers
NT3 Cod livers
NT2 Fish mince
NT2 Fish skin
NT2 Freshwater fish
NT3 Ayu
NT3 Bream
NT3 Burbot
NT3 Carp
NT4 Bighead carp
NT5 *Aristichthys nobilis*
NT4 Crucian carp
NT4 *Cyprinus carpio*
NT4 Grass carp
NT5 White amur
NT4 Rohu
NT5 *Labeo rohita*
NT4 Silver carp
NT3 Catfish
NT4 Channel catfish
NT5 *Ictalurus punctatus*
NT4 *Silurus asotus*
NT3 Chub
NT4 *Leuciscus cephalus*
NT3 *Colossoma macropomum*
NT3 Eels
NT3 Nile perch
NT3 Pacu
NT3 Perch
NT4 *Perca fluviatilis*
NT4 Yellow perch
NT3 Pike
NT3 River fish
NT3 Roach
NT3 Snakehead
NT3 Sunfish
NT3 Tench
NT3 Tilapia
NT4 Nile tilapia
NT5 Bolti
NT5 *Oreochromis niloticus*
NT5 *Tilapia nilotica*
NT4 *Oreochromis*
NT5 *Oreochromis niloticus*
NT3 Vendace
NT4 Coregonus albula
NT3 Walleye
NT2 Lamprey
NT2 Marine fish
NT3 Alaska pollock
NT4 Alaska pollack
NT4 *Theragra chalcogramma*
NT4 Walleye pollack
NT3 Alewife
NT3 Anchovy
NT4 Anchovy pastes
NT4 Budu
NT4 *Engraulis encrasicholus*
NT3 Barracuda
NT3 Barramundi
NT3 Bigeye snapper
NT4 *Priacanthus macracanthus*
NT3 Bluefish
NT3 Blue whiting
NT4 *Micromesistius poutassou*
NT3 Bombay duck
NT3 Capelin
NT3 Coalfish
NT3 Cod
NT4 Cod livers
NT4 *Gadus morhua*
NT4 Rock cod
NT3 Conger eels
NT3 Croakers
NT3 Cutlassfish
NT3 Dogfish
NT3 Dolphinfish
NT4 Mahimahi
NT3 Drum
NT3 Filefish
NT3 Flatfish
NT4 Arrowtooth flounder
NT4 Bastard halibut
NT5 *Paralichthys olivaceus*
NT4 Dab
NT4 Flounders
NT5 Japanese flounders
NT6 *Paralichthys olivaceus*
NT5 *Platichthys flesus*
NT4 Halibut
NT5 Atlantic halibut

NT5 Greenland halibut
NT5 *Reinhardtius hippoglossoides*
NT4 Megrim
NT5 *Lepidorhombus boscii*
NT4 Plaice
NT5 *Pleuronectes platessa*
NT4 Sole
NT4 Turbot
NT3 Flying fish
NT3 Grenadier
NT3 Groundfish
NT3 Grouper
NT4 *Epinephelus guaza*
NT3 Gurnard
NT3 Haddock
NT3 Hagfish
NT3 Hairtail
NT3 Hake
NT4 *Merluccius australis*
NT4 *Merluccius hubbsi*
NT4 *Merluccius merluccius*
NT4 Pacific hake
NT5 *Merluccius productus*
NT5 Pacific whiting
NT4 Red hake
NT3 Herring
NT4 *Clupea harengus*
NT4 Kippers
NT4 Matjes
NT4 Rollmops
NT3 Hilsa
NT3 Hoki
NT3 Kilka
NT3 Kingklip
NT3 Lanternfish
NT3 Ling
NT4 *Molva molva*
NT3 Ling cod
NT4 *Ophiodon elongatus*
NT3 Lizardfish
NT3 Lumpfish
NT4 *Cyclopterus lumpus*
NT3 Mackerel
NT4 Atlantic mackerel
NT5 *Scomber scombrus*
NT4 Chub mackerel
NT5 *Scomber japonicus*
NT4 Frigate mackerel
NT4 Horse mackerel
NT4 Indian mackerel
NT4 Jack mackerel
NT5 *Trachurus japonicus*
NT5 *Trachurus murphyi*
NT4 Pacific mackerel
NT4 Scad
NT4 Seer fish
NT4 Smoked mackerel
NT4 Spanish mackerel
NT3 Marlins
NT3 Menhaden
NT4 *Brevoortia tyrannus*
NT3 Milkfish
NT4 *Chanos chanos*
NT3 Monkfish
NT3 Morwong
NT3 Mullet
NT4 *Mugil cephalus*
NT3 Orange roughy
NT3 Paddlefish
NT4 *Polyodon spathula*
NT3 Pilchards
NT3 Pollack
NT3 Pollock
NT3 Pomfret
NT4 Butterfish
NT3 *Priacanthus tayenus*
NT3 Pufferfish
NT3 Rabbitfish
NT3 Ray
NT3 Redfish
NT3 Redspot emperor
NT4 *Lethrinus lentjan*
NT3 Rockfish
NT3 Sablefish
NT3 Sailfish
NT3 Saithe
NT3 Sand lance
NT3 Sardine
NT4 Monterey sardine
NT4 *Sardina pilchardus*
NT3 *Sardinella*
NT3 Saury
NT3 Sculpin
NT3 Sea bass
NT4 Striped bass
NT5 *Morone saxatilis*
NT3 Sea bream
NT4 Bogue
NT5 *Boops boops*
NT4 Red sea bream
NT5 *Pagrus major*
NT4 *Sparus aurata*
NT3 Sea fish
NT3 Sea perch
NT3 Shad
NT4 Indian shad
NT3 Sharks
NT4 Shark fins
NT3 Sheatfish
NT3 Skate
NT3 Snapper
NT3 Sprat
NT3 Swordfish
NT3 Threadfin bream
NT3 Tuna
NT4 Bigeye tuna
NT4 Bonito
NT4 Skipjack tuna
NT5 Katsuobushi
NT4 White tuna
NT5 Albacore
NT4 Yellowfin tuna
NT3 Whitebait
NT3 White fish
NT3 Whiting
NT3 Wreckfish
NT4 *Polyprion americanus*
NT3 Yellowfin
NT3 Yellowtail
NT2 Oily fish
NT3 Anchovy
NT4 Anchovy pastes
NT4 Budu
NT4 *Engraulis encrasicholus*
NT3 Carp
NT4 Bighead carp
NT5 *Aristichthys nobilis*
NT4 Crucian carp
NT4 *Cyprinus carpio*
NT4 Grass carp
NT5 White amur
NT4 Rohu
NT5 *Labeo rohita*
NT4 Silver carp
NT3 Eels
NT3 Herring
NT4 *Clupea harengus*
NT4 Kippers
NT4 Matjes
NT4 Rollmops
NT3 Hilsa
NT3 Mackerel
NT4 Atlantic mackerel
NT5 *Scomber scombrus*
NT4 Chub mackerel
NT5 *Scomber japonicus*
NT4 Frigate mackerel
NT4 Horse mackerel
NT4 Indian mackerel
NT4 Jack mackerel
NT5 *Trachurus japonicus*
NT5 *Trachurus murphyi*
NT4 Pacific mackerel
NT4 Scad
NT4 Seer fish
NT4 Smoked mackerel
NT4 Spanish mackerel
NT3 Orange roughy
NT3 Pilchards
NT3 Salmon
NT4 Atlantic salmon
NT5 *Salmo salar*
NT4 Pacific salmon
NT5 Cherry salmon
NT6 Masu salmon
NT5 Chinook salmon
NT6 King salmon
NT5 Chum salmon
NT6 Keta salmon
NT6 *Oncorhynchus keta*
NT5 Coho salmon
NT5 Pink salmon
NT5 Sockeye salmon
NT6 Red salmon
NT4 Smoked salmon
NT3 Sardine
NT4 Monterey sardine
NT4 *Sardina pilchardus*
NT3 Sprat
NT3 Swordfish
NT3 Trout
NT4 Brook trout
NT4 Brown trout
NT4 Rainbow trout
NT5 *Oncorhynchus mykiss*
NT4 Sea trout
NT4 Smoked trout
NT3 Tuna
NT4 Bigeye tuna
NT4 Bonito
NT4 Skipjack tuna
NT5 Katsuobushi
NT4 White tuna
NT5 Albacore
NT4 Yellowfin tuna
NT3 Whitebait

NT2 Sturgeon
NT3 Beluga
NT2 Whitefish
NT3 *Coregonus lavaretus*
NT1 Fish products
NT2 Ceviche
NT2 Fish balls
NT2 Fishburgers
NT2 Fish cakes
NT2 Fish crackers
NT2 Fish fingers
NT2 Fish hydrolysates
NT2 Fish in marinades
NT2 Fish in oils
NT2 Fish in sauces
NT2 Fish meal
NT2 Fish noodles
NT2 Fish pastes
NT3 Anchovy pastes
NT2 Fish pates
NT2 Fish preserves
NT2 Fish sauces
NT3 Budu
NT3 Ishiru
NT3 Nuoc-mam
NT3 Patis
NT2 Fish sausages
NT2 Fish soups
NT2 Kamaboko
NT2 Katsuobushi
NT2 Kusaya
NT2 Matjes
NT2 Momoni
NT2 Nukazuke
NT2 Oils fish
NT3 Fish oils
NT4 Anchovy oils
NT4 Cod liver oils
NT4 Fish liver oils
NT4 Menhaden oils
NT4 Salmon oils
NT4 Sardine oils
NT4 Tuna oils
NT2 Pates
NT3 Fish pates
NT3 Liver pates
NT3 Terrines
NT2 Restructured fish products
NT2 Roes
NT3 Caviar
NT3 Caviar substitutes
NT3 Milt
NT2 Rollmops
NT2 Salted fish
NT2 Sashimi
NT2 Smoked fish
NT3 Kippers
NT3 Smoked mackerel
NT3 Smoked salmon
NT3 Smoked trout
NT2 Surimi
NT2 Sushi
NT1 Jellyfish
NT1 Jeotgal
NT1 Plankton
NT1 Sea cucumbers
NT1 Sea food products
NT1 Sea foods industry
NT1 Sea urchins
NT2 Sea urchin gonads
NT1 Seaweeds
NT2 *Caulerpa*
NT2 *Chondrus*
NT3 *Chondrus crispus*
NT2 *Cystoseira*
NT2 Dulse
NT3 *Palmaria palmata*
NT2 *Ecklonia*
NT2 *Eucheuma*
NT2 *Fucus*
NT2 *Furcellaria*
NT2 *Gigartina*
NT2 *Gracilaria*
NT2 *Hizikia*
NT2 *Iridaea*
NT2 *Laminaria*
NT3 Kombu
NT2 Laver
NT2 *Macrocystis*
NT2 Onigusa
NT2 *Phyllophora*
NT2 *Porphyra*
NT3 Nori
NT3 *Porphyra yezoensis*
NT2 *Sargassum*
NT2 *Ulva*
NT3 Sea lettuces
NT3 *Ulva lactuca*
NT2 *Undaria*
NT3 *Undaria pinnatifida*
NT3 Wakame
NT1 Shellfish
NT2 Crustacea
NT3 Crabs
NT4 Blue crabs
NT5 *Callinectes sapidus*
NT4 Crab meat
NT5 Crab legs
NT4 Mud crabs
NT4 Red crabs
NT4 Snow crabs
NT3 Crawfish
NT3 Crayfish
NT3 Krill
NT3 Lobsters
NT4 American lobsters
NT3 Norway lobsters
NT4 Langoustines
NT4 Scampi
NT3 Prawns
NT4 Kuruma prawns
NT4 Prawn crackers
NT3 Shrimps
NT4 *Crangon crangon*
NT4 *Pandalus borealis*
NT4 Tiger shrimps
NT2 Farmed shellfish
NT2 Molluscs
NT3 Bivalves
NT4 Arkshells
NT4 Carpet shells
NT4 Clams
NT5 Freshwater clams
NT5 *Pseudocardium sachalinensis*
NT5 *Tapes philippinarum*
NT4 Cockles
NT4 Mussels
NT5 Blue mussels
NT5 Green mussels
NT5 *Mytilus edulis*
NT5 *Mytilus galloprovincialis*
NT5 *Mytilus trossulus*
NT4 Oysters
NT5 *Crassostrea gigas*
NT5 *Crassostrea virginica*
NT5 Oyster sauces
NT4 Razor shells
NT4 Scallops
NT5 *Patinopecten yessoensis*
NT3 Cephalopods
NT4 Cuttlefish
NT4 Octopus
NT4 Squid
NT5 Ika shiokara
NT5 *Illex argentinus*
NT5 *Ommastrephes bartrami*
NT3 Gastropods
NT4 Abalones
NT4 Limpets
NT4 Periwinkles
NT4 Snails
NT5 Land snails
NT5 Snail meat
NT4 Top shells
NT4 Trumpet shells
NT4 Turban shells
NT4 Whelks
NT1 Shiokara
NT2 Ika shiokara
RT Amnesic shellfish poisoning
RT Aquaculture products
RT Diarrhoetic shellfish poisoning
RT Neurological shellfish poisoning
RT Paralytic shellfish poisoning
UF Sea-foods

Sea-foods
HN heading up to vol. 24 (1992); use Sea foods from vol. 25 (1993)
USE **Sea foods**

Sea foods industry
HN introduced from vol. 39, issue 1 (2007)
BT1 Food industry
BT2 Industries
BT1 Sea foods
BT2 Aquatic foods
BT3 Animal foods
BT4 Foods
RT Fish industry

Sea kale
BT1 Vegetables specific
BT2 Vegetables
BT3 Crops
BT4 Plants
BT3 Plant foods
BT4 Foods

Seal blubber
BT1 Blubber
BT2 Animal fats
BT3 Fats animal

BT4 Animal foods
BT5 Foods
BT4 Fats
BT5 Lipids
BT6 Nutrients
BT1 Seals
BT2 Animals
RT Seal blubber oils
RT Seal oils

Seal blubber oils
BT1 Marine oils
BT2 Oils
BT3 Lipids
BT4 Nutrients
RT Seal blubber
RT Seal oils

Seal carcasses
BT1 Carcasses
BT2 Meat
BT3 Animal foods
BT4 Foods
BT1 Seal meat
BT2 Meat specific
BT3 Meat
BT4 Animal foods
BT5 Foods
BT2 Seals
BT3 Animals

Sea lettuces
BT1 *Ulva*
BT2 Seaweeds
BT3 Algae
BT4 Microorganisms
BT3 Sea foods
BT4 Aquatic foods
BT5 Animal foods
BT6 Foods

Sealing
BT1 Packaging
BT2 Technology
NT1 Seaming
RT Closures

Seal meat
BT1 Meat specific
BT2 Meat
BT3 Animal foods
BT4 Foods
BT1 Seals
BT2 Animals
NT1 Seal carcasses

Seal oils
BT1 Marine oils
BT2 Oils
BT3 Lipids
BT4 Nutrients
RT Seal blubber
RT Seal blubber oils

Seals
BT1 Animals
NT1 Seal blubber
NT1 Seal meat
NT2 Seal carcasses

Seaming
BT1 Sealing
BT2 Packaging
BT3 Technology

Sea mustard
HN used up to vol. 39 (2007)
USE **Wakame**

Sea perch
SN syn. sea bass
BT1 Marine fish
BT2 Fish
BT3 Animals
BT3 Sea foods
BT4 Aquatic foods
BT5 Animal foods
BT6 Foods

Sea slugs
HN used up to vol. 39 (2007)
USE **Sea cucumbers**

Season
RT Climate
RT Environment
RT Weather

Seasonings
BT1 Condiments
BT2 Flavourings
BT3 Additives

Sea squirts
SN syn. ascidians
BT1 Ascidians
BT2 Sea foods
BT3 Aquatic foods
BT4 Animal foods
BT5 Foods

Sea trout
BT1 Trout
BT2 Oily fish
BT3 Fish
BT4 Animals
BT4 Sea foods
BT5 Aquatic foods
BT6 Animal foods
BT7 Foods
RT Brown trout

Sea urchin gonads
BT1 Sea urchins
BT2 Sea foods
BT3 Aquatic foods
BT4 Animal foods
BT5 Foods

Sea urchins
BT1 Sea foods
BT2 Aquatic foods
BT3 Animal foods
BT4 Foods
NT1 Sea urchin gonads
UF Echinoids

Sea water
BT1 Water

Seaweeds
BT1 Algae
BT2 Microorganisms
BT1 Sea foods
BT2 Aquatic foods
BT3 Animal foods
BT4 Foods
NT1 *Caulerpa*
NT1 *Chondrus*
NT2 *Chondrus crispus*
NT1 *Cystoseira*
NT1 Dulse
NT2 *Palmaria palmata*
NT1 *Ecklonia*
NT1 *Eucheuma*
NT1 *Fucus*
NT1 *Furcellaria*
NT1 *Gigartina*
NT1 *Gracilaria*
NT1 *Hizikia*
NT1 *Iridaea*
NT1 *Laminaria*
NT2 Kombu
NT1 Laver
NT1 *Macrocystis*
NT1 Onigusa
NT1 *Phyllophora*
NT1 *Porphyra*
NT2 Nori
NT2 *Porphyra yezoensis*
NT1 *Sargassum*
NT1 *Ulva*
NT2 Sea lettuces
NT2 *Ulva lactuca*
NT1 *Undaria*
NT2 *Undaria pinnatifida*
NT2 Wakame
RT Agar
RT Alginates
RT Carrageenans
RT Fucoidans

Secalins
BT1 Cereal proteins
BT2 Proteins cereal
BT3 Vegetable proteins
BT4 Proteins vegetable
BT5 Proteins
BT6 Nutrients
BT5 Vegetable products
BT6 Plant foods
BT7 Foods
RT Rye

Secretion
HN introduced from vol. 39, issue 1 (2007)
BT1 Physiology
BT2 Science

Sedimentation
BT1 Precipitation

Seed coats
HN introduced from vol. 42, issue 1 (2010)
BT1 Plants
RT Hulls
RT Husks
RT Seeds

Seedless grapes
BT1 Grapes
BT2 Berries
BT3 Fruits specific
BT4 Fruits
BT5 Crops
BT6 Plants
BT5 Plant foods
BT6 Foods

Seeds
BT1 Plant foods
BT2 Foods
NT1 African breadfruit seeds
NT1 Apricot seeds
NT1 Betel nuts
NT1 Cereals
NT2 Acha
NT2 Barley
NT3 Barley fibre
NT3 Barley flour
NT3 Barley starch
NT3 Malting barley
NT3 Pearl barley
NT2 Corn
NT3 Baby corn
NT3 Corn bran
NT3 Corn bread
NT3 Corn chips
NT3 Corn cobs
NT3 Cornflakes
NT3 Corn flour
NT3 Corn masa
NT3 Corn starch
NT4 High amylose corn starch
NT3 Kenkey
NT3 Kwoka
NT3 Popcorn
NT4 Microwave popcorn
NT3 Pozol
NT3 Sweetcorn
NT2 Jobs tears
NT2 Millet
NT3 Bajra
NT3 Common millet
NT3 Finger millet
NT3 Fonio
NT3 Foxtail millet
NT3 Millet flour
NT3 Millet starch
NT3 Pearl millet
NT3 Ragi
NT3 Teff
NT2 Oats
NT3 *Avena fatua*
NT3 Oat bran
NT3 Oat fibre
NT3 Oat flakes
NT3 Oat flour
NT3 Oatmeal
NT3 Oat starch
NT3 Porridge
NT2 Rice
NT3 Arare
NT3 Basmati rice
NT3 Black rice
NT3 Brown rice
NT3 Dosai
NT3 Idli
NT3 Lao-chao
NT3 Paddy
NT3 Puffed rice
NT3 Puto
NT3 Rice bran
NT3 Rice bread
NT3 Rice cakes
NT3 Rice crackers
NT3 Rice flour
NT3 Rice koji
NT3 Rice milk
NT3 Rice noodles
NT3 Rice powders
NT3 Rice starch
NT3 Sikhe
NT3 Tape
NT4 Tape ketan
NT3 Yukwa
NT2 Rye
NT3 Rye bran
NT3 Rye bread
NT3 Rye flour
NT3 Rye starch
NT2 Sorghum
NT3 Jowar
NT3 Milo
NT3 Sorghum flour
NT3 Sorghum starch
NT2 Triticale
NT3 Triticale flour
NT2 Tritordeum
NT2 Wheat
NT3 Atta
NT3 Bulgur
NT3 Durum wheat
NT3 Einkorn
NT3 Emmer
NT3 Maida
NT3 Spelt
NT4 Spelt wheat
NT3 Wheat bran
NT3 Wheat bread
NT3 Wheat breadmaking
NT3 Wheat dough
NT3 Wheat fibre
NT3 Wheat flour
NT3 Wheat germ
NT3 Wheat gluten
NT3 Wheat starch
NT2 Wild rice
NT1 Cycad seeds
NT1 Grain
NT1 Grape seeds
NT1 Ogiri
NT1 Oilseeds
NT2 African locust beans
NT3 Dawadawa
NT3 Iru
NT2 African mango seeds
NT3 Dika nuts
NT2 African oil beans
NT3 Ugba
NT2 Aiele fruits
NT2 Babassu palm kernels
NT2 *Brassica* seeds
NT2 *Camelina sativa*
NT2 Castor beans
NT2 Cottonseeds
NT3 Cottonseed meal
NT3 Cottonseed proteins
NT3 Gossypol
NT2 Crambe seeds
NT3 *Crambe abyssinica*
NT2 Cucumber seeds
NT2 *Cuphea*
NT2 Egusi
NT2 *Euphorbia*
NT2 Evening primrose seeds
NT2 Flax seeds
NT3 Linseeds
NT2 Gourd seeds
NT2 *Guizotia*
NT2 Hemp seeds
NT2 Illipe nuts
NT2 Jojoba seeds
NT2 Jute seeds
NT2 Kenaf seeds
NT2 Kusum
NT2 Lupin seeds
NT3 Lupin meal
NT2 Madhuca seeds
NT2 Meadowfoam
NT2 Melon seeds
NT2 *Moringa*
NT2 Mustard seeds
NT3 Ethiopian mustard
NT4 *Brassica carinata*
NT3 Indian mustard
NT2 Niger seeds
NT2 Nuts
NT3 Acorns
NT3 Almonds
NT4 Sweet almonds
NT3 Australian chestnuts
NT3 Brazil nuts
NT3 Butternuts
NT3 Cashew nuts
NT3 Cedar nuts
NT3 Chestnuts
NT4 Japanese chestnuts
NT4 Sweet chestnuts
NT3 Chilean hazelnuts
NT3 Coconuts
NT4 Bongkrek
NT4 Coconut cream
NT4 Coconut milk
NT4 Coconut water
NT4 Copra
NT4 Desiccated coconut
NT4 Nata
NT3 Cola nuts
NT4 *Cola nitida*
NT3 Conophor nuts
NT3 Ginkgo nuts
NT3 Gorgon nuts
NT3 Hazelnuts
NT3 Hickory nuts
NT3 Macadamia nuts
NT3 Nut pastes
NT4 Peanut pastes
NT3 Nut products
NT3 Peanuts
NT4 Ontjom
NT4 Peanut butter
NT4 Peanut meal
NT4 Peanut milk
NT4 Peanut pastes
NT4 Peanut products

NT4 Peanut proteins
NT4 Roasted peanuts
NT3 Pecan nuts
NT3 Pine nuts
NT3 Pistachio nuts
NT3 Walnuts
NT2 Olives
NT3 Black olives
NT3 Table olives
NT2 Perilla seeds
NT2 Pumpkin seeds
NT2 Rapeseeds
NT3 Bird rape
NT3 *Brassica napus*
NT3 Rapeseed meal
NT2 Raya seeds
NT2 Rubber seeds
NT2 Safflower seeds
NT2 Sal seeds
NT2 Sesame seeds
NT3 Halva
NT3 Sesame
NT3 Sesame seed meal
NT3 Tahini
NT4 Tehineh
NT2 Shea nuts
NT2 Soybeans
NT3 Black soybeans
NT3 Soybean sprouts
NT2 Squash seeds
NT2 Sunflower seeds
NT3 Sunflower meal
NT3 Sunflowers
NT2 Tomato seeds
NT2 *Vernonia*
NT2 Watermelon seeds
NT2 White mustard
NT2 Yellow mustard
NT1 Parthenocarpy
NT1 *Prosopis africana* seeds
NT1 Pseudocereals
NT2 Amaranth grain
NT3 Amaranth flour
NT3 Amaranth starch
NT3 *Amaranthus*
NT3 Grain amaranth
NT2 Buckwheat
NT3 Buckwheat flour
NT3 Buckwheat starch
NT2 Canary grass
NT2 Quinoa
NT3 Quinoa flour
NT1 Psyllium
RT Seed coats
UF Pips
UF Stones

Seer fish
HN under Fish up to vol. 42 (2010)
BT1 Mackerel
BT2 Marine fish
BT3 Fish
BT4 Animals
BT4 Sea foods
BT5 Aquatic foods
BT6 Animal foods
BT7 Foods
BT2 Oily fish
BT3 Fish
BT4 Animals
BT4 Sea foods
BT5 Aquatic foods
BT6 Animal foods
BT7 Foods

Sekts
BT1 Sparkling wines
BT2 Wines sparkling
BT3 Wines
BT4 Alcoholic beverages
BT5 Beverages alcoholic
BT6 Beverages

Selenites
HN introduced from vol. 39, issue 1 (2007)
BT1 Selenium
BT2 Elements
BT3 Minerals
BT4 Nutrients

Selenium
SN symbol Se is also used in the index
BT1 Elements
BT2 Minerals
BT3 Nutrients
NT1 Se
NT1 Selenites
NT1 Selenomethionine
NT1 Selenoproteins

Selenomethionine
HN introduced from vol. 43, issue 1 (2011)
BT1 Methionine
BT2 Amino acids
BT3 Nutrients
BT3 Organic acids
BT4 Acids
BT3 Organic nitrogen compounds
BT2 Organic sulfur compounds
BT1 Selenium
BT2 Elements
BT3 Minerals
BT4 Nutrients

Selenoproteins
HN introduced from vol. 41, issue 1 (2009)
BT1 Proteins
BT2 Nutrients
BT1 Selenium
BT2 Elements
BT3 Minerals
BT4 Nutrients

SEM
BT1 Electron microscopy
BT2 Microscopy
BT3 Analytical techniques
UF Scanning electron microscopy

Semeron
USE **Desmetryn**

Semicarbazide
HN introduced from vol. 39, issue 1 (2007)
BT1 Contaminants
BT2 Contamination
BT1 Organic nitrogen compounds

Semi skimmed milk
BT1 Milk
BT2 Dairy products
BT3 Animal foods
BT4 Foods
RT Skim milk

Semolina
BT1 Cereal products
BT2 Plant foods
BT3 Foods
RT Cereal flours
RT Flours cereal
RT Pasta

Sencor
USE **Metribuzin**

Senegal
BT1 West Africa
BT2 Africa

Senescence
BT1 Ripening

Sensors
BT1 Apparatus
BT2 Technology
BT1 Equipment
BT2 Technology

Sensory analysis
HN heading from vol. 19 (1987); use Organoleptic evaluation up to vol. 18 (1986)
BT1 Analytical techniques
NT1 Consumer panels
NT1 Flavour thresholds
NT1 Olfactometry
NT1 Panellists
NT1 Quantitative descriptive analysis
NT1 Sensory scores
NT1 Sensory thresholds
NT1 Taste panels
NT1 Texture profile analysis
NT1 Time intensity
RT Electronic noses
RT Sensory properties
UF Organoleptic evaluation
UF Sensory evaluation

Sensory evaluation
USE **Sensory analysis**

Sensory perception
HN introduced from vol. 39, issue 1 (2007)
BT1 Human physiology
BT2 Physiology
BT3 Science
RT Propylthiouracil
RT Sensory properties

Sensory properties
HN heading from vol. 19 (1987); use Organoleptic properties up to vol. 18 (1986)
NT1 Appearance

NT1 Aroma
NT2 Aromatization
NT2 Bouquet
NT2 Odour activity values
NT2 Odour threshold values
NT2 Pungency
NT1 Chalkiness
NT1 Chemesthesis
NT1 Dryness
NT1 Eating quality
NT1 Flavour
NT2 Aftertaste
NT2 Astringency
NT2 Bitterness
NT2 Fruitiness
NT2 Rancidity
NT2 Saltiness
NT2 Sharpness
NT2 Soapiness
NT2 Sourness
NT2 Sweetness
NT2 Taints
NT3 Boar taint
NT3 Cork taint
NT3 Off flavour
NT3 Off odour
NT3 Warmed over flavour
NT2 Umami
NT1 Greasiness
NT1 Juiciness
NT2 Succulence
NT1 Mealiness
NT1 Mouthfeel
NT2 Grittiness
NT1 Palatability
NT1 Texture
NT2 Body
NT2 Chewiness
NT2 Consistency
NT3 Consistometers
NT3 Creaminess
NT3 Graininess
NT3 Lumpiness
NT3 Pastiness
NT3 Plasticity
NT3 Smoothness
NT2 Crispness
NT2 Crumbliness
NT2 Crunchiness
NT2 Firmness
NT3 Penetrometers
NT3 *Rigor mortis*
NT3 Rigorometers
NT3 Softening
NT3 Softness
NT2 Spreadability
NT2 Springiness
NT2 Tenderness
NT3 Tenderometers
NT2 Texturometers
NT2 Toughness
NT1 Wateriness
RT Colour
RT Mechanical properties
RT Rheological properties
RT Sensory analysis
RT Sensory perception
UF Organoleptic properties

Sensory scores
BT1 Sensory analysis
BT2 Analytical techniques

Sensory thresholds
BT1 Sensory analysis
BT2 Analytical techniques

Separation
BT1 Processing
BT2 Technology
NT1 Centrifugation
NT2 Bactofugation
NT2 Centrifuges
NT3 Centrifugal separators
NT2 Ultracentrifugation
NT1 Flocculation
NT2 Floc
NT2 Flocculants
NT1 Flotation
NT1 Fractionation
NT2 Foam fractionation
NT1 Immunomagnetic separation
NT1 Partitioning
NT1 Pervaporation
NT1 Separators
NT2 Centrifugal separators
NT1 Sieving
NT2 Sieves
NT2 Sifting
NT3 Sifters
NT1 Strainers
RT Aqueous two phase systems
RT Dialysis

Separators
BT1 Equipment
BT2 Technology
BT1 Separation
BT2 Processing
BT3 Technology
NT1 Centrifugal separators

Septoria
BT1 Fungi
BT2 Microorganisms
RT Diseases plant

Sequencing
BT1 Analytical techniques
RT Amino acids
RT Genes
RT Protein engineering
RT Proteins

Sequestrants
BT1 Additives
RT Chelating agents

Serbia
BT1 Europe

Serine
BT1 Amino acids
BT2 Nutrients
BT2 Organic acids
BT3 Acids
BT2 Organic nitrogen compounds

Serological tests
BT1 Immunological techniques
BT2 Analytical techniques

Serology
BT1 Immunological techniques
BT2 Analytical techniques
BT1 Immunology

Serotonin
SN syn. 5-hydroxytryptamine
BT1 Biogenic amines
BT2 Amines
BT3 Organic nitrogen compounds

Serotype
BT1 Immunology

Serotyping
BT1 Immunological techniques
BT2 Analytical techniques

Serra cheese
BT1 Cheese varieties
BT2 Cheese
BT3 Dairy products
BT4 Animal foods
BT5 Foods

Serrano ham
BT1 Ham
BT2 Meat products
BT3 Animal foods
BT4 Foods

Serratia
HN under Enterobacteriaceae up to vol. 24 (1992); heading from vol. 30 (1998)
BT1 Bacteria
BT2 Microorganisms
NT1 *Serratia liquefaciens*
NT1 *Serratia marcescens*

Serratia liquefaciens
BT1 *Serratia*
BT2 Bacteria
BT3 Microorganisms

Serratia marcescens
BT1 *Serratia*
BT2 Bacteria
BT3 Microorganisms

Serum
USE **Blood**

Sesame
HN heading up to vol. 24
BT1 Sesame seeds
BT2 Oilseeds
BT3 Seeds
BT4 Plant foods
BT5 Foods

Sesame oils
BT1 Vegetable oils
BT2 Oils vegetable
BT3 Oils
BT4 Lipids
BT5 Nutrients

BT3 Vegetable products
BT4 Plant foods
BT5 Foods
RT Sesamol
UF Gingelly oils
UF Til oils

Sesame seed meal
BT1 Flours
BT2 Plant foods
BT3 Foods
BT1 Sesame seeds
BT2 Oilseeds
BT3 Seeds
BT4 Plant foods
BT5 Foods

Sesame seeds
HN heading from vol. 25 (1993); under Sesame up to vol. 24 (1992)
BT1 Oilseeds
BT2 Seeds
BT3 Plant foods
BT4 Foods
NT1 Halva
NT1 Sesame
NT1 Sesame seed meal
NT1 Tahini
NT2 Tehineh
RT Sesamin
RT Sesamolin
UF Gingelly seeds

Sesamin
HN introduced from vol. 39, issue 1 (2007)
BT1 Lignans
BT2 Phenols
BT3 Alcohols
BT3 Aromatic compounds
BT4 Organic compounds
RT Sesame seeds

Sesamol
BT1 Antioxidants
BT2 Additives
BT1 Phenols
BT2 Alcohols
BT2 Aromatic compounds
BT3 Organic compounds
RT Sesame oils

Sesamolin
HN introduced from vol. 39, issue 1 (2007)
BT1 Lignans
BT2 Phenols
BT3 Alcohols
BT3 Aromatic compounds
BT4 Organic compounds
RT Sesame seeds

Sesbania
BT1 Vegetables specific
BT2 Vegetables
BT3 Crops
BT4 Plants
BT3 Plant foods
BT4 Foods

Sesquiterpenes
HN introduced from vol. 43, issue 1 (2011)
BT1 Hydrocarbons
BT2 Organic compounds
BT1 Sesquiterpenoids
BT2 Terpenoids
BT3 Lipids
BT4 Nutrients
NT1 Caryophyllene
NT1 Farnesene
NT1 Humulene

Sesquiterpenoids
BT1 Terpenoids
BT2 Lipids
BT3 Nutrients
NT1 Farnesol
NT1 Ipomeamarone
NT1 Nootkatone
NT1 Sesquiterpenes
NT2 Caryophyllene
NT2 Farnesene
NT2 Humulene

Setting
BT1 Solidification

Sevin
USE **Carbaryl**

Sevruga
USE **Sturgeon**

Sex
SN used for the gender of both livestock and humans
RT Castration
RT Genetics

Seychelles
BT1 Africa

11S Globulins
BT1 Globulins
BT2 Proteins
BT3 Nutrients
BT1 Vegetable proteins
BT2 Proteins vegetable
BT3 Proteins
BT4 Nutrients
BT3 Vegetable products
BT4 Plant foods
BT5 Foods

7S Globulins
HN introduced from vol. 39, issue 1 (2007)
BT1 Globulins
BT2 Proteins
BT3 Nutrients
BT1 Vegetable proteins
BT2 Proteins vegetable
BT3 Proteins
BT4 Nutrients
BT3 Vegetable products
BT4 Plant foods
BT5 Foods

Shad
BT1 Marine fish
BT2 Fish
BT3 Animals
BT3 Sea foods
BT4 Aquatic foods
BT5 Animal foods
BT6 Foods
NT1 Indian shad

Shaddocks
SN syn. pomelos, pummelos
BT1 Pomelos
BT2 Citrus fruits
BT3 Fruits specific
BT4 Fruits
BT5 Crops
BT6 Plants
BT5 Plant foods
BT6 Foods

Shading
BT1 Cultivation
BT2 Agriculture

Shallots
BT1 Vegetables specific
BT2 Vegetables
BT3 Crops
BT4 Plants
BT3 Plant foods
BT4 Foods

Shandy
BT1 Beer
BT2 Alcoholic beverages
BT3 Beverages alcoholic
BT4 Beverages

Shape
BT1 Physical properties

Shaping
BT1 Moulding
BT2 Processing
BT3 Technology

Shark fins
HN introduced from vol. 37, issue 5 (2005)
BT1 Sharks
BT2 Marine fish
BT3 Fish
BT4 Animals
BT4 Sea foods
BT5 Aquatic foods
BT6 Animal foods
BT7 Foods

Sharks
BT1 Marine fish
BT2 Fish
BT3 Animals
BT3 Sea foods
BT4 Aquatic foods
BT5 Animal foods
BT6 Foods
NT1 Shark fins

Sharon fruit
USE **Persimmons**

Sharpness
BT1 Flavour
BT2 Sensory properties

Shashlik
BT1 Meat products
BT2 Animal foods
BT3 Foods

Shea nut butter
BT1 Vegetable fats
BT2 Fats vegetable
BT3 Fats
BT4 Lipids
BT5 Nutrients
BT3 Vegetable products
BT4 Plant foods
BT5 Foods

Shea nuts
BT1 Oilseeds
BT2 Seeds
BT3 Plant foods
BT4 Foods

Shear
HN heading up to vol. 24 (1992)
BT1 Rheological properties
BT2 Mechanical properties
BT3 Physical properties
RT Deformation
RT Shear values
RT Tenderness
RT Toughness

Shear strength
BT1 Mechanical properties
BT2 Physical properties

Shear values
BT1 Rheological properties
BT2 Mechanical properties
BT3 Physical properties
RT Shear

Sheatfish
BT1 Marine fish
BT2 Fish
BT3 Animals
BT3 Sea foods
BT4 Aquatic foods
BT5 Animal foods
BT6 Foods

Sheep
BT1 Animals
NT1 Ewe cheese
NT1 Ewe milk
NT1 Ewe yoghurt
RT Lambs
RT Mutton
UF Ewes
UF Ovine
UF Rams

Sheep carcasses
BT1 Carcasses
BT2 Meat
BT3 Animal foods
BT4 Foods
BT1 Mutton
BT2 Meat specific
BT3 Meat
BT4 Animal foods
BT5 Foods

Sheep cheese
USE **Ewe cheese**

Sheep meat
USE **Mutton**

Sheep milk
USE **Ewe milk**

Sheep milk cheese
USE **Ewe cheese**

Sheep muscles
USE **Mutton**

Shelf life
HN heading from vol. 25 (1993); use Shelf-life up to vol. 24 (1992) or Keeping quality up to vol. 18 (1986)
NT1 Freshness
NT1 Long life foods
NT1 Perishability
RT Spoilage
RT Storage
RT Storage life
UF Keeping quality
UF Shelf-life

Shelf-life
HN heading from vol. 19 (1987) to vol. 24 (1992)
USE **Shelf life**

Shell
HN heading up to vol. 24 (1992)
USE **Shells**

Shellac
BT1 Coatings

Shellfish
BT1 Animals
BT1 Sea foods
BT2 Aquatic foods
BT3 Animal foods
BT4 Foods
NT1 Crustacea
NT2 Crabs
NT3 Blue crabs
NT4 *Callinectes sapidus*
NT3 Crab meat
NT4 Crab legs
NT3 Mud crabs
NT3 Red crabs
NT3 Snow crabs
NT2 Crawfish
NT2 Crayfish
NT2 Krill
NT2 Lobsters
NT3 American lobsters
NT2 Norway lobsters
NT3 Langoustines
NT3 Scampi
NT2 Prawns
NT3 Kuruma prawns
NT3 Prawn crackers
NT2 Shrimps
NT3 *Crangon crangon*
NT3 *Pandalus borealis*
NT3 Tiger shrimps
NT1 Farmed shellfish
NT1 Molluscs
NT2 Bivalves
NT3 Arkshells
NT3 Carpet shells
NT3 Clams
NT4 Freshwater clams
NT4 *Pseudocardium sachalinensis*
NT4 *Tapes philippinarum*
NT3 Cockles
NT3 Mussels
NT4 Blue mussels
NT4 Green mussels
NT4 *Mytilus edulis*
NT4 *Mytilus galloprovincialis*
NT4 *Mytilus trossulus*
NT3 Oysters
NT4 *Crassostrea gigas*
NT4 *Crassostrea virginica*
NT4 Oyster sauces
NT3 Razor shells
NT3 Scallops
NT4 *Patinopecten yessoensis*
NT2 Cephalopods
NT3 Cuttlefish
NT3 Octopus
NT3 Squid
NT4 Ika shiokara
NT4 *Illex argentinus*
NT4 *Ommastrephes bartrami*
NT2 Gastropods
NT3 Abalones
NT3 Limpets
NT3 Periwinkles
NT3 Snails
NT4 Land snails
NT4 Snail meat
NT3 Top shells
NT3 Trumpet shells
NT3 Turban shells
NT3 Whelks
RT Aquaculture

Shelling
BT1 Shells

Shells
HN heading from vol. 25 (1993); use Shell up to vol. 24 (1992)
SN use for shells other than egg shells
NT1 Shelling
NT1 Shucking
RT Cracking
UF Shell

Sherbet
BT1 Sugar confectionery
BT2 Plant foods
BT3 Foods

Sherry
BT1 Fortified wines
BT2 Wines
BT3 Alcoholic beverages

BT4 Beverages alcoholic
BT5 Beverages

Shewanella
BT1 Bacteria
BT2 Microorganisms
NT1 *Shewanella putrefaciens*

Shewanella putrefaciens
BT1 *Shewanella*
BT2 Bacteria
BT3 Microorganisms

Shiga like toxins
BT1 Toxins
BT2 Residues
RT Haemolytic uraemic syndrome
RT Verotoxins

Shiga toxins
BT1 Toxins
BT2 Residues
RT *Shigella*

Shigella
HN heading from vol. 25 (1993); under Enterobacteriaceae up to vol. 24 (1992)
BT1 Bacteria
BT2 Microorganisms
NT1 *Shigella boydii*
NT1 *Shigella dysenteriae*
NT1 *Shigella flexneri*
NT1 *Shigella sonnei*
RT Shiga toxins
RT Shigellosis

Shigella boydii
HN introduced from vol. 39, issue 1 (2007)
BT1 *Shigella*
BT2 Bacteria
BT3 Microorganisms

Shigella dysenteriae
BT1 *Shigella*
BT2 Bacteria
BT3 Microorganisms

Shigella flexneri
BT1 *Shigella*
BT2 Bacteria
BT3 Microorganisms

Shigella sonnei
BT1 *Shigella*
BT2 Bacteria
BT3 Microorganisms

Shigellosis
BT1 Diseases
BT1 Poisoning
RT *Shigella*

Shiitake
USE ***Lentinula edodes***

Shikimic acid
HN introduced from vol. 39, issue 1 (2007)
BT1 Organic acids
BT2 Acids

Shiokara
BT1 Fermented foods
BT2 Processed foods
BT3 Foods
BT1 Sea foods
BT2 Aquatic foods
BT3 Animal foods
BT4 Foods
NT1 Ika shiokara
RT Jeotgal

Shipping
BT1 Transport

Ships
BT1 Transport

Shochu
BT1 Spirits
BT2 Alcoholic beverages
BT3 Beverages alcoholic
BT4 Beverages

Shops
BT1 Marketing
BT2 Economics
RT Supermarkets

Shortbread
BT1 Biscuits
BT2 Bakery products
BT3 Cereal products
BT4 Plant foods
BT5 Foods

Short chain fatty acids
HN introduced from vol. 39, issue 1 (2007)
SN syn. volatile fatty acids
BT1 Volatile fatty acids
BT2 Fatty acids
BT3 Lipids
BT4 Nutrients
BT3 Organic acids
BT4 Acids
BT2 Volatile compounds
NT1 Butanoic acid
NT2 Butyric acid
NT1 Hexanoic acid
NT2 Caproic acid
NT1 Hydroxybutyric acid
NT1 Isobutyric acid
NT1 Isocaproic acid
NT1 Isovaleric acid
NT1 Pentanoic acid
NT2 Valeric acid

Shortening
SN used for shortening of muscles
BT1 Contraction

Shortenings
BT1 Fats
BT2 Lipids
BT3 Nutrients

Shoti
SN syn. zedoary
BT1 Vegetables specific
BT2 Vegetables
BT3 Crops
BT4 Plants
BT3 Plant foods
BT4 Foods

Shoyu
BT1 Soy sauces
BT2 Fermented foods
BT3 Processed foods
BT4 Foods
BT2 Sauces
BT3 Condiments
BT4 Flavourings
BT5 Additives
BT2 Soy products
BT3 Vegetable products
BT4 Plant foods
BT5 Foods

Shredding
BT1 Comminution
BT2 Processing
BT3 Technology

Shrikhand
BT1 Buffalo milk
BT2 Buffaloes
BT3 Animals
BT2 Milk
BT3 Dairy products
BT4 Animal foods
BT5 Foods
BT1 Fermented milk
BT2 Fermented dairy products
BT3 Dairy products
BT4 Animal foods
BT5 Foods
BT3 Fermented foods
BT4 Processed foods
BT5 Foods
BT2 Milk
BT3 Dairy products
BT4 Animal foods
BT5 Foods
UF Srikand
UF Srikhand

Shrimps
BT1 Crustacea
BT2 Shellfish
BT3 Animals
BT3 Sea foods
BT4 Aquatic foods
BT5 Animal foods
BT6 Foods
NT1 *Crangon crangon*
NT1 *Pandalus borealis*
NT1 Tiger shrimps
RT Prawns

Shrinkage
RT Size

Shrink packaging
BT1 Packaging
BT2 Technology

Shubat
BT1 Camel milk
BT2 Camels
BT3 Animals
BT2 Milk
BT3 Dairy products
BT4 Animal foods
BT5 Foods
BT1 Fermented milk
BT2 Fermented dairy products
BT3 Dairy products
BT4 Animal foods
BT5 Foods
BT3 Fermented foods
BT4 Processed foods
BT5 Foods
BT2 Milk
BT3 Dairy products
BT4 Animal foods
BT5 Foods
RT Koumiss

Shucking
BT1 Shells

Shuttle vectors
BT1 Cloning vectors
BT2 Genetic techniques
BT3 Genetics
RT Plasmids

Si
HN under Minerals up to vol. 42 (2010)
BT1 Elements
BT2 Minerals
BT3 Nutrients
UF Silicon

Sialic acid
SN syn. N-acetylneuraminic acid
BT1 Organic acids
BT2 Acids

Side dishes
HN introduced from vol. 41, issue 1 (2009)
BT1 Dishes
BT2 Meals
BT3 Processed foods
BT4 Foods

Sideritis
BT1 Plants

Siderophores
BT1 Microbial proteins
BT2 Microorganisms
BT2 Proteins
BT3 Nutrients
BT1 Virulence factors

Sides
USE **Carcasses**

Sierra Leone
BT1 West Africa
BT2 Africa

Sieva beans
USE **Lima beans**

Sieves
BT1 Equipment
BT2 Technology
BT1 Sieving
BT2 Separation
BT3 Processing
BT4 Technology

Sieving
BT1 Separation
BT2 Processing
BT3 Technology
NT1 Sieves
NT1 Sifting
NT2 Sifters

Sifters
BT1 Equipment
BT2 Technology
BT1 Sifting
BT2 Sieving
BT3 Separation
BT4 Processing
BT5 Technology

Sifting
BT1 Sieving
BT2 Separation
BT3 Processing
BT4 Technology
NT1 Sifters

Sigma factors
USE **σ Factors**

Sikhe
BT1 Beverages
BT1 Rice
BT2 Cereals
BT3 Crops
BT4 Plants
BT3 Seeds
BT4 Plant foods
BT5 Foods

Silage
BT1 Feeds

Silica
HN heading from vol. 43 (2011); under Minerals up to vol. 42 (2010)
BT1 Minerals
BT2 Nutrients
RT Silicic acid

Silica gels
BT1 Gels
BT2 Physical phases
BT3 Chemistry
BT4 Science

Silicates
BT1 Salts
NT1 Zeolites

Silicic acid
BT1 Acids
RT Silica

Silicon
USE **Si**

Siljo
BT1 Fermented foods
BT2 Processed foods
BT3 Foods
BT1 Legumes
BT2 Vegetables specific
BT3 Vegetables
BT4 Crops
BT5 Plants
BT4 Plant foods
BT5 Foods

Silos
BT1 Containers
RT Bins
RT Storage

Silurus asotus
BT1 Catfish
BT2 Freshwater fish
BT3 Fish
BT4 Animals
BT4 Sea foods
BT5 Aquatic foods
BT6 Animal foods
BT7 Foods

Silver
USE **Ag**

Silver carp
HN introduced from vol. 39, issue 1 (2007)
BT1 Carp
BT2 Freshwater fish
BT3 Fish
BT4 Animals
BT4 Sea foods
BT5 Aquatic foods
BT6 Animal foods
BT7 Foods
BT2 Oily fish
BT3 Fish
BT4 Animals
BT4 Sea foods
BT5 Aquatic foods
BT6 Animal foods
BT7 Foods

Silvex
USE **Fenoprop**

Simazine
BT1 Triazine herbicides
BT2 Herbicides
BT3 Pesticides
BT4 Biocides
BT4 Residues
UF Gesatop

Simmering
BT1 Cooking
BT2 Thermal processing
BT3 Processing thermal
BT4 Processing
BT5 Technology

Simmondsin
BT1 Glycosides
BT2 Carbohydrates
BT3 Nutrients

BT3 Organic compounds
RT Jojoba oils

Simplesse
BT1 Fat substitutes
BT2 Fats
BT3 Lipids
BT4 Nutrients

Simulated foods
BT1 Processed foods
BT2 Foods
NT1 Analogues
NT1 Artificial foods
NT1 Butter substitutes
NT1 Cheese substitutes
NT1 Cocoa butter substitutes
NT1 Coffee substitutes
NT1 Imitation foods
NT2 Imitation crab meat
NT2 Imitation dairy products
NT3 Imitation cheese
NT3 Imitation cream
NT1 Meat analogues
NT1 Meat substitutes
NT1 Milk substitutes

Simultaneous distillation-extraction
HN introduced from vol. 41, issue 1 (2009)
BT1 Analytical techniques

Simultaneous saccharification and fermentation
BT1 Fermentation technology
BT2 Biotechnology
BT3 Technology
BT2 Process control
BT3 Technology

Sinapic acid
BT1 Organic acids
BT2 Acids

Sinapine
BT1 Esters
BT2 Organic compounds

Singapore
BT1 Asia

Single cell proteins
HN heading up to vol. 21 (1989)
BT1 Biomass
BT2 Fermentation products
BT3 Biotechnology
BT4 Technology
BT1 Proteins
BT2 Nutrients

Single cream
BT1 Cream
BT2 Dairy products
BT3 Animal foods
BT4 Foods

Single market
BT1 Markets
BT2 Economics

Sinigrin
BT1 Glucosinolates
BT2 Glycosides
BT3 Carbohydrates
BT4 Nutrients
BT4 Organic compounds

Sitao
USE **Asparagus beans**

Site directed mutagenesis
HN mutagenesis site directed also used in the index up to vol. 29 (1997)
BT1 Mutagenesis
BT2 Genetic techniques
BT3 Genetics
BT2 Modification
BT1 Protein engineering
BT2 Genetic techniques
BT3 Genetics
BT2 Modification

Sitophilus
BT1 Insects
BT2 Pests
NT1 Rice weevils
NT2 *Sitophilus oryzae*
NT1 *Sitophilus granarius*
NT1 *Sitophilus zeamais*

Sitophilus granarius
BT1 *Sitophilus*
BT2 Insects
BT3 Pests

Sitophilus oryzae
BT1 Rice weevils
BT2 *Sitophilus*
BT3 Insects
BT4 Pests

Sitophilus zeamais
HN introduced from vol. 39, issue 1 (2007)
BT1 *Sitophilus*
BT2 Insects
BT3 Pests

Sitostanol
BT1 Phytostanols
BT2 Stanols
BT3 Sterols
BT4 Alcohols
BT4 Steroids
BT5 Lipids
BT6 Nutrients

Sitosterol
BT1 Sterols
BT2 Alcohols
BT2 Steroids
BT3 Lipids
BT4 Nutrients

Size
BT1 Physical properties
RT Shrinkage

Size exclusion chromatography
HN introduced from vol. 39, issue 1 (2007)
BT1 Chromatography
BT2 Analytical techniques

Skate
BT1 Marine fish
BT2 Fish
BT3 Animals
BT3 Sea foods
BT4 Aquatic foods
BT5 Animal foods
BT6 Foods
RT Ray

Skatole
BT1 Biogenic amines
BT2 Amines
BT3 Organic nitrogen compounds
BT1 Heterocyclic compounds
RT Taints

Skimmed milk
USE **Skim milk**

Skim milk
HN heading was Skim-milk up to vol. 24 (1992)
BT1 Milk
BT2 Dairy products
BT3 Animal foods
BT4 Foods
NT1 Dried skim milk
NT1 Skim milk powders
RT Semi skimmed milk
UF Skimmed milk
UF Skim-milk

Skim-milk
HN heading up to vol. 24 (1992)
USE **Skim milk**

Skim milk powders
BT1 Powders
BT2 Dried foods
BT3 Processed foods
BT4 Foods
BT2 Instant foods
BT3 Processed foods
BT4 Foods
BT1 Skim milk
BT2 Milk
BT3 Dairy products
BT4 Animal foods
BT5 Foods
RT Dried milk
RT Dried skim milk
RT Milk powders

Skin
HN heading from vol. 25 (1993)
SN use for animal skin; for fruit or vegetable skins use Peel
NT1 Chicken skin
NT1 Fish skin
NT1 Swine skin
RT Hides

Skinning
BT1 Processing
BT2 Technology

Skin prick testing
HN introduced from vol. 39, issue 1 (2007)
BT1 Clinical techniques

Skin spot
BT1 Plant disorders
BT2 Diseases plant
BT3 Diseases

Skipjack tuna
BT1 Tuna
BT2 Marine fish
BT3 Fish
BT4 Animals
BT4 Sea foods
BT5 Aquatic foods
BT6 Animal foods
BT7 Foods
BT2 Oily fish
BT3 Fish
BT4 Animals
BT4 Sea foods
BT5 Aquatic foods
BT6 Animal foods
BT7 Foods
NT1 Katsuobushi

Skyr
BT1 Fermented milk
BT2 Fermented dairy products
BT3 Dairy products
BT4 Animal foods
BT5 Foods
BT3 Fermented foods
BT4 Processed foods
BT5 Foods
BT2 Milk
BT3 Dairy products
BT4 Animal foods
BT5 Foods

Slaughter
NT1 Electrical stimulation
NT1 Electrocution
NT1 Lairage
NT1 Stunning
NT2 Electrical stunning
RT Animal stress
RT Boning
RT Carcasses
RT Evisceration
RT Gutting
RT Slaughterhouses

Slaughter animals
BT1 Animals

Slaughter by-products
USE **Offal**

Slaughterhouses
NT1 Abattoirs
NT1 Butcheries
RT Lairage
RT Slaughter

Sleep
HN introduced from vol. 41, issue 1 (2009)
BT1 Human physiology
BT2 Physiology
BT3 Science

Slicing
BT1 Cutting
BT2 Processing
BT3 Technology

Slime bacteria
BT1 Bacteria
BT2 Microorganisms

Slivovitz
BT1 Fruit brandies
BT2 Brandies
BT3 Spirits
BT4 Alcoholic beverages
BT5 Beverages alcoholic
BT6 Beverages

Sloes
BT1 Fruits specific
BT2 Fruits
BT3 Crops
BT4 Plants
BT3 Plant foods
BT4 Foods

Slovakia
BT1 Europe
BT1 European Union
RT Czechoslovakia
RT Organization for Economic Cooperation and Development

Slovenia
BT1 Europe
BT1 European Union

Slow cooking
HN introduced from vol. 39, issue 1 (2007)
BT1 Cooking
BT2 Thermal processing
BT3 Processing thermal
BT4 Processing
BT5 Technology

Sludges
HN heading up to vol. 24 (1992)
BT1 Wastes

Slugs
BT1 Pests

Small round structured virus
HN introduced from vol. 43, issue 1 (2011); small round structured viruses also used in the index up to vol. 42 (2010)
BT1 Norwalk virus
BT2 Norovirus
BT3 Noroviruses
BT4 Caliciviruses
BT5 Viruses
BT6 Microorganisms
UF Small round structured viruses

Small round structured viruses
HN Small round structured virus used in the index from vol. 43 (2011)
USE **Small round structured virus**

Smear cheese
BT1 Cheese varieties
BT2 Cheese
BT3 Dairy products
BT4 Animal foods
BT5 Foods

Smell
USE **Aroma**

Smen
BT1 Butter
BT2 Dairy products
BT3 Animal foods
BT4 Foods
UF Moroccan smen

Smetana
BT1 Fermented cream
BT2 Cream
BT3 Dairy products
BT4 Animal foods
BT5 Foods
BT2 Fermented dairy products
BT3 Dairy products
BT4 Animal foods
BT5 Foods
BT3 Fermented foods
BT4 Processed foods
BT5 Foods

Smoke
BT1 Smoking
BT2 Preservation
BT3 Technology

Smoke concentrates
HN under Smoking up to vol. 24 (1992)
BT1 Flavourings
BT2 Additives
RT Smoking

Smoked fish
BT1 Fish products
BT2 Sea foods
BT3 Aquatic foods
BT4 Animal foods
BT5 Foods
BT1 Smoked foods
BT2 Processed foods
BT3 Foods
NT1 Kippers
NT1 Smoked mackerel
NT1 Smoked salmon
NT1 Smoked trout

Smoked foods
BT1 Processed foods
BT2 Foods
NT1 Smoked fish
NT2 Kippers

NT2 Smoked mackerel
NT2 Smoked salmon
NT2 Smoked trout
RT Smoking

Smoked mackerel
BT1 Mackerel
BT2 Marine fish
BT3 Fish
BT4 Animals
BT4 Sea foods
BT5 Aquatic foods
BT6 Animal foods
BT7 Foods
BT2 Oily fish
BT3 Fish
BT4 Animals
BT4 Sea foods
BT5 Aquatic foods
BT6 Animal foods
BT7 Foods
BT1 Smoked fish
BT2 Fish products
BT3 Sea foods
BT4 Aquatic foods
BT5 Animal foods
BT6 Foods
BT2 Smoked foods
BT3 Processed foods
BT4 Foods

Smoked salmon
BT1 Salmon
BT2 Oily fish
BT3 Fish
BT4 Animals
BT4 Sea foods
BT5 Aquatic foods
BT6 Animal foods
BT7 Foods
BT1 Smoked fish
BT2 Fish products
BT3 Sea foods
BT4 Aquatic foods
BT5 Animal foods
BT6 Foods
BT2 Smoked foods
BT3 Processed foods
BT4 Foods

Smoked trout
BT1 Smoked fish
BT2 Fish products
BT3 Sea foods
BT4 Aquatic foods
BT5 Animal foods
BT6 Foods
BT2 Smoked foods
BT3 Processed foods
BT4 Foods
BT1 Trout
BT2 Oily fish
BT3 Fish
BT4 Animals
BT4 Sea foods
BT5 Aquatic foods
BT6 Animal foods
BT7 Foods

Smoke flavourings
BT1 Flavourings
BT2 Additives
RT Smoking

Smokehouses
BT1 Smoking
BT2 Preservation
BT3 Technology

Smoking
BT1 Preservation
BT2 Technology
NT1 Smoke
NT1 Smokehouses
RT Curing
RT Hickory smoke
RT Liquid smoke
RT Smoke concentrates
RT Smoked foods
RT Smoke flavourings
RT Wood smoke

Smoothies
HN introduced from vol. 37, issue 5 (2005); under Beverages up to vol. 42 (2010)
BT1 Soft drinks
BT2 Beverages

Smoothness
BT1 Consistency
BT2 Texture
BT3 Sensory properties

Sn
HN under Minerals and Packaging materials up to vol. 42 (2010)
BT1 Tin
BT2 Metals
BT3 Elements
BT4 Minerals
BT5 Nutrients
BT2 Packaging materials

Snack foods
HN heading from vol. 25 (1993); under Snacks up to vol. 24 (1992)
BT1 Processed foods
BT2 Foods
NT1 Canapes
NT1 Dim sum
NT1 Falafel
NT1 Food bars
NT2 Cereal bars
NT3 Muesli bars
NT2 Confectionery bars
NT3 Chocolate bars
NT2 Ice cream bars
NT1 Pakoras
NT1 Popcorn
NT2 Microwave popcorn
NT1 Prawn crackers
NT1 Rice crackers
NT1 Sandwiches
NT1 Yukwa
RT Corn masa
UF Snacks

Snacking
HN introduced from vol. 43, issue 1 (2011)
BT1 Eating habits
BT2 Consumer behaviour
BT3 Consumer response

Snacks
HN heading up to vol. 24 (1992)
USE **Snack foods**

Snail meat
BT1 Meat specific
BT2 Meat
BT3 Animal foods
BT4 Foods
BT1 Snails
BT2 Gastropods
BT3 Molluscs
BT4 Shellfish
BT5 Animals
BT5 Sea foods
BT6 Aquatic foods
BT7 Animal foods
BT8 Foods

Snails
BT1 Gastropods
BT2 Molluscs
BT3 Shellfish
BT4 Animals
BT4 Sea foods
BT5 Aquatic foods
BT6 Animal foods
BT7 Foods
NT1 Land snails
NT1 Snail meat

Snakehead
BT1 Freshwater fish
BT2 Fish
BT3 Animals
BT3 Sea foods
BT4 Aquatic foods
BT5 Animal foods
BT6 Foods

Snakes
BT1 Animals

Snap beans
BT1 Common beans
BT2 Legumes
BT3 Vegetables specific
BT4 Vegetables
BT5 Crops
BT6 Plants
BT5 Plant foods
BT6 Foods

Snapper
BT1 Marine fish
BT2 Fish
BT3 Animals
BT3 Sea foods
BT4 Aquatic foods
BT5 Animal foods
BT6 Foods
UF Snappers

BT5 Nutrients
UF Low sodium foods

Sodium metabisulfite
SN syn. sodium pyrosulfite
BT1 Metabisulfites
BT2 Preservatives
BT3 Additives
BT2 Sulfites
BT3 Salts
BT1 Preservatives
BT2 Additives
UF Sodium metabisulphite

Sodium metabisulphite
HN used for sodium metabisulfite up to vol. 35, issue 6 (2003)
USE **Sodium metabisulfite**

Sodium *o*-phenylphenate
USE **2-Phenylphenol**

Sodium pyrosulfite
SN syn. sodium metabisulfite
BT1 Metabisulfites
BT2 Preservatives
BT3 Additives
BT2 Sulfites
BT3 Salts
BT1 Preservatives
BT2 Additives
UF Sodium pyrosulphite

Sodium pyrosulphite
HN used for sodium pyrosulfite up to vol. 35, issue 6 (2003)
USE **Sodium pyrosulfite**

Sodium tripolyphosphate
BT1 Phosphates
BT2 Salts

Soft cheese
BT1 Cheese varieties
BT2 Cheese
BT3 Dairy products
BT4 Animal foods
BT5 Foods

Soft drinks
HN heading from vol. 24 (1992); under Beverages up to vol. 23 (1991)
BT1 Beverages
NT1 Carbonated beverages
NT1 Coca-cola
NT1 Cola beverages
NT1 Energy drinks
NT1 Fruit cordials
NT1 Fruit juice beverages
NT2 Citrus beverages
NT2 Fruit beverages
NT2 Orange juice beverages
NT1 Fruit juices
NT2 Apple juices
NT3 Apple cider
NT3 Apple juice concentrates
NT2 Apricot juices
NT2 Banana juices
NT2 Barbados cherry juices
NT2 Berry juices
NT3 Bilberry juices
NT3 Blackberry juices
NT3 Blackcurrant juices
NT3 Blueberry juices
NT3 Cranberry juices
NT3 Elderberry juices
NT3 Raspberry juices
NT3 Redcurrant juices
NT3 Strawberry juices
NT2 Cashew apple juices
NT2 Cherry juices
NT2 Citrus juices
NT3 Citrus juice concentrates
NT4 Orange juice concentrates
NT3 Grapefruit juices
NT3 Lemon juices
NT3 Lime juices
NT3 Orange juices
NT4 Mandarin juices
NT5 Tangerine juices
NT4 Orange juice concentrates
NT2 Fig juices
NT2 Fruit juice concentrates
NT3 Apple juice concentrates
NT3 Citrus juice concentrates
NT4 Orange juice concentrates
NT3 Grape juice concentrates
NT2 Fruit nectars
NT3 Apricot nectars
NT3 Mango nectars
NT3 Papaya nectars
NT3 Peach nectars
NT3 Pineapple nectars
NT2 Grape juices
NT3 Grape juice concentrates
NT2 Guava juices
NT2 Hawthorn juices
NT2 Kiwifruit juices
NT2 Mango juices
NT2 Melon juices
NT2 Musts
NT3 Apple musts
NT3 Grape musts
NT4 Concentrated rectified musts
NT2 Noni juices
NT2 Passion fruit juices
NT2 Peach juices
NT2 Pear juices
NT2 Persimmon juices
NT2 Pineapple juices
NT2 Plum juices
NT2 Pomegranate juices
NT2 Prune juices
NT2 Quince juices
NT2 Sea buckthorn juices
NT2 Tomato juices
NT2 Watermelon juices
NT1 Ginger ale
NT1 Ginger beer
NT1 Guarana
NT2 *Paullinia cupana*
NT1 Isotonic drinks
NT1 Lemonade
NT1 Mineral waters
NT2 Bottled mineral waters
NT2 Soda water
NT2 Spring waters
NT1 Orange beverages
NT1 Performance drinks
NT1 Smoothies
NT1 Sports drinks
NT1 Squash
NT1 Tonic waters
NT1 Vegetable juice beverages
NT1 Vegetable juices
NT2 Cabbage juices
NT2 Carrot juices
NT2 Vegetable juice concentrates
NT2 Vegetable nectars

Softeners
BT1 Additives

Softening
BT1 Firmness
BT2 Texture
BT3 Sensory properties

Soft frozen beverages
HN under Soft drinks up to vol. 42 (2010)
BT1 Frozen beverages
BT2 Beverages

Softness
BT1 Firmness
BT2 Texture
BT3 Sensory properties

Soft pet foods
HN introduced from vol. 39, issue 1 (2007)
BT1 Pet foods

Software
USE **Computer software**

Soils
BT1 Cultivation
BT2 Agriculture

Solanidine
BT1 Alkaloids
BT2 Organic nitrogen compounds

Solanine
BT1 Glycoalkaloids
BT2 Alkaloids
BT3 Organic nitrogen compounds
RT Potatoes

Solanum
BT1 Vegetables specific
BT2 Vegetables
BT3 Crops
BT4 Plants
BT3 Plant foods
BT4 Foods

Solanum tuberosum
BT1 Potatoes
BT2 Vegetables specific
BT3 Vegetables
BT4 Crops

BT5 Plants
BT4 Plant foods
BT5 Foods

Solar driers
HN driers solar also used in the index up to vol. 29 (1997)
BT1 Driers
BT2 Drying
BT3 Thermal processing
BT4 Processing thermal
BT5 Processing
BT6 Technology
BT2 Equipment
BT3 Technology
BT1 Solar drying
BT2 Drying
BT3 Thermal processing
BT4 Processing thermal
BT5 Processing
BT6 Technology

Solar drying
BT1 Drying
BT2 Thermal processing
BT3 Processing thermal
BT4 Processing
BT5 Technology
NT1 Solar driers

Solar energy
BT1 Energy

Solar radiation
BT1 Radiation

Sole
BT1 Flatfish
BT2 Marine fish
BT3 Fish
BT4 Animals
BT4 Sea foods
BT5 Aquatic foods
BT6 Animal foods
BT7 Foods

Solidification
NT1 Caking
NT1 Setting
RT Crystallization
RT Gelation

Solid phase extraction
BT1 Analytical techniques

Solid phase microextraction
BT1 Analytical techniques

Solids
BT1 Physical phases
BT2 Chemistry
BT3 Science
NT1 SNF
NT1 Soluble solids
NT1 TS
NT1 TSS
RT Brix values
RT DM
RT Dry matter

Solids not fat
USE **SNF**

Solid state fermentation
BT1 Fermentation technology
BT2 Biotechnology
BT3 Technology
BT2 Process control
BT3 Technology

Solomon Islands
BT1 Oceania

Solubility
BT1 Physical properties
NT1 Solubilization
RT Solvents

Solubilization
BT1 Solubility
BT2 Physical properties

Soluble fibre
HN introduced from vol. 39, issue 1 (2007)
BT1 Dietary fibre
BT2 Fibre

Soluble solids
BT1 Solids
BT2 Physical phases
BT3 Chemistry
BT4 Science

Solvents
NT1 Acetone
NT1 Acetonitrile
NT1 Aqueous two phase systems
NT1 Benzene
NT1 Carbon dioxide
NT2 CO_2
NT2 Dry Ice
NT2 Supercritical CO_2 extraction
NT1 Carbon tetrachloride
NT1 Chloroform
NT1 Decane
NT1 Decanol
NT1 Dichloromethane
NT1 Dimethylformamide
NT1 Dimethyl sulfide
NT2 Methyl sulfide
NT1 Dimethyl sulfoxide
NT1 Dioxane
NT1 Ethanol
NT2 Alcohol
NT2 Alcoholometers
NT1 Ethyl acetate
NT1 Formamide
NT1 Heptane
NT1 Hexane
NT1 Isopropanol
NT1 Isopropyl alcohol
NT1 Methanol
NT1 Methylene chloride
NT1 Organic solvents
NT1 Pentane
NT1 Petroleum
NT1 Propanol
NT2 Chloropropanols
NT1 2-Propanol
NT1 Propanone
NT1 Propyl alcohol
NT1 Pyridine
NT1 Supercritical fluids
NT1 Tetrachloromethane
NT1 Toluene
NT1 Trichloromethane
NT1 Xylene
RT Solubility

Somalia
BT1 East Africa
BT2 Africa

Somatic cells
HN cells somatic also used in the index up to vol. 29(1997)
BT1 Cells
UF Cells somatic

Somatic cells counts
BT1 Cells
BT1 Microbiological techniques

Somatotrophin
USE **Somatotropin**

Somatotropin
BT1 Hormones
BT2 Residues
NT1 Bovine somatotropin
NT1 Porcine somatotropin
UF Growth hormone
UF Somatotrophin

Somen
BT1 Pasta
BT2 Cereal products
BT3 Plant foods
BT4 Foods

Sonication
HN introduced from vol. 37, issue 5 (2005)
BT1 Extraction
BT2 Processing
BT3 Technology
BT1 Sound

SOPP
USE **2-Phenylphenol**

Sorbates
BT1 Preservatives
BT2 Additives
BT1 Salts
RT Sorbic acid

Sorbets
BT1 Desserts
BT2 Processed foods
BT3 Foods

Sorbic acid
BT1 Organic acids
BT2 Acids
BT1 Preservatives
BT2 Additives
RT Sorbates

Sorbitan
BT1 Emulsifiers
BT2 Additives

Sorbitol
BT1 Polyols
BT2 Alcohols
BT2 Carbohydrates
BT3 Nutrients
BT3 Organic compounds
UF Glucitol

Sorbitol dehydrogenases
USE **L-Iditol 2-dehydrogenases**

Sorbose
HN under Sugars up to vol. 42 (2010)
BT1 Monosaccharides
BT2 Sugars
BT3 Carbohydrates
BT4 Nutrients
BT4 Organic compounds
BT3 Plant foods
BT4 Foods

Sorghum
BT1 Cereals
BT2 Crops
BT3 Plants
BT2 Seeds
BT3 Plant foods
BT4 Foods
NT1 Jowar
NT1 Milo
NT1 Sorghum flour
NT1 Sorghum starch
RT Sweet sorghum

Sorghum beer
BT1 Beer
BT2 Alcoholic beverages
BT3 Beverages alcoholic
BT4 Beverages

Sorghum flour
HN introduced from vol. 39, issue 1 (2007)
BT1 Cereal flours
BT2 Flours cereal
BT3 Cereal products
BT4 Plant foods
BT5 Foods
BT1 Sorghum
BT2 Cereals
BT3 Crops
BT4 Plants
BT3 Seeds
BT4 Plant foods
BT5 Foods

Sorghum malt
BT1 Malt
BT2 Cereal products
BT3 Plant foods
BT4 Foods

Sorghum starch
HN introduced from vol. 39, issue 1 (2007)
BT1 Sorghum
BT2 Cereals
BT3 Crops
BT4 Plants
BT3 Seeds
BT4 Plant foods
BT5 Foods
BT1 Starch
BT2 Glucans
BT3 Polysaccharides
BT4 Carbohydrates
BT5 Nutrients
BT5 Organic compounds
BT2 Thickeners
BT3 Additives

Sorgo
SN syn. sweet sorghum
BT1 Sweet sorghum
BT2 Crops
BT3 Plants
RT Sugar crops

Sorption
NT1 Absorption
NT2 Absorbents
NT1 Adsorption
NT2 Adsorbents
NT1 Desorption
NT1 Moisture sorption
NT1 Water sorption
RT Diffusion
RT Humidity
RT Ion exchange
RT Moisture content

Sorrel
HN under Spices up to vol. 42 (2010)
BT1 Herbs
BT2 Spices
BT3 Flavourings
BT4 Additives

Sorting
BT1 Grading

Sotolon
HN introduced from vol. 39, issue 1 (2007)
BT1 Furanones
BT2 Aroma compounds
BT3 Flavour compounds
BT3 Volatile compounds
BT2 Furans
BT3 Heterocyclic compounds
BT2 Ketones
BT3 Carbonyl compounds
BT4 Organic compounds

Soudjouk
BT1 Sausages
BT2 Meat products
BT3 Animal foods
BT4 Foods

Souffles
BT1 Egg products
BT2 Animal foods
BT3 Foods

Sound
NT1 Noise
NT1 Sonication
RT Acoustics
RT Ultrasound

Soup mixes
BT1 Mixes
BT2 Dried foods
BT3 Processed foods
BT4 Foods
BT2 Instant foods
BT3 Processed foods
BT4 Foods
BT1 Soups
BT2 Processed foods
BT3 Foods

Soups
BT1 Processed foods
BT2 Foods
NT1 Borshch
NT1 Bouillon
NT1 Broths
NT1 Consommes
NT1 Fish soups
NT1 Instant soups
NT1 Soup mixes
NT1 Vegetable soups
RT Instant foods

Sour cherries
BT1 Cherries
BT2 Fruits specific
BT3 Fruits
BT4 Crops
BT5 Plants
BT4 Plant foods
BT5 Foods

Sour cream
BT1 Fermented cream
BT2 Cream
BT3 Dairy products
BT4 Animal foods
BT5 Foods
BT2 Fermented dairy products
BT3 Dairy products
BT4 Animal foods
BT5 Foods
BT3 Fermented foods
BT4 Processed foods
BT5 Foods

Sourdough
BT1 Dough
BT2 Bakery products
BT3 Cereal products
BT4 Plant foods
BT5 Foods
RT Sourdough bread

Sourdough bread
HN introduced from vol. 39, issue 1 (2007)
BT1 Bread
BT2 Bakery products
BT3 Cereal products
BT4 Plant foods
BT5 Foods
RT Sourdough

Sour milk
BT1 Fermented milk

BT2 Fermented dairy products
BT3 Dairy products
BT4 Animal foods
BT5 Foods
BT3 Fermented foods
BT4 Processed foods
BT5 Foods
BT2 Milk
BT3 Dairy products
BT4 Animal foods
BT5 Foods

Sourness
BT1 Flavour
BT2 Sensory properties

Soursop
BT1 Fruits specific
BT2 Fruits
BT3 Crops
BT4 Plants
BT3 Plant foods
BT4 Foods

Sous vide
BT1 Cooking
BT2 Thermal processing
BT3 Processing thermal
BT4 Processing
BT5 Technology
BT1 Vacuum
RT Sous vide foods

Sous vide foods
BT1 Processed foods
BT2 Foods
RT Sous vide
RT Sous vide meals

Sous vide meals
BT1 Meals
BT2 Processed foods
BT3 Foods
RT Sous vide foods

South Africa
HN heading up to vol. 24 (1992)
BT1 Southern Africa
BT2 Africa

South America
HN heading up to vol. 24 (1992)
BT1 America
NT1 Argentina
NT1 Bolivia
NT1 Brazil
NT1 Chile
NT1 Colombia
NT1 Ecuador
NT1 Falkland Islands
NT1 French Guiana
NT1 Guyana
NT1 Paraguay
NT1 Peru
NT1 South Georgia
NT1 Surinam
NT1 Uruguay
NT1 Venezuela

Southern Africa
BT1 Africa
NT1 Angola
NT1 Botswana
NT1 Comoros
NT1 Lesotho
NT1 Madagascar
NT1 Malawi
NT1 Mauritius
NT1 Mozambique
NT1 Namibia
NT1 Reunion
NT1 South Africa
NT1 Swaziland
NT1 Zambia
NT1 Zimbabwe

Southern blotting
BT1 Blotting
BT2 Hybridization
BT3 Genetic techniques
BT4 Genetics

Southern peas
BT1 Cowpeas
BT2 Legumes
BT3 Vegetables specific
BT4 Vegetables
BT5 Crops
BT6 Plants
BT5 Plant foods
BT6 Foods

South Georgia
SN full name is South Georgia and the South Sandwich Islands
BT1 South America
BT2 America

South Korea
SN full name is Republic of Korea
BT1 Asia
RT Korea

South West Africa
USE **Namibia**

Sovetskii cheese
BT1 Cheese varieties
BT2 Cheese
BT3 Dairy products
BT4 Animal foods
BT5 Foods

Sowing
BT1 Cultivation
BT2 Agriculture

Sows
USE **Swine**

Soyabeans
USE **Soybeans**

Soybean lecithins
USE **Soy lecithins**

Soybean oils
BT1 Soy products
BT2 Vegetable products
BT3 Plant foods
BT4 Foods
BT1 Vegetable oils
BT2 Oils vegetable
BT3 Oils
BT4 Lipids
BT5 Nutrients
BT3 Vegetable products
BT4 Plant foods
BT5 Foods
UF Soy oils

Soybeans
BT1 Legumes
BT2 Vegetables specific
BT3 Vegetables
BT4 Crops
BT5 Plants
BT4 Plant foods
BT5 Foods
BT1 Oilseeds
BT2 Seeds
BT3 Plant foods
BT4 Foods
NT1 Black soybeans
NT1 Soybean sprouts
UF Soyabeans

Soybean sprouts
BT1 Legume sprouts
BT2 Legumes
BT3 Vegetables specific
BT4 Vegetables
BT5 Crops
BT6 Plants
BT5 Plant foods
BT6 Foods
BT2 Sprouts
BT3 Vegetables specific
BT4 Vegetables
BT5 Crops
BT6 Plants
BT5 Plant foods
BT6 Foods
BT1 Soybeans
BT2 Legumes
BT3 Vegetables specific
BT4 Vegetables
BT5 Crops
BT6 Plants
BT5 Plant foods
BT6 Foods
BT2 Oilseeds
BT3 Seeds
BT4 Plant foods
BT5 Foods

Soy beverages
BT1 Beverages
BT1 Soy products
BT2 Vegetable products
BT3 Plant foods
BT4 Foods
NT1 Soymilk

Soy cheese
BT1 Soy products
BT2 Vegetable products
BT3 Plant foods
BT4 Foods

Soy curd
BT1 Soy products

BT2 Vegetable products
BT3 Plant foods
BT4 Foods

Soy flour
USE **Soy meal**

Soy globulins
BT1 Soy proteins
BT2 Vegetable proteins
BT3 Proteins vegetable
BT4 Proteins
BT5 Nutrients
BT4 Vegetable products
BT5 Plant foods
BT6 Foods

Soy glycinin
BT1 Soy proteins
BT2 Vegetable proteins
BT3 Proteins vegetable
BT4 Proteins
BT5 Nutrients
BT4 Vegetable products
BT5 Plant foods
BT6 Foods

Soy ice cream
BT1 Soy products
BT2 Vegetable products
BT3 Plant foods
BT4 Foods

Soy infant formulas
BT1 Infant foods
BT2 Processed foods
BT3 Foods
BT1 Soy products
BT2 Vegetable products
BT3 Plant foods
BT4 Foods

Soy lecithins
BT1 Lecithins
BT2 Emulsifiers
BT3 Additives
BT2 Phospholipids
BT3 Lipids
BT4 Nutrients
BT1 Soy products
BT2 Vegetable products
BT3 Plant foods
BT4 Foods
UF Soybean lecithins

Soy meal
BT1 Flours
BT2 Plant foods
BT3 Foods
BT1 Soy products
BT2 Vegetable products
BT3 Plant foods
BT4 Foods
UF Soy flour

Soymilk
BT1 Soy beverages
BT2 Beverages
BT2 Soy products
BT3 Vegetable products
BT4 Plant foods
BT5 Foods

Soy oils
USE **Soybean oils**

Soy pastes
BT1 Pastes
BT2 Processed foods
BT3 Foods
BT1 Soy products
BT2 Vegetable products
BT3 Plant foods
BT4 Foods

Soy products
BT1 Vegetable products
BT2 Plant foods
BT3 Foods
NT1 Chungkook-jang
NT1 Doenjang
NT1 Kinema
NT1 Kochujang
NT1 Meju
NT1 Miso
NT1 Natto
NT1 Okara
NT2 Meitauza
NT1 Soybean oils
NT1 Soy beverages
NT2 Soymilk
NT1 Soy cheese
NT1 Soy curd
NT1 Soy ice cream
NT1 Soy infant formulas
NT1 Soy lecithins
NT1 Soy meal
NT1 Soy pastes
NT1 Soy purees
NT1 Soy sauces
NT2 Kanjang
NT2 Kecap
NT2 Shoyu
NT1 Soy yoghurt
NT1 Tempeh
NT1 Tofu
NT2 Sufu
NT1 Yuba

Soy protein concentrates
BT1 Protein concentrates
BT2 Concentrates
BT3 Processed foods
BT4 Foods
BT2 Protein products
BT1 Soy proteins
BT2 Vegetable proteins
BT3 Proteins vegetable
BT4 Proteins
BT5 Nutrients
BT4 Vegetable products
BT5 Plant foods
BT6 Foods

Soy proteins
BT1 Vegetable proteins
BT2 Proteins vegetable
BT3 Proteins
BT4 Nutrients
BT3 Vegetable products
BT4 Plant foods
BT5 Foods
NT1 Conglycinin
NT1 β-Conglycinin
NT1 Glycinin
NT1 Promine
NT1 Soy globulins
NT1 Soy glycinin
NT1 Soy protein concentrates
NT1 Soy 11S globulins
NT1 Soy 7S globulins
RT Textured vegetable proteins

Soy purees
BT1 Soy products
BT2 Vegetable products
BT3 Plant foods
BT4 Foods
BT1 Vegetable purees
BT2 Purees
BT3 Pulps
BT4 Processed foods
BT5 Foods
BT2 Vegetable products
BT3 Plant foods
BT4 Foods

Soy sauces
BT1 Fermented foods
BT2 Processed foods
BT3 Foods
BT1 Sauces
BT2 Condiments
BT3 Flavourings
BT4 Additives
BT1 Soy products
BT2 Vegetable products
BT3 Plant foods
BT4 Foods
NT1 Kanjang
NT1 Kecap
NT1 Shoyu
RT Miso
RT Moromi

Soy 11S globulins
BT1 Soy proteins
BT2 Vegetable proteins
BT3 Proteins vegetable
BT4 Proteins
BT5 Nutrients
BT4 Vegetable products
BT5 Plant foods
BT6 Foods
RT Glycinin

Soy 7S globulins
BT1 Soy proteins
BT2 Vegetable proteins
BT3 Proteins vegetable
BT4 Proteins
BT5 Nutrients
BT4 Vegetable products
BT5 Plant foods
BT6 Foods
RT β-Conglycinin

Soy yoghurt
BT1 Soy products
BT2 Vegetable products

BT3 Plant foods
BT4 Foods

Space flight foods
BT1 Meals
BT2 Processed foods
BT3 Foods
RT Military rations

Spaghetti
BT1 Pasta
BT2 Cereal products
BT3 Plant foods
BT4 Foods

Spain
HN heading up to vol. 24 (1992)
BT1 Europe
BT1 European Union
NT1 Canary Islands
RT Organization for Economic Cooperation and Development

Spanish mackerel
SN syn. chub mackerel; syn. Pacific mackerel
BT1 Mackerel
BT2 Marine fish
BT3 Fish
BT4 Animals
BT4 Sea foods
BT5 Aquatic foods
BT6 Animal foods
BT7 Foods
BT2 Oily fish
BT3 Fish
BT4 Animals
BT4 Sea foods
BT5 Aquatic foods
BT6 Animal foods
BT7 Foods

Sparkling winemaking
BT1 Winemaking
BT2 Processing
BT3 Technology
NT1 Champagnization

Sparkling wines
SN index heading is Wines sparkling
BT1 Wines sparkling
BT2 Wines
BT3 Alcoholic beverages
BT4 Beverages alcoholic
BT5 Beverages
NT1 Cavas
NT1 Champagne
NT1 Sekts

Sparus aurata
BT1 Sea bream
BT2 Marine fish
BT3 Fish
BT4 Animals
BT4 Sea foods
BT5 Aquatic foods
BT6 Animal foods
BT7 Foods

Spearmint
HN under Spices up to vol. 42 (2010)
BT1 Mint
BT2 Herbs
BT3 Spices
BT4 Flavourings
BT5 Additives

Species identification
BT1 Origin

Specifications
RT Standards

Specific conductivity
BT1 Electrical properties
BT2 Physical properties
RT Electrical conductivity

Specific gravity
USE **sp. gr.**

Specific heat
BT1 Thermophysical properties
BT2 Physical properties

Specific rotation
BT1 Optical properties
BT2 Physical properties

Speck
BT1 Meat products
BT2 Animal foods
BT3 Foods

Spectinomycin
BT1 Aminoglycoside antibiotics
BT2 Antibiotics
BT3 Drugs
BT4 Residues
UF Actinospectacin

Spectra
BT1 Spectroscopy
BT2 Analytical techniques

Spectrofluorometry
BT1 Fluorometry
BT2 Analytical techniques
BT1 Spectroscopy
BT2 Analytical techniques
UF Fluorescence spectroscopy

Spectrometry
USE **Spectroscopy**

Spectrophotofluorometry
BT1 Fluorometry
BT2 Analytical techniques
BT1 Spectroscopy
BT2 Analytical techniques

Spectrophotometry
USE **Spectroscopy**

Spectroscopy
BT1 Analytical techniques
NT1 Atomic absorption spectroscopy
NT2 AAS
NT1 Atomic emission spectroscopy
NT2 ICP-AES
NT1 Circular dichroism
NT1 Electron paramagnetic resonance
NT1 Electron spin resonance
NT1 FTIR spectroscopy
NT1 ICP-OES
NT1 IR spectroscopy
NT2 IR analysis
NT2 IR spectra
NT1 Mass spectroscopy
NT2 Electrospray ionization MS
NT2 GC-MS
NT2 ICP-MS
NT2 LC-MS
NT2 MALDI-TOF-MS
NT2 MS
NT1 NIR spectroscopy
NT1 Nuclear magnetic resonance
NT2 Magnetic resonance imaging
NT2 NMR
NT2 Proton magnetic resonance
NT2 Proton resonance
NT1 Raman spectroscopy
NT1 Spectra
NT1 Spectrofluorometry
NT1 Spectrophotofluorometry
NT1 UV spectroscopy
NT1 X-ray fluorescence spectroscopy
RT Fluorometry
UF Spectrometry
UF Spectrophotometry

Spelt
SN syn. spelt wheat
BT1 Wheat
BT2 Cereals
BT3 Crops
BT4 Plants
BT3 Seeds
BT4 Plant foods
BT5 Foods
NT1 Spelt wheat

Spelt wheat
SN syn. spelt
BT1 Spelt
BT2 Wheat
BT3 Cereals
BT4 Crops
BT5 Plants
BT4 Seeds
BT5 Plant foods
BT6 Foods

Spermidine
BT1 Polyamines
BT2 Amines
BT3 Organic nitrogen compounds
RT Spermine

Spermine
BT1 Biogenic amines
BT2 Amines

BT3 Organic nitrogen compounds
BT1 Polyamines
BT2 Amines
BT3 Organic nitrogen compounds
RT Spermidine

sp. gr.
SN syn. relative density
BT1 Density
BT2 Physical properties
NT1 Relative density
RT Gravity
UF Specific gravity

Sphingolipids
BT1 Lipids
BT2 Nutrients
NT1 Sphingomyelin
RT Phospholipids

Sphingomonas
BT1 Bacteria
BT2 Microorganisms
NT1 *Sphingomonas paucimobilis*

Sphingomonas paucimobilis
BT1 *Sphingomonas*
BT2 Bacteria
BT3 Microorganisms

Sphingomyelin
BT1 Sphingolipids
BT2 Lipids
BT3 Nutrients

Spices
BT1 Flavourings
BT2 Additives
NT1 African nutmeg
NT1 *Afromomum danielli*
NT1 Ajowan
NT1 Allspice
NT1 Aniseed
NT1 Asafoetida
NT1 Black cumin
NT1 Capers
NT1 Caraway
NT1 Cardamom
NT1 *Cassia*
NT1 Cayenne pepper
NT1 Celery seeds
NT1 Chilli
NT1 Chopi
NT1 Cinnamon
NT2 *Cinnamomum zeylanicum*
NT1 Cloves
NT1 Coertuek
NT2 *Echinophora tenuifolia*
NT1 Coriander
NT2 Coriander leaves
NT2 Coriander seeds
NT1 Cumin
NT1 Curry powders
NT1 Dill
NT2 Dill leaves
NT2 Dill seeds
NT1 Fennel seeds
NT1 Fenugreek
NT1 Galangal
NT1 Garlic
NT1 Ginger
NT1 Herbs
NT2 *Agastache*
NT2 Angelica
NT2 *Artemisia*
NT2 Basil
NT3 Sweet basil
NT2 Bay
NT3 Bay leaves
NT3 Laurel
NT2 Borage
NT2 *Calamintha*
NT2 Catmint
NT2 Chamomile
NT3 Camomile
NT2 Chervil
NT2 Chives
NT2 Comfrey
NT2 Coriander leaves
NT2 Costmary
NT2 Curry leaves
NT3 *Murraya koenigii*
NT2 Davana
NT2 Dill leaves
NT2 Dittany
NT2 Hyssop
NT2 Lemon balm
NT2 Lemongrass
NT2 Marjoram
NT2 Mint
NT3 Peppermint
NT3 Spearmint
NT2 Mugwort
NT3 *Artemisia vulgaris*
NT2 Oregano
NT2 Palmarosa
NT2 Parsley
NT2 Rosemary
NT2 Rue
NT2 Sage
NT2 Samphire
NT3 Sea fennel
NT4 *Crithmum maritimum*
NT2 Savory
NT3 *Satureja*
NT2 Sorrel
NT2 Tansy
NT2 Tarragon
NT2 Thyme
NT2 Wormwood
NT1 Horseradish
NT1 Japanese pepper
NT1 Juniper
NT1 Kokum
NT1 Lovage
NT1 Mace
NT1 Mustard seeds
NT2 Ethiopian mustard
NT3 *Brassica carinata*
NT2 Indian mustard
NT1 Nutmeg
NT1 Paprika
NT1 Pepper
NT2 Black pepper
NT2 Peppercorns
NT2 *Piper longum*
NT2 White pepper
NT1 Poppy seeds
NT1 Saffron
NT1 Sarsaparilla
NT1 Star anise
NT1 Sumac
NT1 Turmeric
NT1 Wasabi
NT1 White mustard
NT1 Wild garlic
NT1 Yellow mustard

Spina bifida
BT1 Neural tube defects
BT2 Diseases

Spinach
BT1 Vegetables specific
BT2 Vegetables
BT3 Crops
BT4 Plants
BT3 Plant foods
BT4 Foods

Spinal cord tissues
BT1 Central nervous system tissues
BT2 Wastes

Spinning
BT1 Texturization
BT2 Processing
BT3 Technology

Spinosad
BT1 Insecticides
BT2 Pesticides
BT3 Biocides
BT3 Residues

Spiramycin
BT1 Macrolide antibiotics
BT2 Antibiotics
BT3 Drugs
BT4 Residues

Spirits
BT1 Alcoholic beverages
BT2 Beverages alcoholic
BT3 Beverages
NT1 Absinthe
NT1 Aquavit
NT1 Arak
NT1 Awamori
NT1 Brandies
NT2 Armagnac
NT2 Brandy
NT2 Cognac
NT2 Eau de vie
NT2 Fruit brandies
NT3 Apple brandy
NT4 Calvados
NT3 Kirsch
NT3 Rakia
NT3 Slivovitz
NT2 Grappa
NT2 Pisco
NT1 Distillates
NT2 Wine distillates
NT1 Gin
NT1 Grape spirits

NT1 Lambanog
NT1 Mezcal
NT1 Ouzo
NT1 Raki
NT1 Rum
NT1 Schnapps
NT1 Shochu
NT1 Sugar cane spirits
NT2 Cachaca
NT1 Tequila
NT1 Vodka
NT1 Whiskies
NT2 Whiskey
NT3 Bourbon whiskey
NT2 Whisky
NT3 Scotch whisky
RT Liqueurs
UF Grain alcohols

Spirulina
BT1 Cyanobacteria
BT2 Bacteria
BT3 Microorganisms
NT1 *Spirulina maxima*
NT1 *Spirulina platensis*

Spirulina maxima
SN synonymous with Arthrospira maxima
BT1 *Spirulina*
BT2 Cyanobacteria
BT3 Bacteria
BT4 Microorganisms

Spirulina platensis
SN synonymous with Arthrospira platensis
BT1 *Spirulina*
BT2 Cyanobacteria
BT3 Bacteria
BT4 Microorganisms

Spleens
BT1 Offal
BT2 Animal foods
BT3 Foods

Splitting
BT1 Cutting
BT2 Processing
BT3 Technology
BT1 Damage

Spoilage
NT1 Bacterial spoilage
NT1 Biodeterioration
NT1 Bloom
NT1 Blowing
NT1 Chilling injury
NT1 Deterioration
NT1 Microbial spoilage
NT2 Decay
NT1 Putrefaction
NT1 Rotting
NT1 Spoilage bacteria
NT1 Spoilage fungi
NT1 Spoilage yeasts
NT1 Sprouting
NT1 Staling
RT Browning
RT Contamination
RT Damage
RT Defects
RT Diseases plant
RT Oxidation
RT Shelf life
RT Taints
RT Trimethylamine

Spoilage bacteria
BT1 Bacteria
BT2 Microorganisms
BT1 Spoilage
RT Bacterial spoilage

Spoilage fungi
HN introduced from vol. 39, issue 1 (2007)
BT1 Fungi
BT2 Microorganisms
BT1 Spoilage

Spoilage yeasts
BT1 Spoilage
BT1 Yeasts
BT2 Fungi
BT3 Microorganisms

Spondias
BT1 Fruits specific
BT2 Fruits
BT3 Crops
BT4 Plants
BT3 Plant foods
BT4 Foods

Sponge
SN intermediate product of dough making
BT1 Dough
BT2 Bakery products
BT3 Cereal products
BT4 Plant foods
BT5 Foods

Sponge cakes
BT1 Cakes
BT2 Bakery products
BT3 Cereal products
BT4 Plant foods
BT5 Foods

Spores
HN heading up to vol. 24 (1992); heading from vol. 43 (2011); under Microbial spores from vol. 25 (1993) up to vol. 42 (2010)
NT1 Microbial spores
NT2 Bacterial spores
NT2 Fungal spores
NT1 Sporulation

Sporobolomyces
HN under Fungi up to vol. 42 (2010)
BT1 Yeasts
BT2 Fungi
BT3 Microorganisms

Sporotrichum
BT1 Fungi
BT2 Microorganisms

Sports drinks
BT1 Health beverages
BT2 Beverages
BT2 Health foods
BT3 Processed foods
BT4 Foods
BT1 Soft drinks
BT2 Beverages
RT Performance drinks
RT Sports foods
RT Sports nutrition
RT Sports supplements

Sports foods
BT1 Health foods
BT2 Processed foods
BT3 Foods
RT Sports drinks
RT Sports nutrition
RT Sports supplements

Sports nutrition
HN introduced from vol. 41, issue 1 (2009)
BT1 Nutrition
RT Physical activity
RT Sports drinks
RT Sports foods
RT Sports supplements

Sports supplements
HN introduced from vol. 38, issue 8 (2006)
BT1 Food supplements
RT Health beverages
RT Health foods
RT Sports drinks
RT Sports foods
RT Sports nutrition

Sporulation
HN under Microbial spores up to vol. 42 (2010)
BT1 Spores
RT Bacterial spores
RT Fungal spores
RT Microbial spores

Spouted bed processing
HN introduced from vol. 41, issue 1 (2009)
BT1 Processing
BT2 Technology

Sprat
BT1 Marine fish
BT2 Fish
BT3 Animals
BT3 Sea foods
BT4 Aquatic foods
BT5 Animal foods
BT6 Foods
BT1 Oily fish
BT2 Fish
BT3 Animals
BT3 Sea foods
BT4 Aquatic foods
BT5 Animal foods
BT6 Foods
UF Sprats

Sprats
HN used up to vol. 29 (1997)
USE **Sprat**

Spray dried foods
BT1 Dried foods
BT2 Processed foods
BT3 Foods

Spray driers
BT1 Driers
BT2 Drying
BT3 Thermal processing
BT4 Processing thermal
BT5 Processing
BT6 Technology
BT2 Equipment
BT3 Technology
BT1 Spray drying
BT2 Drying
BT3 Thermal processing
BT4 Processing thermal
BT5 Processing
BT6 Technology

Spray drying
HN heading was Spray-drying up to vol. 24 (1992)
BT1 Drying
BT2 Thermal processing
BT3 Processing thermal
BT4 Processing
BT5 Technology
NT1 Spray driers
UF Spray-drying

Spray-drying
HN heading up to vol. 24
USE **Spray drying**

Spraying
HN introduced from vol. 39, issue 1 (2007)
SN foliar sprays also exists in the index
BT1 Processing
BT2 Technology

Spreadability
BT1 Texture
BT2 Sensory properties

Spreads
BT1 Processed foods
BT2 Foods
NT1 Butterine
NT1 Butter spreads
NT1 Calories low spreads
NT1 Cheese spreads
NT1 Dairy spreads
NT1 Fats low spreads
NT1 Peanut butter
RT Margarines
RT Pastes
RT Pates

Springiness
BT1 Texture
BT2 Sensory properties

Spring waters
BT1 Mineral waters
BT2 Soft drinks
BT3 Beverages
BT2 Water

Sprouting
SN used in relation to potatoes and other tubers; for sprouting of seeds use germination
BT1 Spoilage

Sprouting inhibitors
USE **Antisprouting agents**

Sprouts
HN introduced from vol. 39, issue 1 (2007)
SN not used for Brussels sprouts
BT1 Vegetables specific
BT2 Vegetables
BT3 Crops
BT4 Plants
BT3 Plant foods
BT4 Foods
NT1 Legume sprouts
NT2 Alfalfa sprouts
NT2 Bean sprouts
NT2 Soybean sprouts
NT1 Radish sprouts

Squalene
BT1 Triterpenes
BT2 Hydrocarbons
BT3 Organic compounds
BT2 Triterpenoids
BT3 Terpenoids
BT4 Lipids
BT5 Nutrients

Squash
SN use for the beverage; for the plant food use Squashes
BT1 Soft drinks
BT2 Beverages
RT Fruit cordials

Squashes
HN heading from vol. 30 (1998); under Vegetables specific up to vol. 29 (1997)
SN use for the plant food; for the beverage use Squash
BT1 Vegetables specific
BT2 Vegetables
BT3 Crops
BT4 Plants
BT3 Plant foods
BT4 Foods
NT1 *Cucurbita moschata*

Squash seeds
BT1 Oilseeds
BT2 Seeds
BT3 Plant foods
BT4 Foods

Squid
HN heading from vol. 30 (1998); under Molluscs up to vol. 29 (1997)
BT1 Cephalopods
BT2 Molluscs
BT3 Shellfish
BT4 Animals
BT4 Sea foods
BT5 Aquatic foods
BT6 Animal foods
BT7 Foods
NT1 Ika shiokara
NT1 *Illex argentinus*
NT1 *Ommastrephes bartrami*

Squid ika shiokara
USE **Ika shiokara**

Squid oils
BT1 Marine oils
BT2 Oils
BT3 Lipids
BT4 Nutrients

Sr
BT1 Metals
BT2 Elements
BT3 Minerals
BT4 Nutrients
BT1 Radioelements
BT2 Isotopes
BT3 Elements
BT4 Minerals
BT5 Nutrients
BT2 Residues
UF Strontium

Srikand
USE **Shrikhand**

Srikhand
USE **Shrikhand**

Sri Lanka
HN heading up to vol. 24 (1992)
BT1 Asia
UF Ceylon

Stability
BT1 Physical properties
NT1 Colloidal stability
NT1 Freeze-thaw stability
NT1 Heat stability
NT1 Oxidative stability
NT1 Stabilization
NT1 Thermal stability
RT Stabilizers

Stabilization
BT1 Stability
BT2 Physical properties

Stabilizers
BT1 Additives
NT1 Agar
NT2 Agar gels
NT2 Agarose
NT1 Alginates
NT2 Alginate gels
NT2 Alginic acid
NT1 Carrageenans
NT2 Carrageenan gels
NT1 Food stabilizers
NT1 Gums
NT2 Cassia gums
NT2 Furcellaran
NT2 Gellan gums
NT2 Guar gums

NT2 Gum arabic
NT3 Gum acacia
NT2 Gum ghatti
NT2 Gum kondagogu
NT2 Gum tragacanth
NT2 Karaya gums
NT2 Locust bean gums
NT3 Carob gums
NT2 Mesquite seed gums
NT2 Mucilage
NT2 Psyllium gums
NT2 Tara gums
NT2 Xanthan gums
NT1 Sucrose acetate isobutyrate
RT Celluloses
RT Stability
RT Thickeners

Stable isotope techniques
HN introduced from vol. 39, issue 1 (2007)
BT1 Analytical techniques
RT Isotopes

Stachybotrys
BT1 Fungi
BT2 Microorganisms
RT Mycotoxins

Stachyose
HN under Sugars up to vol. 42 (2010)
BT1 Oligosaccharides
BT2 Polysaccharides
BT3 Carbohydrates
BT4 Nutrients
BT4 Organic compounds
BT2 Sugars
BT3 Carbohydrates
BT4 Nutrients
BT4 Organic compounds
BT3 Plant foods
BT4 Foods

Stacking
BT1 Handling

Staining
SN not for staining techniques used in analytical procedures
BT1 Discoloration

Stainless steel
BT1 Steel
BT2 Packaging materials
BT2 Surfaces

Staling
HN heading from vol. 25 (1993); under Spoilage up to vol. 24 (1992)
BT1 Spoilage
RT Retrogradation

Standardization

Standards
RT Certification
RT Legislation
RT Specifications
RT Tolerance

Stanol esters
BT1 Esters
BT2 Organic compounds
BT1 Stanols
BT2 Sterols
BT3 Alcohols
BT3 Steroids
BT4 Lipids
BT5 Nutrients

Stanols
BT1 Sterols
BT2 Alcohols
BT2 Steroids
BT3 Lipids
BT4 Nutrients
NT1 Phytostanols
NT2 Sitostanol
NT1 Stanol esters

Staphylococcus
BT1 Bacteria
BT2 Microorganisms
NT1 *Staphylococcus aureus*
NT1 *Staphylococcus carnosus*
NT1 *Staphylococcus epidermidis*
NT1 *Staphylococcus equorum*
NT1 *Staphylococcus intermedius*
NT1 *Staphylococcus saprophyticus*
NT1 *Staphylococcus sciuri*
NT1 *Staphylococcus simulans*
NT1 *Staphylococcus xylosus*

Staphylococcus aureus
BT1 *Staphylococcus*
BT2 Bacteria
BT3 Microorganisms

Staphylococcus carnosus
BT1 *Staphylococcus*
BT2 Bacteria
BT3 Microorganisms

Staphylococcus epidermidis
HN introduced from vol. 41, issue 1 (2009)
BT1 *Staphylococcus*
BT2 Bacteria
BT3 Microorganisms
RT Epidermin

Staphylococcus equorum
HN introduced from vol. 39, issue 1 (2007)
BT1 *Staphylococcus*
BT2 Bacteria
BT3 Microorganisms

Staphylococcus intermedius
BT1 *Staphylococcus*
BT2 Bacteria
BT3 Microorganisms

Staphylococcus saprophyticus
HN introduced from vol. 42, issue 1 (2010)
BT1 *Staphylococcus*
BT2 Bacteria
BT3 Microorganisms

Staphylococcus sciuri
HN introduced from vol. 39, issue 1 (2007)
BT1 *Staphylococcus*
BT2 Bacteria
BT3 Microorganisms

Staphylococcus simulans
HN introduced from vol. 39, issue 1 (2007)
BT1 *Staphylococcus*
BT2 Bacteria
BT3 Microorganisms

Staphylococcus xylosus
BT1 *Staphylococcus*
BT2 Bacteria
BT3 Microorganisms

Star anise
BT1 Spices
BT2 Flavourings
BT3 Additives

Star apples
BT1 Fruits specific
BT2 Fruits
BT3 Crops
BT4 Plants
BT3 Plant foods
BT4 Foods

Starch
BT1 Glucans
BT2 Polysaccharides
BT3 Carbohydrates
BT4 Nutrients
BT4 Organic compounds
BT1 Thickeners
BT2 Additives
NT1 Amaranth starch
NT1 Amylopectins
NT1 Amyloses
NT1 Arrowroot
NT1 Barley starch
NT1 Buckwheat starch
NT1 Canna starch
NT1 Cassava starch
NT2 Tapioca
NT1 Corn starch
NT2 High amylose corn starch
NT1 Dextrins
NT2 Amylodextrins
NT2 Cyclodextrins
NT2 Maltodextrins
NT2 Pyrodextrins
NT1 Farina
NT1 Legume starch
NT1 Millet starch
NT1 Modified starches
NT1 Mung bean starch
NT1 Oat starch
NT1 Pea starch
NT1 Potato starch
NT1 Resistant starch
NT1 Rice starch
NT1 Rye starch
NT1 Sago
NT1 Sorghum starch
NT1 Starch granules

NT1 Sweet potato starch
NT1 Wheat starch
NT1 Yam starch
RT Retrogradation
UF Starches
UF Starches specific

Starches
HN used as a heading for specific starches from vol. 25 (1993) to vol. 29 (1997); under Starches specific up to vol. 24 (1992)
USE **Starch**

Starches specific
HN used as a heading for specific starches up to vol.24 (1992)
USE **Starch**

Starch granules
BT1 Starch
BT2 Glucans
BT3 Polysaccharides
BT4 Carbohydrates
BT5 Nutrients
BT5 Organic compounds
BT2 Thickeners
BT3 Additives

Starch hydrolysates
BT1 Sugar syrups
BT2 Plant foods
BT3 Foods
UF Hydrolysed starches

Starch synthases
SN EC 2.4.1.21
BT1 Glycosyltransferases
BT2 Transferases
BT3 Enzymes

Starch syrups
BT1 Sugar syrups
BT2 Plant foods
BT3 Foods

Star fruit
SN syn. carambolas
BT1 Carambolas
BT2 Fruits specific
BT3 Fruits
BT4 Crops
BT5 Plants
BT4 Plant foods
BT5 Foods

Starters
BT1 Bacteria
BT2 Microorganisms
NT1 Adjunct cultures
NT1 Butter starters
NT1 Cheese starters
NT1 Dairy starters
NT1 Lactic starters
NT1 Nuruk
NT1 Yoghurt starters
RT Buttermaking
RT Cheesemaking
RT Fermentation

Starvation
HN introduced from vol. 41, issue 1 (2009)
BT1 Physiology
BT2 Science
RT Fasting

Statistical analysis
BT1 Mathematics
BT2 Science
NT1 Chemometrics

Statistics
BT1 Economics

Steaks
BT1 Meat
BT2 Animal foods
BT3 Foods
RT Beef steaks

Steam
BT1 Energy
BT1 Steaming
BT2 Cooking
BT3 Thermal processing
BT4 Processing thermal
BT5 Processing
BT6 Technology

Steamed bread
BT1 Bread
BT2 Bakery products
BT3 Cereal products
BT4 Plant foods
BT5 Foods

Steaming
BT1 Cooking
BT2 Thermal processing
BT3 Processing thermal
BT4 Processing
BT5 Technology
NT1 Steam

Stearic acid
SN syn. octadecanoic acid
BT1 Octadecanoic acid
BT2 Saturated fatty acids
BT3 Fatty acids
BT4 Lipids
BT5 Nutrients
BT4 Organic acids
BT5 Acids
NT1 Hydroxystearic acid

Stearidonic acid
HN introduced from vol. 39, issue 1 (2007)
BT1 ω-3 Fatty acids
BT2 PUFA
BT3 Unsaturated fatty acids
BT4 Fatty acids
BT5 Lipids
BT6 Nutrients
BT5 Organic acids
BT6 Acids

Stearin
BT1 Triglycerides
BT2 Glycerides
BT3 Emulsifiers
BT4 Additives
BT3 Fatty acid esters
BT4 Esters
BT5 Organic compounds
BT3 Lipids
BT4 Nutrients
NT1 Palm stearin

Stearoyl lactylates
BT1 Lactylates
BT2 Emulsifiers
BT3 Additives

Stearyl alcohol
BT1 Alcohols

Steel
BT1 Packaging materials
BT1 Surfaces
NT1 Stainless steel

Steeping
BT1 Soaking
BT2 Processing
BT3 Technology

Steers
HN type of cattle not specified in the index from vol. 25 (1993)
USE **Cattle**

Stems
HN introduced from vol. 39, issue 1 (2007)
BT1 Plants

Stenotrophomonas
BT1 Bacteria
BT2 Microorganisms
NT1 *Stenotrophomonas maltophilia*

Stenotrophomonas maltophilia
BT1 *Stenotrophomonas*
BT2 Bacteria
BT3 Microorganisms

Sterculic acid
BT1 Fatty acids
BT2 Lipids
BT3 Nutrients
BT2 Organic acids
BT3 Acids

Stereoisomers
BT1 Isomers

Sterigmatocystins
BT1 Mycotoxins
BT2 Toxins
BT3 Residues
BT1 Xanthones
BT2 Heterocyclic compounds

Sterilization
BT1 Thermal processing
BT2 Processing thermal
BT3 Processing
BT4 Technology

NT1 Autoclaves
NT1 Ohmic heating
NT1 Retorting
NT1 UHT treatment
RT Canning
RT Fumigation
RT Pasteurization
RT Sterilized milk
RT UHT cream
RT UHT milk

Sterilized milk
BT1 Milk
BT2 Dairy products
BT3 Animal foods
BT4 Foods
RT Sterilization
UF Sterilized milks

Sterilized milks
HN heading up to vol. 24 (1992)
USE **Sterilized milk**

Steroids
BT1 Lipids
BT2 Nutrients
NT1 Brassinosteroids
NT1 Cortisol
NT1 Sapogenins
NT1 Sterols
NT2 Avenasterol
NT2 Brassicasterol
NT2 Campesterol
NT2 Cholesterol
NT3 Cholesterol low foods
NT3 Cholesterol oxidation products
NT4 Cholesterol oxides
NT2 Cucurbitacins
NT2 Desmosterol
NT2 Ergosterol
NT2 Phytosterols
NT2 Sitosterol
NT2 Stanols
NT3 Phytostanols
NT4 Sitostanol
NT3 Stanol esters
NT2 Sterol esters
NT2 Stigmastadienes
NT2 Stigmasterol

Sterol esters
HN introduced from vol. 39, issue 1 (2007)
BT1 Esters
BT2 Organic compounds
BT1 Sterols
BT2 Alcohols
BT2 Steroids
BT3 Lipids
BT4 Nutrients

Sterols
HN heading from vol. 25 (1993); under Steroids up to vol. 24 (1992)
BT1 Alcohols
BT1 Steroids
BT2 Lipids
BT3 Nutrients
NT1 Avenasterol
NT1 Brassicasterol
NT1 Campesterol
NT1 Cholesterol
NT2 Cholesterol low foods
NT2 Cholesterol oxidation products
NT3 Cholesterol oxides
NT1 Cucurbitacins
NT1 Desmosterol
NT1 Ergosterol
NT1 Phytosterols
NT1 Sitosterol
NT1 Stanols
NT2 Phytostanols
NT3 Sitostanol
NT2 Stanol esters
NT1 Sterol esters
NT1 Stigmastadienes
NT1 Stigmasterol

Stevia rebaudiana
BT1 Plants
RT Rebaudiosides
RT Steviol
RT Stevioside

Steviol
HN introduced from vol. 39, issue 1 (2007)
BT1 Diterpenoids
BT2 Terpenoids
BT3 Lipids
BT4 Nutrients
RT *Stevia rebaudiana*

Stevioside
BT1 Diterpenoids
BT2 Terpenoids
BT3 Lipids
BT4 Nutrients
BT1 Glycosides
BT2 Carbohydrates
BT3 Nutrients
BT3 Organic compounds
BT1 Sweeteners
BT2 Additives
RT Rebaudiosides
RT *Stevia rebaudiana*

Stewing
BT1 Cooking
BT2 Thermal processing
BT3 Processing thermal
BT4 Processing
BT5 Technology

St Helena
SN overseas territory of the United Kingdom
BT1 United Kingdom
BT2 Europe
BT2 European Union

Stickiness
BT1 Rheological properties
BT2 Mechanical properties
BT3 Physical properties

Sticking
BT1 Adhesion
BT2 Physical properties

Stiffness
BT1 Rheological properties
BT2 Mechanical properties
BT3 Physical properties

Stigmastadienes
BT1 Sterols
BT2 Alcohols
BT2 Steroids
BT3 Lipids
BT4 Nutrients

Stigmasterol
BT1 Sterols
BT2 Alcohols
BT2 Steroids
BT3 Lipids
BT4 Nutrients

Stilbenes
HN introduced from vol. 39, issue 1 (2007)
BT1 Phenols
BT2 Alcohols
BT2 Aromatic compounds
BT3 Organic compounds
NT1 Piceatannol
NT1 Piceid
NT1 Resveratrol
RT Polyphenols

Stillage
HN under By-products up to vol. 42 (2010)
BT1 Effluents
BT2 Waste water
BT3 Wastes
BT3 Water
RT Brewing
RT Distillation
RT Winemaking

Stilton cheese
BT1 Cheese varieties
BT2 Cheese
BT3 Dairy products
BT4 Animal foods
BT5 Foods

Stink bugs
BT1 Insects
BT2 Pests

Stir frying
BT1 Frying
BT2 Cooking
BT3 Thermal processing
BT4 Processing thermal
BT5 Processing
BT6 Technology

Stirred tank bioreactors
HN introduced from vol. 39, issue 1 (2007)
BT1 Bioreactors
BT2 Fermentation technology
BT3 Biotechnology
BT4 Technology
BT3 Process control
BT4 Technology

Stirring
BT1 Mixing
BT2 Processing
BT3 Technology

Stocking density (aquaculture)
HN introduced from vol. 42, issue 1 (2010)
BT1 Aquaculture

Stocking density (husbandry)
HN introduced from vol. 42, issue 1 (2010)
BT1 Husbandry
BT2 Agriculture

Stocks
BT1 Juices
BT2 Liquids
BT3 Physical phases
BT4 Chemistry
BT5 Science

Stollen
BT1 Cakes
BT2 Bakery products
BT3 Cereal products
BT4 Plant foods
BT5 Foods

Stomachs
BT1 Offal
BT2 Animal foods
BT3 Foods

Stone fruits
BT1 Fruits specific
BT2 Fruits
BT3 Crops
BT4 Plants
BT3 Plant foods
BT4 Foods

Stones
USE **Seeds**

Stoppers
BT1 Closures
BT2 Packaging
BT3 Technology

Storage
NT1 Ambient storage
NT1 Intermittent warming
NT1 Retail display
NT1 Storage cold
NT2 Cold storage
NT3 Cold stores
NT2 Frozen storage
NT1 Storage controlled atmosphere
NT2 Controlled atmosphere storage
NT1 Storage life
NT1 Stores
NT1 Warehouses
RT Preservation
RT Shelf life
RT Silos
RT Tanks
UF Storage fruits
UF Storage vegetables

Storage cold
BT1 Storage
NT1 Cold storage
NT2 Cold stores
NT1 Frozen storage
RT Refrigerated storage
RT Refrigeration

Storage controlled atm
HN used for storage controlled atmosphere up to vol. 24 (1992)
USE **Storage controlled atmosphere**

Storage controlled atmosphere
HN storage controlled atm also used in the index up to vol. 24 (1992)
BT1 Storage
NT1 Controlled atmosphere storage
UF Storage controlled atm

Storage fruits
HN heading up to vol. 24 (1992)
USE **Storage**

Storage life
BT1 Storage
RT Shelf life

Storage proteins
BT1 Vegetable proteins
BT2 Proteins vegetable
BT3 Proteins
BT4 Nutrients
BT3 Vegetable products
BT4 Plant foods
BT5 Foods

Storage vegetables
HN heading up to vol. 24 (1992)
USE **Storage**

Stores
BT1 Storage

Stout
BT1 Beer
BT2 Alcoholic beverages
BT3 Beverages alcoholic
BT4 Beverages

Stoves
USE **Ovens**

Stracchino cheese
BT1 Cheese varieties
BT2 Cheese
BT3 Dairy products
BT4 Animal foods
BT5 Foods

Strainers
BT1 Equipment
BT2 Technology
BT1 Separation
BT2 Processing
BT3 Technology

Strain identification
HN introduced from vol. 39, issue 1 (2007)
BT1 Origin

Strawberries
BT1 Berries
BT2 Fruits specific
BT3 Fruits
BT4 Crops
BT5 Plants
BT4 Plant foods
BT5 Foods
NT1 Strawberry jams
NT1 Strawberry pulps
NT1 Strawberry purees
RT Strawberry juices

Strawberry jams
BT1 Jams
BT2 Fruit preserves
BT3 Fruit products
BT4 Plant foods
BT5 Foods
BT3 Preserves
BT4 Processed foods
BT5 Foods
BT1 Strawberries
BT2 Berries
BT3 Fruits specific
BT4 Fruits
BT5 Crops
BT6 Plants
BT5 Plant foods
BT6 Foods

Strawberry juices
BT1 Berry juices
BT2 Fruit juices
BT3 Fruit products
BT4 Plant foods
BT5 Foods
BT3 Soft drinks
BT4 Beverages
RT Strawberries

Strawberry pulps
HN introduced from vol. 39, issue 1 (2007)
BT1 Fruit pulps
BT2 Fruit products
BT3 Plant foods
BT4 Foods
BT2 Pulps
BT3 Processed foods
BT4 Foods
BT1 Strawberries
BT2 Berries
BT3 Fruits specific
BT4 Fruits
BT5 Crops
BT6 Plants
BT5 Plant foods
BT6 Foods

Strawberry purees
HN introduced from vol. 39, issue 1 (2007)
BT1 Fruit purees
BT2 Fruit products
BT3 Plant foods

BT4 Foods
BT2 Purees
BT3 Pulps
BT4 Processed foods
BT5 Foods
BT1 Strawberries
BT2 Berries
BT3 Fruits specific
BT4 Fruits
BT5 Crops
BT6 Plants
BT5 Plant foods
BT6 Foods

Strawberry tree fruits
BT1 Berries
BT2 Fruits specific
BT3 Fruits
BT4 Crops
BT5 Plants
BT4 Plant foods
BT5 Foods
UF Arbutus berries

Straw mushrooms
BT1 Edible fungi
BT2 Fungi edible
BT3 Vegetables specific
BT4 Vegetables
BT5 Crops
BT6 Plants
BT5 Plant foods
BT6 Foods
RT *Volvariella*

Street foods
BT1 Fast foods
BT2 Processed foods
BT3 Foods

Strength
BT1 Mechanical properties
BT2 Physical properties

Streptococcus
BT1 Bacteria
BT2 Microorganisms
NT1 Lactic streptococci
NT1 *Streptococcus bovis*
NT1 *Streptococcus faecalis*
NT1 *Streptococcus faecium*
NT1 *Streptococcus macedonicus*
NT1 *Streptococcus mutans*
NT1 *Streptococcus pyogenes*
NT1 *Streptococcus salivarius*
NT1 *Streptococcus suis*
NT1 *Streptococcus thermophilus*
NT1 *Streptococcus uberis*
RT *Lactococcus*

Streptococcus bovis
SN synonymous with Streptococcus equinus
BT1 *Streptococcus*
BT2 Bacteria
BT3 Microorganisms

Streptococcus faecalis
SN synonymous with Enterococcus faecalis
BT1 *Streptococcus*
BT2 Bacteria
BT3 Microorganisms

Streptococcus faecium
HN introduced from vol. 41, issue 1 (2009)
SN synonymous with Enterococcus faecium
BT1 *Streptococcus*
BT2 Bacteria
BT3 Microorganisms

Streptococcus macedonicus
HN introduced from vol. 41, issue 1 (2009)
BT1 *Streptococcus*
BT2 Bacteria
BT3 Microorganisms

Streptococcus mutans
BT1 *Streptococcus*
BT2 Bacteria
BT3 Microorganisms

Streptococcus pyogenes
BT1 *Streptococcus*
BT2 Bacteria
BT3 Microorganisms

Streptococcus salivarius
BT1 *Streptococcus*
BT2 Bacteria
BT3 Microorganisms

Streptococcus suis
BT1 *Streptococcus*
BT2 Bacteria
BT3 Microorganisms

Streptococcus thermophilus
BT1 *Streptococcus*
BT2 Bacteria
BT3 Microorganisms

Streptococcus uberis
HN introduced from vol. 41, issue 1 (2009)
BT1 *Streptococcus*
BT2 Bacteria
BT3 Microorganisms

Streptomyces
HN under Actinomycetales up to vol. 24 (1992); heading from vol. 30 (1998)
BT1 Bacteria
BT2 Microorganisms
NT1 *Streptomyces albulus*
NT1 *Streptomyces coelicolor*
NT1 *Streptomyces diastaticus*
NT1 *Streptomyces globisporus*
NT1 *Streptomyces griseus*
NT1 *Streptomyces lividans*
NT1 *Streptomyces murinus*
NT1 *Streptomyces olivaceoviridis*
NT1 *Streptomyces thermoviolaceus*

Streptomyces albulus
BT1 *Streptomyces*
BT2 Bacteria
BT3 Microorganisms

Streptomyces coelicolor
BT1 *Streptomyces*
BT2 Bacteria
BT3 Microorganisms

Streptomyces diastaticus
BT1 *Streptomyces*
BT2 Bacteria
BT3 Microorganisms

Streptomyces globisporus
BT1 *Streptomyces*
BT2 Bacteria
BT3 Microorganisms

Streptomyces griseus
BT1 *Streptomyces*
BT2 Bacteria
BT3 Microorganisms

Streptomyces lividans
BT1 *Streptomyces*
BT2 Bacteria
BT3 Microorganisms

Streptomyces murinus
BT1 *Streptomyces*
BT2 Bacteria
BT3 Microorganisms

Streptomyces olivaceoviridis
BT1 *Streptomyces*
BT2 Bacteria
BT3 Microorganisms

Streptomyces thermoviolaceus
BT1 *Streptomyces*
BT2 Bacteria
BT3 Microorganisms

Streptomycin
BT1 Aminoglycoside antibiotics
BT2 Antibiotics
BT3 Drugs
BT4 Residues

Streptoverticillium
BT1 Bacteria
BT2 Microorganisms
NT1 *Streptoverticillium mobaraense*

Streptoverticillium mobaraense
SN synonymous with Streptomyces mobaraensis
BT1 *Streptoverticillium*
BT2 Bacteria
BT3 Microorganisms

Stresnil
USE **Azaperone**

Stress
NT1 Animal stress
NT1 Osmotic stress
NT1 Oxidative stress
NT1 Stress proteins
NT2 Cold shock proteins
NT2 Heat shock proteins

NT1 Stress relaxation
NT1 Stress resistance
NT1 Yield stress
RT Antifreeze proteins
RT Elicitation
RT σ Factors

Stress proteins
BT1 Proteins
BT2 Nutrients
BT1 Stress
NT1 Cold shock proteins
NT1 Heat shock proteins

Stress relaxation
BT1 Rheological properties
BT2 Mechanical properties
BT3 Physical properties
BT1 Stress

Stress resistance
BT1 Physiology
BT2 Science
BT1 Stress
RT Bacteriocins resistance
RT Heat resistance

Stretch
BT1 Rheological properties
BT2 Mechanical properties
BT3 Physical properties

Stretching
BT1 Processing
BT2 Technology

String beans
BT1 Common beans
BT2 Legumes
BT3 Vegetables specific
BT4 Vegetables
BT5 Crops
BT6 Plants
BT5 Plant foods
BT6 Foods

Striped bass
BT1 Sea bass
BT2 Marine fish
BT3 Fish
BT4 Animals
BT4 Sea foods
BT5 Aquatic foods
BT6 Animal foods
BT7 Foods
NT1 *Morone saxatilis*

Stroke
BT1 Cardiovascular diseases
BT2 Diseases

Strontium
USE **Sr**

Structural genes
BT1 Operons
BT2 Genetics
RT Gene expression
RT Genes

Structure
RT Conformation
RT Physical properties

Structured lipids
BT1 Lipids
BT2 Nutrients

Strudels
BT1 Pastries
BT2 Bakery products
BT3 Cereal products
BT4 Plant foods
BT5 Foods

Stuffings
BT1 Fillings

Stunning
BT1 Slaughter
NT1 Electrical stunning

Sturgeon
BT1 Fish
BT2 Animals
BT2 Sea foods
BT3 Aquatic foods
BT4 Animal foods
BT5 Foods
NT1 Beluga
UF Sevruga

Styrene
BT1 Polystyrene
BT2 Plastics
BT3 Packaging materials
RT Aromatic compounds
RT Hydrocarbons

Subcutaneous fat
HN introduced from vol. 42, issue 1 (2010)
BT1 Animal fats
BT2 Fats animal
BT3 Animal foods
BT4 Foods
BT3 Fats
BT4 Lipids
BT5 Nutrients

Suberin
HN under Polysaccharides up to vol. 42 (2010)
BT1 Biopolymers

Submerged fermentation
HN introduced from vol. 39, issue 1 (2007)
BT1 Fermentation technology
BT2 Biotechnology
BT3 Technology
BT2 Process control
BT3 Technology

Subsidies
HN introduced from vol. 42, issue 1 (2010)
BT1 Economics

Subtilins
BT1 Bacteriocins
BT2 Antibiotics
BT3 Drugs
BT4 Residues
RT *Bacillus subtilis*

Subtilisins
SN EC 3.4.21.62, formerly EC 3.4.21.14
BT1 Proteinases
BT2 Hydrolases
BT3 Enzymes

Succinic acid
BT1 Organic acids
BT2 Acids

Succinylation
BT1 Modification

Succulence
BT1 Juiciness
BT2 Sensory properties

Sucralose
BT1 Sweeteners
BT2 Additives

Sucrases
USE **Sucrose α-glucosidases**

Sucrose
BT1 Disaccharides
BT2 Sugars
BT3 Carbohydrates
BT4 Nutrients
BT4 Organic compounds
BT3 Plant foods
BT4 Foods
RT Sugar
RT Sugar confectionery
RT Sugar processes
UF Saccharose

Sucrose acetate isobutyrate
BT1 Stabilizers
BT2 Additives

Sucrose α-glucosidases
SN EC 3.2.1.48
BT1 Glycosidases
BT2 Hydrolases
BT3 Enzymes
UF Sucrases

Sucrose-phosphate synthases
SN EC 2.4.1.14
BT1 Glycosyltransferases
BT2 Transferases
BT3 Enzymes

Sucrose polyesters
BT1 Additives
BT1 Esters
BT2 Organic compounds
BT1 Fat substitutes
BT2 Fats
BT3 Lipids
BT4 Nutrients
NT1 Olestra

Sucrose synthases
SN EC 2.4.1.13
BT1 Glycosyltransferases

BT2 Transferases
BT3 Enzymes

Sucuk
BT1 Sausages
BT2 Meat products
BT3 Animal foods
BT4 Foods

Sudan
BT1 East Africa
BT2 Africa

Sudan dyes
HN introduced from vol. 41, issue 1 (2009)
BT1 Colorants
BT2 Additives

Suet
BT1 Animal fats
BT2 Fats animal
BT3 Animal foods
BT4 Foods
BT3 Fats
BT4 Lipids
BT5 Nutrients

Suffix
USE **Benzoylprop-ethyl**

Sufu
BT1 Fermented foods
BT2 Processed foods
BT3 Foods
BT1 Tofu
BT2 Soy products
BT3 Vegetable products
BT4 Plant foods
BT5 Foods

Sugar
BT1 Plant foods
BT2 Foods
NT1 Beet sugar
NT2 Beet sugar factories
NT2 Beet sugar industry
NT2 Beet sugar products
NT1 Brown sugar
NT1 Cane sugar
NT2 Bagasse
NT3 Sugar cane bagasse
NT2 Cane sugar factories
NT2 Cane sugar industry
NT2 Cane sugar products
NT2 Sugar cane bagasse
NT1 Granulated sugar
NT1 Honeys
NT2 Honey beverages
NT2 Honeycombs
NT2 Honeydew honey
NT2 Pollen
NT2 Propolis
NT1 Icing sugar
NT1 Jaggery
NT2 Gur
NT1 Molasses
NT2 Beet molasses
NT2 Cane molasses
NT1 Sugar cubes
NT1 Sugar factories
NT1 Sugar industry
NT1 Sugar low confectionery
NT1 Sugar low foods
NT1 Sugar products
NT1 Sugar refineries
NT1 Sugar substitutes
NT1 White sugar
RT Flavour compounds
RT Sucrose
RT Sugar confectionery
RT Sugar processes
RT Sugars
RT Sugar syrups
RT Sweeteners

Sugar alcohols
HN heading from vol. 25 (1993) to vol. 29 (1997)
BT1 Polyols
BT2 Alcohols
BT2 Carbohydrates
BT3 Nutrients
BT3 Organic compounds

Sugar apples
BT1 Fruits specific
BT2 Fruits
BT3 Crops
BT4 Plants
BT3 Plant foods
BT4 Foods

Sugar beet cossettes
BT1 Sugar beets
BT2 Crops
BT3 Plants

Sugar beet juices
USE **Beet sugar juices**

Sugar beet molasses
USE **Beet molasses**

Sugar beet pectins
HN introduced from vol. 39, issue 1 (2007)
BT1 Pectins
BT2 Pectic substances
BT3 Polysaccharides
BT4 Carbohydrates
BT5 Nutrients
BT5 Organic compounds
BT1 Sugar beets
BT2 Crops
BT3 Plants

Sugar beet pulps
HN introduced from vol. 42, issue 1 (2010)
BT1 Sugar beets
BT2 Crops
BT3 Plants
BT1 Wastes

Sugar beets
HN heading from vol. 25 (1993); under Beet sugar up to vol. 24 (1992)
BT1 Crops
BT2 Plants
NT1 Sugar beet cossettes
NT1 Sugar beet pectins
NT1 Sugar beet pulps
RT Beet sugar
RT Sugar crops

Sugar cane
HN heading from vol. 25 (1993); under Cane sugar up to vol. 24 (1992)
BT1 Crops
BT2 Plants
RT Cane sugar
RT Sugar crops

Sugar cane bagasse
BT1 Bagasse
BT2 Cane sugar
BT3 Sugar
BT4 Plant foods
BT5 Foods
BT2 Wastes
BT1 Cane sugar
BT2 Sugar
BT3 Plant foods
BT4 Foods

Sugar cane juices
USE **Cane sugar juices**

Sugar cane molasses
USE **Cane molasses**

Sugar cane spirits
HN introduced from vol. 39, issue 1 (2007)
BT1 Spirits
BT2 Alcoholic beverages
BT3 Beverages alcoholic
BT4 Beverages
NT1 Cachaca
RT Rum

Sugar confectionery
BT1 Plant foods
BT2 Foods
NT1 Aerated confectionery
NT1 Boiled sweets
NT1 Bonbons
NT1 Butterscotch
NT1 Candy
NT2 Chewy candy
NT1 Candy floss
NT1 Caramels
NT1 Chocolate
NT2 Chocolate crumb
NT2 Chocolate factories
NT2 Chocolate industry
NT2 Chocolate liquor
NT2 Chocolate mass
NT2 Chocolate products
NT3 Chocolate bars
NT3 Chocolate beverages
NT4 Drinking chocolate
NT3 Chocolate chips
NT3 Chocolate coatings
NT3 Chocolate confectionery
NT3 Chocolate couverture
NT3 Chocolate desserts
NT3 Chocolate dragees
NT3 Chocolate milk
NT3 Chocolate powders
NT3 Chocolates
NT3 Chocolate truffles

NT3 Dark chocolate
NT3 Milk chocolate
NT3 White chocolate
NT1 Confectionery
NT2 Confectionery bars
NT3 Chocolate bars
NT2 Confectionery industry
NT2 Confectionery products
NT2 Confections
NT2 Frozen confectionery
NT1 Confectionery pastes
NT1 Cotton candy
NT1 Cough drops
NT1 Croquant
NT1 Dragees
NT1 Dulce de leche
NT1 Fondants
NT1 Frappe
NT1 Fudges
NT1 Gum confectionery
NT2 Bubble gums
NT2 Chewing gums
NT3 Polyvinyl acetate
NT1 Halva
NT1 Ice lollies
NT1 Jelly confectionery
NT2 Fruit gums
NT2 Jellies
NT2 Jelly babies
NT2 Wine gums
NT1 Liquorice
NT1 Lollipops
NT1 Lozenges
NT1 Marrons glaces
NT1 Marshmallows
NT1 Marzipan
NT1 Mints
NT1 Nougat
NT1 Pastilles
NT1 Persipan
NT1 Pralines
NT1 Sandesh
NT1 Sherbet
NT1 Sugar confectionery industry
NT1 Sugar low confectionery
NT1 Sweetmeats
NT1 Sweets
NT1 Toffees
NT1 Turkish delight
NT1 Turron
NT1 Yokan
RT Sucrose
RT Sugar

Sugar confectionery industry
BT1 Food industry
BT2 Industries
BT1 Sugar confectionery
BT2 Plant foods
BT3 Foods

Sugar crops
BT1 Crops
BT2 Plants
RT Sorgo
RT Sugar beets
RT Sugar cane
RT Sweet sorghum

Sugar cubes
BT1 Sugar
BT2 Plant foods
BT3 Foods

Sugar factories
BT1 Food factories
BT1 Sugar
BT2 Plant foods
BT3 Foods

Sugar industry
BT1 Food industry
BT2 Industries
BT1 Sugar
BT2 Plant foods
BT3 Foods

Sugar juices
BT1 Plant foods
BT2 Foods
NT1 Beet sugar juices
NT1 Cane sugar juices
NT1 Massecuites
RT Sugar processes

Sugar low confectionery
BT1 Sugar
BT2 Plant foods
BT3 Foods
BT1 Sugar confectionery
BT2 Plant foods
BT3 Foods
UF Low sugar confectionery

Sugar low foods
BT1 Sugar
BT2 Plant foods
BT3 Foods
RT Lite foods
UF Low sugar foods

Sugar manufacture
USE **Sugar processes**

Sugar pans
BT1 Equipment
BT2 Technology
BT1 Sugar processes
BT2 Processing
BT3 Technology

Sugar processes
HN heading from vol. 25 (1993)
SN processes used in preparing sugar
BT1 Processing
BT2 Technology
NT1 Carbonatation
NT1 Liming
NT1 Sugar pans
NT1 Vacuum pans
RT Beet molasses
RT Beet sugar
RT Beet sugar juices
RT Cane molasses
RT Cane sugar
RT Cane sugar juices
RT Massecuites
RT Molasses
RT Sucrose
RT Sugar
RT Sugar juices
UF Sugar manufacture

Sugar products
BT1 Sugar
BT2 Plant foods
BT3 Foods

Sugar refineries
BT1 Sugar
BT2 Plant foods
BT3 Foods

Sugars
SN specific sugars and sugars in general
BT1 Carbohydrates
BT2 Nutrients
BT2 Organic compounds
BT1 Plant foods
BT2 Foods
NT1 Amino sugars
NT2 *N*-Acetylglucosamine
NT2 Furosine
NT2 Hexosamines
NT3 Galactosamine
NT3 Glucosamine
NT1 Disaccharides
NT2 Cellobiose
NT2 Difructose anhydride
NT2 Gentiobiose
NT2 Isomaltose
NT2 Isomaltulose
NT3 Palatinose
NT2 Lactose
NT3 Lactose low foods
NT2 Lactulose
NT2 Maltose
NT2 Melibiose
NT2 Nigerose
NT2 Sucrose
NT2 Trehalose
NT1 Monosaccharides
NT2 Aldoses
NT2 Arabinose
NT2 Fructose
NT2 Fucose
NT2 Galactose
NT2 Glucose
NT3 Glucose-6-phosphate
NT2 Hexoses
NT2 Ketoses
NT2 Mannose
NT2 Pentoses
NT2 Psicose
NT2 Rhamnose
NT2 Ribose
NT2 Sorbose
NT2 Tagatose
NT2 Xylose
NT2 Xylulose
NT1 Nonreducing sugars
NT1 Oligosaccharides
NT2 Chitooligosaccharides
NT2 Fructooligosaccharides
NT3 Kestose
NT3 Nystose
NT2 Galactooligosaccharides
NT2 Glucooligosaccharides
NT3 Isomaltooligosaccharides

NT3 Maltooligosaccharides
NT4 Maltohexaose
NT4 Maltotetraose
NT4 Maltotriose
NT3 Panose
NT2 Lactosucrose
NT2 Melezitose
NT2 Raffinose
NT2 Stachyose
NT2 Verbascose
NT2 Xylooligosaccharides
NT1 Reducing sugars
NT1 Saccharides
NT1 Uronic acids
NT2 Galacturonic acid
NT2 Glucuronic acid
NT2 Polyuronides
RT Dextrose equivalent
RT Flavour compounds
RT Sugar
UF Sugars specific

Sugars nonreducing
HN heading from vol. 25 (1993) to vol. 27 (1995); used in addition to nonreducing sugars up to vol. 29 (1997)
USE **Nonreducing sugars**

Sugars reducing
HN heading from vol. 25 (1993) to vol. 27 (1995); used in addition to reducing sugars up to vol. 29 (1997)
USE **Reducing sugars**

Sugars specific
HN used as a heading for specific sugars up to vol. 24 (1992)
USE **Sugars**

Sugar substitutes
BT1 Sugar
BT2 Plant foods
BT3 Foods
RT Sweeteners

Sugar syrups
BT1 Plant foods
BT2 Foods
NT1 Beet sugar syrups
NT1 Cane sugar syrups
NT1 Corn syrups
NT2 Fructose high corn syrups
NT2 Isoglucose
NT2 Isosyrups
NT1 Fructose syrups
NT1 Glucose syrups
NT1 Hydrolysed lactose syrups
NT1 Hydrolysed starch syrups
NT2 Lycasin
NT1 Invert sugar
NT1 Lactose syrups
NT1 Maltose syrups
NT1 Maple syrups
NT2 Maple saps
NT1 Starch hydrolysates
NT1 Starch syrups
NT1 Syrups
NT2 Fruit syrups
NT1 Treacle
RT Sugar
RT Sweeteners

Sulfadiazine
HN under Drugs up to vol. 42 (2010)
BT1 Sulfonamides
BT2 Antibiotics
BT3 Drugs
BT4 Residues

Sulfadimidine
SN syn. sulfamethazine
BT1 Sulfamethazine
BT2 Sulfonamides
BT3 Antibiotics
BT4 Drugs
BT5 Residues
UF Sulphadimidine

Sulfamates
USE **Cyclamates**

Sulfamethazine
SN syn. sulfadimidine
BT1 Sulfonamides
BT2 Antibiotics
BT3 Drugs
BT4 Residues
NT1 Sulfadimidine
UF Sulphamethazine

Sulfanilamide
BT1 Sulfonamides
BT2 Antibiotics
BT3 Drugs
BT4 Residues
UF Sulphanilamide

Sulfates
BT1 Salts
NT1 SDS
UF Sulphates

Sulfathiazole
BT1 Sulfonamides
BT2 Antibiotics
BT3 Drugs
BT4 Residues
UF Sulphathiazole

Sulfhydryl groups
BT1 Thiols
BT2 Organic sulfur compounds
UF Sulphydryl groups

Sulfides
BT1 Salts
NT1 Allyl sulfides
NT2 Diallyl disulfide
NT1 Dimethyl sulfide
NT2 Methyl sulfide
NT1 Dimethyl trisulfide
NT1 Disulfides
NT2 Carbon disulfide
NT2 Diallyl disulfide
NT2 Dimethyl disulfide
NT1 H_2S
UF Sulphides

Sulfitation
BT1 Processing
BT2 Technology
RT Sulfites
UF Sulphitation

Sulfites
BT1 Salts
NT1 Bisulfites
NT1 Metabisulfites
NT2 Potassium metabisulfite
NT2 Sodium metabisulfite
NT2 Sodium pyrosulfite
RT Desulfitation
RT Sulfitation
RT Sulfur dioxide
UF Sulphites

Sulfolobus
BT1 Archaea
BT2 Microorganisms
NT1 *Sulfolobus solfataricus*

Sulfolobus solfataricus
BT1 *Sulfolobus*
BT2 Archaea
BT3 Microorganisms

Sulfonamides
BT1 Antibiotics
BT2 Drugs
BT3 Residues
NT1 Chloramine T
NT1 Sulfadiazine
NT1 Sulfamethazine
NT2 Sulfadimidine
NT1 Sulfanilamide
NT1 Sulfathiazole
UF Sulphonamides

Sulforaphane
HN introduced from vol. 39, issue 1 (2007)
BT1 Isothiocyanates
BT2 Organic nitrogen compounds
BT2 Organic sulfur compounds
BT2 Volatile sulfur compounds
BT3 Volatile compounds
RT Glucoraphanin

Sulfur
SN symbol S is also used in the index
BT1 Elements
BT2 Minerals
BT3 Nutrients
NT1 S
UF Sulphur

Sulfur dioxide
SN symbol SO2 is also used in the index
BT1 Gases
BT2 Physical phases
BT3 Chemistry
BT4 Science
BT1 Oxides
BT1 Preservatives
BT2 Additives
NT1 SO_2
RT Sulfites
RT Sulfurous acid
UF Sulphur dioxide

Sulfuric acid
USE **H_2SO_4**

Sulfurous acid
BT1 Acids
BT1 Preservatives
BT2 Additives
RT Sulfur dioxide
UF Sulphurous acid

Sulphadimidine
HN used for sulfadimidine up to vol. 35, issue 6 (2003)
USE **Sulfadimidine**

Sulphamates
HN used for sulfamates up to vol. 35, issue 6 (2003)
USE **Cyclamates**

Sulphamethazine
HN used for sulfamethazine up to vol. 35, issue 6 (2003)
USE **Sulfamethazine**

Sulphanilamide
HN used for sulfanilamide up to vol. 35, issue 6 (2003)
USE **Sulfanilamide**

Sulphates
HN used for sulfates up to vol. 35, issue 6 (2003)
USE **Sulfates**

Sulphathiazole
HN used for sulfathiazole up to vol.35, issue 6 (2003)
USE **Sulfathiazole**

Sulphides
HN used for sulfides up to vol. 35, issue 6 (2003)
USE **Sulfides**

Sulphitation
HN used for sulfitation up to vol. 35, issue 6 (2003)
USE **Sulfitation**

Sulphites
HN used for sulfites up to vol. 35, issue 6 (2003)
USE **Sulfites**

Sulphonamides
HN used for sulfonamides up to vol. 35, issue 6 (2003)
USE **Sulfonamides**

Sulphur
HN used for sulfur up to vol. 35, issue 6 (2003)
USE **Sulfur**

Sulphur dioxide
HN used for sulfur dioxide up to vol. 35, issue 6 (2003)
USE **Sulfur dioxide**

Sulphuric acid
HN used for sulfuric acid up to vol. 35, issue 6 (2003)
USE **H_2SO_4**

Sulphurous acid
HN used for sulfurous acid up to vol. 35, issue 6 (2003)
USE **Sulfurous acid**

Sulphydryl groups
HN used for sulfhydryl groups up to vol. 35, issue 6 (2003)
USE **Sulfhydryl groups**

Sultanas
BT1 Dried fruits
BT2 Fruits dried
BT3 Dried foods
BT4 Processed foods
BT5 Foods
BT3 Fruits
BT4 Crops
BT5 Plants
BT4 Plant foods
BT5 Foods

Suluguni cheese
BT1 Cheese varieties
BT2 Cheese
BT3 Dairy products
BT4 Animal foods
BT5 Foods

Sumac
HN introduced from vol. 37, issue 5 (2005)
BT1 Spices
BT2 Flavourings
BT3 Additives

Summer sausages
BT1 Sausages
BT2 Meat products
BT3 Animal foods
BT4 Foods

Sunburn
SN skin blemish of fruits and vegetables due to exposure to the sun
BT1 Damage
BT1 Plant disorders
BT2 Diseases plant
BT3 Diseases

Sunett
BT1 Acesulfame K
BT2 Sweeteners
BT3 Additives

Sunfish
BT1 Freshwater fish
BT2 Fish
BT3 Animals
BT3 Sea foods
BT4 Aquatic foods
BT5 Animal foods
BT6 Foods

Sunflower meal
BT1 Flours
BT2 Plant foods
BT3 Foods
BT1 Sunflower seeds
BT2 Oilseeds
BT3 Seeds
BT4 Plant foods
BT5 Foods

Sunflower oils
BT1 Vegetable oils
BT2 Oils vegetable
BT3 Oils
BT4 Lipids
BT5 Nutrients
BT3 Vegetable products
BT4 Plant foods
BT5 Foods

Sunflowers
HN heading up to vol. 24 (1992)
BT1 Sunflower seeds
BT2 Oilseeds
BT3 Seeds
BT4 Plant foods
BT5 Foods

Sunflower seeds
HN heading from vol. 25 (1993); under Sunflowers up to vol. 24 (1992)
BT1 Oilseeds
BT2 Seeds
BT3 Plant foods
BT4 Foods
NT1 Sunflower meal
NT1 Sunflowers

Sunlight
BT1 Light
BT2 Radiation

Sunset Yellow
BT1 Colorants
BT2 Additives

Supercooling
HN introduced from vol. 41, issue 1 (2009)
BT1 Cooling
BT2 Thermal processing
BT3 Processing thermal
BT4 Processing
BT5 Technology

Supercritical CO_2 extraction
BT1 Carbon dioxide
BT2 Gases
BT3 Physical phases
BT4 Chemistry
BT5 Science
BT2 Inorganic compounds
BT2 Oxides
BT2 Solvents
BT1 Extraction
BT2 Processing
BT3 Technology

Supercritical fluid chromatography
BT1 Chromatography
BT2 Analytical techniques
RT Supercritical fluids

Supercritical fluid extraction
BT1 Extraction
BT2 Processing

BT3 Technology
RT Supercritical fluids

Supercritical fluids
HN introduced from vol. 39, issue 1 (2007)
BT1 Fluids
BT2 Liquids
BT3 Physical phases
BT4 Chemistry
BT5 Science
BT1 Solvents
RT Supercritical fluid chromatography
RT Supercritical fluid extraction

Supercritical HPLC
BT1 High performance liquid chromatography
BT2 Chromatography
BT3 Analytical techniques

Supermarkets
BT1 Marketing
BT2 Economics
RT Shops

Superoxide dismutases
SN EC 1.15.1.1
BT1 Oxidoreductases
BT2 Enzymes

Superoxides
BT1 Oxides
BT1 Reactive oxygen species
BT2 Free radicals
BT3 Radicals

Suppliers
BT1 Food business
BT2 Economics
NT1 Supply chains
NT2 Efficient consumer response

Supplies
BT1 Economics
NT1 Supply chains
NT2 Efficient consumer response

Supply chains
HN introduced from vol. 42, issue 1 (2010)
BT1 Suppliers
BT2 Food business
BT3 Economics
BT1 Supplies
BT2 Economics
NT1 Efficient consumer response

Supracide
USE **Methidathion**

Surface active agents
BT1 Surfactants

Surface active properties
BT1 Functional properties
BT2 Physical properties
RT Surfactants

Surface pasteurization
HN introduced from vol. 41, issue 1 (2009)
BT1 Pasteurization
BT2 Thermal processing
BT3 Processing thermal
BT4 Processing
BT5 Technology

Surface plasmon resonance
HN introduced from vol. 39, issue 1 (2007)
BT1 Analytical techniques

Surfaces
HN heading from vol. 25 (1993)
NT1 Ceramics
NT1 Enamels
NT1 Floors
NT1 Lacquers
NT2 Varnishes
NT1 Paints
NT1 Steel
NT2 Stainless steel
NT1 Worktables
RT Contact Materials
RT Fouling

Surface tension
BT1 Rheological properties
BT2 Mechanical properties
BT3 Physical properties

Surfactants
NT1 Biosurfactants
NT1 Cetavlon
NT1 Cetyltrimethylammonium bromide
NT1 Deoxycholate
NT1 Detergents
NT1 SDS
NT1 Surface active agents
NT1 Surfactin
RT Antiseptics
RT Cleaning
RT Disinfectants
RT Hygiene
RT Surface active properties

Surfactin
BT1 Antibiotics
BT2 Drugs
BT3 Residues
BT1 Surfactants

Surimi
HN heading from vol. 30 (1998); under Fish products or Meat products up to vol. 29 (1997)
BT1 Fish products
BT2 Sea foods
BT3 Aquatic foods
BT4 Animal foods
BT5 Foods
BT1 Meat products
BT2 Animal foods
BT3 Foods

Surinam
SN also known as Suriname
BT1 South America
BT2 America
UF Dutch Guiana

Survival curves
HN introduced from vol. 39, issue 1 (2007)
BT1 Predictive modelling
BT2 Microbiological techniques

Susceptors
USE **Microwave susceptors**

Sushi
BT1 Fish products
BT2 Sea foods
BT3 Aquatic foods
BT4 Animal foods
BT5 Foods

Suspension cultures
BT1 Cell culture

Sustainability
HN introduced from vol. 43, issue 1 (2011)
RT Consumption
RT Environment
RT Food security
RT Production

Swallowing
HN introduced from vol. 41, issue 1 (2009)
BT1 Human physiology
BT2 Physiology
BT3 Science

Swaziland
BT1 Southern Africa
BT2 Africa

Sweden
HN heading up to vol. 24 (1992)
BT1 Europe
BT1 European Union
RT Organization for Economic Cooperation and Development

Swedes
BT1 Vegetables specific
BT2 Vegetables
BT3 Crops
BT4 Plants
BT3 Plant foods
BT4 Foods
UF Rutabagas

Sweet almonds
BT1 Almonds
BT2 Nuts
BT3 Fruits
BT4 Crops
BT5 Plants
BT4 Plant foods
BT5 Foods
BT3 Oilseeds
BT4 Seeds
BT5 Plant foods
BT6 Foods

Sweet basil
HN under Spices up to vol. 42 (2010)
BT1 Basil
BT2 Herbs
BT3 Spices
BT4 Flavourings
BT5 Additives

Sweetbreads
BT1 Offal
BT2 Animal foods
BT3 Foods

Sweet cherries
BT1 Cherries
BT2 Fruits specific
BT3 Fruits
BT4 Crops
BT5 Plants
BT4 Plant foods
BT5 Foods

Sweet chestnuts
BT1 Chestnuts
BT2 Nuts
BT3 Fruits
BT4 Crops
BT5 Plants
BT4 Plant foods
BT5 Foods
BT3 Oilseeds
BT4 Seeds
BT5 Plant foods
BT6 Foods

Sweetcorn
HN heading from vol. 30 (1998); under Corn up to vol.29 (1997)
BT1 Corn
BT2 Cereals
BT3 Crops
BT4 Plants
BT3 Seeds
BT4 Plant foods
BT5 Foods
BT1 Vegetables specific
BT2 Vegetables
BT3 Crops
BT4 Plants
BT3 Plant foods
BT4 Foods

Sweet cream
BT1 Cream
BT2 Dairy products
BT3 Animal foods
BT4 Foods

Sweeteners
BT1 Additives
NT1 Acesulfame K
NT2 Sunett
NT1 Alitame
NT1 Artificial sweeteners
NT1 Aspartame
NT2 NutraSweet
NT1 Cyclamates
NT2 Sodium cyclamate
NT1 Cyclamic acid
NT1 Dipeptide sweeteners
NT1 Dulcin
NT1 Glycyrrhizic acid
NT1 Glycyrrhizin
NT1 Isomalt
NT1 Lycasin
NT1 Monatin
NT1 Natural sweeteners
NT1 Neohesperidin dihydrochalcone
NT1 Neotame
NT1 Rebaudiosides
NT1 Saccharin
NT1 Stevioside
NT1 Sucralose
NT1 Sweet proteins
NT2 Brazzein
NT2 Curculin
NT2 Monellin
NT2 Thaumatin
RT Flavour compounds
RT Flavourings
RT Glycosides
RT Polyols
RT Sugar
RT Sugar substitutes
RT Sugar syrups
UF Raftilose

Sweet limes
BT1 Citrus fruits
BT2 Fruits specific
BT3 Fruits
BT4 Crops
BT5 Plants
BT4 Plant foods
BT5 Foods

Sweetmeats
BT1 Sugar confectionery
BT2 Plant foods
BT3 Foods

Sweetness
BT1 Flavour
BT2 Sensory properties

Sweet peppers
BT1 Capsicums
BT2 Vegetables specific
BT3 Vegetables
BT4 Crops
BT5 Plants
BT4 Plant foods
BT5 Foods

Sweet potatoes
BT1 Vegetables specific
BT2 Vegetables
BT3 Crops
BT4 Plants
BT3 Plant foods
BT4 Foods
NT1 Sweet potato starch
UF *Ipomoea batatas*

Sweet potato starch
BT1 Starch
BT2 Glucans
BT3 Polysaccharides
BT4 Carbohydrates
BT5 Nutrients
BT5 Organic compounds
BT2 Thickeners
BT3 Additives
BT1 Sweet potatoes
BT2 Vegetables specific
BT3 Vegetables
BT4 Crops
BT5 Plants
BT4 Plant foods
BT5 Foods

Sweet proteins
HN introduced from vol. 41, issue 1 (2009)
BT1 Proteins
BT2 Nutrients
BT1 Sweeteners
BT2 Additives
NT1 Brazzein
NT1 Curculin
NT1 Monellin
NT1 Thaumatin
RT Flavour compounds
RT Miraculin

Sweets
BT1 Sugar confectionery
BT2 Plant foods
BT3 Foods

Sweet sorghum
SN syn. sorgo
BT1 Crops
BT2 Plants
NT1 Sorgo
RT Sorghum
RT Sugar crops

Swelling
BT1 Functional properties
BT2 Physical properties

Swine
BT1 Animals
NT1 Swine kidneys
NT1 Swine livers
NT1 Swine skin
RT Bacon
RT Ham
RT Kasseler
RT Pork
RT Rendement Napole genes
UF Boars
UF Hogs
UF Pigs
UF Porcine
UF Sows
UF Wild boars

Swine carcasses
BT1 Carcasses
BT2 Meat
BT3 Animal foods
BT4 Foods
BT1 Pork
BT2 Meat specific
BT3 Meat
BT4 Animal foods
BT5 Foods
UF Boar carcasses

Swine fever
BT1 Animal diseases
BT2 Diseases animal
BT3 Diseases

Swine kidneys
BT1 Kidneys
BT2 Offal
BT3 Animal foods
BT4 Foods
BT1 Swine
BT2 Animals

Swine livers
BT1 Livers
BT2 Offal
BT3 Animal foods
BT4 Foods
BT1 Swine
BT2 Animals

Swine muscles
USE **Pork**

Swine skin
BT1 Skin
BT1 Swine
BT2 Animals

Swiss chard
SN syn. leaf beet
BT1 Vegetables specific
BT2 Vegetables
BT3 Crops
BT4 Plants
BT3 Plant foods
BT4 Foods
NT1 Leaf beet
UF Chard

Swiss cheese
BT1 Cheese varieties
BT2 Cheese
BT3 Dairy products
BT4 Animal foods
BT5 Foods

Swiss rolls
SN syn. jelly rolls
BT1 Cakes
BT2 Bakery products
BT3 Cereal products
BT4 Plant foods
BT5 Foods
UF Jelly rolls

Switzerland
HN heading up to vol. 24 (1992)
BT1 Europe
RT Organization for Economic Cooperation and Development

Sword beans
BT1 Legumes
BT2 Vegetables specific
BT3 Vegetables
BT4 Crops
BT5 Plants
BT4 Plant foods
BT5 Foods
NT1 *Canavalia gladiata*

Swordfish
BT1 Marine fish
BT2 Fish
BT3 Animals
BT3 Sea foods
BT4 Aquatic foods
BT5 Animal foods
BT6 Foods
BT1 Oily fish
BT2 Fish
BT3 Animals
BT3 Sea foods
BT4 Aquatic foods
BT5 Animal foods
BT6 Foods

Syagrus
BT1 Palms
BT2 Plants

Synbiotic foods
HN introduced from vol. 39, issue 1 (2007)
BT1 Novel foods
BT2 Foods
RT Prebiotics

Synechococcus
BT1 Cyanobacteria
BT2 Bacteria
BT3 Microorganisms
UF *Anacystis*

Synechocystis
HN introduced from vol. 39, issue 1 (2007)
BT1 Cyanobacteria
BT2 Bacteria
BT3 Microorganisms

Syneresis
RT Curd
RT Gels

Synthases
SN use for synthases in general; see also specific names for individual synthases
BT1 Enzymes

Syria
SN full name is Syrian Arab Republic
BT1 Middle East

Syringic acid
BT1 Organic acids
BT2 Acids
BT1 Phenols
BT2 Alcohols
BT2 Aromatic compounds
BT3 Organic compounds

Syrups
BT1 Sugar syrups
BT2 Plant foods
BT3 Foods
NT1 Fruit syrups

T

2,4,5-T
BT1 Phenoxy herbicides
BT2 Herbicides
BT3 Pesticides
BT4 Biocides
BT4 Residues

Table grapes
BT1 Grapes
BT2 Berries
BT3 Fruits specific
BT4 Fruits
BT5 Crops
BT6 Plants
BT5 Plant foods
BT6 Foods

Table olives
HN introduced from vol. 41, issue 1 (2009)
BT1 Olives
BT2 Fruits specific
BT3 Fruits
BT4 Crops
BT5 Plants
BT4 Plant foods
BT5 Foods
BT2 Oilseeds
BT3 Seeds
BT4 Plant foods
BT5 Foods

Tacos
BT1 Bakery products
BT2 Cereal products
BT3 Plant foods
BT4 Foods

Taco shells
BT1 Bakery products
BT2 Cereal products
BT3 Plant foods
BT4 Foods

Taenia
BT1 Parasites
BT2 Pests

Tagatose
HN under Sugars up to vol. 42 (2010)
BT1 Monosaccharides
BT2 Sugars
BT3 Carbohydrates
BT4 Nutrients
BT4 Organic compounds
BT3 Plant foods
BT4 Foods

Tagetes maxima
BT1 Plants

Tagetes minuta
BT1 Plants

Tagliatelli
BT1 Pasta
BT2 Cereal products

BT3 Plant foods
BT4 Foods

Tahini
HN under Vegetable products up to vol. 42 (2010)
BT1 Pastes
BT2 Processed foods
BT3 Foods
BT1 Sesame seeds
BT2 Oilseeds
BT3 Seeds
BT4 Plant foods
BT5 Foods
NT1 Tehineh
RT Confectionery pastes
RT Halva
RT Nut pastes

Taints
HN heading from vol. 25 (1993); under Spoilage up to vol. 24 (1992)
BT1 Flavour
BT2 Sensory properties
NT1 Boar taint
NT1 Cork taint
NT1 Off flavour
NT1 Off odour
NT1 Warmed over flavour
RT Acrolein
RT Androstenone
RT Geosmin
RT Guaiacol
RT 2-Methylisoborneol
RT Skatole
RT Spoilage
RT Trichloroanisole

Taiwan
BT1 Asia
UF Formosa

Tajikistan
BT1 Asia

Take away foods
BT1 Fast foods
BT2 Processed foods
BT3 Foods

Takju
BT1 Rice wines
BT2 Cereal wines
BT3 Alcoholic beverages
BT4 Beverages alcoholic
BT5 Beverages

Talaromyces
SN teleomorph of Paecilomyces
BT1 Fungi
BT2 Microorganisms
NT1 *Talaromyces avellaneus*
NT1 *Talaromyces macrosporus*

Talaromyces avellaneus
BT1 *Talaromyces*
BT2 Fungi
BT3 Microorganisms

Talaromyces macrosporus
BT1 *Talaromyces*
BT2 Fungi
BT3 Microorganisms

Taleggio cheese
BT1 Cheese varieties
BT2 Cheese
BT3 Dairy products
BT4 Animal foods
BT5 Foods

Tallow
BT1 Animal fats
BT2 Fats animal
BT3 Animal foods
BT4 Foods
BT3 Fats
BT4 Lipids
BT5 Nutrients

Tamales
BT1 Bakery products
BT2 Cereal products
BT3 Plant foods
BT4 Foods

Tamarillos
BT1 Fruits specific
BT2 Fruits
BT3 Crops
BT4 Plants
BT3 Plant foods
BT4 Foods
UF Tree tomatoes

Tamarinds
BT1 Fruits specific
BT2 Fruits
BT3 Crops
BT4 Plants
BT3 Plant foods
BT4 Foods

Tamper evident closures
BT1 Closures
BT2 Packaging
BT3 Technology

Tamper evident packaging
BT1 Packaging
BT2 Technology

Tanganyika
USE **Tanzania**

Tangelo
BT1 Citrus fruits
BT2 Fruits specific
BT3 Fruits
BT4 Crops
BT5 Plants
BT4 Plant foods
BT5 Foods

Tangerine juices
BT1 Mandarin juices
BT2 Orange juices
BT3 Citrus juices
BT4 Fruit juices
BT5 Fruit products
BT6 Plant foods
BT7 Foods
BT5 Soft drinks
BT6 Beverages
RT Tangerines

Tangerines
BT1 Mandarins
BT2 Oranges
BT3 Citrus fruits
BT4 Fruits specific
BT5 Fruits
BT6 Crops
BT7 Plants
BT6 Plant foods
BT7 Foods
RT Tangerine juices

Tangle
USE ***Laminaria***

Tangor
BT1 Citrus fruits
BT2 Fruits specific
BT3 Fruits
BT4 Crops
BT5 Plants
BT4 Plant foods
BT5 Foods

Tania
BT1 Vegetables specific
BT2 Vegetables
BT3 Crops
BT4 Plants
BT3 Plant foods
BT4 Foods
UF Taniers

Taniers
USE **Tania**

Tankers
BT1 Transport

Tanks
BT1 Containers
RT Storage

Tannases
SN EC 3.1.1.20
BT1 Esterases
BT2 Hydrolases
BT3 Enzymes

Tannic acid
BT1 Tannins
BT2 Aromatic compounds
BT3 Organic compounds
BT2 Glycosides
BT3 Carbohydrates
BT4 Nutrients
BT4 Organic compounds
BT2 Organic acids
BT3 Acids

Tannins
BT1 Aromatic compounds
BT2 Organic compounds
BT1 Glycosides
BT2 Carbohydrates
BT3 Nutrients
BT3 Organic compounds

BT1 Organic acids
 BT2 Acids
NT1 Ellagitannins
NT1 Proanthocyanidins
 NT2 Procyanidins
NT1 Tannic acid
RT Ellagic acid
RT Flavonoids

Tanoor
BT1 Bread
 BT2 Bakery products
  BT3 Cereal products
   BT4 Plant foods
    BT5 Foods

Tanshen
BT1 Plants

Tansy
HN under Spices up to vol. 42 (2010)
BT1 Herbs
 BT2 Spices
  BT3 Flavourings
   BT4 Additives

Tanzania
SN full name is United Republic of Tanzania
BT1 East Africa
 BT2 Africa
UF Tanganyika

Tapazole
USE **Methimazole**

Tape
BT1 Cassava
 BT2 Vegetables specific
  BT3 Vegetables
   BT4 Crops
    BT5 Plants
   BT4 Plant foods
    BT5 Foods
BT1 Fermented foods
 BT2 Processed foods
  BT3 Foods
BT1 Rice
 BT2 Cereals
  BT3 Crops
   BT4 Plants
  BT3 Seeds
   BT4 Plant foods
    BT5 Foods
NT1 Tape ketan

Tape ketan
BT1 Tape
 BT2 Cassava
  BT3 Vegetables specific
   BT4 Vegetables
    BT5 Crops
     BT6 Plants
    BT5 Plant foods
     BT6 Foods
 BT2 Fermented foods
  BT3 Processed foods
   BT4 Foods
 BT2 Rice
  BT3 Cereals
   BT4 Crops
    BT5 Plants
   BT4 Seeds
    BT5 Plant foods
     BT6 Foods

Tapes philippinarum
BT1 Clams
 BT2 Bivalves
  BT3 Molluscs
   BT4 Shellfish
    BT5 Animals
    BT5 Sea foods
     BT6 Aquatic foods
      BT7 Animal foods
       BT8 Foods

Tapeworms
HN introduced from vol. 39, issue 1 (2007)
BT1 Parasites
 BT2 Pests

Tapioca
HN heading up to vol. 24 (1992)
SN syn. cassava starch
BT1 Cassava starch
 BT2 Cassava
  BT3 Vegetables specific
   BT4 Vegetables
    BT5 Crops
     BT6 Plants
    BT5 Plant foods
     BT6 Foods
 BT2 Starch
  BT3 Glucans
   BT4 Polysaccharides
    BT5 Carbohydrates
     BT6 Nutrients
     BT6 Organic compounds
  BT3 Thickeners
   BT4 Additives
UF Tapioca starch

Tapioca starch
USE **Tapioca**

Taps
BT1 Dispensers
 BT2 Equipment
  BT3 Technology

Tap water
BT1 Water

Tarag
BT1 Fermented milk
 BT2 Fermented dairy products
  BT3 Dairy products
   BT4 Animal foods
    BT5 Foods
  BT3 Fermented foods
   BT4 Processed foods
    BT5 Foods
 BT2 Milk
  BT3 Dairy products
   BT4 Animal foods
    BT5 Foods

Tara gums
HN introduced from vol. 41, issue 1 (2009)
BT1 Gums
 BT2 Polysaccharides
  BT3 Carbohydrates
   BT4 Nutrients
   BT4 Organic compounds
 BT2 Stabilizers
  BT3 Additives
 BT2 Thickeners
  BT3 Additives

Tarhana
BT1 Cereal products
 BT2 Plant foods
  BT3 Foods
BT1 Dairy products
 BT2 Animal foods
  BT3 Foods
BT1 Fermented foods
 BT2 Processed foods
  BT3 Foods
RT Kishk
RT Trahanas

Tariffs
BT1 Trade
 BT2 Economics

Taro
HN heading from vol. 30 (1998); under Vegetables specific up to vol. 29 (1997)
BT1 Vegetables specific
 BT2 Vegetables
  BT3 Crops
   BT4 Plants
  BT3 Plant foods
   BT4 Foods
NT1 Poi

Tarragon
HN under Spices up to vol. 42 (2010)
BT1 Herbs
 BT2 Spices
  BT3 Flavourings
   BT4 Additives

Tartaric acid
BT1 Additives
BT1 Organic acids
 BT2 Acids
RT Calcium tartrate
RT Preservatives
RT Tartrates

Tartrates
BT1 Salts
NT1 Calcium tartrate
RT Tartaric acid

Tartrazine
BT1 Colorants
 BT2 Additives

Tarts
BT1 Pies
 BT2 Bakery products
  BT3 Cereal products
   BT4 Plant foods
    BT5 Foods

Tastant
USE **Flavour compounds**

Taste
USE **Flavour**

Taste panels
BT1 Sensory analysis
BT2 Analytical techniques
RT Panellists

Taste thresholds
USE **Flavour thresholds**

Taurine
BT1 Amino acids
BT2 Nutrients
BT2 Organic acids
BT3 Acids
BT2 Organic nitrogen compounds

Taxation
BT1 Food policy
BT2 Economics

Taxonomy
BT1 Science

TBA reactive substances
HN TBARS used in the index from vol. 35, issue 6 (2003)
USE **TBARS**

TBARS
HN TBA reactive substances used in the index up to vol. 35, issue 6 (2003)
RT TBA values
RT Thiobarbituric acid values
UF TBA reactive substances

TBA values
SN heading is Thiobarbituric acid values
BT1 Thiobarbituric acid values
NT1 Malonaldehyde
NT1 Malondialdehyde
RT Oxidation
RT Quality control
RT Rancidity
RT TBARS

TBHQ
BT1 Antioxidants
BT2 Additives
UF *tert*-Butylhydroquinone

Tc
BT1 Radioelements
BT2 Isotopes
BT3 Elements
BT4 Minerals
BT5 Nutrients
BT2 Residues
UF Technetium

TDE
HN under Insecticides up to vol. 42 (2010); under DDT from vol. 43 (2011)
BT1 DDT
BT2 Acaricides
BT3 Pesticides
BT4 Biocides
BT4 Residues
BT2 Organochlorine insecticides
BT3 Insecticides
BT4 Pesticides
BT5 Biocides
BT5 Residues
BT3 Organochlorine pesticides
BT4 Pesticides
BT5 Biocides
BT5 Residues
UF DDD

Te
HN under Minerals up to vol. 42 (2010)
BT1 Elements
BT2 Minerals
BT3 Nutrients
UF Tellurium

Tea
HN heading up to vol. 29 (1997) and from vol. 43 (2011); under Teas from vol. 30 (1998) up to vol. 42 (2010)
BT1 Teas
BT2 Beverages
BT2 Crops
BT3 Plants
BT2 Plant foods
BT3 Foods
NT1 Black tea
NT1 Brick tea
NT1 Decaffeinated tea
NT1 Green tea
NT1 Oolong tea
NT1 Pouchong tea
NT1 Pu-erh tea
NT1 Tea extracts
NT1 Tea leaves
RT Alkaloids
RT Caffeine
RT Theaflavins
RT Thearubigins
RT Withering

Tea bags
BT1 Teas
BT2 Beverages
BT2 Crops
BT3 Plants
BT2 Plant foods
BT3 Foods

Tea beverages
BT1 Teas
BT2 Beverages
BT2 Crops
BT3 Plants
BT2 Plant foods
BT3 Foods
NT1 Chai
NT1 Iced tea
NT1 Kombucha
NT1 Lemon tea

Tea extracts
HN introduced from vol. 42, issue 1 (2010)
BT1 Extracts
BT2 Flavourings
BT3 Additives
BT1 Tea
BT2 Teas
BT3 Beverages
BT3 Crops
BT4 Plants
BT3 Plant foods
BT4 Foods

Tea granules
BT1 Instant foods
BT2 Processed foods
BT3 Foods
BT1 Teas
BT2 Beverages
BT2 Crops
BT3 Plants
BT2 Plant foods
BT3 Foods

Tea leaves
BT1 Tea
BT2 Teas
BT3 Beverages
BT3 Crops
BT4 Plants
BT3 Plant foods
BT4 Foods

Tea powders
BT1 Powders
BT2 Dried foods
BT3 Processed foods
BT4 Foods
BT2 Instant foods
BT3 Processed foods
BT4 Foods
BT1 Teas
BT2 Beverages
BT2 Crops
BT3 Plants
BT2 Plant foods
BT3 Foods

Teas
HN heading from vol. 30 (1998)
BT1 Beverages
BT1 Crops
BT2 Plants
BT1 Plant foods
BT2 Foods
NT1 Fruit tea
NT1 Herb tea
NT2 Honeybush tea
NT2 Mate
NT3 Yerba mate
NT4 *Ilex paraguariensis*
NT2 Rooibos tea
NT2 Tochu tea
NT1 Instant tea
NT1 Tea
NT2 Black tea
NT2 Brick tea
NT2 Decaffeinated tea
NT2 Green tea
NT2 Oolong tea
NT2 Pouchong tea
NT2 Pu-erh tea
NT2 Tea extracts

NT2 Tea leaves
NT1 Tea bags
NT1 Tea beverages
NT2 Chai
NT2 Iced tea
NT2 Kombucha
NT2 Lemon tea
NT1 Tea granules
NT1 Tea powders

Tea seed oils
BT1 Vegetable oils
BT2 Oils vegetable
BT3 Oils
BT4 Lipids
BT5 Nutrients
BT3 Vegetable products
BT4 Plant foods
BT5 Foods

Tea tree oils
BT1 Essential oils
BT2 Flavourings
BT3 Additives
BT2 Vegetable oils
BT3 Oils vegetable
BT4 Oils
BT5 Lipids
BT6 Nutrients
BT4 Vegetable products
BT5 Plant foods
BT6 Foods

Tebuconazole
HN introduced from vol. 41, issue 1 (2009)
BT1 Fungicides
BT2 Pesticides
BT3 Biocides
BT3 Residues

Technetium
USE **Tc**

Technology
HN introduced from vol. 42, issue 1 (2010)
NT1 Antisense technology
NT1 Apparatus
NT1 Automation
NT1 Biotechnology
NT1 Clean room technology
NT1 Cloning technology
NT1 Encapsulation
NT1 Equipment
NT1 Information technology
NT1 Mechanization
NT1 Microfluidic technology
NT1 Nanotechnology
NT1 Packaging
NT1 Preservation
NT1 Process control
NT1 Processing
NT1 Quality control

Tecto
USE **Thiabendazole**

Teenagers
USE **Adolescents**

Teff
BT1 Millet
BT2 Cereals
BT3 Crops
BT4 Plants
BT3 Seeds
BT4 Plant foods
BT5 Foods

Tehineh
SN alternative name for tahini
BT1 Tahini
BT2 Pastes
BT3 Processed foods
BT4 Foods
BT2 Sesame seeds
BT3 Oilseeds
BT4 Seeds
BT5 Plant foods
BT6 Foods
RT Confectionery pastes
RT Halva

Teleme cheese
BT1 Cheese varieties
BT2 Cheese
BT3 Dairy products
BT4 Animal foods
BT5 Foods

Telemetry
BT1 Analytical techniques

Tellurium
USE **Te**

TEM
BT1 Electron microscopy
BT2 Microscopy
BT3 Analytical techniques
UF Transmission electron microscopy

Temephos
BT1 Organophosphorus insecticides
BT2 Insecticides
BT3 Pesticides
BT4 Biocides
BT4 Residues
BT2 Organophosphorus pesticides
BT3 Pesticides
BT4 Biocides
BT4 Residues
UF Abate

Temik
USE **Aldicarb**

Temp.
BT1 Temperature

Temp. abuse indicators
BT1 Temperature

Tempe
USE **Tempeh**

Tempeh
BT1 Fermented foods
BT2 Processed foods
BT3 Foods
BT1 Soy products
BT2 Vegetable products
BT3 Plant foods
BT4 Foods
UF Tempe

Temper
BT1 Tempering
BT2 Thermal processing
BT3 Processing thermal
BT4 Processing
BT5 Technology

Temperature
NT1 Endpoint temp.
NT1 Endpoint temp. indicators
NT1 Temp.
NT1 Temp. abuse indicators
NT1 Thermistors
NT1 Thermocouples
NT1 Thermometers
NT1 Thermostats
NT1 Time temp. indicators
RT Heat

Tempering
BT1 Thermal processing
BT2 Processing thermal
BT3 Processing
BT4 Technology
NT1 Temper
RT Chocolate

Tempura
BT1 Fried foods
BT2 Processed foods
BT3 Foods

Tench
BT1 Freshwater fish
BT2 Fish
BT3 Animals
BT3 Sea foods
BT4 Aquatic foods
BT5 Animal foods
BT6 Foods

Tenderization
BT1 Processing
BT2 Technology
RT Meat

Tenderness
BT1 Texture
BT2 Sensory properties
NT1 Tenderometers
RT Shear

Tenderometers
BT1 Tenderness
BT2 Texture
BT3 Sensory properties

Tenjan
USE **Doenjang**

Tenoran
USE **Chloroxuron**

Tenox
BT1 Antioxidants
BT2 Additives

Tensile strength
BT1 Mechanical properties
BT2 Physical properties

Tensiometry
BT1 Analytical techniques

Tenuazonic acid
BT1 Mycotoxins
BT2 Toxins
BT3 Residues

Tepary beans
BT1 Legumes
BT2 Vegetables specific
BT3 Vegetables
BT4 Crops
BT5 Plants
BT4 Plant foods
BT5 Foods

Tequila
BT1 Spirits
BT2 Alcoholic beverages
BT3 Beverages alcoholic
BT4 Beverages

Teratogenesis
HN heading up to vol. 24
RT Carcinogens
RT Mutagens
RT Teratogenicity

Teratogenicity
BT1 Health
RT Diet
RT Mutagenicity
RT Mutants
RT Mutations
RT Nutrition
RT Teratogenesis

Terbacil
BT1 Herbicides
BT2 Pesticides
BT3 Biocides
BT3 Residues

Terbufos
BT1 Nematocides
BT2 Pesticides
BT3 Biocides
BT3 Residues
BT1 Organophosphorus insecticides
BT2 Insecticides
BT3 Pesticides
BT4 Biocides
BT4 Residues
BT2 Organophosphorus pesticides
BT3 Pesticides
BT4 Biocides
BT4 Residues

Terbuthylazine
BT1 Triazine herbicides
BT2 Herbicides
BT3 Pesticides
BT4 Biocides
BT4 Residues

Terfezia
BT1 Edible fungi
BT2 Fungi edible
BT3 Vegetables specific
BT4 Vegetables
BT5 Crops
BT6 Plants
BT5 Plant foods
BT6 Foods

Terminology
BT1 Nomenclature
RT Definitions

Termites
BT1 Insects
BT2 Pests

Termitomyces
BT1 Edible fungi
BT2 Fungi edible
BT3 Vegetables specific
BT4 Vegetables
BT5 Crops
BT6 Plants
BT5 Plant foods
BT6 Foods

Terpenes
HN heading up to vol. 24; under Terpenoids from vol. 25
SN general use only; see also monoterpenes, sesquiterpenes, diterpenes and triterpenes
BT1 Hydrocarbons
BT2 Organic compounds
BT1 Terpenoids
BT2 Lipids
BT3 Nutrients
RT Aroma compounds

Terpenoids
HN heading from vol. 25; under Terpenes up to vol. 24
BT1 Lipids
BT2 Nutrients
NT1 Carotenoids
NT2 Apocarotenal
NT2 Astacene
NT2 Bixin
NT2 Capsanthin
NT2 Carotenes
NT3 α-Carotene
NT3 β-Carotene
NT3 Provitamin A
NT2 Crocin
NT3 Crocetin
NT2 Lycopene
NT2 Norisoprenoids
NT3 β-Damascenone
NT3 Ionones
NT2 Phytoene
NT2 Phytofluene
NT2 Xanthophylls
NT3 Astaxanthin
NT3 Canthaxanthin
NT3 Cryptoxanthin
NT3 Diatoxanthin
NT3 Fucoxanthin
NT3 Lutein
NT3 Neoxanthin
NT3 Tunaxanthin
NT3 Violaxanthin
NT3 Zeaxanthin
NT1 Diterpenoids
NT2 Cafestol
NT2 Carnosic acid
NT2 Carnosol
NT2 Diterpenes
NT2 Kahweol
NT2 Rebaudiosides
NT2 Steviol
NT2 Stevioside
NT1 Isoprene
NT1 Isoprenoids
NT1 Monoterpenoids
NT2 Borneol
NT2 Camphor
NT2 Carvacrol
NT2 Carveol
NT2 Carvone
NT2 Cineole
NT3 Eucalyptol
NT2 Citral
NT3 Geranial
NT3 Neral
NT2 Citronellal
NT2 Citronellol
NT2 Dill ether
NT2 Geraniol
NT2 Hotrienol
NT2 Linalool
NT2 Menthol
NT2 Menthone
NT2 2-Methylisoborneol
NT2 Monoterpenes
NT3 Camphene
NT3 Limonene
NT3 Myrcene
NT3 Pinenes
NT3 Terpinene
NT2 Nerol
NT2 Safranal
NT2 Terpineol
NT2 Terpinyl acetate
NT2 Thujone
NT2 Thymol
NT1 Rishitin
NT1 Sesquiterpenoids
NT2 Farnesol
NT2 Ipomeamarone
NT2 Nootkatone
NT2 Sesquiterpenes
NT3 Caryophyllene
NT3 Farnesene
NT3 Humulene
NT1 Terpenes
NT1 Triterpenoids
NT2 Amyrin
NT2 Cucurbitacins
NT2 Glycyrrhizic acid
NT2 Glycyrrhizin
NT2 Limonoids
NT3 Limonin
NT3 Limonoid glucosides

NT3 Nomilin
NT2 Oleanolic acid
NT2 Quassin
NT2 Sapogenins
NT2 Triterpenes
NT3 Squalene
NT2 Ursolic acid
NT1 Vitamin E
NT2 Tocols
NT3 Tocopherols
NT4 α-Tocopherol
NT4 Tocotrienol
NT4 Vitamin E acetate
RT Aroma compounds

Terpinene
HN also under Flavour compounds up to vol. 42 (2010)
BT1 Aroma compounds
BT2 Flavour compounds
BT2 Volatile compounds
BT1 Monoterpenes
BT2 Hydrocarbons
BT3 Organic compounds
BT2 Monoterpenoids
BT3 Terpenoids
BT4 Lipids
BT5 Nutrients

Terpineol
HN also under Flavour compounds up to vol. 42 (2010)
BT1 Alcohols
BT1 Aroma compounds
BT2 Flavour compounds
BT2 Volatile compounds
BT1 Monoterpenoids
BT2 Terpenoids
BT3 Lipids
BT4 Nutrients

Terpinyl acetate
HN also under Flavour compounds up to vol. 42 (2010)
BT1 Acetates
BT1 Aroma compounds
BT2 Flavour compounds
BT2 Volatile compounds
BT1 Esters
BT2 Organic compounds
BT1 Monoterpenoids
BT2 Terpenoids
BT3 Lipids
BT4 Nutrients

Terramycin
USE **Oxytetracycline**

Terreic acid
BT1 Mycotoxins
BT2 Toxins
BT3 Residues

Terrines
BT1 Pates
BT2 Fish products
BT3 Sea foods
BT4 Aquatic foods
BT5 Animal foods
BT6 Foods
BT2 Meat products
BT3 Animal foods
BT4 Foods

Terroir
BT1 Winemaking
BT2 Processing
BT3 Technology

tert-Butylhydroquinone
USE **TBHQ**

Testosterone
BT1 Androgens
BT2 Hormones
BT3 Residues

Tetilla cheese
BT1 Cheese varieties
BT2 Cheese
BT3 Dairy products
BT4 Animal foods
BT5 Foods

Tetrachlorodibenzo-*p*-dioxins
BT1 Polychlorinated dibenzo-*p*-dioxins
BT2 Contaminants
BT3 Contamination
BT2 Organic halogen compounds

Tetrachloroisophthalonitrile
USE **Chlorothalonil**

Tetrachloromethane
SN syn. carbon tetrachloride
BT1 Chlorinated hydrocarbons
BT2 Organic halogen compounds
BT1 Fumigants
BT2 Biocides
BT1 Solvents

Tetrachlorvinphos
BT1 Acaricides
BT2 Pesticides
BT3 Biocides
BT3 Residues
BT1 Organophosphorus insecticides
BT2 Insecticides
BT3 Pesticides
BT4 Biocides
BT4 Residues
BT2 Organophosphorus pesticides
BT3 Pesticides
BT4 Biocides
BT4 Residues
UF Gardona
UF Rabon

Tetracyclines
HN heading up to vol. 24 (1992)
BT1 Antibiotics
BT2 Drugs
BT3 Residues
NT1 Chlortetracycline
NT1 Doxycycline
NT1 Oxytetracycline

Tetradifon
HN under Insecticides up to vol. 42 (2010)
BT1 Acaricides
BT2 Pesticides
BT3 Biocides
BT3 Residues

Tetragenococcus
HN introduced from vol. 39, issue 1 (2007)
BT1 Bacteria
BT2 Microorganisms
NT1 *Tetragenococcus halophilus*

Tetragenococcus halophila
USE ***Tetragenococcus halophilus***

Tetragenococcus halophilus
HN introduced from vol. 39, issue 1 (2007)
BT1 *Tetragenococcus*
BT2 Bacteria
BT3 Microorganisms
UF *Tetragenococcus halophila*

Tetrahydrofolate
BT1 Folates
BT2 Vitamin B group
BT3 Vitamins
BT4 Nutrients

Tetrahydrophthalimide
BT1 Captan
BT2 Dicarboximide fungicides
BT3 Fungicides
BT4 Pesticides
BT5 Biocides
BT5 Residues

Tetrazoles
BT1 Organic nitrogen compounds

Tetrodotoxin
BT1 Toxins
BT2 Residues

Texture
BT1 Sensory properties
NT1 Body
NT1 Chewiness
NT1 Consistency
NT2 Consistometers
NT2 Creaminess
NT2 Graininess
NT2 Lumpiness
NT2 Pastiness
NT2 Plasticity
NT2 Smoothness
NT1 Crispness
NT1 Crumbliness
NT1 Crunchiness
NT1 Firmness
NT2 Penetrometers
NT2 *Rigor mortis*
NT2 Rigorometers
NT2 Softening
NT2 Softness
NT1 Spreadability
NT1 Springiness

NT1 Tenderness
NT2 Tenderometers
NT1 Texturometers
NT1 Toughness
RT Compressibility
RT Rheological properties
RT Texturization

Textured vegetable proteins
HN heading up to vol. 24 (1992)
BT1 Vegetable proteins
BT2 Proteins vegetable
BT3 Proteins
BT4 Nutrients
BT3 Vegetable products
BT4 Plant foods
BT5 Foods
RT Soy proteins
RT Texturization

Texture profile analysis
BT1 Sensory analysis
BT2 Analytical techniques

Texturization
BT1 Processing
BT2 Technology
NT1 Spinning
NT1 Texturizers
NT1 Texturizing agents
RT Extrusion
RT Texture
RT Textured vegetable proteins

Texturizers
BT1 Texturization
BT2 Processing
BT3 Technology
RT Texturizing agents

Texturizing agents
BT1 Texturization
BT2 Processing
BT3 Technology
RT Texturizers

Texturometers
BT1 Texture
BT2 Sensory properties

Th
HN under Minerals up to vol. 42 (2010)
BT1 Metals
BT2 Elements
BT3 Minerals
BT4 Nutrients
UF Thorium

Thailand
BT1 Asia

Thallium
USE **Tl**

Thaumatin
BT1 Sweet proteins
BT2 Proteins
BT3 Nutrients
BT2 Sweeteners
BT3 Additives
RT Katemfe

Thawing
BT1 Thermal processing
BT2 Processing thermal
BT3 Processing
BT4 Technology
NT1 Defrosting
NT1 Drip
NT1 Freeze-thaw stability
NT1 Purge loss

Theaflavins
BT1 Flavonoids
BT2 Aromatic compounds
BT3 Organic compounds
BT2 Pigments
RT Tea
RT Thearubigins

Theanine
BT1 Alkaloids
BT2 Organic nitrogen compounds
BT1 Amino acids
BT2 Nutrients
BT2 Organic acids
BT3 Acids
BT2 Organic nitrogen compounds

Thearubigins
BT1 Flavonoids
BT2 Aromatic compounds
BT3 Organic compounds
BT2 Pigments
RT Tea
RT Theaflavins

Theobromine
BT1 Alkaloids
BT2 Organic nitrogen compounds
BT1 Purines
BT2 Heterocyclic compounds
BT2 Organic nitrogen compounds
RT Cocoa

Theophylline
BT1 Alkaloids
BT2 Organic nitrogen compounds
BT1 Purines
BT2 Heterocyclic compounds
BT2 Organic nitrogen compounds

Theragra chalcogramma
HN under Alaska pollack up to vol. 42 (2010)
BT1 Alaska pollock
BT2 Marine fish
BT3 Fish
BT4 Animals
BT4 Sea foods
BT5 Aquatic foods
BT6 Animal foods
BT7 Foods

Therapy
HN introduced from vol. 38, issue 8 (2006); heading
NT1 Diet therapy
NT2 Calories low diet
NT2 Carbohydrates low diet
NT2 Diabetic diet
NT2 Fats low diet
NT2 Ketogenic diet
NT2 Sodium low diet
NT2 Wt. loss diet
NT1 Immunotherapy
RT Clinical techniques
RT Diseases

Thermal capacity
BT1 Thermophysical properties
BT2 Physical properties

Thermal conductivity
HN under Conductivity up to vol. 24 (1992); conductivity thermal also used in the index up to vol. 29 (1997)
BT1 Thermophysical properties
BT2 Physical properties
UF Conductivity

Thermal diffusivity
BT1 Thermophysical properties
BT2 Physical properties

Thermal expansion
BT1 Thermophysical properties
BT2 Physical properties

Thermal processes
HN heading up to vol. 24 (1992)
BT1 Thermal processing
BT2 Processing thermal
BT3 Processing
BT4 Technology

Thermal processing
SN index heading is Processing thermal
BT1 Processing thermal
BT2 Processing
BT3 Technology
NT1 Cook chill processing
NT1 Cooking
NT2 Baking
NT3 Bakeries
NT3 Baking industry
NT3 Baking properties
NT3 Baking quality
NT3 Proofers
NT3 Proofing
NT2 Blanching
NT2 Boiling
NT3 Boilers
NT3 Parboiling
NT2 Braising
NT2 Broiling
NT2 Cookers
NT2 Cooking properties
NT3 Cooking loss
NT2 Frying
NT3 Deep frying
NT3 Frying properties
NT3 Stir frying
NT2 Grilling
NT2 Hard to cook defect
NT2 Microwave cooking
NT2 Roasting

NT2 Sauteing
NT2 Simmering
NT2 Slow cooking
NT2 Sous vide
NT2 Steaming
NT3 Steam
NT2 Stewing
NT2 Toasting
NT1 Cooling
NT2 Air cooling
NT2 Chilling
NT3 Chillers
NT2 Coolers
NT2 Hydrocooling
NT2 Supercooling
NT2 Vacuum cooling
NT1 Drying
NT2 Air drying
NT2 Driers
NT3 Freeze driers
NT3 Solar driers
NT3 Spray driers
NT2 Drum drying
NT2 Freeze drying
NT3 Freeze driers
NT2 Impingement drying
NT2 IR drying
NT2 Osmotic drying
NT2 Parching
NT2 Roller drying
NT2 Solar drying
NT3 Solar driers
NT2 Spray drying
NT3 Spray driers
NT2 Thin layer drying
NT2 Vacuum drying
NT2 Withering
NT1 Evaporation
NT2 Evaporators
NT2 Vacuum evaporation
NT2 Vaporization
NT1 Freezing
NT2 Cryogenics
NT2 Cryopreservation
NT2 Deep freezing
NT2 Freezers
NT2 Freeze-thaw stability
NT2 Ice nucleation activity
NT2 Immersion freezing
NT2 Liquid nitrogen
NT2 Pressure shift freezing
NT1 Heating
NT2 Annealing
NT2 Dielectric heating
NT2 Flaming
NT2 Heat
NT2 Heat distribution
NT2 Heaters
NT2 Heat transfer
NT2 Induction heating
NT2 IR heating
NT2 Reheating
NT2 Thermization
NT2 Warming
NT1 Hydrothermal processing
NT1 Pasteurization
NT2 HTST pasteurization
NT2 LTLT pasteurization
NT2 Pasteurizers
NT2 Surface pasteurization
NT2 Ultrapasteurization
NT1 Refrigeration
NT2 Refrigerants
NT3 Chlorofluorocarbons
NT3 Freons
NT2 Refrigerated storage
NT2 Refrigerated transport
NT2 Refrigerators
NT1 Rendering
NT1 Scalding
NT1 Sterilization
NT2 Autoclaves
NT2 Ohmic heating
NT2 Retorting
NT2 UHT treatment
NT1 Tempering
NT2 Temper
NT1 Thawing
NT2 Defrosting
NT2 Drip
NT2 Freeze-thaw stability
NT2 Purge loss
NT1 Thermal processes

Thermal properties
BT1 Thermophysical properties
BT2 Physical properties

Thermal stability
SN syn. heat stability
BT1 Stability
BT2 Physical properties
BT1 Thermophysical properties
BT2 Physical properties
RT Heat resistance
UF Thermostability

Thermistors
BT1 Temperature

Thermization
BT1 Heating
BT2 Thermal processing
BT3 Processing thermal
BT4 Processing
BT5 Technology

Thermoactinomyces
BT1 Bacteria
BT2 Microorganisms
NT1 *Thermoactinomyces vulgaris*

Thermoactinomyces vulgaris
HN introduced from vol. 43, issue 1 (2011)
BT1 *Thermoactinomyces*
BT2 Bacteria
BT3 Microorganisms

Thermoanaerobacter
BT1 Bacteria
BT2 Microorganisms
NT1 *Thermoanaerobacter brockii*
NT1 *Thermoanaerobacter ethanolicus*

Thermoanaerobacter brockii
BT1 *Thermoanaerobacter*
BT2 Bacteria
BT3 Microorganisms

Thermoanaerobacter ethanolicus
BT1 *Thermoanaerobacter*
BT2 Bacteria
BT3 Microorganisms

Thermoanaerobacterium
BT1 Bacteria
BT2 Microorganisms
NT1 *Thermoanaerobacterium thermosulfurigenes*

Thermoanaerobacterium thermosulfurigenes
HN introduced from vol. 43, issue 1 (2011)
SN synonymous with Clostridium thermosulfurogenes
BT1 *Thermoanaerobacterium*
BT2 Bacteria
BT3 Microorganisms

Thermoascus
BT1 Fungi
BT2 Microorganisms
NT1 *Thermoascus aurantiacus*

Thermoascus aurantiacus
BT1 *Thermoascus*
BT2 Fungi
BT3 Microorganisms

Thermobifida
HN introduced from vol. 43, issue 1 (2011)
BT1 Bacteria
BT2 Microorganisms
NT1 *Thermobifida fusca*

Thermobifida fusca
HN introduced from vol. 43, issue 1 (2011)
SN synonymous with Thermomonospora fusca
BT1 *Thermobifida*
BT2 Bacteria
BT3 Microorganisms

Thermococcus
HN introduced from vol. 41, issue 1 (2009)
BT1 Archaea
BT2 Microorganisms
NT1 *Thermococcus kodakaraensis*

Thermococcus kodakaraensis
BT1 *Thermococcus*
BT2 Archaea
BT3 Microorganisms

Thermocouples
BT1 Temperature

Thermodynamic properties
HN introduced from vol. 39, issue 1 (2007)
BT1 Thermophysical properties
BT2 Physical properties

Thermogenesis
HN introduced from vol. 39, issue 1 (2007)
BT1 Human physiology
BT2 Physiology
BT3 Science
RT Metabolic rate

Thermogravimetric analysis
USE **Gravimetry**

Thermoluminescence
BT1 Fluorescence
BT2 Analytical techniques
BT2 Optical properties
BT3 Physical properties

Thermolysins
SN EC 3.4.24.27, formerly EC 3.4.24.4
BT1 Lysins
BT2 Proteinases
BT3 Hydrolases
BT4 Enzymes

Thermometers
BT1 Temperature

Thermomonospora
BT1 Bacteria
BT2 Microorganisms
NT1 *Thermomonospora fusca*

Thermomonospora fusca
SN synonymous with Thermobifida fusca
BT1 *Thermomonospora*
BT2 Bacteria
BT3 Microorganisms

Thermomyces
BT1 Fungi
BT2 Microorganisms
NT1 *Thermomyces lanuginosus*

Thermomyces lanuginosus
SN synonymous with Humicola lanuginosa
BT1 *Thermomyces*
BT2 Fungi
BT3 Microorganisms

Thermophiles
SN organisms which grow above 45 C
BT1 Microorganisms
RT Mesophiles
RT Psychrophiles
RT Psychrotrophs
UF Thermophilic bacteria

Thermophilic bacteria
USE **Thermophiles**

Thermophysical properties
BT1 Physical properties
NT1 b.p.
NT1 Cryoscopes
NT1 Enthalpy
NT1 Entropy
NT1 f.p.
NT1 Glass transition
NT1 Glass transition temp.
NT1 Heat resistance
NT1 Heat stability
NT1 Melting
NT1 m.p.
NT1 Specific heat
NT1 Thermal capacity
NT1 Thermal conductivity
NT1 Thermal diffusivity
NT1 Thermal expansion
NT1 Thermal properties
NT1 Thermal stability
NT1 Thermodynamic properties

Thermostability
USE **Thermal stability**

Thermostats
BT1 Temperature

Thermotoga
BT1 Bacteria
BT2 Microorganisms
NT1 *Thermotoga maritima*

Thermotoga maritima
BT1 *Thermotoga*
BT2 Bacteria
BT3 Microorganisms

Thermus
BT1 Bacteria
BT2 Microorganisms
NT1 *Thermus aquaticus*
NT1 *Thermus nonproteolyticus*
NT1 *Thermus thermophilus*

Thermus aquaticus
BT1 *Thermus*
BT2 Bacteria
BT3 Microorganisms

Thermus nonproteolyticus
SN unapproved name
BT1 *Thermus*
BT2 Bacteria
BT3 Microorganisms

Thermus thermophilus
BT1 *Thermus*
BT2 Bacteria
BT3 Microorganisms

Thiabendazole
BT1 Benzimidazole
BT2 Fungicides
BT3 Pesticides
BT4 Biocides
BT4 Residues
UF Tecto

Thiamin
SN syn. vitamin B1; syn. vitamin F
BT1 Vitamin B group
BT2 Vitamins
BT3 Nutrients
UF Aneurin
UF Aneurine
UF Thiamine
UF Vitamin B_1
UF Vitamin F

Thiamine
USE **Thiamin**

Thiamphenicol
BT1 Antibiotics
BT2 Drugs
BT3 Residues

Thiazoles
BT1 Aroma compounds
BT2 Flavour compounds
BT2 Volatile compounds
BT1 Organic sulfur compounds
BT1 Volatile sulfur compounds
BT2 Volatile compounds

Thickeners
BT1 Additives
NT1 Agar
NT2 Agar gels
NT2 Agarose
NT1 Alginates
NT2 Alginate gels
NT2 Alginic acid
NT1 Bulking agents
NT2 Methylcellulose
NT1 Carrageenans
NT2 Carrageenan gels
NT1 Food thickeners
NT1 Gums
NT2 Cassia gums
NT2 Furcellaran
NT2 Gellan gums
NT2 Guar gums
NT2 Gum arabic
NT3 Gum acacia
NT2 Gum ghatti
NT2 Gum kondagogu
NT2 Gum tragacanth
NT2 Karaya gums
NT2 Locust bean gums
NT3 Carob gums
NT2 Mesquite seed gums
NT2 Mucilage
NT2 Psyllium gums
NT2 Tara gums
NT2 Xanthan gums
NT1 Starch
NT2 Amaranth starch
NT2 Amylopectins
NT2 Amyloses
NT2 Arrowroot
NT2 Barley starch
NT2 Buckwheat starch
NT2 Canna starch
NT2 Cassava starch
NT3 Tapioca
NT2 Corn starch
NT3 High amylose corn starch
NT2 Dextrins
NT3 Amylodextrins
NT3 Cyclodextrins
NT3 Maltodextrins
NT3 Pyrodextrins
NT2 Farina
NT2 Legume starch
NT2 Millet starch
NT2 Modified starches
NT2 Mung bean starch
NT2 Oat starch

NT2 Pea starch
NT2 Potato starch
NT2 Resistant starch
NT2 Rice starch
NT2 Rye starch
NT2 Sago
NT2 Sorghum starch
NT2 Starch granules
NT2 Sweet potato starch
NT2 Wheat starch
NT2 Yam starch
RT Celluloses
RT Colloids
RT Stabilizers
RT Thickening

Thickening
BT1 Processing
BT2 Technology
RT Thickeners

Thickness
SN used for depth, e.g. of backfat, not viscosity
BT1 Physical properties

Thidiazuron
BT1 Cytokinins
BT2 Plant growth regulators
BT3 Cultivation
BT4 Agriculture

Thielaviopsis
BT1 Fungi
BT2 Microorganisms

Thin layer chromatography
SN abbrev. TLC also used in index
BT1 Chromatography
BT2 Analytical techniques
NT1 HPTLC
NT1 TLC

Thin layer drying
HN introduced from vol. 39, issue 1 (2007)
BT1 Drying
BT2 Thermal processing
BT3 Processing thermal
BT4 Processing
BT5 Technology

Thinning
BT1 Cultivation
BT2 Agriculture

Thiobacillus thiooxidans
BT1 Bacteria
BT2 Microorganisms

Thiobarbituric acid values
SN abbrev. TBA values is also used in the index
NT1 TBA values
NT2 Malonaldehyde
NT2 Malondialdehyde
RT Oxidation
RT Quality control
RT Rancidity
RT TBARS

Thiocyanates
USE **Isothiocyanates**

Thiodan
USE **Endosulfan**

Thioesters
BT1 Aroma compounds
BT2 Flavour compounds
BT2 Volatile compounds
BT1 Esters
BT2 Organic compounds
BT1 Thiols
BT2 Organic sulfur compounds

Thioglucosidases
SN EC 3.2.1.147, formerly 3.2.3.1
BT1 Glycosidases
BT2 Hydrolases
BT3 Enzymes
UF Glucosinolases
UF Myrosinases

Thioglycolic acid
BT1 Organic acids
BT2 Acids
BT1 Thiols
BT2 Organic sulfur compounds

Thioglycosides
BT1 Glycosides
BT2 Carbohydrates
BT3 Nutrients
BT3 Organic compounds
BT1 Thiols
BT2 Organic sulfur compounds

Thiols
SN syn. mercaptans
BT1 Organic sulfur compounds
NT1 Dithiothreitol
NT1 Mercaptans
NT2 Methyl mercaptan
NT1 Mercaptoethanol
NT1 Methanethiol
NT2 Methyl mercaptan
NT1 Methional
NT1 Methionol
NT1 Sulfhydryl groups
NT1 Thioesters
NT1 Thioglycolic acid
NT1 Thioglycosides
RT Alcohols

Thionins
BT1 Cereal proteins
BT2 Proteins cereal
BT3 Vegetable proteins
BT4 Proteins vegetable
BT5 Proteins
BT6 Nutrients
BT5 Vegetable products
BT6 Plant foods
BT7 Foods

Thiophanate
BT1 Benzimidazole
BT2 Fungicides
BT3 Pesticides
BT4 Biocides
BT4 Residues
BT1 Carbamate pesticides
BT2 Pesticides
BT3 Biocides
BT3 Residues
UF Topsin

Thiophanate-methyl
BT1 Benzimidazole
BT2 Fungicides
BT3 Pesticides
BT4 Biocides
BT4 Residues
BT1 Carbamate pesticides
BT2 Pesticides
BT3 Biocides
BT3 Residues
UF Methylthiophanate
UF Pelt 44

Thiophenes
BT1 Organic sulfur compounds
BT1 Volatile sulfur compounds
BT2 Volatile compounds
RT Aroma compounds

Thioredoxin
HN introduced from vol. 39, issue 1 (2007)
BT1 Antioxidants
BT2 Additives
BT1 Proteins
BT2 Nutrients

Thiouracil
BT1 Antithyroid agents
BT2 Drugs
BT3 Residues

Thiourea
BT1 Organic nitrogen compounds
BT1 Organic sulfur compounds

Thiram
BT1 Dithiocarbamate fungicides
BT2 Fungicides
BT3 Pesticides
BT4 Biocides
BT4 Residues
UF TMTD

Thirst
HN introduced from vol. 39, issue 1 (2007)
BT1 Human physiology
BT2 Physiology
BT3 Science

Thistles
BT1 Plants
NT1 *Cynara humilis*

Thixotropy
BT1 Rheological properties
BT2 Mechanical properties
BT3 Physical properties

Thorium
USE **Th**

Thraustochytrium
HN introduced from vol. 41, issue 1 (2009)

BT1 Chromista
BT2 Microorganisms

Threadfin bream
BT1 Marine fish
BT2 Fish
BT3 Animals
BT3 Sea foods
BT4 Aquatic foods
BT5 Animal foods
BT6 Foods

Threonine
HN heading from vol. 25 (1993); under Amino acids up to vol. 24 (1992)
BT1 Amino acids
BT2 Nutrients
BT2 Organic acids
BT3 Acids
BT2 Organic nitrogen compounds

Threshers
BT1 Harvesting
BT2 Agriculture

Thrips
BT1 Insects
BT2 Pests

Thujone
HN also under Flavour compounds up to vol. 42 (2010)
BT1 Aroma compounds
BT2 Flavour compounds
BT2 Volatile compounds
BT1 Ketones
BT2 Carbonyl compounds
BT3 Organic compounds
BT1 Monoterpenoids
BT2 Terpenoids
BT3 Lipids
BT4 Nutrients

Thyme
HN heading from vol. 30 (1998); under Spices up to vol. 29 (1997)
BT1 Herbs
BT2 Spices
BT3 Flavourings
BT4 Additives
RT Thyme oils

Thyme oils
HN introduced from vol. 41, issue 1 (2009)
BT1 Essential oils
BT2 Flavourings
BT3 Additives
BT2 Vegetable oils
BT3 Oils vegetable
BT4 Oils
BT5 Lipids
BT6 Nutrients
BT4 Vegetable products
BT5 Plant foods
BT6 Foods
RT Thyme

Thymine
BT1 Pyrimidines
BT2 Heterocyclic compounds
BT2 Organic nitrogen compounds

Thymol
HN also under Flavour compounds up to vol. 42 (2010)
BT1 Aroma compounds
BT2 Flavour compounds
BT2 Volatile compounds
BT1 Monoterpenoids
BT2 Terpenoids
BT3 Lipids
BT4 Nutrients
BT1 Phenols
BT2 Alcohols
BT2 Aromatic compounds
BT3 Organic compounds

Thyristors
BT1 Process control
BT2 Technology

Thyroxine
BT1 Hormones
BT2 Residues

Ti
HN under Minerals up to vol. 42 (2010)
BT1 Metals
BT2 Elements
BT3 Minerals
BT4 Nutrients
UF Titanium

Tiamulin
BT1 Antibiotics
BT2 Drugs
BT3 Residues

Tibet
BT1 China
BT2 Asia

Tigernuts
SN syn. chufa nuts
BT1 Chufa nuts
BT2 Vegetables specific
BT3 Vegetables
BT4 Crops
BT5 Plants
BT4 Plant foods
BT5 Foods
NT1 *Cyperus esculentus*

Tiger shrimps
BT1 Shrimps
BT2 Crustacea
BT3 Shellfish
BT4 Animals
BT4 Sea foods
BT5 Aquatic foods
BT6 Animal foods
BT7 Foods

Tilapia
BT1 Freshwater fish
BT2 Fish
BT3 Animals
BT3 Sea foods
BT4 Aquatic foods
BT5 Animal foods
BT6 Foods
NT1 Nile tilapia
NT2 Bolti
NT2 *Oreochromis niloticus*
NT2 *Tilapia nilotica*
NT1 *Oreochromis*
NT2 *Oreochromis niloticus*

Tilapia nilotica
BT1 Nile tilapia
BT2 Tilapia
BT3 Freshwater fish
BT4 Fish
BT5 Animals
BT5 Sea foods
BT6 Aquatic foods
BT7 Animal foods
BT8 Foods

Tilmicosin
BT1 Macrolide antibiotics
BT2 Antibiotics
BT3 Drugs
BT4 Residues

Til oils
USE **Sesame oils**

Tilsit cheese
BT1 Cheese varieties
BT2 Cheese
BT3 Dairy products
BT4 Animal foods
BT5 Foods

Timber
BT1 Wood
BT2 Packaging materials

Time intensity
BT1 Sensory analysis
BT2 Analytical techniques

Time temp. indicators
BT1 Temperature

Time temp. integrators
BT1 Quality control
BT2 Technology

Tin
HN heading up to 1992; non-descriptor from 1993 to 2010 (USE Sn); reinstated (as heading) from vol. 43, issue 1 (2011)
BT1 Metals
BT2 Elements
BT3 Minerals
BT4 Nutrients
BT1 Packaging materials
NT1 Sn

Tin plate
BT1 Packaging materials

Tipburn
BT1 Plant disorders
BT2 Diseases plant
BT3 Diseases

Titanium
USE **Ti**

Titin
BT1 Animal proteins
BT2 Proteins animal
BT3 Proteins
BT4 Nutrients
RT Connectin

Title
SN indicates that an FSTA record has no abstract, i.e. bibliographic details and index only

Titratable acidity
HN acidity titratable also used in the index up to vol. 29 (1997)
BT1 Acidity
BT2 Physical properties

Titration
BT1 Analytical techniques
NT1 Titrimetry
NT1 Volumetric analysis
RT Neutralization

Titrimetry
BT1 Titration
BT2 Analytical techniques

Tl
HN under Minerals up to vol. 42 (2010)
BT1 Metals
BT2 Elements
BT3 Minerals
BT4 Nutrients
UF Thallium

TLC
SN index heading is Thin layer chromatography
BT1 Thin layer chromatography
BT2 Chromatography
BT3 Analytical techniques

TMTD
USE **Thiram**

Toast
BT1 Bread
BT2 Bakery products
BT3 Cereal products
BT4 Plant foods
BT5 Foods

Toast bread
BT1 Bread
BT2 Bakery products
BT3 Cereal products
BT4 Plant foods
BT5 Foods

Toasting
BT1 Cooking
BT2 Thermal processing
BT3 Processing thermal
BT4 Processing
BT5 Technology

Tobacco
HN introduced from vol. 39, issue 1 (2007)
BT1 Plants

Tochu tea
BT1 Herb tea
BT2 Teas
BT3 Beverages
BT3 Crops
BT4 Plants
BT3 Plant foods
BT4 Foods
RT *Eucommia ulmoides*

Tocols
BT1 Vitamin E
BT2 Antioxidants
BT3 Additives
BT2 Terpenoids
BT3 Lipids
BT4 Nutrients
BT2 Vitamins
BT3 Nutrients
NT1 Tocopherols
NT2 α-Tocopherol
NT2 Tocotrienol
NT2 Vitamin E acetate

α-Tocopherol
BT1 Tocopherols
BT2 Tocols
BT3 Vitamin E
BT4 Antioxidants
BT5 Additives
BT4 Terpenoids
BT5 Lipids
BT6 Nutrients
BT4 Vitamins
BT5 Nutrients

α-Tocopherol acetate
USE **Vitamin E acetate**

Tocopherols
BT1 Tocols
BT2 Vitamin E
BT3 Antioxidants
BT4 Additives
BT3 Terpenoids
BT4 Lipids
BT5 Nutrients
BT3 Vitamins
BT4 Nutrients
NT1 α-Tocopherol
NT1 Tocotrienol
NT1 Vitamin E acetate

α-Tocopheryl acetate
USE **Vitamin E acetate**

Tocotrienol
BT1 Tocopherols
BT2 Tocols
BT3 Vitamin E
BT4 Antioxidants
BT5 Additives
BT4 Terpenoids
BT5 Lipids
BT6 Nutrients
BT4 Vitamins
BT5 Nutrients

Toddy
BT1 Palm wines
BT2 Wines palm
BT3 Alcoholic beverages
BT4 Beverages alcoholic
BT5 Beverages
BT3 Palms
BT4 Plants

Toffees
BT1 Sugar confectionery
BT2 Plant foods
BT3 Foods

Tofu
BT1 Soy products
BT2 Vegetable products
BT3 Plant foods
BT4 Foods
NT1 Sufu

Togo
BT1 West Africa
BT2 Africa

Tolerance
NT1 Permissible levels
RT Legislation
RT Standards
RT Toxicity

Toluene
BT1 Aromatic compounds
BT2 Organic compounds
BT1 Solvents

Toma cheese
HN introduced from vol. 39, issue 1 (2007)
BT1 Cheese varieties
BT2 Cheese
BT3 Dairy products
BT4 Animal foods
BT5 Foods

Tomatillos
BT1 Fruits specific
BT2 Fruits
BT3 Crops
BT4 Plants
BT3 Plant foods
BT4 Foods

Tomatine
BT1 Alkaloids
BT2 Organic nitrogen compounds
RT Tomatoes

Tomato catsups
SN syn. tomato ketchups
BT1 Catsups
BT2 Ketchups
BT3 Sauces
BT4 Condiments
BT5 Flavourings
BT6 Additives
BT1 Tomato ketchups

BT2 Ketchups
BT3 Sauces
BT4 Condiments
BT5 Flavourings
BT6 Additives
BT2 Tomato products
BT3 Tomatoes
BT4 Fruits specific
BT5 Fruits
BT6 Crops
BT7 Plants
BT6 Plant foods
BT7 Foods
RT Tomato sauces

Tomato concentrates
BT1 Concentrates
BT2 Processed foods
BT3 Foods
BT1 Tomato products
BT2 Tomatoes
BT3 Fruits specific
BT4 Fruits
BT5 Crops
BT6 Plants
BT5 Plant foods
BT6 Foods

Tomatoes
BT1 Fruits specific
BT2 Fruits
BT3 Crops
BT4 Plants
BT3 Plant foods
BT4 Foods
NT1 Cherry tomatoes
NT1 Tomato products
NT2 Tomato concentrates
NT2 Tomato ketchups
NT3 Tomato catsups
NT2 Tomato pastes
NT2 Tomato powders
NT2 Tomato pulps
NT2 Tomato purees
NT2 Tomato sauces
NT1 Tomato skins
RT Tomatine
RT Tomato juices

Tomato juices
BT1 Fruit juices
BT2 Fruit products
BT3 Plant foods
BT4 Foods
BT2 Soft drinks
BT3 Beverages
RT Tomatoes

Tomato ketchups
SN syn. tomato catsups
BT1 Ketchups
BT2 Sauces
BT3 Condiments
BT4 Flavourings
BT5 Additives
BT1 Tomato products
BT2 Tomatoes
BT3 Fruits specific
BT4 Fruits
BT5 Crops
BT6 Plants
BT5 Plant foods
BT6 Foods
NT1 Tomato catsups
RT Tomato sauces

Tomato pastes
BT1 Pastes
BT2 Processed foods
BT3 Foods
BT1 Tomato products
BT2 Tomatoes
BT3 Fruits specific
BT4 Fruits
BT5 Crops
BT6 Plants
BT5 Plant foods
BT6 Foods

Tomato powders
HN introduced from vol. 39, issue 1 (2007)
BT1 Powders
BT2 Dried foods
BT3 Processed foods
BT4 Foods
BT2 Instant foods
BT3 Processed foods
BT4 Foods
BT1 Tomato products
BT2 Tomatoes
BT3 Fruits specific
BT4 Fruits
BT5 Crops
BT6 Plants
BT5 Plant foods
BT6 Foods

Tomato products
BT1 Tomatoes
BT2 Fruits specific
BT3 Fruits
BT4 Crops
BT5 Plants
BT4 Plant foods
BT5 Foods
NT1 Tomato concentrates
NT1 Tomato ketchups
NT2 Tomato catsups
NT1 Tomato pastes
NT1 Tomato powders
NT1 Tomato pulps
NT1 Tomato purees
NT1 Tomato sauces

Tomato pulps
BT1 Fruit pulps
BT2 Fruit products
BT3 Plant foods
BT4 Foods
BT2 Pulps
BT3 Processed foods
BT4 Foods
BT1 Tomato products
BT2 Tomatoes
BT3 Fruits specific
BT4 Fruits
BT5 Crops
BT6 Plants
BT5 Plant foods
BT6 Foods

Tomato purees
BT1 Fruit purees
BT2 Fruit products
BT3 Plant foods
BT4 Foods
BT2 Purees
BT3 Pulps
BT4 Processed foods
BT5 Foods
BT1 Tomato products
BT2 Tomatoes
BT3 Fruits specific
BT4 Fruits
BT5 Crops
BT6 Plants
BT5 Plant foods
BT6 Foods

Tomato sauces
BT1 Sauces
BT2 Condiments
BT3 Flavourings
BT4 Additives
BT1 Tomato products
BT2 Tomatoes
BT3 Fruits specific
BT4 Fruits
BT5 Crops
BT6 Plants
BT5 Plant foods
BT6 Foods
RT Tomato catsups
RT Tomato ketchups

Tomato seed oils
BT1 Vegetable oils
BT2 Oils vegetable
BT3 Oils
BT4 Lipids
BT5 Nutrients
BT3 Vegetable products
BT4 Plant foods
BT5 Foods

Tomato seeds
BT1 Oilseeds
BT2 Seeds
BT3 Plant foods
BT4 Foods

Tomato skins
BT1 Peel
BT1 Tomatoes
BT2 Fruits specific
BT3 Fruits
BT4 Crops
BT5 Plants
BT4 Plant foods
BT5 Foods

Tomography
HN introduced from vol. 39, issue 1 (2007)
BT1 Analytical techniques

Tonga
BT1 Oceania

Tongues
BT1 Offal
BT2 Animal foods
BT3 Foods

Tonic waters
BT1 Soft drinks
BT2 Beverages

Tooth decay
USE **Dental caries**

Top fermenting yeasts
BT1 Brewers yeasts
BT2 Yeasts brewers
BT3 *Saccharomyces*
BT4 Yeasts
BT5 Fungi
BT6 Microorganisms
RT Brewing

Topinambour
USE **Jerusalem artichokes**

Toppings
NT1 Frostings
NT1 Icings

Top shells
BT1 Gastropods
BT2 Molluscs
BT3 Shellfish
BT4 Animals
BT4 Sea foods
BT5 Aquatic foods
BT6 Animal foods
BT7 Foods

Topsin
USE **Thiophanate**

Torak
USE **Dialifos**

Tordon
USE **Picloram**

Torte
USE **Torten**

Tortellini
BT1 Pasta
BT2 Cereal products
BT3 Plant foods
BT4 Foods

Torten
BT1 Cakes
BT2 Bakery products
BT3 Cereal products
BT4 Plant foods
BT5 Foods
BT1 Desserts
BT2 Processed foods
BT3 Foods
BT1 Flans
BT2 Bakery products
BT3 Cereal products
BT4 Plant foods
BT5 Foods
UF Torte

Tortilla chips
BT1 Chips
BT2 Processed foods
BT3 Foods

Tortillas
BT1 Bakery products
BT2 Cereal products
BT3 Plant foods
BT4 Foods

Torulaspora
BT1 Yeasts
BT2 Fungi
BT3 Microorganisms
NT1 *Torulaspora delbrueckii*

Torulaspora delbrueckii
BT1 *Torulaspora*
BT2 Yeasts
BT3 Fungi
BT4 Microorganisms

Torula yeast
SN common name for Pichia jadinii; anamorph is Candida utilis
BT1 *Candida*
BT2 Yeasts
BT3 Fungi
BT4 Microorganisms
RT *Torulopsis*

Torulopsis
SN obsolete genus; synonym of Candida
BT1 Yeasts
BT2 Fungi
BT3 Microorganisms
NT1 *Torulopsis glabrata*
RT Torula yeast

Torulopsis glabrata
SN obsolete species; synonym of Candida glabrata
BT1 *Torulopsis*
BT2 Yeasts
BT3 Fungi
BT4 Microorganisms

Total quality management
BT1 Quality control
BT2 Technology

Total solids
USE **TS**

Total soluble solids
HN TSS used in the index from vol. 35, issue 6 (2003)
USE **TSS**

Toughness
HN heading up to vol. 24 (1992)
BT1 Texture
BT2 Sensory properties
RT Shear

Toxaphene
USE **Camphechlor**

Toxicity
NT1 Cytotoxicity
NT1 Enterotoxicity
NT1 Hepatotoxicity
NT1 Neurotoxicity
NT1 Reproductive toxicity
RT Health
RT Poisoning
RT Tolerance
RT Toxicology
RT Toxins

Toxicology
RT Food safety
RT Toxicity

Toxic substances
USE **Toxins**

Toxins
BT1 Residues
NT1 Aerolysins
NT1 Azaspiracids
NT1 Botulotoxins
NT1 Brevetoxins
NT1 Cereulide
NT1 Ciguatoxin
NT1 Colicins
NT1 Cycasin
NT1 Cytolethal distending toxin
NT1 Cytotoxins
NT1 Diarrhoetic shellfish toxins
NT1 Dinoflagellate toxins
NT1 Domoic acid
NT1 Endotoxins
NT1 Enterotoxins
NT2 Cholera toxin
NT1 Exotoxins
NT1 Goitrogens
NT1 Gonyautoxins
NT1 Hepatotoxins
NT1 Hypoglycine A
NT1 Killer toxins
NT1 Lathyrogens
NT1 Listeriolysins
NT1 Microcystins
NT1 Mycotoxins
NT2 Aflatoxins
NT3 Aflatoxin B_1
NT3 Aflatoxin B_2
NT3 Aflatoxin B_3
NT3 Aflatoxin D_1
NT3 Aflatoxin G_1
NT3 Aflatoxin G_2
NT3 Aflatoxin M_1
NT3 Aflatoxin M_2
NT3 Aflatoxin P_1
NT3 Aflatoxin Q_1
NT2 Agaritine
NT2 Alternariol
NT2 Amatoxins
NT3 Amanitins
NT2 Beauvericin
NT2 Byssochlamic acid
NT2 Citreoviridin
NT2 Citrinin
NT2 Cyclochlorotine
NT2 Cyclopiazonic acid
NT2 Cytochalasins
NT2 Enniatins
NT2 Eremofortin
NT2 F2 toxin

NT2 Fumagillin
NT2 Fumonisins
NT3 Fumonisin B_1
NT3 Fumonisin B_2
NT3 Fumonisin B_3
NT2 Fusaproliferin
NT2 Fusarin C
NT2 Gliotoxin
NT2 Griseofulvin
NT2 Gyromitrin
NT2 Kojic acid
NT2 Luteoskyrin
NT2 Moniliformin
NT2 β-Nitropropionic acid
NT2 Ochratoxins
NT3 Ochratoxin A
NT2 Patulin
NT2 Penicillic acid
NT2 Penitrems
NT2 Polyketides
NT2 Roquefortine
NT2 Rubratoxins
NT2 Rugulosin
NT2 Sterigmatocystins
NT2 Tenuazonic acid
NT2 Terreic acid
NT2 Tremorgens
NT2 Tremortins
NT2 Trichothecenes
NT3 Deoxynivalenol
NT3 Diacetoxyscirpenol
NT3 Fusarenon X
NT3 Nivalenol
NT3 Trichothecin
NT3 T2 toxin
NT3 Vomitoxin
NT2 Verrucosidin
NT2 Verruculogen
NT2 Versicolorin
NT2 Viriditoxin
NT2 Volvatoxins
NT2 Xanthomegnin
NT2 Zearalenol
NT2 Zearalenone
NT1 Neurotoxins
NT2 Anatoxins
NT1 Okadaic acid
NT1 Palytoxin
NT1 Paralytic shellfish toxins
NT1 Pyrrolizidine alkaloids
NT1 Saxitoxin
NT1 Shiga like toxins
NT1 Shiga toxins
NT1 Tetrodotoxin
NT1 Tutin
NT1 Vero cytotoxins
NT1 Verotoxins
NT1 Xanthotoxin
NT1 Yessotoxins
RT Alkaloids
RT Carcinogens
RT Contamination
RT Food safety
RT Glycosides
RT Heterocyclic compounds
RT Linamarin
RT Mycotoxicosis
RT Nitrosamines
RT Nitroso compounds
RT Phytohaemagglutinins
RT Poisoning
RT Poisons
RT Polybrominated biphenyls
RT Polychlorinated biphenyls
RT Ricin
RT Toxicity
UF Toxic substances

Toxoplasma
HN heading from vol. 30 (1998)
BT1 Parasites
BT2 Pests
NT1 *Toxoplasma gondii*
RT Toxoplasmosis

Toxoplasma gondii
BT1 *Toxoplasma*
BT2 Parasites
BT3 Pests

Toxoplasmosis
BT1 Diseases
BT1 Poisoning
RT *Toxoplasma*

2,4,5-TP
USE **Fenoprop**

Traceability
RT Origin
RT Product recalls

Trace elements
HN under Minerals up to vol. 42 (2010)
BT1 Elements
BT2 Minerals
BT3 Nutrients

Trace metals
USE **Metals**

Trachurus japonicus
BT1 Jack mackerel
BT2 Mackerel
BT3 Marine fish
BT4 Fish
BT5 Animals
BT5 Sea foods
BT6 Aquatic foods
BT7 Animal foods
BT8 Foods
BT3 Oily fish
BT4 Fish
BT5 Animals
BT5 Sea foods
BT6 Aquatic foods
BT7 Animal foods
BT8 Foods

Trachurus murphyi
BT1 Jack mackerel
BT2 Mackerel
BT3 Marine fish
BT4 Fish
BT5 Animals
BT5 Sea foods
BT6 Aquatic foods
BT7 Animal foods
BT8 Foods
BT3 Oily fish
BT4 Fish
BT5 Animals
BT5 Sea foods
BT6 Aquatic foods
BT7 Animal foods
BT8 Foods

Trade
BT1 Economics
NT1 EFTA
NT1 Exports
NT1 Fair trade
NT1 Imports
NT1 Mercosur
NT1 Tariffs
NT1 Trade agreements
NT2 GATT
NT2 NAFTA
NT1 World Trade Organization
RT Marketing
RT Markets

Trade agreements
BT1 Trade
BT2 Economics
NT1 GATT
NT1 NAFTA

Trademarks
BT1 Labelling
BT2 Packaging
BT3 Technology

Trahanas
BT1 Cereal products
BT2 Plant foods
BT3 Foods
BT1 Dairy products
BT2 Animal foods
BT3 Foods
BT1 Fermented foods
BT2 Processed foods
BT3 Foods
RT Kishk
RT Tarhana

Training
BT1 Education

Trametes
HN Coriolus also used in the index up to vol. 42 (2010)
BT1 Fungi
BT2 Microorganisms
NT1 *Trametes hirsuta*
NT1 *Trametes versicolor*
UF *Coriolus*

Trametes hirsuta
HN introduced from vol. 43, issue 1 (2011); Coriolus hirsutus also used in the index up to vol. 42 (2010)
BT1 *Trametes*
BT2 Fungi
BT3 Microorganisms
UF *Coriolus hirsutus*

Trametes versicolor
HN Coriolus versicolor also used in the index up to vol. 42 (2010)
BT1 *Trametes*

BT2 Fungi
BT3 Microorganisms
UF *Coriolus versicolor*

Tranquilizers
BT1 Drugs
BT2 Residues

Transaminases
SN EC 2.6.1
BT1 Transferases
BT2 Enzymes
NT1 Aspartate transaminases
RT Aminotransferases

Transcription
BT1 Gene expression
BT2 Genetics
NT1 Transcription factors
RT σ Factors

Transcription factors
HN introduced from vol. 41, issue 1 (2009)
BT1 Transcription
BT2 Gene expression
BT3 Genetics
RT Proteins

Transducers
BT1 Apparatus
BT2 Technology

Transesterification
BT1 Esterification

***trans* Fatty acids**
BT1 Unsaturated fatty acids
BT2 Fatty acids
BT3 Lipids
BT4 Nutrients
BT3 Organic acids
BT4 Acids
NT1 Elaidic acid
NT1 Vaccenic acid

Transferases
SN EC 2
BT1 Enzymes
NT1 Acetolactate synthases
NT1 Acyltransferases
NT2 Acetyltransferases
NT2 Alcohol *O*-acetyltransferases
NT2 Fatty acid synthases
NT2 γ-Glutamyltransferases
NT2 Protein-glutamine γ-glutamyltransferases
NT1 Aminotransferases
NT1 Citrate synthases
NT1 DNA-directed DNA polymerases
NT1 DNA-directed RNA polymerases
NT1 Glucose-1-phosphate adenylyltransferases
NT1 Glutathione transferases
NT1 Glycosyltransferases
NT2 Alternansucrases
NT2 Cyclomaltodextrin glucanotransferases
NT2 Dextransucrases
NT2 Fructosyltransferases
NT2 1,4-α-Glucan branching enzymes
NT2 4-α-Glucanotransferases
NT2 Glucosyltransferases
NT2 Lactose synthases
NT2 Levansucrases
NT2 Starch synthases
NT2 Sucrose-phosphate synthases
NT2 Sucrose synthases
NT2 Transglucosylases
NT1 Methyltransferases
NT1 Phosphorylases
NT1 Phosphotransferases
NT2 Kinases
NT3 Aspartate kinases
NT3 Fructokinases
NT3 Glucokinases
NT3 Hexokinases
NT1 Transaminases
NT2 Aspartate transaminases
NT1 Transpeptidases

Transferrins
BT1 Animal proteins
BT2 Proteins animal
BT3 Proteins
BT4 Nutrients
BT1 Glycoproteins
BT2 Proteins
BT3 Nutrients

Transformation
BT1 Gene transfer
BT2 Gene cloning
BT3 Genetic techniques
BT4 Genetics

Transgenes
BT1 Genes
BT2 Chromosomes
BT3 Genetics
BT2 Genomes
BT3 Genetics
RT Transgenic animals
RT Transgenic plants

Transgenic animals
HN also under Novel foods up to vol. 42 (2010)
BT1 Animals
BT1 Genetics
RT Cloned animals
RT GMO
RT GM organisms
RT Novel foods
RT Transgenes

Transgenic plants
HN also under Novel foods up to vol. 42 (2010)
BT1 Genetics
BT1 Plants
RT GMO
RT GM organisms
RT Novel foods
RT Transgenes

Transglucosylases
SN members of subclass EC 2.4.1; syn. glucosyltransferases
BT1 Glycosyltransferases
BT2 Transferases
BT3 Enzymes

Transglutaminases
USE **Protein-glutamine γ-glutamyltransferases**

Transglycosylation
BT1 Glycosylation
BT2 Modification

Translation
BT1 Gene expression
BT2 Genetics

Translucency
BT1 Optical properties
BT2 Physical properties

Transmissible spongiform encephalopathies
USE **Prion diseases**

Transmission electron microscopy
USE **TEM**

Transmittance
HN introduced from vol. 39, issue 1 (2007)
BT1 Optical properties
BT2 Physical properties

Transparency
BT1 Optical properties
BT2 Physical properties

Transpeptidases
BT1 Transferases
BT2 Enzymes

Transport
NT1 Aircraft
NT1 Lorries
NT1 Refrigerated transport
NT1 Shipping
NT1 Ships
NT1 Tankers
NT1 Trucks
NT1 Vans
NT1 Vehicles
RT Distribution
RT Handling
RT Pallets

Transposable elements
BT1 Genetics
RT Transposition

Transposition
BT1 Genetics
RT Insertion sequences
RT Transposable elements
RT Transposons

Transposons
BT1 Genetics
RT Transposition

Trappist cheese
BT1 Cheese varieties
BT2 Cheese
BT3 Dairy products
BT4 Animal foods
BT5 Foods

Travnik cheese
BT1 Cheese varieties
BT2 Cheese
BT3 Dairy products
BT4 Animal foods
BT5 Foods

Trays
BT1 Containers

Treacle
BT1 Sugar syrups
BT2 Plant foods
BT3 Foods

Treculia africana
BT1 Plants
RT African breadfruit seeds

Trees
BT1 Plants

Tree tomatoes
USE **Tamarillos**

Treflan
USE **Trifluralin**

Trehalases
USE **α,α-Trehalases**

α,α-Trehalases
SN EC 3.2.1.28
BT1 Glycosidases
BT2 Hydrolases
BT3 Enzymes
UF Trehalases

Trehalose
HN under Sugars up to vol. 42 (2010)
BT1 Disaccharides
BT2 Sugars
BT3 Carbohydrates
BT4 Nutrients
BT4 Organic compounds
BT3 Plant foods
BT4 Foods

Trematodes
BT1 Parasites
BT2 Pests

Tremorgens
BT1 Mycotoxins
BT2 Toxins
BT3 Residues

Tremortins
BT1 Mycotoxins
BT2 Toxins
BT3 Residues

Trenbolone acetate
BT1 Anabolic steroids
BT2 Drugs
BT3 Residues

Triacetin
HN introduced from vol. 41, issue 1 (2009)
BT1 Triglycerides
BT2 Glycerides
BT3 Emulsifiers
BT4 Additives
BT3 Fatty acid esters
BT4 Esters
BT5 Organic compounds
BT3 Lipids
BT4 Nutrients

Triacylglycerol lipases
SN EC 3.1.1.3
BT1 Lipases
BT2 Esterases
BT3 Hydrolases
BT4 Enzymes

Triacylglycerols
SN syn. triglycerides
BT1 Triglycerides
BT2 Glycerides
BT3 Emulsifiers
BT4 Additives
BT3 Fatty acid esters
BT4 Esters
BT5 Organic compounds
BT3 Lipids
BT4 Nutrients

Triadimefon
BT1 Fungicides
BT2 Pesticides
BT3 Biocides
BT3 Residues

Tri-allate
BT1 Herbicides
BT2 Pesticides
BT3 Biocides
BT3 Residues

Triazine herbicides
HN introduced from vol. 43, issue 1 (2011)
BT1 Herbicides
BT2 Pesticides
BT3 Biocides
BT3 Residues
NT1 Atrazine
NT1 Cyanazine
NT1 Desmetryn
NT1 Prometryn
NT1 Propazine
NT1 Simazine
NT1 Terbuthylazine

Triazophos
BT1 Acaricides
BT2 Pesticides
BT3 Biocides
BT3 Residues
BT1 Nematocides
BT2 Pesticides
BT3 Biocides
BT3 Residues
BT1 Organophosphorus insecticides
BT2 Insecticides
BT3 Pesticides
BT4 Biocides
BT4 Residues
BT2 Organophosphorus pesticides
BT3 Pesticides
BT4 Biocides
BT4 Residues

Tribolium
BT1 Insects
BT2 Pests

Tribunil
USE **Methabenzthiazuron**

Tributyltin
BT1 Butyltins
BT2 Organotin compounds
BT3 Contaminants
BT4 Contamination
BT3 Organic compounds

Tricaprylin
BT1 Triglycerides
BT2 Glycerides
BT3 Emulsifiers
BT4 Additives
BT3 Fatty acid esters
BT4 Esters
BT5 Organic compounds
BT3 Lipids
BT4 Nutrients

Trichinae
BT1 Parasites
BT2 Pests

Trichinella
BT1 Parasites
BT2 Pests
NT1 *Trichinella spiralis*
RT Trichinosis

Trichinella spiralis
BT1 *Trichinella*
BT2 Parasites
BT3 Pests

Trichinosis
BT1 Diseases
BT1 Poisoning
RT *Trichinella*

Trichlorfon
BT1 Acaricides
BT2 Pesticides
BT3 Biocides
BT3 Residues
BT1 Organophosphorus insecticides
BT2 Insecticides
BT3 Pesticides
BT4 Biocides
BT4 Residues

BT2 Organophosphorus pesticides
BT3 Pesticides
BT4 Biocides
BT4 Residues
UF Chlorophos

Trichloroacetonitrile
BT1 Fumigants
BT2 Biocides
UF Tritox

Trichloroanisole
BT1 Haloanisoles
BT2 Organic halogen compounds
BT1 Volatile compounds
RT Taints

Trichloroethylene
BT1 Fumigants
BT2 Biocides

Trichloromethane
SN syn. chloroform
BT1 Chlorinated hydrocarbons
BT2 Organic halogen compounds
BT1 Fumigants
BT2 Biocides
BT1 Solvents

Trichoderma
HN heading from vol. 25 (1993); under Fungi up to vol. 24 (1992)
BT1 Fungi
BT2 Microorganisms
NT1 *Trichoderma harzianum*
NT1 *Trichoderma koningii*
NT1 *Trichoderma longibrachiatum*
NT1 *Trichoderma reesei*
NT1 *Trichoderma viride*

Trichoderma harzianum
BT1 *Trichoderma*
BT2 Fungi
BT3 Microorganisms

Trichoderma koningii
BT1 *Trichoderma*
BT2 Fungi
BT3 Microorganisms

Trichoderma longibrachiatum
BT1 *Trichoderma*
BT2 Fungi
BT3 Microorganisms

Trichoderma reesei
BT1 *Trichoderma*
BT2 Fungi
BT3 Microorganisms

Trichoderma viride
BT1 *Trichoderma*
BT2 Fungi
BT3 Microorganisms

Tricholoma
BT1 Edible fungi
BT2 Fungi edible
BT3 Vegetables specific
BT4 Vegetables
BT5 Crops
BT6 Plants
BT5 Plant foods
BT6 Foods
NT1 *Tricholoma matsutake*
UF Matsutake

Tricholoma matsutake
BT1 *Tricholoma*
BT2 Edible fungi
BT3 Fungi edible
BT4 Vegetables specific
BT5 Vegetables
BT6 Crops
BT7 Plants
BT6 Plant foods
BT7 Foods

Trichophyton
BT1 Fungi
BT2 Microorganisms

Trichosporon
HN under Fungi up to vol. 42 (2010)
BT1 Yeasts
BT2 Fungi
BT3 Microorganisms
NT1 *Trichosporon cutaneum*
NT1 *Trichosporon pullulans*

Trichosporon cutaneum
HN under Fungi up to vol. 42 (2010)
BT1 *Trichosporon*
BT2 Yeasts
BT3 Fungi
BT4 Microorganisms

Trichosporon pullulans
HN introduced from vol. 39, issue 1 (2007); under Fungi up to vol. 42 (2010)
BT1 *Trichosporon*
BT2 Yeasts
BT3 Fungi
BT4 Microorganisms

Trichothecenes
BT1 Mycotoxins
BT2 Toxins
BT3 Residues
NT1 Deoxynivalenol
NT1 Diacetoxyscirpenol
NT1 Fusarenon X
NT1 Nivalenol
NT1 Trichothecin
NT1 T2 toxin
NT1 Vomitoxin

Trichothecin
BT1 Trichothecenes
BT2 Mycotoxins
BT3 Toxins
BT4 Residues
RT *Trichothecium*

Trichothecium
BT1 Fungi
BT2 Microorganisms
RT Mycotoxins
RT Trichothecin

Tricyclohexyltin hydroxide
USE **Cyhexatin**

Trifluralin
BT1 Herbicides
BT2 Pesticides
BT3 Biocides
BT3 Residues
UF Treflan

Triforine
BT1 Fungicides
BT2 Pesticides
BT3 Biocides
BT3 Residues

Triglycerides
HN heading from vol. 25 (1993); under Glycerides up to vol. 24 (1992)
SN syn. triacylglycerols
BT1 Glycerides
BT2 Emulsifiers
BT3 Additives
BT2 Fatty acid esters
BT3 Esters
BT4 Organic compounds
BT2 Lipids
BT3 Nutrients
NT1 Olein
NT2 Palm olein
NT1 Stearin
NT2 Palm stearin
NT1 Triacetin
NT1 Triacylglycerols
NT1 Tricaprylin
NT1 Trilinolein
NT1 Triolein
NT1 Tripalmitin
NT1 Tristearin

Trigonelline
BT1 Alkaloids
BT2 Organic nitrogen compounds

Trihalomethanes
BT1 Disinfection by-products
BT2 Disinfection
BT3 Hygiene
BT1 Organic halogen compounds

Triiodobenzoic acid
BT1 Plant growth regulators
BT2 Cultivation
BT3 Agriculture

Triiodothyronine
BT1 Hormones
BT2 Residues

Trilinolein
HN introduced from vol. 37, issue 5 (2005)
BT1 Triglycerides
BT2 Glycerides
BT3 Emulsifiers
BT4 Additives
BT3 Fatty acid esters

BT4 Esters
BT5 Organic compounds
BT3 Lipids
BT4 Nutrients

Trilon B
BT1 Additives
RT EDTA

Trimethoprim
HN under Drugs up to vol. 42 (2010)
BT1 Antibiotics
BT2 Drugs
BT3 Residues

Trimethylamine
BT1 Amines
BT2 Organic nitrogen compounds
RT Aroma compounds
RT Off odour
RT Spoilage

Trimming
BT1 Cutting
BT2 Processing
BT3 Technology

Trinidad and Tobago
BT1 West Indies
BT2 America

Triolein
SN syn. olein
BT1 Triglycerides
BT2 Glycerides
BT3 Emulsifiers
BT4 Additives
BT3 Fatty acid esters
BT4 Esters
BT5 Organic compounds
BT3 Lipids
BT4 Nutrients

Tripalmitin
BT1 Triglycerides
BT2 Glycerides
BT3 Emulsifiers
BT4 Additives
BT3 Fatty acid esters
BT4 Esters
BT5 Organic compounds
BT3 Lipids
BT4 Nutrients

Tripe
BT1 Offal
BT2 Animal foods
BT3 Foods

Tripolyphosphates
BT1 Phosphates
BT2 Salts

Trisodium phosphate
BT1 Phosphates
BT2 Salts

Tristearin
BT1 Triglycerides
BT2 Glycerides
BT3 Emulsifiers
BT4 Additives
BT3 Fatty acid esters
BT4 Esters
BT5 Organic compounds
BT3 Lipids
BT4 Nutrients

Triterpenes
HN introduced from vol. 43, issue 1 (2011)
BT1 Hydrocarbons
BT2 Organic compounds
BT1 Triterpenoids
BT2 Terpenoids
BT3 Lipids
BT4 Nutrients
NT1 Squalene

Triterpenoids
HN introduced from vol. 41, issue 1 (2009)
BT1 Terpenoids
BT2 Lipids
BT3 Nutrients
NT1 Amyrin
NT1 Cucurbitacins
NT1 Glycyrrhizic acid
NT1 Glycyrrhizin
NT1 Limonoids
NT2 Limonin
NT2 Limonoid glucosides
NT2 Nomilin
NT1 Oleanolic acid
NT1 Quassin
NT1 Sapogenins
NT1 Triterpenes
NT2 Squalene
NT1 Ursolic acid

Trithion
USE **Carbophenothion**

Triticale
BT1 Cereals
BT2 Crops
BT3 Plants
BT2 Seeds
BT3 Plant foods
BT4 Foods
NT1 Triticale flour

Triticale flour
HN introduced from vol. 39, issue 1 (2007)
BT1 Cereal flours
BT2 Flours cereal
BT3 Cereal products
BT4 Plant foods
BT5 Foods
BT1 Triticale
BT2 Cereals
BT3 Crops
BT4 Plants
BT3 Seeds
BT4 Plant foods
BT5 Foods

Tritium
BT1 Hydrogen
BT2 Elements
BT3 Minerals
BT4 Nutrients
BT1 Radioelements
BT2 Isotopes
BT3 Elements
BT4 Minerals
BT5 Nutrients
BT2 Residues

Tritordeum
BT1 Cereals
BT2 Crops
BT3 Plants
BT2 Seeds
BT3 Plant foods
BT4 Foods
RT Barley
RT Wheat

Tritox
USE **Trichloroacetonitrile**

Tropical fruits
BT1 Fruits specific
BT2 Fruits
BT3 Crops
BT4 Plants
BT3 Plant foods
BT4 Foods

Tropomyosin
BT1 Animal proteins
BT2 Proteins animal
BT3 Proteins
BT4 Nutrients

Troponin
BT1 Animal proteins
BT2 Proteins animal
BT3 Proteins
BT4 Nutrients

Trout
HN heading from vol. 30 (1998); under Fishes up to vol. 29 (1997)
BT1 Oily fish
BT2 Fish
BT3 Animals
BT3 Sea foods
BT4 Aquatic foods
BT5 Animal foods
BT6 Foods
NT1 Brook trout
NT1 Brown trout
NT1 Rainbow trout
NT2 *Oncorhynchus mykiss*
NT1 Sea trout
NT1 Smoked trout
UF Trouts

Trouts
HN heading up to vol. 24 (1992)
USE **Trout**

Trub
BT1 Worts

Trucks
BT1 Transport
RT Lorries

Truffles
USE ***Tuber***

Trumpet shells
BT1 Gastropods
BT2 Molluscs
BT3 Shellfish
BT4 Animals
BT4 Sea foods
BT5 Aquatic foods
BT6 Animal foods
BT7 Foods

Trussing
BT1 Processing
BT2 Technology

Trypsin
HN heading up to vol. 24 (1992)
SN EC 3.4.21.4
BT1 Proteinases
BT2 Hydrolases
BT3 Enzymes

Trypsin inhibitors
BT1 Proteinases inhibitors
BT2 Antinutritional factors
BT3 Nutritional values
BT2 Enzyme inhibitors
BT3 Enzymes

Tryptamine
BT1 Biogenic amines
BT2 Amines
BT3 Organic nitrogen compounds

Tryptophan
BT1 Amino acids
BT2 Nutrients
BT2 Organic acids
BT3 Acids
BT2 Organic nitrogen compounds

Tryptophol
BT1 Alcohols
BT1 Heterocyclic compounds

TS
BT1 Solids
BT2 Physical phases
BT3 Chemistry
BT4 Science
UF Total solids

TSS
HN total soluble solids used in the index up to vol. 35, issue 6 (2003)
BT1 Solids
BT2 Physical phases
BT3 Chemistry
BT4 Science
UF Total soluble solids

T2 toxin
BT1 Trichothecenes
BT2 Mycotoxins
BT3 Toxins
BT4 Residues

Tuba
BT1 Palm wines
BT2 Wines palm
BT3 Alcoholic beverages
BT4 Beverages alcoholic
BT5 Beverages
BT3 Palms
BT4 Plants

Tuber
BT1 Edible fungi
BT2 Fungi edible
BT3 Vegetables specific
BT4 Vegetables
BT5 Crops
BT6 Plants
BT5 Plant foods
BT6 Foods
NT1 Black truffles
NT1 White truffles
UF Truffles

Tuberculosis
BT1 Diseases
RT *Mycobacterium*

Tubers
BT1 Vegetables specific
BT2 Vegetables
BT3 Crops
BT4 Plants
BT3 Plant foods
BT4 Foods

Tubes
BT1 Containers

Tubs
BT1 Containers

Tulum cheese
BT1 Cheese varieties
BT2 Cheese
BT3 Dairy products
BT4 Animal foods
BT5 Foods

Tumbling
BT1 Processing
BT2 Technology
RT Meat

Tumours
USE **Cancer**

Tuna
HN heading from vol. 30 (1998); under Fishes up to vol. 29 (1997)
BT1 Marine fish
BT2 Fish
BT3 Animals
BT3 Sea foods
BT4 Aquatic foods
BT5 Animal foods
BT6 Foods
BT1 Oily fish
BT2 Fish
BT3 Animals
BT3 Sea foods
BT4 Aquatic foods
BT5 Animal foods
BT6 Foods
NT1 Bigeye tuna
NT1 Bonito
NT1 Skipjack tuna
NT2 Katsuobushi
NT1 White tuna
NT2 Albacore
NT1 Yellowfin tuna
UF Tunas
UF Tunny

Tuna oils
BT1 Fish oils
BT2 Oils fish
BT3 Fish products
BT4 Sea foods
BT5 Aquatic foods
BT6 Animal foods
BT7 Foods
BT3 Marine oils
BT4 Oils
BT5 Lipids
BT6 Nutrients

Tunas
HN heading up to vol. 24 (1992)
USE **Tuna**

Tunaxanthin
BT1 Xanthophylls
BT2 Carotenoids
BT3 Pigments
BT3 Terpenoids
BT4 Lipids
BT5 Nutrients

Tungsten
USE **W**

Tunisia
BT1 North Africa
BT2 Africa

Tunny
USE **Tuna**

Turban shells
BT1 Gastropods
BT2 Molluscs
BT3 Shellfish
BT4 Animals
BT4 Sea foods
BT5 Aquatic foods
BT6 Animal foods
BT7 Foods

Turbidimetry
BT1 Analytical techniques

Turbidity
BT1 Optical properties
BT2 Physical properties
NT1 Cloud
NT2 Clouding agents
NT1 Cloudiness
NT1 Haze

Turbot
BT1 Flatfish
BT2 Marine fish
BT3 Fish

BT4 Animals
BT4 Sea foods
BT5 Aquatic foods
BT6 Animal foods
BT7 Foods

Turgor
USE **Osmotic pressure**

Turkey
BT1 Asia
BT1 Europe
BT1 Middle East
RT Organization for Economic Cooperation and Development

Turkey carcasses
BT1 Carcasses
BT2 Meat
BT3 Animal foods
BT4 Foods
BT1 Turkey meat
BT2 Poultry meat
BT3 Meat specific
BT4 Meat
BT5 Animal foods
BT6 Foods
BT2 Turkeys
BT3 Poultry
BT4 Birds

Turkey frankfurters
BT1 Frankfurters
BT2 Sausages
BT3 Meat products
BT4 Animal foods
BT5 Foods
RT Turkey sausages

Turkey ham
BT1 Turkey products
BT2 Turkey meat
BT3 Poultry meat
BT4 Meat specific
BT5 Meat
BT6 Animal foods
BT7 Foods
BT3 Turkeys
BT4 Poultry
BT5 Birds

Turkey livers
BT1 Livers
BT2 Offal
BT3 Animal foods
BT4 Foods

Turkey meat
HN heading from vol. 30 (1998); under Turkeys and Poultry meat up to vol. 29 (1997)
BT1 Poultry meat
BT2 Meat specific
BT3 Meat
BT4 Animal foods
BT5 Foods
BT1 Turkeys
BT2 Poultry
BT3 Birds
NT1 Turkey carcasses
NT1 Turkey mince
NT1 Turkey products
NT2 Turkey ham
NT2 Turkey patties

Turkey mince
BT1 Turkey meat
BT2 Poultry meat
BT3 Meat specific
BT4 Meat
BT5 Animal foods
BT6 Foods
BT2 Turkeys
BT3 Poultry
BT4 Birds
UF Ground turkey

Turkey patties
BT1 Meat patties
BT2 Patties
BT3 Meat products
BT4 Animal foods
BT5 Foods
BT1 Turkey products
BT2 Turkey meat
BT3 Poultry meat
BT4 Meat specific
BT5 Meat
BT6 Animal foods
BT7 Foods
BT3 Turkeys
BT4 Poultry
BT5 Birds

Turkey products
BT1 Turkey meat
BT2 Poultry meat
BT3 Meat specific
BT4 Meat
BT5 Animal foods
BT6 Foods
BT2 Turkeys
BT3 Poultry
BT4 Birds
NT1 Turkey ham
NT1 Turkey patties

Turkeys
BT1 Poultry
BT2 Birds
NT1 Turkey meat
NT2 Turkey carcasses
NT2 Turkey mince
NT2 Turkey products
NT3 Turkey ham
NT3 Turkey patties

Turkey sausages
BT1 Sausages
BT2 Meat products
BT3 Animal foods
BT4 Foods
RT Poultry sausages
RT Turkey frankfurters

Turkish delight
BT1 Sugar confectionery
BT2 Plant foods
BT3 Foods
UF Lokum
UF Lukum
UF Rahat

Turkmenistan
BT1 Asia

Turmeric
BT1 Spices
BT2 Flavourings
BT3 Additives

Turnip rooted celery
USE **Celeriac**

Turnips
BT1 Vegetables specific
BT2 Vegetables
BT3 Crops
BT4 Plants
BT3 Plant foods
BT4 Foods

Turron
BT1 Sugar confectionery
BT2 Plant foods
BT3 Foods

Turtles
BT1 Animals

Tutane
USE **Butylamine**

Tutin
BT1 Toxins
BT2 Residues

Tvaroh
BT1 Quarg
BT2 Cheese varieties
BT3 Cheese
BT4 Dairy products
BT5 Animal foods
BT6 Foods

Tvorog
BT1 Quarg
BT2 Cheese varieties
BT3 Cheese
BT4 Dairy products
BT5 Animal foods
BT6 Foods

Twarog
BT1 Quarg
BT2 Cheese varieties
BT3 Cheese
BT4 Dairy products
BT5 Animal foods
BT6 Foods

Tykmaelk
BT1 Fermented milk
BT2 Fermented dairy products
BT3 Dairy products
BT4 Animal foods
BT5 Foods
BT3 Fermented foods
BT4 Processed foods
BT5 Foods
BT2 Milk

BT3 Dairy products
BT4 Animal foods
BT5 Foods

Tylose
HN introduced from vol. 39, issue 1 (2007)
BT1 Celluloses
BT2 Glucans
BT3 Polysaccharides
BT4 Carbohydrates
BT5 Nutrients
BT5 Organic compounds
BT1 Model foods
RT Meat

Tylosin
BT1 Macrolide antibiotics
BT2 Antibiotics
BT3 Drugs
BT4 Residues

Typhoid
BT1 Diseases
RT *Salmonella* Typhi

Typing
BT1 Genetic techniques
BT2 Genetics

Tyramine
BT1 Biogenic amines
BT2 Amines
BT3 Organic nitrogen compounds

Tyrophagus
BT1 Insects
BT2 Pests

Tyrosinases
SN show activity of catechol oxidases EC 1.10.3.1 and monophenol monooxygenases EC 1.14.18.1
BT1 Phenolases
BT2 Oxidoreductases
BT3 Enzymes

Tyrosine
HN heading from vol. 25 (1993); under Amino acids up to vol. 24 (1992)
BT1 Amino acids
BT2 Nutrients
BT2 Organic acids
BT3 Acids
BT2 Organic nitrogen compounds

Tyrosol
BT1 Phenols
BT2 Alcohols
BT2 Aromatic compounds
BT3 Organic compounds

U

U
BT1 Radioelements
BT2 Isotopes
BT3 Elements
BT4 Minerals
BT5 Nutrients
BT2 Residues
UF Uranium

UASB bioreactors
BT1 Bioreactors
BT2 Fermentation technology
BT3 Biotechnology
BT4 Technology
BT3 Process control
BT4 Technology
UF Upflow anaerobic sludge blanket bioreactors

Ubiquinone
USE **Coenzyme Q**

Udon
BT1 Pasta
BT2 Cereal products
BT3 Plant foods
BT4 Foods

Uganda
BT1 East Africa
BT2 Africa

Ugba
BT1 African oil beans
BT2 Legumes
BT3 Vegetables specific
BT4 Vegetables
BT5 Crops
BT6 Plants
BT5 Plant foods
BT6 Foods
BT2 Oilseeds
BT3 Seeds
BT4 Plant foods
BT5 Foods
BT1 Fermented foods
BT2 Processed foods
BT3 Foods

UHT cream
BT1 Cream
BT2 Dairy products
BT3 Animal foods
BT4 Foods
RT Sterilization

UHT milk
HN under Sterilized milks up to vol. 24
BT1 Milk
BT2 Dairy products
BT3 Animal foods
BT4 Foods
RT Sterilization

UHT treatment
BT1 Sterilization
BT2 Thermal processing
BT3 Processing thermal
BT4 Processing
BT5 Technology

Uji
BT1 Cassava
BT2 Vegetables specific
BT3 Vegetables
BT4 Crops
BT5 Plants
BT4 Plant foods
BT5 Foods
BT1 Fermented foods
BT2 Processed foods
BT3 Foods
BT1 Porridges
BT2 Cereal products
BT3 Plant foods
BT4 Foods
RT Koko

UK
HN used as abbrev. for United Kingdom up to vol. 24 (1992)
USE **United Kingdom**

Ukraine
BT1 Europe

Ulcerative colitis
HN introduced from vol. 39, issue 1 (2007)
BT1 Inflammatory bowel disease
BT2 Diseases
RT Colitis

Ulluco
BT1 Vegetables specific
BT2 Vegetables
BT3 Crops
BT4 Plants
BT3 Plant foods
BT4 Foods

Ultracentrifugation
BT1 Centrifugation
BT2 Separation
BT3 Processing
BT4 Technology

Ultrafiltration
BT1 Filtration
BT2 Processing
BT3 Technology
NT1 Diafiltration
RT Concentration
RT Dialysis
RT Membranes

Ultrapasteurization
BT1 Pasteurization
BT2 Thermal processing
BT3 Processing thermal
BT4 Processing
BT5 Technology

Ultra performance liquid chromatography
USE **UPLC**

Ultrasonics
HN heading up to vol. 24 (1992)
BT1 Ultrasound

Ultrasound
HN heading from vol. 25 (1993); under Ultrasonics up to vol. 24 (1992)
NT1 Ultrasonics
RT Sound

Ultrastructure
RT Physical properties

Ultraviolet
HN heading up to vol. 24 (1992); under Ultraviolet radiation from vol. 25 (1993)
USE **UV**

Ultraviolet irradiation
USE **UV irradiation**

Ultraviolet radiation
HN heading from vol. 25 (1993); under Ultraviolet up to vol. 24 (1992)
SN abbrev. UV is also used in the index
BT1 Radiation
NT1 UV radiation
NT2 UV

Ultraviolet spectrophotometry
USE **UV spectroscopy**

Ulva
HN introduced from vol. 41, issue 1 (2009)
BT1 Seaweeds
BT2 Algae
BT3 Microorganisms
BT2 Sea foods
BT3 Aquatic foods
BT4 Animal foods
BT5 Foods
NT1 Sea lettuces
NT1 *Ulva lactuca*

Ulva lactuca
BT1 *Ulva*
BT2 Seaweeds
BT3 Algae
BT4 Microorganisms
BT3 Sea foods
BT4 Aquatic foods
BT5 Animal foods
BT6 Foods

Umami
BT1 Flavour
BT2 Sensory properties

Ume
USE **Japanese apricots**

UMP
BT1 Nucleotides
UF Uridine monophosphate

Undaria
BT1 Seaweeds
BT2 Algae
BT3 Microorganisms
BT2 Sea foods
BT3 Aquatic foods
BT4 Animal foods
BT5 Foods
NT1 *Undaria pinnatifida*
NT1 Wakame

Undaria pinnatifida
SN Latin name for wakame, also used in the index
BT1 *Undaria*
BT2 Seaweeds
BT3 Algae
BT4 Microorganisms
BT3 Sea foods
BT4 Aquatic foods
BT5 Animal foods
BT6 Foods

Undecanone
BT1 Aroma compounds
BT2 Flavour compounds
BT2 Volatile compounds
BT1 Ketones
BT2 Carbonyl compounds
BT3 Organic compounds

Union of Soviet Socialist Republics
HN heading up to vol. 24 (1992); use individual states from vol. 25 (1993)
UF USSR

United Arab Emirates
BT1 Asia
BT1 Middle East

United Kingdom
HN heading up to vol. 24
BT1 Europe
BT1 European Union
NT1 England
NT1 Northern Ireland
NT1 Scotland
NT1 St Helena
NT1 Wales
RT Organization for Economic Cooperation and Development
UF Great Britain
UF Isle of Man
UF UK

United States of America
HN heading up to vol. 24 (1992)
BT1 North America
BT2 America
RT Organization for Economic Cooperation and Development
UF USA

Unsaponifiable matter
BT1 Lipids
BT2 Nutrients

Unsaturated fats
HN fats unsaturated also used in the index up to vol. 29 (1997)
BT1 Fats
BT2 Lipids
BT3 Nutrients
RT Polyunsaturated fats
RT Unsaturation

Unsaturated fatty acids
HN fatty acids unsaturated also used in the index up to vol. 29 (1997)
BT1 Fatty acids
BT2 Lipids
BT3 Nutrients
BT2 Organic acids
BT3 Acids
NT1 Essential fatty acids
NT1 Monounsaturated fatty acids
NT2 Decenoic acid
NT2 Docosenoic acid
NT3 Erucic acid
NT2 Eicosenoic acid
NT2 Hexadecenoic acid
NT3 Palmitoleic acid
NT2 Octadecenoic acid
NT3 Elaidic acid
NT3 Oleic acid
NT3 Petroselinic acid
NT3 Vaccenic acid
NT2 Ricinoleic acid
NT1 PUFA
NT2 Conjugated fatty acids
NT3 CLA
NT3 Eleostearic acid
NT2 Eicosatetraenoic acid
NT3 Arachidonic acid
NT2 ω-3 Fatty acids
NT3 Docosahexaenoic acid
NT3 Docosapentaenoic acid
NT3 Eicosapentaenoic acid
NT3 α-Linolenic acid
NT3 Stearidonic acid
NT2 ω-6 Fatty acids
NT3 Arachidonic acid
NT3 Linoleic acid
NT4 CLA
NT3 γ-Linolenic acid
NT2 Linolenic acid
NT3 Eleostearic acid
NT3 α-Linolenic acid
NT3 γ-Linolenic acid
NT1 *trans* Fatty acids
NT2 Elaidic acid
NT2 Vaccenic acid
RT Unsaturation

Unsaturation
HN heading up to vol. 24 (1992)
SN includes degree of unsaturation
RT Monounsaturated fatty acids
RT Polyunsaturated fats
RT PUFA
RT Unsaturated fats
RT Unsaturated fatty acids

Upflow anaerobic sludge blanket bioreactors
USE **UASB bioreactors**

UPLC
HN introduced from vol. 43, issue 1 (2011)
BT1 High performance liquid chromatography
BT2 Chromatography
BT3 Analytical techniques
UF Ultra performance liquid chromatography

Upper Volta
USE **Burkina Faso**

Uracil
BT1 Pyrimidines
BT2 Heterocyclic compounds
BT2 Organic nitrogen compounds

Uranium
USE **U**

Urd beans
USE **Black gram**

Urea
SN syn. carbamide
BT1 Amides
BT2 Organic nitrogen compounds

Ureases
SN EC 3.5.1.5
BT1 Hydrolases
BT2 Enzymes

Urethane
SN syn. ethyl carbamate
BT1 Carcinogens
BT2 Mutagens
BT1 Esters
BT2 Organic compounds
BT1 Organic nitrogen compounds

Uric acid
BT1 Purines
BT2 Heterocyclic compounds
BT2 Organic nitrogen compounds

Uridine
BT1 Nucleosides

Uridine monophosphate
USE **UMP**

Uronic acids
BT1 Organic acids
BT2 Acids
BT1 Sugars
BT2 Carbohydrates
BT3 Nutrients
BT3 Organic compounds
BT2 Plant foods
BT3 Foods
NT1 Galacturonic acid
NT1 Glucuronic acid
NT1 Polyuronides

Ursolic acid
HN introduced from vol. 41, issue 1 (2009)
BT1 Organic acids
BT2 Acids
BT1 Triterpenoids
BT2 Terpenoids
BT3 Lipids
BT4 Nutrients

Urticaria
BT1 Diseases

Uruguay
HN heading up to vol. 24
BT1 South America
BT2 America

USA
HN used as abbrev. for United States of America up to vol. 24 (1992)
USE **United States of America**

USSR
HN used as abbrev. for Union of Soviet Socialist Republics up to vol. 24 (1992)
USE **Union of Soviet Socialist Republics**

Utensils
BT1 Equipment
BT2 Technology
NT1 Ceramics
NT1 Scoops

UV
SN heading is Ultraviolet radiation
BT1 UV radiation
BT2 Ultraviolet radiation
BT3 Radiation
UF Ultraviolet

UV irradiation
HN introduced from vol. 43, issue 1 (2011)
BT1 Irradiation
BT2 Processing
BT3 Technology
RT UV radiation
UF Ultraviolet irradiation

UV radiation
SN heading is Ultraviolet radiation
BT1 Ultraviolet radiation
BT2 Radiation
NT1 UV
RT UV irradiation

UV spectroscopy
BT1 Spectroscopy
BT2 Analytical techniques
UF Ultraviolet spectrophotometry

Uzbekistan
BT1 Asia

V

V
HN under Minerals up to vol. 42 (2010)
BT1 Metals
BT2 Elements
BT3 Minerals
BT4 Nutrients
UF Vanadium

Vaccenic acid
BT1 Octadecenoic acid
BT2 Monounsaturated fatty acids
BT3 Unsaturated fatty acids
BT4 Fatty acids
BT5 Lipids
BT6 Nutrients
BT5 Organic acids
BT6 Acids
BT1 *trans* Fatty acids
BT2 Unsaturated fatty acids
BT3 Fatty acids
BT4 Lipids
BT5 Nutrients
BT4 Organic acids
BT5 Acids

Vaccination
HN introduced from vol. 42, issue 1 (2010)
BT1 Immunology

Vaccinia virus
HN introduced from vol. 43, issue 1 (2011)
BT1 Orthopoxvirus
BT2 Viruses
BT3 Microorganisms

Vacuum
NT1 Sous vide
NT1 Vacuum cooling
NT1 Vacuum distillation
NT1 Vacuum drying
NT1 Vacuum evaporation
NT1 Vacuum impregnation
NT1 Vacuum packaging
NT1 Vacuum pans

Vacuum cooling
BT1 Cooling
BT2 Thermal processing
BT3 Processing thermal
BT4 Processing
BT5 Technology
BT1 Vacuum

Vacuum distillation
HN introduced from vol. 42, issue 1 (2010)
BT1 Distillation
BT2 Processing
BT3 Technology
BT1 Vacuum
UF Molecular distillation

Vacuum drying
HN drying vacuum also used in the index up to vol. 29 (1997)
BT1 Drying
BT2 Thermal processing
BT3 Processing thermal
BT4 Processing
BT5 Technology
BT1 Vacuum

Vacuum evaporation
BT1 Evaporation
BT2 Thermal processing
BT3 Processing thermal
BT4 Processing

BT5 Technology
BT1 Vacuum

Vacuum impregnation
HN introduced from vol. 39, issue 1 (2007)
BT1 Processing
BT2 Technology
BT1 Vacuum

Vacuum packaging
HN packaging vacuum also used in the index up to vol. 29 (1997)
BT1 Packaging
BT2 Technology
BT1 Vacuum

Vacuum pans
BT1 Equipment
BT2 Technology
BT1 Sugar processes
BT2 Processing
BT3 Technology
BT1 Vacuum

Valeraldehyde
HN also under Volatile compounds up to vol. 42 (2010)
SN syn. pentanal
BT1 Pentanal
BT2 Aldehydes
BT3 Carbonyl compounds
BT4 Organic compounds
BT2 Aroma compounds
BT3 Flavour compounds
BT3 Volatile compounds

Valeric acid
SN syn. pentanoic acid
BT1 Pentanoic acid
BT2 Aroma compounds
BT3 Flavour compounds
BT3 Volatile compounds
BT2 Saturated fatty acids
BT3 Fatty acids
BT4 Lipids
BT5 Nutrients
BT4 Organic acids
BT5 Acids
BT2 Short chain fatty acids
BT3 Volatile fatty acids
BT4 Fatty acids
BT5 Lipids
BT6 Nutrients
BT5 Organic acids
BT6 Acids
BT4 Volatile compounds

Valine
BT1 Amino acids
BT2 Nutrients
BT2 Organic acids
BT3 Acids
BT2 Organic nitrogen compounds

Valves
BT1 Equipment
BT2 Technology

Vanadium
USE **V**

Vanaspati
BT1 Vegetable fats
BT2 Fats vegetable
BT3 Fats
BT4 Lipids
BT5 Nutrients
BT3 Vegetable products
BT4 Plant foods
BT5 Foods

Vancomycin
BT1 Antibiotics
BT2 Drugs
BT3 Residues

Vanilla
BT1 Flavourings
BT2 Additives
RT Vanilla beans
RT Vanillin

Vanilla beans
HN introduced from vol. 39, issue 1 (2007)
BT1 Crops
BT2 Plants
RT Vanilla

Vanillic acid
BT1 Organic acids
BT2 Acids
BT1 Phenols
BT2 Alcohols
BT2 Aromatic compounds
BT3 Organic compounds

Vanillin
BT1 Flavourings
BT2 Additives
BT1 Phenols
BT2 Alcohols
BT2 Aromatic compounds
BT3 Organic compounds
RT Vanilla

Vans
BT1 Transport

Vapona
USE **Dichlorvos**

Vaporization
BT1 Evaporation
BT2 Thermal processing
BT3 Processing thermal
BT4 Processing
BT5 Technology

Vapours
BT1 Gases
BT2 Physical phases
BT3 Chemistry
BT4 Science
BT1 Physical phases
BT2 Chemistry
BT3 Science
NT1 Water vapour

var
RT Breed
RT cv
RT Genetics
UF Variety

Variety
HN heading from vol. 18 (1986) to vol. 24 (1992)
USE **var**

Varnishes
BT1 Lacquers
BT2 Surfaces

Vats
BT1 Equipment
BT2 Technology
RT Cheesemaking
RT Winemaking

Veal
BT1 Meat specific
BT2 Meat
BT3 Animal foods
BT4 Foods
NT1 Veal calf carcasses
RT Beef
RT Cattle

Veal calf carcasses
BT1 Carcasses
BT2 Meat
BT3 Animal foods
BT4 Foods
BT1 Veal
BT2 Meat specific
BT3 Meat
BT4 Animal foods
BT5 Foods

Vectors
HN heading for vol. 22 (1990) and 23 (1991); under Cloning vectors from vol. 24 (1992)
BT1 Cloning vectors
BT2 Genetic techniques
BT3 Genetics
NT1 Expression vectors

Vegan diet
BT1 Diet
BT2 Nutrition
RT Vegan foods
RT Vegetarian diet
RT Vegetarian foods

Vegan foods
BT1 Processed foods
BT2 Foods
RT Vegan diet
RT Vegetarian diet
RT Vegetarian foods

Vegetable burgers
BT1 Vegetable products
BT2 Plant foods
BT3 Foods

Vegetable fats
SN index heading is Fats vegetable

BT1 Fats vegetable
BT2 Fats
BT3 Lipids
BT4 Nutrients
BT2 Vegetable products
BT3 Plant foods
BT4 Foods
NT1 Borneo tallow
NT1 Cocoa butter
NT2 Cocoa butter equivalents
NT2 Cocoa butter extenders
NT2 Cocoa butter substitutes
NT1 Coconut butter
NT1 Illipe butter
NT1 Kokum
NT1 Sal fats
NT1 Shea nut butter
NT1 Vanaspati
RT Oilseeds
RT Vegetable oils

Vegetable juice beverages
BT1 Soft drinks
BT2 Beverages

Vegetable juice concentrates
HN introduced from vol. 42, issue 1 (2010)
BT1 Concentrates
BT2 Processed foods
BT3 Foods
BT1 Vegetable juices
BT2 Soft drinks
BT3 Beverages
BT2 Vegetable products
BT3 Plant foods
BT4 Foods

Vegetable juices
BT1 Soft drinks
BT2 Beverages
BT1 Vegetable products
BT2 Plant foods
BT3 Foods
NT1 Cabbage juices
NT1 Carrot juices
NT1 Vegetable juice concentrates
NT1 Vegetable nectars

Vegetable nectars
BT1 Vegetable juices
BT2 Soft drinks
BT3 Beverages
BT2 Vegetable products
BT3 Plant foods
BT4 Foods

Vegetable oils
SN index heading is Oils vegetable
BT1 Oils vegetable
BT2 Oils
BT3 Lipids
BT4 Nutrients
BT2 Vegetable products
BT3 Plant foods
BT4 Foods
NT1 Argemone oils
NT1 Avocado oils
NT1 Baobab oils
NT1 Borage oils
NT1 Camelina oils
NT1 Castor oils
NT1 Coffee oils
NT1 Corn oils
NT2 Corn fibre oils
NT1 Cottonseed oils
NT1 Essential oils
NT2 Bitter almond oils
NT2 Buchu oils
NT2 Cinnamon oils
NT2 Citronella essential oils
NT2 Citrus essential oils
NT3 Bergamot essential oils
NT4 Bergamot oils
NT3 Bitter orange essential oils
NT3 Citrus oils
NT3 Lemon essential oils
NT3 Lime essential oils
NT3 Neroli oils
NT3 Orange essential oils
NT2 Clary sage essential oils
NT2 Clove oils
NT2 Garlic oils
NT2 Hop essential oils
NT2 Lemongrass oils
NT2 Mint oils
NT2 Nutmeg oils
NT2 Oleoresins
NT2 Oregano oils
NT2 Peppermint essential oils
NT2 Petitgrain oils
NT2 Rosemary essential oils
NT2 Sage essential oils
NT2 Tea tree oils
NT2 Thyme oils
NT1 Evening primrose oils
NT1 Flax seed oils
NT2 Linseed oils
NT1 Grape seed oils
NT1 Jojoba oils
NT1 Kapok oils
NT1 Lupin seed oils
NT1 Meadowfoam oils
NT1 Millet oils
NT1 Mustard seed oils
NT1 Nut oils
NT2 Almond oils
NT2 Beech nut oils
NT2 Brazil nut oils
NT2 Coconut oils
NT2 Groundnut oils
NT2 Hazelnut oils
NT2 Pecan oils
NT2 Walnut oils
NT1 Oat oils
NT1 Olive oils
NT2 Olive oil mills effluents
NT2 Olive pomace oils
NT3 Sansa oils
NT1 Palm oils
NT2 Babassu oils
NT2 Palm kernel oils
NT2 Palm oil mills effluents
NT2 Palm olein
NT2 Palm stearin
NT1 Perilla oils
NT1 Pumpkin seed oils
NT1 Rapeseed oils
NT1 Rice bran oils
NT1 Rice germ oils
NT1 Safflower oils
NT1 Sea buckthorn oils
NT1 Sesame oils
NT1 Soybean oils
NT1 Sunflower oils
NT1 Tea seed oils
NT1 Tomato seed oils
NT1 Wheat germ oils
RT Oilseeds
RT Vegetable fats

Vegetable pickles
BT1 Pickles
BT2 Fermented foods
BT3 Processed foods
BT4 Foods
BT1 Vegetable products
BT2 Plant foods
BT3 Foods
NT1 Cucumber pickles
NT1 Narazuke
NT1 Pickled onions

Vegetable preserves
BT1 Preserves
BT2 Processed foods
BT3 Foods
BT1 Vegetable products
BT2 Plant foods
BT3 Foods

Vegetable products
BT1 Plant foods
BT2 Foods
NT1 Bean jams
NT2 Ann
NT1 Coleslaw
NT1 Falafel
NT1 Fats vegetable
NT2 Vegetable fats
NT3 Borneo tallow
NT3 Cocoa butter
NT4 Cocoa butter equivalents
NT4 Cocoa butter extenders
NT4 Cocoa butter substitutes
NT3 Coconut butter
NT3 Illipe butter
NT3 Kokum
NT3 Sal fats
NT3 Shea nut butter
NT3 Vanaspati
NT1 Fufu
NT1 Kimchies
NT2 Kakdugi
NT1 Oils vegetable
NT2 Vegetable oils
NT3 Argemone oils
NT3 Avocado oils
NT3 Baobab oils
NT3 Borage oils
NT3 Camelina oils
NT3 Castor oils
NT3 Coffee oils
NT3 Corn oils
NT4 Corn fibre oils
NT3 Cottonseed oils
NT3 Essential oils
NT4 Bitter almond oils
NT4 Buchu oils

NT4 Cinnamon oils
NT4 Citronella essential oils
NT4 Citrus essential oils
NT5 Bergamot essential oils
NT6 Bergamot oils
NT5 Bitter orange essential oils
NT5 Citrus oils
NT5 Lemon essential oils
NT5 Lime essential oils
NT5 Neroli oils
NT5 Orange essential oils
NT4 Clary sage essential oils
NT4 Clove oils
NT4 Garlic oils
NT4 Hop essential oils
NT4 Lemongrass oils
NT4 Mint oils
NT4 Nutmeg oils
NT4 Oleoresins
NT4 Oregano oils
NT4 Peppermint essential oils
NT4 Petitgrain oils
NT4 Rosemary essential oils
NT4 Sage essential oils
NT4 Tea tree oils
NT4 Thyme oils
NT3 Evening primrose oils
NT3 Flax seed oils
NT4 Linseed oils
NT3 Grape seed oils
NT3 Jojoba oils
NT3 Kapok oils
NT3 Lupin seed oils
NT3 Meadowfoam oils
NT3 Millet oils
NT3 Mustard seed oils
NT3 Nut oils
NT4 Almond oils
NT4 Beech nut oils
NT4 Brazil nut oils
NT4 Coconut oils
NT4 Groundnut oils
NT4 Hazelnut oils
NT4 Pecan oils
NT4 Walnut oils
NT3 Oat oils
NT3 Olive oils
NT4 Olive oil mills effluents
NT4 Olive pomace oils
NT5 Sansa oils
NT3 Palm oils
NT4 Babassu oils
NT4 Palm kernel oils
NT4 Palm oil mills effluents
NT4 Palm olein
NT4 Palm stearin
NT3 Perilla oils
NT3 Pumpkin seed oils
NT3 Rapeseed oils
NT3 Rice bran oils
NT3 Rice germ oils
NT3 Safflower oils
NT3 Sea buckthorn oils
NT3 Sesame oils
NT3 Soybean oils
NT3 Sunflower oils
NT3 Tea seed oils
NT3 Tomato seed oils
NT3 Wheat germ oils
NT1 Proteins vegetable
NT2 Vegetable proteins
NT3 Arachin
NT3 Carmin
NT3 Conarachin
NT3 Cottonseed proteins
NT3 Cruciferins
NT3 Dioscorin
NT3 Edestin
NT3 Expansins
NT3 Helianthinin
NT3 Leaf proteins
NT3 Lectins
NT4 Concanavalin A
NT4 Haemagglutinins
NT4 Phytohaemagglutinins
NT4 Ricin
NT3 Legume proteins
NT3 Legumin
NT3 Lupin proteins
NT3 Napins
NT3 Oilseed proteins
NT3 Oleosins
NT3 Patatin
NT3 Peanut proteins
NT3 Pea proteins
NT3 Phaseolins
NT3 Plant proteins
NT3 Proteins cereal
NT4 Cereal proteins
NT5 Avenins
NT5 Friabilins
NT5 Gliadins
NT5 Glutelins
NT5 Gluten
NT6 Gluten low foods
NT7 Gluten low bread
NT6 Vital gluten
NT6 Wheat gluten
NT5 Glutenin
NT5 Hordein
NT5 Hordothionins
NT5 Kafirins
NT5 Opaque 2
NT5 Oryzenin
NT5 Prolamins
NT5 Puroindolines
NT5 Purothionin
NT5 Secalins
NT5 Thionins
NT5 Zein
NT3 11S Globulins
NT3 7S Globulins
NT3 Soy proteins
NT4 Conglycinin
NT4 β-Conglycinin
NT4 Glycinin
NT4 Promine
NT4 Soy globulins
NT4 Soy glycinin
NT4 Soy protein concentrates
NT4 Soy 11S globulins
NT4 Soy 7S globulins
NT3 Storage proteins
NT3 Textured vegetable proteins
NT3 Vicilin
NT1 Soy products
NT2 Chungkook-jang
NT2 Doenjang
NT2 Kinema
NT2 Kochujang
NT2 Meju
NT2 Miso
NT2 Natto
NT2 Okara
NT3 Meitauza
NT2 Soybean oils
NT2 Soy beverages
NT3 Soymilk
NT2 Soy cheese
NT2 Soy curd
NT2 Soy ice cream
NT2 Soy infant formulas
NT2 Soy lecithins
NT2 Soy meal
NT2 Soy pastes
NT2 Soy purees
NT2 Soy sauces
NT3 Kanjang
NT3 Kecap
NT3 Shoyu
NT2 Soy yoghurt
NT2 Tempeh
NT2 Tofu
NT3 Sufu
NT2 Yuba
NT1 Vegetable burgers
NT1 Vegetable juices
NT2 Cabbage juices
NT2 Carrot juices
NT2 Vegetable juice concentrates
NT2 Vegetable nectars
NT1 Vegetable pickles
NT2 Cucumber pickles
NT2 Narazuke
NT2 Pickled onions
NT1 Vegetable preserves
NT1 Vegetable pulps
NT2 Carrot pulps
NT1 Vegetable purees
NT2 Potato purees
NT2 Soy purees
NT1 Vegetable salads
NT2 Potato salads
NT1 Vegetable soups
RT Pickles
RT Salads

Vegetable proteins
SN index heading is Proteins vegetable
BT1 Proteins vegetable
BT2 Proteins
BT3 Nutrients
BT2 Vegetable products
BT3 Plant foods
BT4 Foods
NT1 Arachin
NT1 Carmin
NT1 Conarachin
NT1 Cottonseed proteins
NT1 Cruciferins
NT1 Dioscorin
NT1 Edestin
NT1 Expansins
NT1 Helianthinin
NT1 Leaf proteins

NT1 Lectins
NT2 Concanavalin A
NT2 Haemagglutinins
NT2 Phytohaemagglutinins
NT2 Ricin
NT1 Legume proteins
NT1 Legumin
NT1 Lupin proteins
NT1 Napins
NT1 Oilseed proteins
NT1 Oleosins
NT1 Patatin
NT1 Peanut proteins
NT1 Pea proteins
NT1 Phaseolins
NT1 Plant proteins
NT1 Proteins cereal
NT2 Cereal proteins
NT3 Avenins
NT3 Friabilins
NT3 Gliadins
NT3 Glutelins
NT3 Gluten
NT4 Gluten low foods
NT5 Gluten low bread
NT4 Vital gluten
NT4 Wheat gluten
NT3 Glutenin
NT3 Hordein
NT3 Hordothionins
NT3 Kafirins
NT3 Opaque 2
NT3 Oryzenin
NT3 Prolamins
NT3 Puroindolines
NT3 Purothionin
NT3 Secalins
NT3 Thionins
NT3 Zein
NT1 11S Globulins
NT1 7S Globulins
NT1 Soy proteins
NT2 Conglycinin
NT2 β-Conglycinin
NT2 Glycinin
NT2 Promine
NT2 Soy globulins
NT2 Soy glycinin
NT2 Soy protein concentrates
NT2 Soy 11S globulins
NT2 Soy 7S globulins
NT1 Storage proteins
NT1 Textured vegetable proteins
NT1 Vicilin

Vegetable pulps
BT1 Pulps
BT2 Processed foods
BT3 Foods
BT1 Vegetable products
BT2 Plant foods
BT3 Foods
NT1 Carrot pulps

Vegetable purees
BT1 Purees
BT2 Pulps
BT3 Processed foods
BT4 Foods
BT1 Vegetable products
BT2 Plant foods
BT3 Foods
NT1 Potato purees
NT1 Soy purees

Vegetable rennets
BT1 Rennets
BT2 Milk clotting enzymes
BT3 Enzymes milk clotting
BT4 Proteinases
BT5 Hydrolases
BT6 Enzymes

Vegetables
SN use for vegetables in general
BT1 Crops
BT2 Plants
BT1 Plant foods
BT2 Foods
NT1 Dried vegetables
NT2 Dried peas
NT1 Vegetables specific
NT2 *Allium*
NT2 *Amaranthus*
NT2 Anu
NT2 Arracacha
NT2 Arrowhead
NT2 Artichokes
NT2 Asparagus
NT2 Aubergines
NT2 Avocados
NT3 Guacamole
NT2 Bamboo
NT3 Bamboo shoots
NT2 Baobab
NT2 Beets
NT3 Beetroots
NT4 Beetroot juices
NT3 Red beets
NT2 Black salsify
NT2 Borage
NT2 Boxthorn
NT2 *Brassica*
NT3 *Brassica carinata*
NT3 *Brassica napus*
NT3 *Brassica oleracea*
NT2 Broccoli
NT2 Brussels sprouts
NT2 Burdock
NT2 Butterbur
NT2 Cabbages
NT3 Red cabbages
NT3 Sauerkraut
NT3 Savoy cabbages
NT3 White cabbages
NT2 Canna
NT3 Canna starch
NT2 Capsicums
NT3 Bell peppers
NT3 *Capsicum annuum*
NT3 Chillies
NT4 Jalapeno peppers
NT4 Red chillies
NT3 Green peppers
NT3 Hot peppers
NT3 Kochujang
NT3 Peppers
NT3 Pimento peppers
NT4 Pimiento peppers
NT3 Red peppers
NT3 Sweet peppers
NT2 Cardoons
NT3 *Cynara cardunculus*
NT2 Carrots
NT3 Carrot chips
NT3 Carrot pulps
NT2 Cassava
NT3 Attieke
NT3 Cassava chips
NT3 Cassava meal
NT3 Cassava starch
NT4 Tapioca
NT3 Gari
NT3 Koko
NT3 Manioc
NT3 Tape
NT4 Tape ketan
NT3 Uji
NT2 Cauliflowers
NT2 Celeriac
NT2 Celery
NT2 Ceylon spinach
NT2 Chayote
NT2 Chicory (vegetables)
NT2 Chinese cabbages
NT3 Pak choi
NT2 Chinese chives
NT2 Chinese water chestnuts
NT2 Chufa nuts
NT3 Tigernuts
NT4 *Cyperus esculentus*
NT2 Cocoyams
NT2 *Corchorus olitorius*
NT2 Courgettes
NT2 Cress
NT2 Cruciferae
NT2 Cucumbers
NT3 Cucumber pickles
NT2 Cucurbitaceae
NT2 *Curcuma*
NT2 Dandelions
NT2 Edible flowers
NT3 Day lilies
NT3 Marigolds
NT2 Elephant yams
NT3 Konjac glucomannans
NT2 Endives
NT2 *Eruca sativa*
NT2 Ewedu
NT2 Exotic vegetables
NT2 Fennel
NT2 Fenugreek
NT2 Fungi edible
NT3 Edible fungi
NT4 *Agaricus*
NT5 *Agaricus bisporus*
NT5 *Agaricus blazei*
NT4 *Agrocybe*
NT4 *Amanita*
NT5 *Amanita phalloides*
NT4 *Armillaria*
NT5 *Armillaria mellea*
NT4 *Auricularia*
NT5 *Auricularia auricula*
NT5 *Auricularia polytricha*
NT4 *Boletus*
NT5 *Boletus edulis*
NT4 *Calocybe*
NT4 *Cantharellus*

NT4 Champignons
NT4 *Coprinus*
NT5 *Coprinus comatus*
NT4 *Cordyceps*
NT5 *Cordyceps militaris*
NT5 *Cordyceps sinensis*
NT4 *Flammulina*
NT5 *Flammulina velutipes*
NT4 *Ganoderma*
NT5 *Ganoderma applanatum*
NT5 *Ganoderma lucidum*
NT4 *Grifola frondosa*
NT4 *Gyromitra*
NT4 *Hericium erinaceus*
NT4 Huitlacoche
NT4 *Hydnum*
NT4 *Lactarius*
NT4 *Leccinum*
NT4 *Lentinula edodes*
NT4 *Lentinus*
NT4 *Lepista*
NT5 *Lepista nuda*
NT4 *Lycoperdon*
NT4 *Morchella*
NT5 *Morchella esculenta*
NT4 Mushrooms
NT5 Wild mushrooms
NT4 *Phellinus linteus*
NT4 *Pholiota*
NT4 *Pleurotus*
NT5 *Pleurotus citrinopileatus*
NT5 *Pleurotus eryngii*
NT5 *Pleurotus florida*
NT5 *Pleurotus ostreatus*
NT5 *Pleurotus sajor-caju*
NT5 *Pleurotus tuberregium*
NT4 *Poria cocos*
NT4 *Russula*
NT4 *Sarcodon aspratus*
NT4 *Sarcodon imbricatum*
NT4 *Schizophyllum*
NT5 *Schizophyllum commune*
NT4 Straw mushrooms
NT4 *Terfezia*
NT4 *Termitomyces*
NT4 *Tricholoma*
NT5 *Tricholoma matsutake*
NT4 *Tuber*
NT5 Black truffles
NT5 White truffles
NT4 *Volvariella*
NT5 *Volvariella volvacea*
NT4 *Xerocomus*
NT2 Gherkins
NT2 Globe artichokes
NT2 Godulbaegi
NT2 Gourds
NT3 *Benincasa hispida*
NT3 Bitter gourds
NT3 Buffalo gourds
NT3 Wax gourds
NT2 Green vegetables
NT2 *Houttuynia cordata*
NT2 Indian spinach
NT3 *Basella*
NT2 Jerusalem artichokes
NT2 Jicama
NT2 Kale
NT2 Kohlrabi
NT2 Komatsuna
NT2 Kudzu
NT2 Leafy vegetables
NT2 Leeks
NT2 Legumes
NT3 Adzuki beans
NT3 African oil beans
NT4 Ugba
NT3 African yam beans
NT3 Alfalfa
NT4 Alfalfa seeds
NT4 Lucerne
NT4 *Medicago sativa*
NT3 American groundnuts
NT3 Asparagus beans
NT3 Asparagus peas
NT3 Bambara groundnuts
NT3 Beach peas
NT4 *Lathyrus maritimus*
NT3 Beans
NT4 Bean curd
NT4 Bean pastes
NT3 Black gram
NT4 Dosai
NT3 Carob beans
NT3 Carob pods
NT3 *Cassia* seeds
NT3 Chick peas
NT4 Bengal gram
NT5 Boondi
NT4 Humous
NT3 Common beans
NT4 Anasazi
NT4 Black beans
NT4 Dry beans
NT4 French beans
NT4 Green beans
NT4 Haricot beans
NT5 Baked beans
NT4 Kidney beans
NT4 Navy beans
NT4 Pea beans
NT4 Pinto beans
NT4 Pole beans
NT4 Snap beans
NT4 String beans
NT4 Wax beans
NT4 White beans
NT3 Cowpeas
NT4 Akara
NT4 Blackeyed peas
NT4 Cowpea meal
NT4 Moinmoin
NT4 Southern peas
NT3 *Detarium microcarpum*
NT3 Dhal
NT3 Dhokla
NT3 Djenkol beans
NT3 Faba beans
NT4 Broad beans
NT4 Field beans
NT4 Horse beans
NT3 Grass peas
NT3 Groundbeans
NT3 Guar beans
NT4 Cluster beans
NT3 Horse gram
NT3 Idli
NT3 Jack beans
NT4 *Canavalia ensiformis*
NT3 Kawal
NT3 Koji
NT4 Rice koji
NT3 Lablab beans
NT3 Legume meal
NT3 Legume proteins
NT3 Legume sprouts
NT4 Alfalfa sprouts
NT4 Bean sprouts
NT4 Soybean sprouts
NT3 Legume starch
NT3 Lentils
NT3 *Leucaena*
NT3 Lima beans
NT3 Lupins
NT4 Lupin proteins
NT4 White lupins
NT3 Mesquite pods
NT3 Moth beans
NT3 Mung beans
NT4 Mung bean starch
NT3 Peas
NT4 Dried peas
NT4 Field peas
NT4 Green peas
NT4 Pea meal
NT4 Pea protein concentrates
NT4 Pea proteins
NT4 Pea starch
NT4 Snow peas
NT3 Pigeon peas
NT3 Pulses
NT3 Red beans
NT3 Rice beans
NT3 Runner beans
NT3 Siljo
NT3 Soybeans
NT4 Black soybeans
NT4 Soybean sprouts
NT3 Sword beans
NT4 *Canavalia gladiata*
NT3 Tepary beans
NT3 Velvet beans
NT3 Vetch seeds
NT3 Winged beans
NT3 Yam beans
NT4 *Pachyrhizus ahipa*
NT2 Lettuces
NT2 Lily bulbs
NT2 Lotus roots
NT2 Maca
NT2 Marrows
NT2 *Moringa*
NT2 Mustard greens
NT3 Ethiopian mustard
NT4 *Brassica carinata*
NT3 Indian mustard
NT2 Nettles
NT2 Oca
NT3 *Oxalis tuberosa*
NT2 Okra
NT2 Onions
NT3 Pickled onions
NT3 Red onions
NT2 Palm hearts
NT2 Parsnips
NT2 Perilla

NT2 Potatoes
NT3 Potato peel
NT3 Potato products
NT4 French fries
NT4 Gnocchi
NT4 Mashed potatoes
NT4 Pommes frites
NT4 Potato chips
NT4 Potato crisps
NT4 Potato flakes
NT4 Potato granules
NT4 Potato meal
NT4 Potato purees
NT4 Potato salads
NT4 Potato starch
NT3 *Solanum tuberosum*
NT2 Pumpkins
NT3 Fluted pumpkins
NT2 Purslane
NT2 Radishes
NT3 Dongchimi
NT3 Japanese radishes
NT3 Kakdugi
NT3 Radish sprouts
NT2 Rakkyo
NT2 Rhubarb
NT2 Rocket
NT2 Root crops
NT2 Root vegetables
NT2 Salad vegetables
NT2 Salsify
NT2 Scallion
NT2 Sea kale
NT2 *Sesbania*
NT2 Shallots
NT2 Shoti
NT2 *Solanum*
NT2 Spinach
NT2 Sprouts
NT3 Legume sprouts
NT4 Alfalfa sprouts
NT4 Bean sprouts
NT4 Soybean sprouts
NT3 Radish sprouts
NT2 Squashes
NT3 *Cucurbita moschata*
NT2 Swedes
NT2 Sweetcorn
NT2 Sweet potatoes
NT3 Sweet potato starch
NT2 Swiss chard
NT3 Leaf beet
NT2 Tania
NT2 Taro
NT3 Poi
NT2 Tubers
NT2 Turnips
NT2 Ulluco
NT2 Vine leaves
NT2 Water chestnuts
NT2 Water convolvulus
NT2 Watercress
NT2 Water dropwort
NT2 Water spinach
NT2 Welsh onions
NT2 White mustard
NT2 Wild cabbage
NT2 Wild rice
NT2 Yacon
NT2 Yams
NT3 Amala
NT3 Yam meal
NT3 Yam starch
NT2 Yellow mustard
NT2 Zedoary
NT3 *Curcuma zedoaria*
NT1 Wild vegetables

Vegetable salads
BT1 Salads
BT1 Vegetable products
BT2 Plant foods
BT3 Foods
NT1 Potato salads

Vegetable soups
HN introduced from vol. 39, issue 1 (2007)
BT1 Soups
BT2 Processed foods
BT3 Foods
BT1 Vegetable products
BT2 Plant foods
BT3 Foods

Vegetables specific
SN use for specific types of vegetable
BT1 Vegetables
BT2 Crops
BT3 Plants
BT2 Plant foods
BT3 Foods
NT1 *Allium*
NT1 *Amaranthus*
NT1 Anu
NT1 Arracacha
NT1 Arrowhead
NT1 Artichokes
NT1 Asparagus
NT1 Aubergines
NT1 Avocados
NT2 Guacamole
NT1 Bamboo
NT2 Bamboo shoots
NT1 Baobab
NT1 Beets
NT2 Beetroots
NT3 Beetroot juices
NT2 Red beets
NT1 Black salsify
NT1 Borage
NT1 Boxthorn
NT1 *Brassica*
NT2 *Brassica carinata*
NT2 *Brassica napus*
NT2 *Brassica oleracea*
NT1 Broccoli
NT1 Brussels sprouts
NT1 Burdock
NT1 Butterbur
NT1 Cabbages
NT2 Red cabbages
NT2 Sauerkraut
NT2 Savoy cabbages
NT2 White cabbages
NT1 Canna
NT2 Canna starch
NT1 Capsicums
NT2 Bell peppers
NT2 *Capsicum annuum*
NT2 Chillies
NT3 Jalapeno peppers
NT3 Red chillies
NT2 Green peppers
NT2 Hot peppers
NT2 Kochujang
NT2 Peppers
NT2 Pimento peppers
NT3 Pimiento peppers
NT2 Red peppers
NT2 Sweet peppers
NT1 Cardoons
NT2 *Cynara cardunculus*
NT1 Carrots
NT2 Carrot chips
NT2 Carrot pulps
NT1 Cassava
NT2 Attieke
NT2 Cassava chips
NT2 Cassava meal
NT2 Cassava starch
NT3 Tapioca
NT2 Gari
NT2 Koko
NT2 Manioc
NT2 Tape
NT3 Tape ketan
NT2 Uji
NT1 Cauliflowers
NT1 Celeriac
NT1 Celery
NT1 Ceylon spinach
NT1 Chayote
NT1 Chicory (vegetables)
NT1 Chinese cabbages
NT2 Pak choi
NT1 Chinese chives
NT1 Chinese water chestnuts
NT1 Chufa nuts
NT2 Tigernuts
NT3 *Cyperus esculentus*
NT1 Cocoyams
NT1 *Corchorus olitorius*
NT1 Courgettes
NT1 Cress
NT1 Cruciferae
NT1 Cucumbers
NT2 Cucumber pickles
NT1 Cucurbitaceae
NT1 *Curcuma*
NT1 Dandelions
NT1 Edible flowers
NT2 Day lilies
NT2 Marigolds
NT1 Elephant yams
NT2 Konjac glucomannans
NT1 Endives
NT1 *Eruca sativa*
NT1 Ewedu
NT1 Exotic vegetables
NT1 Fennel
NT1 Fenugreek
NT1 Fungi edible
NT2 Edible fungi
NT3 *Agaricus*
NT4 *Agaricus bisporus*
NT4 *Agaricus blazei*
NT3 *Agrocybe*

NT3 *Amanita*
NT4 *Amanita phalloides*
NT3 *Armillaria*
NT4 *Armillaria mellea*
NT3 *Auricularia*
NT4 *Auricularia auricula*
NT4 *Auricularia polytricha*
NT3 *Boletus*
NT4 *Boletus edulis*
NT3 *Calocybe*
NT3 *Cantharellus*
NT3 Champignons
NT3 *Coprinus*
NT4 *Coprinus comatus*
NT3 *Cordyceps*
NT4 *Cordyceps militaris*
NT4 *Cordyceps sinensis*
NT3 *Flammulina*
NT4 *Flammulina velutipes*
NT3 *Ganoderma*
NT4 *Ganoderma applanatum*
NT4 *Ganoderma lucidum*
NT3 *Grifola frondosa*
NT3 *Gyromitra*
NT3 *Hericium erinaceus*
NT3 Huitlacoche
NT3 *Hydnum*
NT3 *Lactarius*
NT3 *Leccinum*
NT3 *Lentinula edodes*
NT3 *Lentinus*
NT3 *Lepista*
NT4 *Lepista nuda*
NT3 *Lycoperdon*
NT3 *Morchella*
NT4 *Morchella esculenta*
NT3 Mushrooms
NT4 Wild mushrooms
NT3 *Phellinus linteus*
NT3 *Pholiota*
NT3 *Pleurotus*
NT4 *Pleurotus citrinopileatus*
NT4 *Pleurotus eryngii*
NT4 *Pleurotus florida*
NT4 *Pleurotus ostreatus*
NT4 *Pleurotus sajor-caju*
NT4 *Pleurotus tuberregium*
NT3 *Poria cocos*
NT3 *Russula*
NT3 *Sarcodon aspratus*
NT3 *Sarcodon imbricatum*
NT3 *Schizophyllum*
NT4 *Schizophyllum commune*
NT3 Straw mushrooms
NT3 *Terfezia*
NT3 *Termitomyces*
NT3 *Tricholoma*
NT4 *Tricholoma matsutake*
NT3 *Tuber*
NT4 Black truffles
NT4 White truffles
NT3 *Volvariella*
NT4 *Volvariella volvacea*
NT3 *Xerocomus*
NT1 Gherkins
NT1 Globe artichokes
NT1 Godulbaegi
NT1 Gourds
NT2 *Benincasa hispida*
NT2 Bitter gourds
NT2 Buffalo gourds
NT2 Wax gourds
NT1 Green vegetables
NT1 *Houttuynia cordata*
NT1 Indian spinach
NT2 *Basella*
NT1 Jerusalem artichokes
NT1 Jicama
NT1 Kale
NT1 Kohlrabi
NT1 Komatsuna
NT1 Kudzu
NT1 Leafy vegetables
NT1 Leeks
NT1 Legumes
NT2 Adzuki beans
NT2 African oil beans
NT3 Ugba
NT2 African yam beans
NT2 Alfalfa
NT3 Alfalfa seeds
NT3 Lucerne
NT3 *Medicago sativa*
NT2 American groundnuts
NT2 Asparagus beans
NT2 Asparagus peas
NT2 Bambara groundnuts
NT2 Beach peas
NT3 *Lathyrus maritimus*
NT2 Beans
NT3 Bean curd
NT3 Bean pastes
NT2 Black gram
NT3 Dosai
NT2 Carob beans
NT2 Carob pods
NT2 *Cassia* seeds
NT2 Chick peas
NT3 Bengal gram
NT4 Boondi
NT3 Humous
NT2 Common beans
NT3 Anasazi
NT3 Black beans
NT3 Dry beans
NT3 French beans
NT3 Green beans
NT3 Haricot beans
NT4 Baked beans
NT3 Kidney beans
NT3 Navy beans
NT3 Pea beans
NT3 Pinto beans
NT3 Pole beans
NT3 Snap beans
NT3 String beans
NT3 Wax beans
NT3 White beans
NT2 Cowpeas
NT3 Akara
NT3 Blackeyed peas
NT3 Cowpea meal
NT3 Moinmoin
NT3 Southern peas
NT2 *Detarium microcarpum*
NT2 Dhal
NT2 Dhokla
NT2 Djenkol beans
NT2 Faba beans
NT3 Broad beans
NT3 Field beans
NT3 Horse beans
NT2 Grass peas
NT2 Groundbeans
NT2 Guar beans
NT3 Cluster beans
NT2 Horse gram
NT2 Idli
NT2 Jack beans
NT3 *Canavalia ensiformis*
NT2 Kawal
NT2 Koji
NT3 Rice koji
NT2 Lablab beans
NT2 Legume meal
NT2 Legume proteins
NT2 Legume sprouts
NT3 Alfalfa sprouts
NT3 Bean sprouts
NT3 Soybean sprouts
NT2 Legume starch
NT2 Lentils
NT2 *Leucaena*
NT2 Lima beans
NT2 Lupins
NT3 Lupin proteins
NT3 White lupins
NT2 Mesquite pods
NT2 Moth beans
NT2 Mung beans
NT3 Mung bean starch
NT2 Peas
NT3 Dried peas
NT3 Field peas
NT3 Green peas
NT3 Pea meal
NT3 Pea protein concentrates
NT3 Pea proteins
NT3 Pea starch
NT3 Snow peas
NT2 Pigeon peas
NT2 Pulses
NT2 Red beans
NT2 Rice beans
NT2 Runner beans
NT2 Siljo
NT2 Soybeans
NT3 Black soybeans
NT3 Soybean sprouts
NT2 Sword beans
NT3 *Canavalia gladiata*
NT2 Tepary beans
NT2 Velvet beans
NT2 Vetch seeds
NT2 Winged beans
NT2 Yam beans
NT3 *Pachyrhizus ahipa*
NT1 Lettuces
NT1 Lily bulbs
NT1 Lotus roots
NT1 Maca
NT1 Marrows
NT1 *Moringa*
NT1 Mustard greens
NT2 Ethiopian mustard
NT3 *Brassica carinata*
NT2 Indian mustard

NT1 Nettles
NT1 Oca
NT2 *Oxalis tuberosa*
NT1 Okra
NT1 Onions
NT2 Pickled onions
NT2 Red onions
NT1 Palm hearts
NT1 Parsnips
NT1 Perilla
NT1 Potatoes
NT2 Potato peel
NT2 Potato products
NT3 French fries
NT3 Gnocchi
NT3 Mashed potatoes
NT3 Pommes frites
NT3 Potato chips
NT3 Potato crisps
NT3 Potato flakes
NT3 Potato granules
NT3 Potato meal
NT3 Potato purees
NT3 Potato salads
NT3 Potato starch
NT2 *Solanum tuberosum*
NT1 Pumpkins
NT2 Fluted pumpkins
NT1 Purslane
NT1 Radishes
NT2 Dongchimi
NT2 Japanese radishes
NT2 Kakdugi
NT2 Radish sprouts
NT1 Rakkyo
NT1 Rhubarb
NT1 Rocket
NT1 Root crops
NT1 Root vegetables
NT1 Salad vegetables
NT1 Salsify
NT1 Scallion
NT1 Sea kale
NT1 *Sesbania*
NT1 Shallots
NT1 Shoti
NT1 *Solanum*
NT1 Spinach
NT1 Sprouts
NT2 Legume sprouts
NT3 Alfalfa sprouts
NT3 Bean sprouts
NT3 Soybean sprouts
NT2 Radish sprouts
NT1 Squashes
NT2 *Cucurbita moschata*
NT1 Swedes
NT1 Sweetcorn
NT1 Sweet potatoes
NT2 Sweet potato starch
NT1 Swiss chard
NT2 Leaf beet
NT1 Tania
NT1 Taro
NT2 Poi
NT1 Tubers
NT1 Turnips
NT1 Ulluco
NT1 Vine leaves
NT1 Water chestnuts
NT1 Water convolvulus
NT1 Watercress
NT1 Water dropwort
NT1 Water spinach
NT1 Welsh onions
NT1 White mustard
NT1 Wild cabbage
NT1 Wild rice
NT1 Yacon
NT1 Yams
NT2 Amala
NT2 Yam meal
NT2 Yam starch
NT1 Yellow mustard
NT1 Zedoary
NT2 *Curcuma zedoaria*
RT Ferns

Vegetarian diet
BT1 Diet
BT2 Nutrition
RT Vegan diet
RT Vegan foods
RT Vegetarian foods

Vegetarian foods
BT1 Processed foods
BT2 Foods
RT Vegan diet
RT Vegan foods
RT Vegetarian diet

Vehicles
BT1 Transport

Veillonella
BT1 Bacteria
BT2 Microorganisms

Velvet beans
BT1 Legumes
BT2 Vegetables specific
BT3 Vegetables
BT4 Crops
BT5 Plants
BT4 Plant foods
BT5 Foods

Vendace
BT1 Freshwater fish
BT2 Fish
BT3 Animals
BT3 Sea foods
BT4 Aquatic foods
BT5 Animal foods
BT6 Foods
NT1 Coregonus albula

Vending machines
BT1 Marketing
BT2 Economics

Venezuela
BT1 South America
BT2 America

Venison
HN heading from vol. 30 (1998); under Meat specific up to vol. 29 (1997)
BT1 Meat specific
BT2 Meat
BT3 Animal foods
BT4 Foods
NT1 Deer carcasses
RT Deer
UF Deer meat

Ventilation
RT Air

Veratryl alcohol
BT1 Alcohols

Verbascose
HN under Sugars up to vol. 42 (2010)
BT1 Oligosaccharides
BT2 Polysaccharides
BT3 Carbohydrates
BT4 Nutrients
BT4 Organic compounds
BT2 Sugars
BT3 Carbohydrates
BT4 Nutrients
BT4 Organic compounds
BT3 Plant foods
BT4 Foods

Vermicelli
BT1 Pasta
BT2 Cereal products
BT3 Plant foods
BT4 Foods

Vermouths
BT1 Aromatized wines
BT2 Wines
BT3 Alcoholic beverages
BT4 Beverages alcoholic
BT5 Beverages

Vernonia
BT1 Oilseeds
BT2 Seeds
BT3 Plant foods
BT4 Foods

Vero cytotoxins
BT1 Toxins
BT2 Residues
RT Verotoxins

Verotoxins
BT1 Toxins
BT2 Residues
RT *Escherichia*
RT Shiga like toxins
RT Vero cytotoxins

Verrucosidin
BT1 Mycotoxins
BT2 Toxins
BT3 Residues

Verruculogen
BT1 Mycotoxins
BT2 Toxins
BT3 Residues

Versicolorin
BT1 Mycotoxins

BT2 Toxins
BT3 Residues

Verticillium
BT1 Fungi
BT2 Microorganisms

Vessels
BT1 Containers

Vetch seeds
BT1 Legumes
BT2 Vegetables specific
BT3 Vegetables
BT4 Crops
BT5 Plants
BT4 Plant foods
BT5 Foods

Veterinary inspection
BT1 Quality control
BT2 Technology

Viability
HN introduced from vol. 39, issue 1 (2007)
BT1 Physiology
BT2 Science

Vibration

Vibrio
BT1 Bacteria
BT2 Microorganisms
NT1 *Vibrio alginolyticus*
NT1 *Vibrio cholerae*
NT1 *Vibrio fischeri*
NT1 *Vibrio lentus*
NT1 *Vibrio metschnikovii*
NT1 *Vibrio mimicus*
NT1 *Vibrio parahaemolyticus*
NT1 *Vibrio vulnificus*
RT Cholera

Vibrio alginolyticus
HN introduced from vol. 39, issue 1 (2007)
BT1 *Vibrio*
BT2 Bacteria
BT3 Microorganisms

Vibrio cholerae
BT1 *Vibrio*
BT2 Bacteria
BT3 Microorganisms

Vibrio fischeri
BT1 *Vibrio*
BT2 Bacteria
BT3 Microorganisms

Vibrio lentus
BT1 *Vibrio*
BT2 Bacteria
BT3 Microorganisms

Vibrio metschnikovii
BT1 *Vibrio*
BT2 Bacteria
BT3 Microorganisms

Vibrio mimicus
BT1 *Vibrio*
BT2 Bacteria
BT3 Microorganisms

Vibrio parahaemolyticus
BT1 *Vibrio*
BT2 Bacteria
BT3 Microorganisms

Vibrio vulnificus
BT1 *Vibrio*
BT2 Bacteria
BT3 Microorganisms

Vicilin
BT1 Globulins
BT2 Proteins
BT3 Nutrients
BT1 Vegetable proteins
BT2 Proteins vegetable
BT3 Proteins
BT4 Nutrients
BT3 Vegetable products
BT4 Plant foods
BT5 Foods

Vicine
BT1 Glycosides
BT2 Carbohydrates
BT3 Nutrients
BT3 Organic compounds
RT Antinutritional factors
RT Convicine

Video image analysis
BT1 Analytical techniques

Vienna sausages
BT1 Sausages
BT2 Meat products
BT3 Animal foods
BT4 Foods

Vietnam
BT1 Asia

Vinasse
BT1 Effluents
BT2 Waste water
BT3 Wastes
BT3 Water

Vinclozolin
BT1 Dicarboximide fungicides
BT2 Fungicides
BT3 Pesticides
BT4 Biocides
BT4 Residues
UF Ronilan

Vinegar
BT1 Condiments
BT2 Flavourings
BT3 Additives
BT1 Fermented foods
BT2 Processed foods
BT3 Foods
NT1 Balsamic vinegar
NT1 Cider vinegar
NT1 Fruit vinegars
NT2 Apple vinegar
NT1 Malt vinegar
NT1 Rice vinegar
NT1 Wine vinegar
RT Acetic acid

Vine leaves
BT1 Vegetables specific
BT2 Vegetables
BT3 Crops
BT4 Plants
BT3 Plant foods
BT4 Foods

Vines
RT Grapes

Viniculture
BT1 Cultivation
BT2 Agriculture
BT1 Winemaking
BT2 Processing
BT3 Technology

Vinification
USE **Winemaking**

Vintage
HN introduced from vol. 39, issue 1 (2007)
BT1 Winemaking
BT2 Processing
BT3 Technology

Vinyl chloride
BT1 Polyvinyl chloride
BT2 Plastics
BT3 Packaging materials

Vinylidene chloride
BT1 Plastics
BT2 Packaging materials

Violaxanthin
BT1 Xanthophylls
BT2 Carotenoids
BT3 Pigments
BT3 Terpenoids
BT4 Lipids
BT5 Nutrients

Vioxan
USE **Carbaryl**

Virginiamycin
BT1 Antibiotics
BT2 Drugs
BT3 Residues

Viriditoxin
BT1 Mycotoxins
BT2 Toxins
BT3 Residues

Virulence
HN heading from vol. 39 (2007)
RT Pathogenesis
RT Pathogenicity
RT Pathogens
RT Quorum sensing
RT Virulence factors

Virulence factors
HN heading from vol. 39 (2007)
NT1 Adherence
NT1 Adhesins
NT1 Aerolysins
NT1 Chemotaxis
NT1 Colonization
NT2 Colonization factors
NT1 Fimbriae
NT1 Flagella
NT1 Flagellins
NT1 Infectivity
NT1 Intimins
NT1 Invasins
NT1 Invasion
NT1 Motility
NT1 Pili
NT1 Pilins
NT1 Porins
NT1 Siderophores
RT Endotoxins
RT Exotoxins
RT Pathogenesis
RT Pathogenicity
RT Pathogens
RT Virulence

Viruses
BT1 Microorganisms
NT1 Adenoviruses
NT2 Mastadenovirus
NT3 Human adenovirus
NT1 Antiviral activity
NT1 Apthovirus
NT2 Foot and mouth disease virus
NT1 Astroviruses
NT2 Mamastrovirus
NT3 Human astrovirus
NT1 Bacteriophages
NT2 Bacteriophages resistance
NT2 Coliphages
NT1 Caliciviruses
NT2 Noroviruses
NT3 Norovirus
NT4 Norwalk virus
NT5 Norwalk-like virus
NT5 Small round structured virus
NT2 Sapoviruses
NT3 Sapovirus
NT4 Sapporo virus
NT1 Coronavirus
NT1 Coxsackieviruses
NT1 Enteric viruses
NT1 Enterovirus
NT2 Echovirus
NT2 Human enterovirus
NT3 Human coxsackievirus
NT2 Poliovirus
NT1 Hepatitis viruses
NT2 Hepatovirus
NT3 Hepatitis A virus
NT2 Hepevirus
NT3 Hepatitis E virus
NT1 Herpesviruses
NT1 Kobuvirus
NT2 Aichi virus
NT1 Lentivirus
NT2 Bovine immunodeficiency virus
NT2 Human immunodeficiency virus
NT1 Orthopoxvirus
NT2 Vaccinia virus
NT1 Parvoviruses
NT2 Parvovirus
NT1 Rotaviruses
NT2 Rotavirus
RT Prokaryotes

Viscera
BT1 Wastes
RT Evisceration
RT Gutting

Viscoelasticity
BT1 Rheological properties
BT2 Mechanical properties
BT3 Physical properties

Viscometers
BT1 Viscosity
BT2 Rheological properties
BT3 Mechanical properties
BT4 Physical properties

Viscometry
BT1 Analytical techniques

Viscosity
BT1 Rheological properties
BT2 Mechanical properties
BT3 Physical properties
NT1 Viscometers
RT Consistency

Vision
HN introduced from vol. 42, issue 1 (2010)
BT1 Human physiology
BT2 Physiology
BT3 Science
RT Eye disorders
RT Eye health

Vision systems
BT1 Quality control
BT2 Technology

Vital gluten
BT1 Gluten
BT2 Cereal proteins
BT3 Proteins cereal
BT4 Vegetable proteins
BT5 Proteins vegetable
BT6 Proteins
BT7 Nutrients
BT6 Vegetable products
BT7 Plant foods
BT8 Foods

Vitamers
BT1 Vitamins
BT2 Nutrients

Vitamin A
BT1 Retinoids
BT2 Vitamins
BT3 Nutrients
RT Retinol
RT Retinols

Vitamin antagonists
BT1 Antinutritional factors
BT2 Nutritional values
RT Vitamins
UF Antivitamins

Vitamin B_1
HN used in the index up to vol. 35, issue 6 (2003)
USE **Thiamin**

Vitamin B_{12}
SN syn. cyanocobalamin
BT1 Cyanocobalamin
BT2 Corrinoids
BT3 Vitamin B group
BT4 Vitamins
BT5 Nutrients
RT Cobalamins

Vitamin B_{13}
HN used in the index up to vol. 35, issue 6 (2003)
USE **Orotic acid**

Vitamin B_2
HN used in the index up to vol. 35, issue 6 (2003)
USE **Riboflavin**

Vitamin B_6
BT1 Vitamin B group
BT2 Vitamins
BT3 Nutrients
NT1 Pyridoxal
NT1 Pyridoxamine
NT1 Pyridoxine

Vitamin B complex
USE **Vitamin B group**

Vitamin B group
HN heading from vol. 25 (1993); under Vitamins B up to vol. 24 (1992)
BT1 Vitamins
BT2 Nutrients
NT1 Biotin
NT1 Cobalamins
NT1 Corrinoids
NT2 Cyanocobalamin
NT3 Vitamin B_{12}
NT1 Folacin
NT1 Folates
NT2 Tetrahydrofolate
NT1 Folic acid
NT1 Nicotinic acid
NT2 Niacin
NT2 Niacinamide
NT2 Nicotinamide
NT2 Nicotinic acid amide
NT1 Pantothenic acid
NT1 Riboflavin
NT1 Thiamin
NT1 Vitamin B_6
NT2 Pyridoxal
NT2 Pyridoxamine
NT2 Pyridoxine
RT Carnitine

UF Vitamin B complex
UF Vitamins B

Vitamin C
BT1 Ascorbic acid
BT2 Antioxidants
BT3 Additives
BT2 Bakery additives
BT3 Additives
BT2 Vitamins
BT3 Nutrients

Vitamin D
BT1 Vitamins
BT2 Nutrients

Vitamin D_2
SN syn. ercalciol; syn. ergocalciferol
BT1 Vitamins
BT2 Nutrients
UF Calciferol

Vitamin D_3
SN syn. cholecalciferol; syn. calciol
BT1 Cholecalciferol
BT2 Vitamins
BT3 Nutrients

Vitamin E
BT1 Antioxidants
BT2 Additives
BT1 Terpenoids
BT2 Lipids
BT3 Nutrients
BT1 Vitamins
BT2 Nutrients
NT1 Tocols
NT2 Tocopherols
NT3 α-Tocopherol
NT3 Tocotrienol
NT3 Vitamin E acetate

Vitamin E acetate
BT1 Acetates
BT1 Esters
BT2 Organic compounds
BT1 Tocopherols
BT2 Tocols
BT3 Vitamin E
BT4 Antioxidants
BT5 Additives
BT4 Terpenoids
BT5 Lipids
BT6 Nutrients
BT4 Vitamins
BT5 Nutrients
UF α-Tocopherol acetate
UF α-Tocopheryl acetate

Vitamin F
HN used in the index up to vol. 35, issue 6 (2003)
USE **Thiamin**

Vitamin G
HN used in the index up to vol. 35, issue 6 (2003)
USE **Riboflavin**

Vitamin H
HN used in the index up to vol. 35, issue 6 (2003)
USE **Biotin**

Vitamin K
BT1 Vitamins
BT2 Nutrients

Vitamin K_1
HN used in the index up to vol. 35, issue 6 (2003)
USE **Phylloquinone**

Vitamin K_3
HN used in the index up to vol. 35, issue 6 (2003)
USE **Menadione**

Vitamin K_2 series
HN used in the index up to vol. 35, issue 6 (2003)
USE **Menaquinones**

Vitamin P
HN used in the index up to vol. 35, issue 6 (2003)
USE **Bioflavonoids**

Vitamin PP
HN used in the index up to vol. 35, issue 6 (2003)
USE **Niacin**

Vitamins
BT1 Nutrients
NT1 Ascorbic acid
NT2 Dehydroascorbic acid
NT2 Vitamin C
NT1 Cholecalciferol
NT2 Vitamin D_3
NT1 Ergocalciferol
NT1 Menadione
NT1 Menaquinones
NT1 Phylloquinone
NT1 Retinoids
NT2 Retinal
NT2 Retinoic acid
NT2 Retinol
NT2 Retinols
NT2 Retinyl palmitate
NT2 Vitamin A
NT1 Vitamers
NT1 Vitamin B group
NT2 Biotin
NT2 Cobalamins
NT2 Corrinoids
NT3 Cyanocobalamin
NT4 Vitamin B_{12}
NT2 Folacin
NT2 Folates
NT3 Tetrahydrofolate
NT2 Folic acid
NT2 Nicotinic acid
NT3 Niacin
NT3 Niacinamide
NT3 Nicotinamide
NT3 Nicotinic acid amide
NT2 Pantothenic acid
NT2 Riboflavin
NT2 Thiamin
NT2 Vitamin B_6
NT3 Pyridoxal
NT3 Pyridoxamine
NT3 Pyridoxine
NT1 Vitamin D
NT1 Vitamin D_2
NT1 Vitamin E
NT2 Tocols
NT3 Tocopherols
NT4 α-Tocopherol
NT4 Tocotrienol
NT4 Vitamin E acetate
NT1 Vitamin K
RT Micronutrients
RT Vitamin antagonists

Vitamins B
HN heading up to vol. 24 (1992)
USE **Vitamin B group**

Vitamin U
HN used in the index up to vol. 35, issue 6 (2003)
USE ***S*-Methylmethionine**

Vitavax
USE **Carboxin**

Viticulture
BT1 Cultivation
BT2 Agriculture

Vitis vinifera
BT1 Grapes
BT2 Berries
BT3 Fruits specific
BT4 Fruits
BT5 Crops
BT6 Plants
BT5 Plant foods
BT6 Foods

Vitreosity
BT1 Optical properties
BT2 Physical properties

Vitrification
BT1 Processing
BT2 Technology

Vla
BT1 Dairy products
BT2 Animal foods
BT3 Foods

Vocabulary
BT1 Nomenclature

Vodka
BT1 Spirits
BT2 Alcoholic beverages
BT3 Beverages alcoholic
BT4 Beverages

Volatile compounds
NT1 Aroma compounds
NT2 Acetaldehyde
NT3 Ethanal
NT2 Acetals
NT2 Acetoin
NT3 Acetylmethylcarbinol
NT3 3-Hydroxy-2-butanone
NT2 α-Acetolactate
NT2 Acetophenone

NT2 Allicin
NT2 Alliin
NT2 Allyl isothiocyanate
NT2 Allyl sulfides
NT3 Diallyl disulfide
NT2 Amyl alcohol
NT3 Pentanol
NT2 Anethole
NT2 Anisaldehyde
NT2 Anisole
NT2 Benzaldehyde
NT2 Benzothiazole
NT2 Benzyl alcohol
NT2 Benzyl isothiocyanate
NT2 Borneol
NT2 Butanoic acid
NT3 Butyric acid
NT2 Butanol
NT3 Butyl alcohol
NT2 Butanone
NT2 Butyl acetate
NT2 Camphene
NT2 Camphor
NT2 Carvacrol
NT2 Carveol
NT2 Carvone
NT2 Caryophyllene
NT2 Cineole
NT3 Eucalyptol
NT2 Cinnamaldehyde
NT2 Cinnamic acid
NT2 Citral
NT3 Geranial
NT3 Neral
NT2 Citronellal
NT2 Citronellol
NT2 Cuminaldehyde
NT2 Cymene
NT2 Cysteine sulfoxides
NT2 γ-Decalactone
NT2 Decanal
NT2 Decanoic acid
NT3 Capric acid
NT2 Decanol
NT2 Diacetyl
NT3 2,3-Butanedione
NT2 Dill ether
NT2 Dimethyl disulfide
NT2 Dimethyl trisulfide
NT2 Dodecanoic acid
NT3 Lauric acid
NT2 Ethyl acetate
NT2 Ethyl butyrate
NT2 Ethyl caprylate
NT2 Ethyl decanoate
NT2 Ethyl formate
NT2 Ethyl hexanoate
NT3 Ethyl caproate
NT2 Ethyl octanoate
NT2 Ethyl vanillin
NT2 Eugenol
NT2 Farnesene
NT2 Farnesol
NT2 Filbertone
NT2 Furanones
NT3 Furaneol
NT4 2,5-Dimethyl-4-hydroxy-3(2*H*)-furanone
NT3 Sotolon
NT2 Geraniol
NT2 Geranyl acetate
NT2 Gingerols
NT2 Heptanoic acid
NT2 2-Heptanone
NT2 Heptenal
NT2 Hexanal
NT2 Hexanoic acid
NT3 Caproic acid
NT2 Hexanol
NT2 Hexenal
NT2 Hexyl acetate
NT2 Hotrienol
NT2 Humulene
NT2 Isoamyl acetate
NT2 Isoamyl alcohol
NT3 Isopentyl alcohol
NT3 Methyl butanol
NT2 Isobutanol
NT3 Isobutyl alcohol
NT3 Methyl propanol
NT2 Isobutyraldehyde
NT3 2-Methylpropanal
NT2 Isobutyric acid
NT2 Isocaproic acid
NT2 Isovaleric acid
NT2 Lenthionine
NT2 Limonene
NT2 Linalool
NT2 Linalyl acetate
NT2 Maltol
NT2 Menthol
NT2 Menthone
NT2 Methanethiol
NT3 Methyl mercaptan
NT2 Methional
NT2 Methionol
NT2 Methyl benzoate
NT2 3-Methylbutanal
NT3 Isovaleraldehyde
NT2 Myrcene
NT2 Myristicin
NT2 Nerol
NT2 Nonanal
NT2 Nonanone
NT2 Nonenal
NT2 Nootkatone
NT2 Norisoprenoids
NT3 β-Damascenone
NT3 Ionones
NT2 Octanal
NT2 Octanoic acid
NT3 Caprylic acid
NT2 Octanone
NT2 1-Octen-3-ol
NT2 Pentanal
NT3 Valeraldehyde
NT2 Pentanedione
NT3 Acetylacetone
NT2 Pentanoic acid
NT3 Valeric acid
NT2 Phenylacetaldehyde
NT2 Phenylethanol
NT3 Phenethyl alcohol
NT2 Pinenes
NT2 Piperidine
NT2 Piperine
NT2 Propanal
NT3 Propionaldehyde
NT2 Pyrazines
NT2 Safranal
NT2 Safrole
NT2 Terpinene
NT2 Terpineol
NT2 Terpinyl acetate
NT2 Thiazoles
NT2 Thioesters
NT2 Thujone
NT2 Thymol
NT2 Undecanone
NT2 Zingerone
NT1 Butanal
NT1 Butyraldehyde
NT1 Geosmin
NT1 Isoeugenol
NT1 Phenylacetic acid
NT1 Pyridine
NT1 Trichloroanisole
NT1 Volatile fatty acids
NT2 Short chain fatty acids
NT3 Butanoic acid
NT4 Butyric acid
NT3 Hexanoic acid
NT4 Caproic acid
NT3 Hydroxybutyric acid
NT3 Isobutyric acid
NT3 Isocaproic acid
NT3 Isovaleric acid
NT3 Pentanoic acid
NT4 Valeric acid
NT1 Volatile organic compounds
NT1 Volatile sulfur compounds
NT2 Isothiocyanates
NT3 Allyl isothiocyanate
NT3 Benzyl isothiocyanate
NT3 Phenethyl isothiocyanate
NT3 Sulforaphane
NT2 Methanethiol
NT3 Methyl mercaptan
NT2 Thiazoles
NT2 Thiophenes

Volatile fatty acids

HN heading from vol. 43 (2011); under Fatty acids up to vol. 42 (2010); fatty acids volatile also used in the index up to vol. 29 (1997)
SN syn. short chain fatty acids
BT1 Fatty acids
BT2 Lipids
BT3 Nutrients
BT2 Organic acids
BT3 Acids
BT1 Volatile compounds
NT1 Short chain fatty acids
NT2 Butanoic acid
NT3 Butyric acid
NT2 Hexanoic acid
NT3 Caproic acid
NT2 Hydroxybutyric acid
NT2 Isobutyric acid
NT2 Isocaproic acid
NT2 Isovaleric acid
NT2 Pentanoic acid
NT3 Valeric acid
RT Aroma compounds

Volatile organic compounds
BT1 Organic compounds
BT1 Volatile compounds

Volatile sulfur compounds
HN introduced from vol. 39, issue 1 (2007)
BT1 Volatile compounds
NT1 Isothiocyanates
NT2 Allyl isothiocyanate
NT2 Benzyl isothiocyanate
NT2 Phenethyl isothiocyanate
NT2 Sulforaphane
NT1 Methanethiol
NT2 Methyl mercaptan
NT1 Thiazoles
NT1 Thiophenes
RT Aroma compounds

Voltammetry
HN heading from vol. 30 (1998); under Analytical techniques up to vol. 29 (1997)
BT1 Analytical techniques

Volumetric analysis
BT1 Titration
BT2 Analytical techniques

Volvariella
BT1 Edible fungi
BT2 Fungi edible
BT3 Vegetables specific
BT4 Vegetables
BT5 Crops
BT6 Plants
BT5 Plant foods
BT6 Foods
NT1 *Volvariella volvacea*
RT Straw mushrooms
UF Padi straw mushrooms

Volvariella volvacea
BT1 *Volvariella*
BT2 Edible fungi
BT3 Fungi edible
BT4 Vegetables specific
BT5 Vegetables
BT6 Crops
BT7 Plants
BT6 Plant foods
BT7 Foods

Volvatoxins
BT1 Mycotoxins
BT2 Toxins
BT3 Residues

Vomitoxin
SN syn. deoxynivalenol
BT1 Trichothecenes
BT2 Mycotoxins
BT3 Toxins
BT4 Residues

W

W
HN under Minerals up to vol. 42 (2010)
BT1 Metals
BT2 Elements
BT3 Minerals
BT4 Nutrients
UF Tungsten

Wafers
BT1 Bakery products
BT2 Cereal products
BT3 Plant foods
BT4 Foods
NT1 Ice cream wafers

Waffles
BT1 Bakery products
BT2 Cereal products
BT3 Plant foods
BT4 Foods

Wakame
BT1 *Undaria*
BT2 Seaweeds
BT3 Algae
BT4 Microorganisms
BT3 Sea foods
BT4 Aquatic foods
BT5 Animal foods
BT6 Foods
UF Sea mustard
UF Wakami

Wakami
USE **Wakame**

Wales
BT1 United Kingdom
BT2 Europe
BT2 European Union

Wallemia
HN introduced from vol. 43, issue 1 (2011)
BT1 Fungi
BT2 Microorganisms
NT1 *Wallemia sebi*

Wallemia sebi
BT1 *Wallemia*
BT2 Fungi
BT3 Microorganisms

Walleye
BT1 Freshwater fish
BT2 Fish
BT3 Animals
BT3 Sea foods
BT4 Aquatic foods
BT5 Animal foods
BT6 Foods

Walleye pollack
HN under Fish up to vol. 42 (2010)
SN syn. Alaska pollack
BT1 Alaska pollock
BT2 Marine fish
BT3 Fish
BT4 Animals
BT4 Sea foods
BT5 Aquatic foods
BT6 Animal foods
BT7 Foods

Walnut oils
HN introduced from vol. 37, issue 5 (2005)
BT1 Nut oils
BT2 Vegetable oils
BT3 Oils vegetable
BT4 Oils
BT5 Lipids
BT6 Nutrients
BT4 Vegetable products
BT5 Plant foods
BT6 Foods

Walnuts
HN heading from vol. 30 (1998); under Nuts up to vol. 29 (1997)
BT1 Nuts
BT2 Fruits
BT3 Crops
BT4 Plants
BT3 Plant foods
BT4 Foods
BT2 Oilseeds
BT3 Seeds
BT4 Plant foods
BT5 Foods

Walruses
BT1 Animals

Warehouses
BT1 Storage

Warmed over flavour
BT1 Taints
BT2 Flavour
BT3 Sensory properties

Warming
BT1 Heating
BT2 Thermal processing
BT3 Processing thermal
BT4 Processing
BT5 Technology

Wasabi
BT1 Spices
BT2 Flavourings
BT3 Additives

Washing
BT1 Cleaning
BT2 Hygiene
BT2 Processing
BT3 Technology

Wastes
NT1 Bagasse
NT2 Sugar cane bagasse
NT1 Central nervous system tissues
NT2 Brains
NT2 Spinal cord tissues
NT1 Dairies wastes
NT2 Dairies effluents
NT1 Feathers
NT1 Food factories wastes
NT2 Food factories effluents

NT1 Hulls
NT1 Husks
NT1 Pomaces
NT2 Apple pomaces
NT2 Grape pomaces
NT1 Sludges
NT1 Sugar beet pulps
NT1 Viscera
NT1 Waste water
NT2 Effluents
NT3 Breweries effluents
NT3 Dairies effluents
NT3 Distilleries effluents
NT3 Food factories effluents
NT3 Olive oil mills effluents
NT3 Palm oil mills effluents
NT3 Stillage
NT3 Vinasse
RT Biodeterioration
RT Biological oxygen demand
RT By-products
RT Chemical oxygen demand
RT Pollution

Waste water
BT1 Wastes
BT1 Water
NT1 Effluents
NT2 Breweries effluents
NT2 Dairies effluents
NT2 Distilleries effluents
NT2 Food factories effluents
NT2 Olive oil mills effluents
NT2 Palm oil mills effluents
NT2 Stillage
NT2 Vinasse

Water
NT1 Drinking water
NT2 Bottled water
NT2 Potable water
NT2 Well water
NT1 Groundwater
NT1 Lake water
NT1 Mineral waters
NT2 Bottled mineral waters
NT2 Soda water
NT2 Spring waters
NT1 Process water
NT1 Reservoir water
NT1 Sea water
NT1 Tap water
NT1 Waste water
NT2 Effluents
NT3 Breweries effluents
NT3 Dairies effluents
NT3 Distilleries effluents
NT3 Food factories effluents
NT3 Olive oil mills effluents
NT3 Palm oil mills effluents
NT3 Stillage
NT3 Vinasse
NT1 Water hardness
NT1 Water supplies
RT Aqueous two phase systems
RT Humidity
RT Ice
RT Moisture content
RT Water activity
RT Water pollution

Water activity
HN heading from vol. 25 (1993); under Moisture content up to vol. 24 (1992)
SN symbol aw also used in the index
NT1 a_w
NT1 Intermediate moisture foods
NT2 Intermediate moisture pet foods
RT Humidity
RT Moisture content
RT Water

Water binding capacity
BT1 Functional properties
BT2 Physical properties
RT Water holding capacity

Water chestnuts
HN introduced from vol. 39, issue 1 (2007)
SN includes Trapa spp., but not Eleocharis dulcis
BT1 Vegetables specific
BT2 Vegetables
BT3 Crops
BT4 Plants
BT3 Plant foods
BT4 Foods
RT Chinese water chestnuts

Water convolvulus
BT1 Vegetables specific
BT2 Vegetables
BT3 Crops
BT4 Plants
BT3 Plant foods
BT4 Foods

Watercore
BT1 Plant disorders
BT2 Diseases plant
BT3 Diseases

Watercress
BT1 Vegetables specific
BT2 Vegetables
BT3 Crops
BT4 Plants
BT3 Plant foods
BT4 Foods

Water dropwort
BT1 Vegetables specific
BT2 Vegetables
BT3 Crops
BT4 Plants
BT3 Plant foods
BT4 Foods

Waterfowl
BT1 Poultry
BT2 Birds

Water hardness
HN introduced from vol. 39, issue 1 (2007)
BT1 Salts
BT1 Water
RT Hardness

Water holding capacity
BT1 Functional properties
BT2 Physical properties
RT Water binding capacity

Water ices
BT1 Frozen foods
BT2 Processed foods
BT3 Foods
RT Ice lollies

Wateriness
BT1 Sensory properties

Watermelon juices
HN introduced from vol. 41, issue 1 (2009)
BT1 Fruit juices
BT2 Fruit products
BT3 Plant foods
BT4 Foods
BT2 Soft drinks
BT3 Beverages
RT Watermelons

Watermelons
HN heading from vol. 30 (1998); under Fruits specific up to vol. 29 (1997)
BT1 Fruits specific
BT2 Fruits
BT3 Crops
BT4 Plants
BT3 Plant foods
BT4 Foods
NT1 Egusi
RT Watermelon juices

Watermelon seeds
BT1 Oilseeds
BT2 Seeds
BT3 Plant foods
BT4 Foods

Water pollution
BT1 Environmental pollution
BT2 Pollution
BT3 Contamination
RT Water

Water sorption
BT1 Sorption
RT Moisture sorption

Water spinach
HN introduced from vol. 37, issue 5 (2005)
BT1 Vegetables specific
BT2 Vegetables
BT3 Crops
BT4 Plants
BT3 Plant foods
BT4 Foods

Water stress
BT1 Irrigation
BT2 Cultivation
BT3 Agriculture

Water supplies
BT1 Water

Water vapour
BT1 Vapours
BT2 Gases
BT3 Physical phases
BT4 Chemistry
BT5 Science
BT2 Physical phases
BT3 Chemistry
BT4 Science

Wax beans
BT1 Common beans
BT2 Legumes
BT3 Vegetables specific
BT4 Vegetables
BT5 Crops
BT6 Plants
BT5 Plant foods
BT6 Foods

Wax coatings
BT1 Coatings
BT1 Waxes
BT2 Fatty acid esters
BT3 Esters
BT4 Organic compounds

Waxes
BT1 Fatty acid esters
BT2 Esters
BT3 Organic compounds
NT1 Beeswax
NT1 Carnauba wax
NT1 Wax coatings
NT1 Wax esters
RT Coatings
RT Dewaxing
RT Lipids

Wax esters
BT1 Waxes
BT2 Fatty acid esters
BT3 Esters
BT4 Organic compounds

Wax gourds
BT1 Gourds
BT2 Vegetables specific
BT3 Vegetables
BT4 Crops
BT5 Plants
BT4 Plant foods
BT5 Foods

Weaning
BT1 Human physiology
BT2 Physiology
BT3 Science
RT Breast feeding
RT Human lactation

Weaning foods
BT1 Infant foods
BT2 Processed foods
BT3 Foods

Weather
HN introduced from vol. 41, issue 1 (2009)
NT1 Acid rain
RT Climate
RT Environment
RT Season

Weevils
BT1 Insects
BT2 Pests

Weighing
BT1 Weight
BT2 Physical properties

Weighing machines
BT1 Weight
BT2 Physical properties
UF Scales

Weight
BT1 Physical properties
NT1 Weighing
NT1 Weighing machines
NT1 Wt.
RT Density

Weissella
BT1 Bacteria
BT2 Microorganisms
NT1 *Weissella confusa*
NT1 *Weissella kimchii*
NT1 *Weissella paramesenteroides*
NT1 *Weissella viridescens*

Weissella confusa
BT1 *Weissella*
BT2 Bacteria
BT3 Microorganisms

Weissella kimchii
SN synonymous with Weissella cibaria
BT1 *Weissella*
BT2 Bacteria
BT3 Microorganisms

Weissella paramesenteroides
BT1 *Weissella*
BT2 Bacteria
BT3 Microorganisms

Weissella viridescens
SN synonymous with Lactobacillus viridescens
BT1 *Weissella*
BT2 Bacteria
BT3 Microorganisms

Weisswurst
HN introduced from vol. 37, issue 5 (2005)
BT1 Sausages
BT2 Meat products
BT3 Animal foods
BT4 Foods

Well water
BT1 Drinking water
BT2 Water

Welsh onions
BT1 Vegetables specific
BT2 Vegetables
BT3 Crops
BT4 Plants
BT3 Plant foods
BT4 Foods

West Africa
BT1 Africa
NT1 Benin
NT1 Burkina Faso
NT1 Cameroon
NT1 Cape Verde
NT1 Cote d'Ivoire
NT1 Equatorial Guinea
NT2 Bioko
NT1 Gambia
NT1 Ghana
NT1 Guinea
NT1 Guinea-Bissau
NT1 Liberia
NT1 Mali
NT1 Mauritania
NT1 Niger
NT1 Nigeria
NT1 Republic of the Congo
NT1 Senegal
NT1 Sierra Leone
NT1 Togo

West Bank
HN introduced from vol. 39, issue 1 (2007)
BT1 Middle East

Western blotting
BT1 Blotting
BT2 Hybridization
BT3 Genetic techniques
BT4 Genetics

Western Samoa
HN used up to vol. 39, issue 1 (2007)
USE **Samoa**

West Indies
HN under Caribbean from vol. 18 (1986) to vol. 24 (1992)
BT1 America
NT1 Antigua and Barbuda
NT1 Bahamas
NT1 Barbados
NT1 Cayman Islands
NT1 Cuba
NT1 Curacao
NT1 Dominica
NT1 Dominican Republic
NT1 Grenada
NT1 Guadeloupe
NT1 Haiti
NT1 Jamaica
NT1 Martinique
NT1 Puerto Rico
NT1 Trinidad and Tobago
NT1 Windward Islands
UF Caribbean

Wet milling
BT1 Milling
BT2 Processing
BT3 Technology

Wet pet foods
HN introduced from vol. 39, issue 1 (2007)

BT1 Pet foods

Wettability
BT1 Physical properties

Whale carcasses
BT1 Carcasses
BT2 Meat
BT3 Animal foods
BT4 Foods
BT1 Whale meat
BT2 Animals
BT2 Meat specific
BT3 Meat
BT4 Animal foods
BT5 Foods

Whale meat
BT1 Animals
BT1 Meat specific
BT2 Meat
BT3 Animal foods
BT4 Foods
NT1 Whale carcasses

Whale oils
BT1 Marine oils
BT2 Oils
BT3 Lipids
BT4 Nutrients

Whales
BT1 Animals
RT Cetacea

Wheat
BT1 Cereals
BT2 Crops
BT3 Plants
BT2 Seeds
BT3 Plant foods
BT4 Foods
NT1 Atta
NT1 Bulgur
NT1 Durum wheat
NT1 Einkorn
NT1 Emmer
NT1 Maida
NT1 Spelt
NT2 Spelt wheat
NT1 Wheat bran
NT1 Wheat bread
NT1 Wheat breadmaking
NT1 Wheat dough
NT1 Wheat fibre
NT1 Wheat flour
NT1 Wheat germ
NT1 Wheat gluten
NT1 Wheat starch
RT Tritordeum

Wheat beer
BT1 Beer
BT2 Alcoholic beverages
BT3 Beverages alcoholic
BT4 Beverages

Wheat bran
BT1 Bran
BT2 Cereal products
BT3 Plant foods
BT4 Foods
BT1 Wheat
BT2 Cereals
BT3 Crops
BT4 Plants
BT3 Seeds
BT4 Plant foods
BT5 Foods

Wheat bread
BT1 Bread
BT2 Bakery products
BT3 Cereal products
BT4 Plant foods
BT5 Foods
BT1 Wheat
BT2 Cereals
BT3 Crops
BT4 Plants
BT3 Seeds
BT4 Plant foods
BT5 Foods
RT Wheat breadmaking

Wheat breadmaking
BT1 Breadmaking
BT2 Bread
BT3 Bakery products
BT4 Cereal products
BT5 Plant foods
BT6 Foods
BT2 Processing
BT3 Technology
BT1 Wheat
BT2 Cereals
BT3 Crops
BT4 Plants
BT3 Seeds
BT4 Plant foods
BT5 Foods
RT Wheat bread

Wheat dough
BT1 Dough
BT2 Bakery products
BT3 Cereal products
BT4 Plant foods
BT5 Foods
BT1 Wheat
BT2 Cereals
BT3 Crops
BT4 Plants
BT3 Seeds
BT4 Plant foods
BT5 Foods

Wheat fibre
BT1 Fibre
BT1 Wheat
BT2 Cereals
BT3 Crops
BT4 Plants
BT3 Seeds
BT4 Plant foods
BT5 Foods

Wheat flour
BT1 Cereal flours
BT2 Flours cereal
BT3 Cereal products
BT4 Plant foods
BT5 Foods
BT1 Wheat
BT2 Cereals
BT3 Crops
BT4 Plants
BT3 Seeds
BT4 Plant foods
BT5 Foods

Wheat germ
BT1 Germ
BT2 Cereal products
BT3 Plant foods
BT4 Foods
BT1 Wheat
BT2 Cereals
BT3 Crops
BT4 Plants
BT3 Seeds
BT4 Plant foods
BT5 Foods
RT Wheat germ oils

Wheat germ oils
BT1 Vegetable oils
BT2 Oils vegetable
BT3 Oils
BT4 Lipids
BT5 Nutrients
BT3 Vegetable products
BT4 Plant foods
BT5 Foods
RT Wheat germ

Wheat gluten
BT1 Gluten
BT2 Cereal proteins
BT3 Proteins cereal
BT4 Vegetable proteins
BT5 Proteins vegetable
BT6 Proteins
BT7 Nutrients
BT6 Vegetable products
BT7 Plant foods
BT8 Foods
BT1 Wheat
BT2 Cereals
BT3 Crops
BT4 Plants
BT3 Seeds
BT4 Plant foods
BT5 Foods

Wheat malt
BT1 Malt
BT2 Cereal products
BT3 Plant foods
BT4 Foods

Wheat starch
BT1 Starch
BT2 Glucans
BT3 Polysaccharides
BT4 Carbohydrates
BT5 Nutrients
BT5 Organic compounds
BT2 Thickeners
BT3 Additives
BT1 Wheat

BT2 Cereals
BT3 Crops
BT4 Plants
BT3 Seeds
BT4 Plant foods
BT5 Foods

Whelks
BT1 Gastropods
BT2 Molluscs
BT3 Shellfish
BT4 Animals
BT4 Sea foods
BT5 Aquatic foods
BT6 Animal foods
BT7 Foods

Whey
BT1 Dairy products
BT2 Animal foods
BT3 Foods
NT1 Acid whey
NT1 Casein whey
NT1 Cheese whey
NT1 Dried whey
NT1 Whey beverages
NT1 Whey concentrates
NT1 Whey proteins
NT2 Whey protein concentrates

Whey beverages
BT1 Dairy beverages
BT2 Beverages
BT2 Dairy products
BT3 Animal foods
BT4 Foods
BT1 Whey
BT2 Dairy products
BT3 Animal foods
BT4 Foods

Whey cheese
BT1 Cheese varieties
BT2 Cheese
BT3 Dairy products
BT4 Animal foods
BT5 Foods

Whey concentrates
BT1 Concentrates
BT2 Processed foods
BT3 Foods
BT1 Whey
BT2 Dairy products
BT3 Animal foods
BT4 Foods

Whey protein concentrates
BT1 Protein concentrates
BT2 Concentrates
BT3 Processed foods
BT4 Foods
BT2 Protein products
BT1 Whey proteins
BT2 Milk proteins
BT3 Proteins milk
BT4 Animal proteins
BT5 Proteins animal
BT6 Proteins
BT7 Nutrients
BT2 Whey
BT3 Dairy products
BT4 Animal foods
BT5 Foods

Whey proteins
HN proteins whey also used in the index up to vol. 29 (1997)
BT1 Milk proteins
BT2 Proteins milk
BT3 Animal proteins
BT4 Proteins animal
BT5 Proteins
BT6 Nutrients
BT1 Whey
BT2 Dairy products
BT3 Animal foods
BT4 Foods
NT1 Whey protein concentrates

Whipped cream
BT1 Cream
BT2 Dairy products
BT3 Animal foods
BT4 Foods

Whipping
BT1 Processing
BT2 Technology
NT1 Beating
RT Aeration
RT Emulsification
RT Foams

Whipping capacity
BT1 Whipping properties
BT2 Functional properties
BT3 Physical properties

Whipping cream
BT1 Cream
BT2 Dairy products
BT3 Animal foods
BT4 Foods

Whipping properties
BT1 Functional properties
BT2 Physical properties
NT1 Whipping capacity

Whiskey
HN under Spirits up to vol. 42 (2010)
BT1 Whiskies
BT2 Spirits
BT3 Alcoholic beverages
BT4 Beverages alcoholic
BT5 Beverages
NT1 Bourbon whiskey
RT Whisky

Whiskies
HN introduced from vol. 43, issue 1 (2011); heading
BT1 Spirits
BT2 Alcoholic beverages
BT3 Beverages alcoholic
BT4 Beverages
NT1 Whiskey
NT2 Bourbon whiskey
NT1 Whisky
NT2 Scotch whisky

Whisky
HN under Spirits up to vol. 42 (2010)
BT1 Whiskies
BT2 Spirits
BT3 Alcoholic beverages
BT4 Beverages alcoholic
BT5 Beverages
NT1 Scotch whisky
RT Whiskey

White amur
HN under Fish up to vol. 42 (2010)
SN syn. grass carp
BT1 Grass carp
BT2 Carp
BT3 Freshwater fish
BT4 Fish
BT5 Animals
BT5 Sea foods
BT6 Aquatic foods
BT7 Animal foods
BT8 Foods
BT3 Oily fish
BT4 Fish
BT5 Animals
BT5 Sea foods
BT6 Aquatic foods
BT7 Animal foods
BT8 Foods

Whitebait
SN young of herring, sprat or other very small fish
BT1 Marine fish
BT2 Fish
BT3 Animals
BT3 Sea foods
BT4 Aquatic foods
BT5 Animal foods
BT6 Foods
BT1 Oily fish
BT2 Fish
BT3 Animals
BT3 Sea foods
BT4 Aquatic foods
BT5 Animal foods
BT6 Foods

White beans
BT1 Common beans
BT2 Legumes
BT3 Vegetables specific
BT4 Vegetables
BT5 Crops
BT6 Plants
BT5 Plant foods
BT6 Foods

White cabbages
BT1 Cabbages
BT2 Vegetables specific
BT3 Vegetables
BT4 Crops
BT5 Plants
BT4 Plant foods
BT5 Foods

White cheese
BT1 Cheese varieties
BT2 Cheese

BT3 Dairy products
BT4 Animal foods
BT5 Foods

White chocolate
HN introduced from vol. 39, issue 1 (2007)
BT1 Chocolate products
BT2 Chocolate
BT3 Sugar confectionery
BT4 Plant foods
BT5 Foods

Whitecurrants
BT1 Berries
BT2 Fruits specific
BT3 Fruits
BT4 Crops
BT5 Plants
BT4 Plant foods
BT5 Foods

White fish
SN general use only; see also other specified white fishes
BT1 Marine fish
BT2 Fish
BT3 Animals
BT3 Sea foods
BT4 Aquatic foods
BT5 Animal foods
BT6 Foods

Whitefish
BT1 Fish
BT2 Animals
BT2 Sea foods
BT3 Aquatic foods
BT4 Animal foods
BT5 Foods
NT1 *Coregonus lavaretus*

White lupins
BT1 Lupins
BT2 Legumes
BT3 Vegetables specific
BT4 Vegetables
BT5 Crops
BT6 Plants
BT5 Plant foods
BT6 Foods

White mould cheese
BT1 Cheese varieties
BT2 Cheese
BT3 Dairy products
BT4 Animal foods
BT5 Foods

White mustard
SN syn. yellow mustard
BT1 Oilseeds
BT2 Seeds
BT3 Plant foods
BT4 Foods
BT1 Spices
BT2 Flavourings
BT3 Additives
BT1 Vegetables specific
BT2 Vegetables
BT3 Crops
BT4 Plants
BT3 Plant foods
BT4 Foods

Whiteners
HN heading up to vol. 24 (1992)
BT1 Additives
NT1 Coffee whiteners
RT Instant foods

Whiteness
BT1 Optical properties
BT2 Physical properties

White pepper
BT1 Pepper
BT2 Spices
BT3 Flavourings
BT4 Additives

White pickled cheese
BT1 Cheese varieties
BT2 Cheese
BT3 Dairy products
BT4 Animal foods
BT5 Foods

White sugar
BT1 Sugar
BT2 Plant foods
BT3 Foods

White truffles
HN introduced from vol. 37, issue 5 (2005)
BT1 *Tuber*
BT2 Edible fungi
BT3 Fungi edible
BT4 Vegetables specific
BT5 Vegetables
BT6 Crops
BT7 Plants
BT6 Plant foods
BT7 Foods

White tuna
SN syn. albacore
BT1 Tuna
BT2 Marine fish
BT3 Fish
BT4 Animals
BT4 Sea foods
BT5 Aquatic foods
BT6 Animal foods
BT7 Foods
BT2 Oily fish
BT3 Fish
BT4 Animals
BT4 Sea foods
BT5 Aquatic foods
BT6 Animal foods
BT7 Foods
NT1 Albacore

White wines
BT1 Wines
BT2 Alcoholic beverages
BT3 Beverages alcoholic
BT4 Beverages

Whiting
BT1 Marine fish
BT2 Fish
BT3 Animals
BT3 Sea foods
BT4 Aquatic foods
BT5 Animal foods
BT6 Foods

WHO
HN used as abbrev. for World Health Organization up to vol. 24
USE **World Health Organization**

Wholegrain foods
BT1 Cereal products
BT2 Plant foods
BT3 Foods

Wholemeal
BT1 Cereal flours
BT2 Flours cereal
BT3 Cereal products
BT4 Plant foods
BT5 Foods

Whole milk
BT1 Milk
BT2 Dairy products
BT3 Animal foods
BT4 Foods

Wholesale
HN introduced from vol. 42, issue 1 (2010)
BT1 Marketing
BT2 Economics

Wieners
BT1 Frankfurters
BT2 Sausages
BT3 Meat products
BT4 Animal foods
BT5 Foods

Wild boar carcasses
BT1 Carcasses
BT2 Meat
BT3 Animal foods
BT4 Foods
BT1 Wild boar meat
BT2 Pork
BT3 Meat specific
BT4 Meat
BT5 Animal foods
BT6 Foods

Wild boar meat
BT1 Pork
BT2 Meat specific
BT3 Meat
BT4 Animal foods
BT5 Foods
NT1 Wild boar carcasses

Wild boars
USE **Swine**

Wild cabbage
BT1 Vegetables specific
BT2 Vegetables

BT3 Crops
BT4 Plants
BT3 Plant foods
BT4 Foods

Wild garlic
BT1 Spices
BT2 Flavourings
BT3 Additives
RT Garlic
UF Caucas

Wild mushrooms
BT1 Mushrooms
BT2 Edible fungi
BT3 Fungi edible
BT4 Vegetables specific
BT5 Vegetables
BT6 Crops
BT7 Plants
BT6 Plant foods
BT7 Foods

Wild rice
BT1 Cereals
BT2 Crops
BT3 Plants
BT2 Seeds
BT3 Plant foods
BT4 Foods
BT1 Vegetables specific
BT2 Vegetables
BT3 Crops
BT4 Plants
BT3 Plant foods
BT4 Foods

Wild vegetables
BT1 Vegetables
BT2 Crops
BT3 Plants
BT2 Plant foods
BT3 Foods

Wild yeasts
BT1 Yeasts
BT2 Fungi
BT3 Microorganisms
RT Contamination
RT Microbial contamination
RT Microbial spoilage

Windward Islands
BT1 West Indies
BT2 America

Wine coolers
BT1 Aromatized wines
BT2 Wines
BT3 Alcoholic beverages
BT4 Beverages alcoholic
BT5 Beverages

Wine distillates
BT1 Distillates
BT2 Spirits
BT3 Alcoholic beverages
BT4 Beverages alcoholic
BT5 Beverages
RT Brandies

Wine gums
BT1 Jelly confectionery
BT2 Sugar confectionery
BT3 Plant foods
BT4 Foods

Wine industry
HN introduced from vol. 41, issue 1 (2009)
BT1 Food industry
BT2 Industries

Winemaking
BT1 Processing
BT2 Technology
NT1 Chaptalization
NT1 Madeirization
NT1 Oenological properties
NT1 Sparkling winemaking
NT2 Champagnization
NT1 Terroir
NT1 Viniculture
NT1 Vintage
NT1 Wineries
RT Fermentation
RT Grape juices
RT Grapes
RT Killer yeasts
RT Maceration
RT Malolactic fermentation
RT Musts
RT Stillage
RT Vats
RT Winemaking grapes
RT Wines
RT Wine yeasts
RT Yeasts wine
UF Vinification
UF Wines manufacture

Winemaking grapes
HN heading from vol. 30 (1998); under Grapes up to vol. 29 (1997)
BT1 Grapes
BT2 Berries
BT3 Fruits specific
BT4 Fruits
BT5 Crops
BT6 Plants
BT5 Plant foods
BT6 Foods
RT Winemaking

Wineries
BT1 Winemaking
BT2 Processing
BT3 Technology

Wines
BT1 Alcoholic beverages
BT2 Beverages alcoholic
BT3 Beverages
NT1 Alcohol low wines
NT1 Aromatized wines
NT2 Retsina
NT2 Sangria
NT2 Vermouths
NT2 Wine coolers
NT1 Dessert wines
NT1 Fortified wines
NT2 Madeira
NT2 Marsala
NT2 Port
NT2 Sherry
NT1 Ice wines
NT2 Eiswein
NT1 Red wines
NT1 Rose wines
NT1 White wines
NT1 Wines sparkling
NT2 Sparkling wines
NT3 Cavas
NT3 Champagne
NT3 Sekts
RT Fruit wines
RT Killer yeasts
RT Musts
RT Winemaking
RT Wine yeasts
RT Yeasts wine

Wines manufacture
USE **Winemaking**

Wines palm
HN heading from vol. 25 (1993); under Wines up to vol. 24 (1992)
SN palm wines also used in the index
BT1 Alcoholic beverages
BT2 Beverages alcoholic
BT3 Beverages
BT1 Palms
BT2 Plants
NT1 Palm wines
NT2 Coconut toddy
NT2 Toddy
NT2 Tuba

Wines sparkling
HN heading from vol. 25 (1993); under Wines up to vol. 24 (1992)
SN sparkling wines also used in the index
BT1 Wines
BT2 Alcoholic beverages
BT3 Beverages alcoholic
BT4 Beverages
NT1 Sparkling wines
NT2 Cavas
NT2 Champagne
NT2 Sekts

Wine vinegar
BT1 Vinegar
BT2 Condiments
BT3 Flavourings
BT4 Additives
BT2 Fermented foods
BT3 Processed foods
BT4 Foods

Wine yeasts
SN index heading is Yeasts wine
BT1 Yeasts wine
BT2 *Saccharomyces*
BT3 Yeasts
BT4 Fungi
BT5 Microorganisms
NT1 Sake yeasts
RT Winemaking
RT Wines

Winged beans
BT1 Legumes
BT2 Vegetables specific
BT3 Vegetables
BT4 Crops
BT5 Plants
BT4 Plant foods
BT5 Foods

Winnowers
BT1 Equipment
BT2 Technology
RT Cereals
RT Husking

Winterization
BT1 Clarification
BT2 Processing
BT3 Technology

Withering
BT1 Drying
BT2 Thermal processing
BT3 Processing thermal
BT4 Processing
BT5 Technology
RT Tea

Witloof
USE **Chicory**

Wolfberries
HN introduced from vol. 39, issue 1 (2007)
BT1 Berries
BT2 Fruits specific
BT3 Fruits
BT4 Crops
BT5 Plants
BT4 Plant foods
BT5 Foods

Women
BT1 Population groups

Wood
BT1 Packaging materials
NT1 Oak
NT1 Timber

Woodcock
BT1 Birds

Wood pigeons
BT1 Birds

Wood smoke
BT1 Flavourings
BT2 Additives
RT Smoking

Woolliness
BT1 Plant disorders
BT2 Diseases plant
BT3 Diseases

Worcestershire sauces
BT1 Sauces
BT2 Condiments
BT3 Flavourings
BT4 Additives
BT3 Animal foods
BT4 Foods

Worktables
BT1 Surfaces

World
RT Countries
RT International

World Health Organization
HN heading up to vol. 24 (1992)
UF WHO

World Trade Organization
BT1 Trade
BT2 Economics

World Wide Web
BT1 Internet
BT2 Information technology
BT3 Technology

Wormwood
HN under Spices up to vol. 42 (2010)
BT1 Herbs
BT2 Spices
BT3 Flavourings
BT4 Additives

Worts
NT1 Trub
RT Beer
RT Brewing
RT Fermentation
RT Mashing

Wounding
BT1 Damage

Wrapping
BT1 Packaging
BT2 Technology

Wreckfish
BT1 Marine fish
BT2 Fish
BT3 Animals
BT3 Sea foods
BT4 Aquatic foods
BT5 Animal foods
BT6 Foods
NT1 *Polyprion americanus*

Wt.
BT1 Weight
BT2 Physical properties

Wt. loss diet
HN introduced from vol. 39, issue 1 (2007)
BT1 Body wt.
BT2 Anthropometric parameters
BT3 Health
BT1 Diet therapy
BT2 Diet
BT3 Nutrition
BT2 Therapy
RT Obesity

Wuerstel
BT1 Sausages
BT2 Meat products

X

Xanthan
HN heading from vol. 30 (1998); xanthans used in the index up to vol. 42 (2010)
BT1 Polysaccharides
BT2 Carbohydrates
BT3 Nutrients
BT3 Organic compounds
NT1 Xanthan gums
RT Exopolysaccharides
RT *Xanthomonas campestris*
UF Xanthans

Xanthan gums
BT1 Gums
BT2 Polysaccharides
BT3 Carbohydrates
BT4 Nutrients
BT4 Organic compounds
BT2 Stabilizers
BT3 Additives
BT2 Thickeners
BT3 Additives
BT1 Xanthan
BT2 Polysaccharides
BT3 Carbohydrates
BT4 Nutrients
BT4 Organic compounds

Xanthans
HN xanthan used in index from vol. 30 (1998)
USE **Xanthan**

Xanthene dyes
BT1 Colorants
BT2 Additives

Xanthine dehydrogenases
SN EC 1.17.1.4, formerly 1.1.1.204
BT1 Dehydrogenases
BT2 Oxidoreductases
BT3 Enzymes
RT Xanthine oxidases

Xanthine oxidases
SN EC 1.17.3.2, formerly 1.1.3.22
BT1 Oxidases
BT2 Oxidoreductases
BT3 Enzymes
RT Xanthine dehydrogenases

Xanthohumol
HN introduced from vol. 37, issue 5 (2005)
BT1 Chalcones
BT2 Antioxidants
BT3 Additives
BT2 Flavonoids
BT3 Aromatic compounds

BT4 Organic compounds
BT3 Pigments

Xanthomegnin
BT1 Mycotoxins
BT2 Toxins
BT3 Residues

Xanthomonas
HN under Pseudomonadaceae up to vol. 24 (1992); heading from vol. 30 (1998)
BT1 Bacteria
BT2 Microorganisms
NT1 *Xanthomonas campestris*

Xanthomonas campestris
BT1 *Xanthomonas*
BT2 Bacteria
BT3 Microorganisms
RT Xanthan

Xanthones
HN introduced from vol. 42, issue 1 (2010)
BT1 Heterocyclic compounds
NT1 Mangiferin
NT1 Sterigmatocystins

Xanthophyllomyces
HN introduced from vol. 43, issue 1 (2011)
BT1 Yeasts
BT2 Fungi
BT3 Microorganisms
NT1 *Xanthophyllomyces dendrorhous*

Xanthophyllomyces dendrorhous
BT1 *Xanthophyllomyces*
BT2 Yeasts
BT3 Fungi
BT4 Microorganisms

Xanthophylls
BT1 Carotenoids
BT2 Pigments
BT2 Terpenoids
BT3 Lipids
BT4 Nutrients
NT1 Astaxanthin
NT1 Canthaxanthin
NT1 Cryptoxanthin
NT1 Diatoxanthin
NT1 Fucoxanthin
NT1 Lutein
NT1 Neoxanthin
NT1 Tunaxanthin
NT1 Violaxanthin
NT1 Zeaxanthin

Xanthotoxin
BT1 Furocoumarins
BT2 Coumarins
BT3 Lactones
BT4 Esters
BT5 Organic compounds
BT4 Heterocyclic compounds
BT3 Phenols
BT4 Alcohols
BT4 Aromatic compounds
BT5 Organic compounds
BT1 Toxins
BT2 Residues

Xe
HN also under Minerals up to vol. 42 (2010)
BT1 Elements
BT2 Minerals
BT3 Nutrients
BT1 Gases
BT2 Physical phases
BT3 Chemistry
BT4 Science
UF Xenon

Xenobiotics
HN introduced from vol. 37, issue 5 (2005)

Xenon
USE **Xe**

Xerocomus
BT1 Edible fungi
BT2 Fungi edible
BT3 Vegetables specific
BT4 Vegetables
BT5 Crops
BT6 Plants
BT5 Plant foods
BT6 Foods

X-ray absorptiometry
HN introduced from vol. 39, issue 1 (2007)
BT1 Analytical techniques

X-ray crystallography
HN introduced from vol. 39, issue 1 (2007)
BT1 Crystallography
BT2 Analytical techniques
UF X-ray diffraction

X-ray diffraction
USE **X-ray crystallography**

X-ray fluorescence spectroscopy
BT1 Fluorometry
BT2 Analytical techniques
BT1 Spectroscopy
BT2 Analytical techniques

X-rays
BT1 Radiation

Xylan
HN xylans used in index up to vol. 42 (2010)
BT1 Polysaccharides
BT2 Carbohydrates
BT3 Nutrients
BT3 Organic compounds
UF Xylans

Xylanases
USE **Xylan degrading enzymes**
USE **Xylan endo-1,3-β-xylosidases**

Xylan degrading enzymes
SN general use only, see also specific enzymes
BT1 Glycosidases
BT2 Hydrolases
BT3 Enzymes
UF Xylanases

Xylan endo-1,3-β-xylosidases
SN EC 3.2.1.32
BT1 Glycosidases
BT2 Hydrolases
BT3 Enzymes
UF Endo-1,3-β-xylanases
UF Xylanases

Xylans
HN xylan used in index from vol. 30 (1998)
USE **Xylan**

Xylan 1,4-β-xylosidases
SN EC 3.2.1.37
BT1 Glycosidases
BT2 Hydrolases
BT3 Enzymes
UF Exo-1,4-β-xylosidases
UF Xylobiases
UF β-Xylosidases

Xylene
HN introduced from vol. 39, issue 1 (2007)
BT1 Aromatic compounds
BT2 Organic compounds
BT1 Solvents

Xylitol
HN heading from vol. 30 (1998); under Sugar alcohols up to vol. 29 (1997)
BT1 Polyols
BT2 Alcohols
BT2 Carbohydrates
BT3 Nutrients
BT3 Organic compounds

Xylitol dehydrogenases
USE **D-Xylulose reductases**

Xylobiases
USE **Xylan 1,4-β-xylosidases**

Xyloglucans
BT1 Glucans
BT2 Polysaccharides
BT3 Carbohydrates
BT4 Nutrients
BT4 Organic compounds

Xylooligosaccharides
HN under Polysaccharides and Sugars up to vol. 42 (2010)
BT1 Oligosaccharides
BT2 Polysaccharides
BT3 Carbohydrates
BT4 Nutrients
BT4 Organic compounds
BT2 Sugars
BT3 Carbohydrates
BT4 Nutrients
BT4 Organic compounds

BT3 Plant foods
BT4 Foods

Xylose
HN under Sugars up to vol. 42 (2010)
BT1 Monosaccharides
BT2 Sugars
BT3 Carbohydrates
BT4 Nutrients
BT4 Organic compounds
BT3 Plant foods
BT4 Foods

Xylose isomerases
SN EC 5.3.1.5; glucose isomerases (non-current EC term) still widely used for this enzyme
BT1 Isomerases
BT2 Enzymes
RT Glucose isomerases

Xylose reductases
USE **Aldehyde reductases**

β-Xylosidases
USE **Xylan 1,4-β-xylosidases**

Xylulose
HN under Sugars up to vol. 42 (2010)
BT1 Monosaccharides
BT2 Sugars
BT3 Carbohydrates
BT4 Nutrients
BT4 Organic compounds
BT3 Plant foods
BT4 Foods

D-Xylulose reductases
SN EC 1.1.1.9
BT1 Dehydrogenases
BT2 Oxidoreductases
BT3 Enzymes
UF Xylitol dehydrogenases

Y

Y
HN under Minerals up to vol. 42 (2010)
BT1 Metals
BT2 Elements
BT3 Minerals
BT4 Nutrients
UF Yttrium

Yacon
BT1 Vegetables specific
BT2 Vegetables
BT3 Crops
BT4 Plants
BT3 Plant foods
BT4 Foods

Yak carcasses
BT1 Carcasses
BT2 Meat
BT3 Animal foods
BT4 Foods
BT1 Yak meat
BT2 Meat specific
BT3 Meat
BT4 Animal foods
BT5 Foods
BT2 Yaks
BT3 Animals

Yakifu
BT1 Bakery products
BT2 Cereal products
BT3 Plant foods
BT4 Foods

Yakju
BT1 Rice wines
BT2 Cereal wines
BT3 Alcoholic beverages
BT4 Beverages alcoholic
BT5 Beverages

Yak meat
BT1 Meat specific
BT2 Meat
BT3 Animal foods
BT4 Foods
BT1 Yaks
BT2 Animals
NT1 Yak carcasses

Yak milk
BT1 Milk
BT2 Dairy products
BT3 Animal foods
BT4 Foods
BT1 Yaks
BT2 Animals

Yaks
BT1 Animals
NT1 Yak meat
NT2 Yak carcasses
NT1 Yak milk

Yakult
BT1 Fermented milk
BT2 Fermented dairy products
BT3 Dairy products
BT4 Animal foods
BT5 Foods
BT3 Fermented foods
BT4 Processed foods
BT5 Foods
BT2 Milk
BT3 Dairy products
BT4 Animal foods
BT5 Foods

Yam beans
BT1 Legumes
BT2 Vegetables specific
BT3 Vegetables
BT4 Crops
BT5 Plants
BT4 Plant foods
BT5 Foods
NT1 *Pachyrhizus ahipa*

Yam meal
HN introduced from vol. 39, issue 1 (2007)
BT1 Flours
BT2 Plant foods
BT3 Foods
BT1 Yams
BT2 Vegetables specific
BT3 Vegetables
BT4 Crops
BT5 Plants
BT4 Plant foods
BT5 Foods

Yams
BT1 Vegetables specific
BT2 Vegetables
BT3 Crops
BT4 Plants
BT3 Plant foods
BT4 Foods
NT1 Amala
NT1 Yam meal
NT1 Yam starch

Yam starch
BT1 Starch
BT2 Glucans
BT3 Polysaccharides
BT4 Carbohydrates
BT5 Nutrients
BT5 Organic compounds
BT2 Thickeners
BT3 Additives
BT1 Yams
BT2 Vegetables specific
BT3 Vegetables
BT4 Crops
BT5 Plants
BT4 Plant foods
BT5 Foods

Yard-long beans
USE **Asparagus beans**

Yarrow
BT1 Plants
NT1 *Achillea millefolium*

Yarrowia
HN under Fungi up to vol. 42 (2010)
BT1 Yeasts
BT2 Fungi
BT3 Microorganisms
NT1 *Yarrowia lipolytica*

Yarrowia lipolytica
HN under Fungi up to vol. 42 (2010)
SN teleomorph of Candida lipolytica
BT1 *Yarrowia*
BT2 Yeasts
BT3 Fungi
BT4 Microorganisms

Yb
HN under Minerals up to vol. 42 (2010)
BT1 Lanthanides
BT2 Metals
BT3 Elements
BT4 Minerals

BT5 Nutrients
UF Ytterbium

Yeast biomass
BT1 Microbial biomass
BT2 Biomass
BT3 Fermentation products
BT4 Biotechnology
BT5 Technology
BT2 Microorganisms
BT1 Yeasts
BT2 Fungi
BT3 Microorganisms

Yeast extracts
BT1 Extracts
BT2 Flavourings
BT3 Additives
BT1 Yeasts
BT2 Fungi
BT3 Microorganisms

Yeast proteins
HN under Proteins up to vol. 42 (2010)
BT1 Microbial proteins
BT2 Microorganisms
BT2 Proteins
BT3 Nutrients
BT1 Yeasts
BT2 Fungi
BT3 Microorganisms

Yeasts
BT1 Fungi
BT2 Microorganisms
NT1 *Arxula*
NT2 *Arxula adeninivorans*
NT1 *Ashbya*
NT2 *Ashbya gossypii*
NT1 *Brettanomyces*
NT2 *Brettanomyces anomalus*
NT2 *Brettanomyces bruxellensis*
NT2 *Brettanomyces intermedius*
NT1 *Candida*
NT2 *Candida albicans*
NT2 *Candida antarctica*
NT2 *Candida boidinii*
NT2 *Candida bombicola*
NT2 *Candida cylindracea*
NT2 *Candida famata*
NT2 *Candida glycerinogenes*
NT2 *Candida guilliermondii*
NT2 *Candida humilis*
NT3 *Candida milleri*
NT2 *Candida intermedia*
NT2 *Candida kefyr*
NT3 *Candida pseudotropicalis*
NT2 *Candida krusei*
NT2 *Candida lipolytica*
NT2 *Candida magnoliae*
NT2 *Candida maltosa*
NT2 *Candida mogii*
NT2 *Candida molischiana*
NT2 *Candida oleophila*
NT2 *Candida parapsilosis*
NT2 *Candida rugosa*
NT2 *Candida saitoana*
NT2 *Candida sake*
NT2 *Candida shehatae*
NT2 *Candida stellata*
NT2 *Candida tropicalis*
NT2 *Candida utilis*
NT2 *Candida valida*
NT2 *Candida versatilis*
NT2 *Candida wickerhamii*
NT2 *Candida zeylanoides*
NT2 Torula yeast
NT1 Cider yeasts
NT1 *Cryptococcus*
NT2 *Cryptococcus albidus*
NT2 *Cryptococcus curvatus*
NT2 *Cryptococcus laurentii*
NT2 *Cryptococcus nodaensis*
NT1 *Debaryomyces*
NT2 *Debaryomyces hansenii*
NT1 *Dekkera*
NT2 *Dekkera anomala*
NT2 *Dekkera bruxellensis*
NT1 Distillers yeasts
NT1 Dried yeasts
NT1 *Endomycopsis*
NT1 *Eremothecium*
NT1 *Hanseniaspora*
NT2 *Hanseniaspora guilliermondii*
NT2 *Hanseniaspora osmophila*
NT2 *Hanseniaspora uvarum*
NT1 *Hansenula*
NT2 *Hansenula polymorpha*
NT1 *Issatchenkia*
NT2 *Issatchenkia orientalis*
NT1 Killer yeasts
NT1 *Kloeckera*
NT2 *Kloeckera apiculata*
NT1 *Kluyveromyces*
NT2 *Kluyveromyces bulgaricus*
NT2 *Kluyveromyces fragilis*
NT2 *Kluyveromyces lactis*
NT2 *Kluyveromyces marxianus*
NT2 *Kluyveromyces phaffii*
NT2 *Kluyveromyces thermotolerans*
NT1 *Metschnikowia*
NT2 *Metschnikowia pulcherrima*
NT1 *Pachysolen*
NT1 *Phaffia*
NT2 *Phaffia rhodozyma*
NT1 *Pichia*
NT2 *Pichia anomala*
NT2 *Pichia fermentans*
NT2 *Pichia guilliermondii*
NT2 *Pichia heedii*
NT2 *Pichia membranifaciens*
NT3 *Pichia membranefaciens*
NT2 *Pichia methanolica*
NT2 *Pichia pastoris*
NT2 *Pichia stipitis*
NT2 *Pichia subpelliculosa*
NT1 *Rhodosporidium*
NT2 *Rhodosporidium toruloides*
NT1 *Rhodotorula*
NT2 *Rhodotorula glutinis*
NT2 *Rhodotorula gracilis*
NT2 *Rhodotorula mucilaginosa*
NT3 *Rhodotorula rubra*
NT1 *Saccharomyces*
NT2 *Saccharomyces bayanus*
NT2 *Saccharomyces boulardii*
NT2 *Saccharomyces carlsbergensis*
NT2 *Saccharomyces cerevisiae*
NT2 *Saccharomyces diastaticus*
NT2 *Saccharomyces exiguus*
NT2 *Saccharomyces pastorianus*
NT2 *Saccharomyces uvarum*
NT2 Yeasts bakers
NT3 Bakers yeasts
NT2 Yeasts brewers
NT3 Brewers yeasts
NT4 Bottom fermenting yeasts
NT4 Top fermenting yeasts
NT2 Yeasts wine
NT3 Wine yeasts
NT4 Sake yeasts
NT1 *Saccharomycodes*
NT1 *Saccharomycopsis*
NT2 *Saccharomycopsis fibuligera*
NT1 *Schizosaccharomyces*
NT2 *Schizosaccharomyces pombe*
NT1 *Schwanniomyces*
NT1 Spoilage yeasts
NT1 *Sporobolomyces*
NT1 *Torulaspora*
NT2 *Torulaspora delbrueckii*
NT1 *Torulopsis*
NT2 *Torulopsis glabrata*
NT1 *Trichosporon*
NT2 *Trichosporon cutaneum*
NT2 *Trichosporon pullulans*
NT1 Wild yeasts
NT1 *Xanthophyllomyces*
NT2 *Xanthophyllomyces dendrorhous*
NT1 *Yarrowia*
NT2 *Yarrowia lipolytica*
NT1 Yeast biomass
NT1 Yeast extracts
NT1 Yeast proteins
NT1 *Zygosaccharomyces*
NT2 *Zygosaccharomyces bailii*
NT2 *Zygosaccharomyces rouxii*
RT Fermentation

Yeasts bakers
SN bakers yeasts also used in the index
BT1 *Saccharomyces*
BT2 Yeasts
BT3 Fungi
BT4 Microorganisms
NT1 Bakers yeasts
RT Breadmaking

Yeasts brewers
SN brewers yeasts also used in the index
BT1 *Saccharomyces*
BT2 Yeasts
BT3 Fungi
BT4 Microorganisms
NT1 Brewers yeasts
NT2 Bottom fermenting yeasts
NT2 Top fermenting yeasts
RT Beer
RT Brewing

Yeasts wine
SN wine yeasts also used in the index
BT1 *Saccharomyces*
BT2 Yeasts
BT3 Fungi
BT4 Microorganisms
NT1 Wine yeasts
NT2 Sake yeasts
RT Winemaking
RT Wines

Yellowfin
BT1 Marine fish
BT2 Fish
BT3 Animals
BT3 Sea foods
BT4 Aquatic foods
BT5 Animal foods
BT6 Foods
UF Yellowfins

Yellowfins
HN used up to vol. 29 (1997)
USE **Yellowfin**

Yellowfin tuna
BT1 Tuna
BT2 Marine fish
BT3 Fish
BT4 Animals
BT4 Sea foods
BT5 Aquatic foods
BT6 Animal foods
BT7 Foods
BT2 Oily fish
BT3 Fish
BT4 Animals
BT4 Sea foods
BT5 Aquatic foods
BT6 Animal foods
BT7 Foods

Yellow mustard
SN syn. white mustard
BT1 Oilseeds
BT2 Seeds
BT3 Plant foods
BT4 Foods
BT1 Spices
BT2 Flavourings
BT3 Additives
BT1 Vegetables specific
BT2 Vegetables
BT3 Crops
BT4 Plants
BT3 Plant foods
BT4 Foods

Yellow perch
HN introduced from vol. 37, issue 5 (2005)
BT1 Perch
BT2 Freshwater fish
BT3 Fish
BT4 Animals
BT4 Sea foods
BT5 Aquatic foods
BT6 Animal foods
BT7 Foods

Yellowtail
BT1 Marine fish
BT2 Fish
BT3 Animals
BT3 Sea foods
BT4 Aquatic foods
BT5 Animal foods
BT6 Foods
UF Amberjack
UF Yellowtails

Yellowtails
HN used up to vol. 29 (1997)
USE **Yellowtail**

Yemen
BT1 Asia
BT1 Middle East

Yerba mate
HN under Beverages up to vol. 42 (2010)
BT1 Mate
BT2 Herb tea
BT3 Teas
BT4 Beverages
BT4 Crops
BT5 Plants
BT4 Plant foods
BT5 Foods
NT1 *Ilex paraguariensis*

Yersinia
HN heading from vol. 25 (1993); under Enterobacteriaceae up to vol. 24 (1992)
BT1 Bacteria
BT2 Microorganisms
NT1 *Yersinia enterocolitica*
NT1 *Yersinia pseudotuberculosis*
NT1 *Yersinia ruckeri*
RT Yersiniosis

Yersinia enterocolitica
BT1 *Yersinia*
BT2 Bacteria
BT3 Microorganisms

Yersinia pseudotuberculosis
HN introduced from vol. 39, issue 1 (2007)
BT1 *Yersinia*
BT2 Bacteria
BT3 Microorganisms

Yersinia ruckeri
BT1 *Yersinia*
BT2 Bacteria
BT3 Microorganisms

Yersiniosis
BT1 Diseases
BT1 Poisoning
RT *Yersinia*

Yessotoxins
BT1 Toxins
BT2 Residues

Yield stress
BT1 Rheological properties
BT2 Mechanical properties
BT3 Physical properties
BT1 Stress

Ymer
BT1 Fermented milk
BT2 Fermented dairy products
BT3 Dairy products
BT4 Animal foods
BT5 Foods
BT3 Fermented foods
BT4 Processed foods
BT5 Foods
BT2 Milk
BT3 Dairy products
BT4 Animal foods
BT5 Foods

Yoghurt
BT1 Fermented milk
BT2 Fermented dairy products
BT3 Dairy products
BT4 Animal foods
BT5 Foods
BT3 Fermented foods
BT4 Processed foods
BT5 Foods
BT2 Milk
BT3 Dairy products
BT4 Animal foods
BT5 Foods
NT1 Buffalo yoghurt
NT1 Ewe yoghurt
NT1 Flavoured yoghurt
NT1 Frozen yoghurt
NT1 Fruit yoghurt
NT1 Goat yoghurt
NT1 Yoghurt beverages
NT2 Drinking yoghurt

Yoghurt beverages
BT1 Dairy beverages
BT2 Beverages
BT2 Dairy products
BT3 Animal foods
BT4 Foods
BT1 Yoghurt
BT2 Fermented milk
BT3 Fermented dairy products
BT4 Dairy products
BT5 Animal foods
BT6 Foods
BT4 Fermented foods
BT5 Processed foods
BT6 Foods
BT3 Milk
BT4 Dairy products
BT5 Animal foods
BT6 Foods
NT1 Drinking yoghurt

Yoghurt starters
BT1 Starters
BT2 Bacteria
BT3 Microorganisms

Yokan
BT1 Sugar confectionery
BT2 Plant foods
BT3 Foods

Youngberries
BT1 Berries
BT2 Fruits specific
BT3 Fruits
BT4 Crops
BT5 Plants
BT4 Plant foods
BT5 Foods

Ytterbium
USE **Yb**

Yttrium
USE **Y**

Yuba
BT1 Soy products
BT2 Vegetable products
BT3 Plant foods
BT4 Foods

Yucca
BT1 Plants

Yugoslavia
HN heading up to vol. 24 (1992)
SN Bosnia and Herzegovina, Croatia, Macedonia, Montenegro, Serbia and Slovenia are also in index
BT1 Europe

Yukwa
BT1 Rice
BT2 Cereals
BT3 Crops
BT4 Plants
BT3 Seeds
BT4 Plant foods
BT5 Foods
BT1 Snack foods
BT2 Processed foods
BT3 Foods

Yusho
BT1 Diseases
BT1 Poisoning
RT Polychlorinated biphenyls

Yuzu
BT1 Citrus fruits
BT2 Fruits specific
BT3 Fruits
BT4 Crops
BT5 Plants
BT4 Plant foods
BT5 Foods

Z

Zabadi
BT1 Zabady
BT2 Fermented milk
BT3 Fermented dairy products
BT4 Dairy products
BT5 Animal foods
BT6 Foods
BT4 Fermented foods
BT5 Processed foods
BT6 Foods
BT3 Milk
BT4 Dairy products
BT5 Animal foods
BT6 Foods

Zabady
BT1 Fermented milk
BT2 Fermented dairy products
BT3 Dairy products
BT4 Animal foods
BT5 Foods
BT3 Fermented foods
BT4 Processed foods
BT5 Foods
BT2 Milk
BT3 Dairy products
BT4 Animal foods
BT5 Foods
NT1 Zabadi

Zaire
SN former name for the Democratic Republic of the Congo
BT1 Central Africa
BT2 Africa
RT Democratic Republic of the Congo
UF Zaire Republic

Zaire Republic
USE **Zaire**

Zambia
BT1 Southern Africa
BT2 Africa

Zearalenol
BT1 Mycotoxins
BT2 Toxins
BT3 Residues

Zearalenone
SN syn. F2 toxin
BT1 Mycotoxins
BT2 Toxins
BT3 Residues

Zeatin
BT1 Cytokinins
BT2 Plant growth regulators
BT3 Cultivation
BT4 Agriculture

Zeaxanthin
BT1 Xanthophylls
BT2 Carotenoids
BT3 Pigments
BT3 Terpenoids
BT4 Lipids
BT5 Nutrients

Zedoary
SN syn. shoti
BT1 Vegetables specific
BT2 Vegetables
BT3 Crops
BT4 Plants
BT3 Plant foods
BT4 Foods
NT1 *Curcuma zedoaria*

Zefir
BT1 Desserts
BT2 Processed foods
BT3 Foods

Zein
BT1 Cereal proteins
BT2 Proteins cereal
BT3 Vegetable proteins
BT4 Proteins vegetable
BT5 Proteins
BT6 Nutrients
BT5 Vegetable products
BT6 Plant foods
BT7 Foods

Zeleny values
RT Cereals

Zeolites
BT1 Silicates
BT2 Salts

Zeranol
BT1 Drugs
BT2 Residues

Zimbabwe
BT1 Southern Africa
BT2 Africa
UF Rhodesia

Zinc
SN symbol Zn also used in index
BT1 Metals
BT2 Elements
BT3 Minerals
BT4 Nutrients
NT1 Zn

Zinc phosphide
BT1 Rodenticides
BT2 Pesticides
BT3 Biocides
BT3 Residues

Zineb
BT1 Dithiocarbamate fungicides
BT2 Fungicides
BT3 Pesticides
BT4 Biocides
BT4 Residues

Zingerone
HN also under Flavour compounds up to vol. 42 (2010)
BT1 Aroma compounds
BT2 Flavour compounds
BT2 Volatile compounds
BT1 Ketones
BT2 Carbonyl compounds
BT3 Organic compounds
BT1 Phenols
BT2 Alcohols
BT2 Aromatic compounds
BT3 Organic compounds
BT1 Pungent principles

BT2 Flavour compounds
RT Ginger

Ziram
BT1 Dithiocarbamate fungicides
BT2 Fungicides
BT3 Pesticides
BT4 Biocides
BT4 Residues

Zirconium
USE **Zr**

Zn
SN index heading is Zinc
BT1 Zinc
BT2 Metals
BT3 Elements
BT4 Minerals
BT5 Nutrients

Zoalene
USE **Dinitolmide**

Zolone
USE **Phosalone**

Zoonoses
BT1 Diseases
RT Animal diseases

Zr
HN under Minerals up to vol. 42 (2010)
BT1 Metals
BT2 Elements
BT3 Minerals
BT4 Nutrients
UF Zirconium

Z-Trim
BT1 Fat substitutes
BT2 Fats
BT3 Lipids
BT4 Nutrients

Zucchini
USE **Courgettes**

Zucchini squashes
USE **Courgettes**

Zwieback
BT1 Bakery products
BT2 Cereal products
BT3 Plant foods
BT4 Foods

Zygosaccharomyces
HN heading from vol. 30 (1998); under Yeasts up to vol. 29 (1997)
BT1 Yeasts
BT2 Fungi
BT3 Microorganisms
NT1 *Zygosaccharomyces bailii*
NT1 *Zygosaccharomyces rouxii*

Zygosaccharomyces bailii
BT1 *Zygosaccharomyces*
BT2 Yeasts
BT3 Fungi
BT4 Microorganisms

Zygosaccharomyces rouxii
BT1 *Zygosaccharomyces*
BT2 Yeasts
BT3 Fungi
BT4 Microorganisms

Zymomonas
HN under Pseudomonadaceae up to vol. 24 (1992); heading from vol. 30 (1998)
BT1 Bacteria
BT2 Microorganisms
NT1 *Zymomonas mobilis*

Zymomonas mobilis
BT1 *Zymomonas*
BT2 Bacteria
BT3 Microorganisms

Appendix I

New terms added to this edition of the thesaurus

N-Acetyl-L-cysteine
β-*N*-acetylhexosaminidases
Acetyltransferases
Actinobacillus
Actinobacteria
S-Adenosyl-L-methionine
Adiponectin
Adults
Aichi virus
Alaska pollock
Alcohol oxidases
Alcohol-related disorders
Alcopops*
Aldoses
Algal oils
Allyl sulfides
Aloe vera
Altitude
Amidation
Amino acid oxidases
Aminoglycoside antibiotics
Amylomyces
Androgens
Anti-ageing activity
Antiallergic activity
Antioxidant status
Apiculture
Apthovirus
Archaea
Arxula
Ascospores*
Ashbya
Asparaginases
Astroviruses
Avian flu

Banana purees
Barley fibre
Bayberries
Beauty foods
Beauveria
Beijerinckia
Benzimidazole fungicides*
Biofuels
Biosecurity
Birth wt.
Bisphenol F diglycidyl ether
Body composition
Body fats
Bovine immunodeficiency virus
Butyl acetate
Butyrivibrio

Caciocavallo cheese
Calories low beverages
Camelina oils
Camelina sativa
Cameras
Candida kefyr
Capillary electrochromatography
Caramelization
Carcass condemnation
Cardiovascular physiology
Carnobacterium maltaromaticum
Cartridges
Caspases
Cassava meal
Catechins*
CD-ROMs
Cheese rind
Chicory (beverages)
Chicory (vegetables)
Chitooligosaccharides
Chloroanisoles*
Cholesterol low foods
Chromista
Clastogenicity
Cloned animal foods
Cloned animals
Cocoa nibs
Conidia*
Conjugated fatty acids
Consumer behaviour
Cordyceps sinensis
Coriander leaves
Coriander seeds
Coronavirus
Corynebacterium casei
Cryphonectria
Crypthecodinium
Cryptosporidium hominis
Curcuminoids
Cytolethal distending toxin

Dicarboximide fungicides
Diet drinks*
Dill leaves
Dill seeds
Dimethyl trisulfide
Diterpenoids
Dithiocarbamate fungicides
Dried sea foods
Drinking habits

Eating disorders
Echovirus
Ecklonia
Eczema*
Edible inks
EFSA*
Eicosanoids
Electronic publications
Enniatins
Enterococcus casseliflavus
Enterococcus gallinarum
Enterovirus
Essential fatty acids
Etherification
Ethyl caprylate
Ethyl decanoate
Ethyl formate
Ethyl octanoate
Euglena
European Food Safety Authority
Expansins
Eye health

Fasting
Fats high diet
Fetal programming*
Fluorescence spectroscopy*
Food aid
Food stamps
Foot and mouth disease virus
Francisella
Francisella tularensis
Freeze-thaw stability
Fruit pastes
Fruit vinegars
Fusarium solani

Gallocatechin gallate
Gastric cancer
Genetic markers
Geobacillus stearothermophilus
Geobacillus thermoleovorans
Gibberella
Gibberella fujikuroi
Gibberella fujikuroi complex
Glucooligosaccharides
Glutathione peroxidases
Glycitein
Goitre
Grain borers
Growth (human)
Growth promoters (animal)

** denotes a non-descriptor*

Growth promoters (microbial)
Growth promoters (plant)

Haemolysis
Haemolytic uraemic syndrome
Haloanisoles
Hanseniaspora guilliermondii
Healthiness
Health promotion
Healthy eating
Hepatitis A virus
Hepatitis E virus
Hepatovirus
Hepevirus
Hexyl acetate
High fat diet*
High protein diet*
Hot beverages
HPTLC
Human adenovirus
Human astrovirus
Human coxsackievirus
Human enterovirus
Human immunodeficiency virus
Hydration status
Hypoallergenic foods

Ice wines
Indole-3-carbinol
Intake
Integrins
Intramuscular fat
IR heating
Irritable bowel syndrome
Isorhamnetin
Issatchenkia
Issatchenkia orientalis

Keratinases
Ketogenic diet
Kidney stones
Kobuvirus
Kocuria

Lactobacillus lindneri
Lactoferricin
Lactose low foods
LAMP
Legume starch
Lentivirus
α-Linolenic acid
γ-Linolenic acid
α-Lipoic acid
Liquefaction
Liquid phase microextraction
Loop-mediated isothermal amplification*
Low calorie beverages*
Low calorie diet*
Low cholesterol foods*
Low fat diet*
Low lactose foods*
Low sodium diet*
Lupin meal

Macrococcus
Macrolide antibiotics
Macronutrients
Mamastrovirus
Mangiferin
Mashed potatoes
Mastadenovirus
Menus
Microfluidic technology
Micronutrients
Millet flour
Molecular distillation*
Mucor circinelloides
Myocardial infarction
Myostatin

Nanoparticles
Neem
Nitzschia
Noni juices
Norovirus
Norwalk-like virus
Norwalk virus
Nut products
Nutrient density

Odorant*
Oil absorption capacity
Oily fish
Oleanolic acid
Oligopeptides
Organic beverages
Orthopoxvirus
Ovarian cancer
Overweight

Parental response
Parvovirus
Pet chews
Phaeodactylum
Phenoxy herbicides
Phlebia
Physical phases
Piceid
Pichia membranifaciens
Pitting disorders
Poliovirus
Portion sizes
Potassium metabisulfite
Poultry meat industry
Prenatal nutrition
Propionibacterium acidipropionici
Propylthiouracil
Proteins high diet
Pseudoalteromonas
Puerarin
Pycnoporus
Pyranoanthocyanins
Pyrimethanil

Quality of life
Quorum sensing

Rahnella
Recipes
Red chillies
Red clover
Red ginseng
Red onions
Regional foods
Reproduction
Reproductive toxicity
Rhizopus nigricans
Rhodosporidium
Rhodosporidium toruloides
RNA interference
Rotavirus
Rye starch

Saccharomyces boulardii
Sage essential oils
Salmonella Agona
Salmonella Gallinarum
Salmonella Oranienburg
Sandwich bars
Sapovirus
Sapoviruses
Sapporo virus
Saturated fats
Scoops
Scotch whisky
Screw caps
Sea buckthorn juices
Seed coats
Selenomethionine
Selenoproteins
Sesquiterpenes
Side dishes
Simultaneous distillation-extraction
Sleep
Small round structured virus
Snacking
Socioeconomic factors
Sodium benzoate
Sodium low diet
Sports nutrition
Spouted bed processing
Staphylococcus epidermidis
Staphylococcus saprophyticus
Starvation
Stocking density (aquaculture)
Stocking density (husbandry)
Streptococcus faecium
Streptococcus macedonicus

** denotes a non-descriptor*

Streptococcus uberis
Subcutaneous fat
Subsidies
Sudan dyes
Sugar beet pulps
Supercooling
Supply chains
Surface pasteurization
Sustainability
Swallowing
Sweet proteins

Table olives
Tara gums
Tastant*
Tea extracts
Tebuconazole
Technology
Thermoactinomyces vulgaris
Thermoanaerobacterium thermosulfurigenes
Thermobifida
Thermobifida fusca
Thermococcus
Thraustochytrium
Thyme oils
Tooth decay*
Trametes hirsuta
Transcription factors
Triacetin
Triazine herbicides
Triterpenes
Triterpenoids

Ultra performance liquid chromatography*
Ultraviolet irradiation*
Ulva
UPLC
Ursolic acid
UV irradiation

Vaccination
Vaccinia virus
Vacuum distillation
Vegetable juice concentrates
Vision

Wallemia
Watermelon juices
Weather
Whiskies
Wholesale
Wine industry

Xanthones
Xanthophyllomyces

** denotes a non-descriptor*

www.ingramcontent.com/pod-product-compliance
Ingram Content Group UK Ltd.
Pitfield, Milton Keynes, MK11 3LW, UK
UKHW051631300926
15471UKWH00017BA/1046

9 780860 1